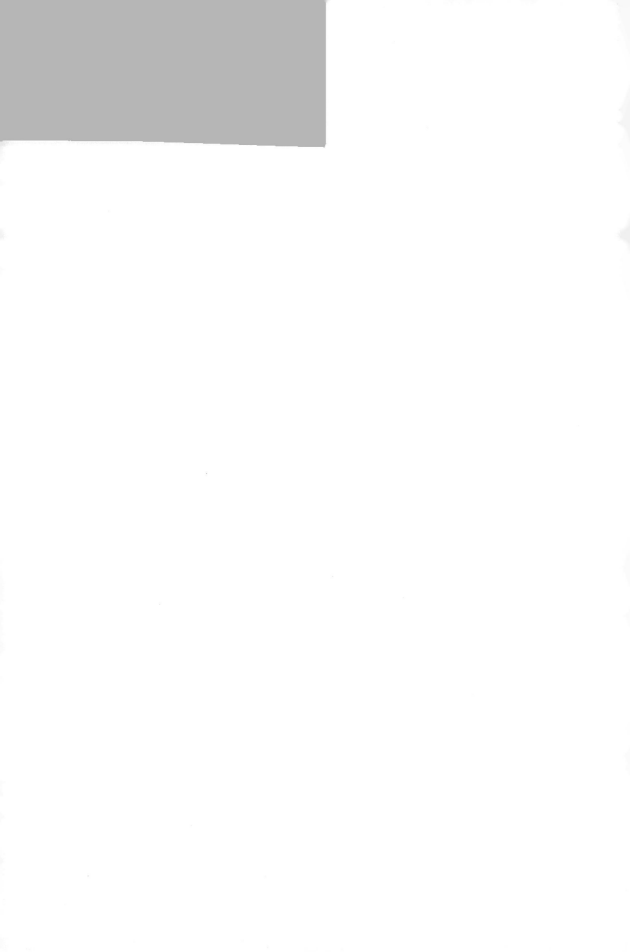

Casebook of Clinical Neuropsychology

Casebook of Clinical Neuropsychology

Edited by

Joel E. Morgan

Ida Sue Baron

Joseph H. Ricker

OXFORD
UNIVERSITY PRESS

2011

OXFORD
UNIVERSITY PRESS

Oxford University Press, Inc., publishes works that further
Oxford University's objective of excellence
in research, scholarship, and education.

Oxford   New York
Auckland   Cape Town   Dar es Salaam   Hong Kong   Karachi
Kuala Lumpur   Madrid   Melbourne   Mexico City   Nairobi
New Delhi   Shanghai   Taipei   Toronto

With offices in
Argentina   Austria   Brazil   Chile   Czech Republic   France   Greece
Guatemala   Hungary   Italy   Japan   Poland   Portugal   Singapore
South Korea   Switzerland   Thailand   Turkey   Ukraine   Vietnam

Published by Oxford University Press, Inc.
198 Madison Avenue, New York, New York 10016

www.oup.com

Oxford is a registered trademark of Oxford University Press, Inc.

Library of Congress Cataloging-in-Publication Data

Casebook of clinical neuropsychology / edited by Joel E. Morgan,
Ida Sue Baron, Joseph H. Ricker.
     p. cm.
  Includes bibliographical references and index.
  ISBN-13: 978-0-19-537425-4
  ISBN-10: 0-19-537425-8
  1. Neuropsychiatry. 2. Clinical neuropsychology.
     I. Morgan, Joel E. II. Baron, Ida Sue. III. Ricker, Joseph H.
  RC341.C37 2010
  616.8—dc22
                                                    2010001853

ISBN-13: 978-0-19-537425-4
ISBN-10: 0-19-537425-8

9 8 7 6 5 4 3 2 1

Printed in the United States of America on acid-free paper

For J. E. M.: To Steffie and Freddie
For I. S. B.: To Peter, David, and Cara
For J. H. R.: To Lance

Foreword

Most will agree that what has now evolved into the field of clinical neuropsychology was initially built on a foundation of single case studies. The unfortunate fates of Phineas Gage, Tan (Broca aphasia), and H. M. have captured imaginations of multiple generations of students entering the field. The value of these famous cases lies well beyond what might be considered answers to a modern game of "neuroscience trivia." Such cases actually serve to provide us with a template for developing a detailed understanding of the effects of brain dysfunction, not only on behavior, but on the person as a whole.

While neuropsychology as a science owes much of its success to findings from studies on patient groups, the individual case study continues to play a significant role in advancing our knowledge in both research and clinical training. Our science will continue to move along with continued descriptions of unusual cases that challenge our theories and lead to paradigm shifts. However, a well-prepared case presentation is equally valuable to our field because it has the potential to not only instruct young students in the use of neuropsychological methods but also to provide seasoned clinicians with a means to refine their understanding of patients seeking their services.

Cognitive scientists have told us for years that categorical learning proceeds through exposure to a series of specific exemplars. The model of clinical training used by neuropsychologists and other health professional fields follows this route

as it is based on a system of providing its novices with exposure to individual cases by observation and through direct clinical contact until they reach a point where they are able to provide the service on their own. This forms the basis of the old adage "watch one, do one, and teach one." Much of our personal knowledge of clinical phenomenology is clearly anchored by the memorable cases we see.

This book provides an insightful look into a number of clinical syndromes through the case presentation method. The editors have assembled an all-star cast of neuropsychologists with expertise in a wide range of clinical subspecialties. While the volume includes descriptions of some relatively rare syndromes, it also includes many excellent examples of the experts' approaches to what might be considered by many to be rather routine cases. The result is an entertaining mix of chapters that provides the reader with the important insights on what is typical in neuropsychology in addition to instruction on how to approach those types of cases seen less frequently. The reader will enjoy these well-written accounts of real-life applications of clinical practice, which provide an inside view of the richness of the data obtained through a comprehensive and evidence-based approach to neuropsychological assessment.

William B. Barr, PhD, ABPP
Departments of Neurology and Psychiatry
New York University School of Medicine

Preface

Clinical evaluation is a basic function of the clinical neuropsychologist, as well as a demonstration of the art of clinical neuropsychology. While there is no substitute for the role of experience, even a novice practitioner may be expected to make astute observations and revealing insights in the service of clinical case formulation. To the dedicated clinician, the hands-on approach of clinical examination has no equal. While scientific revelations concerning brain–behavior relationships often emerge from well-controlled studies of large numbers of subjects, it is the challenge of the singular case that has an extraordinary attraction.

No doubt each clinical neuropsychologist has a profound professional memory related to at least one patient who had a particular disorder, whether it was a condition to be documented or detected. These memorable cases form what is arguably essential knowledge about the profession of clinical neuropsychology, and they underscore the core responsibilities that are basic to examination in the service of the individual.

How many times has a clinician been about to evaluate a patient but wished to preliminarily consult a knowledgeable colleague about what is known about the typical presentation, the most efficacious way to assess the patient, the kinds of recommendations/interventions that have proved useful…or, the solution to the diagnostic befuddlement engendered by the rare, singular case?

Recognizing the importance of these in vivo experiences, we decided to enlist the expertise of our colleagues and produce a casebook. The contributors were encouraged to pull a chart out of their files, one they could not forget or might favor for teaching. The range is from the ordinary to the unique. Authors were asked to detail the key facts related to the diagnosis at issue within a broadly set but logically organized framework and to provide their clinical data and interpretive formulations, with the aim that their case discussion have generalizable utility to colleagues.

Originally conceived as a companion to the *Textbook of Clinical Neuropsychology* (Morgan & Ricker, 2008, New York: Taylor & Francis), it is our intention that the *Casebook of Clinical Neuropsychology* serve as a reference textbook on which the reader may rely in preparation for examination of a patient with a known diagnosis, but whose disorder might not have been previously encountered by this clinician with any frequency. The volume may also prove helpful to compare and contrast one's own clinical findings and observations with those of a colleague who has had experience with the condition of interest. One can learn a good deal about diagnostic considerations and potential intervention strategies when these are described by informed and experienced clinical professionals. We certainly gained these insights as we read each of the contributed chapters.

The chapters are broadly grouped by general diagnostic categories. Child and adult cases are combined within sections, as each age group has lessons for practitioners more commonly exposed to other age groups. The somewhat artificial distinction between child and adult neuropsychology is deliberately blurred in this volume, and hopefully makes for some interesting reading. For example, the child with multiple sclerosis can be compared with the adult with multiple sclerosis, the child with stroke with the adult with stroke, the child with a traumatic brain injury with an adult also injured…there may be valuable lessons about lifespan neuropsychology to be learned from a thorough reading, and that includes perusal of those chapters one might skip if corralled to age-defined sections. We encourage readers to make these leaps into case discussions that do not often come their way.

We wish to thank all of the contributors to this volume for their willingness to join us in this endeavor and for their successful efforts to express their clinical acumen through the case presentation format. We especially want to acknowledge the support and encouragement of Joan Bossert, vice president and editorial director of the Medical Division, Mark O'Malley, production editor, and Aaron van Dorn, editorial assistant, at Oxford University Press. Their support for this project has been fundamental in allowing this volume to be published.

Joel E. Morgan, New Jersey
Ida Sue Baron, Maryland
Joseph H. Ricker, Pennsylvania

Contents

V. Neurodegenerative Disorders

VI.   Vascular Disorders

Contributors

Margot D. Ahronovich, MD
Department of Pediatrics and Neonatology
Fairfax Neonatal Associates at Inova Fairfax
    Hospital for Children
Falls Church, Virginia

Vicki Anderson, PhD
Royal Children's Hospital and Murdoch Childrens
    Research Institute
University of Melbourne
Melbourne, Australia

Jim Andrikopoulos, PhD, ABPP (CN)
Ruan Neurology Clinic
Des Moines, Iowa

Kira Armstrong, PhD, ABPP (CN)
Department of Psychiatry
Cambridge Hospital, and
Harvard Medical School
Cambridge, Massachusetts

Bradley N. Axelrod, PhD, ABN
Psychology Section
Department of Veterans Affairs Medical Center
Detroit, Michigan

Ida Sue Baron, PhD, ABPP (CN)
Department of Pediatrics
Inova Fairfax Hospital for Children
Falls Church, Virginia

Marianne Barton, PhD
Department of Psychology
University of Connecticut
Storrs, Connecticut

John T. Beetar, PhD, ABPP (CN)
Kennedy Krieger Institute
Johns Hopkins University School of Medicine
Baltimore, Maryland

Erin D. Bigler, PhD, ABPP (CN)
Departments of Psychology and Neuroscience and
    The Neuroscience Center
Brigham Young University
Provo, Utah

Alyssa J. Braaten, PhD
Atlanta Veterans Affairs Medical Center and
    Department of Rehabilitation Medicine
Emory University
Atlanta, Georgia

Jason Brandt, PhD, ABPP (CN)
Department of Psychiatry & Behavioral Sciences
and Department of Neurology
Johns Hopkins University School of Medicine
Baltimore, Maryland

Shane S. Bush, PhD, ABPP (CN, RP), ABN
Long Island Neuropsychology, P.C.
Lake Ronkonkoma, New York

Robert Butler, PhD, ABPP (CN)
Departments of Pediatrics, Neurology and Psychiatry
Oregon Health and Sciences University
Portland, Oregon

Deborah Cahn-Weiner, PhD, ABPP (CN)
Department of Neurology
University of California, San Francisco
San Francisco, California

HEATHER CARMICHAEL OLSON, PhD
Department of Psychiatry and Behavioral Sciences
University of Washington School of Medicine
and Seattle Childrens Hospital Child
Research Institute
Seattle, Washington

KATELIN CARR
Department of Psychology
University of Connecticut
Storrs, Connecticut

JAMES P. CHANDLER, MD
Department of Neurological Surgery
Northwestern University Feinberg School of
Medicine and Northwestern Memorial Hospital
Chicago, Illinois

EILEEN L. COOLEY, PhD
Department of Psychology
Agnes Scott College
Decatur, Georgia

DARCY COX, PsyD, ABPP (CN)
Department of Psychiatry
University of British Columbia
Vancouver, British Columbia, Canada

ELLEN M. CROUSE, PhD
Veterans Affairs Medical Center of Memphis and
Department of Psychiatry
University of Tennessee College of Medicine
Memphis, Tennessee

BEN DEERY
Murdoch Childrens Research Institute and
Royal Children's Hospital
Melbourne, Australia

ANDREW T. DeMARCO, MA, SLP
Department of Communication Sciences and
Disorders
Temple University
Philadelphia, Pennsylvania

TANYA DIVER, PhD
Department of Psychiatry
Children's Hospital and Harvard
Medical School
Boston, Massachusetts

JACOBUS DONDERS, PhD, ABPP (CN, RP)
Mary Free Bed Rehabilitation Hospital
Grand Rapids, Michigan

LINDA EWING-COBBS, PhD
Children's Learning Institute and Department of
Pediatrics & Psychiatry and Behavioral Sciences
University of Texas Health Science Center
at Houston
Houston, Texas

JANET E. FARMER, PhD, ABPP (RP)
Department of Health Psychology and
The Thompson Center for Autism and
Neurodevelopmental Disorders
University of Missouri
Columbia, Missouri

PHILIP S. FASTENAU, PhD
Department of Neurology
Case Western Reserve University School
of Medicine and University Hospitals
Neurological Institute
Cleveland, Ohio

DEBORAH FEIN, PhD, ABPP (CN)
Department of Psychology
The University of Connecticut
Storrs, Connecticut

TANIS J. FERMAN, PhD, ABPP (CN)
Department of Psychology and Psychiatry
Mayo Clinic
Jacksonville, Florida

PAUL A. FRIEDMAN, MD
Department of Physical Medicine and
Rehabilitation
Scott & White Hospital
Temple, Texas

JOHN B. FULTON, PhD
Children's Center for Neuropsychological
Rehabilitation
Barrow Neurological Institute
Phoenix, Arizona

JENNIFER C. GIDLEY LARSON, MA
Department of Psychology
University of Utah
Salt Lake City, Utah

DAWN GIUFFRE MEYER, PhD
Department of Psychiatry and Behavioral Sciences
NorthShore University HealthSystem
Evanston, Illinois

Anthony J. Giuliano, PhD
Department of Psychiatry
Beth Israel Deaconess Medical Center and
    Harvard Medical School
Boston, Massachusetts

Miriam T. Goldstein, PhD
Department of Psychiatry
Columbia University College of Physicians and
    Surgeons
New York, New York

Christopher L. Grote, PhD, ABPP (CN)
Department of Behavioral Sciences
Rush University Medical Center
Chicago, Illinois

Kathleen Y. Haaland, PhD, ABPP (CN)
New Mexico VA Healthcare System and
    Departments of Psychiatry and Neurology
University of New Mexico
Albuquerque, New Mexico

Walter J. Hader, MD, FRCS
Division of Neurosurgery
Department of Clinical Neurosciences
University of Calgary
Calgary, Alberta, Canada

Lisa G. Hahn, PhD
Neuropsychology Associates of New Jersey
Madison, New Jersey

Thomas A. Hammeke, PhD, ABPP (CN)
Department of Neurology
Division of Neuropsychology
Medical College of Wisconsin
Milwaukee, Wisconsin

Robin Hanks, PhD, ABPP (CN)
Department of Physical Medicine
    and Rehabilitation
Wayne State University School of Medicine
Detroit, Michigan

Robert E. Hanlon, PhD, ABPP (CN)
Departments of Psychiatry and Neurology
Northwestern University Feinberg School of
    Medicine
Chicago, Illinois

Lauren Herlihy
Department of Psychology
University of Connecticut
Storrs, Connecticut

Mary Iampietro, BS
Department of Psychology
Temple University
Philadelphia, Pennsylvania

Jennifer A. Janusz, PsyD, ABPP (CN)
Department of Neurology
The Children's Hospital
University of Colorado Denver School of Medicine
Denver, Colorado

Benjamin L. Johnson-Markve, PsyD
Neuroscience Research Institute and Department of
    Physical Medicine and Rehabilitation
Florida Hospital
Orlando, Florida

Stephen M. Kanne, PhD, ABPP (CN)
Department of Health Psychology and
    Thompson Center for Autism and
    Neurodevelopmental Disorders
University of Missouri
Columbia, Missouri

Heather L. Katzen, PhD
University of Miami Miller School of Medicine
Miami, Florida and Weill Medical College of
    Cornell University
New York, New York

Lauren Kenworthy, PhD
Departments of Pediatrics, Neurology, and Psychiatry
George Washington University Medical School
Washington, District of Columbia

Kimberly A. Kerns, PhD
Department of Psychology
University of Victoria
Victoria, British Columbia, Canada

Michael W. Kirkwood, PhD, ABPP (CN)
Department of Physical Medicine & Rehabilitation
University of Colorado-Denver and
    The Children's Hospital
Aurora, Colorado

Kelley Knoch
Department of Psychology
University of Connecticut
Storrs, Connecticut

Gregory P. Lee, PhD, ABPP (CN)
Department of Neurology
Medical College of Georgia
Augusta, Georgia

Antolin M. Llorente, PhD
Department of Pediatrics
University of Maryland School of Medicine and
    Mt. Washington Pediatric Hospital
Baltimore, Maryland

David W. Loring, PhD, ABPP (CN)
Department of Neurology
Emory University
Atlanta, Georgia

Sherrill R. Loring, MD
Andrew C. Carlos Multiple Sclerosis Institute
Shepherd Center
Atlanta, Georgia

John A. Lucas, PhD, ABPP (CN)
Department of Psychiatry & Psychology
Mayo Clinic
Jacksonville, Florida

E. Mark Mahone, PhD, ABPP (CN)
Kennedy Krieger Institute
Johns Hopkins University School of Medicine
Baltimore, Maryland

Aaron C. Malina, PhD, ABPP (CN)
Department of Psychiatry
Northshore University Healthsystem
Evanston, Illinois

Robert L. Mapou, PhD, ABPP (CN)
Private Practice, William R. Stixrud and Associates,
LLC, Silver Spring, Maryland
Departments of Psychiatry and Neurology
Uniformed Services University of the Health Sciences
Bethesda, Maryland

Bernice A. Marcopulos, PhD, ABPP (CN)
Western State Hospital and Department of Psychiatry
Neurobehavioral Sciences University of Virginia
    School of Medicine
Charlottesville, Virginia

Ann C. Marcotte, PhD, ABPP (CN)
Department of Psychiatry
Columbia University College of Physicians and
    Surgeons
New York, New York

Maria J. Marquine, PhD
Department of Behavioral Sciences
Rush University Medical Center
Chicago, Illinois

William J. McMullen Jr., PhD, ABPP (CN)
Sutter Pacific Epilepsy Program
California Pacific Medical Center
San Francisco, CA

Kimberly M. Miller, PhD
Mental Health Unit
Veterans Affairs Northern California
    Healthcare System
Martinez, California

Ismail Mohamed, MD, FRCP
Department of Pediatrics and Alberta
    Children's Hospital
University of Calgary
Calgary, Alberta, Canada

Scott Mooney, PhD
Neuroscience & Rehabilitation Center
Dwight D. Eisenhower Army Medical Center
Fort Gordon, Georgia

Anna Bacon Moore, PhD
Atlanta Veterans Affairs Medical Center and
    Department of Rehabilitation Medicine
Emory University
Atlanta, Georgia

Joel E. Morgan, PhD, ABPP (CN)
Department of Neurology & Neurosciences
UMDNJ-New Jersey Medical School
Newark, New Jersey

Thomas Myers, MS
Department of Psychology
Queens College
The City University of New York
Flushing, New York

Marc A. Norman, PhD, ABPP (CN)
Department of Psychiatry
University of California, San Diego
San Diego, California

Marsha J. Nortz, PhD, ABPP (CN)
Department of Pediatrics
Cincinnati Children's Hospital Medical Center and
    University of Cincinnati
Cincinnati, Ohio

Martin D. Oliveira, PsyD,
Northwestern University Feinberg School of
    Medicine and Northwestern Memorial Hospital
Chicago, Illinois

MARYKAY PAVOL, PhD, ABPP (CN)
Neurological Institute
Columbia University College of
    Physicians and Surgeons
New York, New York

MARY R. PRASAD, PhD
Children's Learning Institute and Department of
    Pediatrics
University of Texas Health Science Center
    at Houston
Houston, Texas

RASHMI RASTOGI, PhD
Inpatient Brain Injury Rehabilitation Program
Staten Island University Hospital
Staten Island, New York

LISA D. RAVDIN, PhD, ABPP (CN)
Department of Neurology
Weill Medical College of Cornell University
New York, New York

CELIANE REY-CASSERLY, PhD, ABPP (CN)
Department of Psychiatry
Children's Hospital and Harvard
    Medical School
Boston, Massachusetts

M. DOUGLAS RIS, PhD, ABPP (CN)
Department of Pediatrics and Texas Children's
    Hospital
Baylor College of Medicine
Houston, Texas

TRESA ROEBUCK-SPENCER, PhD, ABPP (CN)
Department of Psychology
University of Oklahoma
Norman, Oklahoma

BRAD L. ROPER, PhD, ABPP (CN)
Memphis Veterans Affairs Medical
    Center and Departments of Psychiatry and
    Neurology
University of Tennessee College of Medicine
Memphis, Tennessee

LESLIE D. ROSENSTEIN, PhD, ABPP (CN)
Neuropsychology Clinic, PC
Austin, Texas

BETH K. RUSH, PhD, ABPP (CN, RP)
Department of Psychology and Psychiatry
Mayo Clinic
Jacksonville, Florida

JOSEPH R. SADEK, PhD
New Mexico Veterans Affairs Healthcare System
    Department of Psychiatry
University of New Mexico
Albuquerque, New Mexico

HARVEY B. SARNAT, MS, MD, FRCPC
Departments of Pediatrics, Pathology
    (Neuropathology), and Clinical Neurosciences
    and Alberta Children's Hospital
University of Calgary
Calgary, Alberta, Canada

ADAM T. SCHMIDT, PhD
Cognitive Neuroscience Laboratory
Department of Physical Medicine and Rehabilitation
Baylor College of Medicine
Houston, Texas

DAVID J. SCHRETLEN, PhD, ABPP (CN)
Departments of Psychiatry & Radiology
Johns Hopkins University School of Medicine
Baltimore, Maryland

MICHAEL SHARLAND, PhD, ABPP (CN)
Department of Neuropsychology
Meritcare Neuroscience
Fargo, North Dakota

ELISABETH M. S. SHERMAN, PhD
Alberta Children's Hospital and Department of
    Pediatrics and Clinical Neurosciences
University of Calgary
Calgary, Alberta, Canada

BARNETT SHPRITZ, MA, OD
Department of Psychiatry & Behavioral Sciences
Johns Hopkins University School of Medicine
Baltimore, Maryland

DANIEL J. SLICK, PhD
Alberta Children's Hospital
University of Calgary
Calgary, Alberta, Canada

BETH S. SLOMINE, PhD, ABPP (CN)
Kennedy Krieger Institute
Johns Hopkins University School of Medicine
Baltimore, Maryland

BRENDA J. SPIEGLER, PhD, ABPP (CN)
Department of Psychology and Division of
    Hematology/Oncology
The Hospital for Sick Children
Toronto, Ontario, Canada

Gerry A. Stefanatos, DPhil
Department of Communication
    Sciences and Disorders
Temple University
Philadelphia, Pennsylvania

Helen A. Steigmeyer, MA
Mt. Washington Pediatric Hospital
Baltimore, Maryland

Esther Strauss[†], PhD
Department of Psychology
University of Victoria
Victoria, British Columbia, Canada

Nikki H. Stricker, PhD
Boston Veterans Affairs Healthcare system
Department of Psychiatry Boston University School
    of Medicine
Boston, Massachusetts

Anthony Y. Stringer, PhD, ABPP (CN), CPCRT
Department of Rehabilitation Medicine
Emory University
Atlanta, Georgia

Jerry J. Sweet, PhD, ABPP (CN, CL)
Department of Psychiatry and
    Behavioral Sciences
NorthShore University HealthSystem and
    University of Chicago Pritzker
    School of Medicine
Evanston, Illinois

Jing E. Tan, MA
Department of Psychology
University of Victoria
Victoria, British Columbia, Canada

Alexander I. Tröster, PhD, ABPP(CN)
Department of Neurology
University of North Carolina School of
    Medicine at Chapel Hill
Chapel Hill, North Carolina

David E. Tupper, PhD, ABPP (CN)
Neuropsychology Section Hennepin Country
    Medical Center, and
Department of Neurology
University of Minnesota Medical School
Minneapolis, Minnesota

Tracy D. Vannorsdall, PhD
Department of Psychiatry
Johns Hopkins University School of Medicine
Baltimore, Maryland

Rebecca C. Williams, BA
Department of Neurology
University of North Carolina at Chapel Hill
    School of Medicine
Chapel Hill, North Carolina

Karen E. Wills, PhD, ABPP (CN)
Psychological Services Department
Children's Hospitals and Clinics of Minnesota
Minneapolis, Minnesota

Ericka L. Wodka, PhD
Kennedy Krieger Institute Johns Hopkins University
    School of Medicine
Baltimore, Maryland

Keith Owen Yeates, PhD, ABPP (CN)
Departments of Pediatrics, Psychology, and
    Psychiatry
The Ohio State University and
Nationwide Children's Hospital
Columbus, Ohio

Ruth E. Yoash-Gantz, PsyD, ABPP (CN)
Salisbury Veterans Affairs Medical Center
    Salisbury, North Carolina and
Department of Psychiatry, Wake Forest University
School of Medicine
Winston-Salem, North Carolina

T. Andrew Zabel, PhD, ABPP (CN)
Kennedy Krieger Institute
Johns Hopkins University School of Medicine
Baltimore, Maryland

[†] Deceased.

Casebook of Clinical Neuropsychology

Part I

Genetic/Developmental Disorders

Genetic and developmental disorders are many and varied. These disorders are common reasons for referral in neuropsychological practice. They may first present in infancy or by early childhood as the neurocognitive and emotional sequelae of abnormal central nervous system development takes its toll on educational performance.

The 13 chapters in this section include both common and rare disorders. These cases are presented to inform both the pediatric and adult neuropsychologist alike, and they illustrate that lifelong challenges are often faced by individuals with these disorders.

I

Fetal Alcohol Spectrum Disorders

Kimberly Kerns and Heather Carmichael Olson

Fetal alcohol spectrum disorders (FASD) is an umbrella term describing a range of outcomes seen among individuals who are born following prenatal exposure to alcohol. Alcohol is a significant neurobehavioral teratogen, which can cause central nervous system (CNS) damage varying from microcellular and neurochemical aberrations to gross structural anomalies. At the functional level, prenatal alcohol exposure can lead to neurodevelopmental disabilities that range from mild developmental delays or learning disabilities to global cognitive deficits. Fetal alcohol spectrum disorders occur in males and females, among all ethnicities, and across all socioeconomic levels. Reported rates of conditions along the fetal alcohol spectrum vary, depending on the population studied and surveillance methods used, with some calculating the rates of the full range of FASD as high as 9 or 10 per 1000 live births (May & Gossage, 2001; Sampson et al., 1997). Current estimates translate to about 40,000 alcohol-affected births in the United States each year (Lupton, Burd, & Hardwood, 2004).

It is important to accurately identify and understand the full range of neurodevelopmental disabilities arising from the effects of prenatal alcohol exposure, so that appropriate services can be provided to affected individuals. Accurate identification and treatment are needed because many individuals with FASD show significant learning problems and/or maladaptive behavior that prevents them from leading productive, independent lives, and this results in significant societal costs (Burd, Cotsonas-Hassler, Martsolfa,

& Kerbeshianb, 2003; Lupton et al., 2004; Stade, Ungar, Stevens, Beyene, & Koren, 2006; Streissguth et al., 2004). Alcohol use during pregnancy, and the issues of offspring born with FASD, are a global public health concern (see http://www.gfmer.ch/Guidelines/Pregnancy_newborn/Fetal_alcohol_syndrome_alcohol_in_pregnancy.htm [accessed 1/10/2009]).

Definitions

The most obvious manifestation of the developmental effects of alcohol is the full fetal alcohol syndrome (FAS). Fetal alcohol syndrome is a permanent birth defect syndrome known to be caused by maternal alcohol consumption during pregnancy. Fetal alcohol syndrome is a medical diagnosis defined by a unique cluster of minor facial anomalies, including short palpebral fissure length, philtrum smoothness, and a thin upper vermillion border (upper lip) (Astley & Clarren, 2001), pre- or postnatal growth deficiency, and CNS dysfunction and/or structural brain abnormalities (IOM, Stratton, Howe, & Battagliam, 1996). The specificity of the FAS facial phenotype to prenatal alcohol exposure supports a clinical judgment that the cognitive and behavioral dysfunction observed among individuals with FAS is due, at least in part, to brain damage caused by a teratogen (Astley, 2004). The U.S. Centers for Disease Control and Prevention (CDC) studies show FAS rates ranging from 0.2 to 1.5 cases per 1000 live births, comparable to other common developmental disabilities such as Down syndrome or spina bifida (Bertrand, Floyd & Weber, 2005; Mirkes, 2003).

Prenatal alcohol exposure, however, is also known to cause a wider spectrum of adverse functional outcomes, whether or not the characteristic facial features occur. Over the years, clinicians and researchers have given a variety of labels to those who lack some or all of the physical features of FAS, but still have neurobehavioral deficits presumed to be related to prenatal alcohol exposure. Labels include descriptive terms used in research such as "prenatal exposure to alcohol" (PEA) (Mattson & Riley, 1998; Sowell et al., 2008) or "prenatally alcohol-exposed" (PAE) (Rasmussen, Talwar, Loomes & Andrew, 2008), and the outdated term "fetal alcohol effects" (FAE), which should no longer be used in clinical or research settings. To label conditions across the spectrum, the Institute of Medicine uses other terms for diagnostic purposes, which are described later in this chapter (IOM et al., 1996).

Indeed, research advances, including neuroimaging research (MRI, MRS, fMRI) and neuropsychological testing, have clarified that not all individuals affected by prenatal exposure to alcohol display the physical features of FAS (e.g., Astley et al., 2009a-d; Mattson, Riley, Gramling, Delis & Jones, 1998; Riley & McGee, 2005). Research has also suggested that the degree and types of neurobehavioral impairments among individuals with heavy prenatal alcohol exposure do not differ between those with and without physical features of FAS (e.g., Fryer, McGee, Matt, Riley & Mattson, 2007; Mattson et al., 1998). While understanding the relationship between the physical and cognitive characteristics is complex and not fully understood (Astley et al., 2009b), what is clear is that no matter what their physical features, those clinically identified with FASD show neurobehavioral impairments.

Diagnosis

Diagnostic systems for clinical and epidemiologic settings are under intensive development. In 1996, the Institute of Medicine (IOM) defined five conditions along the spectrum with categories of: (1) FAS with confirmed prenatal alcohol exposure; (2) FAS without confirmed prenatal alcohol exposure; (3) partial FAS (pFAS); (4) alcohol-related neurodevelopmental disorder (ARND); and (5) alcohol-related birth defects (ARBD). At that time, the IOM made recommendations that research data be gathered to allow refinement and validation of the diagnostic system(s). Since then, national guidelines for diagnosis have been and are now being developed around the world. For example, guidelines for diagnosing FAS (only) were developed in the United States (Bertrand et al., 2004). Enhanced gestalt and checklist methods (e.g., Burd, Cotsonas-Hasslera, Martsolfa, & Kerbeshian, 2003; Kable, Coles, & Taddeo, 2007; McGee, Schonfeld, Roebuck-Spencer, Riley, & Mattson, 2008) (some defining FAS/non-FAS only), case-defined diagnostic systems diagnosing across the fetal alcohol spectrum (e.g., Astley, 2004), and systems designed specifically to operationalize the original IOM diagnostic criteria across the spectrum (e.g., Hoyme et al., 2005) have been developed. These are being used in clinical and research settings in the United States and in collaborative international research. In Canada, national guidelines for diagnosing conditions across the fetal alcohol spectrum "have adapted the method of the 4-Digit Diagnostic Code… to identify(ing) domains and severity of impairment or certainty of brain damage," and thus are meant to operationalize the IOM guidelines (Chudley, Conry, Cook, Loock, Rosales, & LeBlanc, 2005, p. 172).

Currently the criteria for a diagnosis of full FAS (only) are comparable across most systems. First, the individual must display facial dysmorphology in three areas: (1) short palpebral fissures (eye slits); (2) smooth philtrum (the ridges between the nose and lips); and (3) thin upper lip. Second, there must be growth deficiency, typically defined as height, weight, or height-weight ratio less than or equal to the 10th percentile. Third, there must be evidence of CNS involvement, such as be a known structural abnormality or CNS dysfunction in three or more domains. Finally, full FAS is typically diagnosed in the context of a confirmed history of prenatal alcohol exposure, but it may be diagnosed when exposure is unknown and the previous criteria are met.

Streissguth and O'Malley (2000), however, argued that diagnosing conditions along the full fetal alcohol spectrum based on facial features is

Rank	Growth deficiency	FAS facial phenotype	CNS damage or dysfunction	Gestational exposure to alcohol
4	**Significant** Height and weight below 3rd percentile	**Severe** All 3 features: PFL 2 or more SDs below mean Thin lip: rank 4 or 5 Smooth philtrum: rank 4 or 5	**Definite** Structural or neurologic evidence	**High risk** Confirmed exposure to high levels
3	**Moderate** Height and weight below 10th percentile	**Moderate** Generally 2 of the 3 features	**Probable** Significant dysfunction across 3 or more domains	**Some risk** Confirmed exposure. Level of exposure unknown or less than rank 4
2	**Mild** Height or weight below 10th percentile	**Mild** Generally 1 of the 3 features	**Possible** Evidence of dysfunction, but less than 3 domains	**Unknown** Exposure not confirmed present or absent
1	**None** Height and weight at or above 10th percentile	**Absent** None of the 3 features	**Unlikely** No structural, neurologic or functional evidence of impairment	**No risk** Confirmed absence of exposure from conception to birth

Note: PFL = palpebral fissure length; SD = standard deviation. Thin Lip and Philtrum assessed with Philtrum Guide.

Figure I-I. 4-Digit Diagnostic Code criteria for fetal alcohol spectrum disorders. CNS, central nervous system; FAS, fetal alcohol syndrome. (Figure used by permission of Susan Astley, PhD.)

problematic, especially because the FAS face arises from prenatal exposure occurring during only a very short period of vulnerability in embryonic development, and so is quite tied to the timing of prenatal alcohol exposure (Sulik, Johnston, & Webb, 1981; Sulik, 2005). Chudley and his colleagues (2005) stated that "in the wide array of FASDs, facial dysmorphology is often absent and, in the final analysis, has little importance compared with the impact of prenatal alcohol exposure on brain function" (p. 56). Given this debate, there has been increasing recent diagnostic emphasis on the neurobehavioral deficits presumed to be related to prenatal alcohol exposure, as these are of greater functional significance than the physical features.

It is certainly of clinical, epidemiological, and research interest to generate accurate diagnoses of individuals, and to reliably differentiate between meaningful subgroups on the fetal alcohol spectrum. Consensus has not yet been reached on a single diagnostic system for FASD, and while there are many areas of agreement

between the systems in common use, they may sometimes yield different diagnostic classifications when applied to the same alcohol-exposed individual. As data accumulate, diagnostic accuracy will improve.

Diagnostic System Used in Case Studies

The University of Washington Fetal Alcohol Syndrome Diagnostic and Prevention Network (FAS DPN) 4-Digit Diagnostic Code (Astley, 2004; Astley & Clarren, 1997) was used to diagnose the two children in case studies presented in this chapter and so is discussed here in more detail. The 4-Digit Diagnostic Code, now in its third edition, comprises a case-defined set of FASD diagnostic guidelines used by many interdisciplinary teams in the United States and other countries that can be used to define clinical subgroups on the fetal alcohol spectrum. This widely used system aims to reduce classification error. Using this diagnostic system, team members evaluate evidence for the following: *(1)* confirmed prenatal alcohol exposure; *(2)* level of pre- or postnatal growth deficiency; *(3)* specific facial anomalies characteristic of the FAS facial phenotype; and *(4)* presence of neurostructural anomalies or other "hard" evidence of neurological impairment (e.g., seizures, sensorineural hearing impairment, small head circumference, positive findings on a clinical MRI), *and* the presence, type, magnitude and breadth of neuropsychological deficits across multiple developmental domains. Each diagnostic criterion is evaluated on a four-point Likert scale, assessing the evidence confirming presence of and/or similarity to the presentation seen in the full fetal alcohol syndrome (FAS) and assessing severity. This coding scheme provides a simple yet structured way to capture the complex, variable way dysfunction related to prenatal alcohol exposure is expressed. Using this system, interdisciplinary teams can render an accurate and comprehensive diagnosis of a condition on the fetal alcohol spectrum and provide referrals and treatment recommendations. Teams usually include a physician, psychologist, social worker or public health nurse, clinic coordinator, and some combination of additional members (speech-language pathologist, occupational therapist, family advocate, and other discipline(s) as appropriate). In using the 4-Digit Diagnostic Code process, evidence from neuropsychological testing can (and often does) play a pivotal role in diagnosis and in intervention planning.

Areas of Functional Compromise

Research studies of FASD reveal a variety of primary neuropsychological deficits, quite consistent with the diffuse teratogenic effects expected from prenatal alcohol exposure. Group studies of samples with FASD, compared to control samples, yield testing evidence of lowered IQ, deficits in attention, difficulties in working memory, slowed processing speed, problems with cognitive flexibility, memory deficits, impairment in visual spatial abilities, difficulties in language (especially higher-order integrative language abilities), impairment in motor and sensory skills, and deficits in executive functions (Carmichael Olson, Feldman, Streissguth, Sampson, & Bookstein, 1998; Church & Kaltenbach,

1997; Coggins, Olswang, Olson, & Timler, 2003 Hamilton, Kodituwakku, Sutherland, & Savage, 2003; Jirikowic, Olson, & Kartin, 2008; Lee, Mattson, & Riley, 2004; Kodituwakku, 2007; Mattson, Goodman, Caine, Delis, & Riley, 1999; McGee et al., 2008; Rasmussen, 2005; Thorne, Coggins, Olson, & Astley, 2007).

Beyond a list of functional domains that may be affected by prenatal alcohol exposure, more general research-based statements can be made. Evidence so far suggests that, regardless of overall intellectual level, those with FASD show cognitive deficits at a greater rate than anticipated given their IQ (Kerns, Don, Mateer, & Streissguth, 1997; Schonfeld, Mattson, Lang, Delis, & Riley, 2001). Also, there appears to be considerable *individual* variability within the neuropsychological profiles among those with FASD when wide-ranging test batteries are used (e.g., Astley et al., 2009b; Carmichael Olson et al., 1998). While a growing number of studies suggest there are likely some commonalities in functional compromise, to date an accepted "behavioral phenotype" has not emerged.

Reviewing the body of neuropsychological evidence so far, Kodituwakku (2007) makes a compelling argument that individuals with FASD often have intact performance on simple tasks (in all cognitive domains) but have a "generalized deficit in processing complex information" (p. 199). He argues that reduced intellectual skills and slow information processing are consistent with this generalized deficit. Further, he makes the point that when tasks require integration of multiple brain regions, individuals with FASD are not able to integrate the information needed to meet task demands.

Of further importance among individuals with FASD are significant deficits seen in social and adaptive behavior. These have consistently been noted in clinical literature and systematic research, especially in the areas of communication and social skills (e.g., Jirikowic, Kartin, & Olson, 2008; Jirikowic, Olson & Kartin, 2008; O'Connor, & Paley, 2009; Streissguth et al., 2004; Thomas, Kelly, Mattson, & Riley, 1998; Whaley, O'Connor, & Gunderson, 2001); adaptive behavior as reported by parents is often even lower than what might be anticipated based on overall intellectual ability, at least in the area of social skills (Astley et al., 2009b; Thomas et al., 1998).

Research reporting on data from other informants such as teachers, comparison studies with other disability groups, and information on specific deficits in social skills and social communication need further investigation. As a general statement, it could be said that as situations demand more complex adaptive behavior and social interactions—and so require increased integration of information or place higher demands on executive functioning—alcohol-affected individuals show more difficulty (Coggins, Olswang, Olson, & Timler, 2003; Kodituwakku, 2007; Schonefeld, Paley, Frankel, & O'Connor, 2006; Siklos, 2008).

Clinical studies and systematic research also reveal a wide variety of "secondary disabilities" in lifestyle and daily function among those with FASD, such as disrupted school experiences, trouble with the law, inappropriate sexual behaviors, and more. Most frequent among these secondary disabilities are mental health problems. Research data document a high prevalence of psychiatric conditions and elevated behavior problems among children, adolescents, and adults with FASD (e.g., Mattson & Riley, 1999; O'Connor & Paley 2009; Roebuck, Mattson & Riley, 1999; Schonfeld, Mattson, & Riley, 2005; Spohr, Willms & Steinhausen, 2007; Steinhausen & Spohr, 1998; Streissguth et al., 2004; Streissguth, Barr, Kogan & Bookstein, 1997). However, causal interpretation of deficits within social/emotional and psychiatric domains is usually complicated because this disability group also shows a high prevalence of environmental risks leading to life stress such as early neglect, multiple placements (impacting attachment), abuse history, lack of parental supervision, and parental psychopathology. There are also often genetic/family history factors associated with parent(s) who have possible substance abuse, attention-deficit/hyperactivity disorder (ADHD), learning disorders, or other issues (e.g., Lynch, Coles, Corly, & Falek, 2003). Indeed these factors likely play to some extent into all areas of functional compromise seen in children with FASD (cognitive, adaptive, social, and mental health) and warrant further investigation. Few clinical studies so far have had sufficient statistical power or adequate comparison samples to fully address all these confounding factors, though multiple, well-designed longitudinal prospective studies

of prenatal alcohol exposure on offspring development have controlled these variables and confirmed the teratogenic effects of alcohol.

Neuroanatomical and Neuroimaging Findings

There is a growing body of research in the field of FASD confirming permanent anatomical differences in those with FASD on a wide variety of brain structures. In general, findings include greater cortical thickness, smaller brain size, and less white matter density in parietal and posterior temporal regions. Abnormalities have also been noted in the cerebellum, corpus callosum, basal ganglia, hippocampus, and amgydala (Astley et al., 2009a; Riikonen, Salone, Partanen, & Verho, 1999; Sowell et al., 2001, 2002, 2008; Swayze et al., 1997). Variations in cognitive processing as assessed by measures of functional neuroimaging have also been noted. In individuals with FAS, Riikonen et al. (1999) found increased blood supply to the right frontal region, characteristic of children with ADHD. Using functional magnetic resonance imaging (fMRI), a number of authors have found differences in frontal lobe activations in individuals with FASD during tasks of working memory and inhibitory control (Astley et al., 2009d; Connor & Mahurin, 2001; Fryer, McGee, et al., 2007; Malisza et al., 2005). While a comprehensive review of the work in this area is beyond the scope of this chapter, the reader is referred to an excellent review by Spadoni, McGee, Fryer, and Riley (2007). Clearly this work will be important in more specifically elucidating the teratogenic effects of alcohol on brain structure and function.

The Importance of Neuropsychological Assessment and Factors to Consider

While "FASD" is an umbrella term, conditions on the fetal alcohol spectrum are considered medical diagnoses. Current guidelines state that diagnosis is best done within the context of a multidisciplinary or interdisciplinary team. Neuropsychologists can play a unique and important role within these teams, given their training in neuroanatomy and neurology, strong psychometric and assessment skills, and familiarity with measures used to evaluate multiple domains (language, motor, social-emotional functioning, and sensorimotor). With this background, neuropsychologists can bridge disciplines and bring versatile skills to situations where a full diagnostic team is not available (such as in remote locations), providing a multifaceted assessment and diagnostic perspective. Neuropsychologists also play a role in specifying both an individual's deficits and strengths, which can guide rehabilitation, vocational, educational, and social services. They can also shed light on how neurologic and psychiatric factors interact to impact the behavior of an alcohol-affected individual.

Understanding the developmental impact of alcohol as a teratogen is important when conducting neuropsychological assessment. Prenatal alcohol exposure can vary significantly in terms of quantity and pattern (frequency, variability, and timing) of maternal drinking during pregnancy (Aronson, 1997; Maier & West, 2001; Sood et al., 2001; Streissguth, Barr, & Sampson, 1990). There are factors that modify the impact of the alcohol on the fetus, such as the mother's age, nutritional status, use of other substances, and even genetic factors (Delpisheh, Topping, Reyad, Tang, & Brabin, 2008; Gemma, Vichi, & Testai, 2007; Gilliam & Irtenkauf, 1990; Jacobson, Jacobson, Sokol, Chiodo, & Corobana, 2004; McCarver, Thomasson, Martier, Sokol, & Li, 1997; Stoler, Ryan, & Holmes, 2002). Variation in environmental factors during critical developmental periods will also impact the child's outcome. This explains why significant individual variability in level and pattern of CNS dysfunction occurs among alcohol-exposed individuals.

Because marked variability in potential cognitive and behavioral outcomes is to be expected, neuropsychological assessment and standardized testing must encompass a broad range of neurobehavioral capacities. Documenting a profile of deficits and areas of intact abilities is imperative to understanding a child's unique learning (and behavioral) profile. As is standard practice, neuropsychological test results must be taken together with developmental and family history of risks and protective factors, as well as caregiver and teacher reports of functional cognitive, behavioral, social, and academic strengths and weaknesses. Neuropsychological assessment

can provide strong evidence to enable a diagnostic assessment of conditions along the fetal alcohol spectrum—and yield a useful description of function in the alcohol-affected individual with implications for treatment and educational programming. The central importance of neuropsychological assessment is clear in the two case studies that follow.

Case Studies

Provided here are two case studies to illustrate the important fact of the remarkably diverse presentations among individuals with FASD. Both case studies show how a supportive family and appropriate services can result in positive outcomes, even in the face of a child's clear learning and behavioral deficits, and even if a child has experienced high-risk circumstances early in life. The first is a case study of a school-aged child with full FAS, and the second is a case study of an adolescent with ARND. These individuals both have conditions diagnosed on the fetal alcohol spectrum, yet they are different from each other in many ways.

Case 1: A Child with Full Fetal Alcohol Syndrome

Assessment results for Case 1, an 8-year-old male of mixed ethnic ancestry, are from testing obtained as part of a research study as his initial diagnostic testing records were not available. Case 1 was originally seen in an FASD diagnostic clinic at age 5 years, secondary to early developmental and behavioral concerns, and a known history of prenatal alcohol exposure. At that time, he was diagnosed with FAS, with a 4-Digit Diagnostic Code of 3444. The initial (growth) digit of "3" in this child's 4-Digit Code indicates that Case 1 showed moderate growth deficiency, either prenatally or postnatally. The second (facial features) digit of "4" in this child's 4-Digit Code indicates a "severe" level of expression of facial features characteristic of the full FAS (compared to age and Caucasian facial norms: small palpebral fissure lengths, thinned upper lip, smooth philtrum). The third (CNS) digit of "4" in this child's 4-Digit Code indicates there was structural evidence suggesting "definite" CNS damage or dysfunction (very small head size).

The final (alcohol exposure) digit of "4" in the 4-Digit Code indicates confirmed exposure to high levels of alcohol (with an exposure pattern consistent with the medical literature placing the fetus at "high risk," generally high peak blood alcohol concentrations delivered at least weekly in early pregnancy).

Because of early neglect, Case 1 was placed with his current caregivers at 18 months of age. Since then, he has lived in a warm family with multiple siblings. During childhood, Case 1 experienced many protective factors at home and in school. His parents have "reframed" their understanding of their son to appropriately understand Case 1's learning and behavior problems in light of his FAS, provided a stable and developmentally stimulating home, and willingly undertaken behavioral consultation intervention specialized for families raising children with FASD.

Observation and Examination Results. At the time of testing, Case 1 was 8 years, 1 month old with diagnoses of both FAS and ADHD. At the time of testing he was taking Ritalin to treat symptoms of ADHD. Case 1 was qualified for school services under the Health Impaired category and receiving supportive school services, including speech-language therapy, tutoring, and a social skills group, and was placed in a regular classroom.

In interview, Case 1's caregivers described their son as an enjoyable, outgoing, happy boy, who was very helpful with chores and willing to accept direction from adults. However, his mother also described difficulties with Case 1's temper, distractibility, and impulsivity. Behavioral concerns also included physical aggression, apparent lying, difficulties maintaining physical boundaries with peers, and trouble at school. Parent report on the Achenbach System of Empirically Based Assessment, Child Behavior Checklist (ASEBA) (Achenbach & Rescorla, 2001), revealed Internalizing and Externalizing Problem scales both in the clinical range, and scores in the clinical range on the DSM-Oriented scales of Affective Problems, Attention-Deficit/Hyperactivity Problems, and Conduct Problems (above the 97th percentile). Case 1's parents had their son involved in age-appropriate activities (scoring at a remarkably high 92nd percentile on

the Activities subscale), but he struggled with social skills and school performance. As a result, his Total Competence score was quite low for his age, at the 7th percentile.

The tester found Case 1 easy to relate to, and a child who wanted to please and be looked upon positively, yet he was highly distractible, worked very fast, and was impulsive during testing. He did persist, even when frustrated, but was often disorganized and inefficient in his approach to tasks. Case 1 was very talkative (with poor articulation). His talkativeness was both helpful (he talked out loud to help himself do better) and a problem (at times talking may have interfered with getting activities done). Case 1 also displayed some odd behaviors during testing, such as laughing inappropriately, making noises, and showing intense periods of excitement.

Case 1's intellectual skills were assessed using the Differential Ability Scales—2nd Edition (DAS-II) (Elliot, 2007). Compared to others his age, his problem-solving skills showed significant variability. His verbal reasoning was estimated as markedly below average, at the 1st percentile. His nonverbal reasoning was in the low range, at the 4th percentile. In contrast, Case 1's spatial reasoning was relatively higher, at the 12th percentile. Importantly, his speed of information processing was solidly average, at the 82nd percentile (though perhaps he traded faster speed for lower accuracy). Even though this variability makes an overall score hard to interpret, Case 1's overall General Conceptual Ability Score was 69, at the 2nd percentile, in the very low range.

Similarly, Case 1 showed striking variability on measures of attention, memory, and executive function. On the Test of Everyday Attention in Children (TEA-Ch) (Manly, Robertson, Anderson, & Nimmo-Smith, 1999), for example, Case 1 demonstrated average skill in sustaining attention on a simple auditory task (~80th percentile). On a visual search task, he maintained accuracy (~80th percentile) but to do so was rather slow (~10th percentile). He had significant difficulty on attention tasks that required mental flexibility, assessed impulsivity, or required divided attention for concurrent completion of a visual and auditory task. On these TEA-Ch measures, his scores ranged from the 12th to below the 1st percentiles.

Compared to other children his age, Case 1's overall learning score on subtests from the Children's Memory Scale (CMS) (Cohen, 1997) was low average (21st percentile). But this overall score fails to capture the discrepancy between his relatively poor visual and better verbal learning and recall skills, and his complex performance pattern. In the verbal domain, on the Word Pairs subtest, he showed a learning rate and total performance in the high average range (63rd and 75th percentiles). He was able to recall this verbal information quite well across both short and longer delays (91st and 75th percentiles, respectively). In striking contrast to his solid, age-appropriate performance with verbal information, Case 1's learning in the nonverbal domain, on the Dot Locations subtest, was low. His learning rate was at the 5th percentile with total performance in the borderline range (9th percentile). However, he did retain and recall nonverbal information he had learned at an average level for age after both short and longer delays (37th and 25th percentiles, respectively).

In the area of executive function, Case 1 was given the Behavioral Assessment of the Dysexecutive Syndrome for Children (BADS-C) (Emslie, Wilson, Burden, Nimmo-Smith, & Wilson, 2003). He scored in the impaired range overall and had clear difficulty remaining organized and flexible when solving unique problems that required him to plan and organize. He scored far below average (<0.2nd percentile band), on several parts of the test that required him to attend to details and organize a number of materials. He also struggled with a task in which, under timed conditions, he had to learn a rule and then change his strategy (and stop himself from responding the original way) when the rule was changed. These findings were very consistent with his caregiver's report of executive function as assessed by the Behavior Rating Inventory of Executive Function (BRIEF) (Gioia, Isquith, Guy, & Kenworthy, 2000), on which Case 1 had multiple elevated scores (especially those assessing problems in behavioral regulation). He also had clinically elevated scores on scales assessing deficits in working memory and the ability to organize his approach to problem solving. Case 1's BRIEF profile suggests that he has a tendency to lose emotional control when flexibility is required or when his routines are interrupted.

Case 1 was also administered the Test of Narrative Language (TNL) (Gillam & Pearson, 2004). This test of integrative language abilities requires that a child understand a spoken story, remember the content, and then retell the story. On the TNL, he performed at the 5th percentile overall, which is consistent with his intellectual skills.

Case 1's mother completed an interview with the Vineland Adaptive Behavior Scale-2nd Edition (VABS-2) (Sparrow, Cicchetti, & Balla, 2005) as a measure of day-to-day functioning, including communication, daily living skills, and socialization. Her ratings revealed that, overall, Case 1 had moderately low performance for age, with an Adaptive Behavior Composite Score at the 6th percentile. Communication skills were rated at the 6th percentile, a moderately low score. Socialization skills were ranked at the 5th percentile, also a moderately low score. In these areas, his behavior was similar to a child of approximately 3–4 years of age, an estimate with which his mother concurred as she reported on her son's day-to-day behavior. Daily living skills, however, were rated slightly higher at the 13th percentile, likely because of Case 1's excellent home environment, where his parents have provided him with extra support and consistent, repeated opportunities for learning activities of daily living.

Case 2: A Child with Alcohol-Related Neurodevelopmental Disorder

Case 2 is a 15-year-old female born to a mother with a history of significant alcohol abuse throughout pregnancy (especially binge drinking), as well as cigarette smoking and possibly some illicit drug use. Case 2 was a healthy full-term infant. At birth, healthcare personnel saw no indication of growth deficiency or facial features suggestive of prenatal alcohol exposure. Case 2 was removed from her birth home due to severe physical abuse in infancy, at about age 9 months, and placed with the family who eventually adopted her, providing a stable and supportive placement.

As a toddler, Case 2 was seen for evaluation because of developmental and behavioral problems, including sleep disturbances, significant temper tantrums, limited social interaction and play skills, aggressive outbursts, and flat affect. Assessment at the time revealed language and motor skills in the average range, though Case 2 met criteria for several psychiatric conditions, including oppositional defiant disorder and reactive attachment disorder. Because of this, she was considered "at risk." Case 2 received intensive early intervention, including therapeutic preschool, and her parents received supportive family counseling and training to handle Case 2's behavior. Case 2's adoptive parents were described as exceptionally motivated and involved in the preschool treatment milieu.

At just about age 5, Case 2 was seen for an FASD diagnostic visit following advocacy by her family. At that time, she was diagnosed with a 4-Digit Code of 1223. The initial (growth) digit of "1" indicated no apparent growth deficiency, and the second (facial features) digit of "2" indicated only mild expression of characteristic facial features. The third (CNS) digit of "2" indicated evidence of some mild to moderate CNS delay and/or dysfunction. This was based on testing indicating primarily impaired adaptive functioning, behavior and social problems (impulsivity and difficulties with peers), unusual sensory sensitivities, mood volatility, and some difficulty with "higher order" language skills for her age, in spite of being quite talkative. Case 2's behavior problems and subtle signs of neurologic impairment and difficulties with skills requiring more complex information processing—not cognitive deficits—were the clearest sign of compromise. The final (alcohol exposure) digit of "3" indicated confirmed prenatal exposure, though not at a level consistent with placing the fetus at "high risk." A 4-Digit Code of 1223 falls within the fetal alcohol spectrum using the 4-Digit Code diagnostic system. Providers might consider this a "milder" form of ARND, and Case 2's condition may have appeared milder (in terms of standardized testing evidence) at the age of 5 years. But her condition was *not* mild in terms of behavioral challenges. In addition, as this case study reveals, the term "mild" did not

describe the struggles with academic, problem solving, and social issues encountered by this child and family as time went on.

Case 2 entered the school system with behavioral and learning supports in place, qualified as Health Impaired given the FASD diagnosis. However, actually obtaining an appropriate level of services required parent and health-care provider advocacy. Additional testing by a psychologist using a neuropsychological approach was needed to make the case for services. Given Case 2's complex presentation with "layers" of psychiatric diagnoses in addition to FASD, she continued to receive ongoing psychiatric and support services but, over time, Case 2's medical diagnosis on the fetal alcohol spectrum proved essential to an overall understanding of her issues.

At age 10 years, thorough neuropsychological assessment documented overall intellectual abilities within the average range, though with striking variation within subtests (Wechsler Intelligence Scale for Children–Third Edition, Wechsler, 1996) subtest scores ranging from the 1st to 91st percentile). Case 2's lowest scores were on measures of learning, working memory, and recall (Wide Range Assessment of Memory and Learning (Adams & Sheslow, 1990) and NEPSY (Korkman, Kirk, & Kemp, 1997) subtests), with performance ranging from the borderline impaired to the average range. Case 2 also showed difficulties on measures of planning and organization (e.g., Rey-Osterrieth Complex Figure (Waber & Holmes, 1986). She received low average scores on simple measures of visual spatial/motor skills, with increasing difficulty as tasks became more complex or lengthy. At age 10 years, testing evidence revealed overall adequate language skills on tasks such as phonological processing and single-word reading, but she continued to have difficulty when administered tasks assessing integrative or "higher order" language abilities for her age. This important pattern of doing well on more basic tasks, but struggling when presented with increasingly complex information, was reflected in her academic performance. On the Woodcock-Johnson Tests of Achievement–Revised (WJ-R) (Woodcock, McGrew, & Mather, 1989), she scored above average for age in basic reading skills, yet her scores were low average in reading comprehension. Consistent with literature so far in the field of FASD, Case 2 had significant difficulty on measures of mathematics, scoring in the impaired range and qualifying for a specific mathematics learning disability. Even though Case 2 was engaging, curious, alert, and charismatic, parent report on the ASEBA continued to reveal a high degree of overall problem behavior. Specific problems included impulsivity, inattentiveness, rigidity, and a concrete problem-solving style, problems with organization, and—most challenging for Case 2 herself and for her family— oppositional and aggressive behavior. By late elementary school, Case 2's mental health diagnoses included posttraumatic stress disorder and generalized anxiety disorder. Her ongoing and complex medication regimen (well supervised by a child psychiatrist) included antidepressants and sleep medications, with changeable mood and anxiety as the main target symptoms.

At age 15 years, Case 2 was again seen for follow-up testing, including neuropsychological assessment. She was administered the Wechsler Intelligence Scale for Children–Fourth Edition (Wechsler, 2003) and scored overall at the 4th percentile, lower than might be expected from earlier assessment. In addition, Case 2 still showed striking variation on individual subtests ranging from solid performance on tasks of verbal comprehension and reasoning (Verbal Comprehension Index = 45th percentile), to significant difficulty with tasks of working memory (Working Memory Index = 0.31st percentile). Subtests that showed the greatest change from earlier testing revealed difficulties now clearly emerging in the areas of working memory and slowed processing speed.

Academic testing revealed reading and writing skills in the average range, reflecting the success of Case 2's own learning efforts. Yet she continued to struggle with mathematics, with poor performance on the Woodcock-Johnson III Tests of Achievement (WJ-III) (Woodcock, McGrew, & Mather, 2001) both Calculation Skills (WJ-III <1st percentile) and Math Reasoning (WJ-III = 5th percentile). Language assessment (Clinical Evaluation of Language Fundamentals–Fourth Edition; Semel, Wing, & Secord, 2003) revealed an interesting pattern of difficulty on the Receptive Language Index

(3rd percentile), with no difficulty on the Expressive Language Index (91st percentile).

When given behavior problem questionnaires, Case 2's parents continued to report concerns, including clinically significant difficulties on the Behavior Assessment System for Children–Second Edition (BASC-2; Reynolds & Kamphaus, 2005) such as problems with atypicality, hyperactivity, anxiety, depression, withdrawal, and functional communication. Similarly, parent report on the BRIEF revealed deficits in significantly elevated scores on both the Behavioral Regulation and Metacognitive Indices. In the crucial area of adaptive function (Scales of Independent Behavior–Revised; Bruininks, Woodcock, Weatherman, & Hill, 1996), Case 2's overall broad independence measure was at the "limited" level (1.4th percentile), with moderately serious general maladaptive behaviors requiring some ongoing limited support.

Case 2 is certainly a person with many genetic, prenatal, and environmental risk factors, and with "layers" of diagnosable conditions, including FASD and psychiatric concerns. This, however, is balanced by the remarkable protective factors of Case 2's own zest for life, humor and determination, good work ethic, and a supportive and strong family skilled at advocacy. Ongoing assessment and multimodal interventions addressing her evolving picture of target symptoms have given Case 2 and her family useful coping techniques and accommodations. Among others, interventions in the school years and beyond have included individualized educational programming, home schooling efforts that emphasized life skills training and customized tutoring, behavioral consultation provided to her parents, social skills groups, Special Olympics participation, medication, and more. Case 2 has learned to consistently ask for help from supportive adults and to use good coping strategies.

Discussion

As shown by these case studies, children with FASD and their families face many challenges. Not only have these children been affected by a known teratogen, but they typically have complex postnatal environments. Their parents, who are frequently foster or adoptive parents, or birth parents in recovery, are often under a great deal of stress. For many individuals with FASD, early testing may reveal only mild (or perhaps moderate) difficulties in development or cognition (as seen with Case 2). However, ongoing and increasing problems in language, social skills, and behavior (adaptive and maladaptive), many times in the context of other mental health concerns, are often observed across the developmental course. Over time, individuals with FASD frequently function at below age expectations in cognitive, linguistic, and behavioral domains, even when they do not display the full FAS. Significant variation is seen in test performance across a wide battery of cognitive domains, with poorer performance on tasks that require higher levels of self-organization or complexity and integration of information. Unfortunately, given this pattern, children with FASD may not be identified or qualified for learning-related services early on. As a result, they have often experienced repeated difficulty and failure and have been identified as children with challenging behavior before receiving a diagnosis on the fetal alcohol spectrum.

Research review and case studies presented here reveal that children with FASD typically score more poorly across multiple developmental domains, but there is as yet no known specific "cognitive profile" of strength or weakness that clearly discriminates those with FASD. This complicates the diagnosis for children without physical features. While Kodituwakku's (2007) suggestion of declining performance with increasing complexity of material across domains may hold promise, this suggestion is not yet useful for diagnosis for two reasons. First, while the idea of increasing complexity fits generally with clinical findings, complexity has not yet been defined as a measurable construct within or across domains, though recent studies have begun the effort to do so (e.g., Aragon et al., 2008). Second, it is possible that a pattern of increasing difficulty with complexity may simply reflect generally diffuse cognitive disability— which is seen in other developmental disorders and therefore not specific to FASD. Clearly, further research is needed to examine methods of operationalizing complexity and to assess its

impact and specificity on performance among children with FASD.

There is also considerable research support that children with FASD, as a group, show deficits in executive function and working memory using standardized measures. This finding holds true in group studies but, unfortunately, these areas of deficit are not always found at the level of the individual., Indeed, in a carefully diagnosed sample of 20 children with FAS/pFAS who were administered six well-validated tasks of executive function, surprising results showed that on the majority of these measures participants did *not* consistently score in the impaired range (Astley et al. 2009b).

In conclusion, children and adolescents with FASD have cognitive difficulty across a wide number of domains. Those with FAS (as marked by facial features) are more frequently recognized (and perhaps understood as disabled), more easily diagnosed, and thus more likely to be provided with services and educational supports. Research findings show that appropriate services and caregiver understanding function as protective factors—lowering the odds of the secondary disabilities often associated with prenatal alcohol exposure. This could partly explain the surprising research finding that children with FAS actually show fewer problems in lifestyle and daily function than those on the wider spectrum (Streissguth et al., 2004).

It is unfortunate and remarkable that so many alcohol-affected children still go unrecognized and underserved, often even after being seen by mental health or other providers. While early recognition and diagnosis of FASD has been found to be associated with better outcomes over time, diagnosis at any age is key to more appropriate treatment recommendations and to the anticipatory guidance and long-term planning that is essential for a lifelong neurodevelopmental disability such as FASD. Treatment methods appropriate for FASD are beginning to be systematically tested (e.g., Bertrand, J., 2009), which will better guide future intervention recommendations. A thorough neuropsychological assessment, informed by knowledge of FASD and potential treatments, can be crucial in both diagnosis and in defining and obtaining appropriate family, child, and educational services and supports.

References

Achenbach, T. M., & Rescorla, L. A. (2001). *Manual for ASEBA School-Age Forms & Profiles*. Burlington: University of Vermont, Research Center for Children, Youth, & Families

Adams, W., & Sheslow, D. (1990). *Wide Range Assessment of Memory and Learning*. Wilmington, DE: Jastak Associates.

Aragon, A. S., Kalberg, W. O., Buckley, D., Barela-Scott, L. M., Tabachnick, B. G., & May, P. A. (2008). Neuropsychological study of FASD in a sample of American Indian children: Processing simple versus complex information. *Alcoholism: Clinical & Experimental Research, 32*, 2136–2148.

Aronson, M. (1997). Children of alcohol mothers: Results from Göteborg, Sweden. In A. P. Streissguth, J. Kanter, M. Lowry, & M. Dorris (Eds.), *The challenge of Fetal Alcohol Syndrome: Overcoming secondary disabilities*. Seattle: University of Washington Press.

Astley, S. J. (2004). *Diagnostic guide for fetal alcohol spectrum disorders: The 4-digit diagnostic code*, 3rd ed. Seattle: University of Washington Publication Services.

Astley, S. J., & Clarren, S. K. (1997). *Diagnostic guide for fetal alcohol syndrome and Related conditions: The 4-digit diagnostic code*. Seattle: University of Washington Publication Services.

Astley, S. J., & Clarren, S. K. (2001). Measuring the facial phenotype of individuals with prenatal alcohol exposure: Correlations with brain dysfunction. *Alcohol and Alcoholism, 36*, 147–159.

Astley, S.J., Aylward, E.H., Olson, H.C., Kerns, K., Brooks, A., Coggins, T.E., Davies, J. Dorn, S. Gendler, B., Jirikowic, T., Kraegel, P., Maravilla, K. & Richards. T. (2009a). Magnetic resonance imaging outcomes from a comprehensive magnetic resonance study of children with fetal alcohol spectrum disorders, *Alcoholsim: Clinical and Experimental Research, 33*, 1671–1689.

Astley, S.J. Olson, H.C., Kerns, K.A., Brooks, A., Aylward, E.A., Coggins, T.E., Davies, J., Dorn, S., Gender, B., Jirikowic, T., Kragel, P., Maravilla, K., & Richards, T. (2009b). Neuropsychological and behavioral outcomes from a comphrensive magnetic resonance study of children with fetal alcohol spectrum disorders, *Canadian Journal of Clinical Pharmacology, 16*, e178–e201.

Astley, S.J., Richards. T., Aylward, E.H., Carmichael Olson, H., Kerns, K., Brooks, A., Coggins, T.E.,Davies, J. Dorn, S. Gendler, B., Jirikowic, T., Kraegel, P., & Maravilla, K. (2009c). Magnetic resonance spectroscopy outcomes from a comprehensive magnetic resonance study of children with fetal alcohol spectrum disorders, *Magnetic Resonance Imaging, 27*, 760–778.

Astley, S.J., Aylward, E.A., Olson, H.C., Kerns, K.A., Brooks, A., Coggins, T.E., Davies, J., Dorn, S., Gender, B., Jirikowic, T., Kragel, P,, Maravilla, K., & Richards, T. (2009d). Functional magnetic resonance imaging outcomes from a comprehensive magnetic resonance study of children with fetal alcohol spectrum disorders. *Journal of Neurodevelopmental Disorders, 1*, 61–80.

Bertrand, J., Floyd, L. L., & Weber, M. K. (2005). Guidelines for identifying and referring persons with fetal alcohol syndrome. *Morbidity and Mortality Weekly Report: Recommendations and Reports, 54*, 1–14.

Bertrand, J., Floyd, R. L., Weber, M. K., O'Connor, M., Riley, E. P., Johnson, K. A., et al. (2004). *Fetal alcohol syndrome: Guidelines for referral and diagnosis*. Atlanta, GA: Centers for Disease Control and Prevention.

Bruininks, R. H., Woodcock, R. W., Weatherman, R. F., & Hill, B. K. (1996). *SIB-R: Scales of Independent Behavior – Revised*. Itasca, IL: Riverside Publishing Company.

Burd, L., Cotsonas-Hasslera, T. M., Martsolfa, J. T., & Kerbeshian, J. (2003). Recognition and management of fetal alcohol syndrome. *Neurotoxicology and Teratology, 25*, 681–688.

Burd, L., Klug, M. G., Martsolf, J. T., & Kereshian, J. (2003). Fetal alcohol syndrome: Neuropsychiatric phenomics. *Neurotoxicology and Teratology, 25*, 697–705.

Carmichael Olson, H., Feldman, J. J., Streissguth, A. P., Sampson, P. D., & Bookstein, F. L. (1998). Neuropsychological deficits in adolescents with fetal alcohol syndrome: Clinical findings. *Alcoholism: Clinical and Experimental Research, 22*, 1998–2012.

Chudley, A. E., Conry, J., Cook, J. L., Loock, C., Rosales, T., & LeBlanc, N. (2005). Fetal alcohol spectrum disorder: Canadian guidelines for diagnosis. *Canadian Medical Association Journal, 172*, S1–S21.

Church, M. W., & Kaltenbach, J. A. (1997). Hearing, speech, language, and vestibular disorders in the fetal alcohol syndrome: A literature review. *Alcoholism: Clinical and Experimental Research, 21*, 495–512.

Coggins, T. E., Olswang, L. B., Carmichael Olson, H., & Timler, G. R. (2003). On becoming socially competent communicators: The challenge for children with fetal alcohol exposure. In Abbeduto, L. (Ed.), *Language & Communication in Mental Retardation: Vol. 27. International Review in Research on Mental Retardation* (pp. 121–150). New York: Academic Press.

Coggins, T. E., Timler, G. R., & Olswang, L. B. (2007). A state of double jeopardy: Impact of prenatal alcohol exposure and adverse environments on the social communicative abilities of school-age children with fetal alcohol spectrum disorder. *Language, Speech and Hearing Services in the Schools, 38*, 117–127.

Cohen, M. J. (1997). *Children's Memory Scale.* San Antonio, TX: The Psychological Corporation.

Connor, P. D., & Mahurin, R. (2001). A preliminary study of working memory in fetal alcohol damage using MRI. *Journal of the International Neuropsychological Society, 7*, 206.

Delpisheh, A., Topping, J., Reyad, M., Tang, A., & Brabin, B. J. (2008). Prenatal alcohol exposure, CYP17 gene polymorphisms and fetal growth restriction. *European Journal of Obstetrics, Gynecology, and Reproductive Biology, 138*(1), 49–53.

Elliot, C. D. (2007). *Differential Abilities Scales – Second Edition.* San Antonio, TX: Harcourt Assessment, Inc.

Emslie, H., Wilson, F. C., Burden, V., Nimmo-Smith, I., & Wilson, B. A. (2003). *Behavioral assessment of the dysexecutive syndrome for children.* San Antonio, Tex.: Harcourt Assessment, Inc.

Fryer, S. L., McGee, C. L., Matt, G. E., Riley, E. P., & Mattson, S. N. (2007). Evaluation of psychopathological conditions in children with heavy prenatal alcohol exposure. *Pediatrics, 119*, 733–741.

Fryer, S. L., Tapert, S. F., Mattson, S. N., Martin, P. P., Spadoni, A. D., & Riley, E. P. (2007). Prenatal alcohol exposure affects frontal striatal BOLD response during inhibitory control. *Alcoholism: Clinical and Experimental Research, 31*, 1415–1424.

Gemma, S., Vichi, S., & Testai, E. (2007). Metabolic and genetic factors contributing to alcohol induced effects and fetal alcohol syndrome. *Neuroscience and Biobehavioral Reviews, 31*(2), 221–229.

Gilliam, D. M., & Irtenkauf, K. T. (1990). Maternal genetic effects on ethanol teratogenesis and dominance of relative embryonic resistance to malformations. *Alcoholism: Clinical and Experimental Research, 14*(4), 539.

Gillam, R. A. & Pearson, N. A. (2004). *The test of narrative language.* Austin, TX: Pro-Ed, Inc.

Gioia, G. A., Isquith, P. K., Guy, S. C., & Kenworthy, L. (2000). *Behavior Rating Inventory of Executive Function.* Lutz, FL: Psychological Assessment Resources.

Hamilton, D. A., Kodituwakku, P., Sutherland, R. J., & Savage, D. D. (2003). Children with fetal alcohol syndrome are impaired at place learning but not cued-navigation in a virtual Morris water task. *Behavioural Brain Research, 143*, 85–94.

Hoyme, H. E., May, P. A., Kalberg, W. O., Kodituwakku, P., Gossage, J. P., Trujillo, P. M., et al. (2005). A practical clinical approach to diagnosis of fetal alcohol spectrum disorders: Clarification of the 1996 Institute of Medicine criteria. *Pediatrics, 115*, 39–47.

Institute of Medicine (IOM)., U.S. Division of Biobehavioral Sciences and Mental Disorders Committee to Study Fetal Alcohol Syndrome. Stratton, K., Howe, C., & Battagliam, F. (Eds). (1996). *Fetal alcohol syndrome: Diagnosis, epidemiology, prevention and treatment.* Washington, DC: National Academy Press.

Bertrand, J. (2009). Interventions for children with fetal alcohol spectrum disorders (FASDs): Overview of findings for five innovative research projects *Research in Developmental Disabilities, 30*, 986-1006.

Jacobson, S. W., Jacobson, J. L., Sokol, R. J., Chiodo, L. M., & Corobana, R. (2004). Maternal age, alcohol abuse history, and quality of parenting as moderators of the effects of prenatal alcohol exposure on 7.5-year intellectual function. *Alcoholism: Clinical and Experimental Research, 28*, 1732–1745.

Jirikowic, T., Kartin, D., & Olson, H. C. (2008). Children with fetal alcohol spectrum disorders: A descriptive profile of adaptive function. *Canadian Journal of Occupational Therapy, 75*, 238–248.

Jirikowic, T., Olson, H. C., & Kartin, D. (2008). Sensory processing, school performance, and adaptive behavior among young school-aged children with FASD. *Physical and Occupational Therapy in Pediatrics, 2*, 117–136.

Kable, J. A., Coles, C. D., & Taddeo, E. (2007). Socio-cognitive habilitation using the math interactive learning experience program for alcohol-affected children. *Alcoholism: Clinical and Experimental Research, 31*, 425–434.

Kerns, K. A., Don, A., Mateer, C. A., & Streissguth, A. P. (1997). Cognitive deficits in nonretarded adults with fetal alcohol syndrome. *Journal of Learning Disabilities, 30*, 685–693.

Kodituwakku, P. W. (2007). Defining the behavioral phenotype in children with fetal alcohol spectrum disorders: A review. *Neuroscience and Biobehavioral Reviews, 31*, 192–201.

Korkman, M., Kirk, U., & Kemp, S. (1997). *A Developmental Neuropsychological Assessment (NEPSY).* San Antonio, TX: Psychological Corporation.

Lee, K. T., Mattson, S. N., & Riley, E. P. (2004). Classifying children with heavy prenatal exposure using measures of attention. *Journal of the International Neuropsychological Society, 10*, 271–277.

Lupton, C., Burd, L., & Harwood, R. (2004). Cost of fetal alcohol spectrum disorders. *American Journal of Medical Genetics. Part C, Seminars in Medical Genetics, 127*(1), 42–50.

Lynch, M. E., Coles, C. D., Corly, T., & Falek, A. (2003). Examining delinquency in adolescents differentially prenatally exposed to alcohol: The role of proximal and distal risk factors. *Journal of Studies on Alcohol, 64*(5), 678–686.

Maier, S. E., & West, J. R. (2001). Drinking patterns and alcohol-related birth defects. *Alcohol Research and Health, 25*, 168–174.

Malisza, K. L., Allman, A. A., Shiloff, D., Jakobson, L., Longstaffe, S., & Chudley, A. E. (2005). Evaluation of spatial working memory function in children and adults with fetal alcohol spectrum disorders: A functional magnetic resonance imaging study. *Pediatric Research, 58*, 1150–1157.

Manly, T., Robertson, I. H., Anderson, V., & Nimmo-Smith, I. (1999). *TEA-Ch Test of Everyday Attention for Children*. London: Harcourt Assessment.

Mattson, S. N., Goodman, A. M., Caine, C., Delis, D. C., & Riley, E. P. (1999). Executive functioning in children with heavy prenatal alcohol exposure. *Alcoholism: Clinical and Experimental Research, 23*, 1808–1815.

Mattson, S.N. & Riley, E.P. (1999). Implicit and explicit memory functioning in children with heavy prenatal alcohol exposure. *Journal of the International Neuropsychological Society, 5*, 462–471.

Mattson, S. N., & Riley, E. P. (1998). A review of the neurobehavioral deficits in children with fetal alcohol syndrome or prenatal exposure to alcohol. *Alcoholism: Clinical and Experimental Research, 22*, 279–294.

Mattson, S. N., Riley, E. P., Gramling, L., Delis, D. C., & Jones, K. L. (1998). Neuropsychological comparison of alcohol-exposed children with or without physical features of fetal alcohol syndrome. *Neuropsychology, 12*, 146–153.

May, P. A., & Gossage, J. P. (2001). Estimating the prevalence of fetal alcohol syndrome. A summary. *Alcohol Research and Health, 25*, 159–167.

McCarver, D. G., Thomasson, H. R., Martier, S. S., Sokol, R. J., & Li, T. (1997). Alcohol dehydrogenase-2*3 allele protects against alcohol-related birth defects among African Americans. *The Journal of Pharmacology and Experimental Therapeutics, 283*, 1095–1101.

McGee, C. L., Schonfeld, A. M., Roebuck-Spencer, T. M., Riley, E. P., & Mattson, S. N. (2008). Children with heavy prenatal alcohol exposure demonstrate deficits on multiple measures of concept formation. *Alcoholism: Clinical and Experimental Research, 32*, 1388–1397.

Mirkes, P. E. (2003). Congenital malformations surveillance report: A report from the national birth defects prevention network. *Birth Defects Research, 67*, 595–668.

O'Connor, M. J., & Paley, B. (2009). Psychiatric conditions associated with prenatal alcohol exposure,

Developmental Disabilities Research Reviews, 15, 225–234.

Rasmussen, C. (2005). Executive functioning and working memory in fetal alcohol spectrum disorder. *Alcoholism: Clinical and Experimental Research, 29*, 1359–1367.

Rasmussen, C., Talwar, V., Loomes, C., & Andrew, G. M. (2008). Brief report: Lie-telling in children with fetal alcohol spectrum disorder. *Journal of Pediatric Psychology, 33*, 220–225.

Reynolds, C. R., & Kamphaus, R.W. (2005). *Behavior Assessment System for Children – Second Edition*. Circle Pines, MN: AGS Publishing.

Riley, E. P., & McGee, C. L. (2005). Fetal alcohol spectrum disorders: An overview with emphasis on changes in brain and behavior. *Experimental Biology and Medicine, 230*, 357–365.

Riikonen, R., Salonen, I., Partanen, K., & Verho, S. (1999). Brain perfusion SPECT and MRI in fetal alcohol syndrome. *Developmental Medicine & Child Neurology, 41*, 652–659.

Roebuck, T. M., Mattson, S. N., & Riley, E. P. (1999). Behavioral and psychosocial profiles of alcohol-exposed children. *Alcoholism: Clinical and Experimental Research, 23*, 1070–1076.

Sampson, P. D., Streissguth, A. P., Bookstein, F. L., Little, R. E., Clarren, S. K., Dehaene, P., et al. (1997). Incidence of fetal alcohol syndrome and prevalence of alcohol-related neurodevelopmental disorder. *Teratology, 56*, 317–326.

Schonfeld, A. M., Mattson, S. N., Lang, A. R., Delis, D. C., & Riley, E. P. (2001). Verbal and nonverbal fluency in children with heavy prenatal alcohol exposure. *Journal of Studies on Alcohol, 62*, 239–246.

Schonfeld, A. M., Mattson, S. N., & Riley, E. P. (2005). Moral maturity and delinquency after prenatal alcohol exposure. *Journal of Studies on Alcohol, 66*, 545–554.

Schonfeld, A. M., Paley, B., Frankel, F., & O'Connor, M. J. (2006). Executive functioning predicts social skills following prenatal alcohol exposure. *Child Neuropsychology, 12*, 439–452.

Semel, E., Wiig, E. H., & Secord, W. A., (2003). *Clinical Evaluation of Language Fundamentals–Fourth Edition*. San Antonio, TX: Harcourt Assessment.

Siklos, S. (2008). *Emotion recognition in children with fetal alcohol spectrum disorders*. Unpublished doctoral dissertation, University of Victoria, Victoria, British Columbia, Canada.

Sood, B., Delaney-Black, V., Covington, C., Nordstrom-Klee, B., Ager, J., Templin, T., et al. (2001). Prenatal alcohol exposure and childhood behavior at age 6 to 7 years: I. Dose-response effect. *Pediatrics, 108*, E34–E34.

Sowell, E. R., Mattson, S. N., Kan, E., Thompson, P. M., Riley, E. P., & Toga, A. W. (2008). Abnormal cortical thickness and brain-behavior correlation patterns in individuals with heavy prenatal alcohol exposure. *Cerebral Cortex*, *18*, 136–144.

Sowell, E. R., Mattson, S. N., Thompson, P. N., Jernigan, T. L., Riley, E. P., & Toga, A. W. (2001). Mapping callosal morphology and cognitive correlates: Effects of heavy prenatal alcohol exposure. *Neurology*, *57*, 235–244.

Sowell, E. R., Thompson, P. M., Mattson, S. N., Tessner, K. D., Jernigan, T. L., & Riley, E. P. (2002). Regional brain shape abnormalities persist into adolescence after heavy prenatal alcohol exposure. *Cerebral Cortex*, *12*, 856–865.

Spadoni, A. D., McGee, C. L., Fryer, S. L., & Riley, E. P. (2007). Neuroimaging and fetal alcohol spectrum disorders. *Neuroscience and Biobehavioral Reviews*, *31*, 239–245.

Sparrow, S. S., Cicchetti, D. V., & Balla, D. A. (2005). *Vineland Adaptive Behavior Scales–Second Edition*. Circle Pines, MN: AGS Publishing.

Spohr, H-L., Willms, J., & Steinhausen, H-C. (2007). Fetal alcohol spectrum disorders in young adulthood. *Journal of Pediatrics*, *150*, 175–179.

Stade, B., Ungar, W. J., Stevens, B., Beyene, J., & Koren, G. (2006). The burden of prenatal exposure to alcohol: Measurement of cost. *Journal of FAS International*, *4*, 1–14.

Steinhausen, H. C., & Spohr, H. L. (1998). Long-term outcome of children with fetal alcohol syndrome: Psychopathology, behavior, and intelligence. *Alcoholism: Clinical and Experimental Research*, *22*, 334–338.

Stoler, J. M., Ryan, L. M., & Holmes, L. B. (2002). Alcohol dehydrogenase 2 genotypes, maternal alcohol use, and infant outcome. *The Journal of Pediatrics*, *141*, 780–785.

Streissguth, A. P., Barr, H. M., Kogan, J., & Bookstein, F. L. (1997). Primary and secondary disabilities. In A. P. Streissguth & J. Kanter (Eds.), *The challenge of fetal alcohol syndrome: Overcoming secondary disabilities* (pp. 25–39). Seattle: University of Washington Press.

Streissguth, A. P., Barr, H. M., & Sampson, P. D. (1990). Moderate prenatal alcohol exposure: Effects on child IQ and learning problems at age 7½ years. *Alcoholism: Clinical and Experimental Research*, *14*, 662–669.

Streissguth, A. P., Bookstein, F. L., Barr, H. M., Sampson, P. D., O'Malley, K., & Young, J. K. (2004). Risk factors for adverse life outcomes in fetal alcohol syndrome and fetal alcohol effects. *Journal of Developmental and Behavioral Pediatrics*, *25*(4), 228–238.

Streissguth, A. P., & O'Malley, K. (2000). Neuropsychiatric implications and long-term consequences of fetal alcohol spectrum disorders. *Seminars in Clinical Neuropsychiatry*, *5*, 177–190.

Sulik, K. K. (2005). Genesis of alcohol-induced craniofacial dysmorphism. *Experimental Biology and Medicine*, *230*, 366–375.

Sulik, K. K., Johnston, M. C., & Webb, M. A. (1981). Fetal alcohol syndrome: Embryogenesis in a mouse model, *Science*, *214*, 936–938.

Swayze, V. W., Johnson, V. P., Hanson, J. W., Piven, J., Sato, Y., Giedd, J. N., et al., (1997). Magnetic resonance imaging of brain anomalies in fetal alcohol syndrome. *Pediatrics*, *99*, 232–240.

Thomas, S. E., Kelly, S. J., Mattson, S. N., & Riley, E. P. (1998). Comparison of social abilities of children with fetal alcohol syndrome to those of children with similar IQ scores and normal controls. *Alcoholism: Clinical and Experimental Research*, *22*, 528–533.

Thorne, J. C., Coggins, T. E., Carmichael Olson, H., & Astley, S. J. (2007). Exploring the utility of narrative analysis in diagnostic decision making: Picture-bound reference, elaboration, and fetal alcohol spectrum disorders. *Journal of Speech, Language, and Hearing Research*, *50*, 459–474.

Waber, D. P., & Holmes, J. M. (1986). Assessing children's memory productions of the Rey-Osterrieth Complex Figure. *Journal of Clinical and Experimental Neuropsychology*, *8*, 565–580.

Wechsler, D. (1996). *Wechsler Intelligence Scale for Children–Third Edition*. New York: Psychological Corporation.

Wechsler, D. (2003). *Wechsler Intelligence Scale for Children–Fourth Edition*. San Antonio, TX: Psychological Corporation.

Whaley, S. E., O'Connor, M. J., & Gunderson, B. (2001). Comparison of the adaptive functioning of children prenatally exposed to alcohol to a nonexposed clinical sample. *Alcoholism: Clinical and Experimental Research*, *25*, 1018–1024.

Woodcock, R. W., McGrew, K., & Mather, N. (1989). *Woodcock-Johnson Tests of Achievement: Revised*. Allen, TX: DLM Teaching Resources.

Woodcock, R. W., McGrew, K. S., & Mather, N. (2001). *Woodcock-Johnson III Tests of Achievement*. Itasca, IL: Riverside Publishing.

2

Asperger Disorder

Lauren Kenworthy

Autism is a neurogenetic disorder that is behaviorally defined by the presence of a triad of impairments affecting social abilities, communication skills, and flexibility of interests and behaviors. Current theory states that autism occurs along a spectrum of severity, hence the term *autism spectrum disorders* (ASDs). The ASDs include Asperger's Disorder, autism, and pervasive developmental disorder–not otherwise specified (a category for individuals who do not meet full criteria for autism). Recent estimates of the prevalence of autism, strictly defined, are approximately 3–4 out of every 10,000 individuals (Yeargin-Allsopp, Rice, Karapurkar, Doernberg, Boyle, & Murphy, 2003), but this rate rises considerably when including the entire autism spectrum (Chakrabarti & Fombonne, 2001), with a recent estimate from the Centers for Disease Control and Prevention (2007) indicating that 1 in 150 children have an ASD in the United States. The prevalence of ASDs has increased dramatically in the last decade, with the greatest area of increase among high-functioning (borderline or higher intelligence) children. Therefore, it is common for pediatric neuropsychologists to encounter a high-functioning child on the autism spectrum in their clinical practice.

Among high-functioning children with ASD, the *Diagnostic and Statistical Manual of Mental Disorders, Fourth Edition, Text Revision* (2000) distinguishes Asperger's Disorder from high-functioning autism (HFA) based on the presence of intact language milestones and communication skills. Thus, Asperger's Disorder is thought to reflect impairments in only two aspects of the autism triad: social interactions and flexibility of behavior. The distinction between high-functioning autism and Asperger's Disorder is controversial, however, with many researchers and clinicians arguing that the groups are fundamentally the same. Although some have argued that Asperger's Disorder is associated with nonverbal learning disabilities (Klin, Volkmar, Sparrow, Cicchetti, & Rourke, 1995), a review of neuropsychological findings in ASD (Ozonoff & Griffith, 2000) did not find conclusive evidence of differences in the profiles of individuals with HFA and Asperger syndrome. There are some data that indicate that children with Asperger's Disorder may have higher IQ scores than those with HFA, but even here the evidence is inconclusive. This chapter describes the case of boy who is diagnosed with Asperger's Disorder, but it is also relevant to many children with the diagnosis of high-functioning autism.

Medical complications, particularly seizure disorders, are more common in low- than high-functioning individuals with ASD. Psychiatric comorbidities are very common and most prominently include attention-deficit/hyperactivity disorder (ADHD), depression, and anxiety (Leyfer et al., 2006). Learning disabilities are also commonly comorbid, particularly in the area of written language and reading comprehension. Other commonly affected academic abilities include organization, note-taking, and test-taking.

Although there are psychopharmacological interventions to address secondary symptoms in

ASDs, including the use of selective serotonin reuptake inhibitors, central stimulants, and atypical antipsychotic medications, there are no current medical treatments for the core triad of impairments in autism. The primary intervention strategies available to target the social, language, and flexibility impairments in ASDs are linguistic, behavioral, and cognitive. Because children with high-functioning ASD (HF-ASD) are frequently educated in mainstream environments, interventions are best applied in school settings, and the development of an appropriate school program is typically a fundamental step (Klin & Volkmar, 2000). In addition, there is a great deal of variability within the cognitive profiles of children with HF-ASDs. For these two reasons, a neuropsychological evaluation that delineates cognitive strengths and weaknesses and makes specific educational recommendations regarding classroom placement, necessary accommodations, and special education and therapy needs, can serve as the cornerstone of a treatment plan for a school-age child with HF-ASD. The developmental neuropsychological assessment model described by Jane Holmes Bernstein (2000) is ideally suited to the needs of children with HF-ASD because it emphasizes identifying diagnostic behavioral clusters, or domains, which pose specific risks to the developing child in specific contexts (e.g., elementary school). Delineation of those risks then drives practical recommendations for intervention (Baron, 2000). The following case is presented using this assessment model.

Case Presentation: John

Referral/Background

John is an 8-year-old Caucasian boy in the second grade who was referred following difficulties with socialization and schoolwork. He had previously been diagnosed with a sensory integration disorder, motor delay, and anxiety. John is a boy with many strengths, including precocious math and science abilities. His parents also report that he has a good sense of humor, likes to learn, and is devoted to a few important people in his life. Primary concerns are social and academic. John has a best friend who is a member of a family with whom John's whole family socializes, but John generally has difficulty interpreting social information. In school, John rarely initiates social contact and is generally isolated. He is often distracted and silly when required to work cooperatively with other students. In addition, John has difficulty recognizing his teacher's position of authority and sometimes rudely challenges the teacher's requests or responds in a stubborn, inflexible manner. Academically, as a second grader, John generally works above grade level, but he struggles with written language. He has difficulty with both the physical act of writing and with formulating written language. In addition, he has had general problems completing assignments.

John is the product of a full-term pregnancy, complicated by a maternal kidney infection. Fetal distress was noted during delivery, and John received oxygen at birth. There were no further perinatal complications. John's medical history is remarkable for removal of adenoids at age 3 and for allergy problems and ear infections. John has a history of anxiety and sleep difficulty for which he takes Zoloft and Remeron. Developmental history includes age-appropriate attainment of basic fine and gross motor and language milestones. Development of preacademic skills was precocious: he memorized the alphabet at 18 months. Family history is unremarkable for neurological, cognitive, or psychological problems.

John has been evaluated repeatedly in the past. His parents presented a series of reports for review. A physical therapy evaluation just prior to age 4 showed significant delays in fine motor skills, poor postural control, and problems with sensory modulation. Based on these findings, John was given a diagnosis of sensory integration dysfunction. John was given a comprehensive psychological evaluation at age 5 that revealed a large discrepancy between John's average visual and visual-motor skills and his very superior verbal skills on the Wechsler Preschool and Primary Scale of Intelligence–Revised Edition. John demonstrated exceptional verbal reasoning and vocabulary skills, along with well-developed auditory memory skills and math reasoning skills. John was noted to have great difficulty adjusting to changes in routine and to be argumentative and inflexible at times. Speech and language evaluation revealed average to very high receptive and expressive language skills. Finally, John was given a math evaluation at age 7. He was found to have very advanced abilities in math, performing above the 99th percentile relative to other children in the first grade.

Evaluation Findings

Evaluation findings are presented here in an integrated format, which includes relevant parent and teacher reports, as well as behavioral observations and test performance, all of which are organized by neuropsychological domain.

General Intellectual Functioning was evaluated using the Wechsler Intelligence Scale for Children–Third Edition (WISC-III) (see Table 2.1). Consistent with his previous evaluation, there is an unusual discrepancy between John's very superior Verbal Comprehension Index and his average Processing Speed and Perceptual Organization Indices. Qualitative observation of John's relatively weaker performance on measures of Processing Speed and Perceptual Organization revealed interference of dysexecutive processes, such as impulsivity and disorganization, as opposed to visual processing deficits. In addition, John struggled with the Picture Arrangement subtest of the WISC-III, due to social problem-solving weaknesses that were also evident on the Comprehension subtest.

Executive Control Functions are a primary area of weakness for John, who struggles in particular with inhibition, organization, working memory, and flexibility. Like many children with executive dysfunction, John's *attention* and problem-solving capabilities are improved with structure. John is able to focus well in a highly structured environment, such as the neuropsychological assessment setting, but he has greater difficulty

at home, which is inherently less structured. John was verbally and motorically *disinhibited* during this evaluation. He also made a number of impulsive errors on timed tasks. Anxiety appeared to be driving a number of these impulsive errors. He was very sensitive to the timed aspects of the tests and wanted to complete the task correctly. John's *organization* abilities are weak. Despite his excellent vocabulary, John struggled, for example, when asked to access his verbal lexicon efficiently: his performance was in the average range on verbal fluency tasks, which was highly discrepant with his very superior verbal knowledge. He also struggled to organize visual information, as demonstrated by a highly part-oriented approach to the Rey-Osterrieth Complex Figure, which interfered with his ability to copy and remember it accurately (see Figure 2.1; see also the color figure in the color insert section). John's difficulty in being able to see the gestalt or "whole" of things is in direct contrast to his prodigious ability to process discrete units of information, as demonstrated by his precocious mastery of the alphabet. Both organization and *working memory* deficits make John sensitive to load when processing auditory information. He repeated sentences extremely well but had relative difficulty with paragraph-length stories. However, both parent and teacher working memory ratings are within normal limits (see Table 2.2), indicating that John is able to compensate for these relative weaknesses with his superior memory skills. This was directly observed on the Coding subtest of the WISC-III on which he had difficulty keeping track of symbol–number associations until he memorized these associations.

Flexibility is another area of executive weakness for John, who has difficulty shifting from one task or topic to another, making transitions,

Table 2-1. Wechsler Intelligence Scale for Children–Third Edition

Verbal (Scaled Scores)		Performance (Scaled Scores)		Indices (Standard Scores)	
Information	19	Picture Completion	9	Verbal IQ	146
Similarities	19	Coding	10	Performance IQ	95
Arithmetic	19	Picture Arrangement	6	Full Scale IQ	124
Vocabulary	19	Block Design	13	Verbal Comprehension	150
Comprehension	13	Object Assembly	8	Perceptual Organization	94
		Symbol Search	10	Processing Speed	101

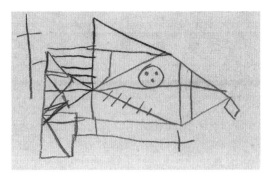

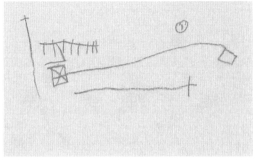

Figure 2-1. (*Top*) Rey-Osterrieth Complex Figure copy condition. (*Bottom*) Rey-Osterrieth Complex Figure delay condition. "See Figure 2.1; see also the color figure in the color insert section."

and who engages in repetitive behaviors, such as pacing obsessively. Thus, although John generally benefits from structure, he has a tendency to become stuck on an idea and is unable to utilize feedback. John demonstrated a number of repetitive routines during testing, including

Table 2-2. Behavior Rating Inventory of Executive Functions (T-scores)

Scale/Index	Parent	Teacher
Inhibit	67	56
Shift	77	79
Emotional Control	61	71
Behavior Regulation Index	70	68
Initiate	58	67
Working Memory	50	54
Plan/Organize	76	**Missing data**
Organization of Materials	46	64
Monitor	79	70
Metacognitive Index	64	
Global Executive Composite	68	

repeatedly using the same phrase. Parent and teacher reports indicate that John can be overly focused and "stubborn" at times, having significant difficulty shifting at school and at home. John was also observed to have difficulty elaborating his answers on portions of testing.

Language-Related Abilities were striking for the contrast between John's phenomenal command of small units of verbal information, including vocabulary and verbal facts, and his relatively poor ability to hold verbal commands in working memory, organize, or flexibly interpret language. During the evaluation, John was initially relatively quiet, which may have reflected test anxiety. As he warmed up, he became more talkative. Articulation, intonation, volume, rate, vocabulary, syntax, and comprehension were generally within normal limits. Consistent with the previous speech and language evaluation, he scored in the average to superior range on basic measures of language expression (Clinical Evaluation of Language Fundamentals III-Screener standard score = 109) and comprehension (Menyuk Syntactic Comprehension Test standard score = 130). John's verbal knowledge for small chunks of information, such as words and facts, is truly remarkable, as he performed at the ceiling of the Information, Similarities, and Vocabulary subtests of the WISC-III. However, executive dysfunction and weak language pragmatics interfered with his ability to apply his linguistic gifts. A relative weakness was observed when John was asked to use his verbal knowledge to solve problems of daily living on the WISC-III Comprehension subtest. This test required John to process longer and more complex questions than asked on other verbal subtests and to apply his general knowledge to generate common-sense solutions to problems. He also struggled on a timed oral formulation task that required him to produce sentences to describe pictures using two or three specific words or phrases, a laboratory finding that was consistent with his teacher's report that John has difficulty formulating his thoughts on written assignments. John also had difficulty with a semantic flexibility task that required him to generate multiple meanings for words.

Visual-Spatial/Visual-Motor performance on a variety of WISC visual-spatial tasks was age appropriate but represented a relative weakness compared to John's verbal abilities. His performance was consistently negatively affected by executive dysfunction. Specifically, John made impulsive errors and was penalized for inefficient, disorganized problem solving on timed tests. John's core visual strengths were evident when he was required to work with abstract visual designs on a structured task. It was a pleasure to watch John copy the abstract visual designs presented on the Block Design subtest, for example. Given a model to copy, he worked quickly, observing visual patterns, and replicating them easily. Consistent with his superlative math skills, John enjoyed working with abstract shapes, angles, and lines in space. His high average score underestimates his abilities, as he made multiple impulsive errors on this task. John had greater difficulty on visual problem-solving tasks that required perception of visual gestalts, organization of visual information, or social problem solving. For example, he had great difficulty assembling a puzzle of a human face.

John's visual-motor capacities have improved since his motor evaluation at 4 years of age. He has benefited from occupational therapy and holds his pencil with an appropriate grasp. John is able to provide appropriate fine motor output over short periods of time, achieving, for example, an average score on the WISC-III Coding subtest. However, ongoing evidence of weakness in this area is provided by his poor bimanual control of pencil and paper and poorly controlled drawing (see Figure 2-1) and letter formation in writing samples. Both teacher and parent report ongoing difficulty with sustained writing. Slowed motor response time was evident on the Test of Variables of Attention, a continuous performance test. Thus, motor difficulties interfered with visual-motor coordination, particularly over time. Executive dysfunction, however, was the primary impediment on visual-motor tasks, as evidenced by the almost two standard deviation drop between his high average performance (standard score = 110) on the structured, relatively simple Beery-Buktenica Developmental Test of Visual-Motor Integration and his low average (standard score = 84) score on his copy of the Rey-Osterrieth Complex Figure. As described earlier, John took an extremely part-oriented approach to the Rey and failed to integrate its component parts.

Learning and Memory was excellent for small units of verbal or visual information, but executive dysfunction interfered with John's ability to learn larger chunks of information and retrieve information from memory. He performed above age expectations in his ability to learn small units of visual or verbal information (Wide Range Assessment of Memory and Learning [WRAML] Sentence Memory standard score = 17; Children's Memory Scale [CMS] Dot Locations scaled score = 15; CMS Number Span scaled scores: Forward = 18, Backward = 19). However, his performance deteriorated as the complexity of information increased due to interference from executive dysfunction (WRAML Story Memory scaled score = 12; Rey-Osterrieth Complex Figure Delay Memory Inventory standard score = 74). John is able to maintain small units of numbers, sentences, and visual data by utilizing his remarkable memory span. He also does very well when given the opportunity to memorize larger chunks of data. For example, on a list-learning task, John was initially overloaded by the large amount of data presented to him, as demonstrated by a major primacy effect in his recall of the list. However, with repetition he was able to compensate with strong rote memorization skills and perform at an above-average level (see CVLT scores below).

California Verbal Learning Test-Children's Version (standard scores)

Total Score **117** Trial 1 **108** Trial 5 **123** Learning Slope **123** Recall Consistency **123** Short Delay Recall Free **100** cued **115** Long Delay Recall Free **123** cued **108** Discriminability **123** (Recognition) Semantic Cluster **77** Primacy **115** Recency **77** Perseverations **92** Interference **100**

John demonstrates weaknesses in the area of *social cognition and social skills*. Social cognition is the ability to make sense of socially relevant information and feelings. It includes interpretation of nonverbal cues, understanding of human relationships, and social problem solving. It also addresses expressive abilities to communicate feelings through nonverbal cues, social motivation, and theory of mind. As noted above, John had difficulty on WISC-III subtests requiring social cognition and even commented after the Picture Arrangement subtest, "I hated that."

Related to this, John had a great deal of difficulty with the Roberts Apperception Test, which required him to tell brief stories describing line drawings of people experiencing emotions or interacting socially. Moreover, he was unable to respond to multiple choice questions about what people in the pictures might be thinking or feeling (e.g., Is this person happy, sad, mad, or scared?). John had great difficulty when describing his own feelings, as well as describing important characteristics of people in his family and human relationships. For example, when asked, "Why do people get married?" his response was "so they can reproduce." During open-ended questions, it was clear that although John wants to have friends, he is more focused on, and motivated by, scientific and mathematical concepts than social interactions.

John's social skills reflect his social cognition profile. Like many children on the autism spectrum, John's best relationships are with the most familiar people in his life: his family. He completed the sentence "I love…" with "…my mommy." Associated with this is his early bonding history, including the development of a social smile, stranger anxiety, recognition of his parents after an absence, physical responsiveness, and engagement in basic interaction games (e.g., peek-a-boo), all of which occurred at appropriate ages. At the same time, his misinterpretation of social information, combined with executive dysfunction, creates significant social difficulties. John is reported to be quite withdrawn both at home and at school. In the one-to-one, highly structured testing situation, John presented as an attractive, cooperative, friendly boy. He has a nice smile, was able to make good eye contact with the examiner, and was good at imitating the examiner's intonation. John had difficulty recognizing socially inappropriate behavior, however. He appeared to be unaware of the impact of his actions on others, not recognizing that imitation of the examiner was inappropriate, for example. The prolonged social interaction required by the assessment was stressful for John, and he responded at times with silliness, raising his voice to answer questions, or answering in pig Latin while sitting underneath the table. John also was unable to pick up on conversational cues from the examiner and respond appropriately, a sign of limited social reciprocity.

Emotional Adjustment is generally appropriate, but John's parents describe a history of anxiety and sleep difficulties. John, like many bright children who struggle with executive dysfunction and social learning problems, was somewhat anxious during this evaluation. Of more concern at the present time are both parent and teacher report on the Behavior Assessment System for Children rating scales of increased dysphoria combined with mild anxiety.

Impression

John's neuropsychological profile is characterized by the following: very superior verbal intelligence; executive dysfunction, including weakness in inhibition, organization, working memory, and flexibility; a social learning disorder; and slowed and poorly controlled motor output. This profile is consistent with, although distinct from, the diagnosis of Asperger Disorder. John meets diagnostic criteria for Asperger Disorder by virtue of his impaired social interaction skills, most notably poor social reciprocity and limited peer interactions; subservience to repetitive behaviors/interests, for example, his repetitive pacing, overfocus on math concepts to the detriment of conversations with others, and extreme rigidity regarding routines; intact early language development and current core language abilities; and lack of general cognitive impairment.

John is a child with remarkable *strengths*. He truly enjoys learning. His performances on measures of vocabulary, verbal reasoning, factual knowledge, and mental arithmetic are at the ceiling of our ability to measure them. He has a powerful memory span, which allows him to memorize small units of information with facility. He can excel at learning larger chunks of information as well, as long as it is presented repeatedly. Moreover, John has superior mathematical and scientific abilities and makes excellent use of his knowledge to support high-level strategic thinking. His ability to think strategically is a prognosticator of his future ability to compensate for areas of difficulty. In fact, John already demonstrates that he makes remarkable compensatory efforts. When John is explicitly taught information that he does not intuitively grasp though rote learning using rules, recipes, and routines, it is predicted that he will make great strides.

John's neuropsychological protocol puts him at *risk* in a variety of situations and with a variety of tasks:

1. John is at risk for being misunderstood and overloaded. His remarkable vocabulary, abstract reasoning, fund of knowledge, and mathematical and scientific abilities are difficult to reconcile with his difficulty completing tasks, learning cooperatively in groups, organizing his thoughts coherently, and flexibility responding to the requests of others. These discrepancies are most readily explained through assumptions of stubborn behavior or inadequate effort on John's part. Moreover, as is the case with many extremely bright children such as John, his compensatory abilities are remarkable and have in many situations masked core deficits. For example, John's remarkable facility at processing words and sentences will lead people to assume that he is a much stronger auditory processor of longer chunks of information than is the case, and to overload him with information. When overwhelmed, the combination of cognitive weakness and anxiety can produce a severely inflexible child.

2. John is also at risk for difficulty with information output. John has difficulty producing work in the classroom because disinhibition, weak working memory, disorganization, and inflexible routines all conspire to limit his ability to work independently. Furthermore, although he has a great store of verbal facts and details, this is not matched by his ability to formulate language and organize ideas. This places John at great risk for frustration over his inability to communicate his ideas. Moreover, while improved, John's long-standing fine motor difficulties continue to hinder his handwriting, which adds a considerable load whenever John is asked to put pencil to paper and thus slows his output.

3. John is susceptible to overfocusing on literal details of instructions and extensive reliance on verbally based, rotely learned rules and approaches to learning. Although this approach may support academic development and is very useful to John in a variety of settings, it may also interfere at times with creative problem solving. More importantly, this style, combined with biologically based inflexibility, may result in apparently rigid behavior when John may simply be having trouble taking in the larger metaphor or meaning of a situation. This thinking style puts John at risk for academic difficulty with expository writing and reading comprehension.

4. John is at high risk for boredom unless he is exposed to a demanding curriculum in math and science.

5. John's difficulty accurately interpreting social information and his constitutional inflexibility places him at risk in his interactions with his teachers and peers. He is likely to miss important information about the expectations of others and get stuck with his own ideas and ways of doing things. Thus, he may not respond appropriately to feedback. He is at particular risk in peer group interactions where he will have the most difficulty controlling the agenda and limiting the amount of information he must process simultaneously. His weakness in organization makes it particularly difficult for him to integrate the information that he receives in such settings. Thus, cooperative learning tasks are very challenging for a child like John.

Recommendations

Recommendations for John use his strengths to combat these risks. They focus on the following: the appropriate school placement for John; the individual therapies and special education supports that he requires; and the accommodations he needs in school. John will require some specialized and individualized services at school; therefore, in a public school setting he must be coded for special education services. The findings of this assessment support coding John as a child with an ASD who is also intellectually gifted. His intellectual abilities make him appropriate for a mainstream classroom if he receives specialized supports.

In order to learn and produce information in cooperative group settings, follow teacher instruction appropriately in class, and maintain appropriate peer relationships, John requires the attention of *a specialized team to support social development.* If appropriately trained, a school psychologist and speech and language therapist can work together to provide counseling, behavior management, and training in social skills and the pragmatics of communication. John requires a "social coach," an adult who genuinely likes and understands him, who can help him learn to improve his ability to pick up on concrete indicators of the feelings of others (e.g., when somebody stands that way, it often means he is angry); logically deconstruct the meaning of social interactions and learn to take the perspective of others (e.g., how do you think he felt when you told him that his math question was "trivial?"); understand the impact of his own actions on others through explicit, concrete, cause–and-effect explanations; and apply social stories and learn associated social rules. Respect John's learning strengths by teaching him in small increments and providing him with discrete social rules, logical and sequential explanations of social events, and routines that he can memorize. Make social skills training intervention an integral part of all activities implemented consistently across the school setting through the use of a behavioral reinforcement system that rewards prosocial behaviors in all children.

John continues to require *occupational therapy* intervention to assist him in becoming comfortable with a keyboard. In addition, John requires helps with fine motor self-care tasks, such as fastening fasteners.

John requires individualized *special education* to improve his written language expression, including teaching him a specific routine for producing written work that is practiced repeatedly and written down in a checklist (e.g.: 1. Brainstorm ideas; 2. Select appropriate ideas for topic matter and length; 3. Put ideas in order, etc….). John also requires special education to improve his executive abilities for working independently and completing tasks. In addition to the use of rules, recipes, routines, and checklists, John needs explicit teaching in order to learn skills that other children may learn on their own. Place specific emphasis on approaches for breaking tasks down into small units, and techniques for identifying the main requirement of an assignment. Provide explicit coaching in strategic planning and goal-oriented problem solving, with an emphasis on consistent routines that can be applied to a variety of independent projects. To be effective, coaches teaching new strategies and routines for tackling work, or demands of daily living, must first model the desired routine and then provide extensive practice with a gradual shift from externally cueing John to having him follow internal cues and written rules or routines.

John's academic and social performance will be improved with familiarity and structure, which can be created through the following *classroom-based accommodations.* Provide John with regularly scheduled down time away from the omnipresent social/executive demands of a standard classroom. Give John free access to his social coach throughout the school day if he needs to address a problem. Provide extra structure for any new experiences or learning, including posting a visual schedule; previewing transitions or unexpected events; providing highly structured routines and frequent one-to-one check-ins to structure independent activities; and using outlines, worksheets, checklists, recipes, written routines, and other interventions to teach John in a step-by-step fashion. Keep oral directions brief or accompany them with a visual reminder, such as a checklist. Take every opportunity to write directions down for John to provide him with visual cues regarding steps he needs to take to carry out work independently. Eliminate handwriting requirements through use of a keyboard or voice-activated software. Apply testing accommodations. Support organizational deficits: Review homework assignments with John before he leaves school each day; assist with the maintenance and organization of a notebook; and provide a daily exchange of information between home and school about assignments and goals.

Finally John's family was encouraged to *engage a psychologist outside of school* to monitor and provide cognitive-behavioral treatment for John's anxiety, in addition to developing a positive behavioral management program at home to target increased flexibility and prosocial behaviors.

Epilogue

John was re-evaluated on two subsequent occasions, when he was 11 and 14 years old. At 11, the presenting problems remained social isolation from peers, inflexibility in conversation and behavior, and poor written expression. His neuropsychological profile was generally consistent with his initial evaluation, although his Verbal Comprehension Index score dropped to 128 on the WISC-IV, while the addition of the Matrix Reasoning subtest to the Performance scale provided him with an opportunity to demonstrate his remarkable visual problem solving in the absence of executive function demands (scaled score = 18). Thus, his overall IQ profile was even, with superior performance in both verbal and nonverbal domains, but there was considerable subtest scatter related to the relative executive demands of the task. John remembered the Block Design subtest from the evaluation conducted almost 4 years previously and requested it when he entered the room for re-evaluation. He continued to be fascinated by and obsessed with mathematical problems. In a further indication of his inflexibility, he appeared for his February evaluation in shorts, because he had been unable to make the transition from fall to winter clothing. John had also developed increased aggressive behavior at home, primarily related to inflexibility.

John's ability to respond to social stimuli had improved, such that he was now able to provide brief stories for the Roberts Apperception cards, but he tended to be very concrete in his responses and often indicated that he did not think the people in the pictures were feeling anything. For example, a picture of a child striding across the floor in anger with a chair over his head was described as "a man asked his son to bring him a chair. His son went to get the chair and carried it back high over his head." When asked explicitly what the person might be thinking or feeling, John said, "not feeling anything substantial."

John's written language remained a major obstacle at school, where he had received handwriting accommodations but no support for the organization of written expression. Conflict between John, his parents, and his teachers had increased, with his teachers insisting that his refusal to write paragraphs was volitional and his parents disagreeing. His performance on a test of written language was discrepant with his Verbal IQ score, and he was given an additional diagnosis of a learning disability affecting written language. Recommendations included the

following: a meeting between the evaluator, John's family, and school personnel to problem solve how to teach John to write; behavior management to target aggressive outbursts; and consideration of stimulant medication.

At 14, John's profile was again highly consistent with previous evaluations. He entered the examination room discussing factorials, which he proceeded to introduce into the conversation whenever it was not structured by the examiner. When presented with the Rey-Osterrieth Complex Figure, he immediately remembered it and a feedback session that occurred when he was 11 in which the effective strategy for copying it was discussed. He described the strategy in some detail while he copied the figure in an entirely part-oriented fashion, directly contradicting what he was saying as he worked. He was fascinated by the strategic possibilities of the Tower of London-Dx, but was unable to hold the two rules governing completion of the tower in mind as he worked. His impulsivity continued to hinder his problem solving.

Although John was now taking Strattera in addition to his other medications, and his family was receiving excellent in-home behavioral management support, he continued to have aggressive, impulsive outbursts, particularly in response to flexibility requirements. He had resisted the help of psychotherapists, firing several. Adaptive daily living and socialization abilities are severely impaired by parent report.

John is placed in a high school for gifted and talented children, which readily accommodates his academic needs, and his writing has improved substantially. He is now producing long works, notably a remarkably insightful autobiography, in which he reported difficulty remembering people's names and noted that he was not connecting with other kids in class the way they were connecting with each other. He is valued by his peers for his remarkable math and science abilities, but he is friendless and isolated during unstructured times. A school observation revealed him to spend his lunch period alone in a darkened classroom turning in a revolving chair.

Recommendations centered on identifying specific goals that would enable John to function independently as he approached adulthood: the ability to make a friend, carry out basic daily living skills, and shape his behavior in response to the requests of others (improve flexibility). Regarding the latter, the examiner recommended explicit cognitive/behavioral training in what flexibility is, what the advantages of being flexible are, and how to be flexible in different situations. A meeting of his treatment team to coordinate these goals and to explicitly pursue John's "buy in" or commitment to pursing these goals was suggested.

Discussion

John is in many ways prototypical of the subset of very high-functioning children with ASD. His profile of poor executive organization and flexibility, social learning impairment, and fine motor weakness, occurring in the context of excellent learning and memory for small chunks of information, is typical of his diagnostic group. Written language learning disabilities, such as those that John has, are also very common. The presence of significant problems with impulsivity is not prototypical, but is common in high-functioning children with ASD. John's difficulty with flexibility is somewhat more severe than is typical, and it may be exacerbated by his remarkable intelligence, which frequently supports his belief that he is smarter than other people. The lack of a family history of an ASD, social learning disorder, or language disorder was unexpected, although subsequent to his first evaluation, John's sister was diagnosed with pervasive developmental disorder–not otherwise specified.

References

American Psychiatric Association (APA). (2000). *Diagnostic and statistical manual of mental disorder* (4th ed., Text rev.). Washington, DC: Author.

Baron, I. S. (2000). Clinical implications and practical applications of child neuropsychological evaluations. In K. O. Yeates, M. D. Ris, & H. G. Taylor (Eds.), *Pediatric neuropsychology: Research, theory, and practice* (pp. 439–456). New York: The Guilford Press.

Bernstein, J. H. (2000). Developmental neuropsychological assessment. In K. O. Yeates, M. D. Ris, & H. G. Taylor (Eds.), *Pediatric neuropsychology: Research, theory, and practice* (pp. 405–438). New York: The Guilford Press.

Center for Disease Control and Prevention (CDC). (2007). *Prevalence of autism spectrum disorders*. Atlanta, GA: U.S. Department of Health and Human Services.

Chakrabarti, S., & Fombonne, E. (2001). Pervasive developmental disorders in preschool children. *The Journal of the American Medical Association*, 285, 3093–3099.

Klin, A., & Volkmar, F.R. (2000). Treatment and intervention guidelines for individuals with Asperger syndrome. In A. Klin, F. Volkmar, & S. S. Sparrow (Eds.), *Asperger syndrome* (pp. 340–366). New York: The Guilford Press.

Klin, A., Volkmar, F. R., Sparrow, S. S., Cicchetti, D. V., & Rourke, B. P. (1995). Validity and neuropsychological characterization of Asperger syndrome. *Journal of Child Psychology and Psychiatry*, 36, 1127–1140.

Leyfer, O. T., Folstein, S. E., Bacalman, S., Davis, N. O., Dinh, E., Morgan, J., et al. (2006). Comorbid psychiatric disorders in children with autism: Interview and development rates of disorders. *Journal of Autism and Developmental Disorders*, 36, 849–861.

Ozonoff, S., & Griffith, E. M. (2000). Neuropsychological function and the external validity of Asperger syndrome. In A. Klin, F. Volkmar, & S. S. Sparrow (Eds.), *Asperger syndrome* (pp. 72–96). New York: The Guilford Press.

Yeargin-Allsopp, M., Rice, C., Karapurkar, T., Doernberg, N., Boyle, C., & Murphy, C. (2003). Prevalence of autism in a US metropolitan area. *The Journal of the American Medical Association*, 289, 49–55.

3

The Identification of Autism Spectrum Disorders in Early Childhood: A Case Report

Marianne Barton, Katelin Carr, Lauren Herlihy, Kelley Knoch, and Deborah Fein

The well-documented benefits of early identification of autism spectrum disorders (ASDs) (for review, see Dumont-Mathieu & Fein, 2005) have led to increased focus on the *earliest manifestations of the disorder, the stability/validity of early diagnosis*, and the *identification of assessment tools suitable for use with very young children*. Equally important, recent recommendations for widespread screening of young children for ASDs (AAP, 2006, 2008) have prompted increased interest in *population-based screening measures* and increased pressure to identify children at risk for the disorder as early as late infancy. All of these efforts have been helpful in permitting the ever-earlier identification and treatment of children with an ASD. At the same time, they highlight the complexity and heterogeneity of the disorder, its interaction with normative variation in developmental trajectories, and our limited understanding of early social and communicative development and its aberrations. We will first discuss some of the literature on these issues and then present a case that illustrates many of them.

A variety of *screening measures* are currently in use or development, including the Checklist for Autism in Toddlers (CHAT; Baron-Cohen, Allen, & Gillberg, 1992), the Modified Checklist for Autism in Toddlers (M-CHAT; Robins, Fein, Barton, & Green, 2001), the Pervasive Developmental Disorders Screening Test-II (PDDST-II; Siegel, 2004), Screening Tool for Autism in Two-Year-Olds (STAT; Stone, Coonrod, & Ousley, 2000), the Checklist for Autism in Toddlers-23 (CHAT-23; Wong et al., 2004)), the Early Screening for Autistic Traits (ESAT; Swinkels et al., 2006, and, most recently, the Infant-Toddler Checklist (ITC; Wetherby & Prizant, 2002). The PDDST-II and the STAT have shown good sensitivity and specificity as stage 2 screeners for use with children in developmental clinics; the authors of the PDDST II have reported good specificity and sensitivity as a stage 1 screener as well (Siegel, 2004), but these data have not yet been replicated in a large community sample (Dumont-Mathieu & Fein, 2005). The STAT is a level-two screen designed to differentiate toddlers with autism from those with other developmental disabilities (Stone et al., 2000; Stone, Coonrod, Turner, & Pozdol, 2004). The validation sample for this measure reported a sensitivity of .83 and a specificity of .86 (Stone et al., 2004).

The CHAT was the first level-one, autism-specific screener and consists of five observation items and nine parent-report items (Baron-Cohen et al., 1992; Baron-Cohen et al., 1996). This measure is currently under revision by the authors due to limited sensitivity (20%–38%) found on follow-up (Baird et al., 2000). The ESAT is a screener for autism in children 14–15 months developed in the Netherlands. The 14-item parent-report questionnaire was reported by the authors to have greater than 90% sensitivity for an ASD but poor specificity for differentiating ASDs from other developmental disorders, a finding that may be related to the fact that the ESAT was tested with especially young children (Swinkels et al., 2006).

Among level-one screeners, the M-CHAT and the ITC currently appear to be most promising. The M-CHAT is a 23-item checklist that asks a parent to provide yes/no responses to questions about his/her toddler's development (Robins et al., 2001). It was adapted from the CHAT by removing the pediatrician observation section and adding parent-report items. The authors report good estimates of specificity and sensitivity, although a follow-up interview was added for children who failed the initial screen to reduce the false-positive rate. Positive predictive value for the M-CHAT has been reported as .36 before and .68–.74 after the follow-up interview (Robins et al., 2001; Kleinman, Robins, et al., 2008). The ITC, a section of the Communication and Symbolic Behavior Scales Developmental Profile (CSBS) has recently been examined as a broadband screener for ASDs (Wetherby et al., 2008). The ITC is composed of 24 items with three to five response choices for questions about social communication milestones, and an additional open-ended question about the parent's developmental concerns (Wetherby et al., 2008). Unique among the screeners reviewed here, the ITC includes standard scores for each month from 6 to 24 based on a large normative sample in addition to a screening cut-off score. The authors report positive predictive values above 70% for children age 9–24 months for communication delays, and 93.3% sensitivity for ASDs in particular, although they caution that a positive screen on the ITC does not distinguish these two groups (Wetherby et al., 2008).

Once children are identified as being at risk for an ASD, they are referred for a more detailed diagnostic evaluation.

In contrast to earlier assertions, it is now clear that *valid and stable diagnoses* of an ASD can be accurately made in children under the age of 3 (Charman et al., 2005, Cox et al., 1999, Eaves & Ho, 2004; Lord, 1995; Moore & Goodson, 2003; Stone et al., 1999). The accuracy of early diagnosis has been further supported by studies investigating the stability of diagnoses given between the ages of 2–3 years with confirmatory diagnoses given 1, 2, and 3 years later (Chawarska, Klin, Paul, & Volkmar, 2007; Cox et al., 1999; Eaves & Ho, 2004; Kleinman et al., 2008; Lord, Storoschuk, Rutter, & Pickles, 1993; Moore & Goodson, 2004; Turner & Stone, 2007). While overall, ASD

diagnoses are considered relatively stable, diagnoses of autism (72%) are more stable than diagnoses of PDD-NOS (42%) (Stone et al., 1999). It is unclear whether the limited diagnostic stability in individuals diagnosed with PDD-NOS at age 2 years is due to higher responsiveness to treatment, the ambiguity in the diagnostic category, or a tendency for the milder symptoms to be transient (Cox et al., 1999; Eaves & Ho, 2004; Stone et al., 1999; Walker et al., 2004).

Some of the earliest manifestations of ASDs have been fruitfully studied with early home movies of diagnosed children, as well as prospective studies of high-risk children (i.e., younger siblings of affected children). These studies have revealed that early signs of autism vary appreciably with age during the period from infancy through early childhood. During the first year of life, children with an ASD are less likely than their typically developing counterparts to orient when their name is called (Osterling & Dawson, 1994; Osterling, Dawson, & Munson, 2002; Werner, Dawson, Osterling, & Dinno, 2000). An absence of social smiling and lack of facial expression have also been identified as early markers of an ASD (Adrien et al., 1992; Zwaigenbaum et al., 2005). Infants with an ASD look at others less frequently than typically developing infants (Osterling & Dawson, 1994; Osterling et al., 2002) show deficits in visual tracking and imitation (Osterling et al., 2002; Zwaigenbaum et al., 2005), and they show fewer social and joint attention behaviors (Osterling & Dawson, 1994; Zwaigenbaum et al., 2005). In the second year of life, children with an ASD show an increased lack of response to name and poor eye contact (Chawarska et al., 2007; Wetherby et al., 2004), as well as failure to point (Chawarska et al., 2007; Cox et al., 1999), delays in functional and symbolic play, and limited response to joint attention prompts (Chawarska et al., 2007). Deficits in sharing enjoyment and interest, lack of facial expression, and lack of showing also characterize this population (Wetherby et al., 2004). Some researchers have found increased frequency of repetitive behaviors in the second year (Wetherby et al., 2004), although others have not (Cox et al., 1999).

Changes in symptom presentation in children with an ASD between the second and third years of life include the emergence of speech

(Charman et al., 2005; Chawarska et al., 2007), in addition to the acquisition of atypical language features, such as echolalia and unusual intonation (Chawarska et al., 2007). Increased bids for joint attention, a lack of pointing, and a marginal increase in communicative gesture use have also been found in children with an ASD during this period, as well as a lack of improvement in coordination of social-communicative behaviors, eye contact, and direction of facial expression toward others (Chawarska et al., 2007).

In the fourth year of life, Cox et al. (1999) found that children with autism continue to exhibit reduced affect sharing and imaginative play relative to children with language disorder. In Charman et al.'s (2005) longitudinal study of children with an ASD, children gained more reciprocal social interaction skills between the ages of 4–5 and 7 years, whereas gains between 3 and 4–5 years were not significant. However, significant gains in communication skills were made in Charman et al.'s (2005) sample from ages 3 through 7.

Communication and social interaction deficits appear to be the most salient characteristics of young children with an ASD, whereas repetitive and stereotyped behaviors in young children have been less fully understood. Repetitive behaviors may be less frequent or less noticeable at younger ages and increase by 42 months (Cox et al., 1999), but other researchers report no changes in the level of repetitive behaviors between the second and third year of life (Charman et al., 2005; Chawarska et al., 2007). Children with an ASD younger than 36 months have been found to exhibit more simplistic repetitive behaviors, such as hand and finger mannerisms and repetitive use of objects, whereas children older than 36 months appear to demonstrate more higher level behaviors, such as resistance to change and circumscribed interests (Mooney, Gray, & Tonge, 2006). Charman et al. (2005) found that repetitive behaviors increased most between the ages of 3 and 4–5 years and then decreased at 7 years. However, Charman et al. (2005) also found significant individual variation in the frequency of repetitive behaviors and other autism symptoms over time.

Variation in the presentation of symptoms of ASDs during early childhood has important implications for the selection of *assessment tools*.

Autism-specific assessment tools currently available to clinicians include measures based on caregiver report, such as the Autism Diagnostic Interview-Revised (ADI-R; Rutter, LeCouteur, & Lord, 1995), and those based on the clinician's behavioral observations of the child, including the Autism Diagnostic Observation Schedule (ADOS; Lord, Rutter, DiLavore, & Risi, 2000) and the Childhood Autism Rating Scale (CARS; Schopler, Reichler, & Renner, 1980). These measures must be supplemented by assessment of developmental level, adaptive skills, and communication skills in order to provide a context in which to evaluate the meaning of atypical social behaviors.

Clinical judgment is considered the "gold standard" for diagnosing ASDs in children less than 5 years old (Volkmar et al, 2005). Both clinicians and the diagnostic measures available rely on criteria from the *Diagnostic and Statistical Manual for Mental Disorders-IV* (*DSM-IV*). Stone and colleagues (1999) have studied the applicability of *DSM-IV* criteria to young children with autism. Their study found the criteria related to social deficits and delayed language to be most prominent in children under 3 years of age. However, other items, such as failure to develop peer relationships, impaired conversational ability, stereotyped and repetitive use of language, and inflexible adherence to routines and rituals, were not as reliably observed in young children with autism.

The stability of diagnoses has been explored based on clinical judgment and commonly used diagnostic instruments. In a study by Kleinman, Ventola, et al. (2008), the initial diagnosis of 77 children (mean age of 2.25 years) was compared with the confirmatory diagnosis made 2 years later (mean age 4.4 years). The authors report high stability for clinical judgment based on the *DSM-IV* (80%), with higher stability for diagnoses of autistic disorder (70%) compared to PDD-NOS (33%). The stability rate for diagnosis was at acceptable levels for diagnosing ASDs in toddlers, with only 15 children moving off the autism spectrum at follow-up and none moving onto the spectrum. Stability was high for diagnosis based on the ADOS (83%) and the CARS (76%), but lower for the ADI-R (67%). Unlike the ADOS and the CARS, the ADI requires the presence of repetitive behaviors or restricted interests to make the diagnosis of autistic disorder. At follow-up, several children who did not originally meet the criteria of repetitive behaviors required for a diagnosis of autistic disorder on the ADI subsequently met criteria after developing restricted interests or repetitive behaviors at age 4. Other studies have also found decreased stability in the ADI-R in 2-year-olds, in part because some children did not develop restricted interests or repetitive behaviors until later in development (Charman et al., 2005; Cox et al., 1999; Turner et al, 2006; Turner & Stone, 2007).

The interrater reliability of diagnostic instruments has also been examined in the early diagnosis of ASDs. When classifying toddlers as spectrum versus nonspectrum, interrater reliability for diagnosis based on clinical judgment, CARS, and *DSM-IV* was considered good, with clinicians agreeing on the diagnosis of 57 out of 65 children (88%). This level of agreement dropped to 64% when distinguishing between autism and PDD-NOS (Stone et al., 1999). High agreement has also been found between clinical judgment based on *DSM-IV* criteria, CARS, and the ADOS-G in a sample of children aged 16–31 months (Ventola et al., 2006). Upon examination of the ADI-R, researchers have found low levels of agreement between the repetitive behaviors domain and other measures (Cox et al., 1999; Saemundsen, Magnusson, Smari, & Sigurdardottir, 2003; Ventola et al., 2006). These studies suggest that a change in the criteria of the ADI-R, namely a decreased cut-off score for the repetitive behaviors and restricted interests domain, may be necessary for the ADI-R to be used reliably in the early diagnosis of ASDs.

The sensitivity and specificity of the diagnostic instruments have been compared to the "gold standard" of clinical judgment. The ADOS-G and CARS have been found to have good sensitivity rates and adequate specificity rates for diagnoses of autism and PDD-NOS (Cox et al, 1999; Ventola et al., 2006). The ADI-R also had adequate specificity rates but relatively poor sensitivity. In one study the ADI-R failed to identify almost half of the children (17 of 36) diagnosed as having autism or PDD-NOS, primarily because these children did not exhibit early repetitive behaviors (Chawarska et al., 2007; Cox et al., 1999; Ventola et al., 2006). Wiggins and Robins (2008) were able to increase the sensitivity rate of the ADI-R, from .33 to .79, with minimal compromise in specificity (.94 to .78) when they excluded the behavioral domain from their analyses.

In addition to consideration of limitations of existing measures for ASD diagnosis, it is important to identify more general developmental concerns related to the assessment of ASDs in toddlers. As noted earlier, there is divergence of autism symptoms from typical behavior changes over the course of early development (Vig & Jedrysek, 1999). Therefore, developmental level or mental age must be considered when interpreting potential autism-related behaviors (Vig & Jedrysek, 1999). Several authors have noted that it is difficult to differentiate global developmental delay (GDD/mental retardation) from ASDs in children with mental ages below 18–24 months (Rutter & Schopler, 1987; Vig & Jedrysek, 1999). The Childhood Autism Rating Scale (CARS) and the Autism Diagnostic Interview-Revised (ADI-R) have been shown to overidentify 2-year-olds and older nonverbal children with mental ages below 18 months (DiLavore, Lord, & Rutter, 1995; Lord et al., 1993; Saemundsen et al., 2003; Vig & Jedrysek, 1999). Specific criteria for ASDs that reference skills and behaviors beyond the toddler's mental age are also problematic. For example, a lack of pretend play skills is a hallmark of ASDs that is assessed by most diagnostic measures; however, the ability to engage in pretend play with dolls or other objects does not typically emerge until 19–22 months (Westby, 1980). Similarly, joint attention typically develops between 9 and 18 months, making this behavior a contentious candidate for autism assessment in children with mental ages less than 12 months (Swinkels et al., 2006). The absence of communication and social skills may be due to delayed development rather than specific to autism. Finally, children with low mental age likely lack sufficient cognitive development to recognize patterns or similarities among objects and events, and therefore they may not experience the distress caused by transitions or by disruptions of habitual routines that is evident in older children with an ASD (Vig & Jedrysek, 1999).

As researchers and clinicians continue their efforts to identify ASDs in younger children, it seems likely that diagnosis will focus increasingly on early forms of social communication and reciprocal interaction, including behaviors evident very early in development which serve those functions, such as gaze shifting, eye contact, gesture, affect sharing, joint attention, and pointing. The following is a brief description of a young child who presented precisely those concerns beginning at about the age of 12 months.

Case Report: Zachary

Zachary lived with his parents, Susan and James, and his 3-year-old brother, Sam. James worked from home as a salesman; Susan was at home full time to care for the children. Zachary's older brother had received Early Intervention services for delayed language acquisition, but he was now developing typically at the age of 39 months.

Zachary was the product of a healthy, planned, and uncomplicated pregnancy. He was born at term after a vaginal delivery and weighed 8 pounds, 10 ounces. He was bottle fed and spit up often. He continued to gag easily as a toddler. When Zachary was 4–5 months old his parents became concerned that his head was unusually large. They had him examined by a neurologist, who found no abnormalities or cause for concern. Zachary was re-evaluated by the same neurologist at 12 months old, and no abnormalities were identified. Other than those issues, Zachary was a healthy and happy infant.

Susan and James report that Zachary was a smiling and responsive baby throughout his first 6 to 8 months of life. He attained motor milestones at the expected times: he sat alone at 9 months and walked at 13 months. At about 10 months, Zachary's parents began to notice a decline in his responsiveness to social play and in his eye contact. They report that until that time, Zachary had enjoyed playing games such as pattycake, made consistent eye contact, and was easily engaged in social play. For the first 11 months of Zachary's life, his older brother had received Speech and Language Therapy services in the family's home. The speech pathologist had frequent contact with Zachary. Neither she nor his parents noted any concerns with his social development or early communication skills.

When Zachary was between the ages of 12 and 15 months, his parents' concerns grew more serious and more focused. Zachary seemed to lose interest in social exchanges and made less frequent eye contact. He began to resist being held and began arching his back when picked up. He lost interest in toys he had previously enjoyed. At 15 months his primary play interest was in pop-up toys. Zachary babbled expressively, but he had no words and used no communicative gestures.

Zachary was nearly 16 months old when he was referred for evaluation following his failure on the Modified Checklist for Autism in Toddlers. This is earlier than the 16–30 month range recommended by the authors of the M-CHAT, but both Zachary's mother and his pediatricians had concerns with his development by 15 months. Zachary's mother spoke to his pediatrician at his 15-month well-baby visit about her concerns that Zachary was slow to develop language and appeared to be more self-absorbed and less interactive over time. The pediatrician referred the family to early intervention services, who subsequently screened Zachary for early signs of autism and referred him for further evaluation.

Zachary was evaluated in two sessions separated by a few weeks. Both of Zachary's parents were present throughout both evaluation sessions. His parents were administered the Autism Diagnostic Interview and the Vineland Adaptive Behavior Scales. Zachary was evaluated using the Mullen Scales of Early Learning and the Autism Diagnostic Observation Schedule. The evaluating clinician also completed the Childhood Autism Rating Scale and a *DSM-IV* autism symptom checklist.

Zachary's parents' responses to the Autism Diagnostic Interview provided further elaboration of their concerns about his atypical development. He communicated primarily by nonspecific crying, although he occasionally pulled his mother's hands to indicate that he wanted food. On occasion he would also pull her hand to request that she activate a favorite toy. He had no conventional gestures, nor did he point at objects outside his reach or follow a point. On occasion he would point to pictures in a book. Zachary appeared to understand very little language directed at him, with the exception of the words *no* and *bottle*. He did respond to a few highly familiar routines: he looked up expectantly if his parents approached him and said, "I'm gonna get you," and he calmed visibly when his mother sang a familiar song. Zachary smiled at his mother occasionally in response to her smile, but this occurred with decreasing frequency; he was more likely to smile in response to television programs.

Zachary also developed several atypical behaviors between the ages of 13 and 15 months. He became very interested in texture and pattern. He began walking on his toes and occasionally banging his head, and he began flapping his hands by his side when he was excited and when he watched television.

Observation of Zachary throughout the evaluation confirmed many of his parents' concerns. With encouragement and visual prompting, Zachary was willing to attempt many of the tasks presented to him, although he did not appear interested in the tasks, and he did not persist at tasks he found difficult. His parents reported that his behavior throughout the evaluation sessions was largely typical of his presentation more generally.

Zachary's scores on the Mullen revealed considerable variability in his skills. On the Gross Motor Scale he attained a T-score of 46, which fell within normal limits for his age. He had more difficulty with the Fine Motor tasks for which he received a T-score of 33. But he had very significant delays in the areas of nonverbal skills (Visual Reception Scale), expressive language, and receptive language, where his skills all fell nearly three standard deviations below the mean. Zachary's ability to communicate intentionally and to understand language was estimated to fall at the 7–9-month level. Zachary was largely disinterested in the tasks presented by the Visual Reception Scale of the Mullen and did not appear to understand the directives. His score on this scale fell at the 6-month level.

Zachary's delays were corroborated by his parents' responses to the Vineland Adaptive Behavior Scale. Zachary's motor skills appeared to be intact, as evidenced by his Standard Score of 119 on this scale. He attained a Standard Score of 81 on the Communication Scale, consistent with an age equivalent of 10 months, and with his scores on the Mullen Language Scales. Zachary's parents described his socialization skills as consistent with those of a 9-month-old, which earned him a Standard Score of 83 on the Socialization Scale. Finally, his Daily Living

Skills earned a Standard Score of 76 and an age equivalent of 8 months.

Clearly both the developmental assessment and Zachary's parents' report of his adaptive skills depicted a highly atypical developmental pattern. Zachary's motor skills appeared to be largely intact, while both his language development and his nonverbal skills were markedly delayed, along with his adaptive skills and play skills as indexed by the Vineland.

Zachary's responses to the play probes of the Autism Diagnostic Observation Schedule corroborated many of the social concerns his parents described. He was briefly interested in many of the toys available to him, but he did not engage in purposeful play with the single exception of pushing buttons on a pop-up toy. He preferred to wander around the room, fingering one toy after another and looking at the pattern in the carpet from a variety of visual angles. It was possible to engage Zachary in interaction for very brief periods of time and in highly familiar routines. For example, he was willing to play a vocal imitation game for two turns with the examiner, before he wandered away from interaction and resumed studying the carpet. Zachary did not respond to his name or to social smiles directed at him by his mother and the examiner. He did respond to his mother singing a familiar song by turning toward her and smiling. He made infrequent and very fleeting eye contact with all of the adults present. Zachary clearly enjoyed some of the toys presented during the ADOS. For example, he watched the bubbles, but he did not make eye contact, nor did he request more bubbles. Instead he wandered away from the table. Zachary had no interest in any pretend play activities, and he did not make any communicative overtures during the course of the ADOS. He did not attempt to call attention to his activity, to direct adult attention to interesting objects, or to share his pleasure or excitement. Zachary received a Total Communication and Social Interaction Score on the ADOS of 20, well above the cutoff for a diagnosis of Autistic Disorder.

Zachary received a score of 32.5 score on the Childhood Autism Rating Scale, which placed him in the mildly-moderately autistic range. He clearly met *DSM-IV* Criteria for a diagnosis of Autistic Disorder. He exhibited marked impairment in reciprocal social interaction, qualitative impairments in communication, and stereotyped and repetitive motor mannerisms and persistent preoccupations with parts of objects.

Zachary's parents were clearly devastated but not surprised by his diagnosis. They also expressed relief that their growing concerns had been validated and that a definitive diagnosis might provide guidelines for effective intervention.

Within weeks of receiving a diagnosis, Zachary was enrolled in intensive early intervention services. He received 20 hours of individual intervention weekly, including weekly speech and language services, weekly occupational therapy and intensive behavioral intervention in his home. At age 2 he began attending a small mother–child play group in addition to his in-home services. At age 3 Zachary began attending a small preschool program for 23 hours weekly. He continued to receive Speech and Language Therapy as well as Occupational Therapy Services, although he no longer received individual behavioral instruction. He did receive individual instructional support designed to facilitate his interactions with peers. Zachary's parents further supplemented his program with intensive work with him at home, and with physical therapy and therapeutic horseback riding.

Zachary was re-evaluated as part of a follow-up study when he was 53 months old. He was administered the same series of measures with the exception of the Vineland Scales and a portion of the Mullen. These were not completed because Zachary became ill.

Zachary's mother completed the Autism Diagnostic Interview and described marked progress in his social and communicative skills. At the age of 24 months Zachary began speaking single words and his language has progressed to full sentences, question forms, and reciprocal conversation. Occasionally Zachary repeated questions directed to him; this was most likely to occur when he was confused by the question. At times Zachary also repeated greetings when people did not respond to him initially.

Zachary's social skills improved dramatically. He made consistent eye contact without prompting and smiled readily in response to smiles. Zachary reportedly played with peers individually and in small groups and initiated play by asking children to join an activity. He was reportedly sad when children left the playground and said good-bye spontaneously. Zachary enjoyed playing with trains, but he could be redirected to other activities. He also enjoyed playing on playground equipment and reading books. He had a preferred friend at school who occasionally visited his home. Zachary engaged somewhat reluctantly in pretend play, most often when initiated by others.

Zachary no longer exhibited stereotypic movements or self-injurious behavior. He continued to struggle with a strong gag reflex and with sensory irregularities. For example, he sometimes sought spinning chairs and he actively resisted having his hair dried.

Zachary's responses to the play probes of the ADOS, Module 2, largely corroborated his mother's description of him. He made consistent eye contact, responded readily to his name, and used language to request desired activities. He showed several objects to his mother and directed her attention to objects he found interesting. He was quick to share his pleasure in preferred activities and to solicit his mother's participation as well as that of the examiners. He willingly engaged in brief periods of reciprocal conversation with the examiners and was able to describe a story depicted in a book. His descriptions were somewhat limited, and while he was able to elaborate conversation following his partners' lead, his responses were more limited than expected of a child of his age. Zachary engaged in brief periods of pretend play. He was most comfortable doing this with adults and did not enjoy play with a series of small figures. Zachary received a score of 3 on both the Communication and the Social Interaction Scales of the ADOS, resulting in a Total score of 6, below the Autism Spectrum Cut-off of 8, but still indicating some residual autistic symptoms.

Taken together, the data from both the ADI and the ADOS suggest that Zachary no longer met criteria for a diagnosis on the autism spectrum. He received a score of 22 on the CARS, which falls in the nonautistic range. He continued to struggle with sensory irregularities and with behavioral regulation, and he may have had relatively subtle language difficulties, but his social development appeared to be progressing on a more typical developmental path. He was inattentive throughout much of the evaluation and occasionally noncompliant, and those behaviors interfered with his performance to a moderate degree.

Zachary demonstrated broadly age-appropriate skills on the Expressive and Receptive Language Scales of the Mullen. He attained T-scores of 45 on the Receptive Language Scale and 44 on the Expressive Language Scale. He communicated in four-word phrases; used pronouns; followed a series of commands; and identified numbers, letters, and number concepts. The Mullen offers a limited assessment, however, of higher order receptive language skills, and some of Zachary's behavior suggested that he should receive further evaluation in this area. Zachary attained a T-score of 35 on the Fine Motor Scale of the Mullen, but he was clearly fatigued and refused to attempt several tasks presented to him. Test administration was suspended at this point and neither the Gross Motor Scale nor the Visual Reception Scale was administered.

Zachary's case, while incomplete, illustrates many of the issues associated with the diagnosis of an ASD in young children. He was identified very early in development and presented readily apparent delays in communication skills and reciprocal social interaction. While his delays were consistent across multiple developmental areas, his age-appropriate scores in motor development, as well as his atypical social presentation, suggest that developmental delay was insufficient to explain his difficulties. His presentation was characterized by a high degree of consistency across measures and across parental report and observation. As a result, a diagnosis of an ASD could be made with a high degree of confidence.

Zachary's difficulties followed a period of apparently typical development and either developed spontaneously between 10 and 15 months, or more likely, emerged as Zachary failed to keep pace with social and communicative milestones. This regressive pattern of emergence of autism is quite common (estimates vary from 15% to 47%; Stefanatos, 2008). Zachary's developmental discontinuities could not be associated with any medical procedures, known risks, or traumatic circumstances. Nor were any underlying neurologic difficulties ever identified. Unlike some children diagnosed with an ASD in the second year of life, Zachary exhibited atypical behaviors and stereotypies as a toddler. These appeared to follow the appearance of social concerns, and they appeared to increase as his social withdrawal increased.

While it is not possible to predict Zachary's progress from this point, his gains thus far bode well for his continued positive trajectory. He may be at risk for attention difficulties, language concerns, or mild social/emotional difficulties, but his progress thus far has been impressive. The minority of children who lose the diagnosis of an ASD do seem to be at risk for attention, subtle difficulties with higher order language functions, and anxiety disorders (Helt et al., 2008; Kelley, Fein, & Naigles, 2006). Careful examination of Zachary's initial presentation reveals little that would have predicted his positive outcome thus far. Clearly, children with autism require, individual intervention services focused on behavioral strategies and functional communication skills beginning as early as possible. The initiation of those services when Zachary was 16 months old, their continuation into the preschool years, and Zachary's family's active involvement in his treatment undoubtedly facilitated his progress, although none of those factors guarantee positive outcomes.

Zachary's case underscores the critical importance of early identification and aggressive early intervention. At the same it reminds us of how much there is yet to learn about the presentation of an ASD in toddlers, the pathways the disorder is likely to take, and those factors that may mediate outcome for young children.

References

Adrien, J., Perrot, A., Sauvage, D., Leddet, I., Larmande, C., Hameury, L., & Barthelemy, C. (1992). Early symptoms in autism from family home movies: Evaluation and comparison between 1st and 2nd year of life using I.B.S.E. scale. *Acta Paedopsychiatrica, 55,* 71–75.

American Academy of Pediatrics, Council on Children With Disabilities, Section on Developmental and Behavioral Pediatrics. (2006). Identifying infants and young children with developmental disorders in the medical home: an algorithm for developmental surveillance and screening. *Pediatrics, 118,* 405–420.

American Academy of Pediatrics. (2008). *Caring for children with autism spectrum disorders: A resource toolkit for clinicians*. Grove Village, IL: American Academy of Pediatrics.

American Psychiatric Association (APA). (1994). *Diagnostic and statistical manual of mental disorders*, (4th ed., Rev. ed.). Washington, DC: APA.

Baird, G., Charman, T., Baron-Cohen, S., Cox, A., Swettenham, J., Wheelwright, S., et al., (2000). A screening instrument for autism at 18 months of age: A 6-year follow-up study. *Journal of American Academy of Child and Adolescent Psychiatry, 39*(6), 694–702.

Baron-Cohen, S., Allen, J., & Gillberg, C. (1992). Can autism be detected at 18 months? The needle, the haystack, and the CHAT. *British Journal of Psychiatry, 161*, 839–843.

Baron-Cohen, S., Cox, A., Baird, G., Swettenham, J., Nightingale, N., Morgan, K., et al., (1996). Psychological markers in the detection of autism in infancy in a large population. *British Journal of Psychiatry, 168*, 158–163.

Charman, T., Taylor, E., Drew, A., Cockerill, H., Brown, J.-A., & Baird, G. (2005). Outcome at 7 years of children diagnosed with autism at age 2: Predictive validity of assessments conducted at 2 and 3 years of age and pattern of symptom change over time. *Journal of Child Psychology and Psychiatry, 46*(5), 500–513.

Chawarska, K., Klin, A., Paul, R., & Volkmar, F. (2007). Autism spectrum disorder in the second year: stability and change in syndrome expression. *Journal of Child Psychology and Psychiatry, 48*(2), 128–138.

Cox, A., Klein, K., Charman, T., Baird, G., Baron-Cohen, S., Swettenham, J., et al., (1999). Autism spectrum disorders at 20 and 42 months of age: Stability of clinical and ADI-R diagnosis. *Journal of Child Psychology and Psychiatry, 40*(5), 719–732.

DiLavore, P. C., Lord, C., & Rutter, M. (1995). The Pre-Linguistic Autism Diagnostic Observation Schedule. *Journal of Autism and Developmental Disorders, 25*, 355–379.

Dumont-Mathieu, T., & Fein, D. (2005). Screening for autism in young children: The Modified Checklist for Autism in Toddlers (M-CHAT) and other measures. *Mental Retardation and Developmental Disabilities, 11*, 253–262.

Eaves, L. C., & Ho, H. H. (2004). The very early identification of autism: Outcome to age 41/2–5. *Journal of Autism and Developmental Disorders, 34*(4), 367–378.

Helt, M., Kelley, E., Kinsbourne, M., Pandey, J., Boorstein, H., Herbert, M., & Fein, D., (2008). Can children with autism recover? If so, how? *Neuropsychology Review, 18*, 339–366.

Kelley, E., Fein, D., & Naigles, L. (2006). Residual language deficits in optimal outcome children with a history of autism. *Journal of Autism and Developmental Disorders, 36*, 807–828.

Kleinman, J., Robins, D., Ventola, P., Pandey, J., Boorstein, H., Esser, E., et al., (2008). The Modified Checklist for Autism in Toddlers: A follow-up study investigating the early detection of autism spectrum disorders. *Journal of Autism and Developmental Disorders, 38*, 827–839.

Kleinman, J., Ventola, P., Pandey, J., Verbalis, A., Barton, M., Hodgson, S., et al., (2008). Diagnostic stability in very young children with autism spectrum disorders. *Journal of Autism and Developmental Disorders, 38*(4), 606–615.

Lord, C. (1995). Follow-up of two-year-olds referred for possible autism. *Journal of Child Psychology and Psychiatry, 36*(8), 1365–1382.

Lord, C., Rutter, M., DiLavore, P., & Risi, S. (2000). *Autism Diagnostic Observation Schedule – WPS edition*. Los Angeles: Western Psychological Services.

Lord, C., Storoschuk, S., Rutter, M., & Pickles, A. (1993). Using the ADI–R to diagnose autism in preschool children. *Infant Mental Health Journal, 14*(3), 234–252.

Mooney, E., Gray, K., & Tonge, B. (2006). Early features of autism: Repetitive behaviours in young children. *European Journal of Child and Adolescent Psychiatry, 15*, 12–18.

Moore, V., & Goodson, S. (2003). How well does early diagnosis of autism stand the test of time? Follow-up study of children assessed for autism at age 2 and development of an early diagnostic service. *Autism, 7*(1), 47–63.

Osterling, J., & Dawson, G. (1994). Early recognition of children with autism: A study of first birthday home videotapes. *Journal of Autism and Developmental Disorders, 24*(3), 247–257.

Osterling, J., Dawson, G., & Munson, J. (2002). Early recognition of 1-year-old infants with autism spectrum disorder versus mental retardation. *Development and Psychopathology, 14*, 239–251.

Robins, D., Fein, D., Barton, M., & Green, J. (2001). The Modified Checklist for Autism in Toddlers: An initial study investigating the early detection of autism and pervasive developmental disorders. *Journal of Autism and Developmental Disorders, 31*, 131–144.

Rutter, M., & Schopler, E. (1987). Autism and pervasive developmental disorders: Concepts and diagnostic issues. *Journal of Autism and Developmental Disorders, 17*, 159–186.

Rutter, M., LeCouteur, A., & Lord, C. (1995). *Autism Diagnostic Interview, revised-WPS edition*. Los Angeles: Western Psychological Services.

Saemundsen, E., Magnusson, P. L., Smari, J., & Sigurdardottir, S. (2003). Autism Diagnostic Interview-Revised and the Childhood Autism Rating Scale: Convergence and discrepancy in diagnosing autism. *Journal of Autism and Developmental Disorders, 33*(3), 319–328.

Schopler, E., Reichler, R. J., & Renner, B. R. (1980). *The Childhood Autism Rating Scales*. Los Angeles: Western Psychological Services.

Siegel, B. (2004). Pervasive Developmental Disorders Screening Test –II (PDDST-II): *Early childhood screener for autistic spectrum disorders*. San Antonio, TX: Pearson, Inc..

Stefanotos, G. (2008) Regression in autism spectrum disorders. *Neuropsychology Review, 18,*, 305–319.

Stone, W., Coonrod, E., & Ousley, O. (2000). Brief report: Screening Tool for Autism in Two-year-olds (STAT): Development and preliminary data. *Journal of Autism and Developmental Disorders*, 30, 607–612.

Stone, W., Coonrod, E., Turner, L., & Pozdol, S. L. (2004). Psychometric properties of the STAT for early autism screening. *Journal of Autism and Developmental Disorders*, 34, 691–701.

Stone, W. L., Lee, E. B., Ashford, L., Brissie, J., Hepburn, S. L., Coonrod, E. E., et al., (1999). Can autism be diagnosed accurately in children under 3 years? *Journal of Child Psychology and Psychiatry, 40*(2), 219–226.

Swinkels, S., Dietz, C., van Daalen, E., Kerkhof, I., van Engeland, H., & Buitelaar, J. (2006). Screening for autistic spectrum in children aged 14 to 15 months. I: The development of the Early Screening for Autistic Traits Questionnaire (ESAT). *Journal of Autism and Developmental Disorders*, 36, 723–732.

Turner, L., Stone, W., Pozdol, S., & Coonrod, E. (2006). Follow-up of children with autism spectrum disorders from age 2 to age 9. *Autism, 10*(3), 243–265.

Turner, L., & Stone, W. (2007). Variability in outcome for children with an ASD diagnosis at age 2. *Journal of Child Psychology and Psychiatry, 48*(8), 793–802.

Ventola, P. E., Kleinman, J., Pandey, J., Barton, M., Allen, S., Green, J., et al., (2006). Agreement among four diagnostic instruments for autism spectrum disorders in toddlers. *Journal of Autism and Developmental Disorders, 36*(7), 839–847.

Vig, S., & Jedrysek, E. (1999). Autistic features in young children with significant cognitive impairment: Autism or mental retardation? *Journal of Autism and Developmental Disorders, 29*(3), 235–248.

Volkmar, F., Chawarska, K., & Klin, A. (2005). Autism in infancy and early childhood. *Annual Review of Psychology, 56*(1), 315–336.

Walker, D. R., Thompson, A., Zwaigenbaum, L., Goldberg, J., Bryson, S. E., Mahoney, W. J., et al., (2004). Specifying PDD-NOS: A Comparison of PDD-NOS, Asperger syndrome, and autism. *Journal of American Academy of Child and Adolescent Psychiatry, 43*(2), 172–180.

Werner, E., Dawson, G., Osterling, J., & Dinno, N. (2000). Brief report: Recognition of autism spectrum disorder before one year of age: A retrospective study based on home videotapes. *Journal of Autism and Developmental Disorders, 30*(2), 157–162.

Westby, C. (1980). Assessment of cognitive and language abilities through play. *Language, Speech, and Hearing Services in Schools, 11*, 154–168.

Wetherby, A., Brosnan-Maddox, S., Peace, V., & Newton, L. (2008). Validation of the Infant-Toddler Checklist as a broadband screener for autism spectrum disorders from 9 to 24 months of age. *Autism, 12*, 487–511.

Wetherby, A., & Prizant, B. (2002). *Communication and Symbolic Behavior Scales Developmental Profile–First Normed Edition*. Baltimore: Brookes.

Wetherby, A., Woods, J., Allen, L., Cleary, J., Dickinson, H., & Lord, C. (2004). Early indicators of autism spectrum disorders in the second year of life. *Journal of Autism and Developmental Disorders, 34*(5), 473–493.

Wiggins, L., & Robins, D. (2008). Brief report: Excluding the ADI-R behavioral domain improves diagnostic agreement in toddlers. *Journal of Autism and Developmental Disorders, 38*(5), 972–976.

Wong, V., Hui, L. H., Lee, W. C., Leung, L. S., Ho, P. K., Lau, W. L., et al., (2004). A modified screening tool for autism (Checklist for Autism in Toddlers (CHAT-23)) for Chinese children. *Pediatrics, 114*, e116–e176.

Zwaigenbaum, L., Bryson, S., Rogers, T., Roberts, W., Brian, J., & Szatmari, P. (2005). Behavioral manifestations of autism in the first year of life. *International Journal of Developmental Neuroscience, 23*, 143–152.

4

Autism Spectrum Disorders: A Case of Siblings

Stephen M. Kanne and Janet E. Farmer

Autism spectrum disorders (ASDs) are characterized by deficits in three core areas: communication skills, social ability, and atypical behaviors. They are considered to be neurologic disorders with a complex genetic origin. Though ASDs share common areas of impairment, they represent a phenotypically heterogeneous group or spectrum of disorders with clinical presentations that differ widely across each affected individual. ASDs vary in core symptom severity, may have other cognitive deficits or other neurological conditions, and often have comorbid emotional, behavioral, and adaptive difficulties that add to their behavioral heterogeneity. Parents and professionals often seek out a neuropsychological evaluation when an ASD is present or suspected for differential diagnosis and to guide treatment recommendations.

Although the specific etiology of autism is unknown, many studies have found evidence of a strong genetic component (Cederlund & Gillberg, 2004; Lauritsen, Pedersen, & Mortensen, 2005; Miles et al., 2005; Muhle, Trentacoste, & Rapin, 2004). If a family member has an ASD, it is not uncommon that another family member has an ASD as well. For example, Cederlund and Gillberg (2004) found that 70% of individuals diagnosed with idiopathic autism had a first- or second-degree relative who also had symptoms of an ASD. The recurrence rate in siblings of children with ASD ranges up to 8%, which is much higher than the prevalence rate in the general population (Muhle et al., 2004). To approach the numbers differently, siblings of children with

ASD are 22 times more likely to have an ASD compared to siblings of children who are typically developing (Lauritsen et al., 2005).

The purpose of this paper is to present cases of two male siblings, 14 months apart in age, whose parents had significant concerns regarding an ASD for both from a very early age. These brothers were raised in the same household and experienced very similar treatments and therapies. Their cases demonstrate how two children, both diagnosed with Autistic Disorder and from nearly identical environmental contexts, can vary considerably in their initial presentation, manifestation of symptoms, symptom progression, and functional skills. First, we briefly describe the components of an autism assessment, then we discuss each of the siblings' first evaluations. A brief synopsis of the 5 years between the evaluations is then offered, followed by a description of the siblings' second evaluations. Finally, we discuss several interesting facets of the cases. Given the behavioral nature of an autism diagnosis, we intentionally focus a great deal on their presentation and behaviors during the evaluations.

Autism Evaluation

In addition to collecting a detailed history reviewing early developmental progression and past symptom presentation, clinicians must assess the core symptoms of an ASD currently presenting through direct observation and interaction with the child. When possible, clinicians should gather information from multiple settings, such as school and home, and include an assessment of other domains that explore alternative etiologies. Cognitive and neuropsychological testing can be helpful in informing differential diagnoses and guiding treatment recommendations for medical and educational professionals (e.g., Klin, Saulnier, Tsatsanis, & Volkmar, 2005; Ozonoff, Goodlin-Jones, & Solomon, 2005).

The Case of AB: Initial Evaluation

Concerns regarding developmental delays and atypical behaviors prompted AB's initial neuropsychological evaluation at 2 years, 3 months of age. The parents noted that AB was often content to play by himself and did not seek out peers (e.g., in Sunday school class). Instead, he appeared aloof and withdrawn. Though he would initiate contact with his parents and would show them some toys, this was typically done "on his own terms," and he easily became hyperfocused on toys and objects. They also had concerns about his speech and language development. AB was only speaking single words at the time of the evaluation, and these were hard to understand. He rarely pointed or gestured and would lead his parents by the hand if he needed something. He often lined toys up, spun objects (e.g., turned toy cars over to watch the wheels), and engaged in repetitive hand motions near his face.

Brief Medical and Developmental History

AB was born weighing 7 lb, 7 ounces after a full-term pregnancy with no prenatal or perinatal complications reported. As noted above, he experienced significant speech and language delays. Motor developmental milestones were achieved within normal limits; he rolled over at 4 months, sat alone at 6 months, crawled at 8 months, and walked at 10 months. He reportedly had three "fainting spells" wherein he lost consciousness after a period of intense crying. During the second episode, he appeared to stop breathing for a brief (15-second) period and his lips turned blue. An electroencephalogram (EEG) at the time was normal.

Behavioral Observations

When greeted in the waiting room, AB did not look at the examiner or return the greeting. He had some difficulty transitioning to the interview as he continued playing with toys. During the interview with his parents, AB played alone quietly, not acknowledging the examiner's presence. He did not use meaningful speech during the interview.

AB willingly left the interview room to begin testing, but he required physical prompting. As soon as the door to the testing room closed, he began to fuss and required a brief visit from his mother until he became interested in playing with foam shapes. He held the shapes up one at a time, telling the examiner the name of each shape (e.g., triangle, square, circle). After a few minutes, he was introduced to pictures to match with a scene. Instead of completing the task or attending to the examiner's instructions, he rotated the pictures, then stood up and left the testing room. After several failed attempts to reengage, the examiner accompanied AB to the waiting room where he played with several toys but did not interact with the examiner. He eventually climbed into the examiner's lap without hesitation and fell asleep.

During the evaluation, AB was observed to flap his hands while standing still and when running. Occasionally, he ran on tiptoes and with his toes slightly turned inward. He also postured his hands in an odd manner. He spoke very little throughout the evaluation. Whereas some of his words were difficult to understand, others were quite clear. He clearly enunciated the names of shapes and counted in English, Spanish, and German. He rarely responded when the examiner called his name. In fact, he appeared to be unaware of the examiner except when toys were mentioned or when he wanted something. At these times, he took the examiner's hand and led to what he wanted.

Evaluation Results

AB was unable to engage in the formal cognitive testing. Given his speech and language delays, the Leiter International Performance Scale, Revised (Leiter-R; Roid & Miller, 1997) was attempted but then discontinued due to his lack of engagement. His results on the Autism Diagnostic Observation Schedule (ADOS; Lord, Rutter, DiLavore, & Risi, 2002) met the criteria for Autism (Module 1, Raw = 19). The ADOS places the child in several situations, or "presses," designed to elicit social and communicative responses allowing the examiner to assess core autism symptoms.

AB's overall adaptive skills were in the impaired range using the Vineland Adaptive Behavior Scale (Sparrow, Cicchetti, & Balla, 2005) by parent report (Adaptive Behavior Composite = 64). Parents also noted clinically significant internalizing behaviors on the Childhood Behavior Checklist (CBCL; Achenbach & Rescorla, 2001). The Childhood Autism Rating Scale (CARS; Tobing & Glenwick, 2002) was completed to better understand AB's history and developmental progression. AB's results were in the mild–moderate autism range (Total Score = 30.0).

As a result of the evaluation, the clinician determined AB met diagnostic criteria for the presence of autistic disorder of at least moderate severity. The parents participated in a comprehensive feedback that explained the results, diagnosis, and answered general questions regarding ASD. Recommendations included a suggestion that AB undergo a full speech/language evaluation with subsequent therapy and receive an evaluation to secure special education services. In addition, the examiner encouraged the family to pursue applied behavior analysis (ABA) therapy for AB, an intense behavioral program proven efficacious for children with ASD (c.f., Myers, Johnson, & Council on Children with Disabilities, 2007). Finally, the parents received information about multiple resources, including contact information for parent support groups and educational resources such as books and Web sites.

The Case of CD: Initial Evaluation

AB's older brother, CD (3 years, 5 months), was evaluated the day after AB. Similar to his brother, CD had several areas of concern. Parents reported that CD was aloof around other children, rarely initiated interactions, and was often withdrawn. He did not engage in parallel play, but he was content to play alone. He was described as affectionate and "connected" to his parents, but he typically had difficulty demonstrating empathy. His eye contact was poor, and he had trouble coordinating his gaze appropriately with his vocalizations. His parents indicated their perception that CD was more "severe" than AB, as he showed similar social difficulties but was more reactive with problematic behaviors.

CD had a history of developmental speech and language delays. Although he was able to speak single words and phrases in a normal developmental time frame, he did not use language for communicative intent. Instead, he used language only to label things or in a rote manner. He engaged in frequent echolalia (i.e., repeating words or phrases he has heard) and did not engage in reciprocal conversation. His parents reported that his nonverbal communication was also poor. He was not gesturing in a typical manner or using facial expressions effectively.

At the time of the evaluation, CD's parents reported that he sometimes banged his head, but not often. However, his play was described as repetitive and mechanical. He tended to be interested in only one main topic at a time. When playing with toys, he often engaged in a repetitive ritual (e.g., turning it in a certain sequence), and he often lined up and categorized his toys. He relied heavily on structure and routines, and they noted he often became upset when making transitions. He had some mild tactile defensiveness (e.g., to textures and clothes, dislikes getting a haircut or feeling the clippings on his skin). He insisted on having his hands cleaned if he perceived them to be dirty.

Brief Medical and Developmental History

CD was born weighing 7 lb, 0 ounces after a full-term and uncomplicated pregnancy. His early motor developmental milestones were reached in a timely manner: rolling over at 4 months, sitting alone at 5 months, crawling at 8 months, and walking at 10 months. In contrast, his parents noted delays in CD's early speech and language developmental milestones. Although he spoke single words at 7 months, his progress from that point forward was described as "slow." They noted that at age 3, he was not speaking in sentences or using speech to communicate in a meaningful way (e.g., he was primarily naming objects).

Two months prior to the evaluation, CD had participated in an evaluation within his school district, wherein his nonverbal intellectual functioning was in the low average range (Leiter-R; standard score [SS] = 85). He performed in the impaired range (SS = 65) on every aspect of the Battelle Developmental Inventory (Newborg et al., 1988), with the exception of the specific subdomain Coping (SS = 100). His preacademic skills were in the superior range (Bracken Basic Concept Scale–Revised; Bracken, 1984). He had an Individualized Educational Program (IEP) and was receiving speech/language therapy with goals addressing his social skills.

Behavioral Observations

When CD was greeted in the waiting room, he made fleeting eye contact but did not maintain it and did not return the greeting. During the interview with his parents, CD explored the room actively and played by himself. He did not acknowledge the examiner's presence or reference others in the room. He spoke using single words and some phrases, though many of his phrases were echolalic. He required prompting to transition to the testing room.

When CD began the testing, he repeated "That silly [examiner's name]" over and over to his father. Upon entering the waiting room during a break in testing, he threw himself to the floor and began crying. His father was able to calm him, after which he accompanied his father back to the testing room. After a brief period with CD on his lap, his father attempted to leave, at which time CD reached for him and began to cry again. Shortly after his father left the room, CD climbed into the examiner's lap and resumed testing. As testing progressed he stopped speaking and crawled to the floor. He was taken back to the waiting room where he had the same reaction as earlier.

Throughout the evaluation, CD rarely produced reciprocal language. He named many things, but primarily echoed the examiner's statements and questions. His many sound substitutions made him difficult to understand. When he appeared to know the answer to a question, he answered quickly. At other times, he looked away from the test material, fell onto the floor, and squirmed. At these times, he did not respond when the examiner asked if he knew the answer. He also did not seem affected when the examiner told him it was "okay" to tell if he did not know an answer. Similarly, he did not show a response to positive statements made by the examiner. Though often difficult to engage, overall, CD was able to be redirected and to complete the testing.

Other notable behaviors included calling his parents by their first names, which they reported was typical. During breaks, he did not interact with the examiner until the end of the day, during a game of imaginative play initiated and maintained by the examiner.

Evaluation Results

CD's overall level of intellectual functioning was in the average range (SS = 103) (Differential Abilities Scales; Elliot, 1990). His performance on the subtests ranged from low average to high average: Block Building SS = 94; Verbal Comprehension SS = 85; Picture Similarities SS = 115; Naming Vocabulary SS = 117. He was also administered a measure of basic language skills, the Clinical Evaluation of Language Fundamentals–Preschool (Wiig, Secord, & Semel, 1992). His receptive language was in the low average range (SS = 81), and his expressive language was in the low end of the average range (SS = 90). As Table 4-1 demonstrates, his individual subtest scores were variable.

Table 4-1. CD's Speech/Language Results on the Clinical Evaluation of Language Fundamentals–Preschool

Index Scores	Standard Scores
Receptive Language Score	81
Expressive Language Score	90
Total Language Score	85

Subtests	Scaled Scores
Linguistic Concepts	5
Basic Concepts	10
Sentence Structure	4
Recalling Sentences in Context	8
Formulating Labels	10
Word Structure	7

Parents reported CD's overall adaptive skills to be in the borderline range on the Vineland Adaptive Behaviour Scale (Adaptive Behaviour Composite = 79) and noted clinically significant internalizing behaviors (CBCL). Teachers also reported a significant degree of internalizing behaviors (Teacher Report Form). Report of his developmental progression met the criteria for mild to moderate autism (CARS; Total Score = 32.5). Of note, on the Gilliam Autism Rating Scale (Gilliam, 1995), his parents did not endorse a significant amount of difficulties, resulting in a "low probability" of autism on this measure. CD's results on the ADOS met criteria for autism (Module 2; Raw = 21).

Similar to his brother, evaluation results indicated that CD met diagnostic criteria for the presence of autistic disorder. Cognitive testing ruled out an overall developmental delay and mental retardation. Results also suggested that a speech/language disorder alone did not account for his presentation. Though his basic language skills appeared relatively intact, his functional and pragmatic language skills were significantly deficient. Recommendations were nearly identical to those for his brother, but with additional suggestions for managing his reactivity.

Comparison of Siblings at Initial Visit

AB and CD both had clear deficits in the three areas necessary for a diagnosis of autistic disorder, reflected in their formal results (e.g., ADOS, CARS); however, they presented in vastly different ways. Table 4-2 presents a comparison of the siblings' results after the initial evaluation. Both boys had significant speech/language delays, but CD's language was better developed, although it was primarily nonfunctional and echolalic. Both boys had significant social deficits, although CD was able to engage better, and even completed

testing; his overall response style was negative and reactive. Both boys also had significant atypical behaviors, though AB demonstrated many more repetitive behaviors, including hand flapping, tip-toe walking, and atypical hand movements, whereas CD adhered more to routines and demonstrated stereotyped language. Both children had difficulty with eye contact; however, AB tended to avoid eye contact, whereas CD had more difficulty coordinating his gaze with his vocalizations. Whereas the parents felt that the older boy, CD, was more severely affected due to the extent of his behavioral difficulties, our results suggested that the younger child was more "severe" due to his degree of aloofness, his inability to engage, and the nature of his repetitive behaviors.

Interim

The parents brought both brothers back for a re-evaluation 5 years after the initial evaluation. In the interim, the parents had moved geographically, actively sought information regarding autism, and proactively involved both brothers in many different types of therapy. In addition to having both children participate in ABA therapy and speech/language therapy, the family also pursued many alternative and biomedical treatments, including a gluten/casein-free diet, vitamin supplements, chelation, and the use of a hyperbolic oxygen chamber. They reported significant improvements for both boys over time.

The Case of AB: Second Evaluation

At the time of the second evaluation, AB was in kindergarten, and 7 years, 3 months of age. He had reportedly made marked improvements in almost every area of concern over the intervening five years. He was receiving speech/language,

Table 4-2. Comparison of Siblings after First Evaluation

	AB	CD
Intellectual Functioning (Leiter-R)	Unable to engage	Average (SS = 103)
Adaptive (Vineland)	Impaired (SS = 64)	Borderline (SS = 79)
Autism Diagnostic Observation Schedule	Total Score = 19	Total Score = 21
Childhood Autism Rating Scale	Total Score = 30	Total Score = 32.5
Speech/Language (CELF-P)	Unable to engage	Low Average (SS = 85)

occupational therapy, and physical therapy as part of his IEP under the special educational eligibility category of Autism. His parents noted that his academic skills were well developed. Both his verbal and nonverbal communication skills were greatly improved, and he now spontaneously initiated conversation with others and responded reciprocally. Though he typically conversed in areas of his special interest, or introduced a conversation with a script specific to a person, he had begun to ask appropriate questions during conversations. Many of his more obvious atypical behaviors had decreased in frequency or intensity.

However, his parents remained concerned regarding AB's ability to communicate effectively. He engaged in echolalia when not fully following a conversation, and his scripting interfered with many interactions. When upset or emotionally charged (even happy), atypical behaviors returned, such as hand flapping and spinning. He hit his head with his fist when he got upset, and, on his "bad days," could be very rigid and reactive. He continued to become self-absorbed and hyper-focused, and he often needed prompting.

Several "splinter skills," or areas of ability well above his other skills had emerged. Some of these were nonfunctional, such as naming all the Presidents of the United States with supporting details. He also had demonstrated a high degree of musical talent. In fact, the parents brought a roll-out keyboard that AB played (with seeming proficiency), though he never had music lessons, and a recording of songs he created using a software program wherein he played each separate instrument himself.

Behavioral Observations

When greeted in the waiting room, AB made eye contact and returned the greeting, but he spoke in a scripted manner with formal intonations. He engaged in some reciprocal conversation, but he did not coordinate his gaze and quickly changed the topic to Presidents of the United States. He demonstrated his ability to recall any President by number.

AB's prosody was exaggerated and had a musical or sing-song quality, particularly when repeating fairly well-rehearsed social responses. He had an extensive vocabulary and mimicked phrases learned from television in stereotyped phrases (e.g., "get out of town... check out our resorts"). He also occasionally made comments that were out of context or possibly paraphasic (e.g. "that looks like a rain job" when referring to an image resembling a planet). He produced sound effects, such as crash sounds, or repeated utterances, such as "tooka took, tooka took, tooka took" or "whoota, whoota, whoota" multiple times during the evaluation. If a question was asked of him, he answered appropriately and spontaneously offered elaborations; however, he rarely asked questions of the examiner.

During testing, AB was able to engage and was pleasant and cooperative. He often used verbal mediation (i.e., talking his way through a problem) during visual tasks. He scanned visual stimuli very carefully, particularly when they were detailed, and was noted to perform quite well on visual-spatial reasoning tasks. However, on items that were timed, he became tense and responded in a more haphazard manner, focusing more on completing the items quickly rather than correctly. AB often created drawings out of words or numbers that he wrote. For example, after spelling the word *look*, he drew a pair of glasses out of the two "Os." After he thought of different types of "silly" high-fives, he suddenly stopped and said "ok, let's concentrate." He also referenced the examiner's facial expressions on multiple occasions. He supported his verbal communication with nonverbal gestures, such as pointing and shrugging. AB exhibited several repetitive behaviors during the evaluation, such as hand flapping and staring at himself in the one-way mirror.

Evaluation Results

AB had many areas of marked improvement compared to his results from 5 years prior. He was able to engage in formal testing, and his overall level of nonverbal intellectual functioning was in the superior range (Leiter-R; SS = 127). His academic skills were also strong (WIAT-II; Wechsler, 2002), with word recognition and spelling in the very superior range, and computational skills in the average range (e.g., Reading SS = 138, Spelling SS = 153, Numerical Operations SS = 103). His visual motor integration was in the average range (SS = 103) (The Beery-Buktenica Developmental Test of Visual-Motor Integration,

Table 4-3. Comparing AB's Diagnostic Algorithm Raw Scores to Current Algorithm Raw Scores on Each ADI-R Subscale

ADI-R Subscale	Diagnostic Algorithm	Current Behavior Algorithm
Reciprocal Social Interaction (Cut-off = 10)	20	7
Communication (Cut-off = 8)	21	10
Repetitive Behaviors and Stereotyped Patterns (Cut-off = 3)	10	8

5th Edition [VMI]; Beery, Buktenica, & Beery, 2004).

A structured interview of past and current autism symptoms, the Autism Diagnostic Interview, Revised (ADI-R; Lord, Rutter, & Le Couteur, 1994), reflected improvements in AB's autism related features. In each domain, as Table 4-3 demonstrates, his current scores indicated improvements compared to his past scores.

On the ADOS, AB's results were now in the range of an Autism Spectrum Disorder rather than meeting criteria for the more severe Autism (Module 3, Raw = 7). Thus, assessment of his current symptoms, in clinic and by parent report, indicated significant improvements in his ASD-related symptoms. However, despite these improvements, his parents' report of his adaptive skills (ABAS-II; Harrison & Oakland, 2003) remained in the impaired range (SS = 69).

AB's diagnosis remained Autistic Disorder. Recommendations targeted improving his pragmatic language and social skills, while continuing to support his need for services in school. Those involved in his care were encouraged to find ways to take advantage of his cognitive strengths and other areas of highly developed skills. Parents were also complimented for their strong advocacy and support.

The Case of CD: Second Evaluation

CD, now 8 years, 5 months of age, had also reportedly made a great deal of progress. His parents noted marked improvements in his communicative/interactive skills, his social skills (e.g., social awareness and perception, ability to understand others' perspective, sense of humor), and his overall mood regulation. They continued to have concerns regarding his tendency to perseverate, his adaptive skills, and his emotional reactivity.

Behavioral Observations

When CD was greeted in the waiting room, he made brief eye contact, smiled, and returned to his play. While transitioning to the interview room, he engaged in casual and reciprocal conversation with appropriate coordination of eye gaze with the examiner. Verbally, he demonstrated slower response latency to questions and his verbal pacing was mildly atypical. During testing, CD was pleasant and cooperative, though he tended to be verbose and tangential. For example, when asked what a number is, he replied "It's a thing that a caveman invented to keep track of things. They were tired of saying, I have a bunch of camels… it can be a tally mark… a symbol, it can be anything, for example, two horses, five golden rings… so we don't have to carry slates and write tally marks." When asked to define an "alligator," he described various types of reptiles and named prehistoric dinosaurs, before providing the correct response. His definition of objects and concepts tended to be functional in nature, as he often provided their various uses, rather than providing a more abstract definition. CD had some difficulty on a measure of visual-spatial construction, in which he was to assemble blocks in a manner similar to that of visual model. He was aware that he was being timed for this task and appeared pressured. For a number of items, he stated that he was finished and then continued to work identifying that something was not quite correct. However, he was usually unable to figure out how to amend his design. On a test of written calculations, CD exhibited significant frustration. He sighed multiple times throughout this task, and on items that were difficult for him, he erased his answers repeatedly before committing to a final answer. It was noted that CD typically did not smile when making a humorous comment, until he saw the examiner smile or laugh, at which point he returned the smile/laugh.

Evaluation Results

On this evaluation, CD demonstrated a significant discrepancy between his level of verbal intellectual functioning, in the superior range (VIQ = 129) (Wechsler Abbreviated Scale of Intelligence; Wechsler, 1999), and his level of visual spatial intellectual functioning, in the average range (PIQ = 97). His academic skills followed the same pattern of stronger performance on verbally related tasks: word recognition in the superior range (WIAT-II; Reading SS = 126), spelling in the very superior range (Spelling SS = 137), and computational skills in the average range (Numerical Operations SS = 97). His ability to learn and recall verbal information (CVLT-C; Delis, Kramer, Kaplan, & Ober, 1994) was in the average range immediately (List A Total SS = 105) and after a delay (e.g., Long Delay Free Recall SS = 93). His visual motor integration was in the superior range (VMI; SS = 122).

Similar to his brother, CD's results on measures specific to autism symptoms reflected improvements. On the ADOS, his total score was now in the range of an autism spectrum disorder rather than the more severe Autism (Module 3; Raw = 7), and, as shown in Table 4-4, his ADI-R results also reflected improvements from the past to his current presentation.

As a result of the evaluation, CD's diagnosis was changed from Autistic Disorder to Pervasive Developmental Disorder–Not Otherwise Specified (PDD-NOS). He did not fully meet the criteria for Autistic Disorder based on his presentation at the time of the second evaluation. We felt that the diagnosis of PDD-NOS accurately captured his continued, though subtle, difficulties associated with his history of an ASD that now

Table 4-4. Comparing CD's Diagnostic Algorithm Raw Scores to Current Algorithm Raw Scores on Each ADI-R Subscale

ADI-R Subscale	Diagnostic Algorithm	Current Behavior Algorithm
Reciprocal Social Interaction (Cut-off = 10)	24	4
Communication (Cut-off = 8)	21	3
Repetitive Behaviors and Stereotyped Patterns (Cut-off = 3)	4	2

did not meet full criteria, while also conveying the progress that he had made. Similar to his brother, despite his improvements, CD's adaptive skills remained problematic and in contrast to his other skills: in the high end of the borderline range by parent report (ABAS-II; SS = 79).

Comparison of Siblings at Second Visit

Both AB and CD had made considerable progress over the intervening 5 years. Table 4-5 presents a comparison of the siblings' results after the second evaluation. AB progressed from being unable to engage in testing to performing in the superior range or above on measures of academic and intellectual functioning. AB's language had improved and he was now using fluent and complex sentences, but he remained echolalic and scripted. He continued to engage in repetitive behaviors, though they had decreased in frequency and intensity.

Table 4-5. Comparison of Siblings after Second Evaluation

	AB	CD
Intellectual Functioning	Superior (Leiter-R; SS = 127)	Superior (WASI; SS = 129)
Adaptive (ABAS-II)	Impaired (SS = 69)	Borderline (SS = 79)
Autism Diagnostic Observation Schedule	Module 3, raw = 7	Module 3, raw = 7
ADI-R; Reciprocal Social Interaction	raw = 7	raw = 4
ADI-R; Communication	raw = 10	raw = 3
ADI-R; Repetitive Behaviors	raw = 8	raw = 2
Reading (WIAT-II)	Very Superior (SS = 138)	Superior (SS = 126)
Spelling (WIAT-II)	Very Superior (SS = 153)	Very Superior (SS = 137)
Numerical Operations (WIAT-II)	Average (SS = 103)	Average (SS = 97)

CD's intellectual functioning results improved from the average range to the high average range and he also demonstrated academic skills well above average. CD's language was now reciprocal though verbose, and he was coordinating the nonverbal aspects of communication better. CD remained reactive, though this was also improved.

Looking solely at their test results fails to convey the striking difference between the siblings from a clinical and behavioral perspective. Both had significant cognitive and academic strengths, and both received the same score on the same module of the ADOS. However, the two boys presented very differently. AB presented with many more atypical behaviors strongly suggesting an ASD. CD's presentation was such that, without knowledge about his prior history or a detailed understanding of his presentation, a diagnosis of an ASD may not appear appropriate. The pattern of differences between the boys at their initial evaluation was maintained, though it increased in magnitude.

Discussion

The evaluations of these siblings utilized the tools appropriate to an ASD evaluation. Core areas associated with an ASD were assessed each time, using instruments such as the ADOS and clinical observation. Developmental history and ASD symptom progression were assessed using the CARS (first visit) and ADI-R (second visit). Several other measures were utilized depending on their age and level of engagement, assessing language (e.g., CELF-P), intellectual ability (e.g., Leiter-R, WASI, DAS), memory (CVLT-C), and adaptive skills (e.g., Vineland, ABAS-II). In addition to supporting diagnostic decisions, these measures provided a framework to guide recommendations for family and educators.

In general, the boys' initial symptom patterns were maintained over the intervening years, though the degree of difference between them had increased. CD demonstrated better levels of engagement and basic social skills, better developed language, and less overt repetitive behaviors compared to his brother. Both improved dramatically between assessments, to the degree that the older brother's symptoms associated with ASD were very subtle. Both had received a

great deal of intense therapy, and both demonstrated many areas of cognitive/academic strength. For both, the symptoms associated with ASD continued to impact their everyday living skills despite the improvements they had made.

The genetics of ASD suggest that there are many parents who have two or more children affected by ASD. The current cases underscore how differently two siblings can present and progress, despite having the same initial diagnosis. This was relevant in the siblings, as the parents initially thought that CD was more severe because of his more externalizing presentation, whereas they perceived AB to be less severe and "low maintenance." Our results suggested that the very factors that gave the impression of lessened severity were actually more impairing and suggestive of a more severe presentation of an ASD, which the later test results confirmed. Research providing a better understanding of autism phenotypes would help in these situations that could prompt better prognosis and treatment planning.

These cases demonstrate the limitations clinicians currently encounter with respect to ASD. The siblings made considerable progress, which was reflected to some extent in the results (ADOS and ADI-R). However, these tools had difficulty capturing the nature and nuances of their improvements. This is understandable as these tools were designed for diagnostic purposes and not designed to be sensitive to change. This is reflected in results wherein both boys scored similarly on the ADOS during the second evaluation, but they were immensely different with respect to their symptom presentation. Another problem is associated with both boys' very strong cognitive test results. Strong cognitive skills are associated with positive prognosis, but they may also cause others to overestimate the extent of difficulty associated with their ASD symptoms. Despite their strong cognitive skills, AB and CD struggle with day-to-day tasks.

AB and CD's cases also underscore how much remains unknown regarding ASD and how clinicians are unable to predict the outcome for children. In the current state of the field, evaluations lead to diagnosis and recommendations, but these recommendations are necessarily general and not finely tuned to each child. Identifying phenotypes can lead to specific treatments tailored for a specific type of ASD. Without this level of specificity, many parents do as AB and CD's parents have done: pursuing multiple treatments and expending a great deal of resources not knowing which is working or why. Future research will also help determine whether their improvements were the result of their natural developmental progression, the therapies they participated in, or some combination of the two.

References

Achenbach, T. M., & Rescorla, L. A. (2001). *Manual for the ASEBA Preschool Forms & Profiles.* Burlington: University of Vermont, Research Center for Children, Youth, & Families.

Beery, K. E., Buktenica, N., & Beery, N. (2004). *Beery – Buktenica Developmental Test of Visual–Motor Integration* (5th ed.). Austin, TX: Pro-Ed.

Bracken, B. A. (1984). *Bracken Basic Concept Scales.* San Antonio, TX: Psychological Corporation.

Cederlund, M., & Gillberg, C. (2004). One hundred males with Asperger syndrome: A clinical study of background and associated factors. *Developmental Medicine and Child Neurology, 46*(10), 652–660.

Delis, D., Kramer, J. H., Kaplan, E., & Ober, B. A. (1994). *California Verbal Learning Test–Children's Version.* San Antonio, TX: The Psychological Corporation.

Elliot, C. (1990). *Differential Ability Scales.* San Antonio, TX: The Psychological Corporation.

Gilliam, J. E. (1995). *Gilliam Autism Rating Scale.* Austin, TX: Pro-Ed.

Harrison, P. L., & Oakland, T. (2003). *Adaptive Behavior Assessment System–Second Edition.* San Antonio, TX: The Psychological Corporation.

Klin, A., Saulnier, C., Tsatsanis, K., & Volkmar, F. R. (2005). Clinical evaluation in autism spectrum disorders: Psychological assessment within a transdisciplinary framework. In F. R. Volkmar, R. Paul, A. Klin, & D. Cohen (Eds.), *Handbook of autism and pervasive developmental disorders, Vol. 2: Assessment, interventions, and policy* (3rd ed., pp. 772–798). Hoboken, NJ: Wiley.

Lauritsen, M. B., Pedersen, C. B., & Mortensen, P. B. (2005). Effects of familial risk factors and place of birth on the risk of autism: A nationwide register-based study. *Journal of Child Psychology and Psychiatry, 46*(9), 963–971.

Lord, C., Rutter, M., DiLavore, P. C., & Risi, S. (2002). *Autism Diagnostic Observation Schedule.* Los Angeles: Western Psychological Services.

Lord, C., Rutter, M., & Le Couteur, A. (1994). Autism Diagnostic Interview–Revised: A revised version of a diagnostic interview for caregivers of individuals with possible pervasive developmental disorders. *Journal of Autism and Developmental Disorders, 24*(5), 659–685.

Miles, J. H., Takahashi, T. N., Bagby, S., Sahota, P. K., Vaslow, D. F., Wang, C. H., et al. (2005). Essential versus complex autism: Definition of fundamental prognostic subtypes. *American Journal of Medical Genetics. Part A, 135*(2), 171–180.

Muhle, R., Trentacoste, S. V., & Rapin, I. (2004). The genetics of autism. *Pediatrics, 113,* e472–e486.

Myers, S. M., Johnson, C. P., & U. S. Council on Children with Disabilities. (2007). Management of children with autism spectrum disorders. *Pediatrics, 120*(5), 1162–1182.

Newborg, J., Stock, J. R., Wnek, L., Guidubaldi, J., Svinicki, J., Dickson, J., et al. (1988). *Batelle Developmental Inventory with recalibrated technical data and norms; Screening test examiner's manual* (2nd ed.). Allen, TX: DLM, Inc.

Ozonoff, S., Goodlin-Jones, B. L., & Solomon, M. (2005). Evidence-based assessment of autism spectrum disorders in children and adolescents. *Journal of Clinical and Adolescent Psychology, 34*(3), 523–540.

Roid, G. H., & Miller, L. (1997). *Leiter International Test of Intelligence–Revised.* Chicago: Stoelting.

Sparrow, S. S., Cicchetti, D., & Balla, D. A. (2005). *Vineland Adaptive Behavior Scales–2nd edition manual.* Minneapolis, MN: NCS Pearson, Inc.

Tobing, L. E., & Glenwick, D. S. (2002). Relation of the Childhood Autism Rating Scale–Parent version to diagnosis, stress, and age. *Research in Developmental Disabilities, 23*(3), 211–223.

Wechsler, D. (1999). *The Wechsler Abbreviated Scale of Intelligence.* San Antonio, TX: The Psychological Corporation.

Wechsler, D. (2002). *Wechsler Individual Achievement Test* (2nd ed.). San Antonio, TX: The Psychological Corporation.

Wiig, E. H., Secord, W., & Semel, E. (1992). *Clinical evaluation of language fundamentals–preschool: Examiner's manual.* New York: The Psychological Corporation.

5

Dyslexia in a Young Adult

Robert L. Mapou

Dyslexia is a developmental reading disorder characterized by difficulty sounding out and reading single words fluently. It is the only developmental learning disability for which there is a research-based definition (Fletcher, Lyon, Fuchs, & Barnes, 2007). This definition is as follows:

Dyslexia is a specific learning disability that is neurobiological in origin. It is characterized by difficulties with accurate and/or fluent word recognition and by poor spelling and decoding abilities. These difficulties typically result from a deficit in the phonological component of language that is often unexpected in relation to other cognitive abilities and the provision of effective classroom instruction. Secondary consequences may include problems in reading comprehension and reduced reading experience that can impede the growth of vocabulary and background knowledge. (Lyon, Shaywitz, & Shaywitz, 2003, p. 1)

Because of early intervention or the development of compensatory strategies, a large proportion of adults with dyslexia can develop average or better ability to decode and read single words in isolation, especially if speed is not stressed. Nonetheless, adults with dyslexia typically struggle with fluency and comprehension when reading text. Even if they can read single words in isolation, they remain slow and inefficient readers. They may also have difficulty on timed measures of decoding and single-word reading. Consequently, assessment must include timed measures of reading (S. Shaywitz, 2003; S. E. Shaywitz & Shaywitz, 2005). Adults with dyslexia can also have associated difficulties in a range of language skills, including word retrieval,

naming speed, verbal working memory, vocabulary, listening comprehension, and semantic knowledge (Mapou, 2009). Moreover, these skills may be more predictive of poor reading in adults than phonological awareness, which appears to be more important for acquisition of reading in early schooling.

Clinically, Wasserstein and Denckla (2009) have proposed three types of reading disorders in adults. The first is a pure phonological subtype, in which reading aloud is impaired, but comprehension is stronger. A case example of a physician with this type of reading disorder was recently presented by the author (See Appendix in Mapou, 2009). The second is a comprehension subtype with the opposite profile: comprehension is impaired, but reading aloud is stronger. The third is a combined subtype, in which both reading aloud and comprehension are impaired. In the case presented here, a young adult college student, comes closest to this third subtype, although his comprehension was still stronger than his decoding and single-word reading skills.

Case Study: Mr. C

Mr. C, a 19-year-old community college freshman working toward an associate's degree, was referred by the disability support service (DSS) coordinator at the college he was attending. Historically, he had developed motor skills normally but had been slow to develop speech and language. He was subsequently slow when learning to recite the alphabet. Because his father had been in the military, he had completed his primary and secondary education in several locations around the world. His problems with reading and writing were identified early in his schooling, and he had an Individualized Education Program (IEP) throughout his schooling. He was also evaluated at regular intervals and was seen for speech/language therapy in elementary school. His father reported that there was never a specific diagnosis and that the family was never given many details about his son's problems. He thought that at one point Mr. C had been diagnosed with dyslexia, but he was unsure. He also reported that there was very limited intervention to improve his son's reading and writing skills. Although Mr. C had received instruction that was appropriate for normal students, he had not received evidence-based intervention that has been shown to be effective for children with dyslexia (e.g., Fletcher et al., 2007). Mr. C had shown no evidence of attention-deficit/hyperactivity disorder (ADHD) in childhood.

Mr. C recalled having been very frustrated in school when younger, especially when his mother made him do his homework. Over time, however, he learned to cope with his difficulties and tried to do his best. Although his math had been at or above grade level throughout his schooling, he was always behind in reading and writing. Consequently, he had been taken out of class for subjects that involved reading and writing, such as English. He also reported having not done well in science, because of the amount of information he had to learn and the similarity among scientific words. From first through ninth grade, Mr. C had been taken out of his classes for tests, so that someone could read the test to him. In 10th grade, however, he began taking tests with the other students, noting that he was able to read key words and answer multiple-choice questions without a reader. He did not repeat any grades and graduated from high school on time.

Mr. C reported no significant medical problems and no significant psychosocial difficulties. His family history was notable for a diagnosed learning disability in his sister.

When seen for evaluation, Mr. C was working part-time while attending community college. He was taking two college classes and reported that he was a B-C student. Although he had

enrolled in an anatomy class, he had dropped it, because he could not retain the information from his readings. Mr. C reported that his main problem in college was with reading. His typical approach when studying was to scan his textbooks, highlighting vocabulary and broad topics. With this approach, he believed he understood 20% to 25% of the material. Writing was another area of difficulty, and Mr. C was working with a tutor for his English class to help him correct and edit his writing. Spelling was particularly difficult; he reported that he often mixed up similarly sounding words and could not sort them out even with a spell-checker. He indicated that it was particularly frustrating when he knew what he wanted to write but could not spell the words. Although Mr. C had been accommodated with extended time on tests in college, an accommodation that he had received previously, he reported that he usually did not need it. He was taking his tests using the Kurzweil 3000 computer program, which, among other functions translated written tests into audio (see http://www.kurzweiledu.com/kurz3000.aspx for information), and had found this very effective. He reported that he had permission to record his classes. Although he had not done that, he was considering it for the future. Mr. C stated that he did not take notes in class, preferring to rely on what he remembered. However, he had just obtained a laptop computer for taking notes and was planning to try this. Mr. C reported strengths in history, because of his memory, and in math. He hoped to eventually work in the finance industry.

Examination Results

In keeping with the author's standard practice, a comprehensive battery was used (Mapou, 2009). Apart from his reading and language difficulties, there was nothing notable about Mr. C's behavior during testing. Intellectual, academic, and neuropsychological testing results are shown in Table 5-1. Mr. C was of average intelligence, with a very slight edge in the visual domain, as might be expected of someone with dyslexia. He had above-average scores on Comprehension, despite the language weaknesses noted below, and on Block Design, with solidly average scores on Information, Arithmetic, Matrix Reasoning, and

Table 5-1. Neuropsychological Test Results

Intellectual Abilities

Wechsler Adult Intelligence Scale-Third Edition
Full Scale IQ 95 (37th percentile)
Verbal IQ 94 (34th percentile)
Performance IQ 97 (42nd percentile)
Verbal Comprehension Index 94 (34th percentile)
Perceptual Organization Index 101 (53rd percentile)

Subtest	SS	Percentile	Subtest	SS	Percentile
Vocabulary	8	25	Picture Completion	8	25
Similarities	8	25	Digit Symbol-Coding	7	16
Arithmetic	10	50	Block Design	13	84
Digit Span	6	9	Matrix Reasoning	10	50
Information	11	63	Picture Arrangement	10	50
Comprehension	12	75	Symbol Search	8	25
Letter-Number Sequencing	8	25			

Visuospatial Constructional Skills

Measure	Raw Score	z-score			
ROCFT Copy	30/36	−1.0			

Learning and Memory
Verbal

CVLT-II Measure	Raw Score	T/ z-score	CVLT-II Measure	Raw Score	z-score
List A, Tr. 1-5 Total	50	48 (T)	List A, Short Delay Free Recall	11	0
List A, Trial 1	5	−1	List A, Short Delay Cued Recall	11	−0.5
List A, Trial 5	13	0	List A, Long Delay Free Recall	13	0.5
List B	4	−1.5	List A, Short Delay Cued Recall	12	−0.5
Total Repetitions	2	0.5	Recognition Total Correct	14	−1
Total Intrusions	4	−0.5	Recognition False-Positive Errors	1	0
Semantic Clustering		0.5	Serial Clustering		0

WMS-III Subtest Measure	Raw Score	SS	Percentile
Logical Memory I Recall Total		9	37
Logical Memory I Learning Slope		5	5
Logical Memory II Recall Total		10	50
Logical Memory Percent Retention	96%	13	84
Logical Memory I Thematic Total		9	37

Table 5-1. Neuropsychological Test Results (*Continued*)

WMS-III Subtest Measure	Raw Score	SS	Percentile
Logical Memory II Thematic Total		10	50
Recognition Story A	10/15 correct		
Recognition Story B (Repeated)	15/15 correct		
Visual			

WMS-III Subtest Measure	Raw Score	SS	Percentile
Family Pictures I Recall Total		13	84
Family Pictures II Recall Total		13	84
Family Pictures Retention	102%	12	75

Measure	Raw Score	z-score	%ile
ROCFT Delayed Recall	27/36	−0.1	
WAIS-III Digit Symbol Incidental Learning			
Pairing	9/9		>50
Free Recall	9/9		>50

Spoken Language Skills

Auditory Phonological Awareness and Rapid Naming
Comprehensive Test of Phonological Processing

Subtest	SS	Percentile	Composite	STD	Percentile
Elision	4	2	Phonological Awareness	67	1
Blending Words	5	5	Phonological Memory	82	12
Memory for Digits	7	16	Rapid Naming	73	3
Rapid Digit Naming	6	9			
Nonword Repetition	7	16			
Rapid Letter Naming	5	5			

Spoken Language Comprehension

Measure	SS/STD	Percentile
WAIS-III Vocabulary	8	25
WJ3ACH Understanding Directions	85	15
OWLS Listening Comprehension	104	61

Spoken Language Production

Measure	STD/SS	Percentile
WJ3ACH Picture Vocabulary	92	29
WJ3COG Rapid Picture Naming	84	15
TLC-E, Level 2 Oral Expression	3	1

(*Continued*)

Table 5-1. Neuropsychological Test Results (*Continued*)

Spoken Language Production

D-KEFS Verbal Fluency Test	SS	Percentile
Letter Fluency: Total Correct	6	9
Category Fluency: Total Correct	9	37
Category Switching: Total Correct	6	9
Category Switching: Total Switching Accuracy	5	5

Span for Verbal Information

Measure	Raw Score	SS	Percentile	Performance Level
WAIS-III Digit Span-Forwards	4–5 digits			Low average
California Verbal Learning Test-II, Trial 1	5 words			Mildly impaired
WMS-III Logical Memory 1st Recall Total		10	50	

Working Memory

Measure	Raw Score	SS/STD	Percentile	Performance Level
WAIS-III Digit Span-Backwards	3–4 digits			Mildly impaired
WAIS-III Arithmetic		10	50	
WAIS-III Letter-Number Sequencing	3–6 items	8	25	
WAIS-III Working Memory Index		88	21	

Reading Skills

Woodcock-Johnson-III Tests of Achievement			*Gates-MacGinitie Reading Test (Level AR)*	
Summary Score/Subtest	STD	Percentile	Score	Percentile
Word Attack	68	2	Comprehension	12
Letter-Word Identification	68	2	Total Time: 24 minutes	
Basic Reading Skills	69	2		
Reading Fluency	74	4		
Passage Comprehension	86	17		
Broad Reading	74	4		

Table 5-1. Neuropsychological Test Results (*Continued*)

Writing Skills

Woodcock-Johnson-III Tests of Achievement

Subtest	STD	Percentile
Spelling	70	2
Writing Fluency	84	15

Wechsler Achievement Test-Second Edition

Subtest	STD	Percentile	Quartile
Written Expression	91	27	
Word Fluency			1

Math Skills

Woodcock-Johnson-III Tests of Achievement

Summary Score/Subtest	STD	Percentile
Math Fluency	79	8
Calculation	93	33
Math Calculation Skills	87	20
Applied Problems	99	47
Broad Mathematics	92	30

Focused Attention/Processing Speed

Measure	SS/STD	Percentile
WAIS-III Digit Symbol-Coding	8	25
WAIS-III Symbol Search	8	25
WAIS-III Processing Speed Index	86	18
WJ3COG Visual Matching	79	8
WJ3COG Decision Speed	84	14
WJ3COG Processing Speed	79	8

Sustained Attention

IVA Continuous Performance Test	STD
Fine Motor Regulation Quotient	70
Full Scale Response Control Quotient (RCQ)	75
Auditory RCQ	82
Auditory Prudence	79
Auditory Consistency	71
Visual RCQ	74
Visual Prudence	80
Visual Consistency	81

(*Continued*)

Table 5-1. Neuropsychological Test Results (*Continued*)

IVA Continuous Performance Test	STD (Raw Score)
Full Scale Attention Quotient (AQ)	84
Auditory AQ	88
Auditory Speed	108 (571 milliseconds)
Auditory Vigilance (Accuracy)	93 (98%)
Auditory Focus	76
Visual AQ	82
Visual Speed	94 (434 milliseconds)
Visual Vigilance (Accuracy)	81 (98%)
Visual Focus	88

CVLT-II, California Verbal Learning Test–Second Edition; D-KEFS, Delis-Kaplan Executive Function System; IVA, Integrated Visual and Auditory; OWLS, Oral and Written Language Scales; ROCFT, Rey-Osterrieth Complex Figure Test; SS, scaled score; STD, standard score; TLC-E, Test of Language Competence, Expanded Edition; WAIS-III, Wechsler Adult Intelligence Scale–Third Edition; WJ3ACH, Woodcock-Johnson–III Tests of Achievement; WJ3COG, Woodcock-Johnson-III Tests of Cognitive Abilities; WMS-III, Wechsler Memory Scale–Third Edition.

Picture Arrangement. Relative weaknesses were seen on Vocabulary, as might be expected due to his not having been a reader, and on Similarities, as well as on Digit Symbol-Coding and Symbol Search, due to slowness, and on Picture Completion. Mr. C did least well on Digit Span, which is consistent with the commonly found weaknesses in span for verbal information and working memory in individuals with dyslexia.

As might have been expected, Mr. C's visuospatial constructional skills were adequate to strong, paralleling the WAIS-III findings. He used the organization effectively when copying the Rey-Osterrieth Complex Figure, shown in Figure 5-1a. His weak score was due to careless reproduction of the details and not to perceptual or organizational problems. He completed all WAIS-III Block Designs correctly, working quickly on most.

Mr. C's learning and memory skills also were normal for verbal material. His skills were stronger for visual material, paralleling the WAIS-III findings and showing the potential for use of visual strategies to assist with verbal learning (e.g., Webbing or Mind Mapping; see Buzan, 1991 and Ellis, 2007).

In contrast, Mr. C had impaired scores in the underlying neuropsychological skills needed for effective reading and writing. Phonological awareness and rapid visual naming were both impaired on the Comprehensive Test of Phonological Processing (CTOPP). Thus, at the most elementary level, he was unable to put together and take apart the sounds that make up words, which, as noted above, is a core deficit in dyslexia. He also showed a double deficit in phonological awareness and rapid naming that is associated with more severe reading disability.

Spoken language comprehension was relatively weak at the single–word level, and there were gaps in Mr. C's word knowledge, as he showed a pattern of missing and passing items across the WAIS-III Vocabulary subtest. At the sentence level, his ability to follow multistep directions on the Understanding Directions subtest of the Woodcock-Johnson-III Tests of Achievement (WJ3ACH) was low average. This likely reflected the demands the task placed on auditory-verbal attention and rapid responding, as Mr. C had difficulty holding each instruction in mind and then carrying it out. In contrast, his comprehension of complex, abstract, and figurative language on the Oral and Written Language Scales was solidly average, showing far better comprehension of oral language, in comparison

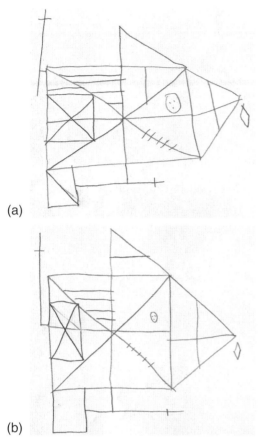

(a)

(b)

Figure 5-1. Rey-Osterreith Complex Figure Test. (*a*) Copy. (*b*) 30-minute delayed recall.

with written language, as can be seen in Table 5-1. This is an important skill needed for books in audio form, which Mr. C had been using for tests but not for reading his textbooks.

Regarding spoken language production, Mr. C's confrontation naming skills were reasonably good, although he made two linguistic errors ("thumbtack for *thimble*, "sundial" for *hourglass*) and used one circumlocution ("telescope building" for *observatory*) on WJ3ACH Picture Vocabulary (the Boston Naming Test was not used because of poor normative data for his age group). A deficit was seen in rapid picture naming on the WJ3ACH, consistent with impaired naming of letters and digits on the CTOPP. On all of these rapid naming tasks, Mr. C worked slowly but made no errors. D-KEFS Verbal Fluency showed a mixed pattern, with below average word generation for letters, but average word generation for categories, a profile that is

commonly associated with weaknesses in verbal organizational skills. Mr. C's ability to generate words from alternating categories was impaired because he lost the correct response set, initially using vegetables instead of fruits, but then correcting himself. It is also possible, given his language impairments, that this was due to semantic confusion between the two categories. Oral formulation of sentences on the Test of Language Competence—Expanded Edition was severely impaired, showing that Mr. C struggled to put his thoughts into words effectively. Speed played a role, as he was unable to complete three of his sentences in the allotted time. Yet he earned full credit on only four items. His other sentences, including the ones completed with extra time, were grammatically awkward (e.g., "Because I work out, it is not hard like him over there," "Before you cross the street, first look across if it's clear"). Impairment in oral sentence formulation typically leads to similar problems with expressive writing, as discussed below.

Impairments in simple span for verbal information and in working memory are common in individuals with dyslexia (Mapou, 2009). Mr. C's skills ranged from mildly impaired to average. His span was weakest for individual items (digits, word list). In contrast, his span was solidly average when he did not have to repeat information word-for-word, despite being presented with a large amount (brief stories). Similarly, with working memory, he did best with context, as his score on WAIS-III Arithmetic was average, with weaker skills on Digit Span-Backwards and Letter-Number Sequencing. Reflecting his difficulties in these skills, Mr. C's WAIS-III Working Memory Index was in the low average range.

As expected, Mr. C's reading was very impaired at the single-word level. When decoding nonsense words on WJ3ACH Word Attack, he missed easy items (e.g., "zup" for *zoop*, "ip" for *ep*, "fowa" for *foy*, "senrick" for *snirk*), never established a basal, and completed less than half the items correctly. He struggled to sound out real words on WJ3ACH Letter-Word Identification, making many errors (e.g., "usual" for *usually*, "scienteest" for *scientist*, "fleece" for *fierce*, "significant" for *sufficient*). He mainly read the easiest words correctly (said "don't know" to *moustache*, *tremendous*, and *urged*, among others) and was not fluent. His reading comprehension was variable, with more impairment seen when speed was stressed. Mr. C read very slowly and made one error on WJ3ACH Reading Fluency, which required a yes-no response to simple sentences. In contrast, the untimed cloze format of WJ3ACH Passage Comprehension proved easier for him, and he achieved a low average score, which was the best among his reading skills. The problem with this task, however, is that it does not adequately reflect the reading comprehension demands of college. These skills are more effectively assessed using a task in which longer passages are read and comprehension is tested with a multiple-choice format, as on the Comprehension section of Gates-MacGinitie Reading Test. On this measure, Mr. C's skills were below average for a community college student. Surprisingly, despite his lack of fluency on other reading measures, he finished the task with 11 minutes to spare. Yet his accuracy was poor, as he answered only 22 of the 48 questions correctly. This was consistent with his report that he did not make much use of extended time on tests and suggested that slowing down might improve his accuracy.

Mr. C's writing skills were somewhat stronger, although the impact of dyslexia and problems with oral formulation were evident. His handwriting was difficult to read and illegible at points. His skills on WJ3ACH Spelling were similar to his single-word reading skills. Again, he made errors reflecting impairment in phonological awareness (e.g., "eraly" for *early*, "gargue" for *garage*, "beutiful" for beautiful, "diffence" for *difference*) and was unable to spell three words at all (*cough, crystal, saucer*). With expressive writing, he had a low average score on WJ3ACH Writing Fluency. Despite the fact that only simple sentences were required, he lost points on three sentences that were incomplete, similar to his problems with oral formulation, and for changing a specified word on a fourth sentence. His strongest score was on Written Expression from the Wechsler Individual Achievement Test—Second Edition. Nonetheless, this score overestimated his skills because the scoring system did not permit penalties for some of the errors he made. Mr. C wrote very few words on the Word Fluency section, with a score that was far below the level of his performance on the Category section of the D-KEFS Verbal Fluency. His single sentences on the second section and essay on the

third section were marred by spelling, punctuation, and grammatical errors. His essay was brief and did not include any supporting evidence for his arguments.

Unlike some individuals with dyslexia, Mr. C had little difficulty with math. Interestingly, he did least well when completing simple math facts on WJ3ACH Math Fluency; in children with dyslexia, lack of automaticity in math fact retrieval is common (Fletcher et al., 2007). His other math skills were in the average range. With harder written calculations on WJ3ACH Calculation, Mr. C completed one algebra problem, but he missed easier subtraction and multiplication problems. He did best when solving math word problems, either in writing (WJ3ACH Applied Problems) or mentally (WAIS-III Arithmetic). This was a bit surprising, as individuals with weaknesses in spoken language can have more difficulty with word problems because of the additional demands on language.

As noted, Mr. C had no history of ADHD. Nonetheless, as shown in Table 5-1, impairments were seen in focused attention/processing speed and sustained attention. His weak scores on measures of focused attention/processing speed, which were due to slow but accurate performances, most likely reflected general slowness on tasks independent of spoken and written language difficulties. In fact, Pennington (2009) has noted that a processing speed deficit is frequent in children with dyslexia, is a cognitive risk factor shared by both dyslexia and ADHD, and may reflect a shared genetic link between the two disorders. Because the IVA Continuous Performance Task used verbal targets (digits), both auditory and visual, this language demand may have affected Mr. C's performance, despite the task's simplicity. In retrospect, it would have been better to have administered a nonverbal sustained attention measure, such as the Test of Variables of Attention.

Some difficulties were evident in the realm of executive functions and problem-solving abilities. Research has shown that these types of difficulties are common in children with learning disabilities, even in the absence of a disorder that directly affects executive functioning, such as ADHD (Wasserstein & Denckla, 2009). Consequently, such difficulties are not surprising in an adult with dyslexia. On the other hand, some of these impairments may have reflected Mr. C's language impairments. First, his verbal organizational skills were weak, as he did not use a strong organizational strategy on the CVLT-II. Yet he still learned and retained the list at an average level. Second, on WAIS-III Similarities, Mr. C could not determine an association on many items and responded that he did not know the answer. It is possible that he was having problems with word retrieval, particularly because he did far better on Comprehension, which permitted a more extended response. Nonetheless and despite his difficulty, he received partial credit on the next-to-the-hardest item. Third, his performance on WAIS-III Picture Completion was at the low end of the average range, as he frequently had difficulty discerning what was missing. Yet he completed the hardest item correctly. On both of these reasoning tasks, Mr. C struggled with "going beyond the obvious" and thinking at a more abstract level. At the same time, because he was able to complete some of the hardest items correctly, his final scores did not reflect the level of item complexity that he reached. Fourth, as noted, Mr. C had initial difficulty establishing the correct response set on the Switching section of D-KEFS Verbal Fluency.

Finally, although Mr. C's verbal learning and memory skills were largely average, an impact of weakness in auditory verbal attention and verbal organization on encoding was seen in his recognition memory performance. On the CVLT-II, he encoded only 14 of the 16 words, which was mildly impaired and weak in comparison with his learning and recall scores. On the WMS-III Logical Memory subtest, he had perfect recognition for Story B, which was presented twice, but missed five questions for Story A, which he had heard only once.

An interview with Mr. C and his father showed no evidence of emotional distress. Although the author usually administers an MMPI-2, this was not completed, because of Mr. C's dyslexia. It was not believed that briefer symptom checklists would have revealed anything more than was learned from the interview and behavioral observations.

Based on Mr. C's history and the results, a dyslexia diagnosis was confirmed. Mr. C showed a classic profile, with impairment in phonological awareness, rapid naming, reading, and writing, in the context of average intelligence and average to above average skills in most other cognitive

realms. His spoken language comprehension was also much stronger than his reading comprehension. Recommendations were made to the DSS for continued accommodations. These included 50% additional time on tests (although the degree of impairment and the potential for improvement if Mr. C learned to slow down and to read more effectively was thought to justify double time), continued use of the Kurzweil 3000 or a reader for tests, use of a computer-based word processor with a spell-checker for essay tests, and use of a calculator for math tests, because of disproportionately slow retrieval of math facts. For the classroom, a note-taker, copies of PowerPoint slides and other visual aids ahead of class, continued permission to record lectures, and preferential seating in class were recommended. For homework, it was recommended that Mr. C apply for audio books from Recording for the Blind and Dyslexic (see http://www.rfbd.org), which he had never done and, if a site license were available, that he be given a copy of the Kurzweil 3000 to use for reading his textbooks at home. In addition, continued access to a proofreader for his written work was recommended. The author's standard accommodations for students with learning disabilities also were recommended. These included taking a reduced course load, priority registration, and access to tutorial support.

Mr. C appeared to have had typical classroom instruction in reading and writing in his early years, but he never had adequate evidence-based intervention for children with dyslexia. Consequently, work with a reading specialist or speech/language pathologist to improve phonological awareness, automaticity of decoding and single-word reading, fluency when reading text, and reading comprehension was recommended. Nonetheless, improving fluency and comprehension in adults with dyslexia can be very difficult when deficits have persisted for many years. Given the linguistic basis of dyslexia, further evaluation of Mr. C's language skills by a speech/language pathologist was recommended, as it was thought that this might direct reading and writing interventions more effectively. Finally, tutoring to improve Mr. C's study skills and expressive writing skills was recommended.

Mr. C was subsequently treated by a speech/language pathologist, who worked at his college, for three semesters. The speech/language pathologist reported that he was cooperative, motivated, accepted needed help, and strove to work independently. He typically arrived for sessions early and rarely missed scheduled sessions. Her treatment focused mainly on Mr. C's English classes and included the following:

- Improving reading at the single-word level, with an emphasis on decoding consonant blends and syllabication
- Clarifying vocabulary, idioms, and other figures of speech with which he was not familiar
- Learning how to analyze literature and poetry critically
- Improving syntax in his sentence structure
- Learning to use clear organization and supporting details when writing essays
- Preparing oral presentations

Mr. C continued to be very interested in the finance field, watched finance shows regularly on television to build his knowledge, and wrote a paper on the organizational structure of a major investment bank. Despite the noted challenges in written language, he was one of only two students who successfully solved a complex problem in his accounting class using Microsoft Excel.

Conclusions

Although Fletcher et al. (2007) have argued that *(1)* that response to intervention is the most effective way to assess learning disabilities in children and that *(2)* only a focused assessment of academic skills should be completed, if deemed necessary, these are not viable approaches for adults for several reasons. First, there are no studies of response-to-intervention paradigms in adults, and colleges and universities do not have response-to-intervention programs. Second, there is far less research on adults with learning disabilities that can guide focused assessment. Third, adults are more complex than children, in terms of educational needs and psychosocial factors. If an adult has not been assessed previously or if the history is unclear, as was the case with Mr. C, a comprehensive assessment is needed to understand the nature of the client's difficulties. In particular, the possibility of an alternate cause or co-occurring disorder (e.g., neurological, ADHD, psychiatric)

must be considered, and focused assessment of academic skills will not be sufficient for this. Fourth, documentation guidelines of colleges, universities, and standardized testing agencies typically require a comprehensive assessment, if one has not been completed recently (Educational Testing Service, 2007).

The case of Mr. C also shows how a comprehensive assessment can answer questions of interest to college DSS personnel. If the only question to be answered is whether a client has dyslexia (or another specific learning disability), then a focused assessment of the specific academic skills and, perhaps, the underlying neuropsychological skills (e.g., phonological awareness, rapid visual naming) is sufficient. On the other hand, comprehensive assessment can answer the following important questions, which should be considered when working with post-secondary education students. These questions are also applicable to adults who are working:

1. *Does the student have the intelligence needed to succeed in college?* In this case, Mr. C was shown to be of at least average intelligence.
2. *Can the student learn and remember information at a normal level?* Mr. C had at least average learning and memory skills, with strength in visual learning and memory.
3. *Are there cognitive strengths that can be used to help the student compensate for weaknesses?* Mr. C showed strengths in the visuospatial realm, which could be used to develop strategies for learning verbal information. He also showed adequate spoken language comprehension, supporting the use of text-to-audio technology for reading.
4. *Are there any other cognitive weaknesses beyond those specific to dyslexia that could impair the student's learning?* Mr. C showed impairment in attention, which could affect him in the classroom. Yet he did not meet diagnostic criteria for ADHD, and so the meaning of this impairment remained unclear. He also showed some relative weaknesses in abstract thinking, which could affect his understanding of certain types of classroom material.
5. *Are there any emotional issues that are affecting classroom performance?* Earlier in his life, Mr. C was very frustrated with his difficulties but, over time, had learned to accept them.

He came across as a well-adjusted young man, and there were no indications that emotional distress was contributing to his problems. If anything, he was a bit unconcerned about his reading difficulties and more resistant than expected to accommodations that might have helped him (e.g., making more effective use of extended time on tests, using text-to-audio technology for his reading assignments rather than reading them on his own, not taking notes in class).

For all of these reasons, comprehensive assessment is believed to be necessary when evaluating adults with learning disabilities.

Acknowledgment

This chapter was presented in slightly different form at the 37th annual meeting of the International Neuropsychological Society, held in February 2009 in Atlanta, GA.

References

Buzan, T. (1991). *Use both sides of your brain* (3rd ed.). New York: Plume.

Educational Testing Service. (2007). Policy statement for documentation of a learning disability in adolescents and adults (2nd ed.). Princeton, NJ: Author.

Ellis, D. (2007). *Becoming a master student* (12th ed.). Boston: Houghton Mifflin.

Fletcher, J. M., Lyon, G. R., Fuchs, L. S., & Barnes, M. A. (2007). *Learning disabilities: From identification to intervention.* New York: Guilford Press.

Lyon, G. R., Shaywitz, S. E., & Shaywitz, B. A. (2003). A definition of dyslexia. *Annals of Dyslexia, 53,* 1-14.

Mapou, R. L. (2009). *Adult learning disabilities and ADHD: Research-informed assessment.* New York: Oxford University Press.

Pennington, B. F. (2009). *Diagnosing learning disorders: A neuropsychological framework* (2nd ed.). New York: Guilford Press.

Shaywitz, S. (2003). *Overcoming dyslexia.* New York: Alfred A. Knopf.

Shaywitz, S. E., & Shaywitz, B. A. (2005). Dyslexia (specific reading disability). *Biological Psychiatry, 57,* 1301-1309.

Wasserstein, J., & Denckla, M. B. (2009). ADHD and learning disabilities in adults: Overlap with executive dysfunction. In T. E. Brown (Ed.), *ADHD comorbidities: Handbook for ADHD complications in children and adults* (pp. 267-285). Washington, DC: American Psychiatric Publishing.

6

Tourette Syndrome

E. Mark Mahone

When a young child begins to make strange movements or sounds, it can be very concerning to parents. Many have heard horror stories about Tourette syndrome and fear that their child will live a life of social rejection (Eivdente, 2000). Often the unusual movements or sounds are *tics*—involuntary, rapid, sudden, nonrhythmic, stereotyped motor movements or vocalizations (Dewey, Tupper, & Bottos, 2004). *Transient tics* are quite common, particularly among children under the age of 10 years, with prevalence estimates ranging from 4% to 24% of all children in this age range (Leckman, 2002; Pringsheim, Davenport, & Lang, 2003), and as high as 27% among children receiving special education (Kurlan et al., 2001). At the other end of the spectrum, Gilles de la Tourette syndrome (TS) represents a more chronic neuropsychiatric disorder, characterized by a pattern of motor and vocal tics that occur for at least 1 year (Singer, 2005a). Tourette syndrome was once considered rare; however, recent estimates suggest that the prevalence may be as high at 3.5% of school-aged children (Singer, 2005a). The symptoms of TS, including spasms, noises, and bursts of obscenities, were first blamed on the devil; in fact, the book/movie *The Exorcist* was reportedly based on a child with TS (Garilick, 1986). Subsequently, until the 1970s, TS was considered to be a form of neurosis; however, current research suggests that it has a neurobiological basis (Olson, Singer, Goodman, & Maria, 2006).

Tics and Tic Disorders

Tics are generally classified as simple or complex, and as motor or vocal (phonic). *Simple motor tics* are focal movements (usually discrete contractions) of small muscle groups, and they can include eye blinks, tongue protrusion, shoulder shrugs, head jerks, nose twitch, or facial grimacing. *Complex motor tics* involve more muscles acting in a coordinated manner to produce more complicated movements that can mimic purposeful motor tasks or gestures (Bradshaw, 2001). Examples include the following: scratching, touching, rubbing, jumping, hand gestures, adjustments for symmetry, imitating the gestures of others (*echopraxia*), or making obscene gestures (*copropraxia*). *Simple vocal tics* are elementary, meaningless noises (Evidente, 2000) such as sniffing, throat clearing, snorting, or squealing. *Complex vocal tics* often include meaningful syllables, words, or phrases (e.g., "okay") and can involve repetition of one's own speech (*palilalia*), repetition of others' speech (*echolalia*), or shouting of obscenities or profanities without provocation (*coprolalia*). Although coprolalia is the behavior most associated with TS on television and in movies (and most feared by parents), it occurs in only about 10% of children with TS (Goldenberg, Brown, & Weiner, 1994). While most tics have a rapid, abrupt time course (i.e., like a sneeze), they can vary and are also classified on the basis of the speed of movement. *Clonic* tics are brief, sudden, and jerk-like; *dystonic* tics involve twisting or posturing, while *tonic* tics involve prolonged or sustained movements or contractions of muscles (e.g., prolonged bending of the trunk; Evidente, 2000).

Onset of tics usually occurs during childhood, with mean age of onset around 6 to 7 years (Evidente, 2000; Singer, 2005b), with peak severity between ages 8 and 12 years (Leckman et al., 1998). Further, most children with TS have onset of motor tics 1 to 2 years before onset of vocal tics. While motor tics often go relatively unnoticed in the classroom, vocal tics can be disruptive, distressing, and embarrassing, as many elementary school students and teachers have had little experience with such behaviors.

Tics can be exacerbated by stress, excitement, fatigue, and acute anxiety, and they can increase following use of central nervous system (CNS) stimulants, caffeine, steroids, and dopaminergic drugs. A child's tics can also increase following inquiry about the movements, or at times as an *echophenomenon*—following observation of a movement or sound in another person (Singer, 2005b). Conversely, tics usually diminish with relaxation, performance of engaging mental or physical activity (e.g., taking neuropsychological tests), and with use of alcohol, marijuana, or nicotine. Tics can be voluntarily suppressed for brief periods and are commonly reduced or absent in sleep, although sleep studies in patients with TS have shown an increased rate of tics during rapid eye movement (REM) sleep (Cohrs et al., 2001). *Premonitory sensations* can precede (and incessantly prompt) tics. These premonitory "urges" are usually sensory events (e.g., itching, tingling, or a feeling of pressure) that occur just prior to tics, with feeling of momentary relief following the tic (Bliss, 1980). Premonitory sensations can occur in over a third of young children with TS (Banaschewski, Woerner, & Rothenberger, 2003). Thus, in some children, tics may represent a voluntary response to an involuntary sensation, introducing a conscious desire to suppress the movements, which can impede concentration and sustained effort.

Differential diagnosis of simple motor tics can include a variety of pathological movements, including tremors, chorea, athetosis, myoclonus, dystonia, akathisia, ballistic movements, paroxysmal dyskinesias, and hyperekplexia (Fahn & Erenberg, 1988). Thus, children with onset of tics should have thorough evaluation by a physician with experience in movement disorders. Complex tics must also be distinguished from *compulsions* and *stereotypies*. Tics and compulsions can share a common presentation, including the pressure to perform some action until the sense of tension is relieved (Hunter, 2007); however, in compulsions, there is usually anxiety surrounding an intrusive thought, and a conscious decision to perform the compulsion to reduce the anxiety. *Stereotypies* are repetitive movements whose form, amplitude, and location are more highly predictable than tics. Motor stereotypies are characterized by their involuntary, patterned, coordinated, repetitive, rhythmic, and nonreflexive features; they typically last for seconds to minutes, occur in clusters, appear many times per day, and are associated with periods of excitement, stress, fatigue, or boredom. In contrast to tics and compulsions, motor stereotypies begin very early in life (usually before age 2 years), are readily suppressed by sensory stimuli or distraction, and are often of little concern to the patient, whose daily activities are rarely affected (Mahone, Bridges, Prahme, & Singer, 2004). While compulsions and stereotypies are distinguished from tics, they often co-occur among individuals with TS (Harris, Mahone, & Singer, 2008).

Diagnosis of Tic Disorders

Diagnosis of TS is based solely on the patient's history and clinical observation. There is no diagnostic laboratory test (Singer, 2005a), and individual magnetic resonance imaging (MRI) scans tend to be unremarkable (Mahone & Slomine, 2008). Since tics wax and wane (and may not be present in the office visit), it is often necessary for the clinician to review a videotape of the child's movements in order to make the diagnosis. The formal diagnostic criteria for TS, as defined by the *Tourette Syndrome Classification Group* (1993) includes the following: *(1)* onset of symptoms before age 21 years; *(2)* presence of multiple motor and at least one vocal tic (not necessarily concurrently); *(3)* waxing and waning course; *(4)* presence of tic symptoms for at least 1 year; *(5)* absence of a precipitating illness; and *(6)* observation of the tics by a knowledgeable individual. The *DSM-IV-TR* (American Psychiatric Association, 2000) recognizes three types of tic disorders. *Transient tic disorders* involve multiple motor and/or vocal tics, many times a day, often in bouts, lasting at least 1 month, but not more than 1 year. *Chronic motor/vocal tic disorders* are identical to transient tic disorders, except that motor *or* vocal tics (but not both) occur for at least 1 year. Finally, *Tourette disorder* (which is similar, but not identical to Tourette syndrome) is characterized by onset by age 18 and presence of motor and vocal tics for at least 1 year that are not caused by a physical illness, injury, or medication. Unlike Tourette syndrome, Tourette disorder requires the presence of functional life impairment or emotional distress caused by the tics. Additionally, there is a requirement for no tic-free intervals of 3 months or more.

Clinical Course and Outcome

Tics spontaneously wax and wane, making ratings of severity and treatment studies difficult to interpret (Singer, 2000). Although outcomes often vary, most research suggests that tics improve in adolescence and young adulthood (Pappert, Guetz, Louis, Blasucci, & Leurgans, 2003). For example, in a naturalistic study of teenagers and young adults who had childhood-onset TS, the tics had disappeared in 26%, diminished considerably in 46%, remained stable in 14%, and increased in severity in 14% (Erenberg, Cruse, & Rothner, 1987). A variety of factors potentially influence the natural course of TS, including adverse prenatal and perinatal events, postinfectious autoimmune reactions, hormonal factors, stress, exposure to drugs, and comorbid medical/psychiatric conditions (Leckman, Peterson, Pauls, & Cohen, 1997).

Etiology and Pathogenesis of Tourette Syndrome

It is generally recognized that TS is a genetic disorder, with much evidence pointing to a single major gene locus with suggestions of autosomal dominant inheritance, although other mechanisms of inheritance have been suggested (Robertson, 2000, 2003). The concordance rate for monozygotic twins is greater than 50%, while

concordance rate among dizygotic twins is around 10% (Hyde, Aaronson, Randolph, Rickler, & Weinberger, 1992). There is substantial evidence that the dopaminergic system is pathophysiologically involved in TS, since dopaminergic medication can induce tics, while blockade of dopaminergic transmission is effective in tic suppression (Robertson, 1989). A variety of investigations have identified anomalous function of the basal ganglia in the pathophysiology of TS (Singer et al., 2002). Increase in dopamine transporter binding is considered a possible, but not necessary alteration and may occur more often among individuals with severe impulse control problems (Muller-Vahl et al., 2000). Binding of antineuronal antibodies (e.g., gamma immunoglobins) has also been suggested as a possible cause for the basal ganglia alterations observed in some children with TS (Hallett, Harling-Berg, Knopf, Stopa, & Kiessling, 2000). Recently, a set of studies has identified a group of children who developed tics and obsessive-compulsive disorder (OCD) following group A ß-hemolytic streptococcal infection (Swedo et al., 1998). The syndrome, labeled the *pediatric autoimmune neuropsychiatric disorders associated with streptococcal infection* (*PANDAS*), has been the source of some controversy, especially since more recent studies have failed to reveal an increased rate of antineuronal antibodies in children with TS (Singer, Hong, Yoon, & Williams, 2005; Singer, Gause, Morris, Lopez, & Tourette Syndrome Study Group, 2008), as well as concern over unwarranted use of antibiotic treatment for tics and/or OCD without evidence of laboratory infection (Gabbbay et al., 2008).

Anatomical and functional disturbances in the cortico-striatal-thalamo-cortical circuits are also thought to be critically involved in the pathogenesis of TS (Albin & Mink, 2006). In adults with TS, aberrant activity in interrelated language, sensorimotor, executive, and paralimbic circuits is associated with tic occurrence, potentially accounting for the execution of motor and vocal tics, as well as the accompanying premonitory urges (Stern et al., 2000). Functionally, *tic suppression* is a highly active, attention-demanding task, requiring constant update of sensory information, and it is associated with increased activity in frontal, superior temporal, and anterior cingulate cortices (Peterson et al., 1998).

Volumetric studies have identified reduced basal ganglia volumes (Peterson et al., 2003), as well as a shift away from normal left-larger-than-right asymmetry of the putamen and lenticular regions of the basal ganglia (Peterson et al., 1993; Singer et al., 1993). Sowell et al. (2008) reported significant thinning of sensorimotor cortex, most prominently over the sensory and motor homunculi that control facial, orolingual, and laryngeal musculature commonly involved in tic symptoms with age interactions, suggesting that cortical thinning in older children with TS could be a sign of persistent illness. Using diffusion tensor imaging (DTI), Plessen et al. (2006) identified reduced interhemispheric white matter connectivity in callosal fibers in all subregions of the corpus callosum among children with TS. At the same time, a variety of other studies have identified *increased* regional brain volumes associated with TS in children, including enlarged right thalamus (Lee et al., 2006), parietal cortex (Peterson et al., 2001), and dorsal prefrontal cortex (Fredericksen et al., 2002), but reduced frontal volumes in adults (Peterson et al., 2001). Thus, while the imaging findings may represent pathological causes of the disease, they may also be related to compensatory changes in the developing nervous system of individuals with TS (Gerard & Peterson, 2003). The inconsistencies among imaging studies also support the case for categorizing children with TS *plus* attention-deficit/hyperactivity disorder (ADHD) separately from those with TS alone (Denckla, 2006). For example, in studies of boys with ADHD with or without TS, researchers noted that the children with ADHD had exactly the same imaging findings as the boys with ADHD plus TS (Aylward et al., 1996; Castellanos, Giedd, Hamburger, Marsh, & Rapoport, 1996). Other studies have shown enlarged corpus callosum in children with "pure" TS, reduced corpus callosum in "pure" ADHD, and (paradoxically) "normal" corpus callosum size in the group with combined TS and ADHD (Baumgardner et al., 1996). Among individuals with TS plus ADHD, correlation of cortical disinhibition with ADHD symptoms is greater than with tic severity, suggesting a more consistent relationship between cortical dysfunction and ADHD symptoms than with tic symptoms (Gilbert et al., 2004) and supporting the argument for subcortical mechanisms in the etiology of TS.

Associated Features and Comorbid Conditions

When a neuropsychologist encounters a child with a history of tics or TS, the next inquiry should be whether the child also has ADHD and/or OCD, since the presence of these comorbidities plays a critical role in treatment and outcome. In fact, the shared etiologic pathways for TS, ADHD, and OCD have led them to be characterized as *developmental basal ganglia disorders* (Grados et al., 2008; Palumbo, Maughan, & Kurlan, 1997). An increased rate of autism has also been observed in TS, with epidemiological research citing 6.5% co-occurrence (Baron-Cohen, Scahill, Hornsey, & Robertson, 1999). Children with TS plus comorbid conditions (especially ADHD and/or OCD) tend to have a more severe neuropsychiatric presentation than children with TS alone (Shin, Chung, & Hong, 2001; Spencer et al., 1998). Like ADHD, the male/female ratio in TS is approximately 4:1, although in TS, males are much more likely to have comorbidities (Freeman et al., 2000). Large-scale studies have shown the overall co-occurrence of ADHD among children with TS to be at least 50% (Spencer et al., 1998), and as high as 64% among boys (Freeman et al., 2000). Obsessive-compulsive disorder occurs in approximately 27% of males and females with TS, with rates of obsessive-compulsive symptoms (short of OCD diagnosis) as high as 40%–60%. Learning disabilities (LDs) are also common in TS (25% of males, 14% of females) but seem to occur in conjunction with other comorbidities (Freeman et al., 2000). In fact, the presence of LDs in children with TS can be accounted for almost entirely by the comorbidities with ADHD, given the 35% overlap between ADHD and LDs (Willcutt, Pennington, Olson, & Defries, 2007). Pure TS is not typically associated with intellectual difficulties or LDs (Singer, Schuerholz, & Denckla, 1994). Rather, just the opposite appears to be true—children with pure TS show unexpectedly high IQ scores (Denckla, 2006; Harris et al., 1996; Mahone et al., 2001) and significantly *increased* IQ when compared to their parents (Casey, Cohen, Schuerholz, Singer, & Denckla, 2000; Schuerholz, Baumgardner, Singer, Reiss, & Denckla, 1996). Nevertheless, based on research evidence suggesting cognitive slowing referable to the basal ganglia in children with pure TS (Harris et al., 1995; Schuerholz et al., 1996), it has been argued that the basal ganglia may account for executive control differences which persist despite higher intellectual functioning in these children (Denckla & Reiss, 1997).

Treatment of Tourette Syndrome

Despite its prevalence, only a minority of children affected by TS come to medical attention, in part because many cases are mild, symptoms are confused with colds or allergies, and because it is often difficult to obtain expert advice (Sandor, 2003). Treatment of TS is based on the functional impairment associated with the tics, as well as the comorbid problems, availability of environmental support, and challenges associated with the stage of development (Singer, 2005a). Prior to initiating treatment, thorough diagnostic assessment should be completed, including medical evaluation to rule out physical conditions that might be causing/contributing to the tics and to ensure that the movements are indeed tics and not some other movement disorder requiring a different treatment. In addition, assessment of comorbidities (especially ADHD, OCD, autism, and LDs) is essential since pharmacological treatments for tics generally do not treat comorbid conditions, and comorbidities can cause greater psychosocial and academic dysfunction than the tics themselves. At this point, referral for neuropsychological consultation is usually indicated.

While a variety of medications have been successful in reducing tics, a conservative approach to pharmacological intervention is usually recommended, with restriction to those patients whose tics cause significant psychosocial or musculoskeletal/physical problems, or are not remediable by nondrug interventions. For many families, education and reassurance about the disorder and its associated features often obviate or delay need for medication (Singer, 2005a). Recent reviews of medication trials for tic suppression identified at least 12 classes of medications that have been used, including stimulants, alpha-2 agonists (e.g., clonidine, guanfacine), classical neuroleptics (e.g., haloperidol, pimozide), atypical neuroleptics (e.g., risperidone, olanzepine), selective serotonin reuptake inhibitors (e.g., fluoxetine), dopamine antagonists (e.g., tetrabenazine), dopamine agonists (e.g., pergolide), benzodiazepines (e.g., clonazepam), botulinum toxin (botox), GABA analogues (baclofen), and anticonvulsants (Gilbert & Lipps, 2005; Robertson, 2000). While the use of stimulants in children with ADHD and tics was once contraindicated, this is no longer the case. The apparent increase in tics with stimulant treatment was confounded by the natural course and onset of tics in TS. When group data were analyzed, there was no significant increase in tics when stimulants were used in patients with tics compared with controls, although some individual patients did experience an increase in tics. Thus, use of stimulants is considered medically appropriate in children with tics where the ADHD symptoms are significantly disturbing their quality of life (Erenberg, 2005).

Although medications are widely prescribed for TS, they are only moderately efficacious and carry the risk of short- and long-term side effects (Himle, Woods, Piacentini, & Walkup, 2006). There is considerable evidence to support the use of behavioral therapy as an alternative to pharmacotherapy, or as an adjunct for those who have obtained maximum benefit from medication. The most rigorously investigated nonpharmacologic treatment for tics is *habit reversal training* (Piacentini & Chang, 2006), which is based on the idea that, despite a biological origin, tics can be worsened, improved, or maintained by environmental events. The behavioral model asserts that tics function to reduce unpleasant premonitory urges (i.e., negative reinforcement) and thus serve to increase or maintain the severity of both the urge and the tic (Himle et al., 2006). This link between urge and tic is considered a learned behavior and habit reversal training seeks to modify that connection. Relaxation training, biofeedback, awareness training, and massed negative practice have also been used with some success to treat motivated children with TS. In contrast, there is little research support for the use of dietary therapies, supplements, or acupuncture (Singer, 2005a).

Neuropsychological Findings in Tourette Syndrome

Neuropsychological function among children with TS varies widely, depending on the presence of comorbidities. Children with "pure" TS tend to have relatively intact profiles, often with unexpectedly high IQ (Schuerholz et al., 1996; Casey et al, 2000; Mahone et al., 2001), strong language skills (Harris et al., 1995), and increased motor speed (Schuerholz, Cutting, Mazzocco, Singer, & Denckla, 1997), compared to controls. Neuropsychological dysfunction among children with pure TS tends to be subtle, including isolated difficulties on measures of inhibition (Cannon, Pratt, & Robertson, 2003), spontaneous intrusions on list-learning trials (Mahone et al., 2001), perseverative errors on card-sorting tasks (Cirino, Chapieski, & Massman, 2000), and visuomotor integration (Schultz et al., 1998). Children with pure TS have also shown slow and variable reaction time on continuous performance tests (Harris et al., 1996; Shucard, Benedict, Tekok-Kilic, & Lichter, 1997) and reduced letter-word fluency (Schuerholz et al., 1996). Reduced output speed in pure TS has not been found to be related to motor slowing (Schuerholz et al., 1997), but rather to mental slowing or "bradyphrenia," considered a feature of subcortical dysfunction and associated with disorders such as Parkinson disease. While a number of studies have identified subtle executive dysfunction among children with pure TS, on most measures, they do not differ from controls, possibly because their somewhat above-average IQ serves to nullify some of the executive control differences (Denckla, 2006; Mahone, Hagelthorn, et al., 2002). For example, one study found that children with pure TS did not differ from controls on performance-based tests of executive function, and they were rated by parents as having greater dysfunction than controls on only one of eight scales from the Behavior Rating Inventory of Executive Function (BRIEF; Gioia, Isquith, Guy, & Kenworthy, 2000). Conversely, children in TS plus ADHD and "pure" ADHD groups were rated as impaired (compared to the control and pure TS groups) on all eight BRIEF scales, but they were not different from each other on any scale (Mahone, Cirino, et al., 2002).

Case Report: Tommy

"Tommy" is a right-handed boy, who was age 7 years, 11 months at the time of initial assessment. Prior to neuropsychological consultation,

he was seen by a pediatric neurologist for evaluation of motor and vocal tics. The neurologist subsequently referred Tommy for neuropsychological assessment to clarify his neurobehavioral functioning and to make recommendations for behavioral, family, and educational intervention. Tommy was subsequently evaluated on two occasions, 2 years apart (age 7 years, 11 months and age 9 years, 11 months).

Relevant History

Throughout the assessments, Tommy lived with his mother, stepfather, two younger half-siblings, and older stepsister. Both biological parents and stepfather were high school graduates with some college. Family medical history was significant for lymphoma, Graves disease, and cerebral palsy, but negative for tics, learning disability, anxiety disorders, or ADHD. In addition to his history of tics, Tommy had been treated for allergies, asthma, and (as a toddler) multiple ear infections. At initial assessment he was taking medication for asthma and allergies, but not for tics. His hearing and vision have consistently been normal.

Tommy was born at full term, following an uncomplicated pregnancy and labor, and has had a generally healthy childhood. Developmental milestones were within normal limits for language, motor, and social skills. Tommy attended a private preschool, and then a public elementary school. At initial assessment, he was in third grade, taking a combination of regular and gifted/talented classes. He had never had special education services. In second grade, teachers reported problems with listening, impulsive behaviors, following written and oral directions, losing school assignments, inability to work independently, careless mistakes, and needing frequent prompting; nevertheless, he received all "Satisfactory" and "Outstanding" marks on his report card that year. Some of Tommy's teachers expressed concern that his movements may have been related to anxiety. He reportedly bit his nails, and he complained of abdominal and back pain as well as occasional headaches. By third grade, Tommy continued to do well, and was very happy with his teacher. Parents reported that he required structure and consistent prompting to complete his homework, which often took 2 to 3 hours per night due to off-task behaviors.

Tommy started having tics about a month after his seventh birthday, which were initially characterized by his eyes moving upwards and to the right bilaterally, occurring several times each day. At initial assessment, these tics had not resolved and additional tics had developed, including tilting his head and neck to one side, covering his mouth with both hands, sniffling, wiggling his nose, sucking in air, puckering/quivering of lips, humming, throat clearing, and several guttural noises. Tommy's tics waxed and waned, and they were exacerbated by lack of sleep, stress, and anxiety. There were no apparent relieving factors for the tics, although the severity decreased during the summer months. His tics had never been present during sleep. Tommy reported that he could sometimes suppress his tics, but it was difficult, felt uncomfortable, and took most of his concentration. Although his friends were aware of his tics, the movements did not appear to be causing any psychosocial difficulties or interfering with play activities. Tommy's neurologist had given the preliminary diagnosis of *probable* Tourette syndrome, since the tics had not yet been present for a full year.

Shortly after his tics began in second grade, Tommy was assessed by his school's special educator, a speech/language pathologist, a school psychologist, and an occupational therapist in the community. He also saw a social worker to address emotional concerns, and an audiologist to evaluate for a central auditory processing disorder. All these assessments were unremarkable, with all test scores at or above age and grade level expectations (i.e., *CELF-III* Total Language standard score [SS] = 136; *WISC-IV* Full Scale IQ = 125; *Beery Developmental Test of Visual Motor Integration* SS = 104, *Visual Perception* SS = 118; *Woodcock-Johnson III* Broad Reading SS = 122, Broad Math SS = 113, Broad Written Language SS = 121). The lone area of relative weakness noted was on the *WISC-IV* Processing Speed Index (SS = 77).

Neuropsychological Examination Results: Age 7 Years, 11 Months

Tommy was seen for initial assessment approximately 10 months after onset of his tics (in September, just after beginning third grade). At that time, he presented as slightly overweight,

with mild twitching and puckering of his lips, and slight twitching of his shoulder and neck, and mildly echopraxic head, eye, and arm movements. Vocal tics were present but difficult to identify due to the frequency of his other vocalizations. Tommy was playful, talkative, and quick to warm up; his mood was consistently happy, although he reported that he becomes angry when other children are mean to him. His activity level was high and he frequently interrupted testing with off-task or humorous comments, and he often disrupted his test performance by singing responses or making his responses more complicated and lengthy than necessary. He was distractible and often missed parts of directions that consisted of more than one or two tasks. He verbalized his problem-solving strategies and kept himself on task by verbally guiding himself. He was nevertheless receptive to verbal and non-verbal redirection, his cooperation was easily elicited, and overall effort was good; thus, the test results were considered to be a valid representation of his skills. Since Tommy had recently undergone multiple school- and community-based assessments of IQ, language, academic achievement, and visuomotor skills, these tests were not repeated at initial assessment; instead, testing focused on skills related to attention, executive function, motor skills, and memory.

Parent ratings on the *Conners' Parent Rating Scale-Revised* yielded elevations on scales assessing criteria for ADHD (*DSM-IV* Inattentive T = 69; *DSM-IV* Hyperactive/Impulsive T = 74). In contrast, teacher ratings on the *Conners' Teacher Rating Scale–Revised* were all within normal limits (T < 60). Tommy was also able to perform adequately on *basic* tasks of sustained attention (i.e., all scores from *Conners' Continuous Performance Test-II*), visual selective attention (*NEPSY* Visual Attention scaled score [ScS] =10; *D-KEFS* Trail Making Visual Scanning ScS = 9), and attentional tasks involving overlearned information (*Children's Memory Scale* Sequences ScS = 13), despite having frequent tics and fidgety behavior during testing.

During the assessment, however, Tommy's performance was adversely impacted by impairments in executive function—including "interfering" behaviors related to independent self-regulation, set maintenance, selective inhibition of responding, response preparation, cognitive flexibility, and organization of time and space. Parent ratings on the *Behavior Rating Inventory of Executive Function (BRIEF)* noted significant concern with executive control (Global Executive Composite T = 68), especially when initiating problem solving and activity, sustaining effort, adjusting to changes in routine or task demands, and planning and organizing activities; however, these observations were not echoed by Tommy's third grade teacher (*BRIEF* Global Executive Composite T = 55). Behaviorally, Tommy also had difficulty on more effortful tests of attentional efficiency (*D-KEFS* Trail Making Letter Sequencing ScS = 6), set-shifting (*D-KEFS* Trail Making Number/Letter Switching ScS = 8, 3 errors), and strategic planning (*D-KEFS* Twenty Questions (ScS = 6).

Even though Tommy had consistently demonstrated strong language skills in prior school assessments, he had inconsistencies in his initial neuropsychological assessment related to executive dysfunction. For example, although his auditory comprehension (*Token Test for Children* Part V Total = 71st percentile), verbal fluency (*NEPSY* Verbal Fluency ScS = 14), and phonological awareness (*CTOPP* Elision ScS = 10) were all intact, his performance on a visual confrontation naming test (*Boston Naming Test*) was well below average (8th percentile) and characterized by impulsive and incorrect answers, as well as phonemic paraphasias. Tommy also had reduced performance on the *Rapid Automatized Naming (RAN)* tests (all trials <10th percentile). He made multiple naming errors (unexpected at his age) and his performance was slowed by his tendency to insert transition words in between items (e.g., "red *and* green *and* blue"), or singing words slowly in order to give him time to think of the name for the next word.

Tommy's visual perceptual (*Hooper Visual Organization* = 94th percentile) and visual motor integration (*NEPSY* Visuomotor Precision ScS = 13) were intact for age, as was his ability to copy a complex visual design (*Rey Complex Figure* copy = 25th percentile). Similarly, Tommy's memory skills were largely intact for verbal and nonverbal information, including basic auditory span (*WISC-IV* Digit Span forward ScS = 13; *WISC-III-PI* Letter Span ScS = 11; *WRAML* Sentence Memory ScS = 16), basic visual span (*WISC-III-PI* Spatial Span forward ScS = 13),

verbal working memory (Digit Span backward ScS = 14), spatial working memory (Spatial Span backward ScS =14), verbal learning and recall (*CVLT-C* Total T = 61; Short delay free z = 1.0, Long delay free z = 0.0; Recognition z = 0.0), and recall of complex visual information (*Rey Complex Figure* delayed recall = 25th percentile; recognition = 94th percentile).

Tommy's motor skills were assessed using the *Revised Physical and Neurological Assessment of Subtle Signs (PANESS)*, which includes a laterality inventory, praxis screening, stressed gaits, balance and hopping tests, and a series of timed motor responses. Tommy's routine gait was within normal limits. He was right-handed for writing and drawing; and his handwriting was uneven, slow, and effortful. There was no evidence of dyspraxia, and his speed on all 12 timed motor tasks was within age-level expectations. In contrast, Tommy had clear bilateral choreiform movements (left greater than right) and motor overflow, as well as difficulties with forward tandem gait and balance tasks (unexpected for his age). On stressed gaits, Tommy had difficulty maintaining a slow steady walking pace, and at times, approached a running pace. He complicated a simple "hopping-on-one-foot" task by flapping his arms like wings, making a sound like a chicken, and spinning around in circles.

Summary of Initial Assessment

By third grade (age 7 years, 11 months), Tommy's educational records and prior testing indicated superior range IQ and core language skills, with largely commensurate academic achievement, and relative weaknesses only when processing speed was required. His tics, while increasing in severity, had not yet impaired his ability to participate in class activities or to form social relationships. Nevertheless, Tommy's neuropsychological profile suggested a neurodevelopmental disorder with the *potential* for marked functional impact on his later academic and social functioning. History, observations, and initial test results indicated that Tommy was having increasing problems with inattention, hyperactivity, and inhibitory control across settings. Although his teacher did not endorse these problems in her ratings (*note*: Tommy had just begun third grade less than 3 weeks earlier), parental report of problems in conjunction with records of past behavior problems from previous teachers suggested that the diagnosis of ADHD, Combined Type, in addition to Tourette syndrome (provisional—assuming symptoms for one more month) was appropriate.

At initial assessment, Tommy's relative weaknesses were observed almost exclusively on tasks with demand for executive control of attention, language, affect, and motor skill. His disinhibition impeded his ability to independently demonstrate his knowledge and complete tasks efficiently, and he was most notable when he was required to work independently, without the aid of external support to keep him on task. From a neuropsychological perspective, these behaviors were very consistent with those encountered by children with disorders impacting the development of frontal-striatal brain systems. As such, this pattern was entirely consistent with Tommy's developmental neurologic history of tics and ADHD—both of which are associated with frontal-striatal brain dysfunction (Denckla, 2006). Furthermore, executive dysfunction can occur independently of IQ. In fact, performance-based tests of executive function may be less sensitive in children with high IQ (Mahone, Hagelthorn, et al., 2002), despite "real-life" dysfunction (Mahone, Cirino et al., 2002). Thus, Tommy's high IQ scores could lead those working with him to have unrealistically high expectations of his *independent* functioning and his need for external support—unfairly attributing his performance deficits to laziness or oppositional behavior.

At this point, Tommy's tics had only begun to emerge. Children with tics have some ability to suppress their tics temporarily, but often find it effortful and uncomfortable. Conscious control of tics is a highly active brain process (Peterson et al., 1998) and occurs at the expense of other cognitive activities—thus interfering with the child's ability to perform academically and socially at age-expected levels in the class setting. Since tics can have a waxing and waning course, academic performance may also vary. During testing, Tommy benefited from being able to express his vocal and motor tics as well as being able to mask his tics through fidgeting movements and verbalizations (e.g., quiet humming, soft verbal commentary on his work, etc.).

These behaviors were actually *helpful* for Tommy. Since he could express his tics freely, he was able to devote more mental effort toward his cognitive tasks, rather than suppressing his tics. This recommendation was communicated to his parents and school.

It was also clear from the history and assessment that Tommy's pattern of difficulties did not fall into the traditional understanding of a learning disability. Tommy did not have a problem with *what* he knew; he had a problem *demonstrating* what he knew. As a result, Tommy was at risk for being less independent than his same-age peers and for having his socially immature and awkward behaviors draw negative attention to him. Initial recommendations focused on family and school education about the nature and course of TS and ADHD, and accommodations for executive control of behavior—especially the idea that managing Tommy's symptoms might require long-term changes in the structure of his environment (home and school), availability of external behavioral support, as well as an understanding that his level of independence may fall behind his age- and IQ-level expectations. Referral for consideration of pharmacological intervention for his ADHD was recommended, but with caution, given the potential for stimulant medications to exacerbate tics. These recommendations were shared with parents, school, and Tommy's neurologist. It was recommended that Tommy have follow-up when he reached fifth grade, in order to reassess his executive skill development when under greater environmental (school) demand and to help prepare for the organizational challenges of middle school.

Follow-up Neuropsychological Examination: Age 9 Years, 11 Months

At follow-up assessment, Tommy was in the fifth grade in a combination of regular education and gifted/talented classes. He had formal diagnoses of TS and ADHD, with a *504 Plan* that provided accommodations for relaxation breaks, teacher education about TS, and assistance with organization. Shortly after initial assessment, Tommy was prescribed Strattera 50 mg/day to treat his comorbid ADHD and had been taking this dose for nearly 2 years (as well as the day of testing), with reports of significant improvement in attentional control. Tommy's grades have been consistently good, and he has not had behavior problems; however, teachers reported increasing difficulty with organization. Parents also described Tommy as being more forgetful, noting that he "constantly" forgot necessary books and materials in his daily transitions between home and school. His motor (face and eye twitching) and vocal tics (humming, stammering, and other noises) had increased, and he seemed more "antsy," despite treatment for ADHD. Parents also reported observing increased signs of worry and anxiousness.

On assessment, Tommy's activity level was within normal expectations, and he showed few signs of inattention. Some motor tics were observed, for example, eye rolling, blinking, lip twitching, and knuckle cracking. Parents endorsed significant concerns with internalizing problems on the *Child Behavior Checklist* (Internalizing Problems scale T = 72), especially fears, worries, feelings of guilt, and the need to be perfect. They also endorsed somatic complaints (T = 78), including frequent headaches, nausea, stomachaches, and fatigue. Despite treatment,

parents also continued to endorse symptoms of ADHD on the *Conners' Parent Rating Scale-Revised* (*DSM-IV* Inattentive T = 71; Hyperactive/Impulsive T = 68); however, as before, teacher ratings on the *Conners' Teacher Rating Scale-Revised* were all within normal limits (all T ≤ 60). In contrast, parents and teachers both endorsed concerns with executive function (*BRIEF* Global Executive Composite: Parent T = 76, Teacher T = 64).

Most performance-based measures from initial assessment were repeated, with additional academic assessment added. At follow-up assessment, *all* performance-based tests of attention, executive function, language, verbal and nonverbal memory, and motor speed were within normal limits, with performance generally equal to or improved from initial assessment. In addition, his spontaneous written expression (*Test of Written Language-3*) was also within normal limits. On motor examination, Tommy no longer had choreiform movements but continued to have motor overflow and dysrhythmia, consistent with the research findings among boys with ADHD (Cole, Mostofsky, Larson, Denckla, & Mahone, 2008).

Table 6-1. Test Scores (Rating Scales)

TEST/Subtest	Score Type	Age 7	Age 9	TEST/Subtest	Score Type	Age 7	Age 9
CPRS				**BRIEF (Parent)**			
Oppositional	T	50	55	Inhibit	T	58	62
Hyperactivity	T	66	60	Shift	T	67	74
Cognitive Problems/	T	66	64	Emotional Control	T	59	58
Inattention				Initiate	T	71	81
Anxious-Shy	T	60	53	Working Memory	T	70	80
Perfectionism	T	64	52	Plan/Organize	T	67	82
Social Problems	T	59	69	Organization	T	72	71
Psychosomatic	T	90	83	of Materials			
DSM-IV Inattentive	T	69	71	Monitor	T	57	56
DSM-IV Hyperactive	T	74	68	Behavior Regulation	T	62	65
DSM-IV Total	T	73	71	Metacognition	T	70	80
ADHD Index	T	65	65	Global Executive	T	68	76
Global Index:	T	68	60	Composite			
Restless-Impulsive				**BRIEF (Teacher)**			
Global Index: Emotional	T	46	41	Inhibit	T	44	60
Lability				Shift	T	50	68
Global Index Total	T	62	55				

(*Continued*)

Table 6-1. Test Scores (Rating Scales) (*Continued*)

TEST/Subtest	Score Type	Age 7	Age 9	TEST/Subtest	Score Type	Age 7	Age 9
CTRS				Emotional Control	T	43	54
Oppositional	T	45	48	Initiate	T	46	48
Hyperactivity	T	48	58	Working Memory	T	55	69
Cognitive Problems/	T	49	51	Plan/Organize	T	59	55
Inattention				Organization	T	57	77
Anxious-Shy	T	42	60	of Materials			
Perfectionism	T	59	64	Monitor	T	51	64
Social Problems	T	45	58	Behavior Regulation	T	45	62
DSM-IV Inattentive	T	49	55	Metacognition	T	55	63
DSM-IV Hyperactive	T	44	60	Global Executive	T	51	64
DSM-IV Total	T	48	58	Composite			
ADHD Index	T	51	55	**ABAS (Parent)**			
Global Index:	T	49	62	General Adaptive	SS	93	
Restless-Impulsive				Composite			
Global Index: Emotional	T	44	50	Communication	ScS	11	
Lability				Community Use	ScS	13	
Global Index Total	T	47	59	Functional Academics	ScS	11	
CBCL				Home Living	ScS	7	
Anxious/Depressed	T		67	Health and Safety	ScS	11	
Withdrawn/Depressed	T		62	Leisure	ScS	9	
Somatic Complaints	T		78	Self-Care	ScS	6	
Social Problems	T		65	Self-Direction	ScS	13	
Thought Problems	T		75	Social	ScS	12	
Attention Problems	T		67	**ABAS (Teacher)**			
Rule-Breaking Behavior	T		50	General Adaptive	SS	119	
Aggressive Behavior	T		55	Composite			
Internalizing Problems	T		72	Communication	ScS	12	
Externalizing Problems	T		51	Community Use	ScS	14	
Total Problems	T		71	Functional Academics	ScS	14	
				Home Living	ScS	11	
				Health and Safety	ScS	12	
				Leisure	ScS	13	
				Self-Care	ScS	12	
				Self-Direction	ScS	11	
				Social	ScS	13	

ABAS, Adaptive Behavior Assessment System; ADHD, attention-deficit/hyperactivity disorder; BRIEF, Behavior Rating Inventory of Executive Function; CBCL, Children's Behavior Checklist; CPRS, Conners' Parent Rating Scale; CTRS, Conners', Teacher Rating Scale; ScS, scaled score (mean = 10 ± 3); SS, standard score (mean = 100 ± 15); T, T-score (mean = 50 ± 10).

Summary of Follow-up Assessment

With family and school support, as well as treatment for his ADHD, Tommy continued to make cognitive and academic progress. His tics, while persistent, were not *directly* impeding his academic functioning. Nevertheless, he was observed to show poor strategic approach characterized by limited judgment of the level of difficulty of different tasks and the amount of effort required to complete them, as well as a tendency to become caught up in details at the expense of efficiency. Parents and teachers noted

Table 6-2. Test Scores (Performance-Based Measures)

TEST/Subtest	Score Type	Age 7	Age 9	TEST/Subtest	Score Type	Age 7	Age 9
WISC-IV				**TOWL-3**			
FSIQ	SS	125		Contextual Conventions	ScS		7
VCI	SS	138		Contextual Language	ScS		12
PRI	SS	112		Story Construction	ScS		11
WMI	SS	116		**CVLT-C**			
PSI	SS	78		List A Total	Z	61	53
Similarities	ScS	17		List A Trial 1 Free Recall	Z	1.5	0.0
Vocabulary	ScS	17		List A Trial 5 Free Recall	Z	0.5	1.0
Comprehension	ScS	15		List A Short Delay Free Recall	Z	1.0	2.0
Block Design	ScS	12		List A Short Delay Cued Recall	Z	1.0	1.5
Matrix Reasoning	ScS	14		List A Long Delay Free Recall	Z	−0.5	1.0
Picture Concepts	ScS	10		List A Long Delay Cued Recall	Z	0.0	1.5
Letter-Number Sequencing	ScS	13		Recognition	Z	0.0	1.0
Digit Span	ScS	13		List B Free Recall	Z	0.0	1.0
Digit Span Forward	ScS	13		Semantic Clustering	Z	−0.5	0.5
Digit Span Backward	ScS	14		Serial Clustering	Z	−0.5	1.5
Coding	ScS	6		Learning Slope	Z	−1.0	1.5
Symbol Search	ScS	6		Perseverations	Z	2.5	1.0
WJ-III				Intrusions	Z	0.0	0.0
Broad Reading	SS	122		**RAN/RAS**			
Letter-Word Identification	SS	120		Letters	Z	−2.3	
Passage Comprehension	SS	128		Numbers	Z	−3.4	
Reading Fluency	SS	108		Colors	Z	−1.5	
Oral Language	SS	115		Object	Z	−1.8	
Story Recall	SS	113		2-Set	Z	−1.7	
Understanding Directions	SS	114		3-Set	Z	−3.3	
Broad Written Language	SS	121		**NEPSY**			
Spelling	SS	109		Verbal Fluency	ScS	14	
Writing Fluency	SS	119		Visuomotor Precision	ScS	13	
Writing Samples	SS	127		Visual Attention	ScS	10	
Broad Mathematics	SS	113		**CMS**			
Calculation	SS	116		Numbers	ScS	13	
Math Fluency	SS	107		Sequences	ScS	13	
Applied Problems	SS	108		**D-KEFS**			
Quantitative Concepts	SS	115		Trails: Visual Scanning	ScS	9	7
Math Calculation Skills	SS	115		Trails: Letter Sequencing	ScS	6	12
Math Reasoning Skills	SS	110		Trails: Number Sequencing	ScS	14	
Written Expression	SS	130		Trails: Number-Letter Switching	ScS	8	14

(*Continued*)

Table 6-2. Test Scores (Performance-Based Measures) (*Continued*)

TEST/Subtest	Score Type	Age 7	Age 9	TEST/Subtest	Score Type	Age 7	Age 9
Academic Skills	SS	119		Twenty Questions	ScS	6	
Academic Fluency	SS	112		Design Fluency: Filled Dots	ScS		9
Academic Applications	SS	123		Design Fluency: Empty Dots	ScS		15
CELF-3				Design Fluency: Switching	ScS		17
Total Language	SS	136		Design Fluency: Total Correct	ScS		15
Receptive Language	SS	131					
Expressive Language	SS	139		**TOKEN TEST FOR CHILDREN**			
Sentence Structure	ScS	14		Part I	Percentile	58	
Concepts and Directions	ScS	17		Part III	Percentile	50	
Word Classes	ScS	12		Part V	Percentile	71	
Word Structure	ScS	17		**REY COMPLEX FIGURE TEST**			
Formulated Sentences	ScS	13		Copy	Percentile	25	
Recalling Sentences	ScS	16		Delayed Recall	Percentile	25	
BOSTON NAMING TEST	Z	−0.80		Recognition	Percentile	92	
PANESS				**HVOT**	Percentile	96	
Foot Tapping - R	Z		0.44	**WISC-III PI**			
Heel-Toe Sequencing -R	Z		3.20	Spatial Span	ScS		14
Hand Patting -R	Z		0.18	Spatial Span Forward	ScS		13
Hand Pronation/ Supination-R	Z		1.98	Spatial Span Backward	ScS		14
Finger Repetition -R	Z		1.42	Letter Span	ScS		11
Finger Sequencing - R	Z		0.64	Symbol Copy	ScS		7
Foot Tapping - L	Z		1.27	**WRAML**			
Heel-Toe Sequencing - L	Z		2.66	Sentence Memory	ScS		16
Hand Patting - L	Z		0.37	**CPT-II**			
Hand Pronation/ Supination - L	Z		1.17	Omissions	T	49	40
Finger Repetition - L	Z		−0.67	Commissions	T	52	38
Finger Sequencing - L	Z		0.58	Mean Response Time	T	40	45
CTOPP				Variability	T	52	39
Elision	ScS	10		D'	T	52	47
VMI	SS	104	114				
VISUAL PERCEPTION	SS						
Verbal Fluency: Letter Fluency	ScS		11				
Verbal Fluency: Category Fluency	ScS		18				
Verbal Fluency: Category Switching	ScS		17				

CELF-3, Clinical Evaluation of Language Fundamentals, Third Edition; CMS, Children's Memory Scale; WISC-III-PI = Wechsler Intelligence Scale, Third Edition, Process Instrument. CPT-II, Conners' Continuous Performance Test II; CTOPP, Comprehensive Test of Phonological Processing; CVLT-C, California Verbal Learning Test–Children's Version; DKEFS, Delis Kaplan Executive Function System; HVOT, Hooper Visual Organization Test; PANESS, Physical and Neurological Assessment of Subtle Signs; ScS, scaled score (mean = 10 ± 3); SS, standard score (mean = 100 ± 15); T, T-Score (mean = 50 ± 10); TOWL-3, Test of Written Language–Third Edition; VMI, Beery Developmental Test of Visual Motor Integration; WISC-IV, Wechsler Intelligence Scale for Children, Fourth Edition; WJ-III, Woodcock Johnson, Test of Achievement, Third Edition; WRAML, Wide Range Assessment of Memory and Learning; Z, z-score (mean = 0 ± 1).

increased deficits in independent implementation of executive functions expected at his age, such as task initiation, working memory, planning, and organization, which appeared to be exacerbated in conjunction with the increased organizational demands of later elementary school. These problems were observed both at home and in the classroom, particularly in managing transitions between these two settings. Thus, family and school recommendations focused on continued external support for his organizational skills. Also, while Tommy appeared to be benefiting from his medication for attention difficulties and disinhibition, his symptoms of anxiety were increasing. It was recommended that Tommy begin working with a therapist around his anxiety, perfectionism, and somatization, and that his parents consult with his prescribing physician about medications that might be able to treat both Tommy's ADHD symptoms as well as alleviate some of his anxiety, and perhaps even address his tics.

Conclusions

Tommy's presentation was quite common among children with TS. As he progressed through elementary school, he faced a number of new risks. It is common for children with symptoms to experience distress and anxiety from the social and academic difficulties caused by the impairments related to the TS and its comorbidities (especially ADHD and anxiety). In addition to working to increase acceptance of his tics, it was important to ensure that the psychosocial consequences of his tics were minimized in the classroom and among his peers. Children with TS can benefit from being involved in active discussion and problem solving on how to best manage their tics within the school and home environments. It is also helpful for families of children with TS to work with a counselor to help minimize the negative consequences of academic and social difficulties, and to maximize positive experiences by capitalizing upon interests and motivation in rewarding activities. Teachers can also help to minimize the social discomfort that children feel as a result of having tics by helping them find ways of discussing it with peers and not allowing the tics to become the focus of classroom activities when they are expressed.

The Role of the Neuropsychologist in Management of Tourette Syndrome

In conclusion, it is important for neuropsychologists working with children with Tourette syndrome to consider the following six guidelines:

1. Make sure the diagnosis is accurate and that the child has been evaluated medically to rule out other conditions that can produce atypical movements. If necessary, help the family locate a physician with experience in pediatric movement disorders.
2. Assist in diagnosis and management of the comorbid conditions, including ADHD, OCD, LDs, and autism spectrum disorders. Recognize that the comorbid conditions may require more significant intervention than the tics and may complicate treatment.
3. Be aware of the acute psychosocial distress that can occur (especially in school) once a child begins to have vocal tics.
4. Educate the family and educational team about the nature and course of TS. Help them understand that tics wax and wane, and that tic-free periods are common. Recognize that parents and teachers may have had misinformation about TS.
5. Take a developmental approach in working with the child—recognizing predictable stress periods in the course of school (e.g., transition to middle school). Also assist with treatment monitoring.
6. Be an informed resource about the research on TS and the support available. Help families interpret conflicting and controversial information they may find on the Web. The national Tourette Syndrome Association (http://www.tsa-usa.org) provides a variety of resources (newsletters, research, videos), as well as links to local chapters. Other Web sites of interest include the National Institute of Neurological Disorders and Stroke (http://www.ninds.nih.gov/disorders/tourette/detail_tourette.htm) and Tourette Syndrome Plus (http://www.tourettesyndrome.net).

References

Albin, R. L., & Mink, J. W. (2006). Recent advances in Tourette syndrome research. *Trends in Neuroscience, 29,* 175–182.

American Psychiatric Association (APA). (2000). *Diagnostic and statistical manual of mental disorders* (4th ed., Text rev.). Washington, DC: Author.

Aylward, E. H., Reiss, A. L., Reader, M. J., Singer, H. S., Brown, J. E., & Denckla, M. B. (1996). Basal ganglia volumes in children with attention deficit hyperactivity disorder. *Journal of Child Neurology, 11,* 112–115.

Banaschewski, T., Woerner, W., & Rothenberger, A. (2003). Premonitory sensory phenomena and suppressibility of tics in Tourette syndrome: Developmental aspects in children and adolescents. *Developmental Medicine and Child Neurology, 45,* 700–703.

Baron-Cohen, S., Scahill, V. L., Hornsey, I. H., & Robertson, M. M. (1999). The prevalence of Gilles de la Tourette syndrome in children and adolescents with autism: A large scale study. *Psychological Medicine, 29,* 1151–1159.

Baumgardner, T. L., Singer, H. S., Denckla, M. B., Rubin, M. A., Abrams, M. T., Colli, M. J., & Reiss, A. L. (1996). Corpus callosum morphology in children with Tourette syndrome and attention deficit hyperactivity disorder. *Neurology, 47,* 1–6.

Bliss, J. (1980). Sensory experiences of Gilles de la Tourette syndrome. *Archives of General Psychiatry, 37,* 1343–1347.

Bradshaw, J. L. (2001). Developmental disorders of the frontostriatal system: Neuropsychological, neuropsychiatric, and evolutionary perspectives. Philadelphia: Psychology Press.

Cannon, S., Pratt, P., & Robertson, M. M. (2003). Executive function, memory, and learning in Tourette's syndrome. *Neuropsychology, 17,* 247–254.

Casey, M. B., Cohen, M., Schuerholz, L., Singer, H. S., & Denckla, M. B. (2000). Language-based cognitive functioning in parents of offspring with ADHD comorbid for Tourette syndrome or learning disabilities. *Developmental Neuropsychology, 17,* 85–110.

Castellanos, F. X., Giedd, J. N., Hamburger, S. D., Marsh, W. L., & Rapoport, J. L. (1996). Brain morphometry in Tourette's syndrome: The influence of comorbid attention-deficit/hyperactivity disorder. *Neurology, 47,* 1581–1583.

Cirino, P., Chapieski, L., & Massman, P. (2000). Card sorting performance and ADHD symptomatology in children and adolescents with Tourette syndrome. *Journal of Clinical and Experimental Neuropsychology, 22,* 245–256.

Cohrs, S., Rasch, T., Altmeyer, S., Kinkelbur, J., Kostanecka, T., Rothenberger, A., Ruther, E., & Hajak, G. (2001). Decreased sleep quality and increased sleep related movements in patients with Tourette's syndrome. *Journal of Neurology, Neurosurgery, and Psychiatry, 70,* 192–197.

Cole, W., Mostofsky, S. H., Larson, J. C. G., Denckla, M. B., & Mahone, E. M. (2008). Age related change in motor subtle signs among girls and boys with ADHD. *Neurology, 71,* 1514–1520.

Denckla, M. B. (2006). Attention-deficit hyperactivity disorder (ADHD) comorbidity: A case for "pure" Tourette syndrome. *Journal of Child Neurology, 21,* 701–703.

Denckla, M. B., & Reiss, A. L. (1997). Prefrontal-subcortical circuits in developmental disorders. In N. A. Krasnegor, G. R. Lyon, & P. S. Goldman-Rakic (Eds.), *Development of the prefrontal cortex: Evolution, neurobiology, and behavior* (pp. 283–293). Baltimore: Brookes.

Dewey, D., Tupper, D. E., & Bottos, S. (2004). Involuntary motor disorders in childhood. In D. Dewey & D. E. Tupper (Eds.), *Developmental motor disorders: A neuropsychological perspective* (pp. 197–210). New York: Guilford.

Erenberg, G. (2005). The relationship between Tourette syndrome, attention deficit hyperactivity disorder, and stimulant medication: A critical review. *Seminars in Pediatric Neurology, 12,* 217–221.

Erenberg, G., Cruse, R. P., & Rothner, A. D. (1987). The natural history of Tourette syndrome: A follow-up study. *Annals of Neurology, 22,* 383–385.

Evidente, V. G. (2000). Is it a tic or Tourette's? *Postgraduate Medicine, 108,* 175–182.

Fahn, S., & Erenberg, G. (1988). Differential diagnosis of tic phenomena: A neurological perspective. In D. J. Cohen, R. D. Bruun, & J. F. Leckman (Eds.), *Tourette's syndrome and tic disorders* (pp. 41–54). New York: John Wiley & Sons.

Fredericksen, K. A., Cutting, L. E., Kates, W. R., Mostofsky, S. H., Singer, H. S., Cooper, K. L., Lanham, D. C., Denckla, M. B., & Kaufmann, W. E. (2002). Disproportionate increases of white matter in right frontal lobe of children with Tourette syndrome. *Neurology, 58,* 85–89.

Freeman, R. D., Fast, D. K., Burd, L., Kerbeshian, J., Robertson, M. M., & Sandor, P. (2000). An international perspective on Tourette syndrome: Selected findings from 3500 individuals in 22 countries. *Developmental Medicine and Child Neurology, 42,* 436–447.

Gabbay, V., Coffey, B. J., Babb, J. S., Meyer, L., Wachtel, C., Anam, S., & Rabinovitz, B. (2008). Pediatric autoimmune neuropsychiatric disorders associated with streptococcus: Comparison of diagnosis and treatment in the community and at specialty clinics. *Pediatrics, 122,* 273–278.

Garelick, G. (1986, December). Exorcising a damnable disease. *Discover,* 74–84.

Gerard, E., & Peterson, B. S. (2003). Developmental processes and brain imaging studies in Tourette syndrome. *Journal of Psychosomatic Research, 55,* 13–22.

Gilbert, D. L., Bansal, A. S., Sethuraman, G., Sallee, F. R., Zhang, J., Lipps, T., & Wasserman, E. M. (2004). Association of cortical disinhibition with tic, ADHD, and OCD severity in Tourette syndrome. *Movement Disorders, 19,* 416–425.

Gilbert, D. L., & Lipps, T. D. (2005). Tourette's syndrome. *Current Treatment Options in Neurology, 7,* 211–219.

Gioia, G.A., Isquith, P.K., Guy, S.C., & Kenworthy, L. (2000). *Behavior rating inventory of executive function.* Odessa Florida: Psychological Assessment Resources.

Goldenberg, J. N., Brown, S. B., & Weiner, W. J. (1994). Coprolalia in younger patients with Gilles de la Tourette syndrome. *Movement Disorders, 9,* 622–625.

Grados, M. A., Mathews, C. A., & Tourette Syndrome Association International Consortium for Genetics. (2008). Latent class analysis of Gilles de la Tourette syndrome using comorbidities: Clinical and genetic implications. *Biological Psychiatry, 64,* 219–225.

Hallett, J. J., Harling-Berg, C. J., Knopf, P. M., Stopa, E. G., & Kiessling, L. S. (2000). Anti-striatal antibodies in Tourette syndrome cause neuronal dysfunction. *Journal of Immunology, 111,* 195–202.

Harris, E. L., Singer, H. S., Reader, M. J., Brown, J. Cox, C. Mohr, J. Schuerholz, L. J. Alyward, E. Reiss, A., Shih, B., Bryan, N., Chase, G. A., & Denckla, M. B. (1995). Executive function in children with Tourette syndrome and/or attention deficit hyperactivity disorder. *Journal of the International Neuropsychological Society, 1,* 511–516.

Harris, K., Mahone, E. M., & Singer, H. S. (2008). Nonautistic motor stereotypies: Clinical features and longitudinal follow-up. *Pediatric Neurology, 38,* 267–272.

Himle, M. B., Woods, D. W., Piacentini, J. C., & Walkup, J. (2006). Brief review of habit reversal training for Tourette syndrome. *Journal of Child Neurology, 21,* 719–725.

Hunter, S. (2007). Pediatric movement disorders. In S. Hunter & J. Donders (Eds.), *Pediatric neuropsychological intervention* (pp. 314–337). Cambridge, UK: Cambridge University Press.

Hyde, T. M., Aaronson, B. A., Randolph, C., Rickler, K. C., & Weinberger, D. R. (1992). Relationship of birth weight to the phenotypic expression of Gilles de la Tourette's syndrome in monozygotic twins. *Neurology, 42,* 652–658.

Kurlan, R., McDermott, M. P., Deeley, C., Como, P. G., Brower, C., Eapen, S., Andresen, E. M., & Miller, B. (2001). Prevalence of tics in schoolchildren and association with placement in special education. *Neurology, 57,* 1383–1388.

Leckman, J. F. (2002). Tourette's syndrome. *Lancet, 360,* 1577–1586.

Leckman, J. F., Peterson, B. S., Pauls, D. L., & Cohen, D. J. (1997). Tic disorders. *Psychiatric Clinics of North America, 20,* 839–861.

Leckman, J. F., Zhang, H., Vitale, A., Lahnin, F., Lynch, K., Bondi, C., Kim, Y. S., & Peterson, B. S. (1998). Course of tic severity in Tourette syndrome: the first two decades. *Pediatrics, 102,* 14–19.

Lee, J-S., Yoo, S-S., Cho, S-Y., Ock., S-M., Lim, M-K., & Panych, L. P. (2006). Abnormal thalamic volume in treatment-naïve boys with Tourette syndrome. *Acta Psychiatry Scandinavia, 113,* 64–67.

Mahone, E. M., Bridges, D., Prahme, C., & Singer, H. S. (2004). Repetitive arm and hand movements (complex motor stereotypies) in children. *Journal of Pediatrics, 145,* 391–395.

Mahone, E. M., Cirino, P. T., Cutting, L. E., Cerrone, P. M., Hagelthorn, K. M., Hiemenz, J. R., Singer, H. S., & Denckla, M. B. (2002). Validity of the Behavior Rating Inventory of Executive Function in children with ADHD and/or Tourette syndrome. *Archives of Clinical Neuropsychology, 17,* 643–662.

Mahone, E. M., Hagelthorn, K. M., Cutting, L. E., Schuerholz, L. J., Pelletier, S. F., Rawlins, C., Singer, H. S., & Denckla, M. B. (2002). Effects of IQ on executive function measures in children with ADHD. *Child Neuropsychology, 8,* 41–51.

Mahone, E.M., Koth, C.W., Cutting, L., Singer, H.S., & Denckla, M.B. (2001). Executive function in fluency and recall measures among children with Tourette Syndrome and ADHD. *Journal of the International Neuropsychological Society, 7,* 102-111.

Mahone, E. M., & Slomine, B. S. (2008). Neurodevelopmental disorders. In J. Morgan & J. Ricker (Eds.), *Textbook of clinical neuropsychology* (pp. 105–128). New York: Taylor and Francis.

Muller-Vahl, K. R., Berding, G., Bruke, T., Kolbe, H., Meyer, G. J., Hundeshagen, H., Dengler, R., Knapp, W. H., & Emrich, H. M. (2000). Dopamine transporter binding in Gilles de la Tourette syndrome. *Journal of Neurology, 247,* 514–520.

Olson, L. L., Singer, H. S., Goodman, W. K., & Maria, B. L. (2006). Tourette syndrome: Diagnosis, strategies, therapies, pathogenesis, and future directions. *Journal of Child Neurology, 21,* 630–641.

Palumbo, D., Maughan, A., & Kurlan, R. (1997). Hypothesis III. Tourette syndrome is only one of several causes of developmental basal ganglia syndrome. *Archives of Neurology, 54,* 475–483.

Pappert, E. J., Goetz, C. G., Louis, E. D., Blasucci, L, & Leurgans, S. (2003). Objective assessments of longitudinal outcome in Gilles de la Tourette's syndrome. *Neurology, 61,* 936–940.

Peterson, B., Riddle, M. A., Cohen, D. J., Katz, L. D., Smith, J. C., Hardin, M. T., & Leckman, J. F. (1993). Reduced basal ganglia volumes in Tourette's syndrome using 3-dimensional reconstruction techniques. *Neurology, 43,* 941–949.

Peterson, B. S., Skudlarski, P., Anderson, A. W., Zhang, H., Gatenby, J. C., Lacadie, C. M., Leckman, J. F., & Gore, J. C. (1998). A functional magnetic resonance imaging study of tic suppression in Tourette syndrome. *Archives of General Psychiatry, 55,* 326–333.

Peterson, B. S., Staib, L., Scahill, L., Zhang, H., Anderson, C., Leckman, J. F., Cohen, D. J., Gore, J. C., Albert, J., & Webster, R. (2001). Regional brain and ventricular volumes in Tourette syndrome. *Archives of General Psychiatry, 58,* 427–440

Peterson, B. S., Thomas, P., Kane, M. J., Scahill, L., Zhang, H., Bronen, R., King, R. A., Leckman, J. F., & Staib, L. (2003). Basal ganglia volumes in patients with Gilles de la Tourette syndrome. *Archives of General Psychiatry, 60,* 415–424.

Piacentini, J., & Chang, S. (2006). Behavioral treatments for tic suppression: Habit reversal training. In J. Walkup, J. Mink, & P. Hollenbeck (Eds.), *Advances in neurology: Tourette syndrome* (pp. 227–233). Philadelphia: Lippincott, Williams, & Wilkins.

Plessen, K. J., Gruner, R., Lundervold, A., Hirsch, J. G., Xu, D., Bansal, R., Hammar, A., Lundervold, A. J., Wentzel-Larsen, T., Lie, S. A., Gass, A., Peterson, B. S., & Hugdahl, K. (2006). Reduced white matter connectivity in the corpus callosum of children with Tourette syndrome. *Journal of Child Psychology and Psychiatry, 47,* 1013–1022.

Pringsheim, T., Davenport, W. J,. & Lang, A. (2003). Tics. *Current Opinion in Neurology, 16,* 523–527.

Robertson, M. M. (1989). The Gilles de la Tourette syndrome: The current status. *British Journal of Psychiatry, 154,* 147–169.

Robertson, M. M. (2000). Tourette syndrome, associated conditions and the complexities of treatment. *Brain, 123,* 425–462.

Robertson, M. M. (2003). Diagnosing Tourette syndrome: Is it a common disorder? *Journal of Psychosomatic Research, 55,* 3–6.

Sandor, P. (2003). Pharmacological management of tics in patients with TS. *Journal of Psychosomatic Research, 55,* 41–48.

Schuerholz, L. J., Baumgardner, T. L., Singer, H. S., Reiss, A. L., & Denckla, M. B. (1996). Neuropsychological status of children with Tourette's syndrome with and without attention deficit hyperactivity disorder. *Neurology, 46,* 958–965.

Schuerholz, L. J., Cutting, L., Mazzocco, M. M., Singer, H. S., & Denckla, M. B. (1997). Neuromotor functioning in children with Tourette syndrome with and without attention deficit hyperactivity disorder. *Journal of Child Neurology, 12,* 438–442.

Schultz, R. T., Carter, A. S., Gladsone, M., Scahill, L., Leckman, J. F., Peterson, B. S., Zhang, H., Cohen, D. J., & Pauls, D. (1998). Visual-motor integration functioning in children with Tourette syndrome. *Neuropsychology, 12,* 134–145.

Shin, M-S., Chung, S-J., & Hong, K-E. M. (2001). Comparative study of the behavioral and neuropsychologic characteristics of tic disorder with or without attention-deficit hyperactivity disorder (ADHD). *Journal of Child Neurology, 16,* 719–726.

Shucard, D. W., Benedict, R. H. B., Tekok-Kilic, A., & Lichter, D. G. (1997). Slowed reaction time during a continuous performance test in children with Tourette's syndrome. *Neuropsychology, 11,* 147–155.

Singer, H. S. (2000). Current issues in Tourette syndrome. *Movement Disorders, 15,* 1051–1063.

Singer, H. S. (2005a). Treatment of Tourette syndrome. In H. S. Singer, E. H. Kossoff, A. L. Hartman, & T. O. Crawford (Eds.), *Treatment of pediatric neurologic disorders* (pp. 125–132). Boca Raton, FL: Taylor & Francis.

Singer, H.S. (2005b). Tourette syndrome: From behaviour to biology. *Lancet Neurology, 4,* 149–159.

Singer, H. S., Gause, C., Morris, C., Lopez, P., & Tourette Syndrome Study Group. (2008). Serial immune markers do not correlate with clinical exacerbations in pediatric autoimmune neuropsychiatric disorders associated with streptococcal infections. *Pediatrics, 121,* 1198–1205.

Singer, H. S., Hong, J. J., Yoon, D. Y., & Williams, P. N. (2005). Serum autoantibodies do not differentiate PANDAS and Tourette syndrome from controls. *Neurology, 65,* 1701–1707.

Singer, H. S., Reiss, A. L., Brown, J. E., Alyward, E. H., Shih. B., Chee, E., Harris, E. L., Reader, M. J., Chase, G. A., Bryan, N., & Denckla, M. B. (1993). Volumetric MRI changes in basal ganglia of children with Tourette syndrome. *Neurology, 43,* 950–956

Singer, H. S., Schuerholz, L. J., & Denckla, M. B. (1994). Learning difficulties in children with Tourette syndrome. *Journal of Child Neurology, 10,* S58–S61

Singer, H. S., Szymnski, S., Giuliano, J., Yokoi, F., Dogan, A. S., Brasic, J. R., Zhou, Y., Grace, A. A.,

& Wong, D. F. (2002). Elevated intrasynaptic dopamine release in Tourette's syndrome measured by PET. *American Journal of Psychiatry*, 159, 1329–1336.

Sowell, E. R., Kan, E., Yoshii, J., Thompson, P. M., Bansal, R., Zu, D., Toga, A. W., & Peterson, B. S. (2008). Thinning of sensorimotor cortices in children with Tourette syndrome. *Nature Neuroscience*, 11, 637–639.

Spencer, T., Biederman, J., Harding, M., O'Donnell, D., Wilens, T., Faraone, S., Coffey, B., & Geller, D. (1998). Disentangling the overlap between Tourette syndrome and ADHD. *Journal of Child Psychology and Psychiatry*, 39, 1037–1044.

Stern, E., Dilbersweig, D. A., Chee, K-Y., Holmes, A., Robertson, M. M., Trimble, M., Frith, C. D., Frackowiak, R. S. J., & Dolan, R. J. (2000). A functional neuroanatomy of tics in Tourette syndrome. *Archives of General Psychiatry*, 57, 741–748.

Swedo, S. E., Leonard, H. L., Garvey, M., Mittleman, B., Allen, A. J., Perlmutter, S., Lougee, L., Dow, S., Zamkoff, J., & Dubbert, B. K. (1998). Pediatric autoimmune neuropsychiatric disorders associated with streptococcal infections: Clinical descriptions of the first 50 cases. *American Journal of Psychiatry*, 155, 264–271.

The Tourette Syndrome Classification Group. (1993). Definition and classification of tic disorders. *Archives of Neurology*, 50, 1013–1016.

Willcutt, E. G., Pennington, B. F., Olson, R. K., & Defries, J. C. (2007). Understanding comorbidity: A twin study of reading disability and attention-deficit/hyperactivity disorder. *American Journal of Medical Genetics: Neuropsychiatric Genetics*, 144B, 709–714.

7

Spina Bifida Myelomeningocele

John Brigham Fulton and Keith Owen Yeates

Spina bifida myelomeningocele (SBM) is the most common neural tube defect compatible with survival, and it occurs at a rate of 0.5–1.0 per 1000 live births. The defect is characterized by protrusion of the spinal cord, meninges, and nerve roots through an opening in the spine at some point along the spinal column. The spinal lesion is evident from the first weeks of gestation and generally requires surgical correction immediately following birth. Investigations into the etiology of SBM have generally examined neural tube defects as a group. Leading theories include genetic influences (Au et al., 2008; Deak et al., 2008) and prenatal maternal factors, such as abnormal levels of folate (Czeizel & Dudas, 1992; Honein, Paulozzi, Matthews, Erickson, & Wong, 2001; Northrup & Volcik, 2000), obesity and diabetes (Northrup & Volcik, 2000), illness (Botto, Moore, Khoury, & Erickson, 1999), and the use of antiepileptic medications (Northrup & Volcik, 2000).

The effect of SBM on the development of the brain occurs through congenital anomalies and frequently via a secondary process of hydrocephalus. Children with SBM almost universally demonstrate a Chiari-II brain malformation, which is a congenital brain distortion characterized by a small and distorted posterior fossa, beaking of the tectum, and herniation of the posterior fossa contents through the tentorial incisure and foramen magnum (Stevenson, 2004; Vinck, Maassen, Mullaart, & Rotteveel, 2006). More than half of children with SBM also demonstrate partial dysgenesis of aspects of the corpus callosum (Hannay, Dennis, Kramer, Blaser, & Fletcher, 2009). In addition to the effects of the malformations, the Chiari-II malformation often obstructs the flow of cerebral spinal fluid, resulting in hydrocephalus in 80%–90% of children with SBM (Charney, 1992). The pathophysiological effects of congenital hydrocephalus include a thinning of the cortical mantle throughout the brain and the stretching of neural fibers, particularly in cerebral commissures such as the corpus callosum (del Bigio, 1993).

Children with SBM have extensive and chronic medical needs that often require long-term care. Spinal disorders such as scoliosis, kyphosis, tethered cord, and syringomyelia are common and often require neurosurgical intervention. Hydrocephalus typically requires shunting, and shunt revision, malfunction, and infection can occur, at times necessitating further surgical intervention. Children with SBM often experience neurogenic bowel and bladder leading to urological intervention. Taken together, these factors increase the risk for difficulties with psychosocial adjustment in children with SBM and place substantial burden on their families (Fletcher & Dennis, 2010).

Neurobehavioral Outcomes

Children with SBM often demonstrate several characteristic cognitive, motor, and behavioral impairments. Despite a common pattern of deficits, significant variability exists between individual children. Likely causes of this variability include the location of the spinal lesion, with more extensive motor and cognitive impairments associated with higher lesions (Fletcher et al., 2005); the presence and severity of the Chiari-II malformation (Vinck et al., 2006); medical complications (Loss, Yeates, & Enrile, 1998); and parental factors (Brown et al., 2008).

Advancements in medical and neurosurgical care have greatly improved the general intellectual outcomes of children with SBM. Despite these improvements, group mean scores on intellectual tests often fall in the low-average range. Children with SBM commonly demonstrate a discrepancy between types of intellectual skills, favoring verbal over nonverbal abilities (Anderson, Northam, Hendy, & Wrenhall, 2001), although this is not true of all ethnic subgroups (Fletcher & Dennis, 2010). Despite stronger verbal reasoning skills, many children with SBM demonstrate deficits in complex language skills, such as phonological awareness, verbal fluency, and comprehension of complex grammatical structures (Anderson et al., 2001; Fletcher, Dennis, & Northrup, 2000), as well as difficulties at the level of text processing and discourse, reflecting problems with pragmatic communication (Barnes & Dennis, 1992, 1998; Dennis, Jacennik, & Barnes, 1994).

Visual-perceptual and visual-motor deficits are well documented in children with SBM and reflect a central area of cognitive impairment. Children with SBM demonstrate the greatest difficulty in skills that require motor output, such as constructional and graphomotor tasks. Nonetheless, performance is also frequently impaired on motor-free measures of visual perceptual skills, particularly when tasks incorporate active perceptual processing, such as visual figure-ground identification and mental rotation. In contrast, performance is often intact on tasks of simple visual perception, such as face recognition, recognition of fragmented objects, and line orientation (Dennis, Fletcher, Rogers, Hetherington, & Francis, 2002; Fletcher et al., 1992).

Several aspects of memory are impacted in children with SBM, with the level of difficulty varying as a function of the kind of information to be remembered and the memory processes involved. In the domain of verbal memory, immediate recall of semantically meaningful information (i.e., story recall) is generally spared. However, delayed recall of stories often falls below expectations, with performance generally returning to the average range for recognition trials. Children with SBM are more prone to memory deficits on tasks that involve learning information that is not as semantically meaningful (i.e., word lists and verbal paired associates), demonstrating diminished encoding, slower learning, and lower spontaneous recall in the context of generally spared recognition and cued recall (Fletcher et al., 1992; Yeates, Enrile, Loss, Blumenstein, & Delis, 1995). The discrepancy between these aspects of verbal learning is thought by some to reflect difficulties developing efficient recall strategies in ambiguous learning situations (Burmeister et al., 2005; Vachha & Adams, 2005). As might be expected given their visual-spatial and visual-motor impairments, children with SBM also demonstrate deficits in nonverbal learning and memory, which have been documented both on tasks requiring graphomotor output and on motor-free tasks (Fletcher et al., 1992; Scott et al., 1998).

Deficits in attention and executive functions have been documented in children with SBM. Approximately one-third of children with SBM meet clinical criteria for attention-deficit/hyperactivity disorder (ADHD), most typically of the inattentive subtype (Burmeister et al., 2005). Despite high rates of ADHD in the population, children with SBM may show different patterns of impairments in attention than those seen in children with ADHD without SBM. More specifically, children with SBM demonstrate greater difficulties with focused attention, whereas their ADHD counterparts demonstrate greater difficulties with sustained attention (Brewer, Fletcher, Hiscock, & Davidson, 2001). In addition to attention difficulties, children with SBM have demonstrated poor performance relative to their peers on tasks measuring other executive functions such as response speed, working memory, cognitive flexibility, and spatial planning (Boyer, Yeates, & Enrile, 2006; Brewer et al., 2001; Fletcher et al., 1996; Rose & Holmbeck, 2007). Beyond performance measures of executive functioning, parents and teachers of children with SBM also report behavioral symptoms of executive function impairments at a higher rate than controls (Brown et al., 2008; Burmeister et al., 2005;

Mahone, Zabel, Levey, Verda, & Kinsman, 2002; Tarazi, Zabel, & Mahone, 2008).

Motor impairments are a core deficit in children with SBM. Paraplegia is common, as are significant difficulties with gross motor coordination in ambulatory children (Dennis et al., 2002; Hetherington & Dennis, 1999). Slowed fine motor speed and diminished dexterity have are also seen in children with SBM (Hetherington & Dennis, 1999), as are impairments in motor timing and the sequencing of motor movements (Dennis et al., 2004).

Given the myriad cognitive and motor difficulties that children with SBM demonstrate, they not surprisingly experience a high rate of deficits in academic skills. More specifically, on measures of academic achievement, children with SBM often demonstrate intact word recognition, but poor reading comprehension, spelling, and arithmetic skills (Anderson et al., 2001; Ayr, Yeates, & Enrile, 2005; Dennis & Barnes, 2002). Various neurocognitive abilities appear to play a role in mediating the degree of academic impairment (Ayr et al., 2005; Barnes, Dennis, & Hetherington, 2004).

Children with SBM also demonstrate higher rates of behavioral and emotional disorders than the general population. As a group, children with SBM are more socially immature, have difficulty establishing friendships, and are less independent relative to their peers. Numerous studies also have shown that children with SBM display a higher rate of behavior problems when compared to controls on standardized rating scales (Fletcher et al., 2000; Holmbeck et al., 2003). These findings are relatively nonspecific, however, in that children with SBM display adjustment problems that do not generally differ from those displayed by children with other chronic physical illnesses that also involve the central nervous system (Lavigne & Faier-Routman, 1992). Moreover, the behavioral difficulties displayed by children with SBM appear to be influenced not only by medical factors, such as hydrocephalus and its treatment, but also by environmental variables that are just as likely to affect children without SBM, such as caregiver and family functioning (Greenley, Holmbeck, Zukerman, & Buck, 2006).

Children with SBM are also likely to demonstrate deficits in adaptive behavior (Holler, Fennel,

Crosson, Boggs, & Mickle, 1995), which typically extend into adulthood. Many adults with spina bifida and hydrocephalus are unable to live independently, instead residing with parents. Although they are often capable of employment, relatively few work in professional or semiskilled occupations (Hunt & Poulton, 1995). Young adults with SBM also demonstrate reductions in certain aspects of quality of life (Hetherington, Dennis, Barnes, Drake, & Gentili, 2006).

Taken together, the modal profile of neurobehavioral outcomes associated with myelomeningocele and shunted hydrocephalus has been likened to what Rourke (1995) termed a nonverbal learning disability. A recent study compared the prevalence of nonverbal learning disabilities in children with SBM to that in a group of healthy siblings (Yeates, Loss, Colvin, & Enrile, 2003). About 50% of the children with SBM displayed a pattern of assets and deficits consistent with nonverbal learning disabilities. However, they also displayed significantly more variability in their patterns of assets and deficits than siblings. The findings suggest a need for caution in making generalizations regarding the presence of nonverbal learning disabilities in children with SBM.

More recent models of neurobehavioral outcomes in SBM have focused on core information processing deficits from a neuroscience perspective and have linked those to the functional assets and deficits shown by children with SBM. Dennis, Landry, Barnes, and Fletcher (2006) proposed that SBM is characterized by core deficits in timing, attention orienting, and movement. They argue that these core deficits prevent the normal development of the ability to assemble and integrate information (i.e., assembled processing), but they have less impact on the ability to activate or categorize information (i.e., associative processing). The combination of intact associative processing and impaired assembled processing results in a cognitive phenotype of assets and deficits within a number of functional domains. For instance, deficits in explicit memory are contrasted with relatively intact implicit memory (Yeates & Enrile, 2005) and deficits in online motor control are contrasted with relatively intact motor adaptation (Colvin, Yeates, Enrile, & Coury, 2003).

Case Presentation: John

History and Behavioral Observations

John was referred for a neuropsychological evaluation by his primary care physician to document his neuropsychological status and to generate recommendations for clinical management. At the time of the evaluation, he was 12 years old and lived at home with his parents. Family history was unremarkable. Birth history was significant for the diagnosis of SBM at birth, followed by surgical repair within the first few days of life. Subsequent magnetic resonance imaging (MRI) documented Chiari-II malformation and hydrocephalus. John promptly underwent surgery for shunt placement and has never required any shunt revisions. John exhibited a neurogenic bowel and bladder that was managed through frequent catheterization and a bowel program. He was not prescribed any medications aside from those prescribed as part of his bowel program.

John was enrolled in the seventh grade at a public middle school. He had been educated with the assistance of an individualized education plan (IEP) since elementary school. He reported that he enjoyed school, but described some frustration because of challenges with ambulation in the school setting. His mother reported that John had a history of difficulties with reading and mathematics, initially described by teachers in the first grade. With the assistance of special education, John's teachers reported substantial academic gains, particularly in reading skills. John also experienced difficulties with writing and received accommodations such as reductions in written work expectations and copies of notes from teachers and peers. In addition to academic difficulties, John's teachers reported difficulties with attention, concentration, and the ability to follow instructions.

Psychosocial functioning more broadly was characterized by attention problems and mild social immaturity. John's mother reported longstanding difficulties with inattention, distractibility, poor compliance with directions, avoidance of work requiring sustained focus, and disorganization. His mother also described John as socially immature for his age, but she denied any substantial emotional or behavioral concerns. Despite his mother's concerns regarding his social functioning, John was a pleasant boy, who was generally well liked by peers and adults. John reported mild self-consciousness related to his ankle-foot orthoses (AFOs) and indicated that he had noticed peers staring at them. He also reported some recent teasing by peers at school that did not appear to focus on his disability.

During the evaluation, John was pleasant and cooperative. His affect was bright. His attention and activity level were well regulated during the structured, one-to-one testing sessions. His response style was impulsive. John easily initiated informal conversation. His language comprehension was intact. His language expression was appropriate in form and content and did not contain overt aphasic errors. Language pragmatics were intact. John demonstrated a satisfactory appreciation of paralinguistic features such as gesture, intonation, and facial expression. John did not demonstrate any unusual physical characteristics. He ambulated independently with the aid of bilateral AFOs. John preferred his right hand for writing and drawing. His graphomotor production was slow, and letters were large and poorly formed.

Test Results

Overall performance on the WISC-IV was in the low-average range, with a Full Scale IQ of 89, at the 23rd percentile (see Table 7.1). Both the Verbal Comprehension and Working Memory Indexes were average, with standard scores of 106 and 91, around the 65th and 25th percentiles, respectively. The Perceptual Organization and Processing Speed Indexes were in the low-average range, with standard scores of 86 and 80, around the 20th and 10th percentiles, respectively. Overall, John's pattern of performance suggested a relative strength in tasks assessing acquired verbal knowledge and relative weaknesses on tasks involving novel nonverbal stimuli or response speed.

Based on observations suggesting his language skills were relatively intact, formal testing in this domain was limited. John demonstrated average retrieval of words to both semantic and phonemic cues on the D-KEFS Verbal Fluency Test.

Verbal memory was below average on list learning tasks, but intact on a story recall task. On the WRAML-2, the Verbal Memory

Table 7-1. Performance on neuropsychological tests by "John"

Wechsler Intelligence Scale for Children-Fourth Edition (WISC-IV)			
Full Scale IQ		Standard Score = 89	%ile = 23
Verbal Comprehension Index = 106		**Perceptual Reasoning Index** = 86	
Similarities	11	Block Design	9
Vocabulary	14	Picture Concepts	8
Comprehension	9	Matrix Reasoning	6
Working Memory Index = 91		**Processing Speed Index** = 80	
Digit Span	7	Coding	6
Letter-Number	10	Symbol Search	7

Wide Range Assessment of Memory and Learning-Second Ed. (WRAML-2)			
Screening Memory Index		Standard Score = 77	%ile = 6
Verbal Memory Index = 80	8	**Visual Memory Index** = 82	8
Story Memory		Design Memory	
Verbal Learning	5	Picture Memory	6

Beery Buktenica Developmental Test of Visual Motor Integration (VMI)		
Subtest	Index Score	Percentile
Visual Motor Integration	75	5
Visual Perception	78	7
Motor Coordination	74	4

Rey-Osterrieth Complex Figure		
Trial	Index Score	Percentile
Copy	77	6
Delayed Recall	78	7

Gordon Diagnostic System			
Delay Task	SS	**Vigilance Task**	SS
Total Efficiency Ratio	81	Total Commissions	89
Total Responses	114	Total Correct	106
Total Correct	70		

Delis Kaplan Executive Function System (D-KEFS)			
Trail Making Test		**Verbal Fluency**	
Visual Scanning	7	Letter Fluency	8
Number Sequencing	7	Category Fluency	11
Letter Sequencing	7	Category Switching	6
Number Letter Switch.	5	Switching Accuracy	8
Motor Speed	8	Tower Test	
		Achievement	6

Grooved Pegboard			
Hand	Raw score		SS
Right	79 seconds		74
Left	77 seconds		83

Wechsler Individual Achievement Test-Second Ed. (WIAT-II)			
Reading Composite = 109		**Mathematics Composite** = 79	
Word Reading	109	Numerical Operations	71
Reading Comprehension	113	Math Reasoning	91
Pseudoword Decoding	106		

Table 7-1. Performance on neuropsychological tests by "John" (*Continued*)

Child Behavior Checklist

	Mother Report (t-score)	Teacher Report (t-score)
Internalizing Problems	34	58
Externalizing Problems	44	53
Total Problems	45	58
Anxious/Depressed	50	57
Withdrawn/Depressed	50	62
Somatic Complaints	50	55
Social Problems	56	59
Thought Problems	50	50
Attention Problems	60	62
Rule-Breaking Behavior	50	50
Aggressive Behavior	50	55

Composite was below average, with a standard score of 80, around the 10th percentile. Memory for verbal narrative was avera ge on the Story Memory subtest. On the Verbal Learning subtest, John's rate of learning was below average, as was his total learning over four trials.

John's nonverbal skills were generally below average. On the VMI, perceptual recognition was below average on the Visual Perception subtest. Constructional skills were below average on the Visual Motor Integration subtest and on the copy trial of the Rey-Osterrieth Complex Figure.

Formal tests of nonverbal memory revealed intact recall of geometric shapes but below average memory for visual details. On the WRAML-2, the Visual Memory Composite was below average, with a standard score of 82, around the 10th percentile. Immediate recall of geometric designs was average on the Design Memory subtest. Immediate recognition of details in pictures was in the low-average range on the Picture Memory subtest. Delayed recall was below average on the Rey-Osterrieth Complex Figure.

Tests of executive functions revealed multiple deficits in this domain. Performance on the Gordon Diagnostic System was characterized by difficulties with sustained attention and response inhibition. Focused attention and response speed were in the low-average range on most trials of the D-KEFS Trail-Making Test, but performance fell below average on the more demanding Number-Letter Switching trial, which involves alternating sequences and cognitive flexibility. Cognitive flexibility was also in the low-average range on the Category Switching trial of the Verbal Fluency Test. Spatial planning was in the low-average range on the Tower Test.

Fine motor speed and dexterity were below average bilaterally on the Grooved Pegboard. Of note, John dropped multiple pegs with both hands on this task.

John's academic achievement was assessed to explore areas of strength and weakness. On the WIAT-II, his Reading Composite of 109 was average, around the 75th percentile. More specifically, word decoding and recognition skills were average on both the Word Reading and Pseudoword Decoding subtests. Performance on the Reading Comprehension subtest was also average, although John required extensive time to read written passages on this task. Performance varied on the subtests that comprise the Mathematics Composite. Understanding of mathematics concepts and completion of word problems were average on the Math Reasoning subtest. In contrast, computational skills were far below average on the Numerical Operations subtest. Errors on this task included incorrect math facts, difficulty regrouping when borrowing for subtraction, and performing the incorrect operation (i.e., subtraction instead of addition).

John's teacher and mother provided ratings of his behavioral and emotional adjustment using the Child Behavior Checklist (CBCL). Neither of the raters reported a significant overall level of behavioral disturbance, but they both noted difficulties with attention and concentration. John's teachers also reported several physical complaints.

Discussion

John demonstrated a pattern of neuropsychological functioning largely consistent with findings from studies of children with SBM. For instance, his general cognitive abilities were in the low-average range, with a discrepancy favoring verbal over nonverbal skills. Within that context, his neuropsychological profile also documented impairments in nonverbal skills, such as perceptual recognition and constructional abilities. He also demonstrated difficulties with a variety of executive functions, such as sustained and focused attention, response inhibition, spatial planning, and cognitive flexibility. John's memory functioning was characterized by specific weaknesses in the recall of word lists and certain aspects of nonverbal memory. His fine motor speed and dexterity were impaired bilaterally. Finally, John demonstrated diminished calculation skills.

John's neuropsychological profile also was characterized by many areas of intact cognitive functioning, some of which reflected strengths relative to other children with SBM. His immediate recall of complex geometric shapes was average, which was somewhat unexpected given his impairments in perceptual recognition and constructional skills. Stimulus size may have accounted for these seemingly discrepant findings, as the perceptual task on the VMI involves increasingly small stimuli. Verbal fluency, an area of difficulty noted in other children with SBM, was also intact. Additionally, John demonstrated globally intact reading skills, including reading comprehension. However, despite average performance within the current evaluation, his history reflected previous difficulties in this domain. Thus, John's better than expected performance relative to other children with SBM likely represents a positive response to academic intervention. Additionally, reading comprehension may vary relative to task demands, as John required extensive time when reading passages, and this did not factor into his overall score. Finally, John appeared to be a well-adjusted young man, who did not demonstrate significant behavioral or emotional difficulties. His mother's description of social immaturity is consistent with research on children with SBM. Nonetheless, these difficulties were reported as mild in severity and were not indicated on parent or teacher rating measures.

Like many children with SBM, John's neuropsychological deficits place him at significant risk for difficulties in school. Nonverbal deficits will likely interfere with new learning, particularly when John is provided visual information without verbal instruction. The nonverbal deficits may also manifest as difficulty learning information that is novel or complex. Difficulties with graphomotor skills may make it challenging for him to manage demands for writing in class. Impaired executive functions, such as attention and response inhibition, will make it difficult for him to work in a systematic and efficient manner. Instead, John is likely to be inattentive, impulsive, and disorganized. He may have difficulty staying on task and completing assignments on time, and the quality of his work may be inconsistent. These difficulties are likely to become especially apparent when academic demands increase and when he is expected to work independently. Finally, John's limitations in mobility, as well as difficulties with bowel and bladder management, present additional challenges in the school setting.

Based on John's cognitive and motor impairments and their detrimental impact on his learning and academic performance, he was recommended for ongoing special education services under the other health impairment (OHI) classification. Given the presence of significant distractibility and inattention, he was also referred to a psychiatrist for medication consultation.

Spina bifida myelomeningocele is a neural tube defect often associated with neuropsychological deficits that place children at risk for academic, social, and behavioral difficulties. The current case of John exemplifies many of the deficits, as well as strengths, that typically occur in association with SBM. Neuropsychological evaluation of children with SBM seeks to provide insight into their neuropsychological functioning and to generate recommendations that address the risks they face, and thereby facilitate their overall development.

References

Anderson, V., Northam, E., Hendy, J., & Wrenhall, J. (2001). *Developmental neuropsychology: A clinical approach*. New York: Psychology Press.

Au, K. S., Tran, P. X., Tsai, C. C., O'Byrne, M. R., Lin, J. I., Morrison, A. C., et al. (2008). Characteristics of a spina bifida population including North American

Caucasian and Hispanic individuals. *Birth Defects Research (Part A)*, 82, 692–700.

Ayr, L. K., Yeates, K. O., & Enrile, B. G. (2005). Arithmetic skills and their cognitive correlates in children with acquired and congenital brain disorder. *Journal of the International Neuropsychological Society*, 11, 249–262.

Barnes, M. A., & Dennis, M. (1992). Reading in children and adolescents after early hydrocephalus and in normally developing age peers: Phonological analysis, word recognition, word comprehension, and passage comprehension skill. *Journal of Pediatric Psychology*, 17, 445–465.

Barnes, M. A., & Dennis, M. (1998). Discourse after early-onset hydrocephalus: Core deficits in children of average intelligence. *Brain and Language*, 61, 309–334.

Barnes, M., Dennis, M., & Hetherington, R. (2004). Reading and writing skills in young adults with spina bifida and hydrocephalus. *Journal of the International Neuropsychological Society*, 10, 655–663.

Botto, L. D., Moore, C. A., Khoury, M. J., & Erickson, J. D. (1999). Neural-tube defects. *New England Journal of Medicine*, 341, 1509–1519.

Boyer, K. M., Yeates, K. O., & Enrile, B. G. (2006). Working memory and information processing speed in children with myelomeningocele and shunted hydrocephalus: Analysis of the Children's Paced Auditory Serial Addition Test. *Journal of the International Neuropsychological Society*, 12, 305–313.

Brewer, V. R., Fletcher, J. M., Hiscock, M., & Davidson, K. C. (2001) Attention processes in children with shunted hydrocephalus versus attention deficit-hyperactivity disorder. *Neuropsychology*, 15, 185–198.

Brown, T. M., Ris, M. D., Beebe, D., Ammerman, R. T., Oppenheimer, S. G., Yeates, K. O., et al. (2008). Factors of biological risk and reserve associated with executive behaviors in children and adolescents with spina bifida myelomeningocele. *Child Neuropsychology*, 14, 118–134.

Burmeister, R., Hannay, H. J., Copeland, K., Fletcher, J. M., Boudousquie, A., & Dennis, M. (2005). Attention problems and executive functions in children with spina bifida and hydrocephalus. *Child Neuropsychology*, 11, 265–283.

Charney, E. (1992). Neural tube defects: Spina bifida and meningomyelocele. In M. Batshaw & Y. Perret (Eds.), *Children with disabilities: A medical primer* (3rd ed., pp. 471–488). Baltimore: Paul H. Brookes.

Colvin, A. N., Yeates, K. O., Enrile, B. G., & Coury, D. L. (2003). Motor adaptation in children with myelomeningocele: Comparison to children with ADHD and healthy siblings. *Journal of the International Neuropsychological Society*, 9, 642–652.

Czeizel, A. E., & Dudas, I. (1992). Prevention of the first occurrence of neural-defects by periconceptional vitamin supplementation. *New England Journal of Medicine*, 327, 1832–1835.

Deak, K. L., Siegel, D. G., George, T. M., Gregory, S., Ashley-Koch, A., & Speer, M. C. (2008). Further evidence for a maternal genetic effect and a sex-influenced effect contributing to risk for human neural tube defects. *Birth Defects Research (Part A): Clinical and Molecular Teratology*, 82, 662–669.

Del Bigio, M. R. (1993). Neuropathological changes caused by hydrocephalus. *Acta Neuropathologica*, 85, 573–585.

Dennis, M., & Barnes, M. A. (2002). Math and numeracy in young adults with spina bifida and hydrocephalus. *Developmental Neuropsychology*, 21, 141–155.

Dennis, M., Edelstein, K., Hetherington, R., Copeland, K., Frederick, J., Blaser, S. E., et al. (2004). Neurobiology of timing in children with spina bifida in relation to cerebellar volume. *Brain*, 127, 1292–1301.

Dennis, M., Fletcher, J. M., Rogers, S., Hetherington, R., & Francis, D. (2002). Object-based and action-based visual perception in children with spina bifida and hydrocephalus. *Journal of the International Neuropsychological Society*, 8, 95–106

Dennis, M., Jacennik, B., & Barnes, M. A. (1994). The content of narrative discourse in children and adolescents after early onset hydrocephalus and in normally developing age peers. *Brain and Language*, 46, 129–165.

Dennis, M., Landry, S. H., Barnes, M., & Fletcher, J. M. (2006). A model of neurocognitive function in spina bifida over the life span. *Journal of the International Neuropsychological Society*, 12, 285–296.

Fletcher, J. M., Brookshire, B. L., Landry, S. H., Bohan, T. P., Davidson, K. C., Francis, D. J., et al. (1996). Attentional skills and executive functions in children with early hydrocephalus. *Developmental Neuropsychology*, 12, 53–76.

Fletcher, J. M., Copeland, K., Frederick, J., Blaser, S. E., Kramer, L. A., Northrup, H., et al. (2005). Spinal lesion level in spina bifida meningomyelocele: A source of neural and cognitive heterogeneity. *Journal of Neurosurgery: Pediatrics*, 102, 268–279.

Fletcher, J. M., & Dennis, M. (2010). Spina bifida and hydrocephalus. In K. O. Yeates, M. D. Ris, H. G. Taylor, & B. Pennington (Eds.), *Pediatric neuropsychology: Research, theory, and practice* (2nd ed., pp. 3-25). New York: Guilford.

Fletcher, J. M., Dennis, M., & Northrup, H. (2000). Hydrocephalus. In K.O. Yeates, M. D. Ris, & H. G. Taylor (2000). *Pediatric neuropsychology: Research, theory, and practice* (pp. 25–46). New York: Guilford.

Fletcher, J. M., Francis, D. J., Thompson, N. M., Brookshire, B. L., Bohan, T. P., Landry, S. H. et al. (1992). Verbal and nonverbal skill discrepancies in hydrocephalic children. *Journal of Clinical and Experimental Neuropsychology, 14,* 593–609.

Greenley, R. N., Holmbeck, G. N., Zukerman, J., & Buck, C. F. (2006). Psychological adjustment and family relationships in children and adolescents with spina bifida. In D. F. Wyszynski (Ed.), *Neural tube defects: From origin to treatment* (pp. 21–55). New York: Oxford University Press.

Hannay, H. J., Dennis, M., Kramer, L., Blaser, S., & Fletcher, J. M. (2009). Partial agenesis of the corpus callosum in spina bifida meningomyelocele and potential compensatory mechanisms. *Journal of Clinical and Experimental Neuropsychology, 31*(2), 180–194.

Hetherington, C. R., & Dennis, M. (1999). Motor function profile in children with early onset hydrocephalus. *Developmental Neuropsychology, 15,* 25–51.

Hetherington, R., Dennis, M., Barnes, M., Drake, J., & Gentili, F. (2006). Functional outcome in young adults with spina bifida and hydrocephalus. *Child's Nervous System, 22*(2), 117–128.

Holler, K. A., Fennell, E. B., Crosson, B., Boggs, S. R., & Mickle, J. P. (1995). Neuropsychological and adaptive functioning in younger versus older children shunted for early hydrocephalus. *Child Neuropsychology, 1,* 63–73.

Holmbeck, G. N., Westhoven, V. C., Phillips, W. S., Bowers, R., Gruse, C., Nikolopoulos, T., et al. (2003). A multimethod, multi-informant, and multidimensional perspective on psychosocial adjustment in preadolescents with spina bifida. *Journal of Consulting and Clinical Psychology, 71,* 782–796.

Honein, M. A, Paulozzi, L. J., Matthews, T. J., Erickson, J. D., &Wong, L. C. (2001). Impact of folic acid fortification of the US food supply on the occurrence of neural tube defects. *Journal of the American Medical Association, 285,* 2981–2986.

Hunt, G. M., & Poulton, A. (1995). Open spina bifida: A complete cohort reviewed 25 years after closure. *Developmental Medicine and Child Neurology, 37,* 19–29.

Lavigne, J. V., & Faier-Routman, J. (1992). Psychological adjustment to pediatric physical disorders: A meta-analytic review. *Journal of Pediatric Psychology, 18,* 667–680.

Loss, N., Yeates, K. O., & Enrile, B. G. (1998). Attention in children with myelomeningocele. *Child Neuropsychology, 4,* 7–20.

Mahone, E. M., Zabel, A., Levey, E., Verda, M., & Kinsman, S. (2002). Parent and self-report ratings of executive function in adolescents with myelomeningocele and hydrocephalus. *Child Neuropsychology, 8,* 258–270.

Northrup, H., & Volcik, K. A. (2000). Spina bifida and other neural tube defects. *Current Problems in Pediatrics, 30,* 313–332.

Rose, B. M., & Holmbeck, G. N. (2007). Attention and executive functions in adolescents with spina bifida. *Journal of Pediatric Psychology, 32,* 983–994.

Rourke, B. P. (Ed.). (1995). *Syndrome of nonverbal learning disabilities: Neurodevelopmental manifestations.* New York: Guilford Press.

Scott, M. A., Davidson, K. C., Fletcher, J. K., Brookshire, B. L., Handry, S. H., Bohan, T. C., et al. (1998). Memory functions in children with early hydrocephalus. *Neuropsychology, 12,* 578–589.

Stevenson, K. L. (2004). Chiari type II malformation: past, present, and future. *Neurosurgery Focus, 16,* 1–7.

Tarazi, R. A., Zabel, A., & Mahone, E. M. (2008). Age-related differences in executive function among children with spina bifida/hydrocephalus based on parent behavior ratings. *Clinical Neuropsychology, 22,* 585–602.

Vachha, B., & Adams, R. C. (2005). Memory and selective learning in children with spina bifida-myelomeningocele and shunted hydrocephalus: A preliminary study. *Cerebrospinal Fluid Research, 2,* (10).

Vinck, A., Maassen, B., Mullaart, R., & Rotteveel, J. (2006). Arnold-Chiari-II malformation and cognitive functioning in spina bifida. *Journal of Neurology, Neurosurgery, and Psychiatry, 77,* 1083–1086.

Yeates, K. O., & Enrile, B. G. (2005). Implicit and explicit memory in children with congenital and acquired brain disorder. *Neuropsychology, 19,* 618–628.

Yeates, K. O., Enrile, B., Loss, N., Blumenstein, E., & Delis, D. (1995). Verbal learning and memory in children with myelomeningocele. *Journal of Pediatric Psychology, 20,* 801–815.

Yeates, K. O., Loss, N., Colvin, A. N., & Enrile, B. G. (2003). Do children with myelomeningocele and hydrocephalus display nonverbal learning disabilities? An empirical approach to classification. *Journal of the International Neuropsychological Society, 9,* 653–662.

8

A Case of Cerebral Palsy (Spastic Diplegia)

T. Andrew Zabel and Adam T. Schmidt

Cerebral palsy (CP) is the most common chronic motor disorder of early childhood, affecting approximately 2/1000 school-aged children (Krageloh-Mann & Horber, 2007; Menkes & Sarnat, 2000). Cerebral palsy refers to a diverse group of motor impairments that arise from numerous acquired and genetic etiologies (Fennell & Dikel, 2001; Korzeniewski, Birbeck, DeLano, Potchen, & Paneth, 2008; Krageloh-Mann & Horber, 2007; Menkes & Sarnat, 2000). It is commonly associated with prematurity, neonatal encephalopathy, and diverse postnatal insults (Fennell & Dikel, 2001; Korzeniewski et al., 2008). The etiology of CP is in great part linked to the concept of *selective vulnerability* (Johnston, 1998). Selective vulnerability refers to susceptibility to injury of specific cells and regions during different periods of brain development. Disruptions in brain development in the early (first trimester) and late (second and third trimesters) prenatal periods, as well as at- or near-term, have been linked with different CP etiologies, including brain malformations, white matter injury around the lateral ventricles, and hypoxic-ischemic encephalopathy (Johnson, Hoon, & Kaufmann, 2008).

The diagnosis of CP is made clinically by the pattern of motor symptoms a child displays (Fennell & Dikel, 2001; Menkes & Sarnat, 2000). Children with motor symptoms of spasticity (e.g., velocity-dependent increased muscle resistance) are often diagnosed according to the extremities involved and/or the extent of asymmetry (e.g., spastic quadriparesis, spastic diplegia, and spast-choreoathetosis are often diagnosed

with dyskinetic CP (Fennell & Dikel, 2001; Menkes & Sarnat, 2000).

One of the most common forms of CP, particularly in preterm infants, is spastic diplegia. Children with spastic diplegia typically exhibit bilateral spasticity of the lower extremities, although involvement of the arms is not uncommon in these children (Menkes & Sarnat, 2000). In addition to motor dysfunction, symptoms such as strabismus, speech difficulties, and seizures are also common in this form of CP (Fennell & Dikel, 2001; Menkes & Sarnat, 2000). White matter disruption commonly referred to as periventricular white matter injury (PWMI) or periventricular leukomalacia (PVL) accounts for a vast majority of the structural anomalies in children with spastic diplegia (Korzeniewski et al., 2008; Krageloh-Mann & Horber, 2007; Volpe, 2003). Periventricular leukomalacia is characterized by bilateral cavitary infarcts in the white matter adjacent to the lateral ventricles, and it is associated with hypoxia/ischemia, infection, and endocrine/metabolic disorders. The developing brain is especially vulnerable to PWMI and PVL from 24–34 weeks gestation when blood vessels serving the periventricular white matter are immature (Johnson, Hoon, & Kaufmann, 2008). During this period of development, oligodendrocyte progenitors that are beginning to form myelin are particularly susceptible to attack by oxygen free radicals, glutamate, and inflammatory cytokines (Hoon et al., 2002; Nagae et al., 2007). While CP is commonly (and possibly erroneously) attributed to factors associated with delivery, there is growing evidence to suggest that a large majority of CP cases with perinatal difficulties (e.g., prematurity) have pre-existing prenatal etiologies such as PWMI or PVL (Nelson & Ellenberg, 1986; Johnson et al., 2008). The lower extremity motor profile of spastic diplegia is likely due in part to the medial lesions associated with PVL, as lumbar motor neurons that innervate the lower extremities are located in a more medial position among the corticospinal fibers (Johnson et al., 2008). Sensory pathways that project broadly to association and visual cortices, however, may also be involved. Using diffusion tensor imaging (DTI), Hoon and colleagues (2002) demonstrated that the posterior thalamic radiations (PTRs), which connect the pulvinar and the lateral geniculate nucleus (LGN) to posterior cortical regions, were especially disrupted in children with CP. In a recent follow-up study of 24 children with PWMI, Hoon and his collaborators (Nagae et al., 2007) reported that both the retrolenticular part of the internal capsule and the posterior thalamic radiations were the white matter tracts with the most frequent and severe injuries, replicating their previous findings.

In addition to motor impairment, children with CP frequently demonstrate a variety of cognitive and learning difficulties. In general, children with spastic quadriparesis tend to exhibit the lowest level of intellectual functioning (Fenell & Dikel, 2001), and there appears to be a modest correlation between severity of motor impairment and intellectual skills in other forms of CP (Fenell & Dikel, 2001). Research also indicates that children with CP and a comorbid seizure disorder are at greater risk for a diagnosis of intellectual disability (i.e., mental retardation) (Fenell & Dikel, 2001). However, it should be emphasized that verbal and perceptual abilities may both be easily underestimated secondary to significant motor difficulties such as fine motor speed/dexterity and oral motor dysfunction (Fenell & Dikel, 2001; Pueyo, Junque, Vendrell, Narberhaus, & Segarra, 2008; Sigurdardottir et al., 2008).

The diverse etiologies of CP combined with the significant difficulties in measuring neuropsychological performance in these individuals has resulted in glacial progress toward defining a "neuropsychological profile" for children with CP.

Nevertheless, the studies that have been completed suggest some general trends especially with regard to spastic cerebral palsy. For example, studies involving children with CP indicate nonverbal reasoning deficits and reduced overall cognitive abilities (i.e., mean IQ in the low average range) (Pirila et al., 2004; Sigurdardottir et al., 2008), difficulties with attention and inhibitory control (Christ, White, Brunstrom, & Abrams, 2003; McDonough & Cohen, 1982), and impairments in visuospatial/visuoperceptual skills (Fazzi et al., 2004; Kozeis et al., 2007; Pirila et al., 2004; Stiers et al., 2002). Many of these neuropsychological features are demonstrated in the case example.

Case Report: Mario

Referral

At the time of the evaluation, Mario was an 8-year-old, left-handed boy who had undergone psychoeducational and neuropsychological assessment on several previous occasions. His medical team followed Mario closely, as he had shown a pattern of early diffuse delays, followed by a pattern of improved articulation and sharp qualitative gains in language ability at age 4 following a trial of Artane. Updated neuropsychological evaluation was requested at age 8 to clarify neurocognitive status for treatment and school planning purposes.

Family History

At the time of this evaluation, Mario was living with his mother and had frequent contact with his father. Mario's parents had high school (mother) and college (father) degrees and came from extended families without overt indication of behavioral, learning, or psychological problems.

Birth and Developmental History

Pregnancy was complicated by maternal hypertension. Magnesium sulfate was administered to delay labor after premature rupture of membranes at 28 weeks gestational age, and Mario was eventually born at 30 weeks. He weighed approximately 3 pounds (1360 grams) at birth, which was considered very low birth weight but also appropriate weight for gestational age. Apgar scores were 8 (at 1 minute) and 9 (at 5 minutes). Mario required ventilatory support for about 1 day, and he used a nasal tube for one additional day. During his 6-week neonatal intensive care unit hospitalization, he was treated for jaundice, apnea, and reflux. His first two cranial ultrasounds performed several days after birth revealed evidence of cystic PVL, and Mario was subsequently diagnosed with CP during his first year of life.

Developmental milestones were reported to be delayed for language acquisition. Although he oriented to sounds and made his own vocalizations, he had no intelligible speech until age 4 years. It is noteworthy that Mario's speech became more intelligible after he began taking an anticholinergic agent (Artane) for general management of athetosis and dystonia. While articulation difficulties persisted, functional expressive vocabulary expanded dramatically at that time.

Early medical history was noteworthy for moderate-to-severe right hip subluxation and moderate left hip subluxation, which significantly disrupted Mario's ability to sit and walk. This problem was surgically treated at age 4 with bilateral osteotomy, adductor lengthening, hamstring tendon lengthening, and spica casting. Later developmental history was noteworthy for moderate equinovarus (clubfoot) that was treated with physical therapy, Botox injections, and casting. At the time of the assessment at age 8, Mario ambulated with a posterior walker and twister cables. In lieu of his family's decision against use of a wheelchair, Mario's community mobility was further augmented by the practice of standing on the back of a stroller propelled by an adult. In response to ongoing speech and motor needs, Mario maintained a high level of speech/language therapy, physical therapy, and occupational therapy, in addition to therapeutic horseback riding.

At age 6, Mario's developmental pediatrician confirmed his diagnosis of asymmetric right spastic diplegia. Neurological exam revealed rigidity, athetosis, and dystonia in the upper extremities, and spasticity in the lower extremities. There was indication of dystonia throughout his upper extremities that negatively impacted upon daily activities. Passive range of motion was within normal limits, but active range of motion was limited. Mario was left hand dominant, with his right upper extremity (flexor posturing) affected greater than his left (patterns of extensor posturing).

As noted above, Mario's first two cranial ultrasounds performed several days after birth showed cystic PVL. Brain MRI performed at approximately 5 years of age (see Figure 8.1; see also the color figure in the color insert section) showed evidence of abnormal enlargement of the occipital horns, diminished white matter, and ventricular scalloping, all of which were suggestive of PVL. Ordinal grading of white matter tracts generated using research-based diffusion tensor imaging (DTI) revealed abnormalities and/or absence of the corpus callosum (body and splenium: see Figure 8.2; see also the color figure in the color insert section), tapetum, internal capsule (posterior and retrolenticular limbs), thalamus, posterior thalamic radiations, superior corona radiata, and superior longitudinal fasciculi.

A recent ophthalmologic appointment performed before the neuropsychological assessment (age 8) suggested age-appropriate visual acuity, with "near 20/20 vision" and no need for corrective lenses. Hearing had been assessed to be within normal limits. Mild sleep difficulties (delayed sleep onset and multiple nighttime wakings) were treated with Melatonin. There was no history of postnatal traumatic brain injury, loss of consciousness, or seizures.

Education

Mario received intensive home, center, and/or school-based therapies beginning at age 2 years. He attended a specialized speech/language program for kindergarten and the beginning of first

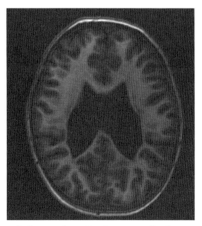

Figure 8-1. Axial MPRAGE image displaying ventricular enlargement and white matter reduction.

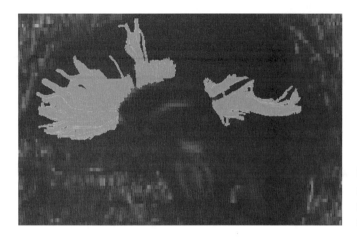

Figure 8-2. Diffusion tensor imaging tractography displaying absent or dysmorphic body and splenium of the corpus callosum.

grade, but he transferred to an inclusion education classroom approximately 2 months into first grade. He had an individualized education plan (IEP) under the Federal Classification Code of Multiple Disabilities. Mario had a one-to-one aide in the classroom to assist him with mobility and curriculum access. By the time of the neuropsychological assessment (age 8), Mario had demonstrated adequate gains in reading but continued to struggle in math.

Mario had completed several developmental/cognitive evaluations in the past. At 20 months of age (prematurity-corrected age of 18 months), performance on the Bayley Scales of Infant Development–Second Edition placed him at an overall age equivalent of 11 months. At approximately 3 years of age, psychoeducational evaluation generated an estimate of intellectual functioning in the low average range (Pictorial Test of Intelligence–Second Edition: Pictorial IQ = 87, percentile = 19).

Validity/Testing Considerations

Multiple potential threats to validity of assessment findings were considered when designing the evaluation at age 8. Based upon observations made during prior assessments (age 6), fatigue was anticipated to be a potentially problematic issue in testing, and a shorter test session/battery with multiple break periods was planned. Additionally, the following variables were considered.

Seating/Positioning. At school, Mario typically sat in a specialized Rifton chair and harness that provided trunk and upper body support, as well as an adjustable footboard, to help him with sitting upright and voicing responses. This chair was not available for testing, and Mario's mother helped the evaluators create a seating arrangement that would provide the necessary level of proximal upper body stabilization. Specifically, Mario was seated in a chair with arms, and several pillows were positioned on either side of him to ensure side support. A wooden box was positioned under his feet so that his legs did not hang from the chair, and stimuli were positioned on a tilt board that sat on the desk in front of him. These seating and positioning accommodations were thought to help manage the potential threats to test score validity posed by effortful/laborious sitting and poor breath support.

Articulation. Due to Mario's persistent articulation problems, it was often difficult to interpret/understand his responses to test questions. For the assessment battery, tests were selected that presented only minimal articulation and verbal formulation demands. Moreover, the assessors included Mario's long-time one-to-one aide in the assessment process to assist with speech interpretation. Specifically, the one-to-one aide was positioned in the testing room, where she could not see the test stimuli, and she used a blank sheet of paper to record what she thought she heard Mario say on tests requiring verbal output. The one-to-one aide's written account of Mario's verbalizations was then used later to confirm and/or correct the evaluator's record of Mario's speech production and test responses.

Motor. Motor limitations and potential for fatigue were taken into account when designing the test battery, with a priority placed upon using untimed measures, tests with limited motor requirements (i.e., tests requiring a general pointing response but not object manipulation), and measures with limited articulation demands.

Behavioral Observations

Mario slowly ambulated to the testing office, requiring great effort and the assistance of his walker and parents. He presented as a friendly, polite, and pleasant boy. Mario readily answered questions with one-word responses, which were periodically difficult to understand due to poor articulation. Although he had to frequently repeat himself to clarify his verbalizations, he persisted with good effort in the test setting and did not show overt signs of frustration. Mario's activity level was within normal expectations throughout the assessment; however, he was easily distracted by extraneous noises in the hallway or objects that he noticed in the testing room. Cooperation was easily elicited and Mario's effort was good. He demonstrated an appropriate range of affect during the session.

Assessment Results

Mario underwent psychoeducational evaluation at age 5 and neuropsychological evaluation at ages 6 and 8. Selected results from the earlier neuropsychological assessment are included for comparison purposes in the narrative below. The neuropsychological evaluation conducted at age 6 was considered comprehensive and broad-based in nature, while the assessment at age 8 was considered a targeted follow-up assessment.

Adaptive Functioning. Parent ratings of independent self-help skills provided at ages 5, 6, and 8 on the Adaptive Behavior Assessment System–Second Edition (ABAS-II) consistently resulted in standard scores well below age-level expectations. Specifically, general adaptive composite (GAC) standard scores were 52, 56, and 67, respectively. Speech and motor limitations were thought to account for many of the low adaptive skill ratings. Of note, qualitative report provided by his parents at the time of the evaluation (age 8) suggested adaptive skill gains that were not reflected in formal parent ratings of ability. For example, Mario had begun to independently identify trash items and *ask* his one-to-one aide to pick them up and throw them away. Moreover, by age 8, ongoing progress in articulation and adapted recreation had resulted in score increases on individual ABAS-II scales of functional communication and leisure activities.

General Intelligence. At age 6, administration of the full Stanford-Binet Intelligence Scale–Fifth Edition (SB-V) yielded a Full Scale IQ score of 68 (VIQ = 76, percentile = 5; PIQ = 64, percentile = 1). At that time, Mario's motor and verbal limitations negatively impacted his performance on most items of the SB-V, and these scores were viewed as likely underestimations of his "true" cognitive abilities, particularly since performance on another common proxy measure of IQ fell within normal limits (Peabody Picture Vocabulary Test–Third Edition [PPVT-III] standard score = 96, percentile = 39).

During the reevaluation performed at age 8, IQ was estimated to range from low average to average based upon performance on several Wechsler Abbreviated Scale of Intelligence (WASI) subtests with limited motor and articulation demands, and Mario obtained the following scores: Similarities T-score = 46, percentile = 34; WASI Matrix Reasoning: T-score = 37, percentile = 9.

Language. Mario presented with significant articulation difficulties during the assessments performed at ages 6 and 8. Formal assessment of language at age 8 was conducted with these speech difficulties in mind, with limited requirements presented for lengthy and/or speeded verbal formulation. Using this approach, Mario demonstrated age-appropriate skills in confrontation naming/expressive vocabulary (Expressive Vocabulary Test–Second Edition [EVT-2] standard score = 89, percentile = 23), verbal repetition (WRAML-2 Sentence Memory scaled score = 9, percentile = 37), single-word receptive vocabulary (PPVT-IV standard score = 93, percentile = 32), and ability to follow verbal directions (NEPSY-II Verbal Comprehension scaled score = 8, percentile = 25). In contrast, Mario's verbal fluency was impaired when informally assessed.

Visual-Perceptual Abilities. Despite ophthalmologic reports of age-appropriate visual acuity, Mario's visual discrimination abilities displayed during testing were well below age-level expectations at age 6 (Beery Test of Visual Perception, SS = 67, 1st percentile). At age 8, Mario's visual-perceptual skills remained in the borderline impaired range when reassessed using the Test of Visual Perceptual Skills–Third Edition [TVPS-3] (Overall: standard score = 72, percentile = 3), with comparable performance on basic visual-discrimination tasks (TVPS-3 Basic: standard score = 70, percentile = 2) and more complex visual-perceptual tasks such as visual closure (TVPS-3 Complex: standard score = 68, percentile = 1). In both assessment instances, symptoms of impulsivity appeared to compound visual-perceptual weaknesses, as Mario appeared distracted by the multiple response options. Of note, Mario had been using a laptop computer at school, and an informal assessment of visual scanning was conducted using the more familiar stimuli of a standard keyboard. On this informal task, Mario's visual search and discrimination were adequate to find letters named by the examiner.

Motor Functioning. At age 6, Mario was unable to place any pegs into a small hole with either upper extremity within a 30-second maximum time limit (Purdue Pegboard), and this task was not readministered at age 8. Performance on the Beery Developmental Test of Visual-Motor Integration–Fifth Edition (VMI-5) was well below age-level expectations at ages 6 (SS = 55, <1st percentile) and 8 (SS = 45, <1st percentile). At each administration, Mario displayed a left-hand preference and was able to produce tremulous copies of vertical and horizontal lines, but he could not produce closed circles.

Memory. At age 6, Mario's immediate recognition of familiar pictures was low average (Differential Ability Scales–Second Edition: Recognition of Pictures T-Score = 37, percentile = 10). At age 8, brief visual attention and memory continued to fall in the low average range when assessed using the Visual Memory subtest of the TVPS-III (scaled score = 7, percentile = 16).

At age 6, Mario's overall verbal recall and learning of items from a word list (Verbal Learning subtest of the Wide Range Assessment of Learning and Memory–Second Edition (WRAML-2) was solidly in the average range (scaled score = 11, percentile = 63), and delayed recall remained in the average range (ScS = 10, percentile = 50). At age 8, verbal learning efficiency remained within normal limits when assessed by way of a 15-item supraspan list-learning task (CVLT-C Trials 1–5 Total T-score = 46, percentile = 34), but spontaneous recall of these items ranged from low average to impaired following short and long delay periods, respectively (CVLT-C: Short Delay Free Recall z-score = –1, percentile = 16; Long Delay Free Recall z-score = –2, percentile = 2). Of note, Mario's performance was within normal limits when presented with a delayed multiple-choice recognition format (CVLT-C: Correct Recognition Hits z-score = 0.5, percentile = 69: Discriminability z-score = –0.5, percentile = 31).

Attention and Executive Functioning. Interestingly, multiple teacher reports obtained at age 6, acquired using the Behavior Assessment System for Children–Second Edition (BASC-2), did not suggest overt symptoms of inattention or hyperactivity at school, although parent report was clinically elevated on the BASC-2 Attention Problems scale. By age 8, however, parent report of Mario's attentional abilities was within normal limits. Qualitative discussion of this finding revealed that both home and school environments managed symptoms of inattention with one-to-one supervision, proactive scheduling of breaks into Mario's routine, and responding as needed to early indicators of fatigue. As such, the ratings provided on the BASC-2 were thought to reflect Mario's attentional functioning when comprehensive accommodations and interventions were in place.

At age 6, performance was in the borderline impaired range on measures of brief attention and memory (SB-V Nonverbal Working Memory scaled score = 5, percentile = 5; Verbal Working Memory scaled score = 4, percentile = 2). Mario's ability to modulate and direct attention was variable throughout both assessments (ages 6 and 8), and his attention was negatively impacted by his susceptibility to fatigue. Mario appeared to respond less impulsively when "fresh" from a break or rest period. After making an impulsive error, Mario would typically provide a correct answer once reminded to "slow down and work carefully." While some tests were more "forgiving" of these types of impulsive errors and spontaneous corrections (e.g., ETV-2; PPVT-IV), fatigue-related symptoms of impulsivity were thought to have a much more deleterious impact upon tests in which visual and verbal stimuli could only be presented once. With this in mind, measures of brief visual and verbal attention administered at age 8 were strategically performed at the beginning of the assessment day, with results falling within normal limits at that time (WRAML-2 Sentence Memory; TVPS-III Visual Memory).

Parental and teacher report of Mario's behavior on a checklist of symptoms of executive dysfunction at ages 6 and 8 generally resulted in scores within normal limits. Consistent at-risk or clinical elevations were noted, however, on a scale assessing cognitive flexibility, rigidity in thinking, and adaptability to transitions (BRIEF Shift scale).

Behavioral and Emotional. At age 6, parent report on the Behavior Assessment System for Children, Second Edition (BASC-2) identified at-risk to clinically significant concern on subscales assessing unusual/atypical behaviors and withdrawn behaviors. His mother indicated that Mario does not always like to play with other children, and he frequently prefers to be with adults because they are more "patient and tolerant" of his limitations. At age 8, parent report resulted in mild "at-risk" elevations on the BASC-2 Anxiety (e.g., worries about what parents think) and Somatization (e.g., complains of being sick when nothing is wrong) scales.

Discussion

Mario's birth history demonstrates a common pattern displayed in youngsters with spastic diplegia. Premature rupture of membranes at 28 weeks gestational age occurred during a key period of prenatal white matter development (i.e., 24 to 34 weeks gestation). This is a critical period of time during which oligodendrocyte progenitors and the early formation of myelin are particularly vulnerable to injury (Hoon et al., 2002; Nagae et al., 2007). The developmental course of the cystic PVL detected on ultrasound shortly after Mario's birth suggests that white matter injury occurred in the weeks prior to delivery. As in many cases of CP, it is unlikely

that an etiology of the PVL will be definitely determined, although hypoxia-ischemia/reperfusion injuries are commonly associated with the occurrence of PVL. Like most children with CP, Mario's developmental history was characterized by intensive medical monitoring, periodic surgery, and frequent therapeutic intervention.

From an assessment perspective, this case demonstrates the utility of planned follow-up assessment when assessing children with CP (Mahone & Slomine, 2008). When originally assessed at age 6 for baseline assessment using a broad-based comprehensive test battery, test results on measures of intellectual and adaptive skill functioning both fell well below age-level expectations. Qualitative observations made throughout the assessment suggested that fatigue, motor limitations, and articulation difficulties all detracted from Mario's test performance at that time. While useful for demonstrating the deleterious impact of these variables upon cognitive functioning (and possibly academic functioning), tests results obtained at age 6 were also considered to be an underestimate of his ability. As such, much of the report summary was dedicated to explaining why Mario did not meet criteria for intellectual disability, and why he might perform higher than test scores might indicate if efforts were made to manage his fatigue, motor issues, and articulation difficulties in the school setting.

In contrast, the planned follow-up assessment performed at age 8 was designed to demonstrate Mario's neurocognitive abilities when appropriate accommodations were proactively introduced. In this case, accommodations included shortening of test battery length, reduction of articulation and motor requirements, presentation of more difficult attentional tasks in the morning when Mario was more rested, and provision of frequent breaks. Using this approach, there was a greater level of confidence that fatigue effects were well managed and that test performance was a valid indicator of Mario's neuropsychological strengths and weaknesses. This proved to be a useful approach to testing for school planning purposes, as it provided additional confirmation of the IEP team's decision to maintain Mario in a mainstream classroom (given evidence of age-appropriate verbal reasoning and receptive language skills) but also provided support for ongoing and/or new accommodation strategies as well.

Mario's case example also demonstrates several additional assessment-related issues for children with CP, including the importance of informal assessment of functional skills and considerations of "real-world" functioning. For instance, documentation of adaptive skill deficits using measures such as the ABAS-II is an important component of assessment, but specific test content may not be sensitive to adaptive skill gains made by children with CP over time. In Mario's case, qualitative parent report suggested an expansion of environmental management and domestic skills (e.g., noticing trash/debris and verbally requesting for its disposal) even though formal parent response continued to indicate that Mario "never" picks up/cleans up after himself. While formal demonstration (i.e., standard scores) of deficits remained necessary to justify multidisciplinary treatment delivery and funding, qualitative description of adaptive and/or cognitive skill gains were considered equally necessary for an ecologically valid assessment of emerging strengths and abilities.

Similarly, we found it useful to consider the realities of Mario's day-to-day functioning when determining actual "abilities" and the importance of formal test findings. While results from the VMI-5 indicated graphomotor deficits that severely limited handwriting, it was our impression that Mario's potential for generating written language would be better predicted by observations regarding his ability to visually scan a keyboard and manipulate a joystick. Once the graphomotor deficit was apparent and related suggestions were made (e.g., 8 x 16 inch wide-lined paper, adapted pencils, wrist weights), the focus of our recommendations could shift to a problem-solving approach in which unconventional approaches could be explored to circumvent the graphomotor difficulty (e.g., informal assessment of keyboard scanning and activation, referral for assistive technology).

From a neuropsychological perspective, Mario's birth history is noteworthy for PVL as well as several additional prematurity-related risk factors often associated with later neurocognitive difficulties, including male gender (Johnson & Breslau, 2000). Several important risk factors linked with prematurity and CP were *not*, however, present in Mario's prenatal and postnatal history, including birth weight <750 grams

(Taylor, Klein, Drotar, Schluchter, & Hack, 2006), seizure disorder (Fenell & Dikel, 2001), bronchopulmonary dysplasia, and/or extended postnatal oxygen requirements (Short et al., 2003; Singer, Yamashita, Lilien, Collin, & Baley, 1997). Herein lies much of the difficulty inherent in predicting cognitive and academic outcomes in children with CP, as various combinations of pre-, peri-, and postnatal risk factors are thought to result in heterogeneity of the neuropsychological profile, even when commonalities in motor presentation may be apparent.

In this case, Mario clearly displayed evidence of visual-perceptual deficits. In terms of specific neuropsychological functions, deficits in visuospatial skills are some of the most frequently cited weaknesses associated with CP (Fazzi et al., 2004). Kozeis and colleagues (2007) noted that most of the children participating in their CP study had immature visual perception skills relative to their age. Specifically, the sample from the Kozeis study performed worse than anticipated on tasks of spatial relationships, visual discrimination, figure-ground perception, visual closure, and visual memory. Fazzi and colleagues (2004) postulated that these types of visual perceptual deficits might occur secondary to disruption of occipital–parietal connections in the "dorsal" visual pathways.

In the case of Mario, visual-perceptual deficits were associated with compelling evidence of disruption of posterior brain systems offered by emerging DTI technology. Specifically, severe abnormalities or complete absence of bidirectional thalamo-cortical (parietal/occipital) fibers such as the postthalamic radiations were detected, as well as severe disruption of the posterior corpus callosum. While this will require further investigation, fiber-tracking methods available via DTI may prove useful for further delineating the injury-related underpinnings of visual-perceptual deficits in children with CP, and they may eventually provide a clinical means for anticipating visual-perceptual difficulties and related need for intervention/accommodations.

With the growing body of evidence suggestive of PVL-related damage to white matter systems that support visual-perceptual abilities, it has become critical that these skills be routinely assessed in children with CP. In the case of Mario, visual perceptual deficits were observed despite recent ophthalmologic assessment indicating "near 20/20 vision" as well as low average range performance on a matrix reasoning task. Stiers and colleagues (2002) noted that, in children with CP, deficits in visuospatial skills are commonly overshadowed by concurrent deficits in (or intact performance on measures of) nonverbal reasoning. While the Stiers et al. cohort of children with CP had generally average-range performance on tasks of nonverbal reasoning, approximately 40% demonstrated additional impairments on at least one task of visuospatial skills. As the functional implications of visual-perceptual deficits are potentially large in children with reduced motor functioning, it is our opinion that comprehensive visual-perceptual assessment should be a central component to the neuropsychological assessment of children with CP. In Mario's case, the test findings helped support the introduction of accommodations designed to assist Mario in his visual analysis of information. For instance, Mario's school team began to magnify his math worksheets using a photocopier, and subsequently they cut the assignment sheets in half vertically in order to reduce both the amount and complexity of visual information being presented.

Finally, Mario demonstrated a high degree of variable attention during assessments performed at ages 6 and 8. While parent and teacher ratings did not indicate overt problems with attention in Mario's day-to-day functioning, conversations with Mario's mother suggested that many of the existing difficulties with sustained attention at home and school were already being addressed by the individualized interventions provided by the one-to-one school and home-health aide. Discussion regarding parent responses on the BRIEF also suggested that potential initiation or organizational issues might be masked by the level of directional support provided by the one-to-one aide. Observing Mario when the familiar routine and behavioral cues of the one-to-one aide were not available allowed the assessors to document the persistence of these attention problems and to provide additional justification for maintaining this effective intervention service. As test results also suggested features of social avoidance and anxiety, recommendations for the one-to-one aide were provided to help in addressing both attentional and social issues while simultaneously reducing Mario's overall level of dependence upon this high level of intervention (e.g., those

recommendations proposed in Zabel, Gray, Gardner, & Ackerman, 2005).

Variable attention and executive dysfunction have been documented in several studies involving children with CP (McDonough & Cohen, 1982). Of note, Christ and colleagues (2003) identified deficits on tasks of inhibitory control in a cohort of children with bilateral spastic CP and postulated that damage to prefrontal white matter tracts secondary to perinatal injury underlie the observed deficits. While overt abnormality was not observed in DTI reconstruction of Mario's frontal white matter, severe structural abnormality was observed in the superior longitudinal fasciculus (SLF). As recent evidence suggests a possible role of SLF abnormalities in disorders of attention (Hamilton et al., 2008; Makris et al., 2008), further investigation will be necessary to determine whether abnormalities of the SLF or nearby fibers connecting posterior and temporal/frontal brain systems underlie attentional difficulties in children with CP.

In conclusion, the neuropsychological assessment of children with CP requires a careful balance of assessment emphases. Comprehensive assessment can document areas of deficit and need for rehabilitation and intervention but also holds considerable potential for the underestimation of ability in this population. Targeted assessment with accommodations, process observations, and informal assessment techniques are often also necessary in order to document areas of intact ability and areas of growth over time. In our opinion, careful assessment design is an essential step in ensuring that a clinically useful picture of both the abilities and treatment/accommodation needs of children with CP emerges from neuropsychological assessment.

References

Christ, S. E., White, D. A., Brunstrom, J. E., & Abrams, R. A. (2003). Inhibitory control following perinatal brain injury. *Neuropsychology, 17*(1), 171–178.

Fazzi, E., Bova, S. M., Uggetti, C., Signorini, S. G., Bianchi, P. E., Maraucci, I., Zoppello, M., & Lanzi, G. (2004). Visual–perceptual impairment in children with periventricular leukomalacia. *Brain and Development, 26*, 506–512.

Fennell, I. P., & Dikel, T. N. (2001). Cognitive and neuropsychological functioning in children with cerebral palsy. *Journal of Child Neurology, 16*, 58–63.

Hamilton, L. S., Levitt, J. G., O'Neill, J., Alger, J. R., Luders, E., Phillips, O. R., Caplan, R., Toga, A. W., McCracken, J., & Narr, K. L. (2008). Reduced white matter integrity in attention-deficit hyperactivity disorder. *Neuroreport, 19*(17), 1705–1708.

Hoon, A. H., Lawrie, W. T., Melhem, E. R., Reinhardt, E. M., van Zijl, P. C. M., Solaiyappan, M., Jiang, H., Johnston, M. V., & Mori, S. (2002). Diffusion tensor imaging of PVL shows affected sensory cortex white matter pathways. *Neurology, 59*, 752–756.

Johnson E. O. & Breslau, N. (2000). Increased risk of learning disabilities in low birth weight boys at age 11 years. *Biological Psychiatry, 47*(6), 490–500.

Johnson, M. W., Hoon, A. H., & Kaufmann, W. E. (2008). Neurobiology, diagnosis, and management of cerebral palsy. In P. J. Accardo (Ed.), Capute & Accardo's neurodevelopmental disabilities in infancy and childhood: Volume II: The spectrum of neurodevelopmental disabilities (3rd ed., pp. 61-81). Baltimore: Paul H. Brookes Publishing.

Johnston, M. V. (1998). Selective vulnerability in the neonatal brain. *Annals of Neurology, 44*, 155–156.

Korzeniewski, S. J., Birbeck, G., DeLano, M. C., Potchen, M. J., & Paneth, N. (2008). A systematic review of neuroimaging for cerebral palsy. *Journal of Child Neurology, 23*(2), 216–227.

Kozeis, N., Anogeianaki, A., Mitova, D. T., Anogianakis, G., Mitov, T., & Klisarova, A. (2007). Visual function and visual perception in cerebral palsied children. *Opthalmic Physiology, 27*, 44–53.

Krageloh-Mann, I., & Horber, V. (2007). The role of magnetic resonance imaging in elucidating the pathogenesis of cerebral palsy: a systematic review. *Developmental Medicine and Child Neurology, 49*, 144–151.

Mahone, E. M., & Slomine, B. S. (2008). Neurodevelopmental disorders. In J. E. Morgan & J. H. Ricker (Eds), *Textbook of clinical neuropsychology* (pp. 105-127). New York: Taylor & Francis.

Makris, N., Buka, S. L., Biederman, J., Papadimitriou, G. M., Hodge, S. M., Valera, E. M., Brown, A. B., Bush, G., Monuteaux, M. C., Caviness, V. S., Kennedy, D. N., & Seidman, L. J. (2008). Attention and executive systems abnormalities in adults with childhood ADHD: A DT-MRI study of connections. *Cerebral Cortex, 18*(5), 1210–1220.

McDonough, S. C., & Cohen, L. B. (1982). Attention and memory in cerebral palsified infants. *Infant Behavior and Development, 5*, 347–353.

Menkes, J. H., & Sarnat, H. B. (2000). Perinatal asphyxia and trauma. In J. H. Menkes & H. B. Sarnat (Eds.), *Child Neurology* (pp. 401-466). Philadelphia: Lippincott, Williams and Wilkins.

Nagae, L. M., Hoon, A. H., Stashinko, E., Lin, D., Zhang, W., Levey, E., Wakana, S., Jiang, H., Leite, C. C., Lucato, L. T., van Zijl, P. C., Johnston, M. V., & Mori, S. (2007). Diffusion tensor imaging in children with periventricular leukomalacia: Variability of injuries to white matter tracts. *American Journal of Neuroradiology, 28*, 1213–1222.

Nelson, K.B., & Ellenberg, J.H. (1986). Antecedents of cerebral palsy: Multivariate analysis of risk. *New England Journal of Medicine, 315*, 81–86.

Pirila, S., van der Meere, J., Korhonen, P., Ruusu-Niemi, P., Kyntaja, M., Nieminen, P., & Korpela, R. (2004). A retrospective neurocognitive study in children with spastic diplegia. *Developmental Neuropsychology, 26*(3), 679–690.

Pueyo, R., Junque, C., Vendrell, A., Narberhaus, A., & Segarra, D. (2008). Raven's Coloured Progressive Matrices as a measure of cognitive functioning in cerebral palsy. *Journal of Intellectual Disability Research, 52*(5), 437–445.

Short, E. J., Klein, N. K., Lewis, B. A., Fulton, S., Eisengart, S., Kercsmar, C., Baley, J., & Singer, L. T. (2003). Cognitive and academic consequences of bronchopulmonary dysplasia and very low birth weight: 8-year-old outcomes. *Pediatrics, 112*(5), e359.

Sigurdardottir, S., Eiriksdottir, A., Gunnarsdottir, E., Meintema, M., Arnadottir, U., & Vik, T. (2008). Cognitive profile in young Icelandic children with cerebral palsy. *Developmental Medicine and Child Neurology, 50*, 357–362.

Singer, L., Yamshita, T., Lilien, L., Collin, M., & Baley, J. (1997). A longitudinal study of developmental outcome of infants with bronchopulmonary dysplasia and very low birth weight. *Pediatrics, 100*(6), 987–993.

Stiers, P., Vanderkelen, R., Vanneste, G., Coene, S., De Rammelaere, M., & Vandenbussche, E. (2002)#. Visual-perceptual impairment in a random sample of children with cerebral palsy. *Developmental Medicine and Child Neurology, 44*, 370–382.

Taylor, H. G., Klein, N., Drotar, D., Schluchter, M., & Hack, M. (2006). Consequences and risks of <1000-g birth weight for neuropsychological skills, achievement, and adaptive functioning. *Journal of Development and Behavioral Pediatrics, 27*(6), 459–469.

Zabel, T. A., Gray, R. M., Gardner, J., & Ackerman, J. (2005). Use of school-based one-to-one aides for children following traumatic brain injury: A proposed practice model. *Physical Disabilities: Education and Related Services, 24*(1), 5–22.

9

Sickle Cell Disease

Karen E. Wills

Sickle cell disease (SCD) is a recessive genetic difference in the gene for globin, part of the hemoglobin (Hb) molecule within red blood cells, which carries oxygen throughout the body (Wang, 2007). It can occur in any population but is most prevalent in people of African and Caribbean descent, including about 70,000 Americans or roughly 1 in 350 African American newborns. The "S" hemoglobin variant has adaptive value in tropical countries because heterozygous SCD trait (the "carrier" status) conveys some resistance to malaria, if joined with typical hemoglobin (Hb-A). Sickle cell trait is not consistently associated with neuropsychological risk, but it does convey increased risk of cardiovascular stenosis and thrombotic stroke among adults (Tsaras, Owusu-Ansah, Boateng, & Amoateng-Adjepong, 2009). The Hb-AS *trait* occurs among 1 in 10 African Americans, but it is much more common in some parts of Africa (occurring among 1 in 25 Nigerians, for example). With increasing migration of people around the world, the prevalence of SCD in the Americas and Europe has increased (Michlitsch, Azimi, Hoppe, Walters, Lubin, et al., 2009; Modell, Darlison, Birgens, Cario, Faustino, et al., 2007).

There are many other hemoglobin variants that can combine with the recessive Hb-S to produce one of the sickle cell diseases (Hb-SS, Hb-SC, Hb-SE, etc.). Different haplotypes are associated with particular profiles of health risk, in part because they produce different proportions of sickled to normal red blood cells. Children with Hb-SS or Hb-S-beta-zero-thalassemia

may have 90% or more of sickled cells in their blood, whereas others (e.g., Hb-SC or Hb-S forms with persistent fetal hemoglobin) have a smaller proportion of sickled cells to normal red blood cells In general, a higher count of sickled blood cells, compared to normal cells, is associated with more severe biomedical complications of SCD. Hb-SS (sickle cell alleles transmitted from both parents) is a high-risk condition in which more than 90% of red blood cells transform to the sickled state. Hb-S-beta-zero-thalassemia also is associated with high risk of vaso-occlusion, particularly acute chest syndrome and pulmonary hypertension (sickle cell obstruction of blood supply to the lungs, causing serious respiratory problems). These patients also are prone to developing bone necrosis in hip and shoulder joints as they move into adulthood. Hb-SC disease (in which one parent contributed the Hb-C allele, and the other an Hb-S) typically has milder complications because only about 50% of red blood cells transform to the sickled state. Hb-S-Beta-plus-thalassemia also tends to be relatively benign. Persisting fetal hemoglobin (PFH, or Hb-F) is a blood anomaly that can occur with any of the sickle cell haplotypes. Fetal hemoglobin provides some protection against SCD complications by interfering with the sickling process; the most effective medication for SCD, hydroxyurea, works by increasing fetal hemoglobin in patients who do not have naturally occurring PFH.

Genetic counseling for African Americans concerned about transmission of SCD typically involves just a simple blood test for presence of sickled cells. It is not very reliable, and it can miss other hemoglobin anomalies that combine with Hb-S to produce one of the serious sickle cell disease variants. Therefore, patients need to be aware of the other genetic subtypes and obtain the more extensive blood tests for Hb-C and beta-thalassemia, in order to make more informed reproductive and newborn screening decisions. There also is need for better counseling about personal health and genetic transmission risks for individuals with Hb-SA sickle cell trait (Michlitsch et al., 2009). Sensitivity to historical, cultural, sociodemographic, racial, and ethnic issues associated with SCD is essential in designing clinical services and research studies (Gustafson, Gettig, Watt-Morse, & Krishnamurti, 2007; Hill, 2003; Neal-Cooper & Scott, 1988; Thompson, 2006).

Sickled cells break down within 10 to 20 days, in contrast to 120 days for normal red blood cells. Thus, sickled cells break down faster than they can be replaced, leading to chronic hemolytic anemia. Sickled cells carry oxygen less efficiently than normal red blood cells, and their more rigid, sticky membranes adhere to vascular endothelium, constricting blood flow. Vaso-occlusive events cause episodes of severe acute pain, chronic aching pain, compensatory increases in blood flow producing pulmonary hypertension (in 40% of patients; Nelson, Adade, McDonough, Moquist, & Hennessey, 2007), and increased cerebrovascular pressure with a greatly increased risk of cerebrovascular ischemia and stroke (Wang, 2007).

Vaso-occlusive pain events commonly are triggered by dehydration, fever, emotional or physical stress, chilling, or sudden changes of body temperature; hence, careful self-management may reduce the frequency of pain events, though it rarely eliminates them completely. Pain events requiring hospitalization are most common in early childhood but continue to average about 1 per year throughout adolescence, typically lasting a few days, usually involving the limbs, back, and abdomen. Priapism (prolonged painful erection), common in adolescence, is embarrassing as well as intensely painful. Pain episodes cause increased school absences; even when children return to school, medications used to manage pain can cause drowsiness and distractibility.

There are lifelong challenges involving nutrition and growth. Children with SCD have to constantly make new red blood cells, expending increased energy and nutrients. Therefore, children may eat a lot yet still feel hungry, and they may remain small for age. Pica (chewing and eating nonfood objects) occurs more commonly among children with SCD than in the general population, though it is unclear whether this is consistently related to nutritional deficiencies (Ivascu, Sarnaik, McCrae, Whitten-Shurney, Thomas, et al., 2001). Short stature, delayed growth, and delayed onset of puberty (by 2 years or more, on average) often are stressful for adolescents and may warrant treatment with growth hormone in adolescence (Wang, 2007). Persistent enuresis is of major concern to youth with SCD, who must stay hydrated to avoid sickling crises, but whose kidneys do not concentrate urine normally (Field, Austin, An, Yan, & DeBaun, 2008). It is not uncommon to find 18-year-old patients worrying that their enuresis will prevent adult intimate relationships. Anecdotally, this problem does not seem to respond well to a standard urine alarm protocol, but controlled studies are lacking.

Managing asthma is particularly important among children and adolescents with SCD because asthma is a significant risk factor for pulmonary hypertension (Nelson et al., 2007) and acute chest syndrome (Boyd, Macklin, Strunk, & DeBaun, 2006); the latter, in turn, is a risk factor for cerebrovascular stroke (Henderson, Noetzel, McKistry, White, Armstrong, & DeBaun, 2003). Acute chest syndrome involves severe pain and oxygen deprivation due to acutely diminished blood flow in the lungs. Pulmonary hypertension (PHT; increased blood pressure in the lungs), which develops to compensate for hypoxia, is a primary cause of death among people with SCD. At less severe levels, PHT contributes to diminished stamina and endurance in sports or physical education, and is associated with neuropsychological impairment (Boyd et al.,2006; Nelson et al., 2007).

At present, there is no risk-free treatment, and no cure, for sickle cell disease. The most promising treatment currently is hydroxyurea, a medication that inhibits sickling and improves cognitive function in children with SCD, but some parents refuse to try it because of the slight increased risk of hematologic cancer (Brawley, Cornelius, Edwards, Gamble, Green, et al., 2008; Puffer, Schatz, & Roberts, 2007). Children with evidence of subclinical stroke who continue to show abnormal cerebral blood flow on TCD screening, together with neuropsychological impairment, may be placed on a chronic blood transfusion protocol (Mazumdar, Heeney, Sox, & Lieu, 2007). Chronic transfusion can cause iron overload, with serious health consequences. In the most severe cases, the child may be referred for bone marrow or stem cell transplant, which can cure SCD but carries high risk of morbidity and mortality (Wang, 2007).

Neuropsychological functioning in children and youth with SCD is affected by their history of chronic anemia, and of cerebrovascular ischemia and infarct (strokes), with specific cognitive and behavioral characteristics related to the size and location of the infarction (Schatz, White, Moinuddin, Armstrong, & DeBaun, 2002). From 10%–15% of children with HbSS will have overt strokes by age 15; another 20%–25% will have "silent strokes"; still more may sustain white matter microinfarct damage not easily measured by current standard neuroimaging (Wang, 2007). Problems with attention, speed of processing, learning and memory, and executive function commonly result; overall IQ and achievement were below those of siblings in the comprehensive center studies (Berkelhammer, Williamson, Sanford, Dirksen, Sharp, et al., 2007; Schatz, Brown, Pascual, Hsu, & DeBaun, 2001), although for most patients, IQ and academic achievement scores were in the average range (Berkelhammer et al., 2007; Wills, Nelson, Nwaneri, & SCD-PLANE Program Team, 2008).

The case presented in this chapter was chosen to illustrate a moderately severe level of neuropsychological impairment due to SCD. It should be emphasized, however, that there is a very wide range of variation in disease characteristics and functional outcome among individuals with SCD. Variation results from individual differences in biomedical and psychosocial characteristics, as discussed in the context of this case (see also Rennie & Panepinto, 2008).

Case Report

Reason for Referral

Troy is an almost-12-year-old, right-handed African American boy with Hb-SS disease, referred by his hematologist to evaluate neurosychological functioning in relation to his history of sickle cell disease (Hb-SS type, ICD 282.60) and associated cerebrovascular disease (ICD 437.1).

Relevant Background

Troy was adopted at 3 weeks following slightly premature birth and diagnosis of sickle cell disease. He was born to a teenage mother who reportedly had adequate prenatal care, with no suspicion of any prenatal substance exposure or major maternal illnesses. Early motor and speech milestones were attained at expected ages. He has had several subclinical strokes including pervasive white matter damage associated with high fever in 2000, at about age 4 years, which resulted in complete unilateral left ear hearing loss. Brain magnetic resonance imaging (MRI) and magnetic resonance angiography (MRA) have documented patchy white matter changes with no progression, but no improvement or resolution of existing damage, since about 2004 (Figure 9.1).

Troy had just completed fifth grade when he was seen for neuropsychological screening in the SCD-PLANE program.[1] He had undergone extensive previous testing, including comprehensive neuropsychological evaluation in 2006 (age 10, grade 4) and a psycheducational evaluation at school in November 2005 (age 9, grade 3). He had an individualized education plan (IEP) in school under the Other Health Disability and Deaf/Hard of Hearing eligibility categories, with goals to improve reading, writing, and math skills and to

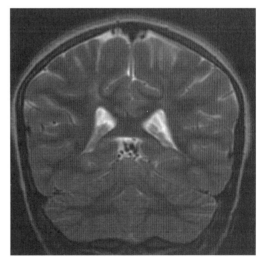

Figure 9-1. Lacunar infarcts in white matter of a 9-year-old boy with sickle cell disease (magnetic resonance image without contrast, T2 coronal image, 2005).

enhance his self-advocacy related to unilateral hearing loss.

Troy was adopted in early infancy by college-educated, English-speaking parents of mixed racial/ethnic heritage who have two biological and three other adopted children, also of a variety of racial/ethnic backgrounds. Troy's father is a clergyman, and his mother is a homemaker. The family is particularly attuned to issues of disability awareness, adoption issues, and tolerance and appreciation of diversity. Parents have provided strong advocacy for Troy's inclusion and, as needed, for support, in his schooling and leisure activities.

Behavioral Observations

Troy presented as a handsome, well-groomed, courteous, cheerful, well-motivated boy. Within this quiet, one-to-one setting with few visual or noise distractions, his unilateral hearing loss did not appear to pose any problems of understanding and responding to test questions. He does not wear any hearing aid. Tests were administered as standardized. Given Troy's good effort and cooperation, the test findings are considered a reliable estimate of functioning in the areas assessed. The present test findings are based on brief outpatient clinic screening (90-minute test battery) but are consistent with findings of the comprehensive neuropsychological evaluation completed 1 year prior to this testing.

Impressions

Average expectations, based on child's age: On all of the tests reported below, unless otherwise noted, all scores are reported as scaled scores (average = 10 ± 2, so the average range is about *8 to 12* points), or as Standard Scores (average = 100 ± 10, so the average range is about *90 to 110* points). The summary of scores, and explanation of test name acronyms, is shown in Table 9.1.

General intellectual functioning is average. Troy's scores are consistent with previous testing showing age-appropriate verbal and nonverbal

Table 9-1. Troy's 2007 Test Score Summary: SCD-PLANE Neuropsychological Screening

Tests Administered/Acronyms

EVT2	Expressive Vocabulary Test, 2nd Ed. (Williams, 2007)
CTOPP	Comprehensive Test of Phonological Processing (Wagner, Torgeson, & Rashotte, 1999)
DKEFS	Delis-Kaplan Executive Function Scales (Delis, Kaplan, & Kramer, 2001)
WISC-IV	Wechsler Intelligence Scales for Children, 4th Ed. (Wechsler, 2003)
WASI	Wechsler Abbreviated Scales of Intelligence (Wechsler, 1999)
WRAML	Wide Range Assessment of Memory and Learning (Adams & Sheslow, 2003)
VMI	Visual-Motor Integration Test (Beery, Buktenica, & Beery, 2006)
WJ3	Woodcock-Johnson Test of Academic Achievement, 3rd Ed. (Woodcock, McGrew, & Mather
BASC2	(2001)
BRIEF	Behavior Assessment System for Children, 2nd Ed. (Reynolds & Kamphaus, 2002)
	Behavior Rating Inventory of Executive Function (Gioia, Isquith, Guy, & Kenworthy, 2000).

Obtained Scores (Average SS range = 100 ± 15; average SS range = 10 ± 3).

Vocabulary (EVT2)	SS
Picture Naming	99
Naming Fluency (CTOPP Rapid Naming)	SS
Objects	5
Colors	9
Letters	7
Numbers	7
Verbal Fluency (DKEFS Semantic and Phonemic Fluency)	SS
Semantic	13
Phonemic	8

Table 9-1. Troy's 2007 Test Score Summary: SCD-PLANE Neuropsychological Screening (*Continued*)

Attention & Working Memory (WISC-IV Digit Span)	SS
Digits Forward	7
Digits Backward	8
Verbal Repetition (WRAML Immediate Memory)	SS
Sentence Recall	5
Story Recall	11
Verbal Memorization (WRAML List Learning)	SS
List Learning	11
Verbal Problem-Solving (DKEFS Twenty Questions)	SS
Twenty Questions	14
Visual-Spatial Reasoning (WASI Matrix Reasoning)	SS
Matrix Reasoning	9
Visual-Motor Construction (VMI Design Copying)	SS
Design Copying	73
Visual-Motor Processing Speed (WISC-IV Coding)	SS
Coding	5
Academic Fluency (TOWRE and WJ3)	SS
TOWRE Sight Words	91
TOWRE Pseudowords	75
WJ3 Reading Fluency	78
WJ3 Math Fluency	72
Motor dexterity and speed (Purdue Pegboard)	SS
Right hand (10 pegs)	55
Left hand (12 pegs)	82
Both hands (10 pegs)	76

SS, standard score.

reasoning abilities. Average scores on the WASI Matrix Reasoning (9) and EVT-2 (99) were consistent with his good ability to generate thoughtful abstract guesses on the D-KEFS Twenty Questions subtest.

Social, behavioral, and emotional adjustment are generally positive. Like most children with sickle cell disease, Troy has more medical concerns, physical pain, and discomfort than children in the general population, resulting in a high score for somatic complaints (BASC-2 T-score = 65; 91st percentile). His parents and teachers do not indicate concerns about mood or conduct, or general adjustment, nor did Troy express any concerns in this brief screening interview.

Parents and teachers express significant concern about inattention, poor working memory, and disorganization. On the BASC-2 parent report, completed by his father, Troy's score for "Attention Problems" is at the lower edge of the clinically significant range (T = 68; 95th percentile compared to same-age boys), suggesting con-

cerns about his ability to focus and sustain concentration. The scores for adaptive functioning are in the average, age-appropriate range except that his father rates Troy as somewhat more disorganized and less self-directed, needing more prompting or reminders than most boys his age (Activities of Daily Living, T = 30; 3rd percentile). On the BRIEF, completed by Troy's father, there is no indication of any problem with impulsivity, inflexibility, or emotional dyscontrol. Troy shows good social awareness, respect for others, and respect for his own and others' possessions. Ratings are clinically problematic on scales of initiating (coming up with an effective approach to solving complex problems, or getting started with tasks); working memory (keeping track of the details while working toward a goal; remembering to do things); and planning/organization (carrying out tasks in a systematic, step-by-step, efficient manner without losing sight of the goal or getting sidetracked). The composite indices for Metacognitive (planning, organization, and study skills) and for General Executive Function are in the clinically significant problem range.

On formal testing, Troy had more difficulty than most children his age when he had to inhibit a well-practiced, automatic reaction, in order to respond in a new or different way. For example, he made a very high number of self-corrected errors on DKEFS color-word inhibition (naming the color of ink in which a color-name is printed, e.g., saying "RED" for the word "blue" printed in red ink). He almost always noticed and corrected his own mistakes, as soon as he made an error; parents and teachers say this is characteristic of Troy in his daily schoolwork. He did not display frustration during testing; but in daily life, he often becomes frustrated because he catches himself making so many mistakes. He is beginning to call himself "stupid" on occasion, his mother says.

Impaired word retrieval (dysnomia) was evident during testing, though less so during informal conversation. Troy struggles to "call to mind" words to label what he sees, even when trying to recall very familiar words such as "key" or "chair" (CTOPP object-naming = 5). He was slower than average on all of the naming tasks, although he had somewhat less difficulty naming symbols that are part of a limited set of words (numbers, letters, and colors) than naming pictures. He did very well with generating a list of items within a meaningful category (e.g., animal names), in contrast to his difficulty with naming a specific object or generating words that begin with a particular letter-sound.

Memory span is normal, but Troy's memorization process is disorganized and inefficient. On the WRAML-2, Troy remembered a normal amount of information from a story or from an unordered list of words (like a shopping list). However, he recalled the information in a haphazard, disorganized way. He repeated story elements out of order, and after a 20-minute delay, he confused elements from the two different stories when recounting them again. He also demonstrated impaired working memory for precise, sequenced information. For example, Troy scored below average on tests of memory for an ordered list of numbers, repeated in either forward or backward order (WISC-4 Digit Span), as well as on a test of word-for-word Sentence Repetition (WRAML-2).

Troy's reading and math skills are markedly deficient, including poor phonological awareness and phonemic processing, as well as slow, inaccurate recall of math facts. Troy's sight-word recognition speed and accuracy were average, but he was very hesitant when sounding out nonsense syllables on the TOWRE. He simplified consonant blends (e.g. "chur" became "cur") and mispronounced vowels unsystematically (ig became "aieg," ni = "nee," fet = "foot"). On his first attempt to read the list quickly, Troy repeatedly slipped into saying a real word that resembled the nonsense word, as if forgetting the rule that "none of these are real words." Retesting after reminding him not to say any "real words" did not improve his score, however. On the WJ3, his performance was very slow on tests of timed reading fluency (understanding short sentences = 75) and timed recall of math facts (math fluency = 72). His scores correspond to the average performance of a typical third-grade student from the WJ3 test standardization sample, whereas Troy has just completed the fifth grade.

Phonological processing skills associated with fluent reading appear underdeveloped, as shown by Troy's difficulty on TOWRE phonemic decoding and DKEFS phonemic verbal fluency. That is, he has limited appreciation for speech sounds, with poor ability to break apart a word into its component sounds and rearrange them to form a different word (e.g., understanding that the three sounds in "tack," "T/A/K," reverse the sounds of "C/A/T"). He did not show automatic mastery of the alphabet letter sequence, on DKEFS Trailmaking, making errors in the "LMNOP" central section of the alphabet. This is a common mistake in the early grades but rare for Troy's age group. He had trouble shifting flexibly back and forth between the alphabet and the number series, to track the sequence "1-A-2-B-3-C..." and so on.

Troy demonstrates average visual-spatial perception and analysis, but poor visual-motor coordination and slow motor speed for drawing, copying, handwriting, and object manipulation. Troy did well with analysis of fine visual details on the WASI Matrix Reasoning test, and with visual scanning and motor speed on the D-KEFS Trailmaking tasks. He scored poorly on the VMI test of design copying, which requires planning and organizing spatial relationships among design elements. There was no sign of tremor (shaky hands) or ataxia (unsteady aim). His handwriting on WJ3 Math Fluency and WISC-4 Coding was large and awkward for his age.

Troy made no errors in copying the WISC-IV Coding symbols, but he was slow to complete this subtest, a timed, repetitive paper-and-pencil task that requires graphomotor speed and accuracy. His visual-motor speed was extremely slow for his age on the Purdue Pegboard for his dominant right hand (55), and below average for the nondominant left hand (82) and for both hands used simultaneously (76).

Summary and Recommendations

Across several evaluations, in the hospital and at school, Troy has demonstrated normal intelligence and memory for familiar, meaningful information, as well as positive social-emotional adjustment. He is beginning to make occasional self-disparaging remarks when frustrated by homework, however, suggesting that Troy's self-esteem and mood may be challenged by the struggle to adapt to increasingly difficult schoolwork and more complex peer relationships as he moves into puberty. Troy consistently has shown clinically significant problems with the following:

1. *Poor graphomotor and fine motor control (handwriting, drawing, copying, manipulating objects).* When younger, Troy benefited from occupational therapy support for penmanship, but this is unlikely to help him succeed in the upper grades. Therefore, current recommendations include increased use of assistive technology (training in keyboarding and voice-to-text technology), decreased demands for unnecessary writing (e.g., copying assignments), tutoring in brief (keyword) note-taking skills, access to teachers' or peers' lecture notes, and extended time to complete tests and written assignments.
2. *Poor concentration, working memory, and ability to divide or shift attention, contributing to poor recall of precise, sequenced information and disorganized recall of narratives (stories, lectures).* Recommendations include considering a trial of low-dose stimulant medication,

which has been helpful (anecdotally) for some children with attentional lapses and slow speed of processing associated with white matter damage from SCD, although the benefit must be weighed against any risk from slightly increased blood pressure. Cognitive remediation strategies, including coaching in memory and executive function strategies, lack empirical support but anecdotally seem to benefit some children (White et al., 2006).

3. *Mild dysnomia (word retrieval difficulty), meaning that Troy often struggles to "call to mind" words or facts that he knows.* Recommendations include teaching him circumlocution strategies, providing a "multiple-choice" question, and waiting longer for Troy to reply to questions.
4. *Slower than average "speed of processing," in general; that is, the pace or tempo of his speech, movement, thought, and action all tend to be slower than average.* He takes more time to formulate his ideas and to express them verbally or in writing. When called on in class, he will need a little more time to answer; he may look blank for a few seconds, even when he has studied and knows the material. Extended time, providing assignments in advance, shortening assignments as possible, and allowing oral rather than written completion of certain assignments will help him keep up with classwork.
5. *Deficient academic achievement.* Currently, Troy has very low scores for Reading Fluency and Math Fluency, as well as poor phonemic decoding on the TOWRE; in October 2005, he had very low scores for Writing Fluency (63) and below-average accuracy on paper-and-pencil math computation (83). More extensive academic achievement testing, done at school in fourth grade, showed that Troy's mastery of basic academic skills was in the low average range for his age and grade placement, with no discrepancy between tested IQ and composite achievement test scores. He had done adequately well with few educational accommodations in the early elementary grades, but his very slow processing speed impeded success in the upper elementary grades, as the volume and complexity of assignments increased. Thus, academic recommendations focused on strengthening his

mastery of phonemically based reading skills, a weakness that may have been associated with his unilateral hearing loss rather than with SCD issues per se, as well as on accommodating and compensating for his slow tempo, variable attention, and poor graphomotor control. Other standard SCD-PLANE

recommendations for school programming are shown in Table 9.2.

Discussion

For infants and preschoolers with SCD, infectious illness is the most serious risk to health and

Table 9-2. Standard SCD-PLANE Recommendations for School-Based Accommodations

Anticipate brief unplanned absences. Allow a higher number of school interruptions for health reasons. Arrange to communicate with parents/student about assignments and missed lectures or tests; if it is a short absence, arrange a time for student to work with teacher or aide to make up missed information without penalty. If it is more than a few days, arrange for someone to work with the student at home, or send home missed information. Extend deadlines for assignments and tests. Keep an extra set of books at home.

Allow for decreased stamina. Adjust physical education expectations and grades to reflect decreased stamina, energy, or endurance. Some students might need to use a wheeled backpack, keep heavy books in the classroom, have more time to pass between classes, or other accommodations if class-to-class transitions are physically demanding.

Manage temperature extremes that can trigger SCD pain crises. Provide protection from exposure to extreme temperatures (weather); bus pick-up in front of home, and alternative plan for recess or P.E., on cold or windy days; and avoid sudden extreme temperature changes (e.g., running into cold weather from a warm room; jumping into a cold pool).

Avoid dehydration that can trigger SCD pain events. Keep a water bottle at desk (and/or free and frequent access to water fountain); if child will not drink water, then provide an alternative noncaloric beverage so the child will stay hydrated.

Many children with SCD will need snacks in addition to school breakfast/lunch. The body works extra hard to make normal blood cells, so metabolism is high and hunger can be distracting: Provide quick, healthy, snack (in locker, or from teacher or nurse) to sustain energy.

High fluid intake means more frequent urination. Provide more frequent, excused, bathroom breaks (children with SCD need increased water intake but do not concentrate their urine, so they need to urinate more often and some cannot "hold it" as well as peers).

Some children have medications, which may cause drowsiness, to be taken during the school day (specify plan; include PRN pain medication appropriate to the child). Pain medications may interfere with alertness, attention, and memory. Children may need repetition and reinforcement of instruction; they may not be able to complete tests at their optimal ability level when they are taking certain pain medication, even if they are able to be present in school. Be prepared to repeat new content material, postpone tests, or allow a retake if necessary.

All children with SCD should have a nursing care plan. Allow for school nurse visit and nurse management if child complains of pain; create a nursing care plan with child's parents and school nurse, so that school and family agree about when to call the parents, and when to call 911. FAST responding is necessary for good health: Teachers, lunchroom and playground supervisors, as well as nurses, should be educated to recognize and know what to do in case of warning signs of stroke, and of pain crisis.

Attention, organization, short-term working memory, and speed of processing often are impaired by SCD especially in cases with stroke (33%) or lung disease (40%). Many have SLD. *(1)* Reduce distractions (preferential seating, study carrels, earphones, etc.). *(2)* Use materials and curricula that engage attention, motivate effort, and aid organization. *(3)* Model, teach, coach, encourage, and reinforce use of organizational and study skills (e.g., Dawson & Guare, 2004). *(4)* Individualize instruction in reading, writing, math, speech skills, as needed. *(5)* Use assistive technology to increase writing/computing speed for students who have slower speed of writing or difficulty quickly retrieving math or spelling facts from memory.

FAST, xxx; PRN, xxx; SCD, sickle cell disease; SLD, xxx.

long-term neuropsychological functioning. In the United States, preschoolers with SCD are maintained on prophylactic penicillin to reduce risk of life-threatening infections that can damage the spleen, brain, kidney, and other organs. Despite state-of-the-art management, however, Troy developed a severe viral illness at age 4 with very high fever that resulted in extensive subcortical and some cortical white matter infarcts (Figure 9.1). These infarcts remained "silent," that is, he never showed classic clinical signs of stroke.

Among children with SCD, IQ scores decrease slightly with age, even in children with normal MRIs, an effect not seen in demographically matched controls. This may be due to the effect of chronic anemia on brain development. The lowest IQ scores are seen in children with SCD, such as Troy, who have both chronically low hematocrit and MRI indicators of subclinical stroke (Hogan, Pit-ten Cate, Vargha-Khadem, Prengler, & Kirkham, 2006Kral MC, Brown RT, Connelly M, Curé JK, Besenski N, et al., 2006). More recent imaging studies indicate cerebral blood perfusion deficits, particularly in the frontal lobes, among children with SCD, including those who have no evidence of MRI abnormalities (Al-Kandari, Owunwanne, Syed, Ar Marouf, Elgazzar, et al., 2007).

A lifetime of brain blood flow insufficiency associated with anemia and cerebrovascular disease typically becomes evident during the elementary school years in the form of slowed speed of processing; difficulty with concentration, working memory, and other aspects of executive dysfunction; and sometimes in deficiencies of language or visuomotor skills. In Troy's case, these difficulties became progressively more apparent and troublesome in the upper elementary grades as he faced increasing demands for multitasking and self-directed project management. Like about 1/4 of children with SCD, Troy had subclinical or "silent" strokes, that is, infarcts visible on MRI/MRA scan, without classic neurologic signs. These children may show slowed reaction times, deterioration in fine motor dexterity or handwriting, or other subtle indicators noticeable to parents and teachers. Neuropsychological tests can differentiate children who have had subclinical strokes from those who have not, with the most sensitive

indicators appearing to be tests of attention and executive function (White et al., 2006).

Subclinical or "silent" strokes (asymptomatic but visible on MRI) tend to occur within the deep frontal white matter, in the borderzone of the anterior and middle cerebral artery distributions, during early childhood, as the result of loss of small vessels in the anterior artery distribution. Recent analysis of MRI data for 23 infants with SCD, ages 10 to 18 months, revealed that 13% already had experienced silent infarcts (Wang, Pavlakis, Helton, McKinstry, Casella, et al., 2008). Neuropsychological deficits may be identifiable on infant intelligence tests (the Bayley Scales; Hogan, Kirkham, Prengler, Telfer, Lane, et al., 2006) or screening measures (Denver Developmental Screening Test; Thompson, Gustafson, Bonner, & Ware, 2002). Longitudinal data from the national comprehensive sickle cell centers suggested that most silent strokes occur before age 6 years in girls and before age 10 years in boys, with no increased incidence among older adolescents (Pegelow, Macklin, Moser, Wang, Bello, et al., 2002). In addition to these small silent strokes, even smaller microinfarcts, too tiny to be visible on MRI scans, may be associated with the observed underdevelopment of the corpus callosum in children with HbSS. Smaller size of the anterior corpus callosum was associated with lower scores on measures of attention and executive function, independent of IQ (Schatz & Buzan, 2006). These changes in white matter integrity are not associated with localization effects but are associated with impaired attention and memorization, as well as lower IQ scores in some cases.

Overt thrombotic strokes (i.e., those causing obvious changes in consciousness and sensory or motor function) tend to occur in subcortical and frontal brain areas and result from stenosis and blockage of major arteries, particularly in the circle of Willis. Hemorrhagic strokes can occur when chronic arterial stenosis results in development, and breakdown, of tiny, fragile, blood vessels (Moyamoya vessels). These types of strokes most often occur among older children (10 years and up) as a result of progressive occlusion of the anterior arteries (Roach, Golomb, Adams, Biller, Daniels, et al., 2008). Anterior infarcts (ACA/MCA borderzone in particular) are more common than posterior infarcts at all ages, though it is possible for infarcts to occur anywhere. A greater amount of tissue loss associated with infarct is associated with lower IQ (Roach et al., 2008; Schatz et al., 2002).

The body compensates for decreased blood flow through narrowed or blocked blood vessels by increasing the pressure and volume of blood flow in other vessels. This can be visualized as increased cerebral blood flow volume (CBFV) in the carotid, middle cerebral, and anterior cerebral arteries, using transcranial Doppler (TCD) testing. Increased CBFV is associated with increased risk of overt cerebrovascular stroke, but it is not a sensitive indicator of silent stroke, for which neuropsychological testing is a better predictor (White et al., 2006). Increased CBFV is associated with lower IQ even in children without evidence of infarcts, perhaps because it signals hemolytic anemia, that is, chronically reduced oxygen-carrying capacity of the blood. Brain cells starved of oxygen do not function or develop properly, and the increased CBFV may not sufficiently compensate for needed oxygen, given the high metabolic demands of a developing brain.

Troy's neuropsychological profile reflects that of many children with SCD in that his IQ and basic academic skills (e.g., reading/decoding, spelling, and mastery of elementary math procedures) scored within the average range. Although children in the large comprehensive center trials have scored lower on IQ tests than their peers or demographically matched controls (Berkelhammer et al., 2007), marked intellectual disability is *not* characteristic of children with SCD, in the absence of severe stroke or MoyaMoya disease. Moreover, Troy had no known prenatal complications that would tend to lower IQ scores, such as drug or alcohol exposure. It is not known whether his mother had sickle cell trait or SCD. The effect of maternal SCD or SC trait on functional outcomes of a developing fetus is not well studied, but maternal Hb-SS presents severe risks to successful pregnancy outcomes, even in developed countries (Howard, Tuck, & Pearson, 1995). Troy's unilateral deafness, which apparently resulted from his high fever and high-dose antibiotic treatment as a 4-year-old, is not typical of children with SCD; it may have contributed to his difficulties with phonological processing, which is also not particularly common among children with SCD in our sample (Lieu, 2004; Wills et al., 2008).

The slow speed of processing, seen across a variety of tasks, and probably contributing to hesitant word finding (dysnomia), is commonly observed in children with SCD who have sustained some white matter damage or dysfunction (Berkelhammer et al., 2007). Slow and awkward graphomotor function also is quite commonly observed. Also characteristic of children with SCD is a pattern of executive dysfunction, resembling the "predominantly inattentive" type of attention-deficit disorder, without problems of hyperactivity, impulsivity, or disruptive conduct. Troy's responding is slow and "spacey," with long latencies and frequent attentional lapses. He has difficulty shifting quickly from one focus of attention to another, on cue, or from one response to the next. These neuropsychological characteristics may reflect dysfunction of frontal-subcortical white matter pathways subserving fine motor control, rapid response output, and executive function (e.g., Brandling-Bennet, White, Armstrong, Christ, & DeBaun, 2003; Christ, Moinuddin, McKinstry, DeBaun, & White, 2007; Hogan, Vargha-Khadem, Saunders, Kirkham, & Baldeweg, 2006).

Troy will enter middle school in another year. He is likely to have delayed onset of puberty, as well as significant growth delay, due to his SCD. Nevertheless, his health-care providers will encourage his family to begin planning now for his transition into adult life. As youth with sickle cell disease (SCD) move into adulthood, they need knowledge, skills, and confidence to manage their own health-care needs and attain a satisfying quality of life; yet there are few resources and no validated programs to train self-advocacy and transition skills for these adolescents.

Certain physical complications of SCD occur more often among adolescents and adults than among younger children. For example, diminished blood supply to the bones can cause an avascular necrosis in which bone deteriorates, necessitating surgeries such as hip replacement. Vascular occlusion to the retina can cause blindness or low vision, and cardiac vasculopathies can cause arrhythmias, which further impair the child's energy and blood circulation. Youth and adults with SCD need ongoing prospective monitoring to detect and promptly treat such late-emerging health issues.

The dedicated, well-informed parenting and comprehensive educational programming that Troy has received clearly support his good psychosocial adjustment, as well as his relatively good physical health status. His affability and good conduct are characteristic of most of the children followed in our clinic, and reported in the literature. A recent study of peer relations described schoolchildren with SCD as somewhat quiet, withdrawn, and often absent due to illness, but likeable and well accepted by peers (Noll, Reiter-Purtill, Vannatta, Gerhardt, & Short, 2007). Family functioning contributes even more than physical disease parameters to individual variability in health outcomes among children with SCD (Thompson, 2006). In this regard, Troy is more fortunate than many youth with SCD, who often have substantial educational, psychosocial, and financial needs. For example, of 82 African American youth with SCD, routinely screened in 2007–2009 by the clinic-embedded neuropsychological testing program at Children's Hospitals and Clinics of Minnesota, nearly two-thirds (63%) required psychosocial or educational interventions for attention, learning, or emotional-behavioral issues (Wills et al., 2008). Adverse psychosocial and educational outcomes, in turn, contribute to poorer self-care and health literacy, and therefore to poorer physical health outcomes (Palermo, Riley, & Mitchell, 2008; Thompson, 2006).

As he moves into the secondary and post-secondary grades, Troy and his family will need to address educational, vocational, social, leisure, and financial issues and resources, as well as SCD-specific health-care concerns. Individual differences related to neuropsychological status, as well as linguistic, socioeconomic, racial, and ethnic differences, may affect how patients access, use, and communicate health-related information (Gustafson et al., 2007). For example, Troy may benefit from emerging on-line interactive media that can engage youth with learning disabilities in strengthening self-understanding and self-advocacy skills.. Transition programming that assumes ongoing parental involvement may be more comfortable and congruent with reality for Troy and his family, as for many patients with SCD, than programs that focus on adolescent "separation and individuation" while ignoring the family and cultural context (Smetana, Campion-Barr, & Metzger, 2006). Given collaborative, individually tailored support from family, school, and hospital, the long-term goals for Troy include post-secondary education, gainful employment, and independent adult living with well-managed SCD. As one successful young adult with SCD said, "I pray for a cure for this disease, but meanwhile, I don't let it hold me down."

Note

1. SCD-PLANE (Program for Learning and Neuropsychological Evaluation) is a joint program of the Hematology-Oncology and Psychology Departments of Children's Hospitals and Clinics of Minnesota that embeds brief screening by a clinical neuropsychologist into the routine annual comprehensive clinic visit for every patient with high-risk forms of SCD. The 90-minute neuropsychological testing, using measures selected to detect the most common SCD-related problems identified by research studies, helps to inform medical management and also provides psychosocial and educational follow-through services to children and their families, as needed. The SCD-PLANE team includes Stephen Nelson, MD; David Slomiany, MD; Jane Hennessey, CPNP; Kristin Moquist, CPNP; Elizabeth McDonough, RN; Linda Litecky, RN; Theresa Huntley, MSW; Jill Swenson, MSW; Karen Wills, PhD; Osita Nwaneri, MD; Joyce Miskowiec, BA; and Josephine Anuforo, BA.

References

Adams, W. & Sheslow, D. (2003). *Wide Range Assessment of Memory and Learning (WRAML2)*. Rolling Meadows, IL: Riverside.

Al-Kandari, F. A., Owunwanne, A., Syed, G. M., Ar Marouf, R., Elgazzar, A. H., Shiekh, M., Rizui, A. M., Al-Ajmi, J. A., & Mohammed, A. M. (2007). Regional cerebral blood flow in patients with sickle cell disease: Study with single photon emission computed tomography. *Annals of Nuclear Medicine*, *21*, 439–445.

Beery, K., Buktenica, N., & Beery, N. (2006). Beery-Buktenica Developmental Test of Visual-Motor Integration, 5th Edition. San Antonio, TX: Pearson.

Berkelhammer, L. D., Williamson, A. L., Sanford, S. D., Dirksen, C. L., Sharp, W. G., Margulies, A. S., &

Prengler, R. A. (2007). Neurocognitive sequelae of pediatric sickle cell disease: A review of the literature. *Child Neuropsychology, 13,* 120–131.

Boyd, J. H., Macklin, E. A., Strunk, R. C., & DeBaun, M. R. (2006). Asthma is associated with acute chest syndrome and pain in children with sickle cell anemia. *Blood, 108,* 2923–2927.

Brandling-Bennett, E. M., White, D. A., Armstrong, M. M., Christ S. E., & DeBaun, M. (2003). Patterns of verbal long-term and working memory performance reveal deficits in strategic processing in children with frontal infarcts related to sickle cell disease. *Developmental Neuropsychology, 24,* 423–434.

Brawley, O. W., Cornelius, L. J., Edwards, L. R., Gamble, V. N., Green, B. L., Inturrisi, C., James, A. H., Laraque, D., Mendez, M., Montoya, C. J., Pollock, B. H., Robinson, L., Scholnik, A. P., & Schori, M. (2008). National Institutes of Health Consensus Development Conference statement: Hydroxyurea treatment for sickle cell disease. *Annals of Internal Medicine, 148,* 932–938.

Christ, S. E., Moinuddin, A., McKinstry, R. C., DeBaun, M., & White, D. A. (2007). Inhibitory control in children with frontal infarcts related to sickle cell disease. *Child Neuropsychology, 13,* 132–141.

Dawson, P., & Guare, R. (2009). Smart But Scattered: The Revolutionary "Executive Skills" Approach to Helping Kids Reach Their Potential. New York: Guilford.

Delis, D., Kaplan, E., & Kramer, J. (2001). *Delis-Kaplan Executive Function Scales (DKEFS).* San Antonio, TX: Pearson.

Field, J. J., Austin, P. F., An, P., Yan, Y., & DeBaun, M. R. (2008). Enuresis is a common and persistent problem among children and young adults with sickle cell anemia. *Urology, 72,* 81–84.

Gioia, G., Isquith, P., Guy, S., & Kenworthy, L. (2000). *BRIEF: Behavior Rating Inventory of Executive Function.* Lutz, FL: Psychological Assessment Resources.

Gustafson, S. L., Gettig, E. A., Watt-Morse, M., & Krishnamurti, L. (2007). Health beliefs among African American women regarding genetic testing and counseling for sickle cell disease. *Genetic Medicine, 9,* 303–310.

Henderson, J. N., Noetzel, M. J., McKinstry, R. C., White, D. A., Armstrong, M., & DeBaun, M. R. (2003). Reversible posterior leukoencephalopathy syndrome and silent cerebral infarcts are associated with severe acute chest syndrome in children with sickle cell disease. *Blood, 15,* 415–419.

Hill, S. (2003). *Managing Sickle Cell Disease in Low Income Families.* Philadelphia: Temple University Press.

Hogan, A. M., Kirkham, F. J., Prengler, M., Telfer, P., Lane, R., Vargha-Khadem, F., & Haan, M. (2006). An exploratory study of physiological correlates of neurodevelopmental delay in infants with sickle cell anaemia. *British Journal of Haematology, 132,* 99–107.

Hogan, A. M., Pit-ten Cate, I. M., Vargha-Khadem, F., Prengler, M., & Kirkham, F. J. (2006). Physiological correlates of intellectual function in children with sickle cell disease: Hypoxaemia, hyperaemia and brain infarction. *Developmental Science, 9,* 379–387.

Hogan, A. M., Vargha-Khadem, F., Saunders, D. E., Kirkham, F. J., & Baldeweg, T. (2006). Impact of frontal white matter lesions on performance monitoring: ERP evidence for cortical disconnection. *Brain, 129,* 2177–2188.

Howard, R. J., Tuck, S. M., & Pearson, T. C. (1995). Pregnancy in sickle cell disease in the UK: Results of a multicentre survey of the effect of prophylactic blood transfusion on maternal and fetal outcome. *British Journal of Obstetrics and Gynaecology, 102,* 947–951.

Ivascu, N. S., Sarnaik, S., McCrac, J., Whitten-Shurney, W., Thomas, R., & Bond, S. (2001). Characterization of pica prevalence among patients with sickle cell disease. *Archives of Pediatric and Adolescent Medicine, 155,* 1243–1247.

Kral, M.C., Brown, R.T., Connelly, M., Curé, J.K., Besenski, N., Jackson, S.M., Abboud, M.R. (2006). Radiographic predictors of neurocognitive functioning in pediatric Sickle Cell disease. *Journal of Child Neurology, 21,* 37–44.

Lieu, J. E. (2004). Speech-language and educational consequences of unilateral hearing loss in children. *Archives of Otolaryngology, Head and Neck Surgery, 130,* 524–530.

Mazumdar, M., Heeney, M. M., Sox, C. M., & Lieu, T. A. (2007). Preventing stroke among children with sickle cell anemia: An analysis of strategies that involve transcranial Doppler testing and chronic transfusion. *Pediatrics, 120,* 1107–1116.

Michlitsch, J., Azimi, M., Hoppe, C., Walters, M. C., Lubin, B., Lorey, F., & Vichinsky, E. (2009). Newborn screening for hemoglobinopathies in California. *Pediatric Blood Cancer, 52,* 486–90.

Modell, B., Darlison, M., Birgens, H., Cario, H., Faustino, P., Giordano, P.C., Gulbis, B., Hopmeier, P., Lena-Russo, D., Romao, L., & Theodorsson, E. (2007). Epidemiology of haemoglobin disorders in Europe: an overview. *Scandinavian Journal of Clinical Laboratory Investigation, 67,* 39–69.

Neal-Cooper, F., & Scott, R. B. (1988). Genetic counseling in sickle cell anemia: Experiences with couples at risk. *Public Health Reports, 103,* 174–178.

Nelson, S. C., Adade, B. B., McDonough, E. A., Moquist, K. L., & Hennessey, J. M. (2007). High prevalence of pulmonary hypertension in children with sickle cell disease. *Journal of Pediatric Hematology and Oncology, 29,* 334–337.

Noll, R. B., Reiter-Purtill, J., Vannatta, K., Gerhardt, C. A., & Short, A. (2007). Peer relationships and emotional well-being of children with sickle cell disease: A controlled replication. *Child Neuropsychology, 13,* 173–187.

Palermo, T. M., Riley, C. A., & Mitchell, B. A. (2008). Daily functioning and quality of life in children with sickle cell disease pain: Relationship with family and neighborhood socioeconomic distress. *Journal of Pain, 9,* 833–840.

Pegelow, C. H., Macklin, E. A., Moser, F. G., Wang, W. C., Bello, J. A., Miller, S. T., Wichinsky, E. P., DeBaun, M. R., Guarini, L., Zimmerman, R. A., Younkin, D. A., Gallagher, D. M., & Kinney, T. R. (2002). Longitudinal changes in brain magnetic resonance imaging findings in children with sickle cell disease. *Blood, 99,* 3014–3018.

Puffer, E., Schatz, J., & Roberts, C. W. (2007). The association of oral hydroxyurea therapy with improved cognitive functioning in children with sickle cell disease. *Child Neuropsychology, 13,* 142–154.

Rennie, K. M., & Panepinto, J. A. (2008). Sickle cell disease. In C. L. Castillo (Ed.), *Children with Complex Medical Issues in Schools* (pp. 367–378). New York: Springer.

Reynolds, C., & Kamphaus, R. (2002). BASC-2 (Behavior Assessment System for Children, Second Edition). San Antonio: Pearson.

Roach, E. S., Golomb, M. R., Adams, R., Biller, J., Daniels, S., Deveber, G., Ferriero, D., Jones, B. V., Kirkham, F. J., Scott, R. M., & Smith, E. R. (2008). Management of stroke in infants and children: A scientific statement from a Special Writing Group of the American Heart Association Stroke Council and the Council on Cardiovascular Disease in the Young. *Stroke, 39,* 2644–2691.

Schatz, J., Brown, R. T., Pascual, J. M., Hsu, L., & DeBaun, M. (2001). Poor school and cognitive functioning with silent cerebral infarcts and sickle cell disease. *Neurology, 56,* 1109–1111.

Schatz, J., & Buzan, R. (2006). Decreased corpus callosum size in sickle cell disease: Relationship with cerebral infarcts and cognitive functioning. *Journal of the International Neuropsychological Society, 12,* 24–33.

Schatz, J., Finke, R. L., Kellett, J. M., & Kramer, J. H. (2002). Cognitive functioning in children with sickle cell disease: A meta-analysis. *Journal of Pediatric Psychology, 27,* 739–748.

Schatz, J., White, D. A., Moinuddin, A., Armstrong, M., & DeBaun, M. R. (2002). Lesion burden and cognitive morbidity in children with sickle cell disease. *Journal of Child Neurology, 17,* 891–895.

Smetana, J. G., Campione-Barr, N., & Metzger, A. (2006). Adolescent development in interpersonal and societal contexts. *Annual Review of Psychology, 57,* 255–284.

Thompson, R. J., Jr. (2006). The interaction of social, behavioral, and genetic factors in sickle-cell disease. In L.M. Hernandez & D.G. Blazer (Eds.), *Genes, Behavior, and the Social Environment: Moving Beyond the Nature-Nurture Debate* (pp. 281–309). Washington, DC: National Academies Press.

Thompson, R. J., Jr., Gustafson, K. E., Bonner, M. J., & Ware, R. E. (2002). Neurocognitive development of young children with sickle cell disease through three years of age. *Journal of Pediatric Psychology, 27,* 235–244.

Torgeson, J., Wagner, R., & Rashotte, C. (1999). *Test of Word Reading Efficiency (TOWRE).* Rolling Meadows, IL: Riverside.

Tsaras, G., Owusu-Ansah, A., Boateng, F. O., & Amoateng-Adjepong, Y. (2009). Complications associated with sickle cell trait: A brief narrative review. *American Journal of Medicine, 122,* 507–512.

Wagner, R., Torgeson, J., & Rashotte, C. (1999). *Comprehensive Test of Phonological Processing (CTOPP).* San Antonio, TX: Pearson.

Wang, W. C. (2007). Central nervous system complications of sickle cell disease in children: An overview. *Child Neuropsychology, 13,* 103–19.

Wang, W. C., Pavlakis, S. G., Helton, K. J., McKinstry, R. C., Casella, J. F., Adams, R. J., & Rees, R. C., & BABY HUG Investigators. (2008). MRI abnormalities of the brain in one-year-old children with sickle cell anemia. *Pediatric Blood and Cancer, 51,* 643–646.

Wechsler, D. (2003). The Wechsler Intelligence Scales for Children, Fourth Edition (WISC-IV). San Antonio, TX: Pearson.

Wechsler, D. (1999). Wechsler Abbreviated Scales of Intelligence (WASI). San Antonio, TX: Pearson.

White, D. A., Moinuddin, A., McKinstry, R. C., Noetzel, M., Armstrong, M., & DeBaun, M. (2006). Cognitive screening for silent cerebral infarction in children with sickle cell disease. *Journal of Pediatric Hematology and Oncology, 28,* 166–169.

Williams, K.T. (2007). *Expressive Vocabulary Test, Second Edition.* San Antonio, TX: Pearson.

Wills, K., Nelson, S., Nwaneri, O., & SCD-PLANE Program Team. (2008, November). *Transition planning for adolescents with sickle cell disease: Medical, neuropsychological, educational-vocational, social-emotional, and ethical considerations*. Paper presented at the State of the Science/Opening Doors Conference, sponsored by Institute for Community Inclusion, American Academy of Pediatrics, and National Institute of Developmental Disabilities and Rehabilitation Research; Bethesda, MD.

Woodcock, R., McGrew, K., & Mather, N. (2001). *Woodcock-Johnson Tests of Achievement, Third Edition (WJ3)*. Rolling Meadows, IL: Riverside.

10

A Case of Neurofibromatosis Type 1

Jennifer A. Janusz

Neurofibromatosis type 1 (NF1) is a common genetic disorder, affecting approximately 1 in 3000 individuals. Neurocutaneous symptoms such as café au lait spots, axillary and inguinal freckling (freckling in the armpit and groin region), cutaneous neurofibromas, and iris hamartomas (Lisch nodules) are the most commonly recognized characteristics of NF1. However, NF1 is a multisystem disorder and diagnostic symptoms also include bony lesions and benign and malignant neural tumors (e.g., optic gliomas and plexiform neurofibromas). Other physical features include headaches, vascular abnormalities, macrocephaly, and scoliosis (North, 2000). Additionally, NF1 is associated with focal areas of hyperintensity seen on T2-weighted magnetic resonance imaging (MRI), sometimes referred to as unidentified bright objects (UBOs; North, 2000), thought to be areas of neural dysplasia or dysmyelination (Hyman et al., 2003). Approximately 60%–70% of children with NF1 have T2 hyperintensities on imaging, most commonly in the basal ganglia, cerebellum, brain stem, and subcortical white matter (North, 2000). T2 hyperintensities are more commonly seen in younger children and typically decrease or disappear by early adulthood (North et al., 1997). Other clinical features include headaches, vascular abnormalities, macrocephaly, and scoliosis (North, 2000). Learning disabilities, attentional problems, and cognitive deficits are also associated with NF1. The diagnostic criteria for NF1 proposed by the National Institutes of Health are outlined in Table 10.1 (National Institutes of Health Consensus Development Conference, 1988). A diagnosis is made when two or more criteria are met.

Neurofibromatosis type 1 is inherited in an autosomal dominant pattern, although the disorder arises from a spontaneous mutation with no family history in approximately 50% of cases (Moore & Denckla, 2000). The NF1 gene, on chromosome 17, is typically classified as a tumor suppressor gene, which helps to explain the frequency of tumors seen in NF1 (North, Hyman, & Barton, 2002). There is no cure for NF1 and treatment is based on presenting symptoms. Plexiform and cutaneous neurofibromas can be disfiguring. While cutaneous neurofibromas can be more easily removed, plexiform neurofibromas are progressive in nature and are not usually treated surgically unless they affect a vital organ. If optic gliomas progress in size or affect vision, they are treated with a combination of surgery, chemotherapy, and cranial radiation (Moore & Denckla, 2000).

Children with NF1 are clearly at risk for significant physical complications. Nonetheless, clinical characteristics are highly variable, even within families. While some individuals with NF1 may have severely disfiguring or life-threatening symptoms, others experience relatively mild symptoms with little impact on their quality of life (Moore & Denckla, 2000). Some studies suggest that only about 20% of children have significant physical complications (Castle, Baser, Huson, Cooper, & Upadhyaya, 2003).

Table 10-1. NIH Diagnostic Criteria for NF1

Two or more of the following features must be present for the diagnosis of NF1:
- Six or more café au lait spots with a diameter greater than 0.5 cm before puberty and 1.5 cm after puberty
- Axillary or inguinal freckling
- Two or more neurofibromas or a single plexiform neurofibroma
- Two or more Lisch nodules (iris hamartomas)
- Optic pathway glioma
- Distinctive osseous lesion such as sphenoid bone dysplasia or thinning of long bone cortex
- A first-degree relative with NF1 by the above criteria

NF1, neurofibromatosis type 1; NIH, National Institutes of Health.

Source: National Institutes of Health Consensus Development Conference, 1988.

Neurobehavioral Profile

Despite the physical risks associated with NF1, parents are often more concerned about cognitive and academic difficulties (North, 2000). Neurobehavioral problems can have lifelong implications, affecting self-esteem, social relationships, educational attainment, and employment (Rosser & Packer, 2003).

Early studies reported mental retardation among a large percentage of children with NF1. However, recent studies suggest that only 4%–8% of children with NF1 meet diagnostic criteria for mental retardation. There does seem to be a "leftward shift" in overall IQ scores, with Full Scale IQ in studies averaging from 89 to 98 (North, 2000). Learning disabilities (LDs), traditionally defined as a significant discrepancy between overall cognitive ability and academic performance, have a higher prevalence in children with NF1 compared to the general population, with rates reported between 30% and 65% (Kayl & Moore, 2000; Mautner, Kluwe, Thakker, & Learke, 2002). One study (Hyman, Shores, & North, 2006) found that while 52% of the sample had scores greater than one standard deviation below the mean on academic measures, only 20% of children met criteria for a specific LD, defined as an IQ-achievement discrepancy. This suggests that while many children with NF1 may demonstrate academic difficulties, fewer may meet traditional definitions of LD.

There is no specific neuropsychological profile of children with NF1 (North, 2000). Early studies suggested that problems with nonverbal skills were predominant in children with NF1, based mostly on research using Verbal and Performance IQ discrepancy data (Rosser & Packer, 2003). While more recent studies have not consistently found VIQ-PIQ discrepancies, performance on the Judgment of Line Orientation test tends to be impaired across studies of children with NF1 (North, 2000). Several studies utilizing functional MRI have also documented recruitment of atypical areas during visuospatial tasks (Billingsley et al., 2004; Clements-Stephens, Rimrodt, Gaur, & Cutting, 2008).

Research that has included more in-depth evaluation of language-based skills has found deficits, including poor performances on measures of both fluency and naming. Problems are also seen on language-based academic tasks, such as reading comprehension and written expression (North et al., 2002). The incidence of dyslexia in NF1 is thought to be about 15%–20% (Watt, Shores, and North, 2008). Functional imaging studies have found that children with NF1 utilize frontal cortices relative to posterior cortices differently than controls when completing phonological processing tasks (Billingsley et al., 2003). Interestingly, one study found that children with NF1 and a reading disability had more global language impairments than children who had only a reading disability (Cutting, Koth et al., 2000), highlighting the importance of investigating broader language functioning beyond just phonologically based deficits in children with NF1.

Attentional deficits have been well described in children with NF1, with deficits documented in sustained attention, selective attention, and divided attention (North et al., 2002). Studies suggest that 30%–50% of children with NF1 are also diagnosed with attention-deficit/hyperactivity disorder (ADHD; Acosta, Gioia, & Silva, 2006). In contrast to the general population, where ADHD is diagnosed more frequently in boys, it seems to occur at equal rates among boys and girls with NF1. Koth, Cutting, and Denckla (2000) compared children with NF1 to their unaffected siblings and parents, finding that ADHD occurred more commonly in children with NF1, suggesting it may be part of the cognitive-behavioral phenotype of this disorder. The use of stimulant medication to address symptoms of ADHD has been shown to be effective in children with NF1 (Mautner et al., 2002).

Few studies have systematically assessed executive functioning skills, although available research suggests that children with NF1 demonstrate both lab-based and everyday executive deficits (Acosta et al., 2006). Hyman and colleagues (2005) documented deficits in planning, organizing, and shifting. Parent-reported deficits in everyday settings have been found in working memory, planning, organizing, problem solving, and self-monitoring (Potter, 2006). This is an important area of ongoing investigation because executive deficits may contribute to poor performance in academics and other functional domains.

Limited research has explored the memory skills of children with NF1. One study found no deficits in visual or verbal memory. In fact, memory performance tended to be stronger than would be expected given overall cognitive ability (Hyman, Shores, & North, 2005). This finding is somewhat unexpected given other deficits noted in the NF1 population, and it is worthy of further exploration.

Deficits in gross and fine motor skills are frequently seen in children with NF1. Studies have documented problems with dexterity, coordination, balance, and gait, as well as psychomotor slowing (Rosser & Packer, 2003). As a result of fine motor deficits, handwriting is frequently affected (Hyman et al., 2005).

A question often posed by parents is whether the neurobehavioral deficits associated with NF1 will continue throughout the child's life. Cutting and colleagues (2002) completed growth curve analyses of neuropsychological profiles of children with NF1. They found that skills that were within the average range at initial testing remained intact, while skills that were impaired on initial evaluation remained impaired across future testings. These findings were supported by another study by Hyman et al. (2003), which documented no improvement in cognitive functioning over an 8-year period. Therefore, it appears that the cognitive deficits associated with NF1 remain relatively stable over time.

From a psychosocial perspective, anxiety and depression are more frequently reported than externalizing problems (Graf, Landolt, Mori, & Botshauser, 2006). Children with NF1 are often socially isolated and not viewed as leaders among their peers (Noll et al., 2007; North et al., 2002). While overall self-concept is not necessarily affected, children with NF1 report negative self-concept regarding physical and sporting abilities. Their limited confidence may also affect their peer relationships (Barton & North, 2006).

On quality-of-life measures, parents of children with NF1 report significant childhood impairment in motor, cognitive, and socioemotional functioning (Graf et al., 2006), as well as poor health perceptions (Oostenbrink et al., 2007). Disease severity, visibility of symptoms, and family history of NF1 have all been found to impact quality of life. However, studies have also identified protective factors, including high family cohesiveness, social support, and knowledge of prognosis (Graf et al., 2006; Oostenbrink et al., 2007).

Neuroanatomic and Genetic Correlates of Cognitive Deficits

Much research has investigated the relationship between T2 hyperintensities and cognitive deficits. The relationship remains controversial because studies have produced mixed findings (Hyman, Gill, Shores, Steinberg, & North, 2007). Several studies suggest that the presence of cognitive deficits is related to the number of sites (Denckla et al., 1996; Hofman, Harris, Bryan, & Denckla, 1994) and location of T2 hyperintensities (Goh, Khong, Leung, & Wong, 2004; Hyman et al., 2007; Moore, Slopis, Schomer, Jackson, & Levy, 1996), with lesions in the thalamus particularly predictive of cognitive dysfunction. On magnetic resonance spectroscopy, children with NF1 demonstrate decreased signal processing in the thalamus, independent of the presence of T2 hyperintensities, and it has been postulated that lesions in this region may further contribute to altered functioning of the thalamus (Hyman et al., 2007). In children with T2 hyperintensities, it does not appear that cognitive functioning improves despite a decrease in the number, size, and intensity of these lesions as the child matures (Hyman et al., 2003).

More recently, research has investigated the role of the NF1 gene in cognitive outcome.

Neurofibromin is the protein product of the NF1 gene. One of the functions of neurofibromin is the downregulation of ras, a protein involved in cellular growth and differentiation. Mutations in the NF1 gene result in inactive neurofibromin, causing excessive ras activity. This leads to unregulated cell growth and is thought to contribute to many of the physical symptoms associated with NF1 (Rosser & Packer, 2003). Using mouse models of NF1, research has suggested that increased ras activity may also underlie cognitive deficits, as treatment with pharmacological agents that inhibit ras improves mouse performance on spatial learning and attentional tasks (Costa et al 2002; Costa & Silva, 2002; Li et al., 2005). This research has recently been translated to humans. Krab and colleagues (2008) treated children with NF1 with simvastatin or a placebo and assessed performance on measures of visual-motor integration, visuospatial analysis, nonverbal memory, speed, and attention. After 12 weeks of treatment, no improvement was noted in cognitive functioning. Despite these results, this remains an important area for future research.

The Case of Patricia M.

Patricia M., an 8-year-old girl, was referred for a neuropsychological evaluation by the geneticist following her through a neurofibromatosis clinic. Patricia was a second grade student, and her parents and teachers had concerns regarding her attention in the classroom as well as her ability to complete more complex tasks independently. Patricia was not receiving special education services at the time of the evaluation.

Patricia was diagnosed with NF1 at approximately 1 year of age after her pediatrician noticed multiple café au lait macules. Her current NF1 characteristics include café au lait spots, bilateral axial and inguinal freckling, and subcutaneous neurofibromas. She also has a plexiform neurofibroma on her left foot. A recent ophthalmology evaluation documented Lisch nodules. Patricia last underwent a brain MRI approximately 1 year ago, which revealed multiple T2 hyperintensities in the basal ganglia, optic radiations, and posterior fossa. There was no evidence of an optic glioma. Patricia's physical symptoms have been stable, and she has not had any surgeries or hospitalizations.

Patricia's mother had no complications during her pregnancy. Patricia was born at 39 weeks gestation, weighing 6 pounds, 8 ounces. The delivery was uncomplicated and Patricia and her mother were discharged home on time. Developmental language and motor milestones were achieved within normal limits.

No problems with the acquisition of early school-related skills were reported during preschool. However, Patricia's kindergarten and first grade teachers both reported that she was fidgety during class and had difficulty staying in her seat. Her current second grade teacher reports similar problems, and that Patricia frequently looks around the classroom, talks to other children, and blurts out answers. After giving the class directions, her teacher finds that she has to spend a few minutes reviewing them with Patricia. Patricia's mother and teacher both report that she has difficulty completing multi-step tasks and requires more structure than others her age. Mrs. M. has to carefully monitor Patricia during homework time. When completing math problems, Patricia has difficulty lining up the numbers. She also inconsistently leaves spaces between words, making her handwriting difficult to read. Mrs. M. describes Patricia's handwriting and pencil control as poor.

Some concerns were also reported regarding anxiety. Since the beginning of second grade, Patricia exhibited anxiety before school, crying and saying she had "butterflies" in her stomach. She seems especially anxious about completing writing and math. Patricia does not like to be the center of attention; for example, she is uncomfortable when people clap for her on her birthday. She also does not like to play group sports because she is concerned that the other children will be too rough. The plexiform neurofibroma on her foot makes running awkward, and she has experienced some teasing by other children in the past. However, her mother reported no significant social problems at present, and that Patricia easily makes and maintains friendships.

Patricia lives with her parents and older brother in a suburban area. Both parents completed college. Her mother is a customer service representative and her father works in sales. There is no family history of NF1. There is an extended maternal family history of depression.

By observation, Patricia appeared her stated age. She was wearing a short-sleeved shirt, so some café au lait spots and small neurofibromas were visible on her arms. Her affect was appropriate to the situation. At first she was hesitant to leave her mother. However, once she started testing, she easily engaged with the examiner and became quite talkative. Attention and self-regulatory problems were apparent during testing. She was observed to be both easily distracted and fidgety. At times, she made unrelated comments in the middle of tasks. She tended to be impulsive and would start tasks before being prompted to do so. During longer or more difficult tasks, she had problems persisting and needed encouragement to keep trying her best. Despite these problems, she was easily redirected, quite likable, and appeared to put forth good effort throughout the evaluation.

Examination Results

On the Differential Ability Scales–Second Edition (DAS-II), Patricia obtained a general conceptual ability (GCA) standard score of 94, at the 34th percentile. However, there was disparity among her cluster scores. While she obtained a Verbal cluster standard score of 115, at the 84th percentile, her Nonverbal Reasoning cluster score was 81 (10th percentile), and her Spatial cluster score was 78 (7th percentile). The DAS-II scores are presented in Table 10.2.

A screening of Patricia's academic skills was completed with the Wechsler Individual Achievement Test–Second Edition (WIAT-II).

She obtained average range scores on all subtests administered (Word Reading SS = 91; Numerical Operations SS = 95; Spelling SS = 91).

Performances on tests of language skills were generally intact. Word knowledge and verbal reasoning were in the average to high-average range on the DAS-II. Expressive vocabulary was also average on the Boston Naming Test. Patricia was able to follow instructions of increasing length and complexity on the Comprehension of Instructions subtest of the NEPSY-II (ss = 12).

Compared to her linguistic skills, relative weaknesses were noted on tasks with greater visuoperceptual and visual-motor demands. Her ability to copy geometric shapes was below average on the VMI (SS = 78). She also had difficulty drawing forms from memory on DAS-II Recall of Designs and accurately orienting blocks on DAS-II Pattern Construction. Although Patricia did relatively better determining patterns and sequences on DAS-II Sequential and Quantitative Reasoning, she had difficulty completing patterns on the Matrices subtest. Her ability to match similar figures and mentally rotate objects was in the low-average range on NEPSY-II Geometric Puzzles (ss = 7). On observation, Patricia appeared to become overwhelmed with tasks that had more complex visual stimuli, such as multiple figures on a page (TEA-Ch Sky Search) or more abstract figures (DAS-II Recall of Designs).

Patricia's performance on memory testing was inconsistent, at least partly due to attention problems. On the California Verbal Learning Test–Children's Version (CVLT-C), Patricia's recall over five learning trials was above average. Her immediate recall of the list was in the low-average range, although she was notably off-task

Table 10-2. Scores on Differential Abilities Scale–Second Edition (DAS-II)

General Conceptual Ability			SS = 89		
Verbal Cluster	SS = 115	Nonverbal Reasoning Cluster	SS = 81	Spatial Cluster	SS =78
Word Definition	T = 56	Matrices	T = 34	Recall of Designs	T = 37
Verbal Similarities	T = 62	Sequential and Quantitative Reasoning	T = 43	Pattern Construction	T = 38

SS, standard score.

during this portion, interrupting herself and wanting to discuss how many more tests were left. In contrast to her immediate recall, delayed recall was in the high-average range. Similarly, on NEPSY-II Memory for Designs, Patricia was inattentive during the immediate recall portion, and she obtained a low-average score; her delayed recall was in the average range.

Significant problems with attention were noted on testing, although Patricia's performance was better on an auditory attention task than a visual attention task. On the Sky Search subtest of the Test of Everyday Attention for Children (TEA-Ch), Patricia had difficulty quickly and accurately identifying specific targets in an array (ss = 6). In contrast, she was able to adequately attend to an auditory stimulus on TEA-Ch Score (ss = 11). Consistent with behavioral observations, Patricia demonstrated impulsive responding on NEPSY Inhibition (ss = 5). In fact, two subtests of the TEA-Ch were discontinued due to Patricia's distractibility, impulsivity, and difficulty staying on task. On the Child Behavior Checklist (CBCL), Mr. and Mrs. M.'s responses yielded an Attention Problems scale in the Clinical range.

Executive functioning deficits were also apparent on testing. On the Tower of London DX, Patricia completed an average number of items correctly (Total Correct SS = 98); however, she tended to use an inefficient strategy, making more moves than necessary to complete items (Total Move Score SS = 80). As a result, she completed several items over the time limit (Total Problem Solving Time SS = 78). She also tended to get "stuck" in her problem solving, and she would subsequently violate a test rule. Problems with working memory were also apparent. She obtained a DAS-II Working Memory cluster standard score of 74, at the 4th percentile. In contrast, verbal reasoning was in the high-average range on the DAS-II, and she had no difficulty generating words to semantic or phonemic prompts on NEPSY-II Word Generation (Word Generation Semantic ss = 12; Word Generation Initial Letter ss = 11). Mr. and Mrs. M. rated Patricia's executive skills in the home environment on the Behavior Rating Inventory of Executive Function (BRIEF). Their ratings yielded significant scores on the Inhibit, Working Memory, Plan/Organize, and Monitor scales.

No problems with gait and balance were noted by observation. Patricia employed a tripod grasp, and she used her right hand for writing and drawing tasks. Writing production yielded poorly formed print letters with limited spacing between letters. Fine motor speed and dexterity were approximately one standard deviation below average bilaterally on the Grooved Pegboard. Patricia made excessive bilateral errors during the fingertip number writing portion of the Sensory Perceptual Examination; however, this may have been due to inattention during this task.

Mr. and Mrs. M. completed the CBCL to provide ratings of Patricia's social, emotional, and behavioral functioning. They reported some characteristics of anxiety, including appearing nervous, feeling she has to be perfect, and worrying, with a score in the Borderline range. No other subscales were elevated.

Discussion

Patricia presents with a neurocognitive profile that is not atypical for a child with NF1. Despite relatively intact linguistic skills, she demonstrates weaknesses in visual-motor and visual-perceptual functioning. Furthermore, she has deficits in attention, regulatory control, and executive functioning skills. Her motor speed is also slow, bilaterally. The neuropsychological profile is suggestive of right hemisphere and frontal-subcortical involvement.

At the time of the evaluation, the greatest concern at school was Patricia's inattention and behavioral dysregulation. Based on the evaluation, a diagnosis of ADHD was made, and it was suggested that her parents consult with the primary physician regarding a trial of stimulant medication. Recommendations for the classroom were provided to the teacher, such as preferential seating, "hands-on" activities, and breaking up the need for sustained attention.

School personnel will need to have a good understanding of Patricia's neurocognitive profile and its effect on her school performance. While the majority of special need students present with language or reading-based learning problems, Patricia displays greater difficulty with visual-motor and visual-perceptual tasks. Teachers will need to be aware of this difference and how it may impact Patricia's math skill development, as well as her ability to interpret visually presented material, such as charts and graphs. As Patricia became easily overwhelmed by complex or increased amounts of visual information, it was suggested that she be presented with only a few problems on a worksheet or that she use a piece of paper to uncover only the area of the assignment sheet in which she needs to be working.

Although Patricia is currently keeping pace academically in school, she may be expected to encounter greater difficulty as she progresses into the upper grades. Patricia's deficits in executive functioning skills will likely interfere with her school performance as tasks become more complex and greater independence is required. To address this, it was recommended that tasks and lessons be presented in a systematic, step-by-step fashion, with more complex or multistep tasks broken down for her. As both her parents and her teacher reported that she has difficulty with complex tasks, using checklists to prompt the individual steps she needs to complete a task may be beneficial. Such lists would also allow teachers to easily prompt her should she have difficulty sustaining effort during a task.

Because of her poor handwriting and slow motor speed, it was recommended that Patricia be provided extra time to complete written tasks. An occupational therapy evaluation was also suggested to determine whether therapy could help to address her handwriting difficulties.

Socioemotionally, Patricia was exhibiting a moderate amount of anxiety. She reported having "butterflies" and feeling anxious about academics, and her parents endorsed worry and perfectionistic tendencies as well. This may suggest that she is working hard to maintain her grades and is beginning to feel anxious about her ability to effectively complete work. It is hoped that with some accommodations in place, her anxiety regarding school will lessen. It was suggested that her parents monitor her anxiety and, should it begin to interfere with her participation in school or social activities, psychotherapy be considered.

At the time of the evaluation, the school was hesitant to provide special education services through an individual education plan (IEP), because Patricia was making adequate academic progress. It was agreed that a Section 504 Plan would likely be sufficient at this time to document the neuropsychological recommendations.

In talking with school personnel, it was emphasized that Patricia's academic progress would need to be closely monitored as her neuropsychological deficits may at some point interfere more with her academic development and, at that point, she may benefit from a more comprehensive IEP. It was also discussed that Patricia may not meet criteria for a traditional learning disability based on discrepancy criteria and that she should qualify for services under the Physical Disability classification, given the impact of her medical disorder on her cognitive functioning.

It was recommended that Patricia return for a neuropsychological evaluation in 2 years to document her progress and make current recommendations. The family was encouraged to return earlier if she should experience greater difficulties in school or if there were any changes in her medical status.

In conclusion, children with NF1 may present with a neurocognitive profile different from "typical" learning disabled students. Testing completed through the school may not explore certain areas of cognitive dysfunction frequently seen in children with NF1 (e.g., executive functions) and a complete neuropsychological evaluation can help to provide a more comprehensive assessment of the strengths and weaknesses of a child with NF1. The neuropsychologist can be helpful to school personnel in understanding a child's neurocognitive profile and how it may manifest in the school setting. The neuropsychologist can also help the school in understanding the physical manifestations of the disease in an effort to help prevent or address any teasing that may occur. As such, working with a neuropsychologist can greatly contribute to the academic, social, and emotional development of the child with NF1.

References

Acosta, M. T., Gioia, G. A., & Silva, A. J. (2006). Neurofibromatosis type 1: New insights into neurocognitive issues. Current Neurology and Neuroscience Reports, 6, 136–143.

Barton, B., & North, K. (2004). Social skills of children with neurofibromatosis type 1. Developmental Medicine and Child Neurology, 46, 553–563.

Barton, B., & North, K. (2006). The self-concept of children and adolescents with neurofibromatosis type 1. *Child: Care, Health, and Development, 33,* 401–408.

Billingsley, R. L., Jackson, E. F., Slopis, J. M., Swank, P. R., Mahankali, S., & Moore, B. D. (2003). Functional magnetic resonance imaging of phonologic processing in neurofibromatosis 1. *Journal of Child Neurology, 18,* 731–740.

Billingsley, R. L., Jackson, E. F., Slopis, J. M., Swank, P. R., Mahankali, S., & Moore, B. D. (2004). Functional MRI of visual-spatial processing in neurofibromatosis, type 1. *Neuropsychologia, 42,* 395–404.

Billingsley, R. L., Schrimsher, G. W., Jackson, E. F., Slopis, J. M., & Moore, B. D. (2002). Significance of planum temporale and planum parietale morphologic features in neurofibromatosis type 1. *Archives of Neurology, 59,* 616–622.

Castle, B., Baser, M. E., Huson, S. M., Cooper, D., & Upadhyaya, M. (2003). Evaluation of genotype-phenotype correlations in neurofibromatosis type 1. *Journal of Medical Genetics, 40,* e109.

Clements-Stephens, A. M., Rimrodt, S. L., Gaur, P., & Cutting, L. E. (2008). Visuospatial processing in children with neurofibromatosis type 1. *Neuropsychologia, 46,* 690–697.

Costa, R. M., Federov, N. B., Kogan, J. H., Murphy, G. G., Stern, J., Ohno, M., et al. (2002). Mechanisms for the learning deficits in a mouse model of neurofibromatosis type 1. *Nature, 415,* 526–530.

Costa, R. M., & Silva, A. J. (2002). Molecular and cellular mechanisms underlying the cognitive deficits associated with neurofibromatosis type 1. *Journal of Child Neurology, 17,* 622–626.

Cutting, L. E., Huang, G. H., Zeger, S., Koth, C. W., Thompson, R. E., & Denckla, M. B. (2002). Growth curve analyses of neuropsychological profiles in children with neurofibromatosis type 1: Specific cognitive tests remain "spared" and "impaired" over time. Journal of the International Neuropsychological Society, 8, 838–846.

Cutting, L. E., Koth, C. W., Burnette, C. P., Abrams, M. T., Kaufmann, W. E., & Denckla, M. B. (2000). Relationship of cognitive functioning, whole brain volumes, and T2-weighted hyperintensities in neurofibromatosis-1. *Journal of Child Neurology, 15,* 157–160.

Cutting, L. E., Koth, C. W., & Denckla, M. B. (2000). How children with neurofibromatosis type 1 differ from "typical" learning disabled clinic attenders: Nonverbal learning disabilities revisited. *Developmental Neuropsychology, 17,* 29–47.

Denckla, M. B., Hofman, K., Mazzocco, M. M., Melhem, E., Reiss, A. L. Bryan, R. N., et al. (1996). Relationship between T2-weighted hyperintensities (unidentified bright objects) and lower IQs in children with neurofibromatosis type 1. *American Journal of Medical Genetics, 67,* 98–102.

Goh, W. H., Khong, P. L., Leung, C. S., & Wong, V. C. (2004). T2-weighted hyperintensities (unidentified bright objects) in children with neurofibromatosis type 1: Their impact on cognitive function. *Journal of Child Neurology, 19,* 853–858.

Graf, A., Landolt, M. A., Mori, A. C., & Botshauser, E. (2006). Qualify of life and psychological adjustment in children and adolescents with neurofibromatosis type 1. *Journal of* Pediatrics, 149, 348–353.

Hofman, K. J., Harris, E. L. Bryan, R. N., & Denckla, M. B. (1994). Neurofibromatosis type 1: The cognitive phenotype. *Journal of Pediatrics, 44,* 878–883.

Hyman, S. L., Gill, D. S., Shores, E. A., Steinberg, A., Joy, P., Gibikote, S. V., et al. (2003). Natural history of cognitive deficits and their relationship to MRI T2-hyperintensities in neurofibromatosis type 1. *Neurology, 60,* 1139–1145.

Hyman, S. L., Gill, D. S., Shores, E. A., Steinberg, A., & North, K. N. (2007). T2 hyperintensities in children with neurofibromatosis type 1 and their relationship to cognitive functioning. *Journal of Neurology, Neurosurgery, and Psychiatry, 78,* 1088–1091.

Hyman, S. L., Shores, A., & North, K. N. (2005). The nature and frequency of cognitive deficits in children with neurofibromatosis type 1. *Neurology, 65,* 1037–1044.

Hyman, S. L., Shores, E. A., & North, K. N. (2006). Learning disabilities in children with neurofibromatosis type 1: Subtypes, cognitive profile, and attention-deficit-hyperactivity disorder. *Developmental Medicine and Child Neurology, 48,* 973–977.

Kayl, A. E., & Moore, B. D. (2000). Behavioral phenotype of neurofibromatosis type 1: Mental retardation and developmental disabilities. *Mental Retardation and Developmental Disabilities Research Review, 6,* 117–124.

Koth, C. W., Cutting, L. E., & Denckla, M. B. (2000). The association of neurofibromatosis type 1 and attention deficit hyperactivity disorder. *Child Neuropsychology, 6,* 185–194.

Krab, L. C., de Goede-Bolder, A., Aarsen, F. K., Pluijm, S. M. F., Bouman, M. J., van der Geest, J. N., et al. (2008). Effect of simvastatin on cognitive functioning in children with neurofibromatosis type 1: A randomized controlled trial. *Journal of the American Medical Association, 300,* 287–294.

Li, W., Cui, Y., Kushner, S. A., Brown, R. A., Jentsch, J. D., Frankland, P. W., et al. (2005). The HMG-CoA reductase inhibitor lovastatin reverses the learning and attention deficits in a mouse model of neurofibromatosis type 1. *Current Biology, 15,* 1961–1967.

Mautner, V. F., Kluwe, L., Thakker, S. D., & Leark, R. A. (2002). Treatment of ADHD in neurofibromatosis type 1. *Developmental Medicine and Child Neurology, 44,* 164–170.

Moore, B., & Denckla, M. B. (2000). Neurofibromatosis. In K. O. Yeates, M. D. Ris, & H. G. Taylor (Eds.), *Pediatric neuropsychology: Research, theory, and practice* (pp. 149–170). New York: Guilford Press.

Moore, B. D., Slopis, J. M., Jackson, E. F., DeWinter, A. E., & Leeds, N. E. (2000). Brain volume in children with neurofibromatosis type 1: Relation to neuropsychological status. *Neurology, 54,* 914–920.

Moore, B. D., Slopis, J. M., Schomer, D., Jackson, E. F., & Levy, B. (1996). Neuropsychological significance of areas of high signal intensity on brain magnetic resonance imaging scans of children with neurofibromatosis. *Neurology, 46,* 1660–1668.

National Institutes of Health Consensus Development Conference. (1988). Neurofibromatosis. Conference statement. *Archives of Neurology, 45,* 575–578.

Noll, R. B., Reiter-Purtill, J., Moore, B. D., Schorry, E. K., Lovell, A. M., Vannatta, K., & Gerhardt, C. A. (2007). Social, emotional, and behavioral functioning of children with NF1. American Journal of Medical Genetics Part A, 143A, 2261–2273.

North, K. (2000). Neurofibromatosis type 1. *American Journal of Medical Genetics, 97,* 119–127.

North, K. N., Hyman, S., & Barton, B. (2002). Cognitive deficits in neurofibromatosis type 1. Journal of Child Neurology, 17, 605–612.

North, K. N., Riccardi, M. D., Samango-Sprouse, C., Ferner, R., Moore, B. D., 3rd, Leguis, E., Ratner, N., & Denckla, M. B. (1997). Cognitive function and academic performance in neurofibromatosis type 1: consensus statement from the NF1 cognitive disorders task force. *Neurology, 48,* 1121–1127.

Oostenbrink, R., Spong, K., de Goede-Bolder, A., Landgraf, J. M., Raat, H., & Moll, H. A. (2007). Parental reports of health-related quality of life in young children with neurofibromatosis type 1: Influence of condition specific determinants. *Journal of Pediatrics, 151,* 182–186.

Potter, B. (2006). Executive functions and psychosocial behavior in children with NF1. Unpublished doctoral dissertation,, Antioch University, Keene, NH.

Rosser, T. L., & Packer, R. J. (2003). Neurocognitive dysfunction in children with neurofibromatosis type 1. *Current Neurology and Neuroscience Reports, 3,* 129–136.

Watt, S. E., Shores, E. A., & North, K. N. (2008). An examination of lexical and sublexical reading skills in children with neurofibromatosis type 1. *Child Neuropsychology, 14,* 401–418.

11

Focal Cortical Dysplasia and Epilepsy Surgery

Elisabeth M. S. Sherman, Harvey B. Sarnat, Ismail Mohamed,
Daniel J. Slick, and Walter J. Hader

The human cortex develops through a series of finely orchestrated, time-dependent, sequential stages that include proliferation of undifferentiated cells, migration, differentiation, postmigratory organization, and programmed cell death (Bentivoglio et al., 2003). Malformations of cortical development (MCDs) are structural abnormalities of the brain caused by alterations of normal development during cortical maturation (Barkovich, Kuzniecky, Jackson, Guerrini, & Dobyns, 2005; Palmini et al., 2004). The type and severity of these developmental abnormalities are critically dependent on the nature and timing of the disruption, as well as on the underlying cause (e.g., genetic, environmental). Malformations of cortical development may range from severe global malformations occurring early in gestation, to milder, more subtle focal cortical disorganization occurring later on (Barkovich, Kuzniecky, Jackson, Guerrini, & Dobyns, 2001). These reflect the different processes that were disrupted during specific stages of normal cortical development, such as neuronal and glial proliferation (e.g., hemimegancephaly), cell migration (e.g., lissencephaly), or cortical organization (e.g., polymicrogyria).

Malformations of cortical development are highly epileptogenic, and seizures secondary to MCDs are often intractable to treatment with antiepileptic medications (AEDs). Because of this, many children and adults with MCDs are referred to epilepsy surgery centers for relief of intractable seizures (Diaz, Sherman, & Hader, 2008). Estimates indicate that 25% of all surgical focal epilepsy cases have focal cortical dysplasia (Tassi et al., 2002). In pediatric series, rates are even higher, with up to 60% of surgical cases presenting with MCDs (Park et al., 2006; Porter et al., 2003). Pathological subtypes may predict surgical outcomes, with better seizure control in milder subtypes in some studies (Fauser et al., 2004) but not others (Krsek et al., 2009). Although about three-quarters of people with focal cortical dysplasia have intractable epilepsy (Semah et al., 1998), exact numbers are difficult to determine because not all people with MCDs present themselves for medical care or receive diagnostic imaging. Malformations of cortical development may occur in many patients, including those with genetic disorders, learning disability, and mental retardation of unknown etiology (Guerrini & Marini, 2006; Humphreys, Kaufman, & Galaburda, 1990; Marin-Padilla, Parisi, Armstrong, Sargent, & Kaplan, 2002; Spalice et al., 2008). Malformations of cortical development may also underlie some of the abnormalities found in fetal alcohol syndrome (Kumada, Jiang, Cameron, & Komuro, 2007), perinatal injury (Marin-Padilla, 1999), and early postnatal head injury (Lombroso, 2000). Because some MCD subtypes involve microscopic abnormalities that are not detectable by magnetic resonance imaging (MRI), a negative MRI does not rule out MCD (Bast, Ramantani, Seitz, & Rating, 2006). Instead, diagnostic confirmation of MCDs relies on histological analysis of resected tissue, such as occurs after epilepsy surgery.

The terms *cortical dysplasia*, *cerebral dysgenesis*, and *neuron migration disorder* have all been

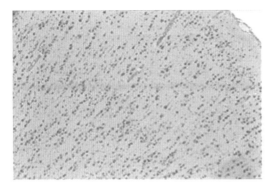

Figure 11-1. Photomicrograph showing fetal-like cortical columnar architecture consistent with focal cortical dysplasia Type IA, as well as heterotopic neurons in the white matter. Hematoxylin and eosin stain; original magnification, 100×.

used interchangeably in the literature to refer to MCDs. Consequently, the general term *MCD* has been proposed to refer to all disorders of cortical development, with more specific terms used for MCD subtypes (Palmini et al., 2004). Malformations of cortical development can therefore be classified according to distinct pathological features, including abnormalities of cell location (heterotopia; see Figure 11.1; see also the color figure in the color insert section), architectural abnormalities in the arrangement of cell layers (columnar vs. the expected laminar arrangement; Figure 11.1), and abnormalities of cell morphology (dysmorphic neurons, balloon cells; see Figure 11.2; see also the color figure in the color insert section).

One of the most widely accepted systems for classifying MCDs of relevance for intractable epilepsy is the classification of Palmini et al. (2004).

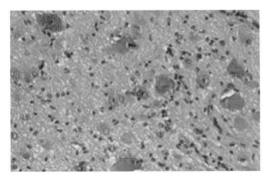

Figure 11-2. Photomicrograph demonstrating balloon cells of the Taylor-type dysplasia (focal cortical dysplasia Type IIB). Hematoxylin and eosin stain; original magnification, 200×.

This system places focal cortical dysplasia (FCD) as a subtype of MCD, and it employs three main classifications: *(1)* Mild MCD, defined as heterotopia occurring in the context of normal architecture; *(2)* FCD Type I, defined as isolated architectural abnormalities with or without giant or immature neurons; and *(3)* FCD Type II, defined as Taylor-type focal cortical dysplasia, or architectural abnormalities and dysmorphic neurons with or without balloon cells (see Table 11.1 for details). Other classification systems also take into account additional factors such as imaging or genetics in addition to pathology (Barkovich et al., 2001; Kuzniecky, 2006; Sarnat & Flores-Sarnat, 2002; Tassi et al., 2002).

We present here a very typical case of a child with a specific MCD who was seen as part of presurgical evaluations in a pediatric epilepsy surgery program. The neuropsychologist's role was to serve as part of the multidisciplinary team comprised of a pediatric epileptologist, neurosurgeon, nurses, radiologists, electroencephalography (EEG) technologists, and neuropathologist. The neuropsychological evaluation's utility was threefold: it served to assist the surgical team in planning surgery and additional investigations needed prior to surgery (such as language mapping), it provided information and recommendations crucial for addressing psychosocial issues, and it provided guidance for school programming and school interventions. We present the case findings in the order in which they occur in an actual surgical work-up: background history and neurological investigations including EEG and imaging first, followed by the neuropsychological evaluation, which was in turn followed by additional investigations involving electrocorticography and language mapping, then the surgery itself, and then finally the neuropathological findings. Consultations with the family throughout this process and specific psychosocial and school recommendations stemming from the neuropsychological evaluation are also described in detail.

Case Report: A. B.

Neurological History

A. B. was a boy born at term weighing 6 lb, 1 oz; maternal gestational diabetes and hypertension

Table 11-1. Classification System for Malformations of Cortical Development

Subtype	Histopathological Features
Mild MCD, Type I	Heterotopic neurons in or adjacent to layer 1
Mild MCD, Type II	With microscopic neuronal heterotopia outside of layer 1
FCD Type IA	Isolated architectural abnormalities (dyslamination, with or without other features of mild MCD)
FCD Type IB	Isolated architectural abnormalities and giant or immature neurons
FCD Type IIA	Taylor-type focal cortical dysplasia: architectural abnormalities with dysmorphic neurons
FCD Type IIB	Taylor-type focal cortical dysplasia: architectural abnormalities with dysmorphic neurons and balloon cells

FCD, focal cortical dysplasia; MCD, malformation of cortical development.

Source: Adapted from Palmini et al. (2004)

were present during the pregnancy. As a baby, he was overactive and a restless sleeper, but he was otherwise healthy, reaching all developmental milestones on time. At age 4, he developed seizures consisting of visual changes in the right visual field, including transient right hemianopia and visual illusions consisting of flashing lights and morphing of objects. These were treated with carbamazepine, but seizures still occurred at least daily. Problems with attention, overactivity, and distractibility were noted upon entry into kindergarten at age 5. At age 8, he was referred to a neurologist because seizures were increasing in frequency. Clinical examination revealed a partial right lower quadrantanopsia. Despite taking two antiepileptic medications (levetiracetam and oxcarbazepine) the patient continued to have five seizures per day. At the time of the assessment, he was in a regular school program but was struggling to maintain his marks. He was right handed and active in several sports and peer activities, and he had a number of friends in the neighborhood and at school. Parents reported no family history of attention-deficit/hyperactivity disorder (ADHD), epilepsy, or learning problems.

Magnetic Resonance Imaging, Electroencephalography, and Single-Photon Emission Computed Tomography

A comprehensive epilepsy surgery evaluation was performed. An MRI demonstrated the presence of a significant malformation in the left parieto-occipital region consisting of a deep cleft with areas of thickened cortex and evidence of polymicrogyria (see Figure 11.3). Inpatient video-EEG monitoring identified occasional epileptiform discharges in the left parietal and temporal lobes with slowing in the left posterior quadrant. Multiple typical partial seizures were recorded with onset in the left posterior quadrant. Ictal single-photon emission computed tomography (SPECT) scanning showed hyperperfusion in the left temporal occipital area adjacent to the malformation.

Neuropsychological Evaluation

Test Results. As part of the presurgical work-up, this child was administered a standard battery that included neuropsychological tests and standardized questionnaires. The battery covered critical cognitive functions necessary in presurgical evaluation of epilepsy patients, including memory and language, and screening for common comorbidities in pediatric epilepsy such as ADHD and depression. Quality-of-life scales were also part of the standard work-up because of the importance of tracking postsurgical changes and real-world impact of treatment, and measures of adaptive functioning were included because of the high base rate of cognitive disability in pediatric epilepsy surgery patients. Specific tests and scales are shown in Tables 11.2 and 11.3.

Behaviorally, the child presented as very friendly and enthusiastic. He had clear difficulty staying on task and was overactive, talkative, and mildly impulsive. However, he was interpersonally appropriate and had a positive mood with good frustration tolerance for challenging tasks. Testing

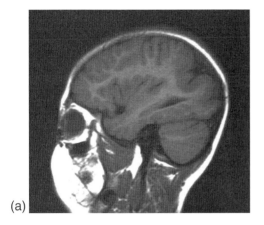

(a)

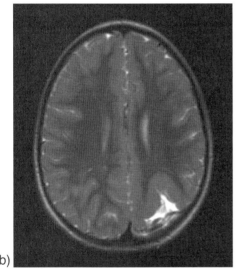

(b)

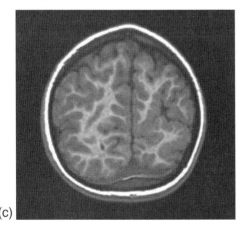

(c)

Figure 11-3. Magnetic resonance image showing left parieto-occipital abnormalities. (*a*) Sagittal T1 image showing abnormal deep parieto-occipital sulcus. (*b*) Axial T2 image showing thickened gray matter along sulcus. (*c*) Coronal 3D GRE T1-weighted image demonstrating evidence of polymicrogyria along deep cleft.

occurred over 2 days. Age-adjusted percentiles are shown in Figure 11.4 for the neuropsychological measures and in Figure 11.5 for the parent, teacher, and self-rated questionnaires.

Overall, A. B. performed well on a number of tests, but he had clear difficulties in certain domains, primarily (*1*) executive functioning and attention, (*2*) verbal memory, (*3*) abstract reasoning, (*4*) math, and (*5*) fine motor function (particularly of the dominant right hand), in the context of IQ in the borderline range (Figure 11.4). He had relative strengths in visual-spatial constructional skills, visual memory, basic language (excluding verbal expression and verbal fluency), and reading. Close examination of memory performance showed difficulties with aspects of verbal rote memory as measured by list-learning tasks such as the CVLT-C and CMS Word Pairs, tasks requiring associative (rather than contextual) learning, with slightly better verbal memory for information presented in context, such as CMS Stories. Visual memory was more consistently strong than verbal memory, but there was some variability in performance, with lower scores obtained on the CMS Faces and RCFT. This was felt to reflect difficulties with attention to visual detail (CMS Faces) and complex visual organization and planning (RCFT), given the task demands of both these tests, rather than to problems with visual encoding and recall per se.

Because determining language dominance is always an important component of the presurgical evaluation, A. B. was also administered a dichotic listening task, along with a lateral dominance examination examining handedness during manipulation of real objects. A dichotic listening test involving detection of phonemes indicated a left-ear superiority in this strongly right-handed child.

Questionnaires indicated clear problems with executive function and attention in daily life consistent with ADHD, and parent and teachers both reported clinically significant problems with behavior at home and at school (Figure 11.5). Depressive symptoms were not evident on self-report. Adaptive behaviour was rated as low, with relative strengths in motor functioning in daily life. Quality-of-life questionnaires indicated very good quality of life overall despite interference from seizures in daily activities (Figure 11.6).

Table 11-2. Neuropsychological Tests for the Presurgical Work-Up

Neuropsychological Domains	Test
IQ	Wechsler Intelligence Scale for Children, Fourth Edition (WISC-IV; Wechsler, 2003)
Attention/ Executive Function	Wisconsin Card Sorting Test–64 (Kongs, Thompson, Iverson, & Heaton, 2000)
	Continuous Attention Test (CAT; Seidel & Joschko, 1991)
	NEPSY Attention and Response Set (Korkman, Kirk, & Kemp, 1998)
	Design Fluency (Jones-Gotman, 1991; Strauss, Sherman, & Spreen, 2006)
	Verbal Fluency (Delis-Kaplan Executive Function System or NEPSY)
	WISC-IV Working Memory Index and Processing Speed Index subtests
Language	Picture Vocabulary Test (Woodcock-Johnson III Tests of Achievement; Woodcock, McGrew, & Mather, 2001)
	Peabody Picture Vocabulary Test, Third Edition (PPVT- III; Dunn & Dunn, 1997)
	Gray Oral Reading Test, Fourth Edition (GORT-4; Weiderholt & Bryant)
	Dichotic Listening (Consonant-Vowel Syllables; Hugdahl, 2000)
	WISC-IV Verbal Comprehension Index subtests
Memory	Children's Memory Scale (CMS; Cohen, 1997)
	California Verbal Learning Test, Children's Version (CVLT-C; Delis, Kramer, Kaplan, & Ober, 1994)
	Rey Complex Figure Test (RCFT; Meyers & Meyers, 1995)
	Continuous Visual Memory Test (CVMT; Trahan & Larrabee, 1999)
Visual-Spatial and Motor	Beery Test of Visuaal-Motor Integration (VMI; Beery & Beery, 2004)
	WISC-IV Perceptual Reasoning Index subtests
	RCFT Copy Trial
	Purdue Pegs (Gardner & Broman, 1979)

Interpretation. One of the challenges in interpreting neuropsychological results and discussing these with the surgical team prior to surgery is that the exact margins of the resection may not be known prior to the surgery itself. In this case, the left-sided surgery was intended to target mainly parietal-occipital lobes. However, surgery could have also potentially included a posterior or mesial temporal resection depending on the results of extraoperative and intraoperative electrocorticography. Because of this, the main risks from a neuropsychological standpoint included the risk of declines in language and/or declines in verbal memory; indeed, risks to language and

Table 11-3. Questionnaires and Scales for the Presurgical Work-Up

Psychosocial Functioning	Child Behavior Checklist (CBCL) and Teacher Rating Form (TRF; Achenbach & Rescorla, 2001)
	ADHD Rating Scale – IV (ADHD-RS-IV; DuPaul, Power, Anastopolous, & Reid, 1998)
	Behavior Rating Inventory of Executive Function (BRIEF; Gioia, Isquith, Guy, & Kenworthy, 2000)
	Child Depression Inventory (CDI; Kovacs & MHS Staff, 2003)
Adaptive Behavior	Adaptive behaviour (Scales of Independent Behaviour–Revised; SIB-R; Bruininks, Woodcock, Weatherman, & Hill, 1997); Parent
	Adaptive Behavior Assessment System II (ABAS-II; Harrison & Oakland, 2003); School
Quality of Life	Impact of Childhood Illness (ICI; Hoare & Russell, 1995)
	The Hague Restrictions in Epilepsy Scale (HARCES; Carpay et al., 1997)
	The Impact of Childhood Neurologic Disability Scale (ICND; Camfield, Breau, & Camfield, 2001)

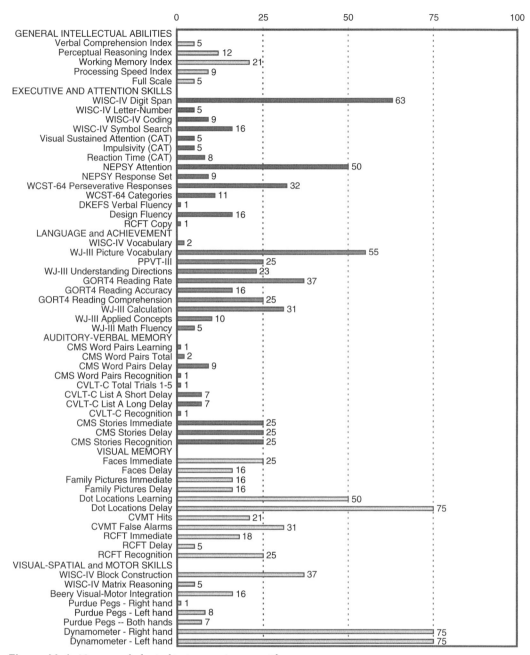

Figure 11-4. Neuropsychological test scores in percentiles.

verbal memory are the most commonly reported neuropsychological side effects of temporal lobe surgery, with base rates of between 30% and 50% (Engman, Andersson-Roswall, Svensson, & Malmgren, 2004; Stroup et al., 2003). In this child's case, language was a relative strength, so there was a definite risk of language decline after

surgery, given the dominant temporal lobe's role in naming and receptive language in most right-handed individuals. The neurosurgeon discussed the likelihood of an expected expansion of the presurgical left quadrantanopsia to a full hemianopsia with left parietal-occipital surgery, and this was felt by the family to be an

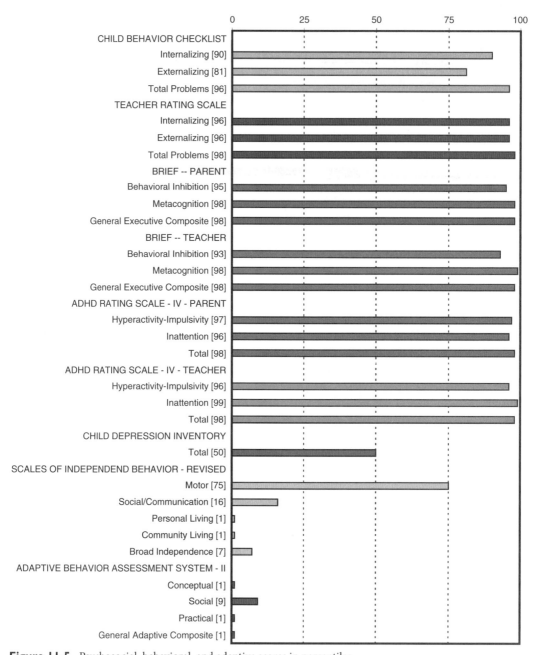

Figure 11-5. Psychosocial, behavioral, and adaptive scores in percentiles.

acceptable risk in light of the possibility of better seizure control.

The dichotic listening results pointed to better language processing in the left ear than in the right ear in a strongly right-handed child. This raised the possibility of atypical language dominance. Language mapping was recommended prior to surgery with an emphasis on mapping receptive language, given the possibility of a left-temporal resection. In this case, determining that the resection zone did not include language sites was important because it may have allowed a more generous resection of epileptogenic tissue, and hence a better chance at seizure control after surgery.

Global QOL

Please rate your child's overall 'Quality of Life' on the scale below: Choose the number which you feel is best and circle it.

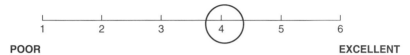

POOR   EXCELLENT

Figure 11-6. Example of global quality-of-life (QOL) item from the Impact of Childhood Neurologic Disability (ICND) Scale.

Because activation of language areas has been reported in dysplastic cortex in some studies (Araujo et al., 2006), it was entirely possible in this case that language and MCD zones might overlap.

The other major factor to determine in his case, in addition to language dominance, was the risk of memory decline with a left-sided surgery, should surgery involve resection of mesial temporal areas. In this case, verbal memory was low preoperatively, which made the risk of verbal memory decline less likely than had high preoperative verbal memory been found (Chelune & Najm, 2001). However, other typical risk factors for verbal memory decline such as the presence of mesial temporal sclerosis on imaging were not present (Martin et al., 2002), and so the risk was not felt to be nil. In addition, it was unclear which cerebral hemisphere was actually subserving memory given the possibility of language reorganization, but strong visual memory and weak verbal memory in the context of lesional epilepsy with left-sided seizure focus seemed to point to the possibility that verbal memory was still being mediated by the left hemisphere, and that visual memory was mediated by the presumably healthy right hemisphere.

Notably, aspects of this case highlight the overlapping but separate sensitivities of different investigations involved in the epilepsy surgery work-up. This child's lesion on imaging was restricted to the occipital and parietal cortex on the left. However, EEG and neuropsychological testing both pointed to dysfunction outside of the lesion zone itself. Specifically, EEGs pointed to a left temporal seizure focus in addition to a parietal focus, and neuropsychology indicated dysfunction in verbal memory, a function presumably also mediated by the left temporal lobe. Neuropsychological testing also pointed to ADHD-type symptoms and thus raised the possibility of other abnormalities outside the identified lesion zone such as the possibility of dysfunction in frontal lobe circuits mediating attention and executive functioning.

Grid Placement and Language Mapping

A. B. then proceeded to a two-stage epilepsy surgery procedure, with grid placement and extraoperative language mapping to be conducted in the first stage. A generous left fronto-temporal-parietal craniotomy was completed followed by insertion of a large subdural grid (see Figure 11.7; see also the color figure in the color insert section) in addition to several subtemporal and occipital subdural strips to record

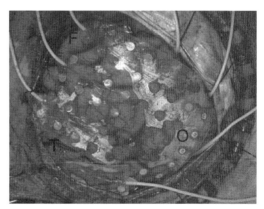

Figure 11-7. Intraoperative view of the left hemisphere and grid. F, frontal lobe; O, occipital lobe; T, temporal lobe.

seizure activity. Multiple typical visual seizures were recorded and found to be arising from the left inferior occipital surface with rapid spread to left mesial and lateral temporal cortices.

Extraoperative language mapping was then carried out by the neuropsychologist using a variety of stimuli and paradigms to capture left-temporal functions of receptive comprehension of language, reading, and naming. Reading level and naming items were determined prior to mapping using results from the neuropsychological assessment as a guide. Baseline testing at the bedside involved developing a series of test items that could be performed error-free, prior to commencing stimulation. In particular, because of the importance of auditory naming sites in the surgical work-up of patients with temporal lobe involvement (Hamberger, Seidel, McKhann, Perrine, & Goodman, 2005), test items were developed using a "riddles" or "guessing game" paradigm, where the child must provide a specific word to a series of spoken clues (e.g., "tell me what cries and wears a diaper"). Because many children feel lethargic or uncomfortable after grid placement, language mapping was carried out in several short sessions using generous praise and reinforcements such as small prizes and stickers. A. B. tolerated the procedure very well. Each stimulation site was stimulated multiple times. No language sites were identified in the left temporal lobe.

Surgical Decision Making

As part of the evaluation, neuropsychological results were discussed in detail with the family, over more than one session. The discussion covered three broad areas: *(1)* A. B.'s overall neuropsychological functioning, with a discussion of specific strengths and weaknesses; *(2)* the factors presumed to underlie any cognitive problems, including the location of the lesion based on imaging and EEG findings, and the combined impact of seizures and AEDs on cognition; *(3)* surgical risks and benefits from a cognitive and psychosocial standpoint; and finally *(4)* implications of test results for school programming and home.

Because no language sites could be identified on language mapping, surgical risks to language were felt to be minimal, and this was reassuring to the family. Risks to memory were also felt to be relatively low because of the low performance on verbal memory tasks. Overall, the family was comfortable with proceeding with surgery after several meetings with the team outlining risks and benefits. Of note, the costs of not proceeding to surgery were also discussed; this included the possibility of cognitive plateauing or decline, which is a risk in chronic epilepsy, as well as the possibility of decreased psychological adjustment and quality of life with continuing chronic seizures of childhood onset (see Elger, Helmstaedter, & Kurthen, 2004; Helmstaedter, Kurthen, Lux, Reuber, & Elger, 2003; Sillanpää, Haataja, & Shinnar, 2004).

Pharmacological and Psychosocial Recommendations

Like many children with chronic seizures, this child had a comorbid ADHD diagnosis (Hermann et al., 2007; Sherman, Slick, Connolly, & Eyrl, 2007). The exact etiology of ADHD symptoms is rarely known in children with epilepsy. At times, the triad of inattention, overactivity, and distractibility might be accounted for by a comorbid, etiologically distinct, non-epilepsy-related ADHD diagnosis. This would not be surprising given the high base rate of ADHD in children seen in tertiary medical settings. Alternatively, ADHD symptoms might be a manifestation of the underlying MCD, which is an equally plausible explanation. Interference from frequent seizures and cognitive effects of AEDs may also contribute to ADHD symptoms in some children, particularly those with a more inattentive profile. Screening for and treating ADHD symptoms in children with epilepsy is important because these symptoms are related to poor quality of life, and they may be overlooked in this patient group (Sherman et al., 2007). In this case, referral to a pediatrician or child psychiatrist was made to review appropriateness of pharmacological interventions (e.g., stimulant medication). Recommendations for specific parent resources for ADHD were provided to the family (e.g., books and audio-visual materials by Russell Barkley, such as the book *Taking Charge of ADHD*; Barkley, 2000), and contact information for the local ADHD support group was provided. A referral to a clinical psychologist was also made to assist the parents in using behavioral techniques for improving the child's self-monitoring, attention to task, and self-control at home and at school, as well as to address externalizing and internalizing behavioral difficulties.

The psychosocial impact of epilepsy was reviewed with the parents, with careful consideration that the child might not become seizure-free after surgery given a lower success of epilepsy surgery in patients with MCD compared to other kinds of etiologies such as mesial temporal sclerosis (MTS) (Alexandre et al., 2006; Diaz, Sherman, & Hader, 2008). The need for parents to resist overprotecting their child and the importance of making sure the child took part in regular peer activities was emphasized, because overprotection and activity restriction are thought to be two factors leading to poor role engagement in adulthood in people with epilepsy (Sherman, in 2009). The importance of not overreinforcing the sick role or the perception of epilepsy as a "disease" was also made, given that some children with intractable epilepsy and multiple hospital admissions receive considerable reinforcement (e.g., parental attention/concern, gifts) for being perceived as being "ill." For children who become seizure-free after surgery but who have no new identity or reinforcement outside the sick role, there is also the risk of the development of non-epileptic seizures. The parents were therefore encouraged to view seizures neutrally and matter of factly; to attempt not to react with fear, overprotection, or anxiety during seizures; and to reinforce the child's strengths and talents rather than overfocusing on seizure-related limitations or medical issues. The importance of addressing caregiver burden was also discussed given that many mothers of children with epilepsy are overwhelmed with care demands and are at risk for psychological disorders (Wood, Sherman, Hamiwka, Blackman, & Wirrell, 2008).

Surgery

The patient then underwent a large left occipital temporal resection, including removal of the parieto-occipital lesion as well as complete removal of the left temporal lobe including mesial temporal structures. There were no complications from the surgery apart from the expected right hemifield deficit from the left occipital resection. Following surgery, the patient became entirely seizure-free. No cognitive declines

were reported by the child or family, and a postoperative neuropsychological assessment was scheduled for 1 year after surgery. Referrals to occupational therapy and to a vision clinic were made to assist with developing recommendations to compensate for the visual field deficit.

Neuropathology

After surgery, surgical specimens were submitted for pathological analysis and evaluated with a standard battery of techniques, including histological, histochemical, immunocytochemical, and electron microscopy studies (Sarnat and Flores-Sarnat, 2009). Three main abnormalities were found: (1) severe cortical dysplasia in the occipital lobe, (2) milder cortical dysplasia in the temporal lobe, and (3) cell loss in the hippocampus. In the left anterior inferior occipital lobe, the cortical gray matter was found to be totally disorganized without the normal pattern of cortical lamination present (see Figure 11.8; see also the color figure in the color insert section). Neurons were disoriented and misplaced, with large pyramidal cells near the molecular zone and small granule cells scattered within the deep layers instead of the normal pattern of organization. There were many heterotopic neurons in the white matter, singly and in clusters (see Figure 11.9; see also the color figure in the color insert section), and these had functional synaptic connections to cortex. No abnormal cells (dysmorphic cells, balloon cells) were found. With

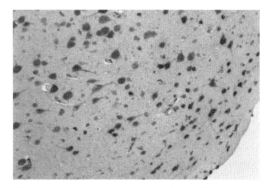

Figure 11-8. Focal cortical dysplasia of left anterior inferior occipital lobe. The cortical architecture is neither columnar as in the fetus nor laminar as in mature brain, but rather neurons of various sizes are arranged and oriented haphazardly.

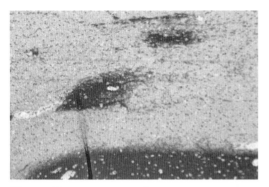

Figure 11-9. Synaptic vesicle reactivity is strong in the deep layers of cortex but not in the white matter beneath the cortex. There are several clusters of heterotopic neurons in the white matter with strong synaptic reactivity within these nodules. Synaptophysin; magnification, 100×.

the milder focal dysplasia in the left posterior temporal cortex, the general architecture of the cortex was well preserved, with normal lamination, but small focal areas of dysplasia were found with loss of lamination and disoriented neurons. A few areas had a fetal-like architecture consisting of columnar rather than laminar arrangement of neurons. There were some heterotopic neurons in the white matter, but not an excessive amount. In the left hippocampus, there was a selective neuronal loss from the CA1 layer, and neurons in CA1 were smaller than in other regions (see Figure 11.10, see also the color figure in the color insert section). There was loss of granule cells focally within the dentate gyrus, without gliosis. The general architecture of the hippocampus was preserved. Overall, the pathological findings were consistent with the presence of FCD Type IA as well as focal neuronal loss in the hippocampus and dentate.

Educational Recommendations

Like many children with significant learning challenges, A. B. required accommodations at school in the form of a modified educational program and specific designation as a child with a severe medical condition affecting learning. All of the following points were included in the neuropsychological report. It was emphasized that his learning challenges were a result of an underlying neurodevelopmental condition (MCD),

as well as epilepsy. As well, it was explained to school staff that because the seizures themselves were a secondary effect of the underlying neurodevelopmental condition, a seizure-free status after surgery would not "cure" his learning problems. This explanation was provided because some schools may remove special programming if a child becomes seizure-free after surgery, mistakenly assuming that seizures are a primary cause of learning challenges rather than a secondary effect of the underlying neurodevelopmental condition that is itself the primary cause of cognitive difficulties. In our experience, it is equally important to emphasize that changes to school programming should not wait until the child has had surgery, but rather need to be instituted as soon as possible; teachers may assume that epilepsy surgery will dramatically reduce

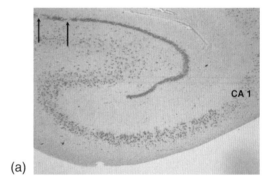

(a)

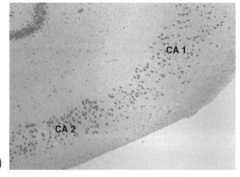

(b)

Figure 11-10. Transverse section of left hippocampus. (*A*) Focal zones of neuronal loss are seen at low magnification in the dentate gyrus (arrows) and in the CA1 sector of Ammon horn (magnification, 40×). (*B*) Higher magnification shows that the CA2 sector is well preserved with a normal compliment of neurons, but the CA1 sector has a reduced number of neurons (magnification, 100×). NeuN, neuronal nuclear antigen.

the need for accommodations or modifications to school programming, which is rarely the case. The most straightforward approach for doing this is to explain that epilepsy surgery is designed to cure seizures, not learning problems. This is important to explain to parents as well. In this case, as is the case for many children with epilepsy, it was explained to the school that like many children with epilepsy, this boy's learning potential could fluctuate from day to day or month to month because of interference from seizures and medication changes, and that his program needed flexibility in order to accommodate time off for medical investigations or postictal recovery.

The school was informed of the need to emphasize visual learning, as well as learning in context, and specific recommendations about one-on-one assistance for complex tasks were made. With regard to general learning approaches, it was emphasized that this boy was primarily a visual learner; specific recommendations for executive function, attention, verbal memory, and motor skills were also provided to the school and parents. These are shown in Table 11.4.

A referral was also made to an educational consultant to explore alternative schooling programs with the family, given the unique challenges of this child with regard to learning, and the fact that the child did not meet criteria for inclusion in special classes for children with frank cognitive disabilities. After consulting with the educational consultant, the parents opted to keep the child in his regular school, with implementation of the recommended changes to his school program.

Discussion

There are few neuropsychological studies of children with MCDs, despite how often these children are referred for neuropsychological or neurological evaluation. Some studies report that a majority of children have developmental and cognitive problems (Lortie, Plouin, Chiron, Delalande, & Dulac, 2002), whereas others report a low prevalence of cognitive limitations (Bast et al., 2006). Other studies find no differences between MCD subgroups (Krsek et al., 2008), or else different cognitive outcomes depending on subtype (Krsek et al., 2009; Lawson et al., 2005). In some reports, cognitive problems relate more to the focality of the MCD than to the MCD subtype (Klein, Levin, Duchowny, & Llabre, 2000). Few studies have used an established neuropathological classification system to classify subtypes, or studied

Table 11-4. Examples of Specific School-Based Recommendations

Executive Function	One-to-one supervision
	Frequent direct feedback
	Immediate reinforcement for goal behaviors
	Routinized environment with clear expectations and warnings for change
	Breaking down complex tasks into manageable mini-tasks
	Use of to-do lists
	Verbal mediation for complex tasks ("Where do I start?" "What's the next step?" "Did I do a good job on this step?" and so on)
Attention	Preferential seating away from distractions
	Quiet work environment
	Distraction-free, uncluttered work environment
	Frequent review and repetition
	Liberal use of incentives to maintain focus (stickers, tokens)
	Frequent breaks between tasks
	Use of short start and stop times to maintain focus and goal-directedness
Verbal Memory	Liberal use of diagrams, charts, pictures, or demonstrations
	Avoidance of learning approaches relying exclusively on lectures, discussions, verbal explanations
	Use of meaningful context to facilitate encoding and retrieval of rote material
Motor	Extra time for writing and fine motor tasks

neuropsychological function in detail. Similarly, information on quality of life is entirely lacking (Sisodiya, 2004), and the prevalence of psychiatric and behavioral comorbities of MCDs is unknown. Studies linking the neuropsychological and neuropathological aspects of MCDs are clearly needed to better understand these conditions for clinical care, but they are also needed to provide answers to fundamental theoretical questions on the cognitive consequences of these specific disruptions in brain development and cognition.

We present here a child who was referred for neuropsychological evaluation prior to epilepsy surgery, a case that in many ways is typical of children seen in tertiary care centers for surgical workups for intractable epilepsy. This child had early seizure onset, pre-existing cognitive difficulties that had not yet been well documented, and a lesion on MRI that was presumed to be a malformation, but the exact subtype and extent was not known until after the resection. Additionally, the underlying pathological substrate was found to involve not a single abnormality or etiology, but rather abnormalities arising during fetal life (severe and milder forms of MCD) as well as acquired pathology (CA1 and dentate cell loss), the latter likely a secondary effect of seizure activity. Of note, the neuropsychological assessment identified prominent verbal memory problems, which raised the possibility of mesial temporal abnormalities that were then confirmed by pathological analysis (CAI and dentate cell loss). In addition, the child had a high-baserate behavioral comorbidity (ADHD) that may or may not have been etiologically related to the underlying MCD, but which was confirmed by the neuropsychological evaluation and which lead to referrals for intervention (both pharmacological and behavioral).

This case illustrates some of the complexities inherent in evaluating children with MCDs who are assessed for epilepsy surgery, and it highlights the important role of the pediatric neuropsychologist as part of the multidisciplinary work-up for pediatric epilepsy surgery. The neuropsychological assessment served to meet several needs, including (1) addressing questions regarding cognitive risks and benefits of surgery for this child; (2) determining whether the cognitive profile was concordant with imaging and other investigations, which may have pointed to the possibility of abnormal areas outside the lesion zones; (3) identifying any additional investigations that could have informed surgical decision making (in this case, language mapping); and (4) addressing additional referrals and recommendations needed for psychosocial and school-based needs. As well, in cases such as this, the neuropsychologist helps families understand the neurologically based nature of their child's cognitive strengths and weaknesses, which can alleviate frustration and help develop realistic expectations and goals with regard to behavior, schooling, and family adjustment. The neuropsychologist also serves as a liaison for implementing school recommendations.

References

Achenbach, T. M., & Rescorla, L. A. (2001). *ASEBA school-age forms and profiles.* Burlington: University of Vermont, Research Center for Children, Youth, & Families.

Alexandre, V., Walz, R., Bianchin, M. M., Velasco, T. R., Terra-Bustamante, V. C., Wichert-Ana, L., Araújo, D., Machado, H. R., Assirati, J. A., Carlotti, C. G., Santos, A. C., Serafini, L. N., & Sakamoto, A. C. (2006). Seizure outcome after surgery for epilepsy due to focal cortical dysplastic lesions. *Seizure, 15*(6), 420–427.

Araujo, D., de Araujo, D. B., Pontes-Neto, O. M., Escorsi-Rosset, S., Simao, G. N., Wichert-Ana, L., Velasco, T. R., Sakamoto, A. C., Leite, J. P., & Santos, A. C. (2006). Language and motor fMRI activation in polymicrogyric cortex. *Epilepsia, 47*(3), 589–592.

Barkley, R. A. (2000). Taking charge of ADHD: The complete, authoritative guide for parents. New York: Guilford.

Barkovich, A. J., Kuzniecky, R. I., Jackson, G. D., Guerrini, R., & Dobyns, W. B. (2001). Classification system for malformations of cortical development. *Neurology, 57,* 2168–2178.

Barkovich, A. J., Kuzniecky, R. I., Jackson, G. D., Guerrini, R., & Dobyns, W. B. (2005). A developmental and genetic classification for malformations of cortical development. *Neurology, 65*(12), 1873–1887.

Bast, T., Ramantani, G., Seitz, A., & Rating, D. (2006). Focal cortical dysplasia: Prevalence, clinical presentation and epilepsy in children and adults. *Acta Neuro Scand, 113,* 72–81.

Beery, K. E., & Beery, N. A. (2004). *Beery-Buktenica Developmental Test of Visual-Motor Integration* (5th ed.). Minneapolis, MN: NCS Pearson.

Bentivoglio, M., Tassi, L., Pech, E., Costa, C., Fabene, P. F., & Spreafico, R. (2003). Cortical development and focal cortical dysplasia. *Epileptic Disorders, 5,* S27–S34.

Bruininks, R. H., Woodcock, R. W., Weatherman, R. F., & Hill, B. K. (1997). *Scales of Independent Behavior–Revised.* Itasca, IL: Riverside Publishing.

Camfield, C. S., Breau, L. M., & Camfield, P. R. (2001). Impact of pediatric epilepsy on the family: A new scale for clinical and research use. *Epilepsia, 41,* 104–112.

Carpay, H., Vermeulen, J., Stroink, H., Brouwer, O. F., Peters, A. C. B., Van Donselaar, C. A., Aldenkamp, A. P., & Arts, W. F. M. (1997). Disability due to restrictions in childhood epilepsy. *Developmental Medicine and Child Neurology, 39,* 521–526.

Chelune, G. C., & Najm, I. (2001). Risk factors associated with postsurgical decrements in memory. In H. Lüders (Ed.), *Epilepsy surgery* (2nd ed., pp. 497–504). Philadelphia: Lippincott, Williams and Wilkens.

Cohen, M. J. (1997). *Children's Memory Scale.* San Antonio, TX: The Psychological Corporation.

Delis, D. C., Kaplan, E., & Kramer, J. H. (2001). *Delis-Kaplan Executive Function System.* San Antonio, TX: The Psychological Corporation.

Delis, D. C., Kramer, J. H., Kaplan, E., & Ober, B. A. (1994). *California Verbal Learning Test – Children's Version.* San Antonio, TX: The Psychological Corporation.

Diaz, J. R., Sherman, E. M. S., & Hader, W. J. (2008). Surgical treatment of intractable epilepsy associated with focal cortical dysplasia. *Neurosurgical Focus, 25*(3), E6.

Dunn, L. M., & Dunn, L. M. (1997). *Peabody Picture Vocabulary Test, Third Edition.* Circle Pines, MN: American Guidance Service.

DuPaul, G. J., Power, T. J., Anastopolous, A. D., & Reid, R. (1998). *ADHD Rating Scale IV.* New York: Guilford Press.

Elger, C. E., Helmstaedter, C., & Kurthen, M. (2004). Chronic epilepsy and cognition. *Lancet Neurology, 3*(11), 663–672.

Engman, E., Andersson-Roswall, L., Svensson, E., & Malmgren, K. (2004). Non-parametric evaluation of memory changes at group and individual level following temporal lobe resection for pharmaco-resistant partial epilepsy. *Journal of Clinical and Experimental Neuropsychology, 26*(7), 943–954.

Fauser, S., Schulze-Bonhage, A., Honegger, J., Carmona, H., Huppertz, H-J., Pantazis, G., et al. (2004). Focal cortical dysplasias: Surgical outcome in 67 patients in relation to histological subtypes and dual pathology. *Brain, 127,* 2406–2418.

Gardner, R. A., & Broman, M. (1979). The Purdue Pegboard: Normative date for 1334 school children. *Journal of Clinical Child Psychology, 8,* 156–162.

Gioia, G. A., Isquith, P. K., Guy, S. C., & Kenworthy, L. (2000). *Behavior Rating Inventory of Executive Function.* Lutz, FL: Psychological Assessment Resources.

Guerrini, R., & Marini, C. (2006). Genetic malformations of cortical development. *Experimental Brain Research, 173,* 322–333.

Hamberger, M. J., Seidel, W. T., McKhann, G. M., Perrine, K., & Goodman, R. R. (2005). Brain stimulation reveals critical auditory naming cortex. *Brain, 128*(11), 2742–2749.

Harrison, P. L., & Oakland, T. (2003). *Adaptive Behavior Assessment System, Second Edition.* San Antonio, TX: The Psychological Corporation.

Helmstaedter, C., Kurthen, M., Lux, S., Reuber, R., & Elger, C. E. (2003). Chronic epilepsy and cognition: A longitudinal study in temporal lobe epilepsy. *Annals of Neurology, 54*(4), 425–432

Hermann, B., Jones, J., Dabbs, K., Allen, C. A., Sheth, R., Fine, J., McMillan, A., & Seidenberg, M. (2007). The frequency, complications and aetiology of ADHD in new onset paediatric epilepsy. *Brain, 130*(12), 3135–3148.

Hoare, P., & Russell, M. (1995). The quality of life of children with chronic epilepsy and their families: Preliminary findings with a new assessment measure. *Developmental Medicine and Child Neurology, 37,* 689–696.

Hugdahl, K. (2000). What can be learned about brain function from dichotic listening? *Revista Española de Neuropsicologia, 2*(3), 62–84.

Humphreys, P., Kaufmann, W. E., & Galaburda, A. M. (1990). Developmental dyslexia in women: Neuro-pathological findings in three patients. *Annals of Neurology, 28,* 727–738.

Jones-Gotman, M. (1991). Localization of lesions by neuropsychological testing. *Neuropsychologia, 15,* 653–674.

Klein, B., Levin, B. E., Duchowny, M. S., & Llabre, M. M. (2000). Cognitive outcome of children with epilepsy and malformations of cortical development. *Neurology, 55,* 230–235.

Kongs, S. K., Thompson, L. L., Iverson, G. L., & Heaton, R. K. (2000). *Wisconsin Card Sorting Test–64 Card Version.* Lutz, FL: Psychological Assessment Resources.

Korkman, M., Kirk, U., & Kemp, S. (1998). *NEPSY: A developmental neuropsychological assessment.* San Antonio, TX: The Psychological Corporation.

Kovacs, M., & MHS Staff. (2003). *Children's Depression Inventory.* Toronto, ON: MHS.

Krsek, P., Maton, B., Korman, B., Pachero-Jacome, E., Jayakar, P., Dunoyer, C., Rey, G., Morrison, G., Ragheb, J., Vinters, H. V., Resnick, T., & Duchowny, M. (2008). Different features of histopatholoigcal subtypes of pediatric focal cortical dysplasia. *Annals of Neurology, 63*, 758–769.

Krsek, P., Pieper, T., Karlmeier, A., Hildebrandt, M., Kolodziejczyk, D., Winkler, P., Pauli, E., Blümcke, I., & Holthausen, H. (2009). Different presurgical characteristics and seizure outcomes in children with focal cortical dysplasia type I or II. *Epilepsia,* 50(1), 125–137.

Kumada, T., Jiang, Y., Cameron, D. B., & Komuro, H. (2007). How does alcohol impair neuronal migration? *Journal of Neuroscience Research, 85*, 465–470.

Kuzniecky, R. I. (2006). Malformations of cortical development and epilepsy, part 1: Diagnosis and classification scheme. *Reviews in Neurological Diseases, 3*, 151–162.

Lortie, A., Plouin, P., Chiron, C., Delalande, O., & Dulac, O. (2002). Characteristics of epilepsy in focal cortical dysplasia in infancy. *Epilepsy Research, 51*(1–2), 133–145.

Lawson, J. A., Birchansky, S., Pacheco, E., Jayakar, P., Resnick, T. J., Dean, P., et al. (2005). Distinct clinicopathologic subtypes of cortical dysplasia of Taylor. *Neurology, 64*, 55–61.

Lombroso, C. T. (2000). Can early postnatal closed head injury induce cortical dysplasia? *Epilepsia, 41*(2), 245–253.

Marrin-Padilla, M. (1999). Developmental neuropathology and impact of perinatal brain damage: III: Gray matter lesions of the neocortex. *Journal of Neuropathology and Experimental Neurology, 58*(5), 407–429.

Marrin-Padilla, M., Parisi, J. E., Armstrong, D. L., Sargent, S. K., & Kaplan, J. A. (2002). Shaken infant syndrome: Developmental neuropathology, progressive cortical dysplasia, and epilepsy. *Acta Neuropathologica, 103*, 321–332.

Martin, R. C., Kretzmer, T., Palmer, C., Sawrie, S., Knowlton, R., Faught, E., et al. (2002). Risk to verbal memory following anterior temporal lobectomy in patients with severe left-sided hippocampal sclerosis. *Archives of Neurology, 59*(12), 1895–1901.

Meyers, J. E., & Meyers, K. R. (1995). *Rey Complex Figure Test and Recognition Trial.* Odessa, FL: Psychological Assessment Resources.

Palmini, A., Najm, I., Avanzini, G., Babb, T., Guerrini, R., Foldvary-Schaefer, N., Jackson, G., Lüders, H. O., Prayson, R., Spreafico, R., & Vinters, H. V. (2004). Terminology and classification of the cortical dysplasias. *Neurology, 62*(6 Suppl 3), S2–S8.

Park, C-K., Kim, S-K., Wang, K-C., Hwang, Y-S., Kim, K. J., Chae, J. H., et al. (2006). Surgical outcome and prognostic factors of pediatric epilepsy caused by cortical dysplasia. *Child's Nervous System, 22*, 586–592.

Porter, B. E., Judkins, A. R., Clancy, R. R., Duhaime, A., Dlugos, D. J., & Golden, J. A. (2003). Dysplasia: A common finding in intractable pediatric temporal lobe epilepsy. *Neurology, 61*, 365–368.

Sarnat, H. B., & Flores-Sarnat, L. (2002). Molecular genetic and morphologic integration in malformations of the nervous system for etiologic classification. *Seminars in Pediatric Neurology, 9*, 335–344.

Sarnat, H. B., & Flores-Sarnat, L. (2009). Neuropathology of paediatric cerebral resections for epilepsy In J.W. Wheless, L.J. Willmore, R.A. Brumback (eds.), *Pediatric epilepsy* (pp. 77-91). Shelton, CT: People's Medical Publishing House.

Semah, F., Picot, M. C., Adam, C., Broglin, D., Arzimanoglou, A., Bazin, B., Cavalcanti, D., & Baulac, M. (1998). Is the underlying cause of epilepsy a major prognostic factor for recurrence? *Neurology, 51*(5), 1256–1262.

Seidel, W. T., & Joschko, M. (1991). Assessment of attention in children. *The Clinical Neuropsychologist, 5*(1), 53–66.

Sherman, E. M. S. (2009). Maximizing quality of life, life satisfaction and wellbeing: Prescriptions for practitioners and people living with epilepsy. *Canadian Journal of Neurological Sciences, 36 (suppl.), s17-s24.*

Sherman, E. M. S., Slick, D. J., Connolly, M. B., & Eyrl, K. L. (2007). ADHD, neurological correlates and health-related quality of life in severe pediatric epilepsy. *Epilepsia, 48*(6), 1083–1091.

Sillanpää, M., Haataja, L., & Shinnar, S. (2004). Perceived impact of childhood-onset epilepsy on quality of life as an adult. *Epilepsia, 45*(8), 971–977.

Sisodiya, S. M. (2004). Scientific commentary: Surgery for focal cortical dysplasia. *Brain, 127*, 2383–2384.

Spalice, A., Parisi, P., Nicita, F., Pizzardi, G., Del Balzo, F., & Iannetti, P. (2008, December 16). Neuronal migration disorders: Clinical, neuroradiologic and genetic aspects. *Acta Paediatrica,* Retreived January 26, 2010, from http://www.ncbi.nlm.nih.gov/pubmed/19120042

Strauss, E., Sherman, E. M. S., & Spreen, O. (2006). *A compendium of neuropsychological tests* (3rd ed.). New York: Oxford University Press.

Stroup, E., Langfitt, J., Berg, M., McDermott, M., Pilcher, W., & Como, P. (2003). Predicting verbal memory decline following anterior temporal lobectomy (ATL). *Neurology, 60*(8), 1266–1273.

Tassi, L., Colombo, N., Garbelli, R., Francione, S., Lo Russo, G., Mai, R., Cardinale, F., Cossu, M., Ferrario, A., Galli, C., Bramerio, M., Citterio, A., & Spreafico, R. (2002). Focal cortical dysplasia: Neuropathological subtypes, EEG, neuroimaging and surgical outcome. *Brain, 125*(Pt 8), 1719–1732.

Trahan, D. E., & Larrabee, G. J. (1999). *Continuous Visual Memory Test*. Lutz, FL: Psychological Assessment Resources.

Weiderholt, J. L., & Bryant, B. R. (2001). *Gray Oral Reading Tests–Fourth Edition*. Austin, TX: PRO-ED.

Wechsler, D. (2003). *Wechsler Intelligence Scale for Children, Fourth Edition*. San Antonio, TX: Harcourt Assessment, Inc.

Wood, L. J., Sherman, E. M. S., Hamiwka, L. D., Blackman, M. A., & Wirrell, E. C. (2008). Maternal depression: The cost of caring for a child with intractable epilepsy. *Pediatric Neurology, 39*(6), 418–422.

Woodcock, R. W., McGrew, K. S., & Mather, N. (2001). *Woodcock-Johnson III Tests of Achievement*. Itasca, IL: Riverside Publishing.

12

Landau-Kleffner Syndrome

Gerry A. Stefanatos and Andrew T. DeMarco

Landau-Kleffner syndrome (LKS) is a disorder of childhood onset characterized by an acquired aphasia that emerges in association with epileptic or epileptiform electroencephalographic abnormalities. The loss of language occurs insidiously or acutely after a period of normal development and typically results in severe impairment of both the comprehension and production of speech. While sporadic seizures are commonly observed some time before or after the regression, 25%–30% of children with LKS do not demonstrate overt seizures. However, electroencephalograms (EEGs) recorded around the time of the regression demonstrate severe epileptic or epileptiform abnormalities, frequently involving generalized high-voltage spike or spike-and-wave discharges with a central or temporal predominance. In their original description, Landau and Kleffner (1957) posited that this abnormal brain electrical activity plays a causal role in the aphasia by disrupting the function of cortical networks required for normal language function.

Designated as a "rare disease" (Office of Rare Diseases, National Institutes of Health), the exact prevalence of LKS is unknown, but it is likely underrecognized and underdiagnosed. The low frequency of the diagnosis (Kramer et al., 1998) has impeded large group studies of the disorder. Consequently, our current understanding of LKS is largely based on more than 300 cases reported in the literature, most within the last 20 years (see reviews by Riviello & Hadjiloizou, 2007; Stefanatos, Kinsbourne, & Wasserstein, 2002).

The syndrome has nevertheless attracted considerable attention and assumed significant conceptual importance. It is the most frequently described form of acquired aphasia in children and is the prototype for a newly defined class of disorder—epileptic encephalopathy—in which a deterioration of cognitive, sensory, and/or motor functions occurs as a result of epileptic or epileptiform activity (Dulac, 2001).

Much of the literature on LKS has focused on the electroencephalographic abnormalities observed in these children. Given that aphasia is a cardinal feature of the syndrome, there are surprisingly few detailed studies directed to understanding the language disorder and associated neuropsychological characteristics of LKS (e.g., Korkman, Granstrom, Appelqvist, & Liukkonen, 1998; Metz-Lutz & Filippini, 2006; Soprano, Garcia, Caraballo, & Fejerman, 1994). In this chapter, we present a comprehensive neuropsychological investigation of a case of LKS. Following a brief history of the diagnosis of LKS and its defining characteristics, key diagnostic issues are discussed and a summary of neuropsychological findings in this case is provided. The results of the evaluation are then discussed in relation to current and emerging conceptions of LKS, its diagnosis and treatment.

Definitional Issues

Landau-Kleffner syndrome first appeared in a standard medical diagnostic manual in the *International Classification of Diseases–9th edition*

Table 12-1. Summary of Diagnostic Criteria for Acquired Aphasia with Epilepsy (Landau-Kleffner syndrome)

- Loss of receptive and expressive language
- Onset usually between 3 and 7 years, regression over days to weeks
- Previously normal progress in language development
- Preservation of general intelligence
- Paroxysmal EEG abnormalities, majority with seizures
- Does not meet criteria for Autistic Disorder (F84.0–F84.1), Disintegrative Disorders of Childhood (F84.2–F84.3), Aphasia Not Otherwise Specified (R47.0)

EEG, electroencephalogram.

Source: Adapted from *International Classification of Diseases, 10th revision.*

(ICD-9) (World Health Organization, 1977) under a nonspecific code for *other forms of epilepsy* (code 345.8). With the release of ICD-10 (World Health Organization, 1992), the syndrome was relabeled *acquired aphasia with epilepsy* (F80.3), although LKS was included parenthetically and has continued to be the most commonly used designation. The diagnostic criteria outlined in ICD-10 (summarized in Table 12-1) are based closely on Landau and Kleffner's original description. Alternative terms referring to the symptom complex have included *acquired auditory verbal agnosia and seizures, epilepsy-aphasia syndrome,* and *acquired epileptiform aphasia,* among others (see Stefanatos et al., 2002 for review).

Landau-Kleffner syndrome has also been incorporated in the International Classification of Epileptic Syndromes (ICES) compiled by the International League Against Epilepsy (ILEA) (1989). Originally labeled *acquired epileptic aphasia* (AEA), it was placed in a category entitled *epilepsies and syndromes undetermined as to whether they are local or generalized.* Subsequently, an ILEA Task Force on Classification and Terminology (Engel, 2001) abandoned the term AEA in favor of LKS and recommended its inclusion, along with a similar condition known as *continuous spike-and-wave during sleep* (CSWS), under a newly described category called the *epileptic encephalopathies.* The syndrome of CSWS is associated with a distinctive electroencephalographic abnormality, *electrical status epilepticus of sleep* (ESES or SES), which is defined by the presence of continuous spike-and-wave activity during a substantial proportion (50%–80%) of non-REM sleep (Tassinari, Bureau, Dravet, Dalla Bernardina, & Rogers, 1992). Comparable but often less severe abnormalities may also be observed in LKS (Genton & Guerrini, 1993), and some have suggested that LKS and CSWS are two behavioral phenotypes associated with the same underlying pathophysiology (Tassinari et al., 2002).

In further revisions of the ICES (Engel, 2006), both LKS and CSWS were subsumed under a single new term *epileptic encephalopathy with continuous spike-and-wave during sleep including Landau-Kleffner syndrome* because it was thought that there were insufficient "mechanistic differences" between the two entities to warrant the delineation of separate syndromes. Unfortunately, this new schema is inappropriate for classifying those children who display typical features of LKS (epileptiform EEG abnormalities and acquired aphasia) but do not have signs of ESES (Panayiotopoulos, 2007). It is also at odds with evidence that, from a clinical standpoint, the two disorders appear dichotomous rather than entities on a continuum (Van Hirtum-Das et al., 2006).

Landau-Kleffner Syndrome Variants

A number of *idiopathic variants* of LKS have been proposed to designate children who display an epileptiform regression of language but who otherwise present with a history or neuropsychological phenotype that does not strictly conform to the criteria in Table 12-1. The terms *epileptiform autistic regression* and *epileptiform disintegrative disorder* (Nass, Gross, & Devinsky, 1998; Tuchman & Rapin, 1997) have been suggested for those children whose epileptiform regression is sufficiently severe and pervasive as to meet criteria for *autistic disorder* (AD) and *childhood disintegrative disorder* (CDD), respectively. *Childhood idiopathic language deterioration*

(ChILD) was proposed (Stefanatos, Kollros, & Rabinovich, 1996) and adopted by some (Holmes & Riviello, 2001) to refer to children whose primary disorder is an idiopathic language deterioration but who otherwise may have additional behavioral involvement that is insufficient in scope and severity to meet criteria for AD or CDD. In addition, *acquired epileptiform opercular syndrome* (Shafrir & Prensky, 1995) describes a condition in which oromotor apraxia (rather than aphasia) is associated with epileptiform EEG abnormalities.

A number of reports have described so-called *symptomatic variants* of the disorder. Unlike the original cases of LKS, the regression and epileptiform abnormalities in these children is associated with identified neuropathology, involving conditions such as tumor (e.g., oligodendroglioma) (Nass, Heier, & Walker, 1993; Solomon, Carson, Pavlakis, Fraser, & Labar, 1993) or demyelinating disease (Perniola et al., 1993). In some cases, childhood diseases such as rubella (Lanzi, Veggiotti, Conte, Partesana, & Resi, 1994) and Hemophilus influenzae meningitis (Ansink, Sarphatie, & van Dongen, 1989) have tentatively been linked to cases of AEA. In addition, parasitic diseases such as neurocysticercosis (Otero, Cordova, Diaz, Garcia-Teruel, & Del Brutto, 1989) and Toxoplasma gondii (Michalowicz, Jozwiak, Ignatowicz, & Szwabowska-Orzeszko, 1988) have been implicated.

Despite wide recognition of significant heterogeneity in both core symptoms and associated symptomology, at present, there are no empirical grounds to inform "lumping" or "splitting" the form of LKS as originally described and the "variants" with identified neuropathology, an atypical history, or a more complicated behavioral phenotype. Some have argued that the boundaries of the disorder should be substantially broadened to include deterioration of any higher cerebral function that occurs in children who exhibit a particular pattern of paroxysmal EEG abnormalities (Hirsch, Maquet, Metz-Lutz, Motte, Finck, & Marescaux, 1995). Others would prefer to maintain the integrity of the original description (Mantovani, 2000) or the "classic" form. Some of this confusion may stem from changes in terminology that have occurred over the years which have made LKS synonymous with acquired epileptic or epileptiform aphasia

when it may be more appropriately considered a subtype of it.

Clinical Manifestations and Diagnostic Considerations

A number of inconsistencies and contradictions surround current conceptions of LKS and its nosological boundaries. The ICD-10 diagnostic criteria attempt to define LKS as a discrete entity with clearly defined boundaries that conform to Landau and Kleffner's original description. However, subsequent observations have revealed substantial variation in onset, temporal course, and associated symptomatology. Given that the criteria have not undergone revision, many children reported in the literature as having LKS show characteristics that deviate from the parameters outlined in ICD-10. In the following subsections, we discuss the clinical manifestations of LKS, taking each of the descriptive guidelines in turn and highlighting relevant deviations that are considered by some to fall within the same spectrum.

Age of Onset

The ICD-10 guidelines suggest that LKS commonly emerges between the ages of 3 and 7 years of age. However, the range of variation is fairly large. Onset as early as 18–22 months (Soprano et al., 1994; Uldall, Sahlholdt, & Alving, 2000) and as late as 14 years (Gerard, Dugas, Valdois, Franc, & Lecendreux, 1993) have been described. Figure 12-1 shows the distribution of age of onset for 208 cases of LKS derived from published reports in the period from 1957 to 2002, supplemented with personal cases. The mean age of onset of aphasia was 4.8 years of age (standard deviation of 2 years). It is noteworthy that nearly one-third (31%) of this sample had an age of onset in the third year of life or earlier.

Loss of Receptive and Expressive Language

Acquired aphasia is the single most prominent defining feature of LKS. Early signs of the disorder commonly entail reduced or inconsistent reactions to spoken communications. Children may

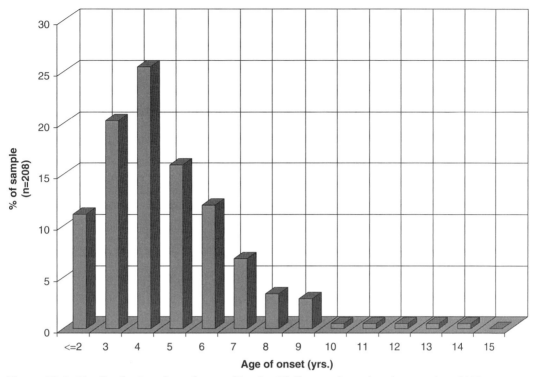

Figure 12-1. The distribution of age of onset of Landau-Kleffner syndrome based on a review of 208 cases from the literature. The mean age of onset of aphasia was 4.8 years with a standard deviation of 2 years. The median age of onset was 4.5 years.

fail to respond consistently to their name being called or otherwise show substantial reductions in their capacity to understand verbally presented information. Diminished responsiveness may extend to environmental sounds, evident in symptoms ranging from a reduction in startle response when exposed to sudden loud noises (Baynes, Kegl, Brentari, Kussmaul, & Poizner, 1998; Dugas, 1982) to a failure to respond appropriately to meaningful environmental sounds (e.g., a doorbell ringing). Receptive language difficulties progressively worsen to the point where children understand little of what is said to them. Comprehension may be limited to only a small number of commonly used words or a restricted range of simple and predictable verbal constructions (Cooper & Ferry, 1978; Kaga, 1999).

Expressive language disturbances emerge in tandem with the receptive decline. Speech production becomes indistinct, marked by phonological disorganization of output. Children have difficulties selecting and combining phonemes into words and phrases, resulting in omissions, distortions, and problems with temporal ordering (Lanzi et al., 1994). Spontaneous speech is often marked by copious phonemic paraphasias, word-finding difficulties, and substantial reductions in mean length of utterance (MLU, the mean number of morphemes in a child's utterances). Children may appear to stutter due to the repeated attempts to output a word. With further syndrome progression, speech may be reduced to recurrent or perseverative production of particular syllables that resembles babbling (e.g., "ta-ta-ta"). It is not uncommon for the language regression to result in a near absence of speech, at least for a period of time (Cooper & Ferry, 1978; Deuel & Lenn, 1977; Hankey & Gubbay, 1987; Msall, Shapiro, Balfour, Niedermeyer, & Capute, 1986; Rapin, Mattis, Rowan, & Golden, 1977). Alterations in voice quality and prosody similar to that associated with hearing impairment have been described (Landau & Kleffner, 1957; Stefanatos, 2008). A proportion of children demonstrate oral dyspraxia, and in some cases, this may be accompanied by a manual dyspraxia (Ansink et al., 1989; Bulteau et al., 1995; Feekery, Parry-Fielder, & Hopkins, 1993).

As the language impairment begins to resolve, children may elicit phonologically more varied verbal productions that are replete with neologisms and jargon (van de Sandt-Koenderman, Smit, van Dongen, & van Hest, 1984). As recovery progresses, neologisms decrease and utterances increase in both frequency and length (van de Sandt-Koenderman et al., 1984). Nevertheless, often children remain reluctant to speak. They seem to demonstrate a "dysbulia of speech", appearing to lack motivation or spontaneity in utilizing their speech to communicate. Verbal productions are frequently marked by syntactically simplified or telegraphic phrases and sentences, lacking in word endings (e.g., tense markers), inflected verbs and function words such as prepositions (e.g., of, to, in, for, with, on), conjunctions (e.g., and, or, but, yet, so, for, nor), and grammatical articles (e.g., the, a, an). Naming and short-term memory difficulties are common (Honbolygo et al., 2006; Majerus et al., 2003; Robinson, Baird, Robinson, & Simonoff, 2001).

Children with LKS often show somewhat greater facility in learning to use signed or written language than in producing and interpreting speech (Baynes et al., 1998; Bishop, 1982; Cooper & Ferry, 1978; Rapin et al., 1977; Worster-Drought, 1971), suggesting that some linguistic representational processes are relatively preserved. The chief impairment underlying the aphasic disturbance in most cases appears to involve mechanisms that mediate the derivation of meaning from sounds of speech (Klein, Kurtzberg, & Brattson, 1995; Rapin et al., 1977; Stefanatos, 1993). As a consequence, the aphasic disturbance is often referred to as a verbal auditory agnosia (VAA) or word deafness, which denotes a severe modality-specific impairment of auditory language comprehension.

While a combination of receptive and expressive deficits is common, approximately 10% of cases demonstrate fairly selective disturbances of expressive language (Feekery et al., 1993; Holmes, McKeever, & Saunders, 1981; Marien, Saerens, Verslegers, Borggreve, & De Deyn, 1993; Sato & Dreifuss, 1973). Some have suggested that an aphasia that primarily involves expressive language is more likely with later onset of the disorder

(Dugas, Gerard, Franc, & Lecendreux, 1995; Gerard et al., 1993). Some reasonably fluent cases have been reported (Chevrie-Muller et al., 1991; Lerman, Lerman-Sagie, & Kivity, 1991). Fluency can vary over the course of the syndrome. Fluent and nonfluent aphasic disturbances can be observed in the same child at different points in syndrome history (van de Sandt-Koenderman et al., 1984).

Previously Normal Progress in Language Development

The ICD-10 guidelines stipulate that children demonstrate normal language development prior to onset of aphasia. This distinguishes LKS from developmental language disorders associated with epileptiform EEG abnormalities. Unfortunately, there are no guidelines as to what constitutes a sufficient deviation from normal language acquisition to preclude the diagnosis of LKS nor how long prior to the regression children should demonstrate normal progress. At least mild delays in early language development are not uncommon. Indeed, review of the literature demonstrates numerous cases described as having LKS who demonstrated regression of language in the context of fairly substantial preexisting and persistent anomalies of language development (e.g., Korkman et al., 1998; Marien et al., 1993; Rossi et al., 1999; Soprano et al., 1994). Delays of early language acquisition might suggest pre-existing anomalies in brain circuitry or connectivity that may relate to their later development of LKS. Consistent with this possibility, several studies have disclosed evidence of anomalies in brain development such as ectopic neurons (Cole et al., 1988; Lou, Brandt, & Bruhn, 1977; Morrell et al., 1995) and perisylvian polymicrogyria (Huppke, Kallenberg, & Gartner, 2005).

Preservation of General Intelligence

In their original description, Landau and Kleffner (1957) demonstrated that LKS is associated with an aphasic disturbance and not a general cognitive decline. Preservation of general intelligence was supported by estimates of nonverbal IQ that were greater than 80 (range from 80 to 137). Unfortunately, the vast majority of subsequent reports of children considered to have LKS are strikingly lacking in information regarding formal intellectual evaluations. Of the reports that have ascertained intelligence levels, a proportion of children (possibly 15%) have fallen below the normal range even when non-verbal IQ measures were employed (Cooper & Ferry, 1978; Deonna, Beaumanoir, Gaillard, & Assal, 1977; Dugas, Masson, Le Heuzey, & Regnier, 1982; Gerard et al., 1993; Kellermann, 1978; Maquet et al., 1995; McKinney & McGreal 1974; Shoumaker, Bennett, Bray, & Curless, 1974). Of five cases reported by Korkman et al. (1998), only one had a nonverbal IQ in the normal range. Assuming the diagnosis of LKS was appropriate in these children, such findings are important as they raise the possibility that the paroxysmal discharges associated with the disorder, while maximally impacting language, can potentially have broader effects on cognition. Estimates obtained in the acute or sub-acute stage of syndrome development may be particularly depressed given the inherent challenges of obtaining optimal performance from a young child with new onset of a severe receptive and expressive communication disorder. These difficulties may be exacerbated by common comorbid problems such as hyperactivity/attentional deficits, low frustration tolerance, emotional disarray, and adjustment issues.

Paroxysmal Electroencephalogram Abnormalities, Majority with Seizures

Approximately 70% to 75% of children with LKS demonstrate overt evidence of seizures within a year or two of the language regression. Seizures are neither frequent nor severe, and onset appears to have little or no temporal relationship to the emergence of the aphasia in the vast majority of cases. Slightly more than half experience a first seizure some time prior to regression (days to years), while the remainder have seizures at the time of or after the onset of aphasia. Importantly, 25% to 30% never demonstrate evidence of clinical seizures (Beaumanoir, 1992; Paquier & Van Dongen, 1996).

Semiology of the seizures includes partial complex (with focal motor and atypical absence symptoms), partial clonic, generalized tonic-clonic, and atonic seizures with head drop. Tonic and myoclonic seizures are rarely seen (Appleton, 1995). Subtle seizures with minor motor or sensory symptomology may often elude detection (Panayiotopoulos, 2007). Seizures are generally easily controlled with standard anticonvulsant treatment (Deuel & Lenn, 1977), often but not invariably without a corresponding improvement in the aphasia (Marescaux et al., 1990).

A cardinal feature of LKS is the presence of epileptic or epileptiform EEG abnormalities (e.g., spike waves, sharp waves, and spike-and-wave complexes). No single epileptiform abnormality encompasses all cases of LKS (Prasad, Stafstrom, & Holmes, 1996). Electroencephalographic manifestations of the disorder in the awake EEG include generalized, bilateral, focal or multifocal spike or spike-wave discharges, usually with a central or temporal lobe predominance (Cole et al., 1988; Hu, Wu, Lin, & Hao, 1989; Rodriguez & Niedermeyer, 1982). Abnormalities can as frequently appear lateralized to the right hemisphere as the left, and commonly, bilateral discharges are present (Cole et al., 1988).

The EEG abnormalities associated with LKS are frequently activated by sleep. During NREM sleep, there may be extended periods of high-amplitude continuous bilateral spike-and-wave discharges occurring 1 to 3 times per second (see Figure 12-2). Abnormalities are thought by some to differ from those seen in CSWS in that they may occupy a lesser percentage of NREM sleep (lower spike-wave index) (Smith & Hoeppner, 2003; Van Hirtum-Das et al., 2006), persist or even increase during REM sleep (Genton et al., 1992; Rossi et al., 1999; Tassinari, Rubboli, Volpi, Billard, & Bureau, 2002), occur at sleep onset (Genton et al., 1992; Rodriguez & Niedermeyer, 1982), or appear maximal in recordings from posterior temporal and parietal rather than frontal electrodes (Hirsch et al., 1995; Lanzi et al., 1994; Paquier, Van Dongen, & Loonen, 1992). Sleep-activated abnormalities can be observed when the awake EEG is unremarkable, so it is critical to obtain recordings throughout at least one full sleep cycle in a child with a history of regression (Genton & Guerrini, 1993). The persistence of ESES appears to correlate with the continuation of language impairment (Rossi et al., 1999; Veggiotti et al., 2002) and, if present for more than 3 years, is associated with long-term language deficits (Robinson et al., 2001).

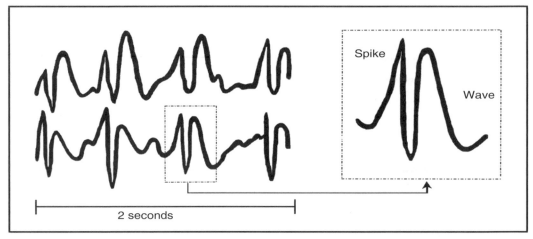

Figure 12-2. (*Left*) Schematic representation of a 2-second segment of an electroencephalogram showing continuous spike and wave activity from a patient with Landau-Kleffner syndrome. (*Right*) Magnification of a single spike-wave complex.

A normal EEG is noncontributory, since in at least 10% of cases, the abnormalities associated with the syndrome are variable and elusive (Beaumanoir, 1985). Abnormalities are known to be highly unstable (Hirsch et al., 1990), variable in the course of syndrome development (Beaumanoir, 1985), and can normalize within months of symptom onset (Humphrey, Knipstein, & Bumpass, 1975; Msall et al., 1986). Since epileptic or epileptiform EEG activity is a fundamental feature of the diagnosis, a significant diagnostic dilemma can emerge if sleep EEGs are not recorded at the time of the regression and later EEGs fail to disclose an epileptiform disturbance. Detecting and localizing abnormalities may require long-term monitoring, and pharmacologic activation protocols have been used in some cases to increase detection probability (Kollros, Stefanatos, Rabinovitch, & Streletz, 1996; Morrell et al., 1995).

Based on the use of intracarotid sodium amytal injection or systemic methohexital injection to localize the source of epileptiform activity, Morrell and colleagues (1995) suggested that while discharges may appear to be bilateral or generalized, they often originate from intrasylvian cortex in the left hemisphere. Magnetoencephalographic studies have also suggested that in a large proportion of children with LKS, epileptiform abnormalities originate in perisylvian cortex (Sobel, Aung, Otsubo, & Smith, 2000).

It has been proposed that these disturbances may arise as a result of aberrations of synaptogenesis or later damage to thalamocortical circuitry (Guzzetta et al., 2005; Morrell et al., 1995).

Does Not Meet Criteria for Autistic Disorder or Pervasive Developmental Disorder

Significant behavioral problems occur in about two-thirds of children diagnosed with LKS, mainly involving attentional deficits, impulsivity, distractibility, hyperactivity, and negative, oppositional, or aggressive behavior (Deonna, Peter, & Ziegler, 1989; Gascon, Victor, & Lombroso, 1973; Humphrey et al., 1975; Lou et al., 1977; Mantovani & Landau, 1980; Shoumaker et al., 1974; Soprano et al., 1994). In addition, avoidant and withdrawn behavior can emerge (Penn, Friedlander, & Saling, 1990). Perseveration and resistance to change in daily activities has also been described (Landau & Kleffner, 1957).

More rarely, behavioral disturbances can also include gestural stereotypies, hyperlexia, echolalia, and echopraxia (Nass & Petrucha, 1990; Rapin et al., 1977). Some children may, at a point in syndrome development, demonstrate symptoms of hyperacusia, finding certain noises (e.g., ambulance siren, vacuum cleaner) to be unusually irritating or noxious (Kellermann,

1978; Stefanatos, 2008). In some cases, the combination of severe communication disorder, stereotypic behaviors, hyperacusia, perseveration, resistance to change, and significant social disabilities can result in a pattern of impairment that resembles a pervasive developmental disorder (e.g., Boyd, Rivera-Gaxiola, Towell, Harkness, & Neville, 1996). Behaviors associated with the autistic spectrum may be more likely to occur with early age of onset (Fejerman & Medina, 1986; Stefanatos et al., 2002). Psychotic-like disturbances have also been described (Dugas, 1982; Hirsch et al., 1990; Nevsimalova, Tauberova, Doutlik, Kucera, & Dlouha, 1992; Roulet, Deonna, & Despland, 1989).

There has been a tendency in the neurological community to view the behavioral abnormalities as a secondary reaction to the communication disorder (Humphrey et al., 1975; Mantovani & Landau, 1980; Tharpe, Johnson, & Glasscock, 1991). While reactive behavioral disturbances may occur, a biological contribution is likely in many if not most cases. There is evidence, for example, to suggest that behavioral disturbances can precede the onset of the aphasia (Beaumanoir, 1985; Boyd et al., 1996; Gerard et al., 1993; Peterson, Koepp, Solmsen, & Villiez, 1978; Roulet Perez, Davidoff, Despland, & Deonna, 1993; Sawhney, Suresh, Dhand, & Chopra, 1988; Soprano et al., 1994; White & Sreenivasan, 1987). Behavioral problems may dissipate with successful pharmacologic treatment of the epileptiform disorder (Kellermann, 1978).

The Diagnostic Process: A Multidisciplinary Approach

The evaluation of children with LKS is necessarily multidisciplinary in nature. In addition to a neurologic examination and sleep-deprived EEG, the neuropsychological evaluation is a central component of this process. Ancillary evaluations may include magnetic resonance imaging (MRI) or computed tomography (CT) to rule out a structural abnormality that may explain the cause of the regression. Consultation with Audiology/Ear, Nose, and Throat (ENT) may be necessary to rule out peripheral hearing impairment (Kale, el-Naggar, & Hawthorne, 1995). In addition, the use of steady-state frequency modulated evoked potentials has been useful in

identifying neurophysiological anomalies associated with verbal auditory agnosia (Riviello & Hadjiloizou, 2007; Stefanatos, 1993, 2008) (see Figure 12-3B). Magnetoencephalography may be used to identify the source of discharges (Paetau et al., 1999; Sobel et al., 2000). Functional neuroimaging methods, including a single-photon emission computed tomography (SPECT) scan (see Figure 12-3C), positron emission tomography (PET), or functional magnetic resonance imaging (fMRI), may be considered to identify anomalies in cerebral activity that may be correlated with functional disturbances related to the epileptiform EEG abnormalities. In addition, evaluation from a speech-language pathologist is a necessary precursor to the development of an appropriate behavioral treatment plan and educational programming.

The Case of B. L.

History

B. L. was a 9-year-old, right-handed, Caucasian male regarded by the child study team of his suburban Philadelphia school district as having global developmental delays. His mother requested this neuropsychological assessment at the suggestion of their pediatric neurologist to assist the diagnostic formulation and guide treatment planning.

B. L. was the 6 lb, 8 oz product of an uneventful full-term pregnancy. Delivery was complicated by bradycardia, prompting an emergency C-section. Apgar scores were 8 and 9 at 1 and 5 minutes, respectively. He was reportedly floppy and was admitted to the intensive care unit for 3 days for monitoring due to meconium aspiration.

Motor milestones were attained in a timely manner. He sat independently at 6 months, stood alone at 10 months, and walked at 11 months. No difficulties were evident in early acquisition of speech. He spoke his first words prior to 1 year, produced word combinations by 17 to 18 months, and formulated short sentences by 21 months of age. He was described as a highly verbal child. At 2 years of age, he had a large vocabulary, (including difficult words such as *astronaut*) and could correctly label all the letters of the alphabet. By 2 years, 3 months, he knew basic color words and could identify shapes by name.

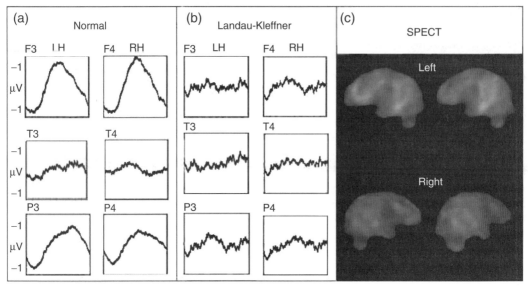

Figure 12-3. (*a*) Steady-state auditory evoked responses to pulsed frequency modulations in a normal 9-year-old child. Responses obtained from frontal (F), temporal (T), and parietal (P) leads are depicted. Each panel displays responses from the left hemisphere (LH) and right hemisphere (RH). (*b*) Representative responses obtained from an age-matched child with Landau-Kleffner syndrome. Comparison indicates clear abnormalities in responses obtained from the Landau-Kleffner syndrome case. Responses are thought to originate in superior temporal cortex. (*c*) Single-photon emission computed tomography scan of left and right hemisphere of a patient with Landau-Kleffner syndrome. Note bilateral perisylvian hypoperfusion.

At 3 years, 8 months of age, in a 6-month period following a severe cold, B. L. suffered a series of three ear infections. During this period he started acting "as if he were deaf". He inconsistently oriented to his name being called and did not respond to loud sounds (e.g., clap) produced immediately behind him. His mother subsequently noted that he ceased to produce words that were previously part of his everyday vocabulary. Multisyllabic words were among the first to be noticeably absent. By the time he was 4 years, 3 months of age, his vocabulary which had been on the order of hundreds of words, diminished to about 10% of its previous size. Intelligibility of his speech also diminished over this period to the point where his speech sounded "garbled". His voice quality became rather monotonic, and he lost his ability to sing on pitch and follow a beat. Eye contact also decreased, and he demonstrated increasing problems with attention and concentration. Otherwise, he remained affectionate and socially interactive. His mother also noted that he started walking on his toes and reportedly had difficulty sleeping through the night.

A hearing evaluation by an ENT specialist at 4 years, 2 months revealed that his audiogram was within normal limits. A month later, he had an episode comprised of several nonfebrile seizures associated with head drop, deviation of the head and eyes to the right, followed by generalized tonic-clonic convulsions. The episode was accompanied by vomiting and loss of bowel control. He was rushed to the emergency room of a large children's hospital, where he underwent a neurological evaluation that included an EEG, as well as brain CT and MRI scans. Structural brain scans failed to reveal anomalies that might explain the onset of these seizures. His EEG was remarkable for frequent left temporal and central sharp waves with rare independent right temporal sharp waves.

At 4 years, 6 months, B.L. returned to the hospital for evaluation of electrical status epilepticus of sleep due to his language regression. The awake EEG demonstrated frequent left temporal-central sharp and slow wave discharges, which alternately showed more spread to the left and then the right parietal area. Throughout the sleep EEG, there was significant activation of these abnormalities with periods where much of the record (from 60% to 100%) was comprised of repetitive, sharp, and slow wave discharges. Most activation occurred during stage I and stage II sleep, although it remained present in stage III sleep. A single subclinical electrographic seizure lasting approximately 40 seconds was observed arising from the left temporal region. B. L. was diagnosed with LKS and was started on an anticonvulsant medication (Depakote). A few months later, Neurontin was added due to a lack of change in his EEG and the emergence of aggressive behavior. However, this caused lethargy and was subsequently discontinued. Around this time, breakthrough absence and febrile seizures were observed. He was then placed on a combination of Lamictal and Depakote.

B. L. had been attending a private preschool program when the regression started but was subsequently asked to leave due to an episode of aggressive behavior. Specifically, an incident occurred where B. L. bit another child, reportedly out of frustration arising from his increasing problems with language comprehension. He was temporarily enrolled in another private program that was inclusive and offered speech-language services.

At 5 years, 1 month of age, a psychoeducational evaluation was completed by the school district's Intermediate Unit. An attempt to administer the Wechsler Preschool and Primary Intelligence Scale of Intelligence–Third Edition was aborted because B. L.'s communication problems, combined with limited attention and distractibility, precluded a valid assessment. However, he was able to complete the Beery Developmental Test of Visual Motor Integration, which yielded an above-average score for his age. By contrast, a speech-language assessment reported deficient scores on both expressive and receptive vocabulary (Test of Early Language Development-3). Similarly, his ability to understand the structure of spoken language fell into the Deficient range.

At 5 years, 5 months of age, B. L. was enrolled in a school for the deaf for approximately 2 years in an effort to facilitate his acquisition of signing skills. He was placed in a hearing-impaired classroom and taught using spoken English with sign language support. At 6 years, he was initiated on a 25-week course of corticosteroid (Prednisone) treatment, starting at 60 mg (2 mg/kg) and titrating down in graded steps every 5 weeks. This was followed by a maintenance dose of 10 mg. After 1 year, this was briefly increased to 20 mg and then reduced to 2.5 mg. According to parent report, positive changes in language ability started to become evident approximately 2 weeks after initiating this course of treatment. Gains were slow but incremental. In the following months, his auditory comprehension improved to the point where he became resistant to learning sign language and this was therefore discontinued.

At age 6 years, 8 months of age, while on Lamictal, Depakote, and low-dose Prednisone, B. L. underwent 24-hour ambulatory EEG monitoring, which indicated that both the awake and sleep EEG were within normal limits. A neuropsychological evaluation revealed a Full Scale IQ of 82, corresponding to the Low Average range. A large discrepancy was evident between his Verbal IQ (77) and his Performance IQ (103). Expressive language problems were evident in poor articulation, paraphasias, and word-finding difficulties. Sentence memory was Deficient and confrontation naming performance corresponded to the Borderline range. Receptive vocabulary fell in the Borderline to Low Average range. Variable problems with attention were also noted. Qualitative problems in social interaction combined with his communication impairment suggested a possible pervasive developmental disorder except he did not display unequivocal patterns of restricted or stereotyped behavior. However, atypical behaviors were evident in perseverative tendencies and highly focused interest in superheroes and dinosaurs. A tentative diagnosis of pervasive developmental disorder, not otherwise specified (PDD-NOS) was suggested should his impairments in social functioning continue.

At the time of the current evaluation, B. L. was enrolled in a special services classroom within the public school system. He was receiving 60 minutes a week of individual/integrated speech therapy. Therapeutic efforts directed to enhancing speech production, word finding, grammar, and vocabulary development were extended and integrated in the classroom environment. His speech was described as "fluent but telegraphic". He could reportedly follow one- or two-step directions with prompting and repetition. The therapist noted that he made poor eye contact and had difficulty with pragmatics (e.g., turn taking). He was reportedly prone to mood swings.

Neuropsychological Evaluation Results

When seen for neuropsychological evaluation at 9 years, 2 months, B. L. appeared to be a happy, well-mannered, and socially forward boy who did not hesitate to introduce himself and converse with others. Despite limitations in the intelligibility of his speech, he was rather loquacious, talking at length to the examiner about his interest in dinosaurs and sharing several books and some fossils he had brought along with him. This narrative mainly entailed recall of basic facts and had a rote quality. His eye contact was often indirect, and social awareness was somewhat limited. Due to variable attention and concentration, the evaluation required several visits to complete.

On intellectual evaluation employing the WISC-IV, B. L. obtained a Full Scale Intelligence Quotient (FSIQ) of 77. Significant scatter was evident among the subscale indices. He performed in the Average to High Average range on subtests

assessing his nonverbal abstract reasoning, ability to employ visual images in thinking, and nonverbal problem solving. Overall, his Perceptual Reasoning Index score of 102 corresponded to the Average range in comparison to other children his age. Similarly, he performed in the Low Average to Average range on subtests assessing rapid graphomotor transcoding skills and speed of visual scanning, obtaining a Processing Speed Index of score of 91. By contrast, his Working Memory Index of 59 corresponded to the Deficient range, suggesting substantial difficulties in holding information in temporary storage while it is being manipulated and processed. In addition, depressed performance on subtests assessing verbal reasoning, word knowledge and verbal formulation resulted in a Verbal Comprehension Index score of 71, corresponding to the Borderline range in comparison to other children his age. A summary of the individual subtest scaled scores (in italics) and subscale indices/standard scores is provided in Table 12-2.

Academically, B. L. demonstrated basic mastery of letter identification on the Wide Range Achievement Test–4th Edition, producing only a single error ("y" for "u"). He stated that he could not read words, but when presented with a word list, he correctly identified "cat". Attempts to read other words on the list revealed a varied pattern of error. He made approximations based on minimal visual cues for some words (e.g., "is"

Table 12-2. Test Results

Wechsler Intelligence Scale for Children-Fourth Edition (WISC-IV)
Full Scale IQ = 77

Verbal Comprehension Index = 71		*Perceptual Reasoning Index = 102*	
Similarities	7	Block Design	13
Vocabulary	2	Picture Concepts	8
Comprehension	6	Matrix Reasoning	10
Working Memory Index = 59		*Processing Speed Index = 91*	
Digit Span	3	Coding	7
Letter-Number	3	Symbol Search	10

Wide Range Achievement Test-Fourth Edition (WRAT-IV)

Subtest	Standard Score	Percentile	Grade Equivalent
Word Reading	55	0.1	<K.0
Spelling	61	0.5	K.2
Math Computation	57	0.2	K.5
Reading Comprehension	N/A		

Table 12-2. Test Results (*Continued*)

Neuropsychological tests				
Domain	Test		Standard Score	Percentile
Motor	**Lateral Dominance**	Right		
	Finger Tapping Test	Left	85	16
		Right	99	48
	Grooved Pegboard Test	Left	75	5
		Right	93	31
Memory	*Verbal*			
	Number Memory (TAPS-3)	Forward - 3	2	<1
	Number Memory (TAPS-3)	Reversed - 2	2	<1
	Word Memory (TAPS-3)		2	<1
	Sentence Memory (TAPS-3)		3	1
	NEPSY Narrative Memory		5	5
	Nonverbal			
	Corsi Blocks Span	Forward - 4	87	19
	Corsi Blocks Span	Backward - 3	80	9
	Rey Complex Figure Test (RCFT)	IMM	89	23
		DEL	94	35
		Recognition	94	35
	NEPSY Memory for Faces	IMM	8	25
		DEL	6	9
Visual spatial	**Perceptual Closure Test**		7	16
	Recognition Discrimination		120	91
	Beery Test/ Visuomotor Integration		111	77
	RCFT (Copy)		97	43
Auditory	**Filtered Words (SCAN)**		3	1
	Auditory Figure-Ground (SCAN)		3	1
	Competing Words (SCAN)		1	1
	SCAN Composite (SCAN)		65	1
	Environmental sounds test		37	1
Language	**ROWPVT**	AE: 6; 3	79	8
	Word Discrimination (TAPS-3)		1	<1
	Phonological Segmentation (TAPS-3)		1	<1
	Phonological Blending (TAPS-3)		1	<1
	Repetition of Nonsense Words (NEPSY)		4	2
	Auditory Comprehension (TAPS-3)		7	16
	Auditory Reasoning (TAPS-3)		1	2
	Test of the Reception of Grammar (TROG)			1-5
	EOWPVT	AE: 7; 7	89	23
	Semantic Fluency Test		108	69-71
	Phonemic Fluency Test		71	3
Attention/ Executive	**Trial-Making A**		102	55
	IVA Full Scale Attention Quotient:		7	
	Visual Attention Quotient		34	
	Vigilance Inattention		15	
	Focus Variability		69	
	Speed Reaction Time		79	

(Continued)

Table 12-2. Test Results (*Continued*)

Neuropsychological tests

Domain	Test	Standard Score
Attention/ Executive	**Auditory Attention Quotient**	44
	Vigilance Inattention	0
	Focus Variability	47
	Speed Reaction Time	87
	IVA Full Scale Response Quotient	43
	Visual Response Control Quotient	61
	Prudence Impulsivity	54
	Consistency Variability	81
	Stamina Fatigue	88
	Auditory Response Control Quotient	38
	Prudence Impulsivity	64
	Consistency Variability	14
	Stamina Fatigue	106

Child Behavior Checklist

Subtests	Mother Report (t-score)	Teacher Report (t-score)
Internalizing Problems	61	61
Externalizing Problems	53	64
Total Problems	63	62
Anxious/Depressed	55	55
Withdrawn	70	66
Somatic Complaints	56	57
Social Problems	68	58
Thought Problems	73	58
Attention Problems	67	55
Rule-Breaking Behavior	50	60
Aggressive Behavior	55	64

ADHD Rating Scale- IV

Subtests	Percentile
Inattention	<75
Hyperactivity/Impulsivity	<50

ADHD, attention-deficit/hyperactivity disorder.

for "in"; "tee" for "tree"), while with other words, his responses bore little or no phonetic or visual resemblance to the target (e.g., "round" for "book"). A somewhat similar pattern was evident on spelling. Overall, B. L. demonstrated significant difficulty in appreciating and applying knowledge of phoneme/grapheme correspondences. His math skills seemed better developed. He was able to manually compute several addition and subtraction problems correctly. However, his score on this measure was lower than expected due to difficulties with word problems. Given his rudimentary word recognition skills,

assessment of reading comprehension could not be completed.

On a modified Edinburgh Handedness Inventory, B. L. demonstrated a preference for his right hand for all fine and gross motor activities examined. Finger tapping speed, assessed with an electronic finger tapper, was within normal limits in both hands with a large performance asymmetry favoring his dominant right hand. On a timed measure of fine motor coordination (Grooved Pegboard Test), B. L.'s left-hand performance corresponded to the Borderline range, while right-hand performance was within normal limits.

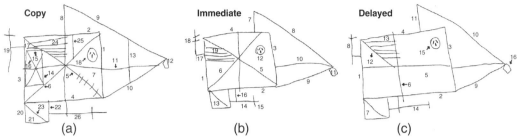

Figure 12-4. Rey-Osterrieth Complex Figure. (*a*) Landau-Kleffner syndrome copy from a model. (*b*) Immediate recall after copy and the model were removed. (*c*) Delayed recall after 30 minutes interspersed with other activities. Numbering on each figure represents the sequential order in which B. L. completed his drawings.

Assessment of memory revealed intact nonverbal/visual memory. His copy of the Rey-Osterrieth Complex Figure (see Figure 12-4) was completed in a timely if mildly disorganized manner. His rendition was characterized by reasonable line quality and adequate preservation of gross spatial relations with the possible exception of elements in the right upper quadrant. His immediate recall was within low normal limits for his age. His delayed recall obtained a half-hour later revealed insubstantial information loss over time, suggesting that processes involved in encoding and consolidating complex visual information in long-term visual memory were fairly intact. Recognition memory was also good. Similarly, on a facial memory task (NEPSY–Memory for Faces; Korkman, Kirk, & Kemp, 1998), both his immediate and delayed recall (30 minutes later) were within normal limits. His nonverbal span of apprehension assessed using the Corsi blocks task corresponded to the Low Average range.

By contrast, B. L.'s span of apprehension for verbal information was relatively limited. Digit span and word span, assessed using the Numerical Memory subtest and Word Memory subtest of the Test of Auditory Perceptual Skills (TAPS-3) (Martin & Brownell, 2005) were both depressed. While his forward Corsi block span was four items, his forward digit span was three items, and his word repetition span was limited to two items. When asked to repeat sentences (Sentence Memory Subtest–TAPS-3), his span was four parts ("Look at the picture and point to the house"), corresponding to the Deficient range. His memory for a narrative material, assessed using the Narrative Memory subtest of the NEPSY (Korkman et al., 1998), was also limited.

B. L.'s performance on measures of visual discrimination (Recognition Discrimination Test; Small, 1968), visuospatial integration (Perceptual Closure subtest; Kaufman & Kaufman, 1983), and visual motor abilities (Beery-Buktenica Developmental Test of Visual-Motor Integration; Beery, Buktenica, & Beery, 2004) corresponded to the Low Average to Superior range in comparison with other children his age. Overall, his visual perceptual and spatial abilities appeared to be well-developed and broadly commensurate with expectations based on his Perceptual Reasoning Index score on the WISC-IV.

Assessment of language and language-related abilities entailed both structured and semi-structured assessment procedures. B. L.'s rate of speech, pitch, intonation, and vocal quality were unremarkable, but he seemed periodically to produce speech at a somewhat elevated volume. This proclivity varied with context and topic. His phonological inventory was age-appropriate with the exception of intermittent w/l and f/th substitutions. Speech intelligibility was reduced by a combination of these typical developmental articulatory substitutions, combined with copious paraphasic errors. Although generally fluent, B. L.'s speech appeared on casual analysis to be distinguished by phonological production problems similar to those seen in apraxia of speech (AoS). However, his productions were not slow or effortful, nor were they characterized by halting and groping for desired articulatory postures as is typical of AoS.

Further analysis confirmed that B. L. had significant difficulty selecting and sequencing phonemes for production. On assessment of diadochokinetic rate, he was able to rapidly repeat the same isolated consonant-vowel (e.g., "ba-ba-ba-ba….", "da-da-da-da-da….", "ga-ga-ga-ga-ga….") at an age-appropriate rate, although with extended production, the vowel drifted ("ba-ba-ba…" became "bo-bo-bo…" and eventually "bu-bu-bu…"). By contrast, he demonstrated a striking inability to correctly and consistently reproduce sequences comprised of different consonant-vowel (CV) syllables such as "ba-da-ga" or "pa-ta-ka", even with repeated modeling from the examiner (repetition). His production of these sound sequences, which necessitate constant repositioning of the oromotor musculature, required inordinate effort and time to output and were either incorrectly ordered or contained sound substitutions. For example, "ba-da-ga" was variously produced as "ma-ga-da", "ba-gu-da", and "ba-ga-dug."

On tests of single word production, he demonstrated sound replacements ("hip" for "ship"), additions ("kokes" for "coat"), and deletions ("ne" for "nest"). These error patterns continued on the Repetition of Nonsense Words subtest (Korkman et al., 1998), which requires that children repeat utterances based on novel phonological information rather than familiar phonological and semantic information present in a known word. Errors included consonant cluster reductions ("foo" for "floo"), cluster distortion combined with vowel centralization ("duh-" for "byoo-"), sound and cluster transposition ("kuh-foo-duh-stroo-skuh" for "skru-floo-nuh-flif-strap"), and errors in place ("kell" for "dell") and manner ("wiss" for "woot") of articulation. His performance on this subtest placed him at the 2nd percentile relative to children his age.

Both spontaneous and elicited verbal productions were marked by phonological, lexical, and "phrasal" paraphasias. For instance, on confrontation naming using the Expressive One-Word Picture Vocabulary Test (Brownwell, 2000a), he produced "check" for "chess", "dasheemz" for "machines", and both "interips" and "intopsis" for "instruments". Phonemic paraphasias were also evident on repetition. He also demonstrated a tendency to produce errors based on poor inhibition of certain lexical associations. For example,

he repeatedly referred to one of his favorite eateries, the sandwich restaurant known as "Subway", as "subway station". Overall, there was marked inconsistency in his verbal productions related to phonological disorganization and word-finding difficulties.

Despite these problems, his intelligibility was at times quite good, both in known and unknown contexts. He produced syntactically simplified sentences. When context called for a complex sentence, he seemed to have trouble organizing it. His attempts to initiate and produce long sentences entailed false starts and recurrent revisions (e.g., "When the boy woke up, the frog was jump… was gone"). At times, he omitted grammatical endings like past tense. His errors marking past tense occurred with both regular and irregular verbs (e.g., "They search everywhere and they say they couldn't find it" for "They searched everywhere and said they couldn't find it"). As evident from the foregoing example, his problems with past-tense markers were not related to difficulties producing terminal consonants.

Phonological deficits were also evident in his performance on tests of phonological awareness. Assessment of his knowledge of sound-based relationships in speech revealed significant impairment of his ability to segment and blend sounds (<1st percentile). When asked to combine the sounds "i" and "t" ("it"), he responded "iz". When asked to blend the sounds in mop (/m/+/o/+/p/), he responded "mcpadpap". He became visibly frustrated with his lack of success on this task. Interestingly, B. L. also had particular difficulty on a measure of word fluency when asked to generate as many words as he could think of in 1 minute given a phonemic prompt ("C", "F", and "L"). By contrast, his ability to retrieve words based on a semantic prompt (foods, animals) fell within normal limits.

On the expressive (EOWPVT) (Brownwell, 2000a) and receptive (ROWPVT) (Brownwell, 2000b) vocabulary tests, B. L. scored in the 23rd and 8th percentiles, respectively. Despite the apparent difficulties he demonstrated on confrontation naming, his performance on the expressive vocabulary test was statistically significantly better than on the receptive portion (*p* = .01).

Evaluation of B. L.'s receptive skills revealed substantial impairments of auditory processing. He was able to discriminate two similar spoken words (e.g., "thing-think") by indicating "same" or "different" only 31% of the time, corresponding to less than the 1st percentile (Martin & Brownell, 2005). Due to concern that his poor performance was in part attributable to the working memory load of this task (given his word span was two), he was administered a separate speech discrimination task requiring that he listen to a single word and choose the corresponding picture from four alternative choices. He performed at a similar level (6th percentile) on this task (Goldman, Fristoe, & Woodcock, 1970). When asked to perform the same task with background noise, his score fell at the 4th percentile in comparison to children his age.

To further examine B. L. 's speech perception problems, he was administered an experimental task requiring that he listen to and repeat individual computer-synthesized CV syllables (/ba/, /da/, /ga/, /pa/, /ta/, or /ka/). He produced a pattern of error suggesting he had particular difficulty with discriminations contingent on place of articulation. He produced most errors when listening to the CV /da/, which he commonly confused with /ga/. In addition, he made an inordinate number of errors in response to /ta/, which he confused with /pa/. He did not make a single error confusing voiced versus unvoiced CVs, suggesting adequate processing of spectral cues such as aspiration which are key to this distinction. With respect to place of articulation, his performance was at or near chance except for velars (back) sounds (/ga/ and /ka/). These sounds have the longest voice-onset time among voiced and unvoiced stop consonants, respectively. Together, these findings suggest an error pattern that may be associated with problems with auditory temporal processing. However, toward the end of this CV repetition task, he demonstrated an inexplicable series of errors (a response of /ha/ in response to presentation of /pa/ and /ta/). These errors seemed out of keeping with the closed set of stop-consonant-vowels he had been hearing. Brief periods of unexpected errors were also evident on a couple of other tasks, including some that were nonverbal in nature. Since he overtly appeared attentive, these errors raised concerns of the possible influence of paroxysmal electrographic activity.

Given the pattern of substantial difficulties with auditory processing, B. L. was also administered an assessment of central auditory processing (Keith, 1986). His ability to discriminate perceptually degraded words (Filtered Words) or words presented in the context of a noisy "cocktail party" background (Auditory Figure-Ground) fell in the Deficient range. On the Competing Words subtest, B. L. was simultaneously presented with different words to each ear (dichotic presentation) and directed to selectively attend and repeat words presented to his right and then his left ear in two separate blocks of trials. He demonstrated profound difficulty attending to and repeating words presented to the right ear compared to the left (2 vs. 21 correct, respectively). This pattern of performance was confirmed on a separate dichotic measure. These findings suggested the possibility of auditory extinction in the right ear, which may reflect neurofunctional deficits in auditory processing of speech in the contralateral (left) hemisphere. His auditory processing problems did not appear to be limited to processing speech. B. L. also had difficulty in correctly identifying environmental sounds, scoring only 66% correct on a 40-item measure (Stefanatos & Madigan, 2000).

B. L. also performed poorly on measures assessing his comprehension of spoken sentences. His ability to understand grammatical contrasts as assessed on the Test of the Reception of Grammar (Bishop, 2003) fell below the 5th percentile in comparison to other children his age. He demonstrated understanding of plural and singular pronouns, reversible action, pronoun gender, comparative constructions, and reversible passive constructions. However, he did not show consistent comprehension of "in" and "on" (possibly related to perception) and the concepts of "above" and "below". In addition, he had difficulty with sentence structures using the form "X but not Y", and those with postmodified subjects ("The boy chasing the horse is fat"). Difficulties in understanding phrase length grammatical information such as postmodified subjects may reflect limitations in working memory.

B. L. exhibited marked inconsistency in his capacity to answer simple WH- questions about short narratives. He performed with about 50% accuracy when answering specific questions about short passages he was read, whether these passages were two or five sentences in length. His performance on the Auditory Comprehension subtest of the TAPS-3 corresponded to the 16th percentile in comparison with other children his age. He also demonstrated depressed accuracy on the Auditory Reasoning subtest of the TAPS-3, which assessed higher-order linguistic processes related to understanding of jokes, riddles, inferences, and abstractions. His responses showed a lack of abstraction and inference. His score corresponded to the 2nd percentile.

On measures of executive control, B. L.'s performance was variable. His score on the Trail Making Test–Part A corresponded to the Average range. He was unable to understand or comply with Trail Making Test–Part B. Problems with attention were apparent on a continuous performance task (Sanford & Turner, 1999). On this measure, B. L. simply had to press a key whenever he saw or heard a particular target (the number "1") presented among a series of distracters (the number "2"). Stimuli were presented both via headphones and a screen computer at a rate of about one per second. He demonstrated a large number of omission and commission errors, suggesting both inattention and impulsivity. His hit rate was poor and the average latency of his responses was significantly delayed. The results from this measure indicated that he had particular difficulty sustaining and focusing attention to targets in the auditory domain, reflected in a disparity between his Visual Attention Quotient (37) and his Auditory Attention Quotient (4).

B. L.'s mother and teacher served as informants for the Achenbach Child Behavior Checklist. Analysis of B. L.'s report profiles revealed clinically significant elevations on the Withdrawn scale and the Thought Problems scale, the latter reflecting some perseverative or rigid thinking. Problems with concentration, inattention, staring blankly, daydreaming, following directions, disturbing other pupils, acting impulsively, sitting still, and seeming confused or "in a fog" were also reported. Despite the greatest number of endorsements of attention-related symptoms, they failed to result in a clinically significant elevation on this measure. It is possible that respondent's observations of some of these behaviors were tempered or confounded by expectations based on the impact of his severe receptive problems.

Discussion

Diagnostic Formulation

B. L. demonstrated an idiopathic acquired aphasia in early childhood associated with epileptiform EEG abnormalities. Around 3 years, 8 months of age, he ceased orienting consistently to his name, and gradually his ability to comprehend and produce speech deteriorated. At 4 years, 2 months of age, B. L. experienced his first seizure. By 4 years, 3 months of age, he had lost approximately 90% of his expressive vocabulary, and his auditory comprehension was severely impaired. An EEG at 4 years, 6 months revealed a pattern of ESES, confirming the diagnosis of LKS. At 6 years, B. L. was initiated on a course of corticosteroid (prednisone) treatment, which reportedly resulted in slow incremental positive changes in language that started at about 2 weeks post treatment onset. A 24-hour ambulatory EEG at age 6 years, 8 months of age, while on Lamictal, Depakote, and a low dose of Prednisone, revealed that both the awake and sleep EEG were within normal limits.

Follow-up at 9 years of age indicated continuing difficulties with communication, although his presentation differed somewhat from the pattern typically associated with LKS. For many children with LKS, speech production is effortful, labored, and sparse. By contrast, B. L. was talkative. He did not demonstrate visible struggle associated with initiating or executing spontaneous speech. Indeed, he was not only interested in but seemed eager to make communicative overtures, despite the fact that the intelligibility of his speech was sometimes limited. However, as is commonly seen in LKS, both spontaneous and elicited speech was characterized by striking disorganization of phonological production. This was evident in cluster reductions, transpositions, additions, substitutions, sound and syllable omissions, and vowel centralization, all marked by conspicuous inconsistency. His diadochokinetic rate for repeating the same syllable (e.g., "ba-ba-ba") was well within normal limits, while selecting, ordering, and outputting sequences of different syllables (e.g., "ba-da-ga") was highly problematic. Analogous problems are common in the spontaneus verbal productions of children with LKS but are often described as articulatory difficulties or are assimilated in descriptions of phonemic paraphasias and jargon. B. L. also produced lexical and "phrasal" paraphasias and had word-finding difficulties, indicating that his problems extended to lexical access. His sentence constructions were rudimentary, and he made errors in grammatical marking that were not secondary to phonological problems.

B. L. also demonstrated deficits in auditory comprehension at multiple levels of analysis (syllable, word, and sentence). At the level of simple auditory discrimination, when listening to syllables and words, he often confused the stop consonants /d/ and /g/ which are distinguished by place of articulation. Several acoustic cues contribute to the differentiation of these stop consonants, and they require resolution of temporal cues lasting several milliseconds (e.g., the release burst: 5 to 15 ms) to tens of milliseconds (e.g., second and third formant frequency transitions: 20 to 50 ms). Similarly, the voiceless stop consonants /t/ and /p/ were also frequently misidentified. This overall pattern of perceptual impairment likely reflects deficits in cortical processes involved in analyzing and encoding rapid temporal acoustic changes in speech signals (see Stefanatos, Gershkoff, & Madigan, 2005). Similar difficulties have been described in many cases of LKS (Baynes et al., 1998; Honbolygo et al., 2006; Klein et al., 1995; Korkman et al., 1998). During the decoding of continuous speech, these problems can impair the accuracy of mapping sound structure to lexical items as well as impede aspects of morphological and syntactic processing (e.g., past tense marking). In addition, the development of phonological processing skills such as phonological awareness and segmentation may be affected.

Auditory temporal processing deficits can often be sufficiently severe in LKS as to amount to a perceptual collapse. In such cases, children have described their phenomenological experience of listening to speech as sounding like rustling leaves or as meaningless chatter ("blah, blah, blah") (Landau & Kleffner, 1957). We have seen a case who, following successful corticosteroid treatment, was able to describe his subjective perception of speech as comparable to the sounds produced by the teacher in animated Charlie Brown cartoons. This sound has the tonal quality of a muted trumpet, with pitch changing in a manner that resembles the prosody of speech. This description suggests some recognition of the slow-frequency changes that cue intonation contours of speech, but little appreciation of the spectro-temporal microstructure necessary to distinguish strings of phonemes, particularly stop consonants. B. L.'s difficulties were not as severe, though they significantly limited not only his perception of single consonant-vowels but also his comprehension of words, phrases, and sentences. At the syntactic level, he demonstrated difficulties in understanding phrase and sentence-length grammatical information (e.g., postmodified subjects), which may also reflect limitations in working memory.

Problems with auditory perception were not limited to processing of speech sounds but were also apparent in difficulties with environmental sound recognition. While environmental sound recognition has rarely been formally assessed in LKS, a few reports have described substantial problems in these children (Denes, Balliello, Volterra, & Pellegrini, 1986; Koeda & Kohno, 1992). Problems may not be obvious in their everyday behavior since, in naturalistic settings, differentiating between many environmental sounds (e.g., a doorbell or a telephone ringing) can be accomplished on the basis of multiple cues such as context and spatial location as well as differences in sound duration, periodicity, and spectral characteristics. In addition, environmental sound recognition may be more robust to problems with auditory temporal processing of the type observed in LKS insofar as normal listeners can often continue to correctly identify these sounds even after they have undergone significant temporal distortion. Formal assessment eliminates contextual and spatial cues and may disclose difficulties that may otherwise elude detection secondary to compensatory masking. Nonverbal sound recognition deficits may be present in as many as half of LKS children at some point in syndrome evolution.

Mechanisms responsible for the auditory analysis of speech are elaborated cortically in a distributed network extending from auditory cortex, to planum temporale, superior temporal sulcus (STS), and anterolateral and posterolateral regions of superior temporal gyrus (Binder et al., 2000; Johnsrude, Zatorre, Milner, & Evans, 1997; Zatorre, Belin, & Penhune, 2002). In the left hemisphere, this network appears to be particularly adept at processing sounds that require the accurate analysis of dynamic acoustic events that unfold or change rapidly over very brief periods of time (5–50 ms) and this may underlie left hemisphere specialization for speech processing (Liegeois-Chauvel, de Graaf, Laguitton, & Chauvel, 1999; Stefanatos, Joe, Aguirre, Detre, & Wetmore, 2008; Tallal, Miller, & Fitch, 1993). That B. L.'s auditory processing problems may be related to anomalies in auditory and auditory association cortex, particularly in the left hemisphere, is consistent with his performance on a task requiring recognition of dichotically presented words. The apparent extinction of words presented to his right ear implicates problems involving left superior temporal cortex or the thalamocortical projections to this area. Based on similar findings of auditory extinction, Metz-Lutz and colleagues (Metz-Lutz & Filippini, 2006; Wioland, Rudolf, & Metz-Lutz, 2001) have suggested that neurofunctional differentiation and refinement of the auditory system in individuals with LKS may be impeded or otherwise negatively influenced by abnormal epileptiform activity during a critical point in their neurodevelopment.

Superior posterior temporal cortex forms part of a network that links left posterior auditory fields and language reception areas (including Wernicke's area) with left frontal articulatory programming systems (Broca's area), which mediate aspects of speech production, including the ability to repeat heard speech. These areas and the pathways that connect them (arcuate and superior longitudinal fasciculus) form part of a auditory-motor integration network that may play an important role in speech development by enabling acoustic-phonetic input to inform the acquisition of language-specific articulatory-phonetic gestures (Hickok, Buchsbaum, Humphries, & Muftuler, 2003). Disruption of components of this circuitry may help explain B. L.'s significant difficulties in sequencing phonemes in speech. A critical area contributing to the function of this network is located in the

region of the posterior Sylvian fissure at the parietal-temporal boundary. B. L.'s last noted electroencephalographic disturbance included this area. The persistence of these difficulties may be related to residual impairment involving posterior superior temporal lobe caused by the epileptiform discharges that occurred earlier in B. L.'s development, or by the pathophysiologic factors that gave rise to them. Alternatively, it remains possible that the function of this area may be influenced by some continuing transient inhibitory or disruptive influences. Concerns were raised during the evaluation of the possibility of subclinical paroxysmal activity, given observations of intermittent unexplained runs of errors on a few simple tasks.

A similarly distributed neural network is involved in working memory (Smith & Jonides, 1997). B. L. demonstrated significant problems with verbal working memory that may contribute to his auditory language comprehension problems. Specifically, limitations of working memory may possibly constrain the ability to analyze the syntactic structure of sentences and use that knowledge to determine sentence meaning (Caplan & Waters, 1999). The presence of short-term memory problems is not uncommon in LKS and may persist into adulthood (Baynes et al., 1998; Honbolygo et al., 2006; Majerus et al., 2003; Robinson et al., 2001).

As previously discussed, the persistence of neuropsychological deficits may reflect the sequelae of prolonged exposure to epileptiform discharges during a critical stage of neurodevelopment. Robinson et al. (2001) have suggested that age at onset may not be as predictive of long-term outcome as the duration of persistence of the sleep-activated epileptiform. Long-term difficulties are likely when ESES has persisted for more than 3 years. The present findings suggest that language and language-related disturbances may continue to be evident in childhood, even when medical treatment with corticosteroids results in apparent resolution of ESES and improvements in language function approximately 2 years post onset. Perhaps, the etiology underlying the emergence of ESES may also play a role in the likelihood of persistence of language deficits.

There is general agreement that temporal lobe dysfunction is critical to syndrome development.

Interestingly, the temporal lobe may also play an important role in mediating some of the social behaviors that appeared to regress along with B. L.'s language. Specifically, parent report stated that along with the loss of his speech, B. L. also diminished his eye contact during social interaction. Recent neuroimaging studies suggest that eye contact is mediated by a widely distributed cortical-subcortical neural network, with areas of the posterior temporal lobe (e.g., STS, superior temporal gyrus, temporoparietal junction) playing a role in the analysis of eye gaze and the interpretation of signals of communicative intent (Senju & Johnson, 2009). Given the contemporaneous onset, the factors that gave rise to B. L.'s language impairment may have also impacted, directly or indirectly, the operation of this gaze processing and social signaling network. Other behavioral abnormalities common in LKS that are potentially linked to temporal lobe pathophysiology include aggressiveness, mood disturbances, anxiety, inattention, impulsivity, and issues with social attention and awareness. (Gascon et al., 1973; Roulet Perez, 1995; Stefanatos, Grover, & Geller, 1995; Stefanatos et al., 2002). This relationship may help explain why features of autism spectrum disorder are not uncommon in children with LKS.

Implications for Treatment

Behavioral/Educational Approaches. Relatively little research has been directed to identifying the most appropriate and effective methods to utilize in therapy for individuals with LKS (Gerard, Dugas, & Sagar, 1991; Pedro & Leisman, 2005; Vance, 1991). The primary focus of the treatment of LKS is on suppressing epileptic or epileptiform activity and enhancing communication. Speech and language therapy plays a central role in the treatment of these children and should be initiated as soon as is feasible. Therapeutic considerations have been discussed by Vance (1991), De Wijngaert (1993), and Lees (2005), so they will not be discussed at length here. Programs need to be integrated into classroom activities and structured to be highly supportive so as to overcome the sense of difficulty and frustration often experienced by these children due to the nature and severity of their disorder.

In the acute stage, when children exhibit profound expressive and receptive deficits, efforts may be well invested in alternative and augmentative communication (AAC) (Gerard et al., 1991). Concerns have been raised that supplemental approaches, such as sign language, have the potential to impede traditional speech and language therapy, which places emphasis on utilizing, improving, and extending residual oral-aural means of communication. However, Perez and Davidoff (2001) suggest that manual sign language can foster the recovery of oral language. B. L. was immersed in an environment that used sign language as a compensatory means of communication. He then declined this approach once his auditory-verbal language abilities reached a certain point of recovery.

Facilitating comprehension may include altering the rate of speech used to communicate with LKS children. It is sometimes helpful to talk more slowly with frequent pauses to allow time to process information (Okada, Hanada, Hattori, & Shoyama, 1963) and to repeat communications. Although very little data is currently available on the effectiveness of this approach specifically in LKS, attempts to directly train auditory discrimination skills may be fruitful. Approaches that temporally condition auditory-verbal input by manipulating (initially slowing) formant transitions in speech have shown some promise in enhancing the auditory processing of language in children with developmental language disorders (Merzenich et al., 1996) and adults patients with acquired aphasia (Dronkers, Husted, & Deutsch, 1999) or word deafness (Stefanatos, Gershkoff, & Madigan, 2005). This approach may benefit children like B. L. who have difficulty processing the rapid spectrotemporal variations that cue phonemic contrasts at the rates that these cue normally occur in natural speech. Certainly, the findings in this case study suggest that auditory temporal processing issues are salient and ought to be considered in developing his therapeutic program. More generally, direct treatment of auditory temporal processing deficits may be unfeasible, frustrating or have limited returns in the acute stage of LKS when auditory agnosia or gross auditory inattention predominates. Correctly timing the initiation of this approach may be critical to its success.

As was evident in this evaluation, children with LKS demonstrate strengths in visual learning and processing skills (Cooper & Ferry, 1978; Jordan, 1980) so the ample use of visual supports such as pictures, outlines, demonstrations, and gesture should be embedded in virtually every facet of the child's educational program. Color and shape coding have been used to facilitate explicit instruction of grammatical rules (Lea, 1970; Ebbels, 2007). With B. L., for example, it was helpful to augment some of the directions given in the course of the assessment with nonverbal gestures and pictures.

It is also potentially beneficial to exploit higher-order processing skills to compensate for speech discrimination difficulties (Maneta, Marshall, & Lindsay, 2001; Morris, Franklin, Ellis, Turner, & Bailey, 1996). This approach attempts to capitalize on the use of relatively intact semantic skills to allow individuals to generate contextual knowledge for incoming communications, which may facilitate the processing of perceptually degraded speech signals.

These practices often form part of a larger effort to develop compensatory strategies or metastrategies, which can include the use of a multimodal communication approaches (Pedro & Leisman, 2005) such as augmenting spoken language with sign language (Perez & Davidoff, 2001; Woll & Sieratzki, 1996), written language (Vance, 1991), or lip reading (Morris, 1997; Shindo, Kaga, & Tanaka, 1991).

Developing appropriate educational programs for children with LKS can be a formidable challenge. Guidelines and suggestions for educational programming are available elsewhere (Chapman, Stormont, & McCathren, 1998; Van Slyke, 2002; Vance, 1991). It is important to consider various ways to enhance the child's capacity to normalize their school life in the face of the newly acquired and often devastating communication impairment. It is often necessary to be proactive in providing a friendly, supportive, secure, and predictable environment to avert children's tendency to become isolated, depressed, and anxious. Staff should be inserviced to understand the nature of the disability and on how to make appropriate use of visual cues and other compensatory strategies in order to effectively communicate with these children and engage them in social interactions.

It is also important to take stock, and if necessary, modify the listening environment by reducing the possible influence of noise sources in the classroom (air vents, street traffic, playground activity, hallway traffic). Several methods to decrease interference resulting from background noise in classrooms, are disussed by Tharpe, Johnson, and Glasscock (1991). In addition, the use of assistive listening devices such as frequency modulation (FM) systems may be considered for this purpose (Flexer, Millin, & Brown, 1990).

Due to the common comorbidity of behavioral problems, a detailed behavior management plan may need to be implemented to address behaviors such as aggressivity and poor impulse control. Effective management may require the cooperation, involvement and training of direct care staff, teachers, and parents in the principles and use of behavioral modification techniques. Deficits in pragmatic skills such as initiating, monitoring, maintaining, and disengaging from conversation, turn taking, poor eye contact, and dealing with difficult social interactions (e.g., losing a game) may be directly addressed in speech-language therapy with extension to the classroom and to naturalistic environments.

Medical Approaches. Corticosteroids and ACTH have gained some acceptance as a treatment of choice for LKS based on case studies. Detailed discussions of treatments with anticonvulsants, ACTH, immunoglobulins, and corticosteriods can be found in Riviello and Hadjiloizou (2007) and Stefanatos et al. (2002). Alternatives to pharmacologic treatment may include the ketogenic diet (Bergqvist, Chee, Lutchka, & Brooks-Kayal, 1999). Surgery may be considered in specific symptomatic cases (Solomon et al., 1993) or as a last resort in those individuals who demonstrate idiopathic LKS associated with medically intractable focal CSWS emanating consistently from a particular identifiable focus (Morrell et al., 1995; Smith & Hoeppner, 2003). Initial reports of success in improving language in idiopathic cases of LKS have been tempered over time with discouraging outcome of language functions in a subsequent series in children with ESES lasting longer than 36 months (Irwin et al., 2001; Robinson et al., 2001).

Psychopharmacologic therapy may be considered for persisting behavioral problems such as difficulties with attention, impulsivity, aggressivity or mood disturbance. Such problems are sometimes ameliorated by controlling the epileptiform activity, but in some instances require adjuvant medical treatment directed to particular symptoms. In evaluating the possible utility of a medication trial for attention problems, it is necessary to exercise prudence in interpreting descriptions of inattentiveness in the classroom, as this may or may not be secondary to their communication disorder. Alternatively, as was seemingly the case in B. L., parents and teachers may underreport attention-deficit disorder symptomology when completing behavioral inventories, because those symptoms may be overshadowed or confounded by the presence of a profound receptive communication disorder. Measures such as continuous performance tests may help tease apart attentional problems from the communication disorder, although care must be taken to ensure that language impairment itself does not impede processing of stimuli used in these tasks.

Long-Term Outcome

Long-term outcome of LKS is highly variable. Dugas et al. reviewed the outcome in 33 of 156 cases published between 1957 in 1989 that had follow-up at 14 years of age or older. Approximately 45% had unfavorable outcomes in which a severe communication deficit continued to be evident in both comprehension and expression. Another 33% had persisting oral and/or written language difficulties but otherwise had good social professional skills and were not substantially impeded in the communication. Approximately 22% had favorable outcomes indexed by independent living and no observable communication difficulties. Bishop (1985) has suggested that earlier age of onset results in poorer long-term outcome. Others have suggested that poor outcome is more likely with longer persistence of the electroencephalographic abnormality and the slower progression of the aphasia at onset (Deonna et al., 1977; Robinson et al., 2001). Boel and Casaer (1989) considered that poor outcome is probable if little to no progress is seen in the first year post onset. If the aphasia is acquired after a child has acquired literacy skills, and literacy is retained, then children

have a better prognosis, at least for educational attainment (Beaumanoir, 1985). Overall, long term outcome studies to date suggest that a majority of cases are left with a lifelong language disability (Deonna et al., 1989; Mantovani & Landau, 1980; Soprano et al., 1994). However, the preponderance of these reports preceded the recent advances in anticonvulsant therapy and the more widespread use of corticosteroid treatment.

Conclusion

In summary, there is disagreement on the boundaries of LKS, and a lack of consensus on underlying mechanisms or treatment. It appears to be a final common pathway of several possible acquired etiologies or the late manifestations of subtle developmental perturbations that may particularly affect posterior temporal cortex and its thalamocortical afferents. Early identification and implementation of appropriate treatment appears to be important to the success of treatment and long-term outcome. While electroencephalographic findings help guide pharmacologic treatment, the long-term well-being of the child is also determined by behavioral treatments. Neuropsychological evaluations therefore play a critical role not only in diagnostic formulation but also in treatment planning. Patterns of strengths and weaknesses derived from these evaluations not only specify the level (phonological, morphological, syntactic, lexical, semantic, pragmatic) and severity of language processing difficulties, but they can also determine the extent of nonverbal cognitive involvement. Information derived from these evaluations provides an important and valid method of monitoring changes in function over time in order to identify whether particular problems are static or resolving. These data are also critical for establishing the efficacy of pharmacological treatment and in identifying other interventions that may be necessary, since pharmacotherapy alone does not address the multidimensional needs of these children. Neuropsychological assessments can further disclose systematic patterns of impairment that are characteristic of the disorder as well as disabilities that may be atypical or unexpected. This information may be helpful in specifying subtypes and in identifying similarities and divergencies between LKS and other epileptiform disorders.

Acknowledgments

The authors gratefully acknowledge the generous contribution of Dr. Peter Kollros for providing some of the historical information and to Kate Tumolo, Michelle Liou, and Tara Brown for their contributions to the preparation of the manuscript.

References

Ansink, B. J., Sarphatie, H., & van Dongen, H. R. (1989). The Landau-Kleffner syndrome–Case report and theoretical considerations. *Neuropediatrics, 20*(3), 170–172.

Appleton, R. E. (1995). The Landau-Kleffner syndrome. *Archives of Disease in Childhood, 72*(5), 386–387.

Baynes, K., Kegl, J. A., Brentari, D., Kussmaul, C., & Poizner, H. (1998). Chronic auditory agnosia following Landau-Kleffner syndrome: A 23 year outcome study. *Brain and Language, 63*(3), 381–425.

Beaumanoir, A. (1985). The Landau-Kleffner syndrome. In C. D. J. Roger & M. Bureau (Eds.), *Epileptic syndromes in infancy, childhood and adolescence* (pp. 181–191). London: John Libbey Eurotext.

Beaumanoir, A. (Ed.). (1992). *The Landau-Kleffner syndrome.* London: John Libbey Eurotext.

Beery, K., Buktenica, N. A., & Beery, N. A. (2004). *Developmental Test of Visual Motor Integration.* San Antonio, TX: Pearson Assessments.

Bergqvist, A. G., Chee, C. M., Lutchka, L. M., & Brooks-Kayal, A. R. (1999). Treatment of acquired epileptic aphasia with the ketogenic diet. *Journal of Child Neurology, 14*(11), 696–701.

Binder, J. R., Frost, J. A., Hammeke, T. A., Bellgowan, P. S., Springer, J. A., Kaufman, J. N., et al. (2000). Human temporal lobe activation by speech and non-speech sounds. *Cerebral Cortex, 10*(5), 512–528.

Bishop, D. V. M. (1982). Comprehension of spoken, written and signed sentences in childhood language disorders. *Journal of Child Psychology and Psychiatry, 23*(1), 1–20.

Bishop, D. V. M. (1985). Age of onset and outcome in "acquired aphasia with convulsive disorder" (Landau-Kleffner syndrome). *Developmental Medicine and Child Neurology, 27*(6), 705–712.

Bishop, D. V. M. (2003). *Test for the Reception of Grammar–Version 2.* San Antonio, TX: Psychological Corporation.

Boel, M., & Casaer, P. (1989). Continuous spikes and waves during slow sleep: A 30 months follow-up study of neuropsychological recovery and EEG findings. *Neuropediatrics, 20,* 176–180.

Boyd, S. G., Rivera-Gaxiola, M., Towell, A. D., Harkness, W., & Neville, B. G. (1996). Discrimination of speech sounds in a boy with Landau-Kleffner syndrome: An intraoperative event-related potential study. *Neuropediatrics, 27*(4), 211–215.

Brownwell, R. (2000a). Expressive One-Word Picture Vocabulary Test. San Antonio, TX: Psychological Corporation.

Brownwell, R. (2000b). Receptive One-Word Picture Vocabulary Test. San Antonio, TX: Psychological Corporation.

Bulteau, C., Plouin, P., Jambaque, I., Renaux, V., Quillerou, D., Boidein, F., et al. (1995). *Aphasia epilepsy: A clinical and EEG study of six cases with CSWS.* London: John Libbey.

Caplan, D., & Waters, G. S. (1999). Verbal working memory and sentence comprehension. *Behavioral and Brain Sciences, 22*(1), 77–94.

Chapman, T., Stormont, M., & McCathren, R. (1998). What every educator should know about Landau-Kleffner syndrome. *Focus on Autism and Other Developmental Disabilities, 13*(1), 39–44.

Chevrie-Muller, C., Chevrie, J. J., Le Normand, M. T., Salefranque, F., Forgue, M., Rigoard, M. T., et al. (1991). A peculiar case of acquired aphasia with epilepsy in childhood. *Journal of Neurolinguistics, 6,* 415–431.

Cole, A. J., Andermann, F., Taylor, L., Olivier, A., Rasmussen, T., Robitaille, Y., et al. (1988). The Landau-Kleffner syndrome of acquired epileptic aphasia: Unusual clinical outcome, surgical experience, and absence of encephalitis. *Neurology, 38*(1), 31–38.

Cooper, J. A., & Ferry, P. C. (1978). Acquired auditory verbal agnosia and seizures in childhood. *Journal of Speech and Hearing Disorders, 43*(2), 176–184.

De Wijngaert, E. A. K. (1993). Language rehabilitation in the Landau-Kleffner syndrome: Considerations and approaches. *Aphasiology, 7,* 475–480.

Denes, G., Balliello, S., Volterra, V., & Pellegrini, A. (1986). Oral and written language in a case of childhood phonemic deafness. *Brain and Language, 29*(2), 252–267.

Deonna, T., Beaumanoir, A., Gaillard, F., & Assal, G. (1977). Acquired aphasia in childhood with seizure disorder: A heterogeneous syndrome. *Neuropadiatrie, 8*(3), 263–273.

Deonna, T., Peter, C., & Ziegler, A. L. (1989). Adult follow-up of the acquired aphasia-epilepsy syndrome in childhood. Report of 7 cases. *Neuropediatrics, 20*(3), 132–138.

Deuel, R. K., & Lenn, N. J. (1977). Treatment of acquired epileptic aphasia. *Journal of Pediatrics, 90*(6), 959–961.

Dronkers, N., Husted, D. A., & Deutsch, G. (1999). Lesion site as a predictor of improvement after "Fast ForWord" treatment in adult aphasic patients. *Brain and Language*, 69, 450–452.

Dugas, M. (1982). The Landau-Kleffner syndrome. Infantile "acquired" aphasia, paroxysmal electroencephalographic changes and epileptic seizures. *La Nouvelle Presse Médicale*, 11(51), 3787–3791.

Dugas, M., Gerard, C. L., Franc, S., & Lecendreux, M. (1995). *Late onset of acquired epileptic aphasia.* London: John Libbey.

Dugas, M., Masson, M., Le Heuzey, M. F., & Regnier, N. (1982). Childhood acquired aphasia with epilepsy (Landau-Kleffner syndrome). 12 personal cases. *Revue Neurologique*, 138(10), 755–780.

Dulac, O. (2001). Epileptic encephalopathy. *Epilepsia*, 42(Suppl. 3), 23–26.

Ebbels, S. (2007). Teaching grammar to school-aged children with specific language impairment using Shape Coding. *Child Language Teaching and Therapy* 23(1), 67–93.

Engel, J. (2001). A proposed diagnostic scheme for people with epileptic seizures and with epilepsy: Report of the ILAE Task Force on Classification and Terminology. *Epilepsia*, 42(6), 796–803.

Engel, J. (2006). Report of the ILAE Classification Core Group. *Epilepsia*, 47(9), 1558–1568.

Feekery, C. J., Parry-Fielder, B., & Hopkins, I. J. (1993). Landau-Kleffner syndrome: Six patients including discordant monozygotic twins. *Pediatric Neurology*, 9(1), 49–53.

Fejerman, N., & Medina, C. S. (1986). *Convulsiones en la infancia* (2nd ed.). Buenos Aires, Argentina: El Ateneo.

Flexer, C., Millin, J., & Brown, L. (1990). Children with developmental disabilities: The effects of sound field amplification in word identification. *Language, Speech and Hearing Service in Schools*, 21, 177–182.

Gascon, G., Victor, D., & Lombroso, C. T. (1973). Language disorders, convulsive disorder, and electroencephalographic abnormalities. Acquired syndrome in children. *Archives of Neurology*, 28, 156–162.

Genton, P., & Guerrini, R. (1993). What differentiates Landau-Kleffner syndrome from the syndrome of continuous spikes and waves during slow sleep? *Archives of Neurology*, 50(10), 1008–1009.

Genton, P., Maton, B., Ogihara, M., Samoggia, G., Guerrini, R., Medina, M. T., et al. (1992). Continuous focal spikes during REM sleep in a case of acquired aphasia (Landau-Kleffner syndrome). *Sleep*, 15(5), 454–460.

Gerard, C. L., Dugas, M., & Sagar, D. (1991). Speech therapy in Landau and Kleffner syndrome. In A. C. I. P. Martins & H. R. V. Dogen (Eds.), *Acquired aphasia in children: Acquisition and breakdown of language in the developing brain* (pp. 279–290). Dordrecht, Netherlands: Kluwer Academic Publishers.

Gerard, C. L., Dugas, M., Valdois, S., Franc, S., & Lecendreux, M. (1993). Landau-Kleffner syndrome diagnosed after 9 years of age: Another Landau-Kleffner syndrome? *Aphasiology*, 7, 463–473.

Goldman, R., Fristoe, M., & Woodcock, R. W. (1970). *Goldman-Fristoe-Woodcock Test of Auditory Discrimination.* Circle Pines, MN: American Guidance Service.

Guzzetta, F., Battaglia, D., Veredice, C., Donvito, V., Pane, M., Lettori, D., et al. (2005). Early thalamic injury associated with epilepsy and continuous spike-wave during slow sleep. *Epilepsia*, 46(6), 889–900.

Hankey, G. J., & Gubbay, S. S. (1987). Acquired aphasia of childhood with epilepsy: The Landau-Kleffner syndrome. *Clinical and Experimental Neurology*, 24, 187–194.

Hickok, G., Buchsbaum, B., Humphries, C., & Muftuler, T. (2003). Auditory-motor interaction revealed by fMRI: Speech, music, and working memory in area Spt. *Journal of Cognitive Neuroscience*, 15(5), 673–682.

Hirsch, E., Maquet, P., Metz-Lutz, M. N., Motte, J., Finck, S., & Marescaux, C. (1995). The eponym 'Landau-Kleffner syndrome' should not be restricted to childhood acquired aphasia with epilepsy. In A. Beaumanoir, M. Bureau, T. Deonna, L. Mira, & C. A. Tassinari (Eds.), *Continuous spikes and waves during slow sleep* (pp. 57–62). London: John Libbey & Company, Ltd.

Hirsch, E., Marescaux, C., Maquet, P., Metz-Lutz, M. N., Kiesmann, M., Salmon, E., et al. (1990). Landau-Kleffner syndrome: A clinical and EEG study of five cases. *Epilepsia*, 31(6), 756–767.

Holmes, G. L., McKeever, M., & Saunders, Z. (1981). Epileptiform activity in aphasia of childhood: An epiphenomenon? *Epilepsia*, 22(6), 631–639.

Holmes, G. L., & Riviello, J. J. (2001). Treatment of childhood idiopathic language deterioration with Valproate. *Epilepsy and Behavior*, 2, 272–276.

Honbolygo, F., Csepe, V., Fekeshazy, A., Emri, M., Marian, T., Sarkozy, G., et al. (2006). Converging evidences on language impairment in Landau-Kleffner Syndrome revealed by behavioral and brain activity measures: A case study. *Clinical Neurophysiology*, 117(2), 295–305.

Hu, S. X., Wu, X. R., Lin, C., & Hao, S. Y. (1989). Landau-Kleffner syndrome with unilateral EEG abnormalities – Two cases from Beijing, China. *Brain Development*, 11(6), 420–422.

Humphrey, I. L., Knipstein, R., & Bumpass, E. R. (1975). Gradually developing aphasia in children.

A diagnostic problem. *Journal of the American Academy of Child Psychiatry, 14*, 652–665.

Huppke, P., Kallenberg, K., & Gartner, J. (2005). Perisylvian polymicrogyria in Landau-Kleffner syndrome. *Neurology, 64*(9), 1660.

International League Against Epilepsy (ILEA). (1985). Commission on Classification and Terminology of the International League against Epilepsy (ILEA). Proposal for classification of epilepsies and epileptic syndromes. *Epilepsia, 26*, 268–278.

ILEA. (1989). Commission on Classification and Terminology of the International League against Epilepsy (ILEA). Proposal for revised classification of epilepsies and epileptic syndromes. *Epilepsia, 30*, 389–399.

Irwin, K., Birch, V., Lees, J., Polkey, C., Alarcon, G., Binnie, C., et al. (2001). Multiple subpial transection in Landau-Kleffner syndrome. *Developmental Medicine and Child Neurology, 43*(4), 248–252.

Johnsrude, I. S., Zatorre, R. J., Milner, B. A., & Evans, A. C. (1997). Left-hemisphere specialization for the processing of acoustic transients. *Neuroreport, 8*(7), 1761–1765.

Jordan, L. S. (1980). Receptive and expressive language problems occurring in combination with a seizure disorder: A case report. *Journal of Communication Disorders, 13*, 295–303.

Kaga, M. (1999). Language disorders in Landau-Kleffner syndrome. *Journal of Child Neurology, 14*(2), 118–122.

Kale, U., el-Naggar, M., & Hawthorne, M. (1995). Verbal auditory agnosia with focal EEG abnormality: An unusual case of a child presenting to an ENT surgeon with "deafness". *Journal of Laryngology Otology, 109*(5), 431–432.

Kaufman, A., & Kaufman, N. (1983). *Kaufman Assessment Battery for Children*. Shoreview, MN: American Guidance Service.

Keith, R. W. (1986). *Screening Test for Auditory Processing Disorders in Children*. San Antonio, TX: Psychological Corporation.

Kellermann, K. (1978). Recurrent aphasia with subclinical bioelectric status epilepticus during sleep. *European Journal of Pediatrics, 128*(3), 207–212.

Klein, S. K., Kurtzberg, D., & Brattson, A. (1995). Electrophysiologic manifestations of impaired temporal lobe auditory processing in verbal auditory agnosia. *Brain and Language, 51*, 383–405.

Koeda, T., & Kohno, Y. (1992). Non-verbal auditory agnosia with EEG abnormalities and epilepsy. An unusual case of Landau-Kleffner syndrome. *Brain and Development, 24*(3), 262–267.

Kollros, P., Stefanatos, G. A., Rabinovitch, H., & Streletz, L. J. (1996). Sleep and amitriptyline enhance the sensitivity of electroencephalograms in children with a pervasive developmental disorder and language regression. *Annals of Neurology, 40*(2), 70.

Korkman, M., Granstrom, M. L., Appelqvist, K., & Liukkonen, E. (1998). Neuropsychological characteristics of five children with the Landau-Kleffner syndrome: Dissociation of auditory and phonological discrimination. *Journal of the International Neuropsychological Society, 4*(6), 566–575.

Korkman, M., Kirk, U., & Kemp, S. (1998). *NEPSY: A Developmental Neuropsychological Assessment*. San Antonio, TX: Psychological Corporation.

Kramer, U., Nevo, Y., Neufeld, M. Y., Fatal, A., Leitner, Y., & Harel, S. (1998). Epidemiology of epilepsy in childhood: A cohort of 440 consecutive patients. *Pediatric Neurology, 18*(1), 46–50.

Landau, W. M., & Kleffner, F. R. (1957). Syndrome of acquired aphasia with convulsive disorder in children. *Neurology, 7*, 523–530.

Lanzi, G., Veggiotti, P., Conte, S., Partesana, E., & Resi, C. (1994). A correlated fluctuation of language and EEG abnormalities in a case of the Landau-Kleffner syndrome. *Brain Development, 16*(4), 329–334.

Lea, J. (1970). *The Color Pattern Scheme: A Method of Remedial Language Teaching*. Oxted Surrey: Moor House School.

Lees, J. (2005). *Children with acquired aphasias* (2nd ed.). London: Whurr Publishers.

Lerman, P., Lerman-Sagie, T., & Kivity, S. (1991). Effect of early corticosteroid therapy for Landau-Kleffner syndrome. *Developmental Medicine and Child Neurology, 33*(3), 257–260.

Liegeois-Chauvel, C., de Graaf, J. B., Laguitton, V., & Chauvel, P. (1999). Specialization of left auditory cortex for speech perception in man depends on temporal coding. *Cerebral Cortex, 9*(5), 484–496.

Lou, H. C., Brandt, S., & Bruhn, P. (1977). Aphasia and epilepsy in childhood. *Acta Neurologica Scandinavica, 56*(1), 46–54.

Majerus, S., Laureys, S., Collette, F., Del Fiore, G., Degueldre, C., Luxen, A., et al. (2003). Phonological short-term memory networks following recovery from Landau and Kleffner syndrome. *Human Brain Mapping, 19*(3), 133–144.

Maneta, A., Marshall, J., & Lindsay, J. (2001). Direct and indirect therapy for word sound deafness. *International Journal of Language and Communication Disorders, 36*(1), 91–106.

Mantovani, J. F. (2000). Autistic regression and Landau-Kleffner syndrome: Progress or confusion? *Developmental Medicine and Child Neurology, 42*(5), 349–353.

Mantovani, J. F., & Landau, W. M. (1980). Acquired aphasia with convulsive disorder: Course and prognosis. *Neurology, 30*(5), 524–529.

Maquet, P., Hirsch, E., Metz-Lutz, M. N., Motte, J., Dive, D., Marescaux, C., et al. (1995). Regional cerebral glucose metabolism in children with deterioration of one or more cognitive functions and continuous spike-and-wave discharges during sleep. *Brain*, *118*(6), 1497–1520.

Marescaux, C., Hirsch, E., Finck, S., Maquet, P., Schlumberger, E., Sellal, F., et al. (1990). Landau-Kleffner syndrome: A pharmacologic study of five cases. *Epilepsia*, *31*(6), 768–777.

Marien, P., Saerens, J., Verslegers, W., Borggreve, F., & De Deyn, P. P. (1993). Some controversies about type and nature of aphasic symptomatology in Landau-Kleffner's syndrome: A case study. *Acta Neurologica Belgica*, *93*(4), 183–203.

Martin, N. A., & Brownell, R. (2005). *Test of Auditory Processing Skills, Third Edition (TAPS-3)*. Novato, CA: Academic Therapy Publications.

McKinney, W., & McGreal, D. A. (1974). An aphasic syndrome in children. *Canadian Medical Association Journal*, *110*(6), 637–639.

Merzenich, M. M., Jenkins, W. M., Johnston, P., Schreiner, C., Miller, S. L., & Tallal, P. (1996). Temporal processing deficits of language-learning impaired children ameliorated by training. *Science*, *271*(5245), 77–81.

Metz-Lutz, M. N., & Filippini, M. (2006). Neuropsychological findings in Rolandic epilepsy and Landau-Kleffner syndrome. *Epilepsia*, *47*(Suppl. 2), 71–75.

Michalowicz, R., Jozwiak, S., Ignatowicz, R., & Szwabowska-Orzeszko, E. (1988). Landau-Kleffner syndrome—epileptic aphasia in children—possible role of toxoplasma gondii infection. *Acta Paediatr Hungarica*, *29*(3–4), 337–342.

Morrell, F., Whisler, W. W., Smith, M. C., Hoeppner, T. J., de Toledo-Morrell, L., Pierre-Louis, S. J., Kanner, A. M., Buelow, J. M., Ristanovic, R., Bergen, D. (1995). Landau-Kleffner syndrome. Treatment with subpial intracortical transection. *Brain*, *118* (Pt. 6), 1529–1546.

Morris, J. (1997). Remediating auditory processing deficits in adults with aphasia. In S. Chiat, J. Law, & J. Marshall (Eds.), *Language disorders in children and adults* (pp. 42–63) London: Whurr.

Morris, J., Franklin, S., Ellis, A. W., Turner, J. E., & Bailey, P. J. (1996). Remediation a speech perception deficit in an aphasic patient. *Aphasiology*, *10*, 137–158.

Msall, M., Shapiro, B., Balfour, P. B., Niedermeyer, E., & Capute, A. J. (1986). Acquired epileptic aphasia. Diagnostic aspects of progressive language loss in preschool children. *Clinical Pediatrics*, *25*(5), 248–251.

Nass, R., Gross, A., & Devinsky, O. (1998). Autism and autistic epileptiform regression with occipital spikes. *Developmental Medicine and Child Neurology*, *40*(7), 453–458.

Nass, R., Heier, L., & Walker, R. (1993). Landau-Kleffner syndrome: Temporal lobe tumor resection results in good outcome. *Pediatric Neurology*, *9*(4), 303–305.

Nass, R., & Petrucha, D. (1990). Acquired aphasia with convulsive disorder: A pervasive developmental disorder variant. *Journal of Child Neurology*, *5*(4), 327–328.

Nevsimalova, S., Tauberova, A., Doutlik, S., Kucera, V., & Dlouha, O. (1992). A role of autoimmunity in the etiopathogenesis of Landau-Kleffner syndrome? *Brain Development*, *14*(5), 342–345.

Okada, S., Hanada, M., Hattori, H., & Shoyama, T. (1963). A case of pure word-deafness (About the relation between auditory perception and recognition of speech-sound). *Studie Phonologica*, *14*, 58–65.

Otero, E., Cordova, S., Diaz, F., Garcia-Teruel, I., & Del Brutto, O. H. (1989). Acquired epileptic aphasia (the Landau-Kleffner syndrome) due to neurocysticercosis. *Epilepsia*, *30*(5), 569–572.

Paetau, R., Granstrom, M. L., Blomstedt, G., Jousmaki, V., Korkman, M., & Liukkonen, E. (1999). Magnetoencephalography in presurgical evaluation of children with the Landau-Kleffner syndrome. *Epilepsia*, *40*(3), 326–335.

Paetau, R., Kajola, M., Korkman, M., Hamalainen, M., Granstrom, M. L., Hari R. (1991). Landau-Kleffner syndrome: Epileptic activity in the auditory cortex. *Neuroreport*, *2*(4), 201–204.

Panayiotopoulos, C. P. (2007). *A clinical guide to epileptic syndromes and their treatment* (2nd ed.). London: Springer.

Paquier, P. F., & Van Dongen, H. R. (1996). Review of research on the clinical presentation of acquired childhood aphasia. *Acta Neurologica Scandinavica*, *93*(6), 428–436.

Paquier, P. F., Van Dongen, H. R., & Loonen, C. B. (1992). The Landau-Kleffner syndrome or "acquired aphasia with convulsive disorder". Long-term follow-up of six children and a review of the recent literature. *Archives of Neurology*, *49*(4), 354–359.

Pedro, V. M., & Leisman, G. (2005). Hemispheric integrative therapy in Landau-Kleffner syndrome: Applications for rehabilitation sciences. *International Journal of Neuroscience*, *115*(8), 1227–1238.

Penn, C., Friedlander, R. I., & Saling, M. M. (1990). Acquired childhood aphasia with convulsive disorder (Landau-Kleffner syndrome). A case report. *South African Medical Journal*, *77*(3), 158–161.

Perez, E. R., & Davidoff, V. (2001). Sign language in childhood epileptic aphasia (Landau-Kleffner syndrome). *Developmental Medicine and Child Neurology*, *43*(11), 739–744.

Perniola, T., Margari, L., Buttiglione, M., Andreula, C., Simone, I. L., & Santostasi, R. (1993). A case of Landau-Kleffner syndrome secondary to inflammatory demyelinating disease. *Epilepsia, 34*(3), 551–556.

Peterson, U., Koepp, P., Solmsen, M., & Villiez, T. H. (1978). Aphasie im Kindesalter mit EEG-Veranderungen [Childhood aphasia with EEG changes]. *Neuropadiatrie, 9,* 84–96.

Prasad, A. N., Stafstrom, C. F., & Holmes, G. L. (1996). Alternative epilepsy therapies: The ketogenic diet, immunoglobulins, and steroids. *Epilepsia, 37* (Suppl. 1), S81–95.

Rapin, I., Mattis, S., Rowan, A. J., & Golden, G. G. (1977). Verbal auditory agnosia in children. *Developmental Medicine and Child Neurology, 19*(2), 197–207.

Riviello, J. J., & Hadjiloizou, S. (2007). The Landau-Kleffner syndrome and epilepsy with continuous spike-wave during sleep. In S. C. Schachter, G. L. Holmes, & D. Kasteleijn-Nolst Trenité (Eds.), *Behavioral aspects of epilepsy* (pp. 377–382). New York: Demos Medical Publishing.

Robinson, R. O., Baird, G., Robinson, G., & Simonoff, E. (2001). Landau-Kleffner syndrome: course and correlates with outcome. *Developmental Medicine and Child Neurology, 43*(4), 243–247.

Rodriguez, I., & Niedermeyer, E. (1982). The aphasia-epilepsy syndrome in children: Electroencephalographic aspects. *Clinical EEG, 13*(1), 23–35.

Rossi, P. G., Parmeggiani, A., Posar, A., Scaduto, M. C., Chiodo, S., & Vatti, G. (1999). Landau-Kleffner syndrome (LKS): Long-term follow-up and links with electrical status epilepticus during sleep (ESES). *Brain Development, 21*(2), 90–98.

Roulet, E., Deonna, T., & Despland, P. A. (1989). Prolonged intermittent drooling and oromotor dyspraxia in benign childhood epilepsy with centrotemporal spikes. *Epilepsia, 30*(5), 564–568.

Roulet Perez, E. (1995). Syndromes of acquired epileptic aphasia and epilepsy with continuous spike-waves during sleep: models for prolonged cognitive impairment of epileptic origin. *Seminars in Pediatric Neurology, 2*(4), 269–277.

Roulet Perez, E., Davidoff, V., Despland, P. A., & Deonna, T. (1993). Mental and behavioural deterioration of children with epilepsy and CSWS: Acquired epileptic frontal syndrome. *Developmental Medicine and Child Neurology, 35*(8), 661–674.

Sanford, J. A., & Turner, A. (1999). *Integrated Visual and Auditory Continuous Performance Test.* Richmond, VA: BrainTrain.

Sato, S., & Dreifuss, F. E. (1973). Electroencephalographic findings in a patient with developmental expressive aphasia. *Neurology, 23,* 181–185.

Sawhney, I. M., Suresh, N., Dhand, U. K., & Chopra, J. S. (1988). Acquired aphasia with epilepsy – Landau-Kleffner syndrome. *Epilepsia, 29*(3), 283–287.

Senju, A., & Johnson, M. H. (2009). The eye contact effect: Mechanisms and development. *Trends in Cognitive Sciences, 13*(3), 127–134.

Shafrir, Y., & Prensky, A. L. (1995). Acquired epileptiform opercular syndrome: A second case report, review of the literature, and comparison to the Landau-Kleffner syndrome. *Epilepsia, 36*(10), 1050–1057.

Shindo, M., Kaga, K., & Tanaka, Y. (1991). Speech discrimination and lip reading in patients with word deafness or auditory agnosia. *Brain and Language, 40*(2), 153–161.

Shoumaker, R. D., Bennett, D. R., Bray, P. F., & Curless, R. G. (1974). Clinical and EEG manifestations of an unusual aphasic syndrome in children. *Neurology, 24,* 10–16.

Small, N. (1968). *Levels of perceptual functioning in children: A developmental study.* Unpublished master's thesis, University of Florida, Gainsville.

Smith, E. E., & Jonides, J. (1997). Working memory: A view from neuroimaging. *Cognitive Psychology, 33,* 5–42.

Smith, M. C., & Hoeppner, T. J. (2003). Epileptic encephalopathy of late childhood: Landau-Kleffner syndrome and the syndrome of continuous spikes and waves during slow-wave sleep. *Journal of Clinical Neurophysiology, 20*(6), 462–472.

Sobel, D. F., Aung, M., Otsubo, H., & Smith, M. C. (2000). Magnetoencephalography in children with Landau-Kleffner syndrome and acquired epileptic aphasia. *American Journal of Neuroradiology, 21*(2), 301–307.

Solomon, G. E., Carson, D., Pavlakis, S., Fraser, R., & Labar, D. (1993). Intracranial EEG monitoring in Landau-Kleffner syndrome associated with left temporal lobe astrocytoma. *Epilepsia, 34*(3), 557–560.

Soprano, A. M., Garcia, E. F., Caraballo, R., & Fejerman, N. (1994). Acquired epileptic aphasia: Neuropsychologic follow-up of 12 patients. *Pediatric Neurology, 11*(3), 230–235.

Stefanatos, G. A. (1993). Frequency modulation analysis in children with Landau-Kleffner syndrome. *Annals of the New York Academy of Sciences, 682,* 412–414.

Stefanatos, G. A. (2008). Speech perceived through a damaged temporal window: Lessons from word deafness and aphasia. *Seminars in Speech and Language, 29*(2), 239–252.

Stefanatos, G.A., Gershkoff A., Madigan S. (2005). On pure word deafness, temporal processing and the left hemisphere. *Journal of the International Neuropsychological Society 11(4),* 456–470.

Stefanatos, G. A., Gershkoff, A., & Madigan, S. (2005). Computer-mediated tools for the investigation and rehabilitation of auditory and phonological processing in aphasia. *Aphasiology, 19*(10/11), 955–964.

Stefanatos, G. A., Grover, W., & Geller, E. (1995). Case study: Corticosteroid treatment of language regression in pervasive developmental disorder. *Journal of the American Academy of Child and Adolescent Psychiatry*, 34(8), 1107–1111.

Stefanatos, G. A., Joe, W. Q., Aguirre, G. K., Detre, J. A., & Wetmore, G. (2008). Activation of human auditory cortex during speech perception: Effects of monaural, binaural, and dichotic presentation. *Neuropsychologia*, 46(1), 301–315.

Stefanatos, G. A., Kinsbourne, M., & Wasserstein, J. (2002). Acquired epileptiform aphasia: A dimensional view of Landau-Kleffner syndrome and the relation to regressive autistic spectrum disorders. *Child Neuropsychology*, 8(3), 195–228.

Stefanatos, G. A., Kollros, P., & Rabinovich, H. (1996). Childhood idiopathic language deterioration: Positive treatment responses associated with improved steady stated auditory evoked potential. *Annals of Neurology*, 40, 301.

Stefanatos, G. A., & Madigan, S. (2000). *The Environmental Sounds Perception Test*. Philadelphia: PA. (available from the author)

Tallal, P., Miller, S., & Fitch, R. H. (1993). Neurobiological basis of speech: A case for the preeminence of temporal processing. *Annals of the New York Academy of Sciences*, 682, 27–47.

Tassinari, C. A., Bureau, M., Dravet, C., Dalla Bernardina, B., & Rogers, J. (1992). Epilepsy with continuous spikes and waves during slow sleep—otherwise described as ESES (epilepsy with electrical status epilepticus during slow sleep). In J. Rogers, M. Bureau, C. Dravet, F. E. Dreifuss, A. Perret, & P. Wolf (Eds.), *Epileptic syndromes in infancy, childhood and adolescence, 2nd Edition* (pp. 245–256). London: John Libbey.

Tassinari, C. A., Rubboli, G., Volpi, L., Billard, C., & Bureau, M. (2002). Electrical status epilepticus during slow sleep (ESES or CSWS) including acquired epileptic aphasia (Landau Kleffner syndrome). In J. Rogers, M. Bureau, C. Dravet, P. Genton, C. A. Tassinari, & P. Wolf (Eds.), *Epileptic syndromes in infancy, childhood and adolescence, 3rd Edition* (pp. 265–283). London: John Libbey.

Tharpe, A. M., Johnson, G. D., & Glasscock, M. E., 3rd. (1991). Diagnostic and management considerations of acquired epileptic aphasia or Landau-Kleffner syndrome. *American Journal of Otology*, 12(3), 210–214.

Tuchman, R. F., & Rapin, I. (1997). Regression in pervasive developmental disorders: Seizures and epileptiform electroencephalogram correlates. *Pediatrics*, 99(4), 560–566.

Uldall, P., Sahlholdt, L., & Alving, J. (2000). Landau-Kleffner syndrome with onset at 18 months and an initial diagnosis of pervasive developmental disorder. *European Journal of Paediatric Neurology*, 4(2), 81–86.

van de Sandt-Koenderman, W. M., Smit, I. A., van Dongen, H. R., & van Hest, J. B. (1984). A case of acquired aphasia and convulsive disorder: Some linguistic aspects of recovery and breakdown. *Brain and Language*, 21(1), 174–183.

Van Hirtum-Das, M., Licht, E. A., Koh, S., Wu, J. Y., Shields, W. D., & Sankar, R. (2006). Children with ESES: Variability in the syndrome. *Epilepsy Research*, 70(Suppl. 1), S248–258.

Van Slyke, P. (2002). Classroom instruction for children with Landau-Kleffner Syndrome. *Child Language Teaching and Therapy*, 18(1), 23–42.

Vance, M. S. (1991). Educational and therapeutic approaches used with a child presenting with acquired aphasia with convulsive disorder (Landau-Kleffner syndrome). *Child Language Teaching and Therapy*, 7, 41–60.

Veggiotti, P., Termine, C., Granocchio, E., Bova, S., Papalia, G., & Lanzi, G. (2002). Long-term neuropsychological follow-up and nosological considerations in five patients with continuous spikes and waves during slow sleep. *Epileptic Disorders*, 4(4), 243–249.

White, H., & Sreenivasan, U. (1987). Epilepsy-aphasia syndrome in children: An unusual presentation to psychiatry. *Canadian Journal of Psychiatry*, 32(7), 599–601.

World Health Organization (WHO). (1977). *Ninth Revision of the International Classification of Diseases and Related Health Problems (ICD-9)*. Geneva: WHO.

World Health Organization (WHO). (1992). *Tenth Revision of the International Classification of Diseases and Related Health Problems (ICD-10)*. Geneva: WHO.

Wioland, N., Rudolf, G., & Metz-Lutz, M. N. (2001). Electrophysiological evidence of persisting unilateral auditory cortex dysfunction in the late outcome of Landau and Kleffner syndrome. *Clinical Neurophysiology: Official Journal of the International Federation of Clinical Neurophysiology*, 112(2), 319–323.

Woll, B., & Sieratzki, J. S. (1996). Sign language for children with acquired aphasia. *Journal of Child Neurology*, 11(4), 347–349.

Worster-Drought, C. (1971). An usual form of acquired aphasia in children. *Developmental Medicine and Child Neurology*, 13(5), 563–571.

Zatorre, R. J., Belin, P., & Penhune, V. B. (2002). Structure and function of auditory cortex: Music and speech. *Trends in Cognitive Sciences*, 6(1), 37–46.

13

A Case of Liver Transplantation in Maple Syrup Urine Disease

Lisa G. Hahn and Joel E. Morgan

Approximately 4% of infants born in the United States have some genetic anomaly, and many of these are disorders of metabolism (Enns, Cowan Klein, & Packman, 2006). One such metabolic disorder is maple syrup urine disease (MSUD), a fairly uncommon autosomal recessive disorder, first identified in 1954 (Menkes, Hurst, & Craig, 1954). The incidence of MSUD has variously been reported between 1 per 150,000–185,000 in the general population (Chuang & Shih, 2001), but the disorder is much more common among the Old Order Mennonites of Pennsylvania (1 in 176 births; Marshall & DiGeorge, 1981). Clinically, these infants appear healthy and normal at birth but within 3 to 5 days after birth, if untreated, they begin to develop a cerebral degenerative disease and their urine is characterized by a sweet smell, similar to the smell of maple syrup. Failure to thrive is common. The disorder is caused by an inherited enzymatic defect, a branched-chain alpha-keto acid dehydrogenase complex (BCKDH) deficiency, which results in inability to digest and metabolize certain proteins. Because proteins cannot be properly metabolized as a result of this enzyme deficiency, there is an accumulated buildup of branched-chain amino acids, particularly leucine, isoleucine, and valine, common in meat, eggs, and milk, among other foods. This buildup and their by-products, found in blood and urine, are toxic. As a consequence of these toxins in the central nervous system (CNS), a severe neonatal cerebral encephalopathy develops with prominent cerebral edema (Brismar et al., 1990). If left untreated, children with MSUD will die of edema resulting in herniation (Riviello, Rezvani, DiGeorge, & Foley, 1991).

In the classic form of the disease, the most severe form, untreated neonates develop symptoms by the end of the first week of life and the characteristic maple syrup aroma of the urine by the fifth-to-seventh day. When diagnosed and treated early, typically with nutritional control, children with MSUD have overall better outcomes. Kaplan et al. (1991) found that children diagnosed and treated at a mean age of 3.5 days had overall higher IQ than children diagnosed at a later age (day 10 of life) whose intellectual functions typically fell within the mentally retarded range (Kaplan et al., 1991). Undiagnosed/untreated children typically die within the first month of life. Hilliges, Awiszus, and Wendel (1993) found that early treated MSUD patients had a mean IQ of 74, while those treated late were mentally retarded (Chuang & Shih, 2001).

Though few studies addressing the cognition of MSUD patients appear in the literature and unfortunately many are replete with flawed methodology, the limited research on cognitive functions among these children suggests greater preservation of verbal skills relative to visualspatial skills within an overall context of generalized cognitive impairment (Walsh & Scott, 2010). Walsh and Scott (2010) presented a case study of a 7-year-old girl, first diagnosed with MSUD on day 7 of life, who had significantly poorer visual perceptual and spatial skills relative to verbal skills. Although on a special diet with appropriate restrictions and supplements, her course of MSUD was said to be only "partially controlled." Wechsler scales revealed a Verbal Comprehension Index at the 16th percentile and a Perceptual Reasoning Index at the 8th percentile, with WRAML2 Story Memory at the 91st percentile, but Picture Memory at the 5th percentile. Rey-Osterrieth Complex Figure copy fell below the 1st percentile, and immediate and delayed recall were at the 2nd percentile. Visual perception fell at the 2nd percentile and left-sided fine motor skills (nondominant; Grooved Pegboard) were at the 4th percentile. Academic achievement ranged between the 12th and 83rd percentile. The authors concluded that their case study was consistent with reports in the literature underscoring weaker nonverbal than verbal cognitive functions in these patients.

More recently, "metabolic cure" has been reported in MSUD after liver transplantation. In a serendipitous case of an 8.5-year-old child with MSUD requiring liver transplantation for another disorder (hypervitaminosis A), metabolic features associated with MSUD were alleviated after transplant surgery (Strauss et al., 2006) and liver transplantation has become more common as a treatment for this condition. But while some studies of children who receive traditional nutritional therapy, as noted above, reported neurocognitive test results, to the best of our knowledge there have been no reports in the literature of cognitive function in MSUD patients who have received liver transplantation. We report such a case.

Case Presentation: J. H.

J. H. was a 10-year, 5-month-old male born to college-educated parents. He was the eldest of three children and resided in a suburban metropolitan area.

Medical and Psychiatric History

J. H. was the product of a normal, spontaneous vaginal birth with labor induced at 35 weeks after his 30-year-old mother was placed on bed rest from 32 through 35 weeks due to a calcified placenta. His Apgar scores reportedly were normal. His mother reported difficulty with feeding during his initial days after birth and he remained hospitalized. He lapsed into a coma from day 7 through day 12 and required a ventilator to assist with breathing. He was diagnosed with MSUD on day 12 and was hospitalized for a total of 7 weeks following birth. He required several hospitalizations throughout his first year of life to assist with treatment and control of MSUD. A nasogastric (NG) tube was placed although he was periodically bottle fed. At the age of 10 months a gastronomy tube (g-tube) was placed due to failure to thrive. The g-tube was used primarily during the first year after placement and then during illness. Although food was introduced later than usual, the child reportedly did well transitioning to regular oral intake. The child followed a low-protein, MSUD diet until he underwent a liver transplant in 2006. He tolerated the transplant well and subsequently a regular diet was introduced.

In addition to a historical diagnosis of MSUD, the client's medical history is notable for an "underdeveloped" hypothalamus reported by the mother. Imaging records were not available to confirm this diagnosis. He also suffered from seizures and reportedly his most recent seizure was a year prior to the evaluation. He suffered from respiratory syncytial virus (RSV) and pneumonia during early childhood. His mother noted he was underweight and had speech articulation problems for which he received speech and language services.

Family medical history is notable for MSUD (younger brother), cancer, hypertension, heart disease, stroke, migraine headaches, and psychiatric disorders (autism and bipolar disorder).

The child's psychiatric history was notable for a diagnosis of attention-deficit/hyperactivity disorder (ADHD) at age 4. He was described as lacking self-control, having a short attention span at times, and being impulsive. His mother noted that J. H. was hyperactive, and she spent a great deal of time attending to him. She reported he was unable to self-soothe or calm himself when upset. He was described as hiding his feelings and at times acted immature and silly. He had a long-standing history of difficulty initiating and maintaining friendships. He preferred to play with younger children or alone, and tended to be a follower. He was enrolled in a social skills group and psychotherapy.

His current medication regimen at the time of the evaluation consisted of Concerta, Ritalin,

Wellbutrin, an immunosuppressant, and an anti-epileptic medication (names were unknown).

Educational History

At the time of the evaluation, the child was enrolled in a public school in New Jersey and had been receiving accommodations under an individual education plan IEP since second grade. He was evaluated during the summer and was entering the fifth grade in the fall. He had participated in resource room services since third grade. In second grade he was in an inclusion class. During fourth grade he participated in resource room services for language arts and math and an inclusion class for science and social studies. For the upcoming year, fifth grade, he was to be enrolled in general education classes for all academic subjects and receive in-class assistance for language arts and math. He also participated in speech and language therapy twice a week.

He completed a psychoeducational evaluation conducted by the school district approximately two-and-a-half years prior to the current evaluation. At that time, his WISC-IV Full Scale IQ was reported to be 78 (7th percentile), with a Verbal Comprehension index score of 89 (23rd percentile), Perceptual Reasoning index score of 65 (1st percentile), Working Memory index score of 99 (47th percentile), and Processing Speed index score of 83 (13th percentile). His academic achievement based on the Woodcock–Johnson–Third Edition Tests of Achievement was generally in the average range except for Math Calculation Skills (17th percentile), Calculation (16th percentile), Math Fluency (23rd percentile), Writing Samples (24th percentile), and Reading Vocabulary (22nd percentile), which were all in the low-average range.

Behavioral Observations

J. H. easily transitioned from sitting in the waiting room with his mother to the evaluation room with the examiner. He readily answered the examiner's questions about school and his home life; however, when testing began he engaged in immature and silly behavior. He often struggled to follow the instructions. Despite taking Concerta the day of the evaluation, he was impulsive,

often responding before questions were completed or providing answers and then changing them. He also consistently interrupted the examiner. Even though he was impulsive, he worked very slowly on most tasks. In fact, he required an hour and a half to complete the WISC-IV. He frequently replied, "I don't know" to questions and refused to guess, even when encouraged to do so. He frequently complained about the testing tasks. He was very fidgety. He appeared to be more interested and invested in completing visual tasks versus verbal ones. He requested two breaks during the morning session. His physical stature was noted to be small, and he was very thin. His speech was notable for difficulties with articulation. Aside from these observations, his spontaneous speech was fluent, grammatical, and free of paraphasic errors. There was no evidence for clinically significant aphasia or an underlying thought disorder. Further, there was no evidence of frank neurobehavioral anomalies such as dysphasia, dystaxia, or gait or balance disturbance.

Neurocognitive Results

J. H. was administered a neuropsychological battery while his mother was interviewed and completed a developmental history questionnaire and standardized behavioral rating scale. The neuropsychological battery consisted of the following measures: Wechsler Intelligence Test for Children–Fourth Edition (WISC-IV); Woodcock-Johnson Tests of Achievement–Third Edition (WJ-III), selected subtests; California Verbal Learning Test for Children (CVLT-C); Rey-Osterrith Complex Figure Test (ROCFT); Wechsler Memory Test–Revised (WMS-R), selected subtests; Boston Naming Test (BNT); Controlled Oral Word Association Test (COWAT); Beery Buktenica Development Test of Visual-Motor Integration (VMI); Trail Making Test Part A and B; Stroop; Connors' Continuous Performance Test–Second Edition (CPT-II); Auditory Consonant Trigrams Test (ACT); Grooved Pegboard Test; Behavior Assessment System for Children–Second Edition, Parent Report.

General Intellectual Functioning. The child's overall Full Scale IQ based on the WISC-IV fell at the

4th percentile (SS = 73). His Verbal Comprehension was at the 10th percentile (SS = 81), Perceptual Organization was at the 3rd percentile (SS = 71), Working Memory was at the 13th percentile (SS = 83), and Processing Speed was at the 9th percentile (SS = 80). Overall, his intellectual profile is generally low average with borderline perceptual reasoning abilities.

Academic Achievement. His academic achievement ranged from low average to average in reading, math, and writing. However, difficulty with passage comprehension and math fluency was noted. His ability in these areas was in the borderline range and significantly below grade expectation.

Language. As noted above, his verbal abilities from the WISC-IV were low average. His vocabulary was low average, verbal abstract reasoning was average, and verbal comprehension was borderline. Confrontation naming was low average.

Executive Functioning. Testing revealed poor sustained visual attention and impulsivity as well as difficulty with divided attention, selective inhibition, and letter fluency. The child's simple visual and psychomotor attention and category fluency were intact. Working Memory from the WISC-IV was low average. His performance on the ACT was also low average.

Fine Motor Skills. His fine motor dexterity was severely impaired bilaterally.

Visual-Spatial/Perceptual Abilities. Abilities in this domain were significantly below expectation, falling in the borderline to severely impaired range based on the ROCFT and the VMI. His copy of the Complex Figure revealed that he failed to appreciate the overall gestalt of the figure. Rather his copy was extremely piecemeal and detail oriented. However, the details did not provide any sense of the original figure. His perceptual abilities from the WISC-IV were in the borderline range. His nonverbal abstract reasoning was variable, ranging from low average to borderline, and visual-motor integration was borderline. His visual scanning also was variable on the WISC-IV, ranging from average to borderline.

Learning/Memory. The child's memory skills were quite variable. Consistent with his poor perceptual skills on other tasks, his visual memory for both the ROCF and WMS-R Visual Reproduction subtest was severely impaired. His verbal memory for stories from the WMS-R was also below expectation, falling in the mildly impaired range. However, his rote (list) learning and memory were intact. In fact, his learning slope was high average and his recall was average and improved to superior when he was provided with cues.

Summary of Neurocognitive Results. The neurocognitive profile revealed low-average to borderline intellectual functioning with weaknesses in executive functioning, visual-spatial abilities, visual learning and memory, prose (story) learning and memory, and fine-motor skills. When compared to his previous test results from 2007, his WISC-IV scores are generally consistent. The results indicate a drop in his working memory ability, yet his perceptual reasoning abilities improved slightly from extremely low to borderline. His academic achievement performance revealed he continued to struggle to make academic gains and in fact had fallen further behind his peers in reading, passage comprehension, and reading and math fluency. See Table 13-1 for neuropsychological data.

Behavioral Rating Scales. The mother completed the *Behavioral Assessment System for Children–2*. Her responses indicate that her son is withdrawn and struggles to initiate friendships. He shies away from group activities and spends his time alone. She did not endorse symptoms of hyperactivity, inattention, depression, or anxiety, even though he carries a diagnosis of ADHD, and she described him as an anxious child during the clinical interview.

Discussion

The literature on MSUD and its neurocognitive profile is quite limited at this time. Numerous variables confound results of available studies,

Table 13-1. Neurocognitive Test Results

Neurocognitive Domain/Instrument	Raw Score	Percentile	Grade Level
Intellectual Functioning			
Wechsler Intelligence Scale for Children–IV			
Full Scale IQ	63	4	
Verbal Comprehension Index	20	10	
Perceptual Reasoning	16	3	
Working Memory	14	13	
Processing Speed	13	9	
Subtests			
Similarities	18	37	
Vocabulary	22	9	
Comprehension	13	5	
Block Design	13	5	
Picture Concepts	12	9	
Matrix Reasoning	12	5	
Digit Span	14	37	
Letter-Number Sequencing	10	5	
Coding	28	5	
Symbol Search	19	25	
Academic Achievement			
Woodcock Johnson Tests of Achievement–III Form A			
Cluster			
Broad Reading		14	3.0
Basic Reading Skills		38	4.0
Math Calculation Skills		25	3.8
Academic Skills		39	4.3
Academic Fluency		19	3.5
Tests			
Letter-Word Identification	48	33	3.8
Reading Fluency	29	16	3.1
Calculation	16	36	4.1
Math Fluency	39	7	2.9
Spelling	35	49	5.4
Writing Fluency	15	41	4.6
Passage Comprehension	18	5	1.9
Word Attack	20	43	4.3
Language			
Boston Naming Test	39	9	
Visuomotor/Visuospatial			
VMI	15	1	
ROCFT Copy	2	<1	
Attention/Executive Function			
Trail Making Test Part A	22	46	
Trail Making Test Part B	33	11	
Stroop			
Word	55	27	

Table 13-1. Neurocognitive Test Results (*Continued*)

Neurocognitive Domain/Instrument	Raw Score	Percentile
Color	40	18
Color-Word	22	17
Interference Score	18	35
Auditory Consonant Trigrams Test		
0"	15	
3"	8	
9"	7	
18"	4	
Total	34	24
CPT		
Clinical Confidence Level	99.90	
Omissions	99.00	
Commissions	76.87	
Hit RT	96.22	
Hit RT Std. Error	96.97	
Variability	95.64	
Detectability	97.78	
Response Style	94.54	
Perseverations	98.95	
Hit RT Block Change	99.00	
Hit SE Block Change	98.29	
Hit RT ISI Change	61.93	
Hit SE ISIS Change	65.99	
Letter Fluency	13	10
Category Fluency	13	36
Fine-Motor Dexterity		
Grooved Pegboard		
Dominant Hand	155	<1
Non-Dominant Hand	176	<1
Learning/Memory		
California Verbal Learning Test for Children		
Total	53	79
Trial 1	7	69
Trial 5	12	69
List B Free Recall	6	50
SD Free Recall	9	50
SD Cued Recall	12	84
LD Free Recall	11	69
LD Cued Recall	14	91
Semantic		84
Serial		16
Slope		50
Perseverations		50
Intrusions		16
Hits	15	84
Recognition Discrimination	100	84
False Positives	0	16

(*Continued*)

Table 13-1. Neurocognitive Test Results (*Continued*)

Neurocognitive Domain/Instrument	Raw Score	Percentile	Grade Level
ROCFT			
Delay	0	<1	
Wechsler Memory Test–Revised			
Logical Memory I	7	3	
Logical Memory II	5	<1	
Visual Reproduction I	1	<1	
Visual Reproduction II	2	<1	

such as age at diagnosis and severity of neonatal course, treatment compliancy, available measures, and so on. One recent study examined the neurocognitive profile of a child diagnosed with MSUD (Walsh et al., 2010) and served as a comparison for the current case study.

The current case study provides additional information about the neurocognitive profile of this rare disease. There are several similarities and differences between the two studies, however, that must be noted. Both cases were diagnosed late, although Walsh and colleagues' case study did not lapse into coma. Both children evidenced cerebral abnormalities on imaging. The current study differs given the implementation of a relatively new treatment approach of a liver transplant. The child presented in this chapter no longer required the traditional MSUD-specific leucine-limiting diet unlike the earlier case study.

Comparison of the neurocognitive profile revealed the generally noted weaker visual-perceptual abilities and attention/executive function deficits, although the current study also revealed deficits in auditory semantic (prose) memory and academic achievement in select areas (i.e., reading and fluency tasks). Both cases required special education services. This is consistent with the available although limited research findings on MSUD.

Although MSUD is a rare disease, the recent treatment advance of liver transplant and the limited understanding of the effects of the disease on neurocognitive abilities indicate further research is necessary to understand and provide appropriate interventions. In the future, using a pre- and postevaluation approach for children who undergo transplantation will be useful.

Research that incorporates more than an "*n* of 1" and uses a well-designed neuropsychological battery is also needed.

References

Brismar, J., Aqeel, A., Brismar, G., Coates, R., Gascon, G., & Ozand, P. (1990). Maple syrup urine disease: Findings on CT and MR scans of the brain in 10 infants. *American Journal of Neuroradiology, 11,* 1219–1228.

Chuang, D. T., & Shih, V. E. (2001). Maple syrup urine disease (branched-chain ketoaciduria). In C. R. Scriver, A. L. Beaudet, & D. Valle (Eds.), *The metabolic and molecular basis of inherited diseases* (8th ed.). New York: McGraw-Hill.

Enns, G. M., Cowan, T. M., Klein, O., & Packman, S. (2006). Aminoacidemias and organic acidemias. In K. F. Swaiman, S. Ashwal, & D. M. Ferriero (Eds.), *Pediatric neurology: Principles and practice* (4th ed.). Philadelphia: Mosby-Elsevier.

Hilliges, C., Awiszus, D. & Wendel, U. (1993). Intellectual performance of children with maple syrup urine disease. *European Journal of Pediatrics, 152,* 144–147.

Kaplan, P., Mazur, A., Field, M., Berlin, J. A., Berry, G. T., Heidenreich, R., Yudkoff, M., & Segal, S. (1991). Intellectual outcome in children with maple syrup urine disease. *Journal of Pediatrics, 119,* 46–50.

Marshall, L., & DiGeorge, A. (1981). Maple syrup urine disease in the Old Order Mennonites. *American Journal of Genetics Supplement, 33,* 139A.

Menkes, J. H., Hurst, P. L., & Craig, J. M. (1954). A new syndrome: Progressive familial infantile cerebral dysfunction associated with an unusual urinary substance. *Pediatrics, 14,* 462.

Riviello, J. J., Rezvani, I., DiGeorge, A. M., & Foley, C. M. (1991). Cerebral edema causing death in children with maple syrup urine disease. *Journal of Pediatrics, 119,* 42–45.

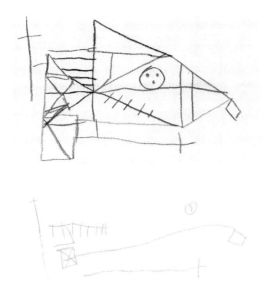

Figure 2-1. (*Top*) Rey-Osterrieth Complex Figure copy condition. (*Bottom*) Rey-Osterrieth Complex Figure delay condition.

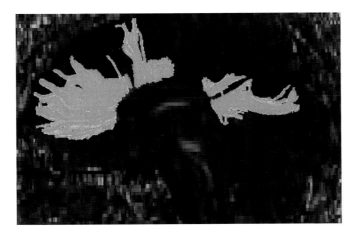

Figure 8-2. Diffusion tensor imaging tractography displaying absent or dysmorphic body and splenium of the corpus callosum.

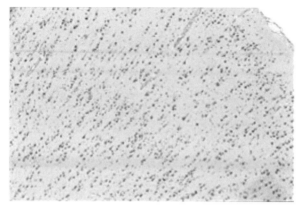

Figure 11-1. Photomicrograph showing fetal-like cortical columnar architecture consistent with focal cortical dysplasia Type IA, as well as heterotopic neurons in the white matter. Hematoxylin and eosin stain; original magnification, 100×.

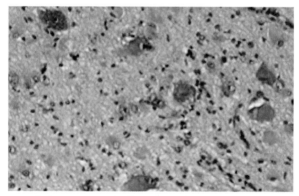

Figure 11-2. Photomicrograph demonstrating balloon cells of the Taylor-type dysplasia (focal cortical dysplasia Type IIB). Hematoxylin and eosin stain; original magnification, 200×.

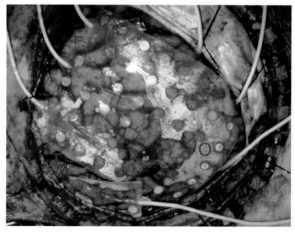

Figure 11-7. Intraoperative view of the left hemisphere and grid. F, frontal lobe; O, occipital lobe; T, temporal lobe.

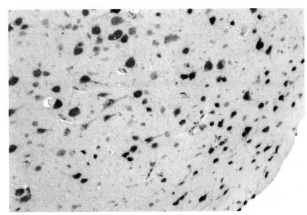

Figure 11-8. Focal cortical dysplasia of left anterior inferior occipital lobe. The cortical architecture is neither columnar as in the fetus nor laminar as in mature brain, but rather neurons of various sizes are arranged and oriented haphazardly.

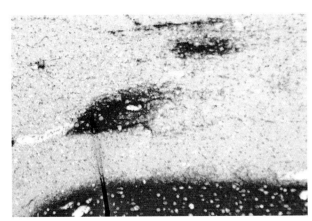

Figure 11-9. Synaptic vesicle reactivity is strong in the deep layers of cortex but not in the white matter beneath the cortex. There are several clusters of heterotopic neurons in the white matter with strong synaptic reactivity within these nodules. Synaptophysin; magnification, 100×.

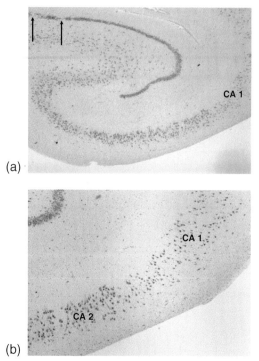

Figure 11-10. Transverse section of left hippocampus. (*a*) Focal zones of neuronal loss are seen at low magnification in the dentate gyrus (arrows) and in the CA1 sector of Ammon horn (magnification, 40×). (*b*) Higher magnification shows that the CA2 sector is well preserved with a normal compliment of neurons, but the CA1 sector has a reduced number of neurons (magnification, 100×). NeuN, neuronal nuclear antigen.

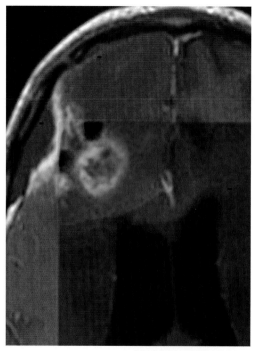

Figure 37-2. A positron emission tomography scan obtained after two resections demonstrating hypometabolism in the right frontal lobe indicative of recurrent glioblastoma multiforme.

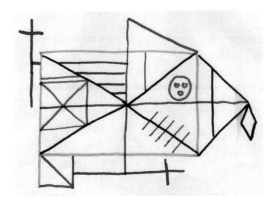

Figure 45-3. Copy of the Rey-Osterrieth Figure, 1999.

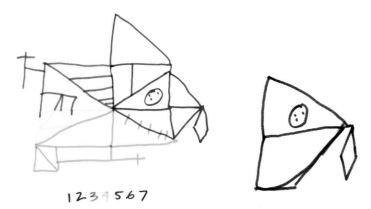

Figure 46-2. S. J.'s Rey-Osterreith Complex Figure copy (*left*) and delayed recall (*right*). Note the very piecemeal and poorly planned/organized approach for his age, which later appears to influence his recall ability.

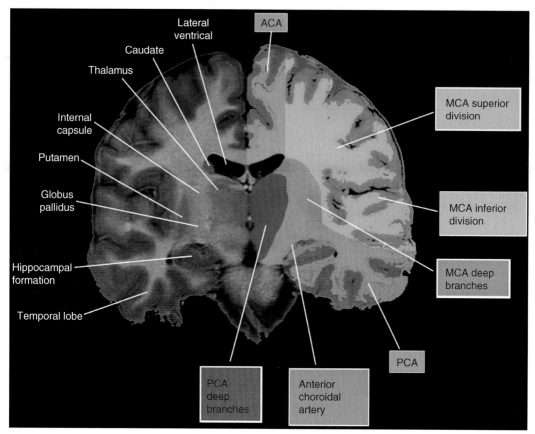

Figure 58-1. Coronal image through the midsection of the thalamus showing different major brain structures and the distribution of the three main cerebral arteries: anterior cerebral artery, blue; middle cerebral artery, mustard yellow; posterior cerebral artery, red-flesh tone. Note the extensiveness of the distribution of the middle cerebral artery, which covers a larger territory than any other cerebral artery.

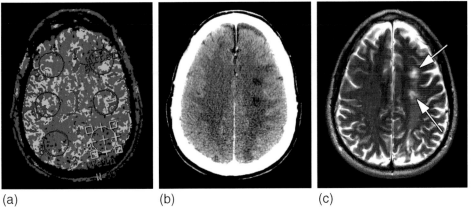

Figure 58-3. All scans are in radiological perspective where the left is on the viewer's right, with the computed tomography (CT) being done 2 days post symptom onset and the magnetic resonance imaging 1 year post stroke. (*a*) Perfusion CT showing subtle asymmetry of blood flow, consistent with ischemia in the left the middle cerebral artery (MCA). (*d*) CT scan showing focal areas of ischemia (dark regions) and reduced density within the white matter of the left hemisphere (note the central white matter of the left hemisphere is darker, reflecting less density). (*c*) T2-weighted focal left hemisphere signal abnormalities (arrows) reflective of old ischemic changes associated with the history of left MCA infarction. Notice the subtle signal differences throughout the entirety of the central white matter of the left hemisphere. Also note that the areas of chronic infarction in the left hemisphere match very closely with the acute areas of infarction.

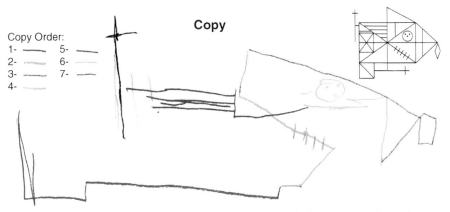

Figure 60-2. Patient's copy of the Rey-Osterreith Complex Figure with the target stimulus in the top right corner.

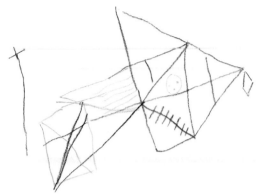

Figure 61-1. Rey-Osterreith Complex Figure copy drawing.

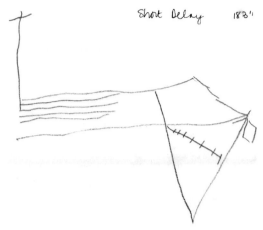

Figure 61-2. Rey-Osterreith Complex Figure 3-minute delay drawing.

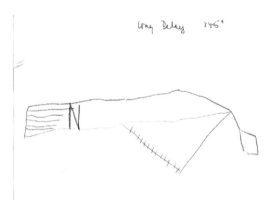

Figure 61-3. Rey-Osterreith Complex Figure 30-minute delay drawing.

Strauss, K. A., Mazariegos, G. V., Sindhi, R., Squires, R., Finegold, D. N., Vockley, G., Robinson, D. L., Hendrickson, C., Virji, M., Cropcho, L., Puffenberger, E. G., McGhee, W., Seward, L. M., & Morton, D. H. (2006). Elective liver transplantation for the treatment of classical maple syrup urine disease. *American Journal of Transplantation*, 6, 557–564.

Walsh, K., & Scott, M. (2010). Neurocognitive profile in a case of maple syrup urine disease. *The Clinical Neuropsychologist*, 24, 689–700.

Part II

Traumatic and Accidental

Traumatic and accidental brain injuries are the leading cause of disability in children and adolescents, and the leading cause of disability in working-age adults. Although not entirely randomly distributed throughout the population, brain injuries can occur at any point in the life span. Thus, these injuries have been major clinical and research topics for neuropsychologists. In particular, the effects of trauma or accidents on the developing brain pose unique considerations for the neuropsychologist. The eight chapters in this section span the range of development from childhood through adulthood. In addition to looking at diagnostic issues, several of these chapters also examine related topics such as recovery and the potential for symptom exaggeration following unequivocal traumatic brain injury.

14

Pediatric Mild Traumatic Brain Injury: All Cases Are Not Complicated Equally

Michael W. Kirkwood

In the United States, pediatric traumatic brain injury (TBI) has an estimated annual incidence of 180 cases per 100,000 and accounts for nearly half a million hospital visits each year (Kraus, 1995; Langlois, Rutland-Brown, & Thomas, 2006). Traumatic brain injury is conventionally graded on a severity continuum ranging from mild to severe. Injuries on the more severe end of this continuum have been well demonstrated to cause significant morbidity and mortality. Mild TBI has historically received less scientific investigation in children, despite the fact that mild injury accounts for at least 80% to 90% of all TBI cases, is clearly significant from a public health perspective, and is a frequent reason for neuropsychological referral.

Following mild TBI, nonhuman animal research indicates that the brain responds with a multilayered metabolic response (Giza & Hovda, 2001). This physiologic disruption can include unchecked ionic shifts, abrupt neuronal depolarization, widespread release of excitatory neurotransmitters, alteration in glucose metabolism, reduced cerebral blood flow, and disturbed axonal function. The pathophysiological effects of mild TBI most often result in temporary cellular and neural system dysfunction, rather than permanent cell damage or destruction (Iverson, Lange, Gaetz, & Zasler, 2007). Thus, dynamic restoration over time typically occurs as the system re-regulates. Of course, as injury at the cellular level becomes more severe, the expectation for slow or incomplete recovery or cell death increases. A number of newer biochemical, electrophysiological, and neuroimaging techniques have potential for characterizing the pathological effects, although none has yet accumulated sufficient evidence to warrant routine clinical deployment. Computed tomography (CT) remains the predominant technology used in acute clinical care because of its ability to readily identify surgically significant lesions. Approximately 5% of individuals presenting to hospital settings with a Glasgow Coma Scale (GCS) score of 15 have intracranial abnormalities identified by CT scan, with percentages considerably higher if the GCS score is 13 or 14, or magnetic resonance imaging (MRI) is utilized (Borg et al., 2004).

Loss of consciousness has traditionally been considered the cardinal sign of mild TBI. However, sport-related concussion data have clearly indicated that many cases of mild TBI do not involve a witnessed period of unresponsiveness. Other acute signs and symptoms of mild TBI include headache, dizziness, confusion, visual disturbance, mental slowing, amnesia, and emesis. With or without a period of unconsciousness, in the first days and weeks after injury, a constellation of neurobehavioral changes can be seen in children, not unlike those apparent in adult populations. These changes are often referred to as "postconcussive symptoms" and can involve a combination of somatic, cognitive, and emotional/behavioral difficulties. Frequently reported subjective symptoms include headache, dizziness, fatigue, sensitivity to light and noise, difficulty concentrating, trouble remembering, and increased anxiety.

The expected duration of postconcussive problems after mild TBI is a topic of considerable scientific controversy. Most methodologically rigorous studies with children indicate that by 2 to 3 months post injury, and oftentimes much sooner, deficits are not apparent when measured by standardized performance-based neurocognitive or academic tests (Carroll et al., 2004; Satz et al., 1997). Fewer pediatric studies have systematically examined outcomes using subjective postconcussive symptom reports from parents or children, though available data suggest that a minority of pediatric patients may display more persistent problems than might be expected if examining test-based results alone (Yeates & Taylor, 2005). Understanding the nature of subjective postconcussive symptoms is confounded by the fact that the symptoms are nonspecific and may reflect premorbid problems, postinjury difficulties unrelated to the trauma, the emotional or physical effects of trauma more generally, or particular fears and expectations associated with cerebral injury. Accurate estimates of lingering postconcussive symptomatology will require additional research that focuses on the relative risk of persistent change following mild TBI in comparison to non–head injury control groups, while accounting for baseline levels of symptomatology and a variety of other noninjury factors.

Research has yet to precisely establish which variables are most important in predicting individual recovery and presentation following pediatric mild TBI. Extant literature suggests that both noninjury and injury variables likely play a role. Noninjury factors that may be influential include age at injury, history of previous concussions, family expectations and functioning, motivation to improve, existence of comorbid conditions such as postinjury stress or pain, and type of postinjury management. Injury-related influences have primarily focused on injury severity. The presence of intracranial abnormalities on conventional neuroimaging has been identified as one marker of severity that negatively affects neurobehavioral outcome. In adult populations, a number of studies have found that visible intracranial pathology after mild TBI increases the risk for select neuropsychological problems during the initial months post injury, as well as for more persistent functional difficulties

(Iverson, 2006; Kashluba, Hanks, Casey, & Millis, 2008). These injuries are now thought to be similar to moderate TBI in their functional outcomes and are generally classified as such or referred to as "complicated mild TBI." Distinguishing between complicated and uncomplicated mild TBI has received less attention in pediatric populations, though initial work supports this intuitively sensible distinction (Levin et al., 2008).

The Case of D. M.

At the time of neuropsychological contact, D. M. was a 14-year-old Caucasian male who had recently been involved in a motor vehicle crash. The primary care physician referred D. M. to a pediatric concussion program for neuropsychological assessment because of parental concerns about lingering postconcussive symptomatology and school problems. He was seen for an abbreviated neuropsychological assessment to assist with medical and educational management. D. M. and his mother participated in the evaluation session. D. M. and both of his parents attended a feedback session. The evaluation was conducted for clinical purposes, with the family disclosing no current or intended legal action relevant to the case.

When D. M. was seen, his parents were in the process of divorcing. They had been separated for about 6 months. The parents described their relationship as reasonably amicable, but the family situation as a whole was stressful. Since the separation, D. M. and his younger sister lived primarily with their mother but also maintained regular contact with their father. Both parents were high school educated. D. M.'s mother was an administrative assistant at a school, and his father worked as a construction foreman. Familial-genetic history was said to be unremarkable for learning and psychiatric problems. Maternal migraines were reported. D. M.'s birth and early developmental history were unremarkable. Educationally, D. M. had never repeated a grade or received any special education services. He did not display any developmental learning or attention problems, although he was described as never being particularly interested in academics. D. M. was in ninth grade at a public high school, historically earning academic marks in the B to

C range. From a psychosocial perspective, he was said to be a sensitive and shy youngster who had always been fairly well adjusted and well behaved. D. M.'s parents had observed increased stress and sadness in D. M. since their separation. He had not participated in any behavioral health services. Socially, he had a small but solid group of friends and was liked by both peers and adults. Extracurricular activities included skateboarding and snowboarding. He was not involved in any team-based sports or other activities that would be considered high risk for concussion.

Medical history was unremarkable until a month prior to the neuropsychological contact, when D. M. was traveling as a belted rear seat passenger in a vehicle driven by a friend. Their slow-moving vehicle was struck by another vehicle traveling about 30 mph, causing air bag deployment and substantial damage to the rear of the vehicle. D. M. was thought to have hit his head on the back of the front seat, though this was not known definitively. He did not lose consciousness. At the scene, he reportedly appeared dazed but was talking and ambulating independently. D. M. reported no memory for the crash itself or for the few minutes before. He described his memory as "fuzzy" for about 15 minutes after the crash. He recalled only a few isolated events about the accident scene and ambulance transport to a local hospital but had continuous memories thereafter. Upon evaluation at the hospital about 45 minutes after the crash, medical records indicated that D. M. was alert, oriented, and in no acute distress. His GCS score was 15. Neurological examination was unremarkable. No neuroimaging was conducted. A few abrasions on the upper extremities were documented. D. M. was also noted to be complaining of a headache and nausea. He was discharged after several hours of monitoring and told to follow-up with his primary physician.

Over the next couple of days (a weekend), D. M. took it easy in the home environment. He reported experiencing headache, fatigue, nausea, and mild dizziness. By parent report, he also seemed "out of it." He went to see his primary care physician a few days after injury. Neurological examination remained unremarkable, and postconcussive symptomatology continued to be documented. He missed 1 day of school and then resumed a normal academic schedule. During the next several weeks, he displayed more difficulty managing educational demands. He had trouble keeping up with the workload, remembering information, and paying attention in class and during completion of homework. His grades began to drop, primarily because of multiple missed assignments. No special support or accommodations had been provided in the school setting.

During a structured postconcussive symptom interview at the time of the neuropsychological contact, D. M. reported that he no longer experienced any dizziness or nausea, although daily headaches were still endorsed. He was also reporting fatigue, trouble with concentration and memory, and feeling slower than normal. His parents were also reporting that D. M.'s personality continued to seem different than before the crash, including that he was more lethargic and less affectively expressive. D. M. had not yet participated in any physical activities that would have increased his concussion risk, but he was expressing a strong desire to snowboard during the upcoming winter sport season.

Observational Data

D. M. presented as a likable young man with blunted affect. He displayed no overt dysmorphology. He was cooperative throughout the evaluation session. No concerns were apparent about his motivation to perform well. He was oriented in all spheres. He displayed occasional lapses in attention and needed several examiner-provided prompts to reengage with the task at hand. Response style was generally systematic, though lack of attention to detail was occasionally noted. Informal conversation was easily elicited. Comprehension was judged intact during conversation, as were form and content of language expression. Speech was well articulated and intelligible. D. M. demonstrated a satisfactory appreciation of paralinguistic features such as gesture, intonation, and facial expression. There were no reported or observed difficulties with basic visual-perceptual processes such as the appreciation of visual fields, gaze patterns, or face/object recognition. D. M. used his preferred right hand for writing and drawing, employing a dynamic tripod grasp.

Test Results and Child Interview

D. M. was administered a focused neuropsychological test battery, consistent with the tiered mild TBI management model outlined by Kirkwood et al. (2008) linking service expenditure to time post injury. The battery was designed to tap areas potentially sensitive to the effects of TBI (e.g., attention, speed) but also those expected to be less sensitive (e.g., single word reading). Though most individuals recover fairly quickly after a mild TBI, the abbreviated neuropsychological evaluation was thought to be justifiable and cost effective, because it would help to identify reasons for D. M.'s lingering problems, assist in the creation of an appropriate clinical management plan, and reduce the risk of prolonged distress and secondary psychosocial problems.

Green's Medical Symptom Validity Test was administered to help evaluate motivation to perform well. No concerns were apparent. D. M. earned perfect scores on the three primary effort indices.

On the two-subtest Wechsler Abbreviated Scale of Intelligence, D. M.'s performance fell in the Average range, with an estimated overall IQ of 95, around the 35th percentile. His Vocabulary subtest T-score was 50, and his Matrix Reasoning subtest T-score was 44. Of note, response style on Matrix Reasoning appeared to reflect occasional inattention to detail. Single-word reading on the Woodcock-Johnson III Letter-Word Identification subtest was average (SS = 97).

The California Verbal Learning Test–Children's Version was administered to evaluate verbal learning and memory. Performance was within normal limits. D. M. earned a Total Trials T-score of 55, with adequate learning slope. List A Short-Delay Free Recall z-score was 0.0 and Long-Delay Free recall was 0.5. Recognition Discriminability z-score was 0.5.

Selected subtests from the Test of Everyday Attention for Children (TEA-Ch), Wechsler Intelligence Scale for Children–Fourth Edition (WISC-IV), and Delis-Kaplan Executive Function System (D-KEFS) were administered to evaluate attention, processing speed, and basic executive functioning. On the TEA-Ch, performance on the Sky Search subtest was average, whereas sustained attention problems were identified on the Code Transmission subtest (ss = 6).

Performance on the WISC-IV Digit Span subtest was average. Performance on the WISC-IV Coding subtest fell in the Low Average range (ss = 7), suggesting modestly decreased processing speed. Performance on the D-KEFS subtests was average, including on the Trail Making Test, Color-Word Interference, and Letter Fluency. D. M.'s mother also rated his executive functioning in everyday settings using the Behavior Rating Inventory of Executive Function; Working Memory was the only significantly elevated subscale.

Fine-motor speed and dexterity were reduced bilaterally on the Grooved Pegboard, with a right-sided z-score of –1.65 and a left-sided z-score of –1.89.

During a brief clinical interview with D. M., he reported loving relationships with his parents. He described some typical disagreements with his younger sister but also said that they had grown a bit closer recently as they both were dealing with the effects of their parents' separation. Socially, he stated that he was comfortable with his peer relationships. Emotionally, he initially reported that his mood was "okay." However, when questioned further, he became teary eyed and acknowledged that he had been feeling sad about his parents' separation over the last few months. Since his injury, he also described feeling particularly stressed and overwhelmed at school and that he might as well just "give up." No suicidal ideation or intent was endorsed. Posttraumatic stress symptomatology was denied.

To help assess his current behavioral/emotional adjustment further, D. M. completed the Children's Depression Inventory, which revealed a moderate level of depressive symptomatology overall (T = 62). His mother completed the Behavior Assessment System for Children–Second Edition; no scales were significantly elevated.

Case Discussion

When evaluating youth suspected of having sustained a mild TBI, one of the first considerations needs to be establishing that a mild TBI actually occurred. Evidence of sufficient biomechanical force applied to the head and neurologic disturbance apparent soon after are typically used to define such injury. In D. M.'s case, he experienced significant acceleration-deceleration forces in

Table 14-1. Test Scores from D. M.'s Abbreviated Neuropsychological Battery

Test	Standardized Score	Performance Description
Green's Medical Symptom Validity Test		
Immediate Recall	100%	Pass
Delayed Recall	100%	Pass
Consistency	100%	Pass
Wechsler Abbreviated Scale of Intelligence		
Estimated 2-subtest IQ	SS = 95	Average
Vocabulary	T = 50	Average
Matrix Reasoning	T = 44	Average
Woodcock-Johnson III Tests of Achievement		
Letter-Word Identification	SS = 97	Average
California Verbal Learning Test – Children's Version		
Total Trials 1-5	T = 54	Average
Short-Delay Free Recall	z = 0.0	Average
Long-Delay Free Recall	z = 0.5	Average
Recognition Discriminability	z = 0.5	Average
Wechsler Intelligence Scale for Children–Fourth Edition		
Digit Span	SS = 11	Average
Coding	SS = 7	Low average
Test of Everyday Attention for Children		
Sky Search Attention score	SS = 8	Average
Code Transmission	SS = 6	Below average
Delis-Kaplan Executive Function System		
Trail Making Visual Scanning	SS = 9	Average
Trail Making Number Sequencing	SS = 11	Average
Trail Making Letter Sequencing	SS = 13	High average
Trail Making Switching	SS = 10	Average
Letter Fluency	SS = 11	Average
Color-Word Color Naming	SS = 10	Average
Color-Word Word	SS = 11	Average
Color-Word Interference	SS = 9	Average
Grooved Pegboard		
Right (preferred)	z = −1.65	Below average
Left	z = −1.89	Below average

the motor vehicle crash and displayed a number of acute injury characteristics suggestive of neurologic insult.

At the time of the neuropsychological contact 1 month post injury, D. M. and his parents were still reporting that he was experiencing daily headaches, attention and memory problems, and personality changes. The results of the abbreviated neuropsychological test battery revealed average overall cognitive ability and commensurate single-word reading, consistent with his unexceptional preinjury academic history. Performance on tests of verbal memory and basic executive

functions were secure as well. Within this context, the neuropsychological profile highlighted problems with response speed and aspects of attention (e.g., sustained attention, working memory). Since the injury, a decline in school functioning was also reported. Psychiatrically, moderate depressive symptomatology was apparent.

Compared with other youth who sustain mild TBI, D. M.'s presentation was similar in some respects but different in others. Immediately after the motor vehicle crash, he displayed several of the most common acute injury characteristics, including appearing dazed and experiencing a headache and memory disturbance. Though some might view the fact that he did not lose consciousness as unusual, the majority of people who sustain mild TBI are likely to display an alteration in consciousness not unlike D. M. rather than a frank period of witnessed unresponsiveness. In the initial days and weeks after injury, D. M. also displayed some classic postinjury symptoms such as headache, fatigue, and attention and memory complaints. However, he also displayed affective blunting and lethargy, which are much less characteristic of mild TBI and more often seen after severe injury. Moreover, in contrast to many other mild TBI patients who display a resolving symptom course over the initial postinjury days and weeks, D. M. continued to display fairly persistent and significant symptomatology (e.g., daily headaches) when seen for neuropsychological evaluation 1 month post injury. On testing, he was also found to have attention problems and response slowing. D. M. additionally displayed moderate depressive symptomatology, likely at least in part attributable to feelings related to his parents' separation several months prior to his injury and increased difficulty managing school demands since his injury.

The neuropsychological impressions and concerns were shared with primary medical personnel, and a brain MRI was ordered 1 month post injury. The imaging documented several nonspecific punctate T2-weighted hyperintensities in the bilateral frontal subcortical white matter, which were thought to represent nonhemorrhagic shear injury. In D. M.'s case, common indices used to determine injury severity, including the GCS score and duration of posttraumatic amnesia, indicated that his injury would be conventionally graded as a mild TBI. Yet he displayed intracranial pathology on neuroimaging. As such, D. M.'s injury was more involved than many mild TBI cases and would generally be referred to as a "complicated mild TBI," as discussed earlier in the introduction section. The prognostic significance of complicated mild TBI in children is not entirely established empirically, but multiple adult studies and initial pediatric work suggest that D. M. would be at increased risk for both educational and psychosocial difficulties.

Recommendations for D. M. included a number of medical follow-up considerations and suggestions to improve his functioning at home and at school. Medically, it was recommended that D. M. consult with a physician with particular expertise in TBI, to help address his ongoing posttraumatic headaches. If pharmacological intervention was deemed medically warranted, it was thought that a medication that could potentially benefit both headache pain and mood (e.g., the antidepressant Amitriptyline) might be worth an initial trial. If D. M.'s attentional problems persisted, it was also recommended that the physician team consider the benefits of a stimulant medication trial. Another recommendation was to consult with the medical specialists about the safety and sensibility of allowing D. M. to pursue his desire to snowboard in the months ahead. Research does not provide an evidenced-based answer as to exactly how long a youth should be restricted from sports after a mild TBI, but most consensus guidelines would recommend a restriction from high-risk activities at least until the individual is asymptomatic and neuroimaging and neurological examinations are unremarkable (Kirkwood, Yeates, & Wilson, 2006).

To help address the difficulties D. M. was having at school, additional support through a formalized Section 504 Plan was recommended. A primary point person was identified (i.e., counselor), who was to provide assistance in carefully monitoring D. M.'s academic and socioemotional progress during the upcoming months and in ensuring that appropriate accommodations were implemented by classroom teachers. The counselor was also to provide some general organizational support, to help D. M. make up missing work and stay on track when managing future assignments and preparing for tests. His teachers agreed to waive noncritical missing assignments that were completed in the weeks after his injury.

D. M.'s school schedule was also rearranged so that he could finish earlier in the day and have some downtime at home before he was expected to complete any homework. In terms of workload over the next few months, it was recommended that D. M., his parents, counselor, and teachers develop an individualized plan whereby he would be expected to complete enough of the work to continue to progress with his peers and allow him to demonstrate an understanding of the underlying principles or skills that would be covered, but not so much that he would become overwhelmed or overly frustrated. More flexibility with regard to assignment due dates and scheduling tests was also recommended.

Within the classroom setting, D. M. was encouraged to sit in a position toward the front of the room, where he would be more engaged with activities and where his teachers could keep a closer eye on him to ensure that he was remaining focused and on task. For tests, extra time was recommended, as was allowing him to take tests in the resource room, which was reportedly quieter and less distracting than the classroom setting. As needed, D. M. was also to be allowed to take short breaks from classroom activities if he became fatigued or developed a headache during class time.

To help address D. M.'s psychosocial needs, he and his parents were provided with general education around the effects of TBI. The cognitive difficulties and personality changes that had been observed since his injury were explained to be not unexpected after the type of injury he sustained, though a return to his baseline level with additional recovery time was said to be a realistic hope as well. A neuropsychological follow-up evaluation in 6 to 12 months was recommended to help document D. M.'s recovery and update the management plan. To directly address D. M.'s current mood, psychological services were strongly recommended. Further evaluation of his reported depressive symptomatology was considered important, as was support in adjusting to the effects of the TBI and the school and family stressors he had been facing.

Conclusion

Few neurologic disorders have engendered as much historical controversy as mild TBI. Though select topics continue to be debated, scientific opinion has begun to converge in recent years. Rigorous research has mostly confirmed that the effects of a single uncomplicated mild TBI are likely to be self-limiting and fairly benign for the majority of school-aged children. At the same time, neurobehavioral outcomes of pediatric mild TBI are apt to be more complex than assumed historically. Because mild TBI is by definition a condition with both neurological and psychological features, neuropsychologists,

who are dually trained in the neurological principles of brain injury and the psychological principles of emotion and behavior, are uniquely positioned to play an important role in its clinical management. As the case of D. M. illustrates, optimal management of pediatric mild TBI requires a sophisticated biopsychosocial conceptualization, because both injury and non-injury-related factors are apt to contribute to a child's postinjury presentation. Clearly, when functional problems or lingering difficulties are apparent after a mild TBI, neuropsychological assessment can help to ensure all relevant domains have been evaluated and appropriate follow-up and intervention have been implemented.

References

Borg, J., Holm, L., Cassidy, J. D., Peloso, P. M., Carroll, L. J., von Holst, H., et al. (2004). Diagnostic procedures in mild traumatic brain injury: Results of the WHO Collaborating Centre Task Force on Mild Traumatic Brain Injury. *Journal of Rehabilitation Medicine, 36*(Suppl. 43), 61–75.

Carroll, L. J., Cassidy, J. D., Peloso, P. M., Borg, J., von Holst, H., Holm, L., et al. (2004). Prognosis for mild traumatic brain injury: Results of the WHO Collaborating Centre Task Force on Mild Traumatic Brain Injury. *Journal of Rehabilitation Medicine, 36*(Suppl. 43), 84–105.

Giza, C. C., & Hovda, D. A. (2001). The neurometabolic cascade of concussion. *Journal of Athletic Training, 36*(3), 228–235.

Iverson, G. L. (2006). Complicated vs uncomplicated mild traumatic brain injury: Acute neuropsychological outcome. *Brain Injury, 20*(13–14), 1335–1344.

Iverson, G. L., Lange, R. T., Gaetz, M., & Zasler, N. D. (2007). Mild TBI. In N. D. Zasler, D. I. Katz, & R. D. Zafonte (Eds.), *Brain injury medicine* (pp. 333–371). New York: Demos.

Kashluba, S., Hanks, R. A., Casey, J. E., & Millis, S. R. (2008). Neuropsychologic and functional outcome after complicated mild traumatic brain injury. *Archives of Physical Medicine and Rehabilitation, 89*(5), 904–911.

Kirkwood, M. W., Yeates, K. O., Taylor, H. G., Randolph, C., McCrea, M., & Anderson, V. A. (2008). Management of pediatric mild traumatic brain injury: A neuropsychological review from injury through recovery. *Clinical Neuropsychology, 22*(5), 769–800.

Kirkwood, M. W., Yeates, K. O., & Wilson, P. E. (2006). Pediatric sport-related concussion: A review of the

clinical management of an oft-neglected population. *Pediatrics, 117*(4), 1359–1371.

Kraus, J. F. (1995). Epidemiological features of brain
injury in children: Occurrence, children at risk,
causes, and manner of injury, severity, and outcomes. In S. H. Broman & M. E. Michel (Eds.),
Traumatic head injury in children (pp. 22–39). New
York: Oxford University Press.

Langlois, J. A., Rutland-Brown, W., & Thomas, K. E.
(2006). *Traumatic brain injury in the United States:
Emergency department visits, hospitalizations, and
deaths.* Atlanta, GA: Centers for Disease Control
and Prevention, National Center for Injury Prevention and Control.

Levin, H. S., Hanten, G., Roberson, G., Li, X., Ewing-
Cobbs, L., Dennis, M., et al. (2008). Prediction of
cognitive sequelae based on abnormal computed
tomography findings in children following mild
traumatic brain injury. *Journal of Neurosurgery:
Pediatrics, 1*(6), 461–470.

Satz, P., Zaucha, K., McCleary, C., Light, R., Asarnow,
R., & Becker, D. (1997). Mild head injury in children and adolescents: A review of studies (1970–
1995). *Psychological Bulletin, 122*(2), 107–131.

Yeates, K. O., & Taylor, H. G. (2005). Neurobehavioural outcomes of mild head injury in children and
adolescents. *Pediatric Rehabilitaton, 8*(1), 5–16.

15

Pediatric Traumatic Brain Injury: Effects of Questionable Effort

Jacobus Donders

Traumatic brain injury (TBI) occurs when there is an acute, external force to the skull with an associated alteration in level of consciousness and the potential to compromise the underlying brain matter. Although many cases of TBI can be prevented (e.g., by means of proper use of restraints or infant seats in automobiles), it remains one of the most common acquired neurological conditions in children, with incidence rates being relatively higher in boys, and predominant causes ranging from falls in young children to motor vehicle accidents in adolescents (Kraus, 1995; Rivara, 1994). The pathophysiology of TBI involves both primary or direct mechanisms, such as accelerating–decelerating or rotational forces that can lead to focal lesions or diffuse axonal stretching, and secondary or indirect mechanisms such as disruptions of intracranial pressure, cerebral perfusion, and cellular homeostasis that can result in ischemia, edema, and neuronal excitotoxicity (Hackbarth et al., 2002; Statler et al., 2001).

The most common classification of injury severity in pediatric TBI involves consideration of a combination of the duration of coma, which is typically defined as the length of time until the child reacts to verbal commands, and findings on neuroimaging. Children who do not have prolonged loss of consciousness and who do not have evidence for acute intracranial abnormalities on computed tomography (CT) or magnetic resonance imaging (MRI) can be classified as having mild TBI, and these account for more than 80% of all cases of pediatric TBI. Although they may be symptomatic for the first few weeks or months

after injury, the vast majority of children who incur an uncomplicated mild TBI in the absence of any premorbid confounding psychosocial history have unremarkable long-term neurobehavioral outcomes (Bijur & Haslum, 1995; Light et al., 1998; Satz et al., 1997).

The risk for long-term sequelae of TBI increases with prolonged coma and when there are intracranial lesions, particularly if those involve prefrontal regions and the associated subcortical white matter projections (Dennis, Guger, Roncadin, Barnes, & Schachar, 2001; Levin et al., 2004; Sera-Grabulosa et al., 2005). It is important to realize that there is no unique, invariant profile of neuropsychological test scores after pediatric TBI and also that some of the relatively more common sequelae are not specific to this condition. That being said, with the more severe forms of pediatric TBI, a number of neurobehavioral problems are known to be relatively common (see Donders, 2007 for a review). From a cognitive point of view, these include deficits in speed of information processing, attention, and novel learning, as well as the pragmatic and inferential aspects of communication. Emotional and behavioral sequelae often include affective instability and impaired social problem solving. A mix of cognitive and behavioral sequelae, such as can be seen in "secondary" attention-deficit/hyperactivity disorder (ADHD) that develops after severe TBI in children without such a premorbid history, has also been described (Max et al., 2004; Slomine et al., 2005).

The cognitive sequelae of severe TBI in children tend to show partial recovery within the first year after injury, with a subsequent relative plateau, but the behavioral and psychosocial residuals tend to persist longer and have less favorable recovery (Anderson, Morse, Catroppa, Haritou, & Rosenfeld, 2004; Taylor et al., 2002; Yeates et al., 2002). Outcomes are also moderated by a number of variables, including most prominently age and family environment. Severe TBI in early childhood interferes with vulnerable skills that are still in a stage of rapid development, and it is therefore associated with an increased risk for long-term deficits (Ewing-Cobbs, Prasad, Landry, Kramer, & DeLeon, 2004). In addition, increased levels of family stress or burden, and associated maladaptive coping and communication dynamics, are a significant risk factor for worse outcomes, particularly from a psychosocial point of view (Anderson et al., 2006; Kinsella, Ong, Murtagh, Prior, & Sawyer, 1999; Ponsford et al., 1999; Yeates et al., 2004). A number of studies have also suggested that the psychosocial consequences of severe pediatric TBI tend to persist in adulthood (Cattelani, Lombardi, Brianti, & Mazzuchi, 1998; Donders & Warschausky, 2007; Nybo, Sainio, & Müller, 2004).

There are clear, evidence-based guidelines for the acute care management of children with severe TBI, including transportation to a pediatric trauma center, aggressive treatment of any hypoxia or hypotension, and maintenance of adequate cerebral perfusion pressure (Adelson et al., 2003). Computed tomography is still the most appropriate technique to guide acute care interventions, but MRI is more appropriate in the subacute and long-term phases (see Bigler, 2007 for a review). There is modest support for the use of agents like methylphenidate and amantadine in the management of the longer term cognitive and behavioral sequelae of pediatric TBI (Beers, Skold, Dixon, & Adelson, 2005; Jin & Schachar, 2004). Recent randomized clinical trials have also provided encouraging findings with regard to the benefits of some forms of cognitive rehabilitation (Van't Hooft et al., 2005), Web-based family problem solving (Wade, Carey, & Wolfe, 2006), and use of parents as primary therapy providers (Braga, Da Paz Júnior, & Ylvisaker, 2005).

There is no standard set of neuropsychological tests that "must" be given to all children with pediatric TBI. However, given the aforementioned prevalence of deficits in attention, novel problem solving, processing speed, and other functions, it is important to examine those areas thoroughly. For example, measures of list verbal learning and speeded performance have considerable criterion validity in the assessment of children with TBI (for a review, see Donders, 2007). Consideration of premorbid school records is also important, especially in those children with prior complicating histories such as learning disability or depression (Donders & Strom, 2000). A number of recent studies have also suggested that it may be important to evaluate effort and motivation during pediatric neuropsychological evaluations (Constantinou & McCaffrey, 2003; Donders, 2005; Green & Flaro, 2003). The following case study is intended to illustrate all of these potentially important assessment considerations.

Case Presentation: John Doe

John Doe was 13 years old when he was referred for outpatient neuropsychological evaluation in late August, 2007. The referral question from the primary care physician pertained to his readiness to resume school. Review of available medical records revealed that John had been involved as the nonrestrained passenger in a motor vehicle accident approximately 4 months previously, about 3 weeks prior to completion of the seventh grade. He had sustained fractures of the left clavicle and right femur, as well as a TBI. Emergency room records indicated that his pupils reacted only sluggishly to light. An acute CT scan of the brain revealed a nondepressed right frontal skull fracture with underlying hemorrhagic contusion. There was an isolated brief seizure within the first 24 hours but none after that. He did not respond to verbal commands until about 36 hours after injury. After a 3-day stabilization in the pediatric intensive care unit, he was transferred to a rehabilitation wing, where he spent another 10 days before being discharged home.

By the time of his appointment for the neuropsychological evaluation, John had completed a course of outpatient physical therapy for his fractures. He was still seeing a speech pathologist once per week, to get help in getting caught up on school work that he had missed at the end of the preceding academic year. John was on no routine prescription medications. His mother accompanied him to the appointment (his father, a long-haul truck driver, was out of state at the time) and she provided informed consent for the assessment to proceed. Although John was visibly displeased with the need to come in for a whole day of tests, he did agree to participate. The mother brought with her a copy of his academic transcript, which showed grades mostly in the B–C range throughout the sixth and seventh grades, with his worst performance in Language Arts (two D grades). She also provided a copy of a psychoeducational evaluation that had been completed at the beginning of the sixth grade. At that time, there was a question whether John might qualify for special education services under the "Other Health Impairment" qualification because of the potential of ADHD in light of the fact that several teachers had concerns about lack of motivation as well as distractibility in class. Scores on measures of psychometric intelligence and academic achievement were consistently in the low-average to average range during that evaluation (see Table 15-1), and he was considered ineligible for special support services. His primary care physician had also decided that there was not sufficient justification for a trial of stimulant medication.

At the time of the neuropsychological evaluation in the summer for 2007, John denied that there was anything wrong with him as the result of his accident. He expressed resentment about the fact that his mother had not allowed him to

Table 15-1. Premorbid Psychological Test Scores

Variable	SS
WISC–IV	
Verbal Comprehension	93
Perceptual Reasoning	88
Working Memory	91
Processing Speed	94
Full Scale IQ	88
WIAT–II	
Word Reading	94
Reading Comprehension	88
Numerical Operations	90
Math Reasoning	89

SS, standard score ($M = 100$, $SD = 15$; higher scores reflect better performance); WIAT–II, Wechsler Individual Achievement Test–Second Edition; WISC–IV, Wechsler Intelligence Scale for Children–Fourth Edition.

sign up for football in the fall, but he did not endorse any other emotional or physical distress. He also stated that he did not want to be placed in any "retard classes," which is how he referenced any special education services. His mother expressed concern about what she perceived to be increased difficulties with staying on task (e.g., to do his chores) as well as somewhat more frequent irritability, although she considered the latter to be manageable within the home. She described his early developmental history as entirely unremarkable and did not endorse any other prior complicating neurological or psychiatric issues. She did mention that John had an older brother with type 1 diabetes, but family medical history was otherwise described as fairly benign. Both John and his mother denied any other recent, unrelated psychosocial stressors.

John presented for the neuropsychological evaluation in casual dress and with adequate grooming. He used corrective contact lenses but no other assistive devices. His affect was somewhat constricted in range but not entirely flat. He did not appear to have any difficulties understanding instructions or questions and although he tended to be terse in his answers, his speech was at all times fluent and coherent. He preferred his right hand for all tasks involving the manipulation of a pencil.

The first few tests that were administered to John yielded unusual findings (see Table 15-2). For example, his very poor performance on WIAT–II Word Reading stood in marked contrast to his premorbid ability, as documented in the psychoeducational evaluation from almost 2 years ago. This task measures an overlearned skill that is rarely affected to this degree by TBI in older children (Ewing-Cobbs, Barnes et al., 2004). In addition, he made an unusually large number of perseverations (i.e., hitting the response key multiple times in response to a single stimulus) on the CPT–II, in an apparent display of irritation with the task. This pattern is often seen in the context of a conduct problem (Fischer, Barkley, Smallish, & Fletcher, 2005). Finally, he clearly violated empirically established and cross-validated criteria for sufficient effort on the TOMM. Previous research has established that there is no statistically significant correlation between severity of TBI and performance on that test (Donders, 2005).

Table 15-2. First Set of Neuropsychological Test Results

Variable	Result
WIAT–II[*]	
Word Reading	73
CPT–II[†]	
Errors of omission	56
Errors of commission	79
Hit reaction time	41
Variability of reaction time	59
Perseverations	93
TOMM[‡]	
Trial 1 correct	35
Trial 2 correct	39
Retention trial correct	38

CPT–II, Conners' Continuous Performance Test–Second Edition; TOMM, Test of Memory Malingering; WIAT–II, Wechsler Individual Achievement Test–Second Edition.

[*]Standard score ($M = 100$, $SD = 15$; higher scores reflect better performance).

[†]T score ($M = 50$, $SD = 10$; higher scores reflect worse performance).

[‡]Raw score.

Following this set of initial test findings, John was gently confronted (in the presence of his mother) about their atypical nature. Specifically, he was told that the results were unusually poor and that they stood in stark contrast with his verbal assertion that there was nothing wrong with him. John then admitted that he had not done his best because he was angry about the need to have to take tests that he considered to be "for retards." He was then advised that he was essentially shooting himself in the foot—that by performing poorly, he would give his parents and school professionals more reason to place him in a categorical special education program. It was then agreed that he would be given an opportunity to start over, as long as he consistently put forth his best effort. He then completed the remainder of the evaluation, in the absence of any third persons, without further incident.

The second set of neuropsychological test results is presented in Table 15-3. These included an embedded measure of effort and motivation, the Reliable Digit Span index, which yielded a raw score of 8, which is in the valid range—even by standards originally developed for adults (for a review, see Babikian & Boone, 2007). In addition,

the CPT–II was repeated about halfway through the afternoon. At that time, his performance suggested considerable accuracy and consistency in his responses, which was considered important information, for two reasons: (1) it showed how much better John was able to do when he put forth good effort, and (2) the findings were not suggestive of a major deficit in sustained attention, which had been raised as a potential concern premorbidly. For these reasons, the second set of neuropsychological test results were considered to be valid.

The findings in Table 15-3 reflect potentially important information about the sequelae of John's TBI. Although his overall Full Scale IQ on the WISC–IV was not necessarily significantly different from its premorbid level, there was a marked decrease in his performance on the Processing Speed index, which has been shown to be selectively sensitive to the effects of TBI (Donders & Janke, 2008). In addition, John demonstrated selective sensori-motor impairment with the left hand on the Grooved Pegboard, which was consistent with the right anterior cerebral involvement on neuroimaging. Thus, there was tangible evidence for a compromise of his neuropsychological status as the result of his TBI.

These neuropsychological test results also provided important information about the circumstances under which John would likely function best when learning new things in school, and under what conditions he could be expected to run into difficulties. For example, the discrepancy between his adequate performance on the WCST–64 (including four categories completed) and his considerable difficulties on the TOL–Dx (including three time violations) suggested that John was able to engage in problem solving as long as the task was interactive with frequent informative feedback and immediate redirection, but that he was quite inefficient in planning ahead independently more than two or three steps. In addition, his performance across the subtests of the WRAML–II suggested that he was relatively less efficient with learning visual material opposed to verbally presented information. This difference may also have been augmented by the fact that on one of the visual subtests (Design Memory), the stimuli were presented for only a very brief (5 sec) period of time; John's deficit in speed of information processing may have

Table 15-3. Second Set of Neuropsychological Test Results

Variable	Result
WISC–IV*	
Verbal Comprehension	95
Perceptual Reasoning	84
Working Memory	88
Processing Speed	78
Full-Scale IQ	83
WIAT–II*	
Reading Comprehension	86
Numerical Operations	88
Trail-Making Test	
Seconds to completion, part A	17
Seconds to completion, part B	41
Grooved Pegboard Test	
Seconds to completion, right hand	70
Seconds to completion, left hand	84
CPT–II[†]	
Errors of omission	38
Errors of commission	49
Hit reaction time	61
Variability of reaction time	54
Perseverations	53
WRAML–II[‡]	
Story Memory	9
Design Memory	6
Verbal Learning	11
Picture Memory	7
WCST–64*	
Perseverative errors	109
Nonperseverative errors	102
TOL–Dx*	
Total moves	72
Total correct	78
Total problem solving time	62
YSR[†]	
Internalizing	35
Externalizing	36
CBC[†]	
Internalizing	51
Externalizing	61
BRIEF Self-Report[†]	
Behavioral Regulation	48
Metacognition	46
BRIEF Informant Report[†]	
Behavioral Regulation	62
Metacognition	58

*Standard score ($M = 100$, $SD = 15$; higher scores reflect better performance).

[†]T score ($M = 50$, $SD = 10$; higher scores reflect worse performance).

[‡]Scaled score ($M = 10$, $SD = 3$; higher scores reflect better performance).

BRIEF, Behavior Rating Inventory of Executive Function; CBC, Achenbach Child Behavior Checklist; CPT–II, Conners' Continuous Performance Test–Second Edition; TOL–Dx, Tower of London–Drexel Version; WCST–64, Wisconsin Card Sorting Test—64 Card Version; WIAT–II, Wechsler Individual Achievement Test–Second Edition; WISC–IV, Wechsler Intelligence Scale for Children–Fourth Edition; WRAML–II, Wide Range Assessment of Memory and Learning–Second Edition; YSR, Achenbach Youth Self-Report contributed to his poor performance. Another noteworthy finding was that he seemed to benefit greatly from the repeated practice of the items on one of the language-based subtests (Verbal Learning), whereas he was only given a one-time exposure to the information on the tasks involving visual materials.

Findings from standardized rating scales that were completed by, respectively, John and his mother about his day-to-day adjustment and functioning were also considered. As can be seen in Table 15-3, John did not endorse any significant problems on either the BRIEF or the YSR, possibly in an attempt at presenting himself in a favorable light. However, his mother described some mild difficulties with emotional reactivity on both the BRIEF and the CBC, although those did not rise to the level that they could be classified as clinically significant.

Because of the aforementioned pattern of neuropsychological test findings, it was possible to make some recommendations with regard to John's upcoming school re-entry. Given the quantitative evidence for compromise of his neurobehavioral abilities as a direct consequence of the injuries sustained in his car accident, an individual education plan for consideration of eligibility for special education support under the TBI qualification was requested. Keeping in mind his adversity to being placed in a categorical or departmentalized program, and also considering the fact that there were a variety of strengths identified in the findings, a combination of teacher consultant services and leaving the last hour open as a study hall (with access to individual assistance on an as-needed basis) was recommended. In light of John's apparent difficulties with independent novel learning and problem solving, in concert with his relatively preserved overlearned verbal skills, an interactive, step-by-step approach to learning new material, possibly with inclusion of a "think-aloud" approach along with more frequent review, was suggested.

Discussion

Children like John can be challenging for the pediatric neuropsychologist, for a number of reasons. First of all, there was a premorbid history about possible concerns about attention and motivation. It is well known that children with suspected ADHD may present with difficulties in novel learning and problem solving, in the absence of any acquired neurological injury. John's case illustrates the importance of reviewing all available records in this regard. The ability to identify a clear decrement in performance as compared to premorbid data was crucial in giving credence to the overall impression that despite whatever pre-existing limitations he may have had, this child had an additional compromise of his cognitive status as the direct consequence of his TBI. Of course, in the vast majority of cases that present in clinical practice, a premorbid WISC–IV is not going to be available. In those cases, it is still important to use an evidence-based approach to the data, such as relating the findings in a dose–response manner to what is known from the literature about the effect of TBI on specific cognitive functions and also what makes sense in terms of brain–behavior relationships (e.g., the selective impairment on the Grooved Pegboard in relation to the right frontal hemorrhagic contusion).

A second challenge that was evident in this case was the influence of effort and motivation. John was not enthused about the appointment and was not doing his best at first. If no attempt had been made to formally evaluate and address this test-taking behavior, the findings would likely have been invalidated or, even worse, they might have been misinterpreted as evidence for more severe cognitive problems than he really had. The latter possibility would likely have resulted in special education recommendations that might alienate him even further.

The final challenge was to integrate all the findings in a manner that led to specific, feasible recommendations for school support services. Just saying that a child has cognitive impairment as the result of brain damage, or where the lesion might be, is not necessarily helpful. Instead, the neuropsychologist should provide the reader with information he or she does not yet know from other sources, such as how the findings inform about the circumstances under which the child can be most successful. In this context, it behooves the neuropsychologist to be aware of federal and state special education criteria and procedures, and also to phrase the recommendations in a manner that is not only intelligible to the non-psychologist but also comes across as not overly prescriptive. For example, the decision about the eligibility for services and the specific nature thereof will be made by the school district in consultation with the parents, so it is typically better to "suggest consideration" of a range of possible solutions as opposed to demanding a narrow range of very specific arrangements.

In conclusion, children with severe TBI can present with a wide range of neurobehavioral problems that may lead to significant challenges to their parents and school teachers. The pediatric neuropsychologist can play an important role in providing improved understanding of the interplay between premorbid, injury-related, and reactive factors that all influence the presentation of the child. As this case illustrates, consideration of test-taking behavior and especially effort and motivation is an integral component of this process.

References

Adelson, P. D., Bratton, S. L., Carney, N. A., Chesnut, R. M., du Coudray, H. E. M., Goldstein, B., et al. (2003). Guidelines for the acute medical management of severe traumatic brain injury in infants, children, and adolescents. *Critical Care Medicine*, 31, 419–491.

Anderson, V. A., Catroppa, C., Dudgeon, P., Morse, S. A., Haritou, F., & Rosenfeld, J. V. (2006). Understanding prediction of functional recovery and outcome 30 months following early childhood head injury. *Neuropsychology*, 20, 42–57.

Anderson, V. A., Morse, S. A., Catroppa, C., Haritou, F., & Rosenfeld, J. V. (2004). Thirty month outcome from early childhood head injury: A prospective analysis of neurobehavioral recovery. *Brain*, 127, 2608–2620.

Babikian, T., & Boone, K. B. (2007). Intelligence tests as measures of effort. In K. B. Boone (Ed.), *Assessment of feigned cognitive impairment: A neuropsychological perspective* (pp. 103–127). New York: Guilford

Beers, S. R., Skold, A., Dixon, C. E., & Adelson, P. D. (2005). Neurobehavioral effects of Amantadine after pediatric traumatic brain injury: A preliminary report. *Journal of Head Trauma Rehabilitation*, 20, 450–463.

Bigler, E. D. (2007). Neuroimaging and its role in developing interventions. In S. J. Hunter & J. Donders (Eds.), *Pediatric neuropsychological intervention* (pp. 415–443). New York: Cambridge.

Bijur, P. E., & Haslum, M. (1995). Cognitive, behavioral, and motoric sequelae of mild head injury in a national birth cohort. In S. H. Brown & M. E. Michel (Eds.), *Traumatic head injury in children* (pp. 147–164). New York: Oxford.

Braga, L. W., Da Paz Júnior, A. C., & Ylvisaker, M. (2005). Direct clinician-delivered versus indirect family-supported rehabilitation of children with traumatic brain injury: A randomized controlled trial. *Brain Injury*, 19, 819–831.

Cattelani, R., Lombardi, F., Brianti, R., & Mazzucchi, A. (1998). Traumatic brain injury in childhood: Intellectual, behavioural and social outcome into adulthood. *Brain Injury*, 12, 183–296.

Constantinou, M., & McCaffrey, R. J. (2003). Using the TOMM for evaluating children's effort to perform optimally on neuropsychological measures. *Child Neuropsychology*, 9, 81–90.

Dennis, M., Guger, S., Roncadin, C., Barnes, M., & Schachar, R. (2001). Attentional-inhibitory control and social-behavioral regulation after childhood closed head injury: Do biological, developmental, and recovery variables predict outcome? *Journal of the International Neuropsychological Society*, 7, 683–692.

Donders, J. (2005). Performance on the Test of Memory Malingering in a mixed pediatric sample. *Child Neuropsychology*, 11, 221–227.

Donders, J. (2007). Traumatic brain injury. In S. J. Hunter & J. Donders (Eds.), *Pediatric neuropsychological intervention* (pp. 91–111). New York: Cambridge.

Donders, J., & Janke, K. (2008). Criterion validity of the WISC–IV after pediatric traumatic brain injury. *Journal of the International Neuropsychological Society*, 14, 651–655.

Donders, J., & Strom, D. (2000). Neurobehavioral recovery after pediatric head trauma: Injury, pre-injury, and post-injury issues. *Journal of Head Trauma Rehabilitation*, 15, 792–803.

Donders, J., & Warschausky, S. (2007). Neurobehavioral outcomes after early versus late childhood traumatic brain injury. *Journal of Head Trauma Rehabilitation*, 22, 296–302.

Ewing-Cobbs, L., Barnes, M., Fletcher, J. M., Levin, H. S., Swank, P. R., & Song, J. (2004). Modeling of longitudinal academic achievement scores after pediatric traumatic brain injury. *Developmental Neuropsychology*, 25, 107–133.

Ewing-Cobbs, L., Prasad, M. R., Landry, S. H., Kramer, L., & DeLeon, R. (2004). Executive functions following traumatic brain injury: A preliminary analysis. *Developmental Neuropsychology*, 26, 487–512.

Fischer, M., Barkley, R. A., Smallish, L., & Fletcher, K. (2005). Executive functioning in hyperactive children as young adults: Attention, inhibition, response perseveration, and the impact of comorbidity. *Developmental Neuropsychology*, 27, 107–133.

Green, P., & Flaro, L. (2003). Word Memory Test performance in children. *Child Neuropsychology*, 9, 189–207.

Hackbarth, R. M., Rzeszutko, K. M., Sturm, G., Donders, J., Kuldanek, A. S., & Sanfilippo, D. J. (2002). Survival and functional outcome in pediatric traumatic brain injury: A retrospective review and analysis of predictive factors. *Critical Care Medicine, 30*, 1630–1635.

Jin, C., & Schachar, R. (2004). Methylphenidate treatment of attention-deficit/hyperactivity disorder secondary to traumatic brain injury: A critical appraisal of treatment studies. *CNS Spectrums, 9*, 217–226.

Kinsella, G., Ong, B., Murtagh, D., Prior, M., & Sawyer, M. (1999). The role of the family for behavioral outcome in children and adolescents following traumatic brain injury. *Journal of Consulting and Clinical Psychology, 67*, 116–123.

Kraus, J. F. (1995). Epidemiological features of brain injury in children: Occurrence, children at risk, causes, and manner of injury, severity, and outcomes. In S. H. Broman & M. E. Michel (Eds.), *Traumatic head injury in children* (pp. 22–39). New York: Oxford.

Levin, H. S., Zhang, L., Dennis, M., Ewing-Cobbs, L., Schachar, R., Max, J., et al. (2004). Psychosocial outcome of TBI in children with unilateral frontal lesions. *Journal of the International Neuropsychological Society, 10*, 305–316.

Light, R., Asarnow, R., Satz, P., Zaucha, K., McCleary, C., & Lewis, R. (1998). Mild closed-head injury in children and adolescents: Behavior problems and academic outcomes. *Journal of Consulting and Clinical Psychology, 66*, 1023–1029.

Max, J. E., Lansing, A. E., Koele, S. L., Castillo, C. S., Bokura, H., Schachar, R., et al. (2004). Attention deficit hyperactivity disorder in children and adolescents following traumatic brain injury. *Developmental Neuropsychology, 25*, 159–177.

Nybo, T., Sainio, M., & Müller, K. (2004). Stability of vocational outcome in adulthood after moderate to severe preschool brain injury. *Journal of the International Neuropsychological Society, 10*, 719–723.

Ponsford, J., Willmott, C., Cameron, P., Ayton, G., Nelms, R., Curran, C., et al. (1999). Cognitive and behavioral outcome following mild traumatic head injury in children. *Journal of Head Trauma Rehabilitation, 14*, 360–372.

Rivara, F. P. (1994). Epidemiology and prevention of pediatric traumatic brain injury. *Pediatric Annals, 23*, 12–17.

Satz, P., Zaucha, K., McCleary, C., Light, R., Asarnow, R., & Becker, D. (1997). Mild head injury in children and adolescents: A review of studies (1970–1995). *Psychological Bulletin, 122*, 107–131.

Serra-Grabulosa, J. M., Junqué, C., Verger, K., Salgado-Pineda, P., Mañeru, C., & Mercader, J. M. (2005). Cerebral correlates of declarative memory dysfunctions in early traumatic brain injury. *Journal of Neurology, Neurosurgery, and Psychiatry, 76*, 129–131.

Slomine, B. S., Salorio, C. F., Grados, M. A., Vasa, R. A., Christensen, J. R., & Gerring, J. P. (2005). Differences in attention, executive functioning, and memory in children with and without ADHD after severe traumatic brain injury. *Journal of the International Neuropsychological Society, 11*, 65–653.

Statler, K. D., Jenkins, L. W., Dixon, C. E., Clark, R. S. B., Marion, D. W., & Kochanek, P. M. (2001). The simple model versus the super model: Translating experimental traumatic brain injury research to the bedside. *Journal of Neurotrauma, 18*, 1195–1206.

Taylor, H. G., Yeates, K. O., Wade, S. L., Drotar, D., Stancin, T., & Minich, N. (2002). A prospective study of short- and long-term outcomes after traumatic brain injury in children: Behavior and achievement. *Neuropsychology, 16*, 15–27.

Van't Hooft, I., Anderson, K., Bergman, B., Sejersen, T., Von Wendt, L., & Bartfai, A. (2005). Beneficial effect from a cognitive training programme on children with acquired brain injuries demonstrated in a controlled study. *Brain Injury, 19*, 511–518.

Wade, S. L., Carey, J., & Wolfe, C. R. (2006). The efficacy of an online cognitive-behavioral, family intervention in improving child behavior and social competence following pediatric brain injury. *Rehabilitation Psychology, 51*, 179–189.

Yeates, K. O., Swift, E., Taylor, H. G., Wade, S. L., Drotar, D., Stancin, T., et al. (2004). Short- and long-term social outcomes following pediatric traumatic brain injury. *Journal of the International Neuropsychological Society, 10*, 412–426.

Yeates, K. O., Taylor, H. G., Wade, S. L., Drotar, D., Stancin, T., & Minich, N. (2002). A prospective study of short- and long-term neuropsychological outcomes after traumatic brain injury in children. *Neuropsychology, 16*, 514–523.

16

From Preschool to College: Consequences of Traumatic Brain Injury Sustained during Early Childhood

Linda Ewing-Cobbs and Mary R. Prasad

Despite the high incidence of moderate to severe traumatic brain injury (TBI) in infants and young children, very little is known about their long-term developmental outcomes and academic course. Young children who sustain significant TBI are at high risk for lifelong reduction in both cognitive abilities and behavioral competencies. Outcome studies examining a variety of neuropsychological tasks have identified widespread alteration in functioning after moderate to severe TBI in diverse outcome areas, including general cognitive, expressive and receptive language, academic, attention, working memory, inhibitory control, social participation, adaptive behavior, and psychological adjustment domains. Therefore, even with the extensive array of changes in neural processes that occur in normal development during infancy and early childhood, sequelae of early injury are significant and persistent, reflecting incomplete recovery of function.

Although recovery is generally favorable following focal brain lesions sustained during childhood (Stiles, 2000), recovery appears to be less favorable following conditions producing diffuse brain insult, such as TBI (Anderson, Catroppa, Morse, Haritou, & Rosenfeld, 2005; Ewing-Cobbs et al., 1997; Ewing-Cobbs et al., 2006). Traumatic brain injury typically reflects a combination of focal and diffuse brain insults. The primary pathophysiological consequence of TBI is traumatic axonal injury (Gennarelli, Thibault, & Graham, 1998). In contrast to focal injuries in which the brain sustains a direct impact, axonal

injury results from angular and rotational head movements of high magnitude that occur with or without impact (Gennarelli et al., 1998). Diffuse pathologic changes reflect the impact of direct injury to both axons and cell bodies as well as effects of secondary reactive pathology related to anoxic, contusion, hemorrhagic, perfusion and reperfusion mechanisms, and cascades of excitatory neurotransmitters (Singleton & Povlishock, 2004). Pathologic studies of diffuse TBI have revealed microscopic features corresponding to Wallerian-type axonal degeneration that most prominently affect the subcortical white matter, corpus callosum, and dorsolateral aspect of the upper brain stem (Adams, Mitchell, Graham, & Doyle, 1977). Focal insults commonly occurring in TBI include space-occupying or mass lesions, including contusions, intracerebral hematomas, and extra-axial hematomas. These lesions produce behavioral changes due to direct tissue damage in addition to remote mass effects, such as midline shift and herniation.

Across the first few years after TBI, infants and preschool-aged children with moderate to severe TBI show lower initial general cognitive scores and less recovery over time than school-aged children or adolescents (Anderson et al., 2005; Anderson et al., 2006; Ewing-Cobbs, Barnes, & Fletcher, 2003; Ewing-Cobbs, Miner, Fletcher, & Levin, 1989). In young children, curves depicting the posttraumatic recovery of IQ scores across time are either flat, indicating no improvement in scores after the initial injury

(Ewing-Cobbs et al., 2003) or show a decline across time (Anderson et al., 2005), indicating failure to develop new skills at age-appropriate rates. In particular, brain injury sustained early in life may interfere with the acquisition of later-developing cognitive, academic, and adaptive behavior skills due to the combined impact of reduced general cognitive functioning and reduced learning efficiency.

In cases of severe TBI, there is significant heterogeneity in both injury characteristics and in behavioral outcomes. Using the model developed by Dennis and colleagues, this heterogeneity can be explained in part by reference to several variables, including the type, timing, and severity of injury, time since injury, and reserve (Dennis, Yeates, Taylor, & Fletcher, 2006). L. G., the child with TBI discussed in this chapter, was evaluated seven times across 15 years, extending from preschool to junior college. In the next section, we present highlights of serial evaluations, followed by brief discussion of how some of the heterogeneity in L. G.'s profile may be explained by the model.

Case Study: L. G.

L. G. sustained a very severe TBI at age 3 years, 5 months in a motor vehicle collision. Her preinjury developmental history suggested average to accelerated acquisition of milestones. Her parents had college degrees and were employed in financial services professions. At the time of hospital admission, she had a Glasgow Coma Scale (Teasdale & Jennett, 1974) score of 3, indicating no spontaneous eye opening, no vocalization, and no response to pain. During the first week post injury, CT scans revealed an extensive infarction of the left hemisphere and diffuse cerebral swelling. She was unable to follow a one-stage request for 5 weeks. Neurological symptoms persisting at discharge included a dense right hemiparesis, right homonomyous hemianopsia, diplopia due to a third cranial nerve injury, and aphasia. L. G. received intensive inpatient and outpatient rehabilitation. Follow-up magnetic resonance imaging (MRI) several years post injury indicated cystic encephalomalacia of the left hemisphere, primarily in the temporal and parietal lobes but extending into the frontal and occipital lobes with associated significant compensatory enlargement of

the left lateral ventricle. The posterior body and splenium of the corpus callosum ranged from thin to partially absent. Abnormalities were not visualized in the right hemisphere.

Preschool Assessments

Initial neuropsychological evaluation 3 months after TBI at age 38 months indicated severely restricted expressive language (Sequenced Inventory of Communication Development; Expressive Communication Age = 18 months, < 0.1%) and significantly reduced receptive language (Receptive Communication Age = 30 months, 1%). Verbal IQ assessment was deferred due to severe expressive aphasia. Based on the McCarthy Scales of Children's Abilities, Perceptual-performance abilities were below expected levels for visual-spatial, visual-motor, and sequencing activities. Figure 16-1 depicts longitudinal verbal and non-verbal estimates of general cognitive abilities from serial assessments.

Following intensive outpatient rehabilitation and participation in an Early Childhood Education program through the public school system, re-evaluation was completed 9 months after injury at 44 months of age. Despite a dense right hemiparesis, L. G. ambulated using a brace on the right lower leg and a shoe guard on the left foot. Speech was telegraphic and consisted primarily of utterances containing two to three nouns and verbs. L. G. received a McCarthy Scale of Children's Abilities General Cognitive Index of 77 (8th percentile), which was considered an underestimate given continuing expressive language difficulty and reduced frustration tolerance. Receptive language was an area of relative strength (Receptive Communication Age = 40 months; IQ equivalent = 82). Despite significant recovery of expressive language abilities, overall performance reflected severe residual expressive aphasia (Expressive Communication Age = 28 months; IQ equivalent = 57). L. G. was very socially engaging but very slow in her response speed. It was recommended that L. G. continue to receive intensive speech/language, physical, and occupational therapies. She received services from her school as well as privately. Her parents were highly involved in her rehabilitation and often worked with her at home on preacademic skills.

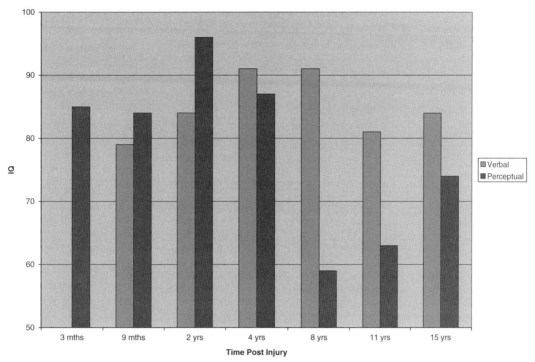

Figure 16-1. Relative performance on longitudinal age-appropriate Verbal and Perceptual-Performance IQ scores is depicted. Despite loss of left hemisphere function, LG showed extensive recovery of verbal skills by 9 months after traumatic brain injury (TBI). By 4 years after TBI, verbal scores were consistently higher than performance-based scores. This pattern is due in part to the format of the Wechsler scales, which emphasize speeded tasks for performance but not verbal subtests. Instruments employed at each interval: McCarthy Scales of Children's Abilities (3 months to 2 years), Stanford-Binet Intelligence Scale IV (4 years), Wechsler Intelligence Scale for Children III (8 and 11 years), and Wechsler Adult Intelligence Scale III (15 years).

Elementary School Assessment

L. G. was re-evaluated at 7 years of age and 4 years post injury. She continued to receive intensive speech/language, physical, and occupational therapies. Interim medical history indicated that anticonvulsant medication had been prescribed due to onset of partial and complex partial seizures. L. G. received instruction in a regular education classroom with extended time for completion of tests and assignments.

The Stanford-Binet Intelligence Scale–Fourth Edition yielded a composite score of 82 (13th percentile). On the Stanford-Binet, which placed less emphasis on speeded tasks, L. G.'s scores in verbal and abstract/visual reasoning areas were similar, ranging from the 21st to 29th percentiles. Quantitative (SS = 78, 8th percentile) and short-term memory (SS = 85, 17th percentile) scores were also significantly below estimated

preinjury potential, indicating fairly widespread lowering of intellectual abilities. Academic achievement scores on the Woodcock-Johnson Revised Tests of Achievement were uniformly in the average range for basic reading, broad reading, broad math, and broad written language. In contrast, neuropsychological evaluation identified persisting difficulties in fine motor speed on the left hand (Grooved Pegboard, <0.1%); the right hand was not testable. Visual-motor integration was age appropriate (Beery VMI, 58%). Despite average comprehension of one-stage requests containing multiple descriptive words, her comprehension of grammatically complex sentences was well below expected levels. She had difficulty understanding prepositions and linguistic concepts such as inclusion/exclusion, temporal relations, spatial relations, and modifiers. This finding is quite common in children with extensive injury to the left hemisphere, for whom comprehension of prepositions and other function words frequently present particular challenges (Dennis & Whitaker, 1976). Oral fluency, based on generating words beginning with specific letters, was average. Rapid naming of pictured objects remained slow and effortful. Assessment of memory using a selective reminding task identified low-average learning and retention of new verbal information (22nd percentile). The Vineland Adaptive Behavior Scales yielded a composite Adaptive Behavior score of 93 (32nd percentile). Once again, scores ranged from above average (socialization domain, 70th percentile) to well below expected levels (motor skills, 2nd percentile). Parent report on behavior checklists was within normal limits in all areas, suggesting good adjustment. It is important to note that although L. G.'s mother rated her very highly in socialization, L. G.'s preferred to play with children much younger than herself, some as young as 3 years of age. It was recommended

that L. G. continue receiving intensive speech/language services to address dysarthria and hypophonia, in addition to receptive, expressive, and pragmatic language skills.

Evaluation 7 years after severe TBI revealed slow, dysarthric speech. Dysnomia was evident, as L. G. frequently struggled to produce a specific word or to generate answers to abstract questions. The Full Scale WISC-III IQ score was 73 (4th percentile). Despite loss of left hemisphere function and resultant aphasia, the WISC-III Verbal Comprehension score remained in the Average range (SS = 95), while the Perceptual-Organization score was Deficient (SS = 64). Figure 16-2 depicts longitudinal performance on Wechsler factor scores on evaluations obtained from 8 to 15 years after the injury.

Academic scores from the Woodcock-Johnson Revised Tests of Achievement indicated average performance in reading, math, and written language, with percentile scores ranging

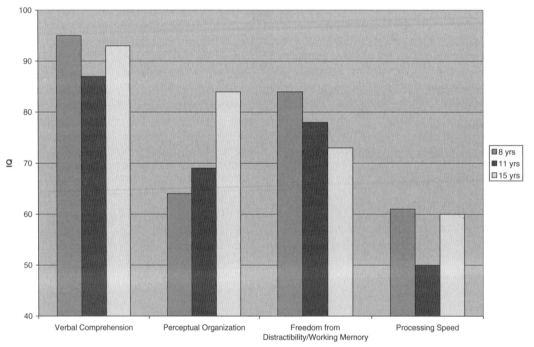

Wechsler Factor Scores Obtained Eight to Fifteen Years After Early TBI

Figure 16-2. Longitudinal factor scores from Wechsler Intelligence Scale for Children III scores (8 and 11 years) and Wechsler Adult Intelligence Scale III (15 years post injury) suggest that Verbal Comprehension scores were significantly higher than other factor scores across the interval tested. However, the Perceptual Organization subtest content of the WAIS-III may be more oriented to assessing power than speed relative to the WISC-III due to inclusion of fewer timed subtests. Processing Speed remained markedly impaired throughout the extended follow-up.

from 34 to 50. In contrast, the Gray Oral Reading Test-3 yielded an Oral Reading Quotient of 64 (<1st percentile), revealing significant difficulties in reading fluency (1st percentile) and comprehension (5th percentile) of connected text.

High School Assessment

At age 14, re-evaluation was requested to assist in preparing for high school entrance. The Wechsler Intelligence for Children–III yielded a Full Scale IQ score of 71. A significant discrepancy was evident between her Verbal IQ (83, 13th percentile) and Performance IQ (63, 1st percentile) scores. The Verbal IQ score was regarded as the best estimate of her learning potential. Calculation of factor scores underlying L. G.'s performance on individual subtests identified strengths in areas requiring predominantly verbal skills and weakness in speeded nonverbal processing skills. Once again, verbal comprehension was an area of relative strength (SS = 87, 19th percentile), while perceptual organization subtest scores were in the deficient range (SS = 69, 2nd percentile). Allowing completion of perceptual organization items beyond time limits revealed significantly better reasoning skills than predicted using standard assessment practices. Difficulties were evident for holding and manipulating information in working memory (7th percentile) and for processing speed (<0.1 percentile). Academic achievement was evaluated using the Woodcock-Johnson III Tests of Achievement. Collapsing across content areas, L. G. showed average development of basic skills across reading, mathematics, and written language areas (45th percentile) as well as the ability to apply these skills (30th percentile). In contrast, academic fluency was deficient (1st percentile), reflecting the continued impact of slowed processing speed on reading speed, math fact retrieval, and fluency of production of written text.

Standardized assessment using the Wide Range Assessment of Memory and Learning yielded a General Memory score of 71 (3rd percentile). Relative strength was noted for recalling details of pictures that were briefly shown (37%); other subtest scores assessing drawing geometric designs from memory, rote learning of words, and story memory were below expected levels (5%). Although parent report identified average levels of both internalizing and externalizing behaviors, both psychological evaluation and teacher report suggested significant elevation of symptoms of anxiety and depression. L. G. was a very sensitive adolescent who was anxious, perfectionistic, and socially immature. L. G.'s social difficulties were strikingly apparent. She had no same-aged friends and continued to prefer interacting with young children. Slowed production and comprehension of language contributed to difficulty interacting comfortably with peers.

Specific academic interventions included using voice transcription software, scribing in lieu of writing or typing, employing taped textbooks, and preloading information prior to its presentation in class to improve retention. An aide was responsible for assisting with transportation of materials for each class, scribing when necessary, highlighting text and curriculum sheets, and assuring implementation of standard accommodations in the regular education setting.

Junior College Assessment

Re-assessment was requested at age 18 to provide recommendations for academic accommodations within a junior college setting. On the Wechsler Adult Intelligence Scale-III (WAIS-III), L. G. received a Full Scale IQ score of 77, which indicates overall intellectual functioning in the Borderline range at the 6th percentile (Verbal IQ = 84, 14th percentile; Performance IQ = 74, 4th percentile). As shown in Figure 16-2, scores underlying L. G.'s performance in different areas revealed average verbal comprehension and low-average perceptual organization scores. These scores reflected L. G.'s reasoning abilities and were regarded as the best estimates of her overall level of cognitive ability. She scored lower on measures of working memory and processing speed, reflecting her continuing difficulties holding and manipulating information in auditory working memory and in rapidly completing paper-and-pencil tasks.

Across different content areas on the WJ-III, L. G.'s performance was average on measures of basic academic skills (35th percentile) and low average on measures of applying skills in new contexts involving reasoning (21st percentile). She showed continued, very significant weakness overall on measures of academic fluency

(0.1 percentile). Despite impressive development of reading and written language abilities given the loss of left hemisphere function, oral language and listening comprehension scores identified very significant continuing difficulties in both receptive (0.05 percentile) and expressive (8th percentile) areas. Reading connected text was characterized by globally reduced fluency (1st percentile) and comprehension (2nd percentile; GORT-4 Oral Reading Quotient = 55, <0.1 percentile).

Neuropsychological evaluation revealed significant variability in performance in different areas. L. G. continued to show significant slowing with her left hand (<1st percentile). In addition, visual-motor integration, as indicated by drawing geometric designs, dropped from average to below expected levels (1st percentile). L. G.'s speed of information processing when she had to visually track one sequence of information was slow (Trail Making A, <1st percentile; one error). Similarly, when she was asked to divide attention between two sequences of information, her performance remained extremely slow (Trail Making B, <1st percentile) but was accurate.

Evaluation of attention included a computerized continuous performance test. L. G.'s performance suggested difficulty focusing attention, some impulsivity, and average ability to sustain attention over time. L. G. made a large number of errors of omission (failing to respond when a letter was on the screen, 3rd percentile) and commission errors (responding to nontarget letters, 2nd percentile). Her reaction time was average for correct responses; however, she showed more variability than expected (7th percentile).

The Wechsler Memory Scale–III yielded an Immediate Memory score of 63 (1st percentile), indicating difficulty retaining recently presented auditory and visual information. Delayed recall of the same information yielded a General Memory quotient of 59 (0.3 percentile); L. G. had difficulty recalling both auditory and visual information following a 30-minute delay. In contrast, her working memory score indicated low-average ability to hold and manipulate auditory verbal and visual spatial information in working memory systems (21 percentile).

Tasks from the Delis-Kaplan Executive Function System were selected to highlight performance in fluency, switching, inhibitory control, and planning areas. Verbal and Design Fluency subtests evaluate the ability to initiate and produce specific words and visual designs according to specific rules that change. L. G.'s verbal fluency for words beginning with specific letters was an area of strength (25th percentile). She had more difficulty retrieving the names of words belonging to specific categories (1st percentile) and in alternating retrieval from different categories (<0.1 percentile). L. G.'s ability to draw designs according to specific criteria was in the average range (25th percentile). She showed less difficulty on visual than verbal material when switching from one set of rules to another (9th percentile). On tests evaluating planning and problem solving, L. G. showed good ability to employ a hypothesis-testing approach to solve novel problems (25th percentile).

L. G.'s mother completed a Child Behavior Checklist. Her ratings of L. G.'s behavior yielded significant elevations (>90th percentile) on the anxious/depressed, somatic complaints, social problems, and attention problems scales. It was recommended that L. G. attend junior college with reduced load (1–2 classes per semester), note-taking assistance, extended time for test completion, and tutoring. Her mother attended class with her and provided additional tutorial support.

Discussion

The Dennis model posits that brain reserve capacity (genetic factors and preinsult status) and cognitive reserve (preinjury and postinjury cognition, socioeconomic status, and family function) have bidirectional influences on each other and directly influence functional plasticity, which then impacts functional outcomes in physical, cognitive, academic, and psychosocial domains. Factors such as age at insult, age at assessment, and characteristics of the brain injury may mediate or moderate the influence of reserve characteristics on specific outcomes. The apparent impact of a brain injury on a given skill may depend on the developmental stage at which the lesion is sustained and at which the skill is evaluated (Goldman, 1974; Kolb, Pellis, & Robinson, 2004) Some skills may show a stable deficit over time, others may show a transient lag and partial catch-up growth, while others may show increasing deficit as the damaged substrate required for mature expression of a given skill cannot support the skill and the child falls farther behind age expectations. L. G.'s case demonstrates the devastating impact of severe early brain injury on development but also illustrates how positive factors, including brain reserve and cognitive reserve, can shape outcomes. Clearly, L. G. had high preinjury potential, in addition to an optimal family environment and provision of extensive rehabilitation therapies for years after the injury.

Type of brain insult, age at injury, and location of damage may influence outcome in several ways. First, L. G.'s injury is best characterized as both diffuse, due to the severe TBI, and focal, given the infarction of the left hemisphere. Although the MRI scan was read as normal for the right hemisphere, test data suggest significant injury did occur to right hemisphere structures, based on the impairment of fine motor speed and coordination in using the left hand and slow processing speed.

Diffuse brain injury from a variety of etiologies is associated with poorer outcomes in younger than in older children (Ewing-Cobbs et al., 2003). L. G.'s early age at injury may have allowed greater reorganization of language abilities than a similar injury sustained later during childhood. Given her age and the extent of left hemisphere injury, her damaged right hemisphere likely provided the substrate for language development. Despite initial mutism and severe aphasia, L. G. developed adequate conversational speech. Her receptive language skills remained impaired with difficulty understanding syntax and complex directions, which are common findings in children who sustained left hemisphere injuries involving language areas. Although at first glance it would appear that L. G.'s visuospatial skills were impaired to a greater degree than her language skills, on untimed visual-perceptual tasks, L. G.'s performance was within the low-average range, comparable to her verbal skills. The lack of a significant difference in verbal and performance scores is consistent with findings from children with nonprogressive unilateral perinatal lesions, in whom laterality of lesion does not affect the pattern of IQ test scores when tested at school age (Ballantyne, Spilkin, Hesselink, & Trauner, 2008). In light of these findings, care should be taken when making inferences about the functional status of cerebral hemispheres and specific brain regions based on neuropsychological test data.

Although L. G. made remarkable gains in her language skills over time, her overall level of intellectual functioning was essentially unchanged from her initial assessment to her last assessment at the age of 18. Across the first few years after TBI, infants and preschool-aged children with moderate to severe TBI show lower initial general cognitive scores and less recovery over time than in school-aged children or adolescents. In young children, curves depicting the posttraumatic recovery of IQ scores across time are either flat, indicating no improvement in scores after the initial injury (Ewing-Cobbs et al., 2003), or show a decline across time (Anderson et al., 2005), indicating failure to develop new skills at age-appropriate rates. In particular, brain injury sustained early in life may interfere with the acquisition of later-developing skills due to the combined impact of reduced general cognitive functioning and reduced learning efficiency. The less complete recovery in young children may reflect damage to mechanisms involved in learning and memory, which interferes with the acquisition of new information and skills (Taylor & Alden, 1997). L. G.'s language skills showed transient lag and partial catch-up growth, while IQ scores showed a relatively stable deficit. Other skills, such as visual motor integration, showed a decline over time, suggesting increased deficit and failure to develop skills at the level expected based on initial assessments and general level of cognitive functioning.

Several caveats regarding assessment of children with severe TBI are indicated by L. G.'s profile. Despite the devastating left hemisphere injury, L. G. mastered basic academic skills as indicated by Woodcock-Johnson achievement test scores in the average range. Although she was able to acquire basic reading and math skills, she struggled with higher order academic skills such as reading comprehension for connected text. Assessments that examine more contextual skills may reveal more significant posttraumatic difficulties than those that assess more concrete skills that can be taught. Another consequence of L. G.'s injury was extremely slow processing speed. Simple reaction time was within normal limits; however, slow processing speed affected all complex cognitive tasks and made the assessments extremely lengthy. Use of testing approaches that incorporate testing of limits strategies can be informative regarding the degree to which requirements for speed, as opposed to cognitive ability, impact performance.

Social integration remained one of L. G.'s greatest areas of difficulty. Although she was very pleasant, engaging, and interacted very well with adults and younger children, she had difficulty interacting with her peers. As a young child, her social integration issues were underappreciated by her parents. As she aged, her social difficulties became more apparent. Her social discourse skills were weak and she had difficulty engaging same-age peers in conversation. Her interests were immature and her slowed language production and comprehension interfered with daily interactions. During adolescence, L. G. became more aware of her areas of difficulty and experienced increased anxiety, which is a common sequelae of significant TBI (Gerring et al., 2002). Direct assessment, rather than sole reliance upon parental report, may reveal concerns with adjustment in general, and with internalizing difficulties in particular.

The sum of the neurological and neuropsychological sequelae of L. G.'s traumatic brain injury limits her educational and occupational opportunities. Hemiparesis, hemianopsia, residual aphasia, low-average reasoning abilities, and slow processing speed reduce the options for competitive employment. With assets that include motivation, tenacity, appropriate social skills, good problem solving, functional literacy and numeracy skills, and outstanding family support, L. G. can be successful in a supported employment environment.

Acknowledgments

Preparation of this chapter was supported in part by the National Institutes of Health-National Institute for Neurological Diseases and Stroke grant R01-NS046308. The authors wish to thank L. G. and her family for the many insights into enhancing life after TBI that they have shared over the years.

References

Adams, J. H., Mitchell, D. E., Graham, D. I., & Doyle, D. (1977). Diffuse brain damage of the immediate impact type. *Brain, 100*, 489–502.

Anderson, V. A., Catroppa, C., Dudgeon, P., Morse, S. A., Haritou, F., & Rosenfeld, J. V. (2006). Understanding predictors of functional recovery and outcome 30 months following early childhood head injury. *Neuropsychology, 20*, 42–57.

Anderson, V., Catroppa, C., Morse, S., Haritou, F., & Rosenfeld, J. (2005). Functional plasticity or vulnerability after early brain injury? *Pediatrics, 116*, 1374–1382.

Ballantyne, A. O., Spilkin, A. M., Hesselink, J., & Trauner, D. (2008). Plasticity in the developing brain: Intellectual, language and academic functions in children with ischaemic perinatal stroke. *Brain, 131*, 2975–2985.

Dennis, M., & Whitaker, H. A. (1976). Language acquisition following hemidecortication: Linguistic superiority of the left over the right hemisphere. *Brain and Language, 3*, 404–433.

Dennis, M., Yeates, K. O., Taylor, H. G., & Fletcher, J. M. (2006). Brain reserve capacity, cognitive reserve capacity, and age-based functional plasticity after congenital and acquired brain injury in children. In Y. Stern (Ed.), *Cognitive reserve* (pp. 53–83). New York: Psychology Press.

Ewing-Cobbs, L., Barnes, M. A., & Fletcher, J. M. (2003). Early brain injury in children: Development and reorganization of cognitive function. *Developmental Neuropsychology, 24*(2–3), 669–704.

Ewing-Cobbs, L., Fletcher, J. M., Levin, H. S., Francis, D. J., Davidson, K., & Miner, M. E. (1997). Longitudinal neuropsychological outcome in infants and preschoolers with traumatic brain injury. *Journal of the International Neuropsychological Society, 3*, 581–591.

Ewing-Cobbs, L., Miner, M. E., Fletcher, J. M., & Levin, H. S. (1989). Intellectual, motor, and language sequelae following closed head injury in infants and preschoolers. *Journal of Pediatric Psychology, 14*, 531–547.

Ewing-Cobbs, L., Prasad, M., Kramer, L., Cox, C., Baumgartner, J., Fletcher, S. et al. (2006). Late intellectual and academic outcomes following traumatic brain injury sustained during early childhood. *Journal of Neurosurgery, 105*(Suppl. 4), 287–296.

Gennarelli, T. A., Thibault, L. E., & Graham, D. I. (1998). Diffuse axonal injury: An important form of traumatic brain damage. *Neuroscientist, 4*, 202–215.

Gerring, J. P., Slomine, B. S., Vasa, R., Grados, M. A., Chen, A., Rising, W. et al. (2002). Clinical predictors of posttraumatic stress disorder after closed head injury in children. *Journal of the American Academy of Child Adolescent Psychiatry, 41*, 157–165.

Goldman, P. S. (1974). An alternative to developmental plasticity: Heterology of CNS structures in infants and adults. In D. G. Stein, J. J. Rosen, & N. Butters (Eds.), *Plasticity and recovery of function in the central nervous system* (pp. 149–174). New York: Academic.

Kolb, B., Pellis, S., & Robinson, T. E. (2004). Plasticity and functions of the orbital frontal cortex. *Brain and Cognition, 55,* 104–115.

Singleton, R. H., & Povlishock, J. T. (2004). Identification and characterization of heterogeneous neuronal injury and death in regions of diffuse brain injury: Evidence for multiple independent injury phenotypes. *The Journal of Neuroscience, 24,* 3543–3553.

Stiles, J. (2000). Neural plasticity and cognitive development. *Developmental Neuropsychology, 18,* 237–272.

Taylor, H. G., & Alden, J. (1997). Age-related differences in outcomes following childhood brain insults: An introduction and overview. *Journal of the International Neuropsychological Society, 3,* 555–567.

Teasdale, G., & Jennett, B. (1974). Assessment of coma and impaired consciousness: A practical scale. *Lancet, 2,* 81–84.

17

Well-Documented, Serious Brain Dysfunction Followed by Malingering

Jerry J. Sweet and Dawn Giuffre Meyer

Some patients have such clear histories of neurological disturbance that it can be quite tempting to simply assume that all abnormal behaviors, symptoms, and problems in living are attributable to the well-documented disorder. The present case provides a good example of the erroneous conclusions that could result from an uncritical acceptance of past history as explanation for present behavior. To elaborate further, the present case is testament to the position that the logical error represented by the well-known Latin phrase *post hoc ergo propter hoc* (i.e., after this, therefore because of this) remains a worthy dictum. As is true for many other health-care specialists, a large proportion of cases evaluated by clinical neuropsychologists is in fact referred at the instance of some event, whether an insidious or sudden spontaneous medical event (e.g., cerebrovascular accident) or an acquired injury (e.g., accident-related traumatic brain injury). At times, it can be tempting to infer a causal connection between the known event A and symptom B provided by the patient and behavior C demonstrated on formal testing. Such a conclusion requires that the clinician critically evaluate pre- and post-event history, moderator and confounding variables that can affect test performance, and determine not only the validity of the symptoms and behaviors but also whether there is a probable causal connection with event A.

Neuropsychologists as Clinicians and Forensic Experts

More so than other specialties within clinical psychology, the specialty of clinical neuropsychology has strongly aligned itself with the scientist-practitioner approach. In a broader sense, it has been suggested repeatedly in relevant literature that the relative success of clinical psychologists in medical settings derives from scientific training that is directly translated into clinical application. This is what Sheridan and Choca (1991) described as "the scientifically minded clinician." The following quote from Rozensky, Sweet, and Tovian (1991) elaborates this viewpoint:

The clear presentation of organized clinical data, diagnostic impressions, treatment plans, and, ultimately, positive treatment outcomes is the product offered by the clinical psychologist within the medical milieu. It is training as a hypothesis tester…with an orientation to accountability, comfort with and training in measuring the effectiveness of interventions, and an objectivity in presenting data, that forms the foundation of the field of clinical psychology in medical settings. (p. 288)

Nowhere in clinical psychology's specialties is this viewpoint more apparent among practitioners than in clinical neuropsychology. Sweet (1999) argued that this strong scientist-practitioner orientation is a predominant factor in explaining the substantial growth of the overall specialty, as well as the substantial increase over time of involvement in forensic activities by clinical neuropsychologists. In reviewing the practice area of forensic neuropsychology, Sweet, Ecklund-Johnson, and Malina (2008) specifically noted similarities between good scientists and good expert witnesses. These observers concluded, in part, that clinical neuropsychology's deep scientific roots appeared salient in making practitioners attractive to triers-of-fact and attorneys, probably explaining the growth of forensic practice by neuropsychologists in the last two decades.

An evolution of legal standards has also increased the demand for expert witnesses who are scientifically grounded. Commonly known as evidentiary standards, legal decisions in cases such as *Daubert vs. Merrell Dow Pharmaceuticals* (1993), *General Electric Co. vs. Joiner* (1997), and *Kumho Tire vs. Carmichael* (1999), along with the Federal Rules of Evidence, have augured for exclusion or restriction of witnesses whose opinion bases are not scientific. In many instances currently, the attempt by an expert witness to justify opinions on the basis of simply having considerable experience is no longer sufficient. As might be expected, a review of all available evidentiary challenges to the inclusion of testimony by neuropsychologists from 1994 to 2005 failed to detect a pattern of exclusion (Sweet et al., 2008). That is, as might be expected in a specialty that is based in science, exclusions of expert neuropsychologist witnesses occurred as a result of individual practitioner judgments that strayed from a scientific basis or from relevance, rather than being en bloc or as a whole group. The case description that follows provides a good example of the importance of an empirically-based and research-supported approach to determining the effects of a neurological disorder, especially when a court would otherwise err in its judgments without expert opinions from a clinical neuropsychological perspective.

Case Presentation

Symptom Onset and Relevant History

Mr. F., a man in his mid-30s, presented at his local hospital with dizziness, vomiting, photophobia, and severe headache pain that had lasted for 2 days

following sudden onset. His neurological examination was normal. A computerized tomography (CT) scan was interpreted as showing no signs of neurological abnormality, other than sinusitis. Mr. F. was discharged with medication to treat sinus problems, and he was advised to follow up with a doctor.

Four days later, Mr. F. was admitted to a different medical center because of persistent severe headache pain. The presenting concerns of his family at that time also included bilateral leg weakness, weakness in his right arm, garbled speech, and disorientation. A CT scan was again interpreted as consistent with sinusitis. Presenting symptoms and other diagnostic procedures resulted in a diagnosis of meningitis, initially thought to be arising from the sinus condition. Mr. F. underwent endoscopic sphenoethmoidectomy (i.e., surgery to decompress his sinuses), and during the procedure a possible pituitary tumor was identified. A subsequent magnetic resonance imaging (MRI) scan was consistent with pituitary macroadenoma, which had compressed the optic chiasm, as well as evidence of new pituitary apoplexy hemorrhage. Additional imaging findings included acute infarction in the inferior medial aspects of the frontal lobes bilaterally (more severe in the left hemisphere), the posterior aspect of the left Sylvian fissure, and the left posterior temporoparietal region in the cortex and subcortical white matter. Mr. F. immediately underwent surgery; the pituitary tumor was removed without additional complications. For the remainder of his inpatient surgical recovery, Mr. F. displayed right hemiparesis and severe receptive and expressive language deficits. Pharmacotherapy was initiated for seizure activity and panhypopituitarism. After approximately two weeks in the hospital, Mr. F. was transferred to a rehabilitation center for further treatment.

Mr. F. received inpatient services with the rehabilitation center for a period of approximately three weeks, and by the end of his stay he was able to eat, dress, walk, and complete orofacial hygiene independently. His cognitive status, language deficits, and hemiparesis were noted to have "improved considerably," but residual impairments remained. Mr. F. had limited insight into the degree of his own impairments. Following discharge, he continued rehabilitative services through the center's day treatment program. Upon entrance into that program, Mr. F. identified speech as his most significant concern, and the services he received included speech/language and cognitive rehabilitation. Nine months following pituitary resection, a neurologist and physical therapist documented that ambulation was normal and coordination was intact. Eleven months post operation, Mr. F. performed in the average range on Boston Diagnostic Aphasia Examination subtests of auditory and reading comprehension. However, he had persistent difficulty comprehending complex information, and he exhibited moderate to severe Broca's aphasia. Nineteen months after onset, Mr. F. denied difficulty with word finding or speech to his neurosurgeon and none was observed by the neurosurgeon.

Mr. F. also received vocational rehabilitation services at intervals. While receiving these services two years after his surgeries, he applied and was hired for a job in direct, face-to-face customer support. However, he did not appear for his first day of work and subsequently was not employed. At the time of his discharge from vocational rehabilitation nearly 2.5 years after his pituitary resection, Mr. F. was noted by staff members to have made gains in independent living, communication, organization, and financial management. Also, he had apparently secured a part-time position relevant to a long-standing interest of his, which he had pursued prior to illness onset.

Mr. F. had no prior history of major medical or psychiatric illnesses, significant injuries or accidents, or educational concerns. He was a high school graduate and had held a variety of unskilled jobs throughout his adulthood, in addition to several positions related to his particular vocational interest, none of which had specific educational requirements. Prior to the illness onset, he had been engaged to be married. The engagement dissolved in the months following his surgeries. Mr. F. lived with his parents, and his family was very dedicated to his care.

Mr. F. initiated a lawsuit against the original hospital, physicians, and radiologist for negligence related to failure to diagnose the pituitary adenoma. He also sued the second medical center, several of its physicians, and a radiologist for negligence relating to their failure to rule out pituitary adenoma promptly.

Initial Neuropsychological Assessment (Conducted by a Local Neuropsychologist as the Plaintiff's Expert)

Interview and Behavioral Observations. Approximately 3.5 years following the pituitary resection, Mr. F. was referred to and evaluated by a neuropsychologist, hired by the plaintiff's attorney as the plaintiff's expert. During interview and testing, which was conducted on two days approximately eight weeks apart, Mr. F. exhibited notable apparent memory deficits and appeared confused and disoriented numerous times. For example, he did not seem to realize the purpose of the evaluation. Also, he reported that he could not remember his inpatient care with the medical or rehabilitation centers. He provided an inaccurate guess regarding his own age, and he was consistently disoriented to time, once providing a date two years earlier. Mr. F. was unemployed and continued to live with his parents. His parents reported that they helped him with dressing, showering, cooking, monitoring his medications, and managing his finances. They expressed concern that their son was continuing to drive even though he had been in several accidents recently. Mr. F. had few concerns regarding depression or mood, describing only occasional bouts of sadness related to limitations following his illness.

Test Findings. Effort was assessed using standalone effort tests and embedded measures during both days of testing. On the short form of the California Verbal Learning Test-II (CVLT-II; Delis, Kramer, Kaplan, & Ober, 2000) forced recognition, he identified only three of nine target words. The Rey 15-Item Test with Recognition Trial (Boone, Salazar, Lu, Warner-Chacon, & Razani, 2002) was given twice. On the first administration, he recalled only five items and identified 2 of 15 items during the recognition portion of the task. During the second administration, he recalled only five items and identified 6 of 15 items during recognition. The Test of Memory Malingering (TOMM; Tombaugh, 1996) was also administered; Mr. F. attained scores of 20 and 21 of 50 on the two learning trials, and 21 of 50 on the delay trial. All of these performances are far below expectation and are indicative of insufficient effort.

On tests of his cognitive abilities, Mr. F. displayed impairment across a number of domains. He performed in the severely impaired range on tests of mathematics and reading, and he attained an even lower reading score when the test was readministered on the second day of testing. Scores were in the impaired range for immediate recall of stories, word list, and visual designs; retention was also poor, with 0% for stories, 0% for word list, and 50% for visual designs. For motor testing, times were in the impaired range for Grooved Pegboard (Lafayette Instrument, 2002), bilaterally. He could not complete the practice trials for Judgment of Line Orientation (JLO; Benton, Hamsher, Varney, & Spreen, 1983) and Trail Making Test (TMT; Reitan & Wolfson, 1993). His performance was markedly impaired on the Wisconsin Card Sorting Test (WCST; Heaton, Chelune, Talley, Kay, & Curtiss, 1993). When given a visual cancellation task, he drew responses in the middle third of the paper only. He also expressed confusion and did not complete a number of tasks when asked, such as developing and writing a simple sentence, reading the time from a clock face, and pointing to his city of residence on a map of the United States.

Conclusions of the Plaintiff's Neuropsychologist. Results indicated performance levels that were considerably worse than at the end of his participation in outpatient rehabilitation services. Results were interpreted by the plaintiff's neuropsychologist as indicating that Mr. F. may have had difficulty comprehending directions at times and that it was also clear that he had put forth less than optimal effort on testing. It was suggested that his reduced effort may have been related to a feeling of "resignation," as no significant positive changes had occurred in his life. Also, recommendations were made that Mr. F. may need to have his medications and sleep re-evaluated, as these factors may have contributed to his difficulties.

Second Neuropsychological Assessment (Conducted by First Author as the Defense's Expert)

Interview. Mr. F. was evaluated approximately 4.5 years following pituitary resection; he was seen for two testing sessions, which occurred 3 days apart. On the first day of the evaluation, he arrived 45 minutes late, accompanied by his mother and his attorney (who did not remain). He was 90 minutes late on the second day, accompanied by his mother.

Mr. F. was unemployed and stated that he could not work due to fatigue and memory problems. His mother noted that speech therapy had been helpful to her son, but his speech had not returned to normal. She provided information regarding his current functioning, reporting that her son had a stutter at times and an intermittent limp. His memory was noted to be quite poor. Mr. F.'s mother retired from her job at an earlier age than she had intended to assist her son. She organized and monitored his medications, cleaned up after him, reminded him to maintain proper hygiene, and handled his finances. Mr. F. and his mother described visual problems, which included absent visual fields when looking up or to the left. Even though these problems occasionally caused Mr. F. to trip over objects lying in his path, he continued to drive. Mr. F.'s mother also discussed personality changes that her son had undergone, which included stubbornness, irritability, depression, and agitation.

Observations. During the evaluation, Mr. F. was observed to walk with a limp at times. He bumped into a chair with his left leg and explained that he had visual limitations in his left field of vision. He told the examiner that he had learned to compensate for his visual field problems during rehabilitative treatment, and he described using these strategies throughout testing.

During a portion of the testing session, Mr. F. read aloud and spelled several simple words during achievement testing. He answered several items on the Minnesota Multiphasic Personality Inventory-2 (MMPI-2; Butcher, Dahlstrom, Graham, Tellegren, & Kaemmer, 1989) without assistance, then he read aloud several more items when asking the examiner for their meaning. However, Mr. F. was not willing to complete the MMPI-2. Moreover, later in the testing session he would not attempt to read or spell on other tests, saying that he could not read and could not remember how to spell even simple words. By his report, he could not remember how to spell his own name. Trail Making Test Part B (Reitan & Wolfson, 1993) could not be completed, as Mr. F. said that he could not complete the practice trial. Later, when several self-report mood inventories were placed on the table before him and read aloud, he appeared to read them to himself and responded to several items by pointing to the written response that he preferred (which had not been read to him).

Test Findings. Mr. F. was given a number of formal tests of motivation and effort (Table 17-1). On all measures from both evaluation sessions, his performance was below expected levels,

Table 17-1 Mr. F.'s Scores on Effort Measures

Word Memory Test

	Percentage Correct
Immediate Recall	52.5
Delayed Recall	45.0
Consistency	52.5

Test of Memory Malingering

	Raw
Trial 1	25
Trial 2	22
Retention	22

Rey 15-Item Test with Recognition Trial

	Correct	z score
Recall Total	6	−3.66
Recognition	6	−3.35
False Positives	0	−0.68
Combination	12	−3.26

Victoria Symptom Validity Test

Day 1 Administration	Correct	Latency
Easy	12	5.26
Difficult	8	7.06
Total	20	6.16
Day 2 Administration	Correct	Latency
Easy	21	2.98
Difficult	1	4.89
Total	22	3.93

Reliable Digit Span

	Forward/ Backward	Total
First administration	3/2	5
Second administration	3/2	5

CVLT-II Forced-Choice Recognition

Words recognized	9

Wisconsin Card-Sorting Test

Index	Regression Outcome	(Probability of) Malingering
Bernard et al. (1996)		
Traumatic brain injury	7.944	
Malingering	13.393	
Suhr & Boyer (1999)	3.16	90%
King et al. (2002)	1.474	80%

indicating insufficient effort. For example, on the Word Memory Test (WMT; Green, 2003) during the immediate recall trial, he correctly identified 52.5% of the previously displayed words. During the delayed recall trial, he chose 45.0% of the target words, and consistency between the immediate and delay trials was 52.5%. During the TOMM (Tombaugh, 1996), Mr. F. correctly recalled 25 items on the first trial, 22 items on the second trial, and 22 items following a delay. On the Rey 15-Item Test with Recognition Trial (Boone et al., 2002), Mr. F. recalled 6 items and on the recognition portion identified only those items that he had recalled. His effort was assessed on both days with the Victoria Symptom Validity Test (VSVT; Slick, Hopp, Strauss, & Thompson, 1997). During the first administration, he accurately identified 20 of 48 target numeric sequences, 12 of 24 easy and 8 of 24 difficult. On the second day of testing, the VSVT was introduced as a test completed the day before, which, when taken again, would very likely be better performed. The rationale provided for expected improvement was that the examiner believed he was capable of a better performance than that seen on the first day of testing, and he was now familiar with the test. However, on the second administration, he correctly chose a total of 22 of 48 targets, with 21 of 24 easy items and only 1 of 24 difficult items correct.

The validity of Mr. F.'s performance was also assessed using several embedded indicators of effort. Digit span was administered twice, and he did not attain a reliable digit span during either administration (RDS = 5 for both). Performance on the CVLT-II (Delis et al., 2000) forced-choice recognition task was quite poor (9 of 16 words). On the WCST (Heaton, Chelune, Talley, Kay, & Curtiss, 1993), three of three validity indicators were above threshold and therefore considered not credible in a brain injury context.

Table 17-2 includes Mr. F.'s scores from neuropsychological measures given during the first and second sessions. Mr. F. scored in the impaired range in all domains of ability tested. He was oriented to person and situation, but he provided an incorrect response when identifying the city in which the testing occurred. Also, he gave inaccurate answers for the year, day of the week, and approximate time of day. When asked his age

and birth date, he responded that he could not remember. On tests of general attention, processing speed, and working memory, his performances ranged from mildly to moderately impaired (e.g., Wechsler Memory Scale-III [WMS-III] Mental Control subtest; Wechsler, 1997) to severely impaired (e.g., Stroop Color and Word Test, Golden & Freshwater, 2002; TMT Part A, Reitan & Wolfson, 1993). Overall indices of working memory and processing speed were severely impaired. In contrast, he performed in the average range on the Spatial Span subtest of the WMS-III.

With few exceptions, scores on verbal and visual memory tests were impaired. For example, immediate and delayed recall for stories (WMS-III Logical Memory subtest; Wechsler, 1997) was severely impaired and Mr. F. responded correctly to only 13 of 30 forced-choice questions on the recognition task. On the CVLT-II (Delis et al., 2000), he was able to recall a maximum of three words during each of the trials, and his overall total words recalled from all five learning trials was severely impaired. Performances during short-delay free and cued recall trials and long-delay free and cued recall trials were moderately to severely impaired. Though he accurately identified 12 of 16 words during the delayed recognition trial, he also misclassified 21 words as targets (i.e., false positives), which resulted in a severely impaired discrimination index score. Immediate and delayed recall of designs (WMS-III Visual Reproduction; Wechsler, 1997) was mildly to moderately impaired, with moderately to severely impaired performance on the recognition task.

Performance on the Wechsler Adult Intelligence Scale-III (WAIS-III; Wechsler, 1997) was in the "Extremely Low" range (FSIQ = 52), with worst scores on Picture Completion and Arithmetic (SS = 1) and best performances on Information, Matrix Reasoning, and Picture Arrangement (SS = 4). On the Wide Range Achievement Test-4 (Wilkinson & Robertson, 2006), he attained scores in the severely impaired range on measures of word reading, spelling, and mathematical computation.

He performed poorly on several tests of executive functioning. For example, he did not complete any categories on the WCST (Heaton et al., 1993) and made 95 perseverative responses. On the

Table 17-2 Mr. F.'s Scores on Tests of Cognitive Ability

Stroop Color and Word Test

	Raw	T
Word reading	40	<20
Color naming	35	20
Color-Word	2	20

Trail-Making Test

	Completion time	T
Trail Making Part A	94"	16
Trail Making Part B	Failed to complete practice	

Wechsler Memory Scale – III
Primary indexes

	Index score (SS)
Auditory Immediate	65
Auditory Delayed	55
Auditory Recognition Delayed	55

Subtest scores

	Raw	SS
Information and Orientation	5	
Spatial Span	16	10
Forward span total score	9	11
Backward span total score	7	10
Mental Control	12	4
Digit Span	6	3
Forward span total score	4	
Backward span total score	2	
Logical Memory (LM)		
LM I	13	2
LM II	1	1
LM Retention	10%	1
LM Recognition	13/30	
Verbal Paired Associates (VPA)		
VPA I	7	6
VPA II	1	4
VPA Retention	33%	3
VPA Recognition	20/24	
Visual Reproduction (VR)		
VR I	63	4
VR II	17	4
VR Retention	27%	5
VR Recognition	31/48	3
VR Copy	102	14

Auditory process composite scores

	Percentile rank
Single trial learning	1
Learning slope	17
Retention	1
Retrieval	21

California Verbal Learning Test-II

	Raw	z
Trial 1	3	−2.0
Trial 2	3	−2.5

(Continued)

Table 17-2 Mr. F.'s Scores on Tests of Cognitive Ability (*Continued*)

California Verbal Learning Test-II

	Raw	z
Trial 3	3	−3.0
Trial 4	3	−3.5
Trial 5	1	−4.5
Trials 1–5	13	T=13
Trial B	3	−1.5
Short free	2	−3.0
Short cued	3	−3.0
Long free	2	−3.0
Long cued	3	−3.0
Recognition hits	12	−2.5
Recognition false positives	21	5.0
Discrimination	0.3	−3.5
Repetitions	0	−1.5
Intrusions	5	0.5
Semantic clustering	0.3	0
Forced choice recognition	9/16	

Wechsler Adult Intelligence Scale–III

IQ and Index scores	SS	
Verbal IQ	57	
Performance IQ	55	
Full-Scale IQ	52	
Verbal Comprehension	61	
Perceptual Organization	56	
Working Memory	51	
Processing Speed	57	

Subtest Scores	Raw	SS
Vocabulary	11	3
Similarities	6	2
Arithmetic	4	1
Digit Span	6	3
Forward span total score	4	
Backward span total score	2	
Information	5	4
Comprehension	5	2
Letter-Number Sequencing	3	2
Picture Completion	3	1
Digit Symbol Coding	8	2
Block Design	5	2
Matrix Reasoning	4	4
Picture Arrangement	2	4
Symbol Search	0	1

(*Continued*)

Table 17-2 Mr. F.'s Scores on Tests of Cognitive Ability (*Continued*)

Wide Range Achievement Test–4

	Raw	Age-SS/Grade Equivalent
Word Reading	34	63/3.0
Spelling	22	61/2.4
Math Computation	21	55/1.9

Wisconsin Card-Sorting Test

	Raw	T or Percentile
Categories completed	0	≤1 percentile
Total errors	85	T < 20
Perseverative responses	95	T < 20
Perseverative errors	70	T < 20
Failure to maintain set	0	>16 percentile
Percent conceptual response	9%	T < 20

Behavioral Dyscontrol Scale

	Raw	z
Total	13	−2.5
Motor Performance Factor	8	
Environmental Independence Factor	4	
Fluid Intelligence Factor	2	

Ruff Figural Fluency

	Raw	T
Unique designs	46	37
Perseverative errors to designs ratio	.107	56.8

Multilingual Aphasia Examination[a]

Visual Naming	Raw	Percentile
Items correct	22	0

Controlled Oral Word Association	Raw	Percentile
Total words	16	1
Perseverations	1	

Animal Naming[b]

	Raw	z
Total animals	13	−1.09

Grip Strength[c]

	Raw Mean	T
Dominant	13.0	0
Nondominant	33.5	31

Finger Tapping Test[c]

	Raw Mean	T
Dominant	34.2	27
Nondominant	39.4	36

Grooved Pegboard Test

	Raw Time	T
Dominant	97"	35
Nondominant	87"	43

(*Continued*)

Table 17-2 Mr. F.'s Scores on Tests of Cognitive Ability (*Continued*)

Reitan-Indiana Aphasia Screening Test Spatial Relations[c]

	Raw	T
Copy score	2	57

Reitan-Klove Sensory Perceptual Examination

Visual	Left Visual Field	Right Visual Field
Above eye level—errors	0	0
Eye level—errors	0	0
Below eye level—errors	0	0

Behavioral Inattention Test[d]

	Raw	Total Possible
Line cancellation	24	36
Letter cancellation	22	40
Star cancellation	37	54
Figure/shape copy	1	4
Line bisection	4	9

Judgment of Line Orientation

	Raw	Percentile
Items correct	4	<1

[a]Benton, Hamsher, & Sivan, 2000.

[b]Tombaugh, Kozak, & Rees, 1999.

[c]Reitan & Wolfson, 1993.

[d]Wilson, Cockburn, & Halligan, 1987.

SS, standard score

Behavioral Dyscontrol Scale (BDS; Grigsby & Kaye, 1996), a general measure of executive functioning involving motor programming, response inhibition, and mirroring tasks, he performed in the moderately to severely impaired range. However, for the Ruff Figural Fluency test (Ruff, 1988) he obtained a score in the low-average range for generation of unique designs, exhibited average planning efficiency, and thus did not demonstrate an abnormal number of perseverative errors.

Mr. F.'s performance on a measure of confrontation naming was severely impaired. Some responses were noteworthy; for example, he identified a picture of a fork as a shovel for dirt and snow. When asked to name an elephant's tusk, he responded, "I don't know, but they're ivory, right?" Phonemic and semantic fluency were also severely impaired, though he made no perseverative errors.

On gross and fine motor tests, scores obtained with his dominant (right) hand were worse than his left; all except for Grooved Pegboard

(Lafayette Instrument, 2002) with his nondominant hand were borderline to severely impaired. Constructional ability was an area of strength for Mr. F. Ability to copy a simple figure was high average and performance on the WMS-III Visual Reproduction subtest (Wechsler, 1997) copy trial was superior. He identified all stimuli correctly on the visual portion of the Reitan-Klove Sensory-perceptual Exam (Reitan & Wolfson, 1993), but he had significant difficulty with letter and line cancellation tasks and performed in the severely impaired range on JLO (Benton et al., 1983).

Conclusions of the Defense's Neuropsychologist. Consistent with results from the first neuropsychological evaluation, Mr. F.'s test results clearly indicated insufficient effort. Moreover, findings from both neuropsychological evaluations were strongly suggestive of deliberate malingering. Mr. F. performed in the insufficient range on all effort measures administered throughout the first and second neuropsychological evaluations.

During the second neuropsychological evaluation, following insufficient performance on the first day of testing, the VSVT (Slick et al., 1997) was readministered on the second day of testing in the context of new instructions that strongly encouraged better performance and strongly suggested he was capable of better performance. Notably, in terms of judging intent, he obtained worse scores on the "difficult" items during the second administration. In fact, his performance was well below chance level, with only 1 of 24 items correctly identified, strongly suggesting that he deliberately chose incorrect answers.

Contributing to the appearance of deliberate malingering, Mr. F. displayed different reading levels on the same task administered on two days of testing during the first neuropsychological evaluation, with worse scores on the second day. During the second neuropsychological evaluation, Mr. F. stated that he could not remember his own birth date, which is known not to occur even in individuals who have acquired dense amnesia (Wiggins & Brandt, 1988).

Additionally, there was a marked contrast in Mr. F.'s presentation demonstrated during examinations with his neurosurgeon and his presentation and performance during both neuropsychological evaluations. He was at times barely able to communicate during the evaluations by the neuropsychologists. Mr. F.'s neurosurgeon described Mr. F. as neurologically intact with only mild word-finding difficulty, and he testified during deposition that Mr. F. was capable of being employed.

Discrepancies that defy neuropsychological explanation also occurred across the neuropsychological evaluations. Whereas the plaintiff's neuropsychologist reported that Grooved Pegboard (Lafayette Instrument, 2002) performance was unattainable in the nondominant hand, the defense evaluation obtained a low-average performance. Dominant-hand Grooved Pegboard performance was four times faster during the defense evaluation! Further, a reading test was administered three times, twice by the plaintiff neuropsychologist and once by the defense neuropsychologist. Both the second and third administrations resulted in lower performances, both of which were well below a similar reading measure obtained during his rehabilitative treatments. Related, though unable to read even simple words when formally tested, Mr. F had

read a complex sentence during his deposition. During the defense neuropsychological evaluation, he was shown the same sentence and again was able to read it out loud and normally. Memory testing comparisons showed substantially better, though still impaired, performances on Logical Memory and Visual Reproduction of the WMS-III (Wechsler, 1997) on the defense neuropsychological evaluation.

The above examples are only the most glaring indications that strongly suggest Mr. F.'s level of impairment during both neuropsychological evaluations had been grossly exaggerated. By comparison, the detailed records from the rehabilitation professionals had described a much higher functioning individual. Given Mr. F.'s well-documented medical course following pituitary resection, it was recommended that the results from the two neuropsychological evaluations should not be used to inform litigation proceedings, as they were not credible. Rather, the extensive records from his rehabilitation treatment were recommended as a more reliable means of determining the neuropsychological sequelae of his illness, which were unquestionably present.

Conclusion of the Case

Deposition occurred 10 months following the second evaluation of Mr. F. By this point in the proceedings, a number of additional health-care professionals had been retained as experts, with some, including a physical medicine and rehabilitation physician, also expressing concern regarding the validity of Mr. F.'s ongoing symptom presentation. Unusual for a protracted litigation case, the lawsuit against both medical centers and all of the health-care providers involved was ultimately voluntarily withdrawn by the plaintiff's own attorney.

Contrast of Clinical Versus Forensic Context for Presentation of Poststroke Sequelae

In a routine clinical context, following a cerebral vascular accident there is a high risk of neuropsychological sequelae, which can be either temporary or in many cases permanent. The presence and nature of these sequelae are determined by such factors as neuroanatomic location, mechanism of cerebrovascular disorder (i.e., thrombosis, embolism, decreased perfusion, hemorrhage), as well as age and education of the patient (Festa, Lazar, & Marshall, 2008). Absent the effects of additional cerebrovascular disease or additional brain disorder, the recovery course typically shows improvement in function in many cases, most often during the months of rehabilitation efforts that follow neurological stabilization. In some individuals, little recovery of function occurs.

In a forensic context, it is most common to evaluate individuals whose medical and neurological status is stable. That is, if an acquired neurological disorder is present, it is most often the case that related litigation occurs long after the condition occurs. Thus, it is not only possible to compare the litigant's neuropsychological findings to those known to occur from the known or alleged neurological disorder, but also possible to compare the litigant's neuropsychological findings to extensive medical documentation that occurred closer in time to the onset of the disorder. In the instance of cerebrovascular accident, it is not expected that the litigant should be far worse than when discharged from extensive rehabilitation. It is also not expected that well-researched thresholds of effort tests and validity indicators will be surpassed, as these have commonly been put into practice only after research has demonstrated that genuine neurological disorders do not result in false positives. Thus, even though factors such as pain, depression, and anxiety are not uncommon in litigants, careful research has found that they do not explain effort test failure (e.g., Ashendorf, Constantinou, & McCaffrey, 2004; Greve, Ord, Curtis, Bianchini, & Brennan, in press; Iverson, Le Page, Koehler, Shojania, & Badii, 2007; Yanez, Fremouw, Tennant, Strunk, & Coker, 2006). In the instance of Mr. F, his findings were far worse than expected based on prior extensive medical records, and within both neuropsychological evaluations that were performed years after his cerebrovascular accident there were clear indications of insufficient effort and nonsensical findings.

Within forensic settings there has been an increasing demand of expert witnesses to render opinions that have scientific foundations. Though not substantially impacting removal of experts from cases whose opinions are not presented in a scientifically based manner (Dahir et al., 2005) or grossly changing the behavior of judges

(Cheng & Yoon, 2005), neuropsychologists likely have noticed an increase in pointed queries during depositions, whether as a treater or as a retained expert, that are aimed at establishing or identifying the lack of scientific bases for opinions (Groscup, Penrod, Studebaker, Huss, & O'Neil, 2002). Vague allusions to "clinical experience" as a basis for expert opinion are decreasingly of interest to attorneys and triers-of-fact. As noted previously in the introduction of this chapter, the strong scientist-practitioner approach in clinical neuropsychology is compatible with the evidentiary trends in the American legal system, and in part explains the increased demand for the services of clinical neuropsychologists with forensic cases. Importantly, a scientist-practitioner approach does not comport with post hoc ergo propter hoc reasoning, but rather seeks to examine the 'goodness of fit' of the cause-and-effect relationship at issue and in the course of doing so considers a full differential diagnosis, rather than simply seeking data that will confirm a favorite a priori hypothesis of a litigant or attorney. The present case provides a clear example in which gross brain dysfunction from a well-documented cause was subsequently confounded by malingering.

References

Ashendorf, L., Constantinou, M., & McCaffrey, R. (2004). The effect of depression and anxiety on the TOMM in community-dwelling older adults. *Archives of Clinical Neuropsychology, 19*, 125–130.

Benton, A., Hamsher, K. deS., & Sivan, A. (2000). *Multilingual Aphasia Examination: Manual of instructions* (3rd Ed.). Iowa City, IA: AJA Associates, Inc.

Benton, A. L., Hamsher, K. deS., Varney, N. R., & Spreen, O. (1983). *Judgment of line orientation*. New York: Oxford University Press.

Bernard, L., McGrath, M. & Houston, W. (1996). The differential effects of simulating malingering, closed head injury, and other CNS pathology on the Wisconsin Card Sorting Test: Support for the "pattern of performance" hypothesis. *Archives of Clinical Neuropsychology*, 11, 231–245

Boone, K. B., Salazar, X., Lu, P., Warner-Chacon, K., & Razani, J. (2002). The Rey 15-Item Recognition Trial: A technique to enhance sensitivity of the Rey 15-Item Memorization Test. *Journal of Clinical and Experimental Neuropsychology*, 24, 561–573.

Butcher, J. N., Dahlstrom, W. G., Graham, J. R., Tellegren, A., & Kaemmer, B. (1989). *MMPI-2: Manual for administration and scoring*. Minneapolis: University of Minnesota.

Cheng, E. K., & Yoon, A. H. (2005). Does *Frye* or *Daubert* matter? A study of scientific admissibility standards. *Virginia Law Review, 91*, 471–513.

Dahir, V. B., Richardson, J. T., Ginsburg, G. P., Gatowski, S. I., Dobbin, S. A., & Merlino, M. L. (2005). Judicial application of Daubert to psychological syndrome and profile evidence: A research note. *Psychology, Public Policy, and Law, 11*, 62–82.

Daubert vs. Merrell Dow Pharmaceuticals, 113 S. Ct. 2786 (1993).

Delis, D. C., Kramer, J. H., Kaplan, E., & Ober, B. A. (2000). *California Verbal Learning Test manual* (2nd ed.). San Antonio, TX: The Psychological Corporation.

Festa, J., Lazar, R., & Marshall, R. (2008). Ischemic stroke and aphasic disorders. In J. Morgan and J. Ricker (Eds.) *Textbook of clinical neuropsychology* (pp. 363-383). New York: Psychology Press.

General Electric Co. vs. Joiner, 522 U.S. 136 (1997).

Golden, C. J., & Freshwater, S. M. (2002). *Stroop Color and Word Test: Revised examiner's manual*. Wood Dale, IL: Stoelting Co.

Green, P. (2003). *Green's Word Memory Test for Windows: User's manual*. Seattle, WA: Green's Publishing, Inc.

Greve, K. W., Ord, J., Curtis, K. L., Bianchini, K. J., & Brennan, A. (2008). Detecting malingering in traumatic brain injury and chronic pain: A comparison of three forced-choice symptom validity tests. *The Clinical Neuropsychologist. 22*, 896-918.

Grigsby, J., & Kaye, K. (1996). *Behavioral Dyscontrol Scale manual* (2nd ed.). Unpublished Test Manual.

Groscup, J. L., Penrod, S. D., Studebaker, C. A., Huss, M. T., & O'Neil, K. M. (2002). The effects of Daubert on the admissibility of expert testimony in state and federal criminal cases. *Psychology, Public Policy, and Law, 8*, 339–372.

Heaton, R. K., Chelune, G. J., Talley, J. L., Kay, G. G., & Curtiss, G. (1993). *Wisconsin Card Sorting Test manual: Revised and expanded*. Lutz, FL: Psychological Assessment Resources, Inc.

Iverson, G. L., Le Page, J., Koehler, B. E., Shojania, K, & Badii, M. (2007). Test of Memory Malingering (TOMM) scores are not affected by chronic pain or depression in patients with fibromyalgia. *The Clinical Neuropsychologist, 21*, 532–546.

Kumho Tire vs. Carmichael, 526 U.S. 137 (1999).

King, J. H., Sweet, J. J., Sherer, M., Curtiss, G., & Vanderploeg, R. (2002). Validity indicators within the Wisconsin Card Sorting Test: Application of new and previously researched multivariate procedures in multiple traumatic brain injury samples. *The Clinical Neuropsychologist, 16*, 506–523.

Lafayette Instrument. (2002). *Grooved Pegboard Test: User instructions*. Lafayette, IN: Author.

Reitan, R. M., & Wolfson, D. (1993). *The Halstead-Reitan Neuropsychological Test Battery* (2nd ed.). Tucson, AZ: Neuropsychology Press.

Rozensky, R., Sweet, J., & Tovian, S. (1991). Toward program development: An integration of science and service. In J. Sweet, R. Rozensky, & S. Tovian (Eds.), *Handbook of clinical psychology in medical settings* (pp. 285–289). New York: Plenum.

Ruff, R. (1988). *Ruff Figural Fluency Test: Administration manual*. San Francisco: Neuropsychological Resources.

Sheridan, E., & Choca, J. (1991). Educational preparation and clinical training within a medical setting. In J. Sweet, R. Rozensky, & S. Tovian (Eds.), *Handbook of clinical psychology in medical settings* (pp. 45-58). New York: Plenum.

Slick, D., Hopp, G., Strauss, E., & Thompson, G. B. (1997). *Victoria Symptom Validity Test* (Version 1.0). Odessa, FL: Psychological Assessment Resources, Inc.

Suhr, J. A. & Boyer, D. (1999). Use of the Wisconsin Card Sorting Test in the detection of malingering in student simulator and patient samples. *Journal of Clinical and Experimental Neuropsychology, 21*, 701–708.

Sweet, J. (Ed.) (1999). *Forensic neuropsychology: Fundamentals and practice*. New York: Psychology Press.

Sweet, J., Ecklund-Johnson, E., & Malina, A. (2008). Overview of forensic neuropsychology. In J. E. Morgan & J. H. Ricker (Eds.) *Textbook of clinical neuropsychology* (pp. 869–890). New York: Taylor & Francis.

Tombaugh, T. N. (1996). *Test of Memory Malingering*. North Tonawanda, NY: Multi-Health Systems, Inc.

Tombaugh, T. N., Kozak, J., & Rees, L. (1999). Normative data stratified by age and education for two measures of verbal fluency: FAS and Animal Naming. *Archives of Clinical Neuropsychology, 14* (2), 167–177.

Wechsler, D. (1997). *Wechsler Adult Intelligence Scale: Administration and scoring manual* (3rd Ed.). Chicago: The Psychological Corporation.

Wechsler, D. (1997). *Wechsler Memory Scale: Administration and scoring manual* (3rd Ed.). Chicago: The Psychological Corporation.

Wiggins, E., & Brandt, J. (1988). The detection of simulated amnesia. *Law and Human Behavior, 12*, 57–78.

Wilkinson, G. S. & Robertson, G. J. (2006). *Wide Range Achievement Test: Professional manual* (4th Ed.). Lutz, FL: Psychological Assessment Resources, Inc.

Wilson, B. A., Cockburn, J., & Halligan, P. W. (1987). *Behavioral Inattention Test manual*. Oxford, England: Thames Valley Test Company.

Yanez, Y. T., Fremouw, W., Tennant, J., Strunk, J., & Coker, K. (2006). Effects of severe depression on TOMM performance among disability-seeking outpatients. *Archives of Clinical Neuropsychology, 21*, 161–166.

18

Moderate to Severe Traumatic Brain Injury

Tresa Roebuck-Spencer

Traumatic brain injury (TBI) describes the condition when a person acquires direct damage to brain tissue due to an external event, as opposed to brain insult from a developmental disorder or disease process. Estimates of the incidence of TBI within the United States include over 1.5 million new cases a year (Rutland-Brown, Langlois, Thomas, & Xi, 2006). Traumatic brain injury most commonly results from motor vehicles and falls, but it can occur from a wide range of causes. Rates of TBI are generally higher for men than women (Langlois, Rutland-Brown, & Wald, 2006) and peak between the ages of 15–24 and for persons greater than 64 (Kraus & Chu, 2005). Alcohol consumption (Smith & Kraus, 1988), prior brain injury (Salcido & Costich, 1992), and low socioeconomic status (Kraus, Fife, Ramstein, Conroy, & Cox, 1986) are also risks for TBI. The case within this chapter will focus on the expected effects of TBI and assessment of an individual with moderate to severe TBI.

The severity of TBI is best understood as falling on a continuum from mild to moderate to severe. Severity of injury is typically determined by level of consciousness at the time of injury as assessed by the Glasgow Coma Scale, with lower scores representing decreased responsiveness and more severe injury (Teasdale & Jennett, 1974). However, other frequently used classification schemes include duration of unconsciousness (e.g., time it takes to follow commands) and duration of posttraumatic amnesia (for review, see Roebuck-Spencer & Sherer, 2008). Indication of initial injury severity is valuable because it is strongly related to short- and long-term outcome and allows one to set general expectations about level of impairment and future recovery. For instance, individuals with moderate to severe TBI are more likely than those with mild TBI to require extensive rehabilitation services and to present with significant and persisting cognitive impairment affecting their ability to return to previous levels of functioning (Dikmen, Reitan, & Temkin, 1983; Harrison-Felix, Newton, Hall, & Kreutzer, 1996).

Moderate to severe TBI is almost always accompanied by observable damage to the brain and is often categorized as a closed versus open or penetrating brain injury. By definition, a closed brain injury involves no penetration of the skull or dura. This could include cases of blunt trauma from a fall or object striking the head and cases of acceleration/deceleration injuries from motor vehicle or other high-speed accidents. Open or penetrating brain injury occurs when an object penetrates the dura and causes direct damage to the brain (e.g., stab wounds, gun shot wounds, penetrating or comminuted skull fracture).

Because conditions resulting in a brain injury are so varied, there is no specific pattern of insult to the brain. Focal injury to the brain is most common after penetrating brain injury, blunt trauma, and acceleration/deceleration related coup-contra-coup injuries. Diffuse injury to the brain is typical following TBI with some of the most common findings including contusions, hematomas, and diffuse axonal injury. Because of abrasion of the brain against bony ridges of the skull, parenchymal contusions are common and often occur in a characteristic distribution involving the frontal and temporal poles, the lateral and inferior aspects of the frontal and temporal lobes, and less commonly the inferior aspects of the cerebellum (Levin, Williams, Eisenberg, High, & Guinto, 1992). Intracranial hematomas often result from tearing of bridging veins and arteries and include subarachnoid, epidural, and subdural hematomas. Hematomas often account for clinical deterioration in patients who initially present well (Rockswold, Leonard, & Nagib, 1987). Diffuse axonal injury refers to stretching and tearing of white matter tracts within the brain. Particularly vulnerable are the cerebral commissures and other white matter tracts of the brain stem (Gennarelli & Graham, 2005). Secondary or delayed complications can also occur following TBI, including swelling/edema, hypoxia/ischemia, raised intracranial pressure, and associated vascular changes (Gennarelli & Graham, 2005).

Individuals with moderate to severe TBI pass through a series of predictable stages of recovery. However, not all individuals will experience all stages, and length of time in each stage varies widely across individuals. By definition, the individual with moderate to severe TBI will experience some loss of consciousness as a result of his/her injury. When this loss of consciousness is prolonged, the individual is described as being in coma. Coma is defined as a period of time in which a person is unresponsive to all stimuli (Teasdale & Jennett, 1974). Following coma, individuals may progress to slightly more responsive states, defined as persistent vegetative state or minimally conscious state (Giacino et al., 2002; Jennett, 2002). Some individuals may not progress past these stages, but those who do typically progress to a responsive but confused state, commonly referred to as a period of posttraumatic amnesia (PTA) or posttraumatic confusion in which the individual is disoriented, confused, responds inappropriately to stimuli, has poor attention, and is generally unable to form new memories (Levin, 1992). Often, the individual with TBI will retain few if any memories while in this stage. Typically, a person is considered to have progressed past this stage once he or she is consistently oriented and can learn and recall events in a continuous fashion.

Following resolution of these initial recovery stages, individuals with moderate to severe TBI typically continue to present with a diverse range of cognitive changes. The magnitude and pattern of cognitive impairment varies as a function of severity of injury, time since injury, and mechanism of injury. Early following injury, almost all areas of cognitive functioning can be affected (Dikmen, McLean, Temkin, & Wyler, 1986) with severity of injury predicting greater severity of cognitive impairment (Dikmen & Machamer, 1995; Tabaddor, Mattis, & Zazula, 1984). Over time cognitive functioning typically improves, with less complex areas of cognition (simple attention) improving prior to more complex areas (problem solving, judgment, etc.) (Dikmen et al., 1983). Diffuse cognitive impairment is generally the rule, particularly following closed brain injuries or acceleration/deceleration injuries. However, individuals with blunt trauma or penetrating brain injury may present with focal as well as diffuse cognitive impairments. Although a specific pattern of cognitive impairment following TBI is typically not observed, the most commonly described impairments occur in the domains of attention, processing speed, learning and memory, and executive functioning (Roebuck-Spencer & Sherer, 2008). It is not uncommon to see less-affected or spared intellectual functioning (Johnstone, Hexum, & Ashkanazi, 1995). Individuals are expected to continue to show cognitive recovery over the first 2 years following injury (Dikmen, Machamer, Temkin, & McLean, 1990; Dikmen et al., 1983; Tabaddor et al., 1984) with some showing evidence of improvement even after this point (Millis et al., 2001).

In addition to cognitive impairments, individuals with TBI also show a range of neurobehavioral and emotional changes. The most common neurobehavioral changes include impulsivity, disinhibition, decreased initiation, decreased self-awareness, poor social judgment, and impaired emotional regulation (all associated with frontal systems dysfunction; for review, see Roebuck-Spencer, Banõs, Sherer, & Novack, 2010). Additionally, rates of depression and anxiety can be quite high following moderate to severe TBI (Kim et al., 2007; Rogers & Read, 2007). Rates of affective disorders may be a result of symptom overlap with other neurobehavioral syndromes (e.g., apathy, fatigue, etc), changes in brain function as a result of the injury, or psychosocial stressors related to the injury and emerging awareness of impairments. Although the most severe neurobehavioral problems tend to improve with time, they are often enduring and can place a greater burden on caregivers than other physical or cognitive impairments following TBI (Riley, 2007). They are often the primary reason individuals with TBI have difficulty returning to previous family roles and community activities such as employment, education, driving, and engagement in leisure activities (Winkler, Unsworth, & Sloan, 2006).

With such a range of cognitive and neurobehavioral changes, neuropsychologists are well suited to provide evaluation and treatment of patients with moderate to severe TBI. Neuropsychologists are often called upon in inpatient settings to evaluate stage of recovery, assist with behavioral management plans, and provide family education and planning. At later stages of recovery and in outpatient settings, neuropsychologists are often asked to address referral questions, including supervision/guardianship needs, ability to return to work or school, and need for additional treatments/psychotropic medication. Notably, it is not always cognitive problems that initiate a referral and many times a patient may present for evaluation due to concerns about emotional and behavioral functioning.

Case of M. R.

M. R. is a 48-year-old, Caucasian, male with history of TBI who presented for an outpatient comprehensive neuropsychological evaluation. He was referred by his treating neurologist to document current level of cognitive functioning and to provide recommendations about treatment options and supervision needs. This question was prompted by a recent medication change that led to an adverse reaction (e.g., obvious mental status changes) and concerns from the family about the patient's ability to continue to live independently. Information for the present evaluation was obtained from a clinical interview with M. R., a telephone interview with the patient's brother, and review of available medical records.

M. R. sustained a TBI as a result of a motor vehicle accident 3 years prior to the evaluation.

Medical records related to acute aspects of this injury were not available. Telephone interview with the patient's brother (with appropriate consents) revealed that directly following his accident, M. R. was in a coma for approximately 4–6 weeks and required comprehensive inpatient rehabilitation for several months. He subsequently received outpatient physical and cognitive rehabilitation for several more months. By patient's independent recall, he had retrograde posttraumatic amnesia for an unspecified time prior to the accident and recalled no events for several months following the accident. Although an estimate, reported length of coma and posttraumatic amnesia indicates that M. R. most likely sustained a severe TBI.

M. R.'s brother reported that initial magnetic resonance imaging (MRI) of the brain demonstrated "shear injury" (i.e., diffuse axonal injury). Records of an MRI of the brain conducted 7 months following his accident revealed mild focal atrophy of the left perisylvian area and asymmetric dilation of the left lateral ventricle consistent with left side head laceration. These findings were read as consistent with TBI and considered improved compared with initial neuroimaging (not available for review).

Following discharge from the hospital, M. R. initially required 24-hour supervision from his family and slowly recovered to the extent that he could live alone. At the time of the current neuropsychological evaluation, he had returned to living alone with the support of daily 5-hour visits from a care provider to assist with household chores and cooking. Additionally, he had court-appointed personal and financial guardians. He had not worked since his accident and was receiving disability benefits. Just prior to this evaluation, M. R. had been prescribed Amantadine with resulting behavioral and cognitive changes, including confusion, poor attention, and disorganized behavior. His brother noted that his cognitive abilities and behavior had improved to baseline levels since discontinuation of this medication.

At the time of the evaluation, M. R. was in good health. His medical history was significant only for asthma. Surgical history prior to his accident was unremarkable. There was no reported history of other neurological disorders, including previous significant brain injuries, strokes, or seizures. Current medications included Zoloft (100 mg q.d.). He reported no side effects of Zoloft, but he was unsure why he was taking this medication. Recent clinic notes from his neurologist indicated near-normal neurological exam with a mini-mental state examination (MMSE) of 27/30 (lost points for orientation and memory recall). Cranial nerves were reported as normal. Reported gait was wide based with ataxia in the right leg. He performed toe/heel walk with difficulty and was slow to perform rapid alternating movements. Muscle tone, bulk, and strength were normal. Sensory exam was normal for all modalities tested. Reflexes were normal with the exception of brisk reflexes at the right knee. He showed a bilateral extensor plantar response. His neurologic exam was considered unchanged since his previous visit 1 year prior with the exception of an improved MMSE.

With regard to psychiatric history, M. R. denied any prior diagnoses or hospitalization. However, he did report a suicide attempt at age 18 over a breakup with a girlfriend. He denied any other past or current episodes of suicidal ideation. His brother reported a suspicion that he was depressed throughout his life. M. R. reported consuming approximately six beers per week and occasional marijuana use prior to his accident but denied abuse or dependence on these substances. In contrast, his brother reported periods of heavy drinking throughout his adult life and believed that M. R. was likely an alcoholic. He reported drinking binges at family gatherings but was unaware whether his drinking ever interfered with vocational responsibilities. He denied knowledge of him ever receiving substance abuse treatment. At the time of the evaluation, M. R. reported that he drank alcohol and consumed marijuana on an infrequent basis and smoked just under a pack/day of cigarettes.

M. R. worked as a computer support technician for a major computer company for 15 years prior to his accident. He was a "C" student and completed high school and 2 years toward an associate's degree. He denied any history of learning disabilities or need for special classes in school. He was divorced prior to his accident and has three adult children. He had recently broken up with a long-term girlfriend just prior to the accident. At the time of the evaluation, M. R. was living alone with supports described above. He had few friends and his family lived in a separate state. He had not returned to driving, and public transportation was limited due to the remote location of his home. He spent most of his time alone rebuilding computers in his basement.

Behavioral Observations

M. R. was brought to his appointment by his brother. He was appropriately groomed, made good eye contact, and was very talkative. He was able to present basic biographical information accurately, but he was not oriented to month, date, or day of the week. He was also not oriented to city, but it is notable that he had traveled from his place of residence to a different state to complete the evaluation. Reported mood was "mediocre," and he displayed a full range of affect appropriate to conversation topic. Speech was slightly accelerated in rate but normal in volume and rhythm. No evidence of confusion or thought disorder was observed; however, the content of his conversational speech was tangential and repetitive. He tended to perseverate on what appeared to be paranoid thoughts that his family and others have stolen from him and may be trying to control his life. These concerns were voiced both during the interview and at inappropriate times during the testing, requiring frequent redirection to task. Decreased self-awareness was also evident. He acknowledged needing help with some household tasks, but he lacked appreciation of his impaired functioning and the severity of his brain injury. He frequently stated that he did not need help or supervision and would, if allowed, be able to return to work and educational endeavors without problem. Gait was unsteady and he walked with a cane. There was no evidence of abnormal motor movements or tremor in his extremities.

M. R.'s behavior during testing was pleasant and cooperative. Auditory comprehension was intact, and he generally understood all task directions without problem. His attention skills were variable, with a tendency to become easily distracted from task, requiring redirection from the examiner. He reported no visual or auditory problems that might have interfered with testing. He attempted all tasks presented and appeared to be motivated to perform his best at all times. There was no obvious behavioral evidence of poor effort or impulsivity, and his frustration tolerance was good.

Test Results

All test names and scores are included in Table 18-1. Overall intellectual functioning was assessed to be in the average range of functioning, consistent with average estimates of his premorbid intellectual functioning.

Despite evidence of greater left than right hemisphere damage on MRI scans, focal language impairments were not evident on testing. Spontaneous speech was fluent and prosodic with no evidence of word-finding problems or paraphasias. Formal assessment of confrontation

Table 18-1. Summary Table of Neuropsychological Test Scores

Global Functioning	Scores	Percentiles
WAIS-III FSIQ (prorated)	StS = 97	42nd percentile
Reading Subtest of the WRAT-3	StS = 96	39th percentile
Language Tests		
Boston Naming Test (57/60 correct)	z = +0.54	71st percentile
WAIS-III Vocabulary	ScS = 10	50th percentile
WAIS-III Similarities	ScS = 8	25th percentile
WAIS-III Information	ScS = 8	25th percentile
Visual Spatial Tests		
Rey Complex Figure–Copy	34/36 points	43rd percentile
Judgment of Line Orientation		22nd percentile
WAIS-III Block Design	ScS = 9	37rd percentile
WAIS-III Matrix Reasoning	ScS = 13	84th percentile
Attention/Concentration		
WAIS-III Digit Span	ScS = 12	75th percentile
WAIS-III Arithmetic	ScS = 9	37rd percentile
Auditory Consonant Trigrams		
9 second	z = −1.59	6th percentile
18 second	z = −1.45	7th percentile
36 second	z = −.95	17th percentile
Learning and Memory		
WMS-III Subtests		
Logical Memory I	ScS = 8	25th percentile
Logical Memory II	ScS = 7	16th percentile
Logical Memory retention (57%)	ScS = 7	16th percentile
Visual Reproduction I	ScS = 5	5th percentile
Visual Reproduction II	ScS = 3	1st percentile
Visual Reproduction Retention (0%)	ScS = 2	<1st percentile
Visual Reproduction Recognition	ScS = 4	2nd percentile
Rey Auditory Verbal Learning**		
Trial 1 (6/15 words)	z = −.22	41st percentile
Trial 5 (8/15 words)	z = −1.45	7th percentile
Total Learning	z = −1.27	10th percentile
Immediate delay (4/15 words)	z = −2.28	<1st percentile
Long Delay (0/15 words)	z = −3.89	<1st percentile
Yes/No Recognition	11 hits; 4 FPs	
Rey Complex Figure Delay		
Short Delay	T = 25	1st percentile
Long Delay	T = <20	<1st percentile

(Continued)

Table 18-1. Summary Table of Neuropsychological Test Scores (*Continued*)

Global Functioning	Scores	Percentiles
Fine Motor Skills		
Tapping DH*	T = 50	50th percentile
Tapping NDH*	T = 38	12th percentile
Grooved Pegboard DH*	T = 21	<1st percentile
Grooved Pegboard NDH*	T = 23	<1st percentile
Processing Speed		
Trail-Making Test, Part A* (45 sec; 0 errors)	T = 35	7th percentile
Symbol Digit Modalities Test		
Written	z = −2.0	2nd percentile
Oral	z = −2.35	1st percentile
Stroop Color Word Test		
Word Reading	T = 27	1st percentile
Color Naming	T = 26	<1st percentile
Executive Functioning		
Verbal Fluency		
Phonemic fluency (FAS)	z = −.78	22nd percentile
Semantic fluency (Animals)	z = −.91	18th percentile
Trail-Making Test, Part B* (105 sec; 0 errors)	T = 39	14th percentile
Stroop Color Word Test–Color Word Condition	T = 29	2nd percentile
Wisconsin Card Sorting Test*		
Total Errors	T = 32	4th percentile
Perseverative Errors	T = 31	3rd percentile
Total Categories	5	11–16th percentile
Symptom Validity		
Test of Memory and Malingering		
Trial 1	49/50	
Trial 2	50/50	
Emotional Functioning		
Beck Depression Inventory–II	10	
Carroll Depression Scale	12	

Note. All standardized scores were corrected for age.

*Scores are corrected for age, sex, and education.

**Scores are corrected for age and sex.

ScS, scaled Score; z, z score; StS, standard score; T, T score; WAIS-III, Wechsler Adult Intelligence Scale–Third Edition; WMS-III, Wechsler Memory Scale–Third Edition; WRAT-3, Wide Range Achievement Test–Third Edition.

naming was in the average range. Verbal subtests of the WAIS-III measuring vocabulary, verbal abstraction, and general fund of knowledge were average to low average.

Performance on tests of spatial-perceptual skills was within normal limits overall. Construction of the Rey-Osterrieth Complex Figure was in the average range with no gross distortions. Perception of spatial relationships was low average (Judgment of Line Orientation 22nd percentile). His command and copy drawings of

a clock were spatially and conceptually accurate. On WAIS-III nonverbal tests, he performed in the average to high-average range on tests of block construction and visual spatial problem solving.

Performance on tests of attention and concentration varied considerably. He recalled six digits forward and seven digits backward on WAIS-III Digit Span. He performed in the average range on a test of mental arithmetic and concentration. On the Auditory Consonant Trigrams test, which required him to perform two tasks concurrently, his performance ranged from the low average to mildly to moderately impaired range across trials.

There was clear evidence of learning and memory impairment with worsening performance as tests became more complex in nature or required more active organization of information. Memory for short stories was low average for his age after immediate and delayed recall trials. He retained only 57% of initially recalled information over time. Initial learning on a word-list task was in the low-average range, and his responses were notable for a large number of perseverative and intrusion errors. Learning slope was decreased over subsequent trials. Performance was impaired following an interference trial and worsened following a long delay. Recognition memory on a yes/no forced-choice task was also impaired, with correct recall of only 11/15 words and four false-positive errors.

Memory impairments were also present on tests of visual memory. Recall of geometric designs was impaired after immediate and long delays, with 0% retention of information over time. His performance showed little improvement on a yes/no recognition trial. Memory for the Rey-Osterrieth Complex Figure was impaired following short and long delays with only 21% retention of information over time. This pattern of performance across tests of verbal and visual memory was indicative of problems both learning and retaining new information.

No gross sensory deficits were observed. Consistent asymmetries in motor performance were not observed on tests of fine motor skills. Finger-tapping speed was average with his dominant (right) hand but mildly impaired with his non-dominant hand. Fine-motor speed and coordination on the Grooved Pegboard Test was moderately to severely impaired bilaterally.

Speed and efficiency of information processing was impaired across all tests assessing this domain. Processing speed and sequencing ability was mildly impaired. On the Symbol Digit Modalities Test, he performed in the impaired range. Based on comparison of the written and oral versions, impairments cannot be attributable to slowed motor speed alone. He also performed in the impaired range on tests of word reading and color naming.

Performance on complex executive reasoning tasks was generally lower than expected based on assessed intellectual functioning. Phonemic and semantic verbal fluency were in the low-average range. On Part B of the Trailmaking Test, psychomotor speed and cognitive flexibility were mildly impaired. Response inhibition was impaired. Impairments were also seen on a test of novel problem solving measuring complex reasoning and mental flexibility. He had difficulty switching strategies in response to feedback and perseverated on incorrect strategies for many trials before attempting a new solution.

M. R. endorsed few symptoms of depression in the clinical interview and on a self-report mood measure. Evidence of mild depression symptoms were evident based on his responses to a less face-valid depression measure. He endorsed symptoms of anhedonia, cognitive and physical difficulties, and feelings of worthlessness and hopelessness. Completion of a more extensive personality measure, such as the MMPI-2 was decided against, given fluctuating level of attention throughout the testing day and a continual need to redirect him to task.

On a test of effort or symptom validity, M. R. performed above threshold for suspected poor effort or malingering. There was no behavioral indication of poor effort or obvious evidence of secondary gain. Thus, aforementioned test results are believed to accurately reflect his current level of cognitive functioning. In contrast to many individuals attempting to exaggerate cognitive impairment, it was clear that M. R. believed he had minimal cognitive impairment, required less supervision than he was receiving, and should be allowed more independence with functional activities.

Conclusions

M. R.'s neuropsychological testing revealed average intellectual abilities consistent with the literature demonstrating that overall IQ is often preserved following TBI (Johnstone et al., 1995). Despite evidence of relatively focal injury to the left hemisphere on early MRI scans, M. R.'s basic language and visual spatial skills were generally preserved with no strong evidence of focal or lateralized impairment. Consistent with the literature on moderate to severe TBI, M. R. presented with diffuse cognitive impairment concentrated in the areas of working memory, speed of information processing, learning and memory, and executive functioning. Variable attention skills were evident on testing and behavioral observation, with worsening attention on more complex tasks. Slowed psychomotor speed was prominent across all tests administered in this domain. Learning and memory of verbal and visual information was impaired with evidence of both recall and encoding difficulties. Notably, performance improved when information was presented in an organized or contextual format. Finally, he demonstrated significant difficulties across tests of executive functioning, including difficulties on tests of novel problem solving, response inhibition, and cognitive flexibility.

In addition to above cognitive impairments, M. R. also demonstrated a range of neurobehavioral changes commonly associated with moderate to severe TBI. Decreased self-awareness was evident, illustrated by discrepancies between his description of his own abilities in comparison to test findings and life situation and by discrepancies between his and his brother's perception of his impairments and abilities. Awareness of social situations and judgment also were impaired. For instance, not described earlier were reports from his brother of a tendency to trust individuals that had taken advantage of him financially in the past. M. R. was also very candid in describing his continued use of alcohol and marijuana without appreciation for the potential hazards of this behavior. Also observed in the evaluation were behavioral regulation problems such as difficulty consistently maintaining attention, difficulty maintaining appropriate conversational topics, and some paranoid ideation.

Neurobehavioral changes, particularly decreased self-awareness, present significant challenges to caregivers and treating health professionals working with patients with TBI. Despite areas of intact cognition, neurobehavioral changes will limit M. R.'s ability to independently make decisions and be aware of his own limitations. Thus, it is essential to consider results of cognitive testing in combination with neurobehavioral changes. Impaired memory and self-awareness will limit a patient's ability to independently provide accurate information about history and current functioning. These problems will also limit a patient's

ability to remember, appreciate, and follow through with recommendations. Therefore, the clinician must carefully assess for the presence of neurobehavioral change through behavioral observation and interview with a collateral source that knows the patient well both before and after injury. It may also be necessary, with permission of the patient or guardian, to provide feedback and recommendations to a caregiver to maximize benefit to the patient.

Neuropsychologists are frequently asked to provide opinions about prognosis for future recovery and the likelihood of a patient's ability to return to work or other functional activities. Based on M. R.'s brother's description of cognitive impairment shortly after his injury and a neurology note documenting improved MMSE scores over the previous year, it is very likely that he has already shown significant cognitive recovery over time. Given that his injury occurred 3 years prior to the evaluation, M. R.'s cognitive functioning and overall clinical presentation is not expected to improve substantially. However, while neurological impairments typically plateau over time, functional status, including return to social and community activities, can occur over many years (Sander, Roebuck, Struchen, Sherer, & High, 2001).

Functional implications of neuropsychological test results are important to address to assist with determination of supervision level. It was predicted that M. R. would have difficulty performing unstructured tasks or projects without some external support. He was also expected to have trouble completing tasks that required speeded performance or deadlines. While his simple attentional skills were quite good, it was predicted that he would likely have trouble maintaining attention over time, when in a distracting or stressful environment, or when required to perform multiple tasks at one time. He will likely have trouble learning new information and remembering important information over time without reminders or compensatory aids. Due to executive dysfunction and problems with decision making, awareness, and judgment, he will likely have trouble planning and implementing optimal responses when confronted with difficult social situations or problems. Despite these problems, the impacts of his impairments on everyday functioning could be reduced with continued utilization of external supports (e.g., home health aid, financial guardian, etc.) and utilization of compensatory strategies (e.g., memory notebooks, calendars, check-in calls from family, pill boxes for medications, etc.), allowing him to maintain his current level of independence.

Recommendations also included provision of feedback to the patient, his family, and personal guardian. It is important that feedback include an opportunity to ask questions and receive psychoeducation about TBI. This can be particularly helpful for families by putting problematic behaviors into perspective and helping families to understand that some behaviors are related to the injury and are not due to decreased motivation or defiance. It also helps the patient and family make plans for the future and determine needed levels of supervision.

M. R.'s family and personal guardian were particularly interested in whether his current level of supervision was appropriate and whether he should move closer to family. M. R. expressed a clear desire to remain in his current living situation. Given test results and that the patient was living alone far from family with limited social supports, continued guardianship and home health-care services were recommended. Alternatively, it was not believed that safety risks were present to a strong enough degree to outweigh M. R.'s personal preference to remain in his current living situation. While it was clear that M. R.'s cognitive and neurobehavioral impairments would limit his ability to accurately manage financial affairs in a timely manner, it was acknowledged that he had the cognitive ability to understand and be informed of his financial status and be included in important decisions regarding his medical and financial affairs. It was suggested that inclusion in such decisions may reduce his paranoid thinking and concerns that others are trying to steal from him and "control" his life. Finding an appropriate balance between safety concerns and respect for the patient's independent choices can be a challenge in these cases.

Rates of substance abuse prior to TBI and risk for continued substance abuse following TBI are high, placing these individuals at risk for exacerbation of impairments, poorer outcome, ongoing safety risks, and future injuries (Corrigan, 1995; Corrigan, Rust, & Lamb-Hart, 1995). In this case,

it was recommended that M. R. abstain from alcohol and marijuana use because such use may exacerbate impairments in cognition, decision making, and judgment. Removal of alcohol and other substances from the home was recommended. M. R. did not have access to a personal vehicle, so concerns for driving unsafely or driving to acquire such substances were abated.

Consideration of comorbid psychiatric issues should also be addressed. Given history of depression, current report of mild depression symptoms, and social isolation, it was recommend that M. R. continue with his current antidepressant medication and that his emotional status be followed regularly by a neurologist or psychiatrist. It was also suggested that he might benefit from a support group with TBI survivors. Given his decreased self-awareness, individual psychotherapy was not recommended.

M. R.'s family and referring physician were particularly interested in potential treatment options. Unfortunately, treatment options decrease as the time since injury increases. Outpatient postacute rehabilitation programs can be beneficial for TBI survivors, particularly those programs that incorporate cognitive rehabilitation and decreased self-awareness into the treatment program. A program with a focus on community reintegration and social skills training would be ideal for M. R. Although postacute rehabilitation programs typically treat patients early in the recovery course (i.e., initially following discharge from inpatient rehabilitation), there is support in the literature that such programs can also improve the functional outcome of individuals at more chronic phases as well (High, Roebuck-Spencer, Sander, Struchen, & Sherer, 2006). However, given that needs for physical and occupational therapy decrease over time, funding for such programs can be limited. Alternatively, M. R. would benefit from participation in a vocational rehabilitation program that would increase his opportunities for vocational training, return to employment, volunteer work, etc. These programs can also help to decrease social isolation. Such services are often available through regional disability programs, but availability and funding opportunities differ from state to state. Unfortunately dwindling access to and funding for these types of services is fast becoming the norm. M. R. and his family were encouraged to explore such brain injury resources within his community and through local chapters of the brain injury association (http://www.biausa.org).

Because TBI frequently occurs as a result of an unexpected event or accident, litigation is often involved or often becomes an issue subsequent to the evaluation. Other secondary gain issues can be prominent as well. Thus, measurement of effort and symptom validity is essential in these cases. While this issue is often more prominent in mild TBI (Iverson, 2005; Mooney, Speed, & Sheppard, 2005), it should not be overlooked in the evaluation of moderate to severe TBI. Documentation of injury severity and current cognitive impairment is not enough to support a claim of TBI-related cognitive changes given that individuals typically improve over time, other medical or psychiatric conditions may be comorbid with the injury, and individuals with true impairment are not immune to exaggeration of deficits.

In summary, this case illustrates a fairly typical presentation of a patient with moderate to severe TBI presenting several years post injury. This case is unique in that this individual was able to return to independent living with external supports in place. Highlighted by this case is the importance of considering comorbid issues, assessing neurobehavioral problems, and being aware of the literature on treatment options and outcome following TBI. Because of the unique problems encountered by these patients and their families, neuropsychologists have the potential to make a strong impact on their care and overall quality of life.

References

Corrigan, J. D. (1995). Substance abuse as a mediating factor in outcome from traumatic brain injury. *Archives of Physical Medicine and Rehabilitation, 76*(4), 302–309.

Corrigan, J. D., Rust, E., & Lamb-Hart, G. L. (1995). The nature and extent of substance abuse problems in persons with traumatic brain injury. *Journal of Head Trauma Rehabilitation, 10*(3), 29–46.

Dikmen, S., & Machamer, J. (1995). Neurobehavioral outcomes and their determinants. *Journal of Head Trauma Rehabilitation, 10*, 74–86.

Dikmen, S., Machamer, J., Temkin, N., & McLean, A. (1990). Neuropsychological recovery in patients with moderate to severe head injury: 2 year follow-up.

Journal of Clinical and Experimental Neuropsychology, 12*(4), 507–519.

Dikmen, S., McLean, A., Jr., Temkin, N. R., & Wyler, A. R. (1986). Neuropsychologic outcome at one-month postinjury. *Archives of Physical Medicine and Rehabilitation, 67*(8), 507–513.

Dikmen, S., Reitan, R. M., & Temkin, N. R. (1983). Neuropsychological recovery in head injury. *Archives of Neurology, 40*(6), 333–338.

Gennarelli, T. A., & Graham, D. I. (2005). Neuropathology. In J. M. Silver, T. W. McAllister, & S. C. Yudofsky (Eds.), *Textbook of traumatic brain injury* (pp. 27–50). Washington, DC: American Psychiatric Publishing, Inc.

Giacino, J. T., Ashwal, S., Childs, N., Cranford, R., Jennett, B., Katz, D. I., et al. (2002). The minimally conscious state: Definition and diagnostic criteria. *Neurology, 58*(3), 349–353.

Harrison-Felix, C., Newton, C. N., Hall, K. M., & Kreutzer, J. S. (1996). Descriptive findings from the traumatic brain injury model systems national data base. *Journal of Head Trauma Rehabilitation, 11*(5), 1–14.

High, W. M., Jr., Roebuck-Spencer, T., Sander, A. M., Struchen, M. A., & Sherer, M. (2006). Early versus later admission to postacute rehabilitation: impact on functional outcome after traumatic brain injury. *Archives of Physical Medicine and Rehabilitation, 87*(3), 334–342.

Iverson, G. L. (2005). Outcome from mild traumatic brain injury. *Current Opinion in Psychiatry, 18*(3), 301–317.

Jennett, B. (2002). The vegetative state. *Journal of Neurology, Neurosurgery and Psychiatry, 73*(4), 355–357.

Johnstone, B., Hexum, C. L., & Ashkanazi, G. (1995). Extent of cognitive decline in traumatic brain injury based on estimates of premorbid intelligence. *Brain Injury, 9*(4), 377–384.

Kim, E., Lauterbach, E. C., Reeve, A., Arciniegas, D. B., Coburn, K. L., Mendez, M. F., et al. (2007). Neuropsychiatric complications of traumatic brain injury: A critical review of the literature (a report by the ANPA Committee on Research). *Journal Neuropsychiatry and Clinical Neurosciences, 19*(2), 106–127.

Kraus, J. F., & Chu, L. D. (2005). Epidemiology. In J. M. Silver, T. W. McAllister, & S. C. Yudofsky (Eds.), *Textbook of traumatic brain injury* (pp. 3–26). Washington, DC: American Psychiatric Publishing, Inc.

Kraus, J. F., Fife, D., Ramstein, K., Conroy, C., & Cox, P. (1986). The relationship of family income to the incidence, external causes, and outcomes of serious brain injury, San Diego County, California. *American Journal of Public Health, 76*(11), 1345–1347.

Langlois, J. A., Rutland-Brown, W., & Wald, M. M. (2006). The epidemiology and impact of traumatic brain injury: A brief overview. *Journal of Head Trauma Rehabilitation, 21*(5), 375–378.

Levin, H. S. (1992). Neurobehavioral recovery. *Journal of Neurotrauma, 9*(Suppl. 1), S359–S373.

Levin, H. S., Williams, D. H., Eisenberg, H. M., High, W. M., Jr., & Guinto, F. C., Jr. (1992). Serial MRI and neurobehavioural findings after mild to moderate closed head injury. *Journal of Neurology, Neurosurgery and Psychiatry, 55*(4), 255–262.

Millis, S. R., Rosenthal, M., Novack, T. A., Sherer, M., Nick, T. G., Kreutzer, J. S., et al. (2001). Long-term neuropsychological outcome after traumatic brain injury. *Journal of Head Trauma Rehabilitation, 16*(4), 343–355.

Mooney, G., Speed, J., & Sheppard, S. (2005). Factors related to recovery after mild traumatic brain injury. *Brain Injury, 19*(12), 975–987.

Riley, G. A. (2007). Stress and depression in family carers following traumatic brain injury: The influence of beliefs about difficult behaviours. *Clinical Rehabilitation, 21*(1), 82–88.

Rockswold, G. L., Leonard, P. R., & Nagib, M. G. (1987). Analysis of management in thirty-three closed head injury patients who "talked and deteriorated". *Neurosurgery, 21*(1), 51–55.

Roebuck-Spencer, T. M., Banõs, J., Sherer, M., & Novack, T. (2010). Neurobehavioral aspects of traumatic brain injury sustained in adulthood. In S. Hunter & J. Donders (Eds.), *Principles and practice of lifespan developmental neuropsychology* (pp. 328–344). New York: Cambridge University Press.

Roebuck-Spencer, T. M., & Sherer, M. (2008). Moderate and severe traumatic brain injury. In J. E. Morgan & J. H. Ricker (Eds.), *Textbook of clinical neuropsychology* (pp. 411–429). New York: Taylor & Francis Group.

Rogers, J. M., & Read, C. A. (2007). Psychiatric comorbidity following traumatic brain injury. *Brain Injury, 21*(13–14), 1321–1333.

Rutland-Brown, W., Langlois, J. A., Thomas, K. E., & Xi, Y. L. (2006). Incidence of traumatic brain injury in the United States, 2003. *Journal of Head Trauma Rehabilitation, 21*(6), 544–548.

Salcido, R., & Costich, J. F. (1992). Recurrent traumatic brain injury. *Brain Injury, 6*(3), 293–298.

Sander, A. M., Roebuck, T. M., Struchen, M. A., Sherer, M., & High, W. M., Jr. (2001). Long-term maintenance of gains obtained in postacute rehabilitation by persons with traumatic brain injury. *Journal of Head Trauma Rehabilitation, 16*(4), 1–19.

Smith, G. S., & Kraus, J. F. (1988). Alcohol and residential, recreational, and occupational injuries: A review of the epidemiologic evidence. *Annual Review of Public Health, 9*, 99–121.

Tabaddor, K., Mattis, S., & Zazula, T. (1984). Cognitive sequelae and recovery course after moderate and severe head injury. *Neurosurgery, 14*(6), 701–708.

Teasdale, G., & Jennett, B. (1974). Assessment of coma and impaired consciousness. A practical scale. *Lancet, 2*(7872), 81–84.

Winkler, D., Unsworth, C., & Sloan, S. (2006). Factors that lead to successful community integration following severe traumatic brain injury. *Journal of Head Trauma Rehabilitation, 21*(1), 8–21.

19

Why Would He Do It? A Case of Probable Malingering in the Context of Severe Traumatic Brain Injury

Daniel J. Slick, Jing E. Tan, and Esther Strauss[†]

This chapter presents a case of probable malingering. The subject is a young adult male who sustained a severe traumatic brain injury (TBI) and was subsequently seen by one of the authors (D. J. S.) for independent examination. Topics covered include *(1)* a brief general review of TBI; *(2)* differential diagnosis of malingering and related conditions; *(3)* methods for detecting noncompliance during neuropsychological assessment; and finally *(4)* an individual case that raises a number of the issues covered.

Traumatic Brain Injuries

Injuries to the brain are defined as *traumatic* when they occur as a result of external physical forces, including any combination of acceleration/deceleration/rotational forces, impact by or against an object, or penetration of the skull by an object. It is now well recognized that TBIs can occur in the absence of any impact or penetration of the skull (see Gaetz, 2004 for an excellent review of TBI pathophysiology). Traumatic brain injuries result in a very substantial number of deaths and cases of permanent disability annually. The U.S. Centers for Disease Control and Prevention (CDC) estimates that approximately 1.4 million people sustain a TBI each year in the United States. Of these, roughly 50,000 die, 235,000 are hospitalized, and 1.1 million are treated and released from an emergency department. It is estimated that 1.6–3.8 million

sports- and recreation-related TBIs occur in the United States each year, most of which are mild TBIs that are not treated in a hospital or emergency department. About 2% of the U.S. population—at least 5.3 million people—have long-term or permanent disabilities as a result of a TBI. The total direct and indirect costs associated with TBIs in the United States in 2000 have been estimated at $60 billion (Langlois, Rutland-Brown, & Thomas, 2006).

There are a number of well-established risk factors for TBI, including sex, age, race, occupation, and socioeconomic status. Overall, males are about twice as likely as females to sustain a TBI. Children between 0 to 4 years of age and adolescents and young adults between 15 to 19 years of age are at the highest risk for sustaining a TBI, while adults age 75 years or older have the highest rates of TBI-related hospitalization and death. Certain occupations, such as active duty military service, are associated with increased TBI risk. TBI-related hospitalization rates are highest among African Americans and American Indians/Alaska Natives, while African Americans have the highest TBI-related mortality rate (Langlois et al., 2006).

In the United States, the leading causes of TBI are falls (28%), motor vehicle collisions (20%), struck by/against events, including sports injuries (19%), and assaults (11%). Motor vehicle accidents result in the greatest number of TBI-related hospitalizations. However, like the incidence, the frequency of causes of TBIs varies by sex, age, race, occupation, and socioeconomic status.

[†] Deceased

224

For example, the TBI rate from falls is highest among children ages 0 to 4 years and adults ages 75 years and older, while the TBI rate from motor vehicle accidents and assaults is highest among adolescents and young adults ages 15 to 19 years (Langlois et al., 2006).

A number of systems for grading severity of TBI are in common use. Most are based on depth and duration of alteration/loss of consciousness. Other factors that are considered in some TBI severity grading systems are injury type, length of posttraumatic amnesia, and neurological and neuroradiological findings (see Sherer & Madison, 2005 for a review). Most medical, neuropsychological, and psychosocial outcome variables and indicators that have been investigated are correlated with TBI severity; more severe injuries are associated with worse outcomes. In addition to this factor, a number of other important prognostic factors have been identified, including age, trajectory of early post-acute recovery, and prior medical, neurological, and psychiatric history (see Larrabee, 2005 and Sherer & Madison, 2005 for reviews of outcomes in mild and moderate-severe brain injuries, respectively).

Persons with TBIs are probably the single most common type of examinee referred by third parties for independent assessment in private practice neuropsychology. The vast majority of such examinees are either personal injury litigants referred by lawyers or disability claimants referred by claims managers. Patients with TBIs are also a major referral type for neuropsychologists in hospital and clinic settings, and a significant proportion of these patients are actively litigating or seeking compensation at the time of assessment.

Malingering among Compensation-Seeking Examinees

Surveys of neuropsychologists in active practice have found that as many as 30%–40% of adults who present for evaluation in the context of litigation are thought to be feigning impairments (Larrabee, 2003, 2007a; Mittenberg, Patton, Canyock, & Condit, 2002; Slick, Tan, Strauss, & Hultsch, 2004). It is therefore highly likely that most neuropsychologists who routinely conduct such assessments will at least occasionally encounter examinees who malinger. The remainder of

this chapter focuses on the detection of malingering in adults within the neuropsychological context. The next section considers the diagnosis of malingering and some related diagnoses, conditions, and constructs. The following section describes methods used to detect malingering and other forms of noncompliance. The final section presents a case of a patient who suffered a severe TBI and in whom the issue of malingering proved to be a significant concern.

Differential Diagnosis of Malingering and Other Related Conditions

According to Slick, Sherman, and Iverson (1999), *malingered neurocognitive dysfunction* (MND) is defined as:

the volitional exaggeration or fabrication of cognitive dysfunction for the purpose of obtaining substantial material gain, or avoiding or escaping formal duty or responsibility. Substantial material gain includes money, goods, or services of nontrivial value (e.g., financial compensation for personal injury). Formal duties are actions that people are legally obligated to perform (e.g., prison, military, or public service, or child support payments or other financial obligations). Formal responsibilities are those that involve accountability or liability in legal proceedings (e.g., competency to stand trial).

Basic elements of the Slick et al. criteria for MND are presented in Table 19-1.

There are no survey data available concerning the extent to which these criteria have been adopted by clinicians, but an informal survey of the literature suggests that they have been adopted by a significant number of researchers in the field.

The Slick et al. criteria were put forth as a first attempt to bring a coherent, standards-based approach to the field of malingering research and clinical practice, and it was expected that they would evolve over time in light of new developments in the field and feedback from clinicians and researchers. Along these lines, a recent thoughtful and detailed analysis and criticism by Larrabee, Greiffenstein, Greve, and Bianchini (2007) provides a number of useful recommendations for revisions. Among other things, Larrabee et al. point out that the Slick et al. criteria employ a relatively crude, nonactuarial method of aggregating indicators for

Table 19-1. Criteria for Diagnosing Malingered Neurocognitive Dysfunction

A.	Clear and substantial external incentive
B1.	Definite response bias
B2.	Probable response bias
B3.	Discrepancy between known patterns of brain function/dysfunction and test data
B4.	Discrepancy between observed behavior and test data
B5.	Discrepancy between reliable collateral reports and test data
B6.	Discrepancy between history and test data
C1.	Self-reported history is discrepant with documented history
C2.	Self-reported symptoms are discrepant with known patterns of brain functioning
C3.	Self-reported symptoms are discrepant with behavioral observations
C4.	Self-reported symptoms are discrepant with information obtained from collateral informants
C5.	Evidence of exaggerated or fabricated psychological dysfunction on standardized measures
D.	Behaviors satisfying Criteria B and/or C were volitional and directed at least in part towards acquiring or achieving external incentives as defined in Criteria A
E.	The patient adequately understood the purpose of the examination and the possible negative consequences of exaggerating or fabricating cognitive deficits
F.	Test results contributing to Criteria B are sufficiently reliable and valid

Definite MND

1. Presence of a substantial external incentive [Criterion A]
2. Definite negative response bias [Criterion B1]
3. Behaviors meeting necessary criteria from group B are not fully accounted for by Psychiatric, Neurological, or Developmental Factors [Criterion D]

Probable MND

1. Presence of a substantial external incentive [Criterion A]
2. Two or more types of evidence from neuropsychological testing, excluding definite negative response bias [two or more of Criteria B2–B6]
   Or
   One type of evidence from neuropsychological testing, excluding definite negative response bias, and one or more types of evidence from Self-Report [one of Criteria B2–B6 and one or more of Criteria C1–C5]
3. Behaviors meeting necessary criteria from groups B or C are not fully accounted for by Psychiatric, Neurological, or Developmental Factors [Criterion D]

Possible MND

1. Presence of a substantial external incentive [Criterion A]
2. Evidence from Self-Report [one or more of Criteria C1–C5]
3. Behaviors meeting necessary criteria from groups B or C are not fully accounted for by Psychiatric, Neurological, or Developmental Factors [Criterion D]
   Or
   Criteria for Definite or Probable MND are met except for Criterion D (i.e., primary psychiatric, neurological, or developmental etiologies cannot be ruled out). In such cases, the alternate etiologies that can not be ruled out should be specified.

Source: Slick, Sherman, & Iverson, 1999.

determining diagnostic certainty, rather than relying on more sophisticated methods for weighing evidence such as derivation of likelihood ratios and predictive power values associated with test results, particularly when such results are chained or otherwise combined across multiple psychometric measures or indices.

Larrabee et al. also point out that the distinction drawn between performance measures and self-report measures with respect to diagnostic value (i.e., data from self-report measures are given less weight) is one that has not been supported by research. Others have taken exception to fundamental conceptual-semantic aspects of the Slick et al. criteria. For example, Boone (2007b) asserts, inter alia, that malingering cannot and should not be diagnosed by neuropsychologists and instead asserts that all that can be reasonably determined is the degree to which an examinee's presentation and test performance is "credible" or "noncredible."

As a further development of the conceptual underpinnings of malingering, we propose a model in which four fundamental dimensions underlying examinee behaviors during assessment must be considered when making a differential diagnosis of malingering: *(1)* volition/ conscious awareness, *(2)* level of effort, *(3)* immediate goal, and *(4)* long-term goal. In this framework, malingering occurs when an examinee *(1)* consciously chooses to *(2)* expend at least some effort during an assessment toward *(3)* a short-term goal of feigning deficits, in the service of *(4)* a long-term goal of obtaining a substantial secondary gain such as a financial settlement. Among adults, financial gain or other material compensation and avoidance of legal liability and criminal responsibility are likely the most common goals of malingering. The situation is somewhat different and more complicated in children, and it will not be discussed here (see Slick, Tan, Sherman, & Strauss, in press).

Malingering by Proxy. In children, the diagnosis *malingering by proxy* may be applied when exaggeration or fabrication of neurocognitive deficits occurs primarily in response to implicit or explicit encouragement/direction by others in positions of influence or authority (Slick et al., in press). This diagnosis may also be applicable to adults with limited or diminished intellectual capacity (i.e., persons who, due to intellectual impairment, are unable to appreciate the implications and possible consequences of feigning impairment) who exaggerate or fabricate neurocognitive deficits in the same circumstances. As with children, malingering by proxy may occur in response to explicit encouragement (i.e., being told to fake impairment) and/or coaching (e.g., being told how to fake impairment), or in response to indirect encouragement such as repeated comments from a significant other about the need for a large settlement, the need for people to see how impaired the examinee is, or the need to punish the plaintiff. Also as with malingering by proxy in children,

some type of reward is typically implicitly or explicitly offered for successful dissimulation, *but the offer of a reward is not necessary for a diagnosis.* All that is required is that an examinee with diminished capacity exaggerates or fabricates deficits in response to implicit or explicit encouragement or direction of someone else. Note, however, that in addition to psychological rewards such as approval or acceptance, proxy malingering can occur in response to the promises of material rewards. Thus, an examinee *with diminished capacity* who exaggerates or fabricates deficits at neuropsychological assessment in order to obtain a financial settlement *at the direction of someone else* is malingering by proxy.

The diagnosis of malingering by proxy turns in part on establishing that an examinee who otherwise meets criteria for malingering (e.g., multiple SVT failure in the context of litigation) does not have sufficient intellectual capacity to fully appreciate the nature and possible consequences of feigning impairment. The question necessarily arises as to how one can determine that an examinee has limited intellectual capacity when the test results normally used to inform such a determination cannot be trusted? Unfortunately there is no easy answer to this question. In some cases, intellectual limitations may be documented prior to injury, as in the case of developmental disabilities. In other cases, acquired intellectual disabilities may be documented after a brain injury, but *before* litigation began. In addition, to diagnose malingering by proxy, one must be reasonably certain that an examinee was acting under the influence of another person when he or she feigned impairment, which may be difficult if not impossible to clearly ascertain, let alone convincingly demonstrate in most cases. When proxy malingering is suspected, it is particularly important to systematically obtain and carefully evaluate collateral informant reports.

Coerced Malingering. In some cases, examinees may exaggerate or fabricate deficits in order to avoid or escape informal or extra-legal punishment by others; that is, in order to avoid explicit or implied physical, sexual, or psychological harm or abuse. For example, a person in an abusive relationship may exaggerate or fabricate deficits at neuropsychological assessment in response to explicit or implied directions from the abuser, with implied or explicit threats associated with failure to comply. These are cases of *coerced malingering*. In some cases, exaggerated or fabricated deficits may occur in the context of both promises of reward and threats of punishment from one or more adults, and the individual may then be viewed as having a combined *malingering by proxy/coercion* presentation. As with malingering by proxy, a diagnosis of coerced malingering requires a reasonable certainty that an examinee was acting under the influence of another person when he or she feigned impairment, and therefore it is particularly important to systematically obtain and carefully evaluate collateral informant reports whenever such a presentation is suspected. In addition, both proxy and coerced malingering cases are complicated in that they raise ethical issues with respect to reporting abuse.

Conversion Disorder. According to the *DSM-IV* (APA, 2000), *conversion disorder* is the dissimulation of sensory or motor deficits that is not conscious or volitional, but rather a manifestation of unconscious psychological process. Thus, unconsciously fabricated cognitive deficits do not fall within the *DSM-IV* definition of conversion disorder (but see Boone & Lu, 1999). In fact, apart from dissociative amnesia, there is no diagnosis in *DSM-IV* that specifically includes unconscious fabrication of *any* type of cognitive deficits. Regardless, true conversion disorder is a relatively rare phenomenon (and dissociative amnesia much rarer still), the actual existence of which continues to be a subject of some debate (c.f., Miller, 1999; Turner, 1999). Although some of the earliest forced-choice symptom validity tests were developed to detect conversion disorders (Brady & Lind, 1961), the detection and diagnosis of conversion cases has received little research interest in neuropsychology (but see Lamberty, 2007).

Factitious Disorder. According to the *DSM-IV* (APA, 2000), *factitious disorder* is defined by the conscious and volitional production of feigned physical or psychological signs or symptoms, the underlying motivation for which is the assumption of the sick role. Factious disorder cannot occur when external incentives such as economic gain, avoiding legal responsibility, or improving physical well-being are present. As with conversion disorder, a number of substantial criticisms have been raised about the *DSM-IV* definition of and criteria for factitious disorder (e.g., Bass & Halligan, 2007), not the least of which is the exclusion of factious disorder in cases where an external incentive is present, making malingering and factitious disorder mutually exclusive. No explanation as to why both external and psychological incentives cannot simultaneously influence behavior is provided, despite the fact that elements of both factitious disorder and malingering are seen in some patients (i.e., feigning directed toward *both* psychological and external gains).

Cogniform Disorder and Cogniform Condition. Unconsciously feigned cognitive deficits do not fit well, if at all, into conceptualizations and diagnostic criteria for conversion, factitious, and somatoform disorders as found in the *DSM-IV*. However, it has been suggested that those with somatoform disorder may in some cases present with feigned cognitive deficits (Boone & Lu, 1999; Stone, et al., 2006), with the implication that this could be incorporated as a formal diagnostic feature. Rather than broadening the definition of somatoform disorder, Delis and Wetter (2007) proposed two new diagnoses, *cogniform disorder* and *cogniform condition*. These diagnostic categories were created to "encompass cases of excessive cognitive complaints and inadequate test-taking effort in the absence of sufficient evidence to diagnose malingering" (p. 589). As would be expected from the titles, Delis and Wetter define cogniform disorder as the more pervasive form of the two diagnoses, in which individuals exhibit excessive cognitive symptoms in widespread areas of their lives. More specifically, Delis and Wetter define *cogniform disorder* as:

a pattern of cognitive complaints or low scores on psychometric cognitive tests that are considered to be excessive because they cannot be fully explained by a neurological disorder, by another mental disorder that is associated with CNS dysfunction (e.g., Schizophrenia), by a general medical condition known to affect CNS function (e.g., renal disease), by the direct effects of a substance (e.g., opioid medications), or by other factors known to affect cognitive functioning (e.g., developmental learning disorder; insomnia; normal aging process). If the cognitive complaints or poor test performances occur in the presence of a known neurological or mental disorder or any other factor known to affect CNS function (e.g., medication), the cognitive symptoms are in excess of what would be expected from the history, physical examination, laboratory tests, or psychometric validity testing." (p. 595)

Whereas in *cogniform condition*,

The essential features of Cogniform Condition are the same as those of Cogniform Disorder in every respect, with the exception of the degree to which the individual exhibits cognitive dysfunction in widespread areas of his or her everyday life. That is, in Cogniform Condition, there is (a) a lack of reasonable evidence that the individual presents as cognitively dysfunctional in many areas of his or her life and (b) evidence of significant inconsistencies between the individual's excessive cognitive complaints or poor test performances in an evaluation and his or her higher level of everyday functioning. (p. 597)

Delis and Wetter also provide detailed criteria for diagnosing Cogniform Disorder and Cogniform Condition. According to Delis and Wetter, both Cogniform Disorder and Cogniform Condition share many diagnostic features with malingering, including presentation with excessive cognitive complaints and/or "evidence of inadequate effort and exaggeration on formal neuropsychological testing," but are differentiated from the latter by a "lack of sufficient evidence of conscious intent." Delis and Wetter do not necessarily consider symptom validity test failure or other strong evidence of noncompliance in the presence of a substantial external incentive as prima fascia evidence of intent to feign deficits. In such cases, a specifier of *with evidence of external incentive* may be applied. Delis and Wetter's proposed diagnoses and associated diagnostic criteria have been met with a mixed reaction, generally positive, but with some significant caveats concerning conceptual/diagnostic formulations and clinical applicability, particularly with respect to how these fit with other similar conceptual and diagnostic entities (Binder, 2007c; Boone, 2007; Larrabee, 2007b).

Neurocognitive Hypochondriasis. Boone (2009) presents a case study illustrative of a proposed diagnosis of *neurocognitive hypochondriasis*: cases in which persons seen for neuropsychological assessment present with reports of "dysfunction in daily life activities secondary to cognitive deficits, but are found on formal testing to have no objective abnormalities." That is, neurocognitive hypochondrias is defined by the presence of a fixed belief in neurologically based cognitive impairment, in the absence of any real impairment. This distinguishes it from both factitious disorder and malingering, in which persons are aware that they are feigning impairment. The absence of abnormal neuropsychological test results also distinguishes neurocognitive hypochondriasis from factitious disorder, malingering, and cogniform disorder. However, as in the latter three diagnoses, the cognitive "dysfunction" in neurocognitive hypochondriasis serves to address a life problem, and it is in that sense an adaptive response. Unlike Slick et al.'s MND and (1999) and Delis and Wetter's (2007) cogniform disorder, Boone does not provide specific detailed diagnostic criteria.

According to Boone, characteristics of individuals prone to neurocognitive hypochondriasis include "hypervigilance to bodily sensations and processes, including minor cognitive malfunctions, which are pathologized as indicative of significant dysfunction and vulnerability" (p.14). Boone speculates that neuropsychological hypochondriasis typically develops in the context of other psychiatric/adjustment problems and problematic interpersonal relationships, and is often precipitated by a real illness or injury.

One issue not addressed by Boone is the generality of normal function in neurocognitive hypochondriasis. That is, as well as not manifesting any deficits on objective testing, must persons with this diagnosis also not manifest any neurocognitive deficits in daily life? What diagnosis would be applicable to examinees who present with claims of dysfunction in daily life that are backed up by reliable collateral reports, but nevertheless obtain normal neuropsychological test results? In addition, Boone's model does not address the role of validity indices on self-report measures. For example, what is the diagnosis in cases where examines present with complaints of cognitive deficits in daily life, normal neurocognitive functioning on objective performance measures, but elevated validity scales on self-report measures (e.g., FBS from the MMPI-2)?

Stereotype Threat. A final category of explanatory constructs for noncompliance on neuropsychological tests is *stereotype threat,* a reduction in performance to match pre-existing low expectations (Kit, Tuokko, & Mateer, 2008; Steele, 1997; Suhr & Gunstad, 2002, 2005). There is evidence that this construct explains some age-related differences in cognitive test performance. For example, Levy (1996) demonstrated that older adults' performance on cognitive tests can be affected by priming with positive and negative stereotypes about aging. Suhr and Gunstad (2002, 2005) further demonstrated a similar effect which they termed "diagnosis threat" in young adults who had suffered mild head injuries. They found that neuropsychological test performance was worse among individuals who were informed about the potential effects of head injury on cognition in comparison to those who were not reminded of their head injury history. Therefore, it is conceivable that expectations of poor performance due to head injury may negatively impact performance on cognitive tests, although the existence and possible mechanisms of such an effect (e.g., conscious vs. unconscious) have not been fully elucidated let alone empirically tested.

Summary

The exaggeration or fabrication of neurocognitive deficits and dysfunction arises out of complex interactions between multiple individual and environmental factors operating at various intensities over time, including internal psychological processes of which a person may or may not be fully aware, external incentives such as potential financial compensation, psychological reinforcement from others such as positive attention and affection, social pressure and coercion, and explicit direction to feign from others. In cases where exaggerated or fabricated cognitive impairments are seen during neuropsychological assessment, more than one of these factors is often present. When this is the case, the relative contributions of each factor cannot be easily estimated, if even teased apart at all. Although

some current diagnostic models for malingering include the possible coexistence of other diagnostic entities such as factious and conversion disorders (e.g., Slick et al., 1999), clinicians are hampered in their approach to cases of feigned deficits by the absence of a comprehensive nosological model that incorporates and integrates all of the critical underlying factors, that adequately operationally defines specific diagnoses, and that allows for multiple primary and secondary diagnoses.

Measures and Methods Used to Inform the Differential Diagnosis of Malingering

From a virtual void only three decades ago has sprung a seemingly exponential proliferation of neuropsychological research on malingering. Both a cause and consequence of this growth has been the development over the same time period of a number of new measures designed specifically for use in detecting and diagnosing malingering, as well as the development of a number of new validity indices for existing tests. The new tests and indices have at least partially filled what was in hindsight a glaring gap in the neuropsychological armamentarium. Such measures are certainly needed, as unaided clinical judgments concerning validity of test results are often erroneous (Faust & Guilmette, 1990; Faust, Hart, & Guilmette, 1988; Faust, Hart, Guilmette, & Arkes, 1988; Heaton, Smith, Lehman, & Vogt, 1978). Recent survey studies have found that clinicians have come to appreciate this problem and have responded by using such measures with increasing frequency (Sharland & Gfeller, 2007), though perhaps still not as often as they should.

A Brief Discussion of Problems with Terminology

A variety of labels are currently applied to tests used to detect and/or aid in differential diagnoses of malingering, including *measures of response bias, effort tests, symptom validity tests,* and *measures for detecting suboptimal performance.* The choice of test terminology is not just a trivial issue of semantics, as it can lead to potentially serious problems with respect to how test results are interpreted and understood, particularly in legal settings. For example, tests used for aiding in differential diagnoses of malingering and other related conditions are often referred to as *tests of effort* or *effort tests*, when they do not in fact directly measure effort at all, but rather may detect *noncompliance with test-taking instructions*. That is, such tests are designed to detect instances in which an examinee does not comply with instructions to put maximum effort toward maximum performance on neuropsychological tests.

An examinee's place along the compliance–noncompliance continuum is a function of both level of effort expended *and* the goal toward which effort was directed on tests. Examinees are fully compliant with assessment when they exert maximum effort toward producing the highest or best possible score in accordance with specific directions for all tests administered. Noncompliance occurs when less than maximal effort is put forth and/or when specific test directions are not followed (e.g., not telling the examiner everything that is remembered on a memory test as instructed).[1] Examinees who put forth minimal effort are substantially noncompliant, but so too are examinees who put maximal effort toward exaggerating or fabricating dysfunction. The dissociation between effort and the goal toward which effort is directed can be illustrated by a hypothetical example in which *greater* effort is probably required to feign deficits than is required for maximal performance: imagine a forced-choice recognition test on which almost all normal adults obtain perfect or near-perfect scores, suggesting that the task is relatively undemanding in terms of cognitive resources. However, the nature of the test is fundamentally changed when taken with intent to malinger; in addition to normal task demands with respect to attention, stimulus processing, encoding, and later recognition, the malingering task set introduces the need to consciously maintain a feigning strategy (e.g., monitoring item difficulty to determine when to make errors), inhibit correct responses, and keep track of performance over time (e.g., maintain a target error rate). Additional cognitive resources must therefore be deployed in order to successfully meet these increased task demands. That is, greater effort must be expended to do poorly than to do well.

In light of these considerations, any tests used for detecting/diagnosing malingering or any other type of noncompliance should more properly be referred to as *noncompliance detection measures*,[2] rather than effort measures. Although the focus in this section has been on performance-based noncompliance detection measures, the designation can be extended to include self-report-based measures, the difference being that the latter detect noncompliance with directions to respond honestly.

Qualities of Effective Noncompliance Detection Measures

Hartman (2002) detailed a number of qualities that effective noncompliance detection measures should or must have. Extrapolating from this, a good measure for detecting noncompliance *must* have the following characteristics: *(1)* be sensitive to noncompliance but insensitive to cognitive dysfunction; *(2)* have *false* face validity, that is, appear to be a legitimate measure of a cognitive ability likely to be exaggerated by persons who feign brain damage; *(3)* be adequately norm-referenced and validated to satisfy clinical and legal (e.g., Daubert) standards; *(4)* be difficult to fake and resistant to coaching; *(5)* be relatively easy to administer and score; and *(6)* be supported by continuing research. For more in-depth discussions about some critical psychometric and diagnostic aspects of detecting noncompliance, see, for example, Boone (2007a), Franklin, (2003), Larrabee (2007a, 2008), Mackinnon (2000), McKenzie (1997), Millis (2001), Mossman (2000a-b, 2003), Mossman and Hart (1996), Pepe (2003), Slick et al. (1999), and Strauss, Sherman, and Spreen (2006).

Types of Noncompliance Detection Measures

There are two basic types of noncompliance detection measures: those derived from conventional neuropsychological tests (i.e., measures originally designed to measure various aspects of cognition, adjustment, and psychopathology), and those developed specifically for detecting noncompliance. Within the category of noncompliance indices developed from conventional measures, there are three basic subtypes. The first type is the simple cutoff. These are usually derived by setting a limit for unusually poor performance for a nonmalingering sample on a test that has a very low floor. For example, a cutoff for a conventional test might be set at the 1st percentile for nonlitigating, severely brain injured patients. Scores below this level obtained by persons with mild head injuries may then be considered pathognomic of noncompliance. A good example of a cutoff type of index is Reliable Digit Span (Greiffenstein, Baker, & Gola, 1994; Heinly, Greve, Bianchini, Love, & Brennan, 2005).

The second type of conventional test noncompliance index is derived by identification of patterns of performance within or across tests that are atypical in legitimate brain injury cases but common in independently classified cases of noncompliance (Larrabee, 2003). For example, unusually poor performance on easier versus more difficult items or tests, inconsistency across tests tapping similar cognitive domains, unusually high numbers of errors on items that are rarely missed by most examinees, a high rate of endorsement of unusual responses, and atypical recall or recognition relative to serial-position at study are all patterns of performance that have been associated with noncompliance. A good example of a pattern of performance type of index is the Vocabulary-Digit Span Index (Mittenberg, Theroux-Fichera, Zielinski, & Heilbronner, 1995). The F, Fb, and Symptom Validity Scale (FBS; Greiffenstein, Fox, & Lees-Haley, 2007; Lees-Halely, English, & Glenn, 1991) developed from the MMPI-2 are other examples of such indices. Marked inconsistency in test scores across multiple testing sessions or assessments in the absence of sufficient medical or situational explanations (e.g., change in neurological status, illness such as flu at the time of testing, extreme fatigue due to atypical sleep depravation, etc.) is another indicator that falls within pattern of performance domain.

The third type of conventional noncompliance index is developed by combining multiple scores using a statistical weighting formula (e.g., derived from logistic regression or Bayesian analyses). These formulae take a number of test scores (and also prior probability of malingering in some types of models) as input and give a probability or likelihood of "malingering" as an output. Statistical models that include only a few variables may essentially equate to a pattern of performance models in that only one or two specific test score patterns result in a high probability of malingering, but in more complex models with many variables, a large number of possible score patterns may result in a high probability of malingering. Examples of this approach can be found in Strauss et al. (2006) and Larrabee (2008).

Until very recently, conventional cognitive tests were developed under the assumption that the examinees to which they would be administered would put forth adequate effort to do well. The possibility of noncompliance was not considered during test design, let alone included as an additional variable that needed to be measured. Similarly, traditional validation models did not account for validity threats from malingering and other forms of noncompliance, and how tests might allow for this to be detected and/or distinguished from legitimate impairment. It is therefore not surprising that with few exceptions, the better noncompliance indices derived from conventional tests that have been developed to date have only moderate diagnostic utility. In response to this problem, and in light of the challenges of developing measures that are effective at measuring both cognitive functions and detecting noncompliance, considerable effort has been expended over the last two decades on the development of measures specifically designed to detect noncompliance.

In comparison to indices derived from conventional tests (so-called embedded indices), measures designed specially for detecting noncompliance are often more accurate, but typically have little to no utility for any other purpose. There are two general types of specific noncompliance detection measures, forced-choice and non-forced-choice measures, although this distinction is somewhat trivial as scores from both types of measures are primarily interpreted by reference to norms due to the limited utility of binomial probability-based analyses of forced-choice scores. More recently, specific psychophysical methods and neuroimaging techniques for detecting noncompliance have been developed (e.g., Kingery & Schretlen, 2007; Rosenfeld et al., 1998) and appear to have considerable potential. However, these methods are currently not available for use outside of research settings and thus will not be described here.

Most measures developed specifically for detecting noncompliance are designed to capitalize on examinee naivety regarding the effects of brain injuries and the absolute/relative difficulty of items/tasks for persons with brain injuries. *False face validity* is created by carefully selecting items and tasks that most people will perceive as very challenging for brain-injured persons, but which are in fact easily passed by most or all patients with legitimate brain injuries. Incorrect assessments of difficulty lead persons who seek to malinger to identify themselves by scoring below the level of legitimate brain-injured patients and/ or by other atypical aspects of their performance (e.g., unusually long response latencies). More sophisticated noncompliance detection measures make use of one or more manipulations of apparent item/task difficulty to increase sensitivity, such as presentation of items that differ in apparent, but not actual difficulty (e.g., trivial increases in delay interval on forced-choice delayed recognition measures). The effectiveness of this tactic is often enhanced by suggesting to examinees that some items or tasks are easier and others more difficult. The Victoria Symptom Validity Test (VSVT; Slick, Hopp, Strauss, & Thompson, 1997) is an example of a test that employs this method.

Although the first forced-choice noncompliance detection measures were originally developed for diagnosing conversion disorder (Brady & Lind, 1961), all such measures that are now in widespread use in neuropsychology have been designed primarily for detecting noncompliance in cases of malingering, as opposed to noncompliance of other kinds (e.g., factitious or conversion disorders, other mental illnesses). As such, the primary place of use of forced-choice measures is in medical-legal assessments. Most forced-choice tests use a two-choice response format, where success by guessing alone should approximate 50% even in the most severe cases of impairment. High or low scores (i.e., above or below chance at $p < .05$) are highly unlikely to occur by chance alone and are thus assumed to reflect purposeful selection of correct or incorrect answers, with the latter being suggestive of noncompliance. Analog and known groups studies (see following section) have shown that most individuals instructed to feign cognitive deficits or believed to be malingering

do not suppress their performance on forced-choice tests below chance levels. Accordingly, reliance on probability derived cutoffs results in very conservative decisions (i.e., very low hit rates). By testing groups of healthy individuals as well as nonlitigants with significant cognitive deficits, investigators have provided data upon which to base empirical cutoffs for noncompliance detection measures that greatly improve sensitivity while maintaining adequate specificity. These results reflect the very low floors typical of most noncompliance detection measures.

Validity of Noncompliance Detection Measures

A review of the validity properties of specific noncompliance detection measures and indices is beyond the scope of this chapter (see instead Boone, 2007a; Larrabee, 2007a; Strauss et al., 2006). However, there is now a considerable research base that supports the utility of the most commonly used forced choice measures, including the Test of Memory Malingering (TOMM; Tombaugh, 1996), Victoria Symptom Validity Test (VSVT; Slick et al., 1997) and Word Memory Test (WMT; Green, Allen, & Astner, 1996) for detecting noncompliance. As well as supporting the validity of specific uses, the research base provides a relatively good basis for interpreting scores from these measures. Among the indices of noncompliance derived from conventional cognitive measures, there is good support for Reliable Digit Span (RDS). Among indices derived from self-report measures, there is very strong support for the Fake Bad Scale (FBS) of the MMPI-2.

The Case of G. W.

The case presented here provides a real-world example of some of the complexities and issues involved in the use and interpretation of noncompliance detection measures and differential diagnosis of malingering.

Background: Injury

G. W., a previously very physically fit young man in excellent health, sustained a severe TBI in a motor vehicle collision 3 months after his

21st birthday. He was the restrained (three-point) right front passenger in a subcompact car that was struck on his side by a truck traveling at highway speed. The main area of impact was just behind where he was sitting, causing severe damage to the car and killing the right rear passenger. His head struck the passenger door, breaking the window glass. G. W. had been drinking prior to the collision and was mildly to moderately intoxicated at the time. He sustained the following bodily injuries: *(1)* fractures of the right leg, right arm, right collarbone, right shoulder, right ribs, and hip; *(2)* right pneumothorax; *(3)* right kidney laceration; and *(4)* multiple bruises, contusions, and lacerations.

According to a witness, G. W. was initially unresponsive, but he opened his eyes after 2–3 minutes. On arrival of the ambulance crew, he was noted by them to be disoriented, combative, and in considerable pain. His Glasgow Coma Score (GCS) was 11. He was found to have a large scalp laceration above the right ear, and a laceration of the right ear. He was bleeding from the right ear canal. He had some difficulty breathing. He had to be extracted from the car, which was severely damaged. He was then transported via helicopter to the hospital, during which time he lapsed back into unconsciousness (GCS = 3). A computed tomography (CT) scan shortly after arrival at the hospital showed a small right posterior epidural hematoma, a small amount of intraventricular blood, and a right basal skull fracture. He underwent emergency surgeries for drainage of the epidural hematoma, multiple orthopedic repairs, and placement of a chest tube. A postsurgical magnetic resonance imaging (MRI) scan showed a number of small areas of parenchymal contusions with mild surrounding edema in lateral and inferior fronto-temporal areas bilaterally. The rest of his brain appeared normal. There was no delay in regaining consciousness after the surgeries, but G. W. became quite agitated and was therefore heavily sedated. Sedation was weaned over a period of several days, but he remained on a substantial amount of opiod pain medication, which was weaned more slowly over the course of his 3-week inpatient stay. G. W. was confused and disoriented as sedation was weaned, and he did not fully clear posttraumatic amnesia—as assessed by the Galveston Orientation and Amnesia Test—until 8 days post injury. A second MRI at 1 week post injury showed substantial resolution of parenchymal contusions and edema, but a scattering of small traumatic white matter lesions was seen throughout the right hemisphere and a small lesion was also seen in the splenium of the corpus callosum.

Apart from early agitation, G. W.'s hospital course was uneventful, and he made an excellent physical recovery. He was released from the hospital to home 3 weeks after the accident, attended a comprehensive outpatient rehabilitation program for 6 weeks, and thereafter continued with additional outpatient physiotherapy for 6 more months after that. During outpatient rehabilitation, he demonstrated difficulties with processing speed, attention, working memory, learning and memory, and executive functions (insight, mental flexibility, planning, organization, initiation, and self-monitoring). His affect was initially quite flat, but punctuated by occasional irritability and outbursts of anger. On discharge from outpatient rehabilitation (8 months post injury), physical recovery was described as excellent, with only mild persisting reductions in leg and arm mobility. Persisting complaints of pain were noted, which were not fully medically explainable. Some concerns regarding ongoing use of pain medications were noted, and a referral was made to a multidisciplinary pain program. Substantial recovery in attention, memory, and executive functions were noted, though some mild difficulties were still seen. He was described as independent with all basic activities of daily living (ADLs). Affect was described as still somewhat flat, but with increased irritability.

Background: Prior History

G. W.'s prior neurological history is remarkable for a sports concussion with a brief loss of consciousness at age 16. Symptoms (headache, dizziness, irritability, inattentiveness, and forgetfulness) persisted for several weeks. He was held out of play for 3 months after this event. There were no persisting symptoms or problems. He also sustained a number of more minor sports head injuries that were associated with brief alterations in consciousness and/or dizziness, both before and after the concussion sustained at age 16 years. His prior medical history was otherwise unremarkable. Early physical development was reportedly precocious. G. W. was a highly talented athlete.

Prior psychiatric and psychosocial history was unremarkable. G. W. was popular in school and had a large group of friends. He consumed alcohol socially. There was no reported history of alcohol abuse. He smoked marijuana occasionally, but he had not tried any other drugs. He had three older sisters. His parents divorced relatively amicably when he was 5 years old, and he lived with his mother thereafter but spent time with his father. Family medical, psychiatric, and psychosocial history was unremarkable. His father had academic difficulties in childhood, completed high school in a nonacademic trade program, and became a successful tradesman who worked his way up to foreman. His mother completed high school and a postsecondary administrative assistant program and was an office manager. His sisters all completed high school. One sister was a homemaker, one worked for his mother as a clerk, and one was attending nursing school.

With respect to academic history, records indicated that G. W. received speech therapy for delayed development of articulation in kindergarten. He was described in early school records as a slow learner who had some difficulties with conceptual thinking. He was never formally assessed for or diagnosed with any learning disabilities, but he received assistance with reading and math throughout grade school. He was also described as more restless and inattentive than most peers but was never formally diagnosed with or treated for attention-deficit/hyperactivity disorder (ADHD). He obtained mostly Cs and a few Bs in grade school. Achievement test scores from grade six were at grade level for math and below grade level in language arts and social studies. In high school, his attendance dropped off and his grades declined to mostly Cs and Ds in core academic courses. His work was often incomplete and of poor quality, and his exam scores were generally below average. His achievement scores in grade nine were below grade level in language arts, math, science, and social studies. He took less academically rigorous course options and received some formal and informal learning supports, including blocks of time in a resource classroom, but nevertheless failed math in grade 11 and again in grade 12 and therefore did not graduate from high school. Teacher comments in his school records note that G. W.'s low performance was felt to be reflective of both low motivation and effort and actual difficulties with reading, mathematics, and attention. However, as in grade school, he was never formally assessed or diagnosed with any learning disabilities or ADHD.

Following high school, G. W. worked at a number of different unskilled/manual labor jobs. Some of these were temporary, but he never held any potentially permanent job for more than 5 months before quitting and was unemployed roughly half of the 3 years between the end of high school and his injury. At the time of his injury, he had been working for 5 months at an assembly plant. His work performance had been satisfactory, and he had been given a raise in wage at 3 months. According to G. W., his plan at the time of his injury was to continue working at the factory for another year while taking evening classes to upgrade his language arts and math and then enter the electrician's program at a local technical college.

G. W. was living with his mother at the time of injury. He had never lived on his own. He was independently managing his finances and was independent in all other ADLs, although his mother continued to do some cooking, cleaning, and laundry for him.

First Neuropsychological Assessment

At 8 weeks post injury, an assessment was conducted by the staff neuropsychologist at the hospital where G. W. was receiving outpatient rehabilitation. He was not litigating at the time of this assessment. At that time, G. W.'s main complaints concerned pain and mobility difficulties stemming from his orthopedic injuries. He did not have any complaints concerning cognition, mood, or personality. However, collateral reports from therapists and G. W.'s family indicated that very substantial cognitive changes/problems were present. Selected scores from this assessment are presented in Table 19-2. Based on these reports, direct observations, and test scores, the primary conclusions drawn in the report from this assessment were that G. W. demonstrated reduced attention, working

Table 19-2. Selected Test Scores from G. W.'s
Three Assessments

Test Score	Time Post Injury		
	2 Months	18 Months	24 Months
VSVT			
Easy raw	23	20	24
Hard raw	18	12	21
TOMM			
T2 raw	45	41	47
Delay raw	40	38	44
RDS	7	6	8
MMPI-2			
F T score	63	61	66
F_B T score	75	64	62
FBS raw	17	23	27
WTAR			
WTAR			80
*VC**	—	—	89
*PO**	—	—	93
*WM**	—	—	92
*PS**	—	—	90
WAIS-III Index scores			
VC	82	76	80
PO	87	81	88
WM	75	74	74
PS	72	79	82
WMS-III Index scores			
Auditory- Immediate	78	82	85
Auditory- Delay	81	75	72
Visual - Immediate	92	85	98
Visual - Delay	90	79	95
CVLT-II			
Total T	—	—	45
SDFR z-score	—	—	−.5
LDFR z-score	—	—	−1
Recognition (Hits) z-score	—	—	−2
Recognition (FA) z-score	—	—	0
FC Recognition z-score	—	—	87.5%
WJ-III Index scores			
Broad Math	—	—	9
Broad Reading	—	—	12
Listening Comprehension	—	—	25

*WTAR-Demographics Predicted Score

memory, processing speed, and verbal memory. He was also described as having significant executive deficits, including difficulties with abstraction, inferential reasoning, impulse control, mental flexibility, planning, organization, initiation, self-monitoring/awareness, and insight. Lastly, significant mood and personality changes were also noted, including flat affect, anhedonia, abulia, irritability, and anger outbursts. No problems with validity of test results were noted in the report, although it can be seen that the VSVT hard item score is at the lower end of the acceptable range and the TOMM delay trial score is below the recommended noncompliance cutoff.

Second Neuropsychological Assessment

At 18 months post injury, G. W. was seen for independent examination by a neuropsychologist retained by his lawyer, hereinafter referred to as the plaintiff's expert (PE). At that time, he was still living at his mother's home and had not returned to work. He was continuing to take prescription pain medications and had not yet attended the pain program that he had been referred to on outpatient rehabilitation discharge. G. W. presented for the assessment with the following complaints: *(1)* moderate to severe chronic daily multifocal pain (shoulder, back, hip, and leg), *(2)* moderate to severe daily headaches, *(3)* moderate to severe daily fatigue, *(4)* anhedonia, *(5)* episodes of depression, *(6)* recurrent distressed suicidal ideation, *(7)* severely slowed thinking, *(8)* severe difficulty sustaining attention, and *(9)* severe difficulty learning and retaining new information, prospective memory deficits, and forgetfulness for events. Collateral reports from G. W.'s family corroborated his self-report and added concerns about irritability and anger outbursts, insight, foresight and judgment, impulse control, and initiation.

Interestingly, although the PE's report noted a prior history of concussion, it did not mention that G. W. remained symptomatic for several weeks afterward and that he was withheld from play for 3 months, nor was the history of multiple minor head injuries with transient symptoms mentioned. The PE accurately summarized G. W.'s academic history with respect to grades and achievement scores, but this was presented in the context of G. W.'s self-report that his low marks were due entirely to lack of interest and effort and distraction from socializing and playing sports. Although school records were reportedly reviewed, no mention was made of the provision of learning supports in grade school and high school and that teachers felt that G. W.'s poor grades were due in part to real difficulties with reading, math, and attention.

With respect to observations, the PE's report noted that G. W.'s affect was generally flat during the assessment, but he demonstrated some irritability during testing. He was described as lacking insight into his cognitive deficits and mood/personality changes. His appearance and behavior were apparently otherwise unremarkable. He was described as cooperative with the assessment and as demonstrating "good effort" on all tests.

With respect to validity of test data, the PE concluded that while G. W. obtained a small number of scores that "might indicate less than optimal effort on some measures," these most likely reflected "a combination of factors secondary to his brain injury, including impairments of attention and memory, and fatigue, and thus the assessment results could be considered valid." The PE's opinion with respect to the etiology of G. W.'s low scores on the VSVT, TOMM, and RDS is not supported by the cumulative literature on these measures (e.g., Strauss et al., 2006), which strongly supports an interpretation that he was substantially noncompliant with the assessment. An additional factor that is strongly in favor of the noncompliance interpretation is the marked decline in scores on multiple cognitive measures and particularly on the noncompliance measures. This is highly inconsistent with the natural course of recovery from TBI, and in the absence of adequate medical or situational explanations, which were absent in this case, is strongly suggestive of problems with compliance at the second assessment. In his report, the PE noted that some of G. W.'s scores had declined relative to the prior assessment, but downplayed the magnitude of the decline and did not offer any opinion as to why the decline had occurred.

The PE concluded that G. W. presented with deficits in multiple domains of cognition secondary to his brain injury, including verbal and visual-spatial intelligence, processing speed, working memory, attention, executive functions, and verbal and visual-spatial memory. No tests of achievement were administered, but the PE concluded that G. W.'s reading and math skills had very likely declined substantially based on G. W.'s self-report. The PE also concluded that G. W. was suffering from depression and posttraumatic stress.

Lastly, the PE concluded that in the absence of his head injury, G. W. would have had no difficulty upgrading his academics and would almost certainly have been able to complete training as an electrician and work successfully in that trade.

Third Neuropsychological Assessment

G. W. was seen by one of us (D. J. S.) at the request of the defense lawyer at 2 years post injury. At that time, G. W. was employed full time as a construction worker. Collateral information was obtained from his mother, with whom he was continuing to live. Except where noted, collateral information obtained from G. W.'s mother was consistent with the information that he provided. At the time of assessment, he had been working for 2 months, and despite ongoing problems with pain and fatigue, was satisfactorily meeting job demands, which were primarily physical. He was fully independent in activities of daily living, at the same level as prior to his brain injury, including banking and driving. His medical status was stable and he was well. He had still not attended the multidisciplinary pain program that he had been referred to, but was no longer using prescription pain medications. His vision and hearing were reportedly normal. He had not sustained any new injuries or serious illnesses in the 2 years since his brain injury. After the second neuropsychological assessment, he had been referred to a psychiatrist who prescribed an SSRI antidepressant, which G. W. took for several weeks and then discontinued on his own. He had not followed up with the psychiatrist. He denied any suicidal ideation over the last 4 months. He described his mood as up and down, with one or two periods of depression lasting a day or two every month. He had not received any counseling or psychotherapy for his depression and was not interested in such services, preferring to "handle it on his own". G. W. reported that he had become aware of problems with irritability and anger over time, but that these were improving. By contrast, G. W.'s mother indicated that while he had recently begun acknowledging problems with irritability and anger, these had not improved over time and were still causing some interpersonal stress and difficulties in daily life at home, but apparently not at work. No symptoms of posttraumatic stress disorder (PTSD) were reported by him. He had not resumed competitive sports due to problems with pain and fatigue, but he had recently resumed occasional play at a recreational level. He was having some ongoing difficulties adjusting to his inability to play competitive sports, which he described as his biggest loss from the accident.

G. W. reported significant changes in his social life. At the time of the accident, he had a large group of friends and spent most of his free time in sports, socializing and engaging in various social activities. In contrast, his social life was extremely limited during the first year after the accident. After he returned home from hospitalization, he mostly just slept and sat around watching TV. Initially, his friends visited frequently, but he did not go out at all due to lack of interest, pain, and fatigue; visits tailed off considerably over time as most of his friends "moved on." He was also embarrassed by his cognitive difficulties and had lost his self-confidence. His mother added that G. W.'s friends were put off by his irritability, lack of motivation and interest, and difficulties appreciating humor and sustaining conversations. Over the year prior to assessment, his social life had picked up; he had re-established some friendships, started going out with friends occasionally, and had a steady female companion for 3 months.

As at the previous assessment, G. W. complained of chronic daily multifocal pain, headaches, and fatigue, with only some slight improvement over time. He also reported ongoing moderate to severe cognitive difficulties in a number of domains, including processing speed, attention, and memory, and that these had not improved appreciably since the previous assessment. He denied any difficulties with thinking, reasoning, or problem-solving skills. Apart from difficulties with attention control, he denied any executive function deficits. Overall, G. W. described his cognitive problems in general terms (e.g., "I think slower"; "I have trouble focusing"; "I forget things all the time, it's a big

problem") and was quite vague when asked to provide more specific details and examples from daily life, tending to repeat more general descriptions and state that he had difficulty recalling and/or describing specific examples. In contrast, he was able to provide relatively detailed and precise descriptions of physical and emotional problems. Collateral report information obtained from his mother supported G. W.'s complaints of cognitive problems in daily life insofar as domain (i.e., processing speed, attention, and memory), but at a much more mild level of severity than he reported, as judged by the specific examples given. However, in contrast to G. W.'s denial of executive function problems, his mother reported mild ongoing dysexecutive symptoms, including difficulties with impulse control, mental flexibility, insight, judgment, abstraction, inferential reasoning, planning and organization, and initiative. Overall, G. W. depicted himself as moderately to severely impaired in a few cognitive domains (processing speed, attention, and memory), while collateral informants described him as having broader but milder cognitive difficulties.

When asked about his litigation status, G. W. stated that he had become quite frustrated with the process in terms of how long it was taking to obtain a settlement and also all of the examinations and assessments he had been obliged to undergo. He voiced strong expectations of a very substantial amount of money in final settlement and expressed considerable frustration and anger at the defendant's insurance carrier and lawyers for holding up payment that he could use and was rightfully owed for having his life "ruined." G. W. also reported that his lawyer had informed him that the results from the previous independent neuropsychological assessment had confirmed severe brain damage that would prevent attainment of his preinjury academic and career goals. Not surprisingly, G. W. stated that because of this, he was no longer planning on attempting to upgrade his education or to pursue training as an electrician. G. W. added that while he still had some anger, he had come to accept that his academic and occupational options would be permanently limited.

With respect to the accident itself, G. W. reported approximately 3 hours of retrograde amnesia and only a few fragmentary, mostly vague memories from his time as an inpatient. His recollection of events from outpatient therapy was somewhat better, but still quite impoverished for the next 5–6 months.

With respect to preinjury academic history, G. W.'s recollection was quite vague, and the details that he did produce were inconsistent with the documented history in that he denied any history of learning difficulties and also reported higher grades than he actually obtained according to the school transcripts. When given some feedback concerning the contents of his academic transcript, G. W. stated that he had a hard time remembering much about school. He attributed his poor performance in school entirely to lack of interest and motivation and preoccupation with sports and socializing, and stated that he never had any learning difficulties whatsoever and could easily have obtained above-average marks had he wanted to. He explained the provision of learning assistance and accommodations with the comment "they didn't know what else to do with me." In contrast, G. W.'s mother gave a rather different academic history. She reported that he was a "lazy" student who was more interested in sports and having fun than studies. She also felt that he could have done much better at school, but on further questioning admitted that he struggled quite a bit early in grade school, never quite caught up after that, and always found school challenging, which was part of the reason he avoided it.

With respect to occupational history, G. W. reported that he was more focused on sports and did not have to work consistently after high school because his mother supported him. He worked when he had to but found it boring and did not like being a "peon." However, he eventually realized that he would need to obtain a regular, high-paying job to support himself and so obtained a position assembling furniture in a factory. This was still "peon" work, but it paid well, and he planned to go back to school and become an electrician, as one of his friends was doing this and had highly recommended it. G. W.'s mother reported that after high school, apart from continued participation in sports and socializing, he "lacked direction" and continued to be lazy until she finally demanded that he obtain steady work to pay his share of household expenses. She

supported his plan to become an electrician, but she had concerns about his ability to put in the required effort to complete training.

With respect to his presentation, G. W.'s appearance, behavior, and demeanor were largely unremarkable. Some *mild* word-finding difficulties, inattentiveness, and distractibility, and slowing of cognition were observed during the assessment. Otherwise no significant cognitive deficits were obvious in conversation or by close observation of other aspects of extra test behavior. His language use was consistent with expectations given his reported academic achievement level. The overall impression was of a young man possessing broadly low-average to average cognitive abilities with somewhat limited education. Although G. W. reported at several points—in response to questions, but not spontaneously—that he was experiencing significant somatic pain, headache and fatigue, only occasional pain behaviors were observed. These appeared quite natural and not in any way manufactured or exaggerated. He appeared somewhat fatigued at the end of the assessment but not markedly so. G. W. reported that his affect was neutral to negative and that he was unhappy about having to attend the assessment. He was somewhat hostile and guarded initially and verbally challenged the qualifications of the examiner and the validity of the assessment early on. After some discussion, during which the examiner suggested calling his lawyer (this was not followed up on), he appeared to become relatively comfortable and was not overtly hostile or oppositional thereafter. He still appeared somewhat guarded during the interview, however. Some flashes of irritability and anger were seen, particularly when asked for clarifications or challenged about some facets of his history during the interview and also at times during testing. He became quite animated when discussing his preinjury sporting achievements. He appeared tearful when talking about the loss of participation in competitive sports. He appeared to find the testing onerous, frequently sighing, occasionally expressing frustration with testing and also some concerns regarding his performance. In between these reactive vacillations of emotion, his affect appeared somewhat dulled. He was not spontaneously interactive or social. He never appeared anxious, and no signs of thought disorder were seen.

Discussion and Case Formulation

Regardless of assessment context, noncompliance should always be considered as a possible explanation for any abnormal test results. In the case of G. W., a number of findings suggest that he was possibly exaggerating some cognitive problems during his first assessment, and very likely exaggerating some cognitive deficits at his second and third assessments, with malingering being the most appropriate diagnosis in latter two instances according to the Slick et al. criteria (1999). The relevant aspects of G. W.'s case leading to these conclusions are reviewed next.

Premorbid History. G. W.'s claims that he could have done much better in school had he been more motivated notwithstanding, both parent report and school records support a conclusion that he had significant learning difficulties in reading and math, bordering on disabilities. There is no documented evidence that he demonstrated a high level of intellectual ability inside or outside of school, and apart from his prowess at sports, there is no indication of any splinter skills or any type of giftedness. The history is therefore consistent with preinjury intellectual abilities in the mid-average to below-average range. His expected preinjury achievement scores would certainly be below grade 12 level in mathematics and likely below grade 12 level in reading. Although there is no evidence that G. W. possessed any above-average cognitive abilities, it would not be unusual if he obtained a few scattered above-average scores across an extensive neuropsychological test battery had he been tested prior to his brain injury (see Strauss et al., 2006 for a review of normal variability). On the other hand, consistently above-average scores in any domain would not have been expected. In this regard, his WTAR score and WTAR-demographics predicted WAIS-III index scores are consistent with expectations.

Taking the full preinjury history into consideration, the PE's opinion that G. W. would have *definitely* been able to complete academic upgrading and complete electrician's training can be called into serious question. Further to this issue, an independent educational/occupational consultation report obtained by the defense included an analysis of statistical trends which demonstrated that persons with academic backgrounds similar to G. W.'s have only a moderate success rate for academic upgrading, and furthermore, that it is relatively rare to find an academic background like G. W.'s among persons who successfully complete electrician training.

TBI and Post-TBI History. From the documented history, it is clear that G. W. sustained a severe traumatic brain injury. Long-term outcomes from such injuries vary considerably across individuals. Nearly complete neurocognitive recoveries are seen in a few such cases, but most persons who survive severe TBIs demonstrate at least some permanent decrements in cognition with associated functional implications (Dikmen, Machamer, Powell, & Temkin, 2003). In G. W.'s case, factors predictive of a relatively good long-term outcome included his youth, excellent physical health at the time of injury, and negative premorbid psychiatric history. In addition, his excellent early neurological recovery was a positive prognostic sign for long-term neurocognitive outcome. In keeping with these predictions, reports of rehabilitation staff were indicative of a substantial neurocognitive recovery, with only relatively mild deficits seen at 8 months post injury. In the absence of new neurological injuries or conditions, there was no basis to expect to see a lower level of function at any assessments subsequent to this point in time (i.e., his second and third assessments). The persistence of significant medically unexplained pain and excessive use of narcotic pain medications at discharge from outpatient rehabilitation at 8 months post injury, in conjunction with persisting changes in mood and irritability, raise concerns about psychiatric TBI sequelae, however, such as substance abuse and somatoform problems.

Presentation and Self-Report. At the second and third assessments, G. W. presented with complaints of significant cognitive dysfunction. While his complaints were not unusual with respect to *possible* sequelae of the type of TBI that he sustained, they were substantially inconsistent with other relevant data. G. W. reported substantially greater impairments of processing speed, attention and memory than would be expected given: *(1)* his initial neuropsychological assessment results and reports of staff concerning his functional level at discharge from outpatient rehabilitation; (2) his level of function demonstrated by extra-test behaviors during the latter two assessments;[3] (3) his level of function in daily life, particularly at the third assessment; and (4) the severity of deficits reported by his mother at the third assessment. Admittedly, G. W. also denied some deficits that were reported by his mother, but the additional cognitive problems she reported were described as only relatively mild in severity.

In addition to apparent exaggeration of cognitive deficits, G. W. also presented with exaggerated somatic complaints. As with his cognitive deficits, G. W. reported a substantially greater severity of pain and fatigue than was *(1)* apparent from his behavior during the assessment, *(2)* reported by his mother, and *(3)* expected given his ability to work.

In addition to apparent exaggeration of symptoms reported during the interview, G. W.'s scores on the MMPI-2 also called the veracity of his complaints into serious question. In particular, his FBS score increased substantially across all three assessments. At the first assessment, at which point he was not yet a litigant, it fell within the normal range. At the second assessment, at which point he had become a litigant, it fell within the borderline range. At the third assessment, at which time G. W. was continuing with litigation and his statements indicated that obtaining a large financial settlement was very important, his FBS score was unambiguously within the symptom exaggeration range. This increase in FBS score strongly suggests that litigation played a role in G. W.'s presentation over time.

Test Performance. With respect to his scores on performance-based noncompliance measures, an interesting pattern emerged across the three assessments. At the first assessment, G. W. obtained scores within the questionable range on VSVT hard items and within the noncompliant range on the TOMM Delay. However, he was not litigating or otherwise actively seeking compensation at that time and there were no other reported indicators of possible noncompliance with the assessment or other information to suggest any other possible reasons for noncompliance with cognitive testing. These data are enigmatic, but nevertheless suggest that G. W.'s

other test scores from that assessment should be interpreted with considerable caution.

In contrast to his scores at the first assessment, G. W.'s scores on the VSVT, TOMM, and RDS from the second assessment—at which time he was actively seeking financial compensation—were all substantially lower, and all very strongly suggestive of noncompliance. For example, with respect to his performance on the VSVT, his scores on both the easy and hard items were lower than those obtained by the vast majority of non-compensation-seeking brain injured individuals, including a small sample of patients with dense amnesia (Slick et al., 2003). In addition, if the unusualness of G. W.'s VSVT scores relative to comparable nonlitigants is set aside and his hard items score accepted at face value, then the implications of chance level performance as a legitimate indicator of ability would have to be accepted. This would imply profound cognitive impairment, with commensurate disabilities in daily life. While G. W. reportedly demonstrated cognitive deficits in daily life at the second assessment, they were not of the magnitude expected if his VSVT scores from that assessment were legitimate. Such profound deficits would also certainly have to be obvious even on informal observation, but they were not noted in the PE's report. One would also expect to see more severe impairment on conventional memory measures than he demonstrated. Furthermore, the large drop in VSVT scores does not makes sense in the context of G. W.'s neurological history and status at the second assessment. A substantial decline in function over time is inconsistent with the natural history of recovery from TBI and there were no new injuries or neurological conditions that could explain such a marked decline in cognitive function, particularly on a test as easy as the VSVT. In addition, a significant decline in cognitive function over this time period was not reported by G. W. or anyone else who knew him. Most critically, the VSVT hard item score obtained by G. W. is much more common among malingerers than nonmalingers, and it is therefore associated with a high positive predictive value for malingering, unless a very low base rate (not applicable to this case) can be assumed. Similar comments apply to G. W.'s scores on the TOMM and RDS from the second assessment.

The picture is somewhat different at the third assessment. G. W. obtained substantially higher scores on performance-based noncompliance measures, though still within a range consistent with exaggeration on the Delay Trial of the TOMM. In addition, there are indicators of noncompliance on the CVLT-II, which was not previously administered, including much poorer delayed recognition than delayed recall (he in fact failed to recognize some items that were recalled right before), and an unusually low score on forced-choice recognition. Altogether, though not as strong on performance-based measures, the evidence of noncompliance (including the elevated FBS scale) was still ample. One possible explanation of G. W.'s better performance on noncompliance detection measures at the third assessment was that he received coaching or information that he was able to utilize with some success. Alternatively, variability of performance on noncompliance detection measures over multiple assessments may also be characteristic of the performance of some uncoached malingerers (e.g., Strauss et al., 2002).

As well as his scores on noncompliance detection measures, G. W.'s profile of test scores across time is also suggestive of compliance problems. His scores declined substantially from the first to second assessments on a number of measures, including the VC and PO indices from the WAIS-III and the Auditory Delayed and Visual Immediate/Delayed indices from the WMS-III. As with the declines seen on the VSVT and TOMM, his reduced performance on conventional measures over time is not consistent with the natural course of recovery from traumatic brain injury. There was no other medical explanation for the decline in scores, and no decline in function was reported over the same time period. With the exception of his Delayed Auditory Memory Index score from the WMS-III, G. W.'s memory scores were all substantially higher on the third than at the second assessment. There is no neurological explanation for this pattern. Given the data from noncompliance detection measures and other information available, the fluctuation in scores is best explained by deliberate but variable suppression of test performance over time. Similar variability over time in performance on conventional measures of cognition among malingerers

has been reported in the literature (e.g., Strauss et al., 2002).

Summary. Given that he had no apparent reason to be noncompliant, one must very seriously consider the possibility that G. W.'s low TOMM and VSVT scores at his first assessment were both false positives. On the other hand, if those scores were true indicators of noncompliance, then malingering would normally have to be ruled out as a diagnosis because G. W. was not formally seeking compensation at the time of testing. However, given that he was very likely malingering at both subsequent assessments, one could speculate that although G. W. had not yet entered into litigation at the time of his first assessment, he was by then already aware of the prospect of financial compensation and suppressed his performance with this goal in mind.

There is much less uncertainty about G. W.'s presentation on his second and third assessments; at both of these, he clearly met Slick et al. criteria for *probable malingering*. This conclusion is based on the following data: *(1)* a substantial external incentive to malinger was present, *(2)* reported symptoms were inconsistent with collateral reports and level of function in daily life, *(3)* his performance on multiple noncompliance detection measures was consistent with negative response bias, and *(4)* changes in his test score profile over time were substantially inconsistent with the natural history of his neurological condition and inconsistent with his level of function in daily life. This does not rule out the presence of some real cognitive TBI sequelae. Indeed, given the severity of his injury, it is quite likely that G. W. had some acquired deficits. However, given the very high likelihood that he was malingering, the type and magnitude of any such deficits cannot be ascertained from his test data. In this case, collateral information from his mother probably provides a more accurate gauge of the real TBI sequelae, which are less functionally severe overall than G. W. reported, but certainly not inconsequential.

With respect to differential diagnosis, collateral reports were indicative of continuing mild dysexecutive problems in daily life, and it is certainly possible that G. W.'s presentation and test scores may have in part reflected some difficulties with insight, judgment, foresight, and inhibitory control. However, there was no evidence from test results (his scores on executive function tests fell within the low average to below average range at all assessments, with no scores in the impaired range), observations, or collateral reports of a level of executive dysfunction sufficient to fully account for his presentation and thus rule out malingering.

With regard to other diagnostic considerations, neurocognitive hypochondriasis can be ruled out because some of his scores were abnormal. Although he likely had some real cognitive deficits, G. W.'s high level of function in daily life indicates that these were not of a magnitude consistent with diminished capacity for purposes of diagnosing malingering by proxy. There was no indication of coercion, though there is really no way to rule out such a possibility. With his documented history and presentation, a somatoform component to G. W.'s pain and fatigue complaints is certainly possible. With respect to the cogniform spectrum, G. W.'s relatively normal level of function in daily life at the time of the third assessment rules out cogniform disorder, but given his complaints and test performance a diagnosis of cogniform condition could be considered. The difficulty in this case is that cogniform condition, as is currently proposed, can be diagnosed when financial incentive is present and there are no criteria for differentiating if from malingering. In the case of G. W., there was no basis to assume that his behavior was not in any way directed toward obtaining a financial settlement and so a diagnosis of probable malingering is still supported, even if there may have been a cogniform component to his presentation. Lastly, although G. W. may have received some interpersonal reinforcement for sustaining a "sick" role (e.g., from his mother), there was no evidence of a major factitious component to his presentation. Reports from his mother suggested that he did not particularly play up or exaggerate his cognitive or somatic symptoms in her presence, nor did he do so in the presence of other family members, with friends, or at work.

One of the questions raised by this case is why G. W. chose to exaggerate his cognitive deficits. The severity of his injuries was indisputable, and he was certainly due compensation. It is doubtful that he believed he might not get any compensation at all unless he exaggerating. Therefore, the most likely reason for exaggerating is a belief that this would increase the amount of compensation that he received. G. W.'s comments during the assessment suggest that he likely felt his behavior was in some way justified by the length of time he had waited for a settlement, the things that he had been forced to endure in the litigation process, and the perception that the insurance company was intending attempting to deny him what he was owed. His anger and frustration, and likely sense of justification for malingering are certainly not unique, as most neuropsychologists who see these types of cases can attest. In any case, such musings are necessarily speculative and fortunately nonessential for the differential diagnosing of malingering. These issues are nevertheless very worthwhile to ponder and study if possible, particularly if one is concerned with *preventing* malingering.

Closing Remarks

When conducting neuropsychological assessments, the first step after all the data have been collected should be an evaluation of the reliability and validity of test results and any other information obtained, as any subsequent interpretations must necessarily be informed by assumptions about validity. This process should always include a consideration of examinee compliance with various aspects of the assessment, including self-report and test performance. Regardless of context, noncompliance should always be considered as an explanation for abnormal test results. Assessment of compliance is facilitated by inclusion of multiple noncompliance detection measures within a test battery. A number of well-validated tests and indices of this type are readily available, and there is no justification for not employing them in most assessments.

When the data suggest that an examinee has been noncompliant with the assessment, then consideration necessarily turns to the underlying reasons for such behavior, and from there to differential diagnosis. Unfortunately, despite considerable progress on development of conceptual/diagnostic models over the last decade, the field of neuropsychology still lacks a single coherent differential diagnostic system for malingering and related behaviors or conditions. To some extent, this state of affairs reflects substantial differences in perspective on malingering among neuropsychologists. Regrettably, the passion with which disparate points of view on malingering are held by some groups and individuals has led to unnecessary polarization and some outright acrimony. Hopefully, the difficulties encountered to date will not substantially discourage or hinder ongoing and increasingly productive efforts to achieve consensus, and an adequate differential diagnostic system acceptable to the majority of neuropsychologists will be in place before end of the coming decade.

Notes

1. Except when failure to follow directions is due to comprehension problems.
2. One would *not* refer to such tests as measure of *compliance*, because a passing score does not necessarily indicate that an examinee was compliant. For example, a well-coached examinee might pass symptom validity tests such as the VSVT, TOMM, WMT, and so on but also purposefully suppress his or her performance on other measures. Only by careful and thorough assessment in which test scores are integrated with other information is it possible to come to some conclusion regarding the reason(s) that an examinee was noncompliant.
3. One must of course be careful in interpreting informal observational data gathered over a short period of time in an atypical setting (e.g., during an assessment), but in G. W.'s case the observational impressions were fully consistent with other information concerning his relatively high level of function in daily life, as subsequently discussed.

References

American Psychiatric Association. (2000). *Diagnostic and statistical manual of mental disorders* (4th ed., Text rev.). Arlington, VA: Author.

Bass, C., & Halligan, P. W. (2007). Illness related deception: Social or psychiatric problem? *Journal of the Royal Society of Medicine, 100,* 81–84.

Binder, L. M. (2007). Comment on "Cogniform disorder and cogniform condition: Proposed diagnoses for excessive cognitive symptoms." *Archives of Clinical Neuropsychology, 22*(6), 681–682.

Boone, K. B. (2007a). Assessment of feigned cognitive impairment: A neuropsychological perspective. New York: Guilford Press.

Boone, K. B. (2007b) A reconsideration of the Slick et al. (1999) criteria for malingered neurocognitive

dysfunction. In K. B. Boone, (Ed.), *Assessment of feigned cognitive impairment: A neuropsychological perspective* (pp. 29–49). New York: Guilford Press.

Boone, K. B. (2007c). Commentary on "Cogniform disorder and cogniform condition: Proposed diagnoses for excessive cognitive symptoms" by Dean C. Delis and Spencer R. Wetter. *Archives of Clinical Neuropsychology, 22*(6), 675–679.

Boone, K. B. (2009). Fixed belief in cognitive dysfunction despite normal neuropsychological scores: Neurocognitive hypochondriasis? *The Clinical Neuropsychologist, 23*(6), 1016–1036.

Boone, K., & Lu, P. (1999). Impact of somatoform symptomatology on credibility of cognitive performance. *Clinical Neuropsychologist, 13*(4), 414–419.

Brady, J. P., & Lind, D. L. (1961). Experimental analysis of hysterical blindness. *Archives of General Psychiatry, 4,* 331–339.

Delis, D. C., & Wetter, S. R. (2007). Cogniform disorder and cogniform condition: Proposed diagnoses for excessive cognitive symptoms. *Archives of Clinical Neuropsychology, 22*(5), 589–604.

Dikmen, S. S., Machamer, J. E., Powell, J. M., & Temkin, N. R. (2003). Outcome 3 to 5 years after moderate to severe traumatic brain injury. *Archives of Physical Medicine and Rehabilitation, 84,* 1449–1457.

Faust, D., & Guilmette, T. J. (1990) To say it's not so doesn't prove that it isn't: Research on the detection of malingering: Reply to Bigler. *Journal of Consulting and Clinical Psychology, 58*(2), 248–250.

Faust, D., Hart, K., & Guilmette, T. J. (1988). Pediatric malingering: The capacity of children to fake believable deficits on neuropsychological testing. *Journal of Consulting and Clinical Psychology, 56,* 578–582.

Faust, D., Hart, K., Guilmette, T. J., & Arkes, H. R. (1988). Neuropsychologists' capacity to detect adolescent malingerers. *Professional Psychology: Research and Practice, 19,* 508–515.

Franklin, R. (Ed.) (2003). Prediction in forensic and neuropsychology: Sound statistical practices. Mahwah, NJ: Erlbaum.

Gaetz, M. (2004). The neurophysiology of brain injury. *Clinical Neurophysiology, 115*(1), 4–18.

Green, P., Allen, L. M., & Astner, K. (1996). The Word Memory Test: A user's guide to the oral and computer-administered forms, US version 1.1. Durham, NC: CogniSyst, Inc.

Greiffenstein, M. R., Baker, W., & Gola, T. (1994). Validation of malingered amnesia measures with a large clinical sample. *Psychological Assessment, 6*(3), 218–224.

Greiffenstein, M. F., Fox, D., & Lees-Haley, P. R. (2007). The MMPI-2 Fake Bad Scale in detection of noncredible brain injury claims. In K. B. Boone, (Ed.), *Assessment of feigned cognitive impairment: A neuropsychological perspective* (pp. 210–235). New York: Guilford Press.

Hartman, D. (2002). The unexamined lie is a lie worth fibbing. Neuropsychological malingering and the Word Memory Test. *Archives of Clinical Neuropsychology, 17*(7), 709–714.

Heaton, R. K., Smith, H. H., Jr., Lehman, R. A., & Vogt, A. T. (1978). Prospects for faking believable deficits on neuropsychological testing. *Journal of Consulting and Clinical Psychology, 46*, 892–900.

Heinly, M. T., Greve, K. W., Bianchini, K., Love, J. M., & Brennan, A. (2005) WAIS digit span-based indicators of malingered neurocognitive dysfunction: Classification accuracy in traumatic brain injury. *Assessment, 12*(4), 429–444.

Kingery, L. R., & Schretlen, D. J. (2007). Functional neuroimaging of deception and malingering. In K. B. Boone, (Ed.), *Assessment of feigned cognitive impairment: A neuropsychological perspective* (pp. 13–25). New York: Guilford Press.

Kit, K. A., Tuokko, H. A., & Mateer, C. A. (2007). A review of the stereotype threat literature and its application in a neurological population. *Neuropsychology Review, 18*(2), 132–148.

Lamberty, G. (2007). Understanding somatization in the practice of neuropsychology. New York: Oxford University Press.

Langlois, J. A., Rutland-Brown, W., & Thomas, K. E. (2006). *Traumatic brain injury in the United States: Emergency department visits, hospitalizations, and deaths.* Atlanta, GA: Centers for Disease Control and Prevention, National Center for Injury Prevention and Control.

Larrabee, G. (2003). Detection of malingering using atypical performance patterns on standard neuropsychological tests. *Clinical Neuropsychologist, 17*(3), 410–425.

Larrabee, G. (2005). Mild traumatic brain injury. In G. J. Larrabee, (Ed.), *Forensic neuropsychology: A scientific approach* (pp. 237–270). New York: Oxford University Press.

Larrabee, G. J. (2007a). *Assessment of malingered neuropsychological deficits.* New York: Oxford University Press.

Larrabee, G. J. (2007b). Commentary on Delis and Wetter, "Cogniform disorder and cogniform condition: Proposed diagnoses for excessive cognitive symptoms." *Archives of Clinical Neuropsychology, 22*(6), 683–687.

Larrabee, G. J. (2008). Aggregation across multiple indicators improves the detection of malingering: Relationship to likelihood ratios. *Clinical Neuropsychologist, 22*(4), 666–679.

Larrabee, G. J., Greiffenstein, M. F., Greve, K. W., & Bianchini, K. J. (2007). Refining diagnostic criteria for malingering. In G. J. Larrabee, (Ed.), *Assessment of malingered neuropsychological deficits* (pp. 334–371). New York: Oxford University Press.

Lees-Haley, R., English, L. T., & Glenn, W. J. (1991). A Fake Bad Scale on the MMPI-2 for personal injury claimants. *Psychological Reports, 68*(1), 203–210.

Levy, B. (1996). Improving memory in old age through implicit self-stereotyping. *Journal of Personality and Social Psychology, 71*(6), 1092–1107.

Mackinnon, A. (2000). A spreadsheet for the calculation of comprehensive statistics for the assessment of diagnostic tests and inter-rater agreement. *Computers in Biology and Medicine, 30*(3), 127–134.

McKenzie, D. P., Vida, S., Mackinnon, A. J., Onghena, P., & Clarke, D. M. (1997). Accurate confidence intervals for measures of test performance. *Psychiatry Research, 69*(2), 207–20.

Miller, E. (1999). Conversion hysteria: Is it a viable concept? *Cognitive Neuropsychiatry, 4*(3), 181–191.

Millis, S.R. and Volinsky, C.T. (2001). Assessment of Response Bias in Mild Head Injury: Beyond Malingering Tests. *Journal of Clinical and Experimental Neuropsychology, 23*(6), 809–828.

Mittenberg, W., Patton, C., Canyock, E. M., & Condit, D. (February, 2002). *A national survey of symptom exaggeration and malingering baserates.* Poster presented at the Annual Meeting of the International Neuropsychological Society, Toronto, Canada.

Mittenberg, W., Theroux-Fichera, S., Zielinski, R., & Heilbronner, R. (1995). Identification of malingered head injury on the Wechsler Adult Intelligence Scale—Revised. *Professional Psychology: Research and Practice, 26*(5), 491–498.

Mossman, D. & Hart, K.J. (1996). Presenting evidence of malingering to courts: Insights from decision theory. *Behavioral Sciences & the Law, 14*(3) 1996, 271–291.

Mossman, D. (2000a). Interpreting clinical evidence of malingering: A Bayesian perspective. *Journal of the American Academy of Psychiatry and the Law, 28*(3), 293–302.

Mossman, D. (2000b). The meaning of malingering data: Further applications of Bayes' theorem. *Behavioral Sciences and the Law, 18*(6), 761–779.

Mossman, D. (2003). Daubert, cognitive malingering, and test accuracy. *Law and Human Behavior, 27*(3), 229–249.

Mossman, D., & Hart, K. J. (1996). Presenting evidence of malingering to courts: Insights from decision theory. *Behavioral Sciences and the Law, 14*(3), 271–291.

Pepe, M. S. (2003). The statistical evaluation of medical tests for classification and prediction. New York: Oxford University Press.

Rosenfeld, R. J., Reinhart, A. M., Bhatt, M., Ellwanger, J., Gora, K., Sekera, M., & Sweet, J. (1998). P300 correlates of simulated malingered amnesia in a matching-to-sample task: Topographic analyses of deception versus truthtelling responses. *International Journal of Psychophysiology, 28*(3), 233–247.

Sharland, M. J., & Gfeller, J. D. (2007). A survey of neuropsychologists' beliefs and practices with respect to the assessment of effort. *Archives of Clinical Neuropsychology, 22*(2), 213–223.

Sherer, M., & Madison, C. F. (2005). Moderate and severe traumatic brain injury. In G. J. Larrabee (Ed.), *Forensic neuropsychology: A scientific approach* (pp. 237–270). New York: Oxford University Press.

Slick, D. J., Hopp, G., Strauss, E., & Thompson G. B. (1997). *Victoria Symptom Validity Test.* Odessa, FL: Psychological Assessment Resources.

Slick, D. J., Sherman, E., & Iverson, G. (1999). Diagnostic criteria for malingered neurocognitive dysfunction: Proposed standards for clinical practice and research. *Clinical Neuropsychologist, 13*(4), 545–561.

Slick, D .J., Tan, J. E., Sherman, E. M. S., & Strauss, E. (in press). Assessing malingering, effort and motivation. In A. S. Davis, (Ed.), *Handbook of pediatric neuropsychology.* New York: Oxford University Press.

Slick, D. J., Tan, J. E., Strauss, E., & Hultsch, D. (2004). Detecting malingering: A survey of experts' practices. *Archives of Clinical Neuropsychology, 19*(4), 465–473.

Slick, D. J., Tan, J. E., Strauss, E., Mateer, C. A., Harnadek, M., & Sherman, E. M. S. (2003). Victoria Symptom Validity Test scores of patients with profound memory impairment: NonLitigant case studies. *Clinical Neuropsychologist, 17*(3), 390–394.

Steele, C. (1997). A threat in the air: How stereotypes shape intellectual identity and performance. *American Psychologist, 52*(6), 613–629.

Stone, D.C., Boone, K.B., Back-Madruga, C, & Lesser, I.M. (2006). Has the rolling uterus finally gathered moss? Somatization and malingering of cognitive deficit in six cases of "toxic mold" exposure. *The Clinical Neuropsychologist, 20,* 766–785.

Strauss, E., Sherman, E., & Spreen, O. (2006). *A compendium of neuropsychological tests: Administration, norms, and commentary* (3rd ed.). New York: Oxford University Press.

Strauss, E., Slick, D. J., Levy-Bencheton, J., Hunter, M., MacDonald, S. W. S., & Hultsch, D. F. (2002). Intraindividual variability as an indicator of malingering in head injury. *Archives of Clinical Neuropsychology, 17,* 423–444.

Suhr, J., & Gunstad, J. (2002). "Diagnosis threat": The effect of negative expectations on cognitive performance in head injury. *Journal of Clinical and Experimental Neuropsychology, 24*(4), 448–457.

Suhr, J., & Gunstad, J. (2005). Further exploration of the effect of "diagnosis threat" on cognitive performance in individuals with mild head injury. *Journal of the International Neuropsychological Society, 11*(1), 23–29.

Tombaugh, T. M. (1996). *Test of Memory Malingering (TOMM).* North Tonawanda, NY: Multi-Health Systems.

Turner, M. (1999). Malingering, hysteria, and the factitious disorders. *Cognitive Neuropsychiatry, 4*(3), 193–201.

20

Recovery following Mild Traumatic Brain Injury

Scott Mooney, Ph.D. and Robin Hanks, Ph.D., ABPP (CN)

According to the Centers for Disease Control and Prevention (CDC), it is estimated that upwards of 1.5 million Americans receive a brain injury annually (Centers for Disease Control and Prevention, 2003). Approximately 70%–90% of the 700,000 persons who present annually to an emergency room related to a presumed brain injury are believed to have experienced a mild traumatic brain injury (mTBI; Centers for Disease Control and Prevention, 2003; Holm, Cassidy, Carroll, & Borg, 2005) and are subsequently discharged home the same day. The highest morbidity of mTBI is found in young adolescent or adult males (Holm et al., 2005).

The World Health Organization's (WHO) Neurotrauma Task Force has operationally defined mTBI, or concussion, as an acute injury to the brain that is a result of mechanical energy applied to the head from an external source, such as blunt trauma, or acceleration/deceleration inertia motion at high velocity (Holm et al., 2005). Various biomechanical models have examined the minimal biomechanical threshold for traumatic brain injury (Brolinson et al., 2006; Zhang, Yang, & King 2004), with resulting suggestion of a minimum threshold for linear forces of 80–100 g, although rotational forces may mediate a lower threshold and raise the likelihood of an mTBI, as linear gravitational acceleration impacts of this magnitude can result in a lack of injury as well. In laymen's terms, 100 g translational force can be equated with a 25 mile-per-hour motor vehicle collision against a brick wall, hitting one's head against the dashboard (McCrae, 2008).

Clinically, mTBI is accompanied by altered mental status (e.g., disorientation, confusion) above and beyond the initial emotional reaction or psychological shock of the traumatic event, loss of consciousness of less than 30 minutes, posttraumatic confusion of less than 24 hours, Glasgow Coma Scale scores of 13–15 that are optimally measured within the first 30 minutes of injury, focal neurological signs, and/or positive head imaging findings not requiring surgical intervention (Holm et al., 2005; Teasdale & Jennett, 1974). Mild traumatic brain injury associated with positive head imaging findings consistent with intracranial hemorrhage, not epidural hemorrhage, are termed "complicated mTBI" (Iverson, 2005; Kashluba, Hanks, Casey, & Millis, 2008). Mild traumatic brain injury associated with positive brain imaging findings (Levine et al., 2006) occurs in approximately 5%–30% of cases and frequently in the presence of skull depressions/fractures, but not whiplash injuries (Holm et al., 2005). Importantly, these aforementioned difficulties should not be accounted for by confounding factors, such as substance intoxication, medications, other bodily injuries and/or treatments, psychological factors, or medical problems such as penetrating head injury (Holm et al., 2005).

The initial pathophysiology of mTBI is thought to be due to mechanical forces applied to the head resulting in several possible outcomes, including skull fracture and/or movement and possible rotation of the cerebrum about the relatively stationary brain stem within the skull (Shaw, 2002).

The result of these forces include possible focal contusions or hemorrhages with increased intracranial pressure arising from diffuse axonal injury (DAI) as neuronal tracts undergo stretching or shearing (Shaw, 2002). Diffuse axonal injury is thought to be a major factor in accounting for altered mental status or loss of consciousness following a head injury (Levine et al., 2006), although it does not account for all of the pathophysiology as microhemorrhages may also play a role. Diffuse axonal injury is presumed to deleteriously impact cortical-subcortical-brainstem neurotransmission initially through the result of these mechanic effects, after which secondary processes, including a cascade of axonal ionic and metabolic changes, diminished cerebrovascular blood flow, and reduced neurotransmission, may result in axonal dis connection/apoptosis (Iverson, 2005; Levine et al., 2006).

Objective cognitive deficits are commonly observed in persons who are recovering following a recent brain injury, typically in a dose–response type relationship (Dikmen et al., 1995; Rohling, Meyers, & Millis, 2003). That is, as the severity of the brain injury increases, as evidenced by duration of loss of consciousness, there is a greater probability for more objective cognitive impairment with a slower resolution of symptoms over time. In mTBI, common areas of dysfunction evidenced early on in recovery include attention-concentration, speed of information processing, and/or memory performances (e.g., Dikmen, Machamer, & Temkin, 2001; Dikmen, McLean, & Temkin, 1986; Levin et al., 1987). Fortunately, well-controlled studies generally show resolution of cognitive deficits following uncomplicated mTBI within a week to 3 months post injury in the vast majority of cases (e.g., Belanger & Vanderploeg, 2005; Carroll et al., 2004; Dikmen et al., 1986; Levin et al., 1987; Macciocchi, Barth, Alves, Rimel, & Jane, 1996; McCrea et al., 2003). Persons with a complicated mTBI may show slower resolution of symptoms following a recovery curve that is consistent with what is expected in moderate brain injury patients (Kashluba et al., 2008).

Postconcussion syndrome or postconcussional disorder can be a common diagnosis following a brain injury (Boake et al., 2005; Shaw, 2002). The DSM-IV-TR includes post concussional disorder in its "criteria sets and axes provided for further study" appendix. The research criteria provided includes the following: "A history of head trauma that causes significant cerebral concussion; evidence from neuropsychological testing or quantified cognitive assessment of difficulty in attention or memory; and three or more of a variety of symptoms that have lasted for at least three months including becoming fatigued easily, disordered sleep, headache, vertigo or dizziness, irritability or aggression on little or no provocation, affective lability, changes in personality, and apathy or lack of spontaneity" (APA, 2000 p. 761). Even though many clinicians make this diagnosis, it is formally a research diagnosis and several criticisms have been offered against postconcussional disorder as a diagnostic category. For example, the constellation of symptoms occurs at a fairly high base rate in the normal population (Iverson & Lang, 2003; Wang, Chan, & Deng, 2006), and the symptoms are shared by several other disorders that generally contain medically unexplained symptoms (Binder, 2005). It is a nonspecific cluster of symptoms that overlaps with chronic pain and emotional distress such as depression and/or anxiety (Iverson, 2005). Some of the strongest criticisms against postconcussion syndrome arise from the expanding scientific knowledge base about the natural course of recovery from mild traumatic brain injuries. The consensus emerging from reviews of the empirical literature is that the expected outcome following an uncomplicated mild traumatic brain injury for the majority of patients is full recovery (Belanger & Vanderploeg, 2005; Carroll et al., 2004). Depending on whether the more stringent provisional DSM-IV-TR or inclusive ICD-10 criteria are used, between 11% and 64% of persons will acknowledge continued or worsening subjective changes in their thinking skills and physical and emotional difficulties beyond the expected time frame of cognitive recovery following brain injury (Boake et al., 2005). Additionally, no studies have shown that the severity of TBI is consistently related to postconcussion syndrome (Holm et al., 2005; Iverson, 2005). Instead, continuance of symptoms is most strongly associated with compensation or litigation involvement (Carroll et al., 2004; Holm et al., 2005).

Case Presentation

A 39-year-old, right-handed, Caucasian woman was referred by her physiatrist for an outpatient neuropsychological evaluation secondary to her persisting memory complaints following involvement in a motor vehicle accident approximately 2 months preceding the evaluation. The patient was a restrained driver who was struck on the driver's side by an oncoming vehicle. Her airbag was deployed and she required extrication by emergency medical service. The patient reportedly struck her head several times during the accident and remembered feeling dazed for a few minutes, but she denied losing consciousness. No retrograde amnesia was reported and she recalled some details of the accident. Head imaging studies at the time of arrival to the emergency room were negative. She was discharged home from the emergency room the same day of the accident.

A few days after the accident she began to experience headaches, and her primary care physician referred her to a neurologist. Brain magnetic resonance imaging (MRI) and electroencephalogram (EEG) performed approximately 1 week after the accident were read as normal. The MRI of the left ankle showed mild subcutaneous edema and joint effusion. Computed tomography (CT) of the spine revealed a small disc-spur at C5/C6. She then began seeing a physiatrist secondary to concerns about the need for outpatient rehabilitation. She was also scheduled to see an ear, nose, and throat (ENT) physician secondary to temporomandibular joint (TMJ) and balance problems.

The patient returned to work as a teacher's aide after 3 weeks, but her headaches reportedly interfered with her ability to continue working. She was a single mother who lived in a house with her teenage son, and she was able to take care of her medications, finances, and personal care independently. She was able to complete most household chores, but would clean in short spurts due to her headaches. Difficulties with balance when cleaning were also noted. She was independent when driving, despite having some anxiety while doing so. She was not currently involved in litigation regarding the motor vehicle collision, but she had hired an attorney and was scheduled to meet with him in the near future.

Past medical history included cholescytectomy. Mental health history included emotional distress and depression secondary to a recent divorce, which resulted in brief outpatient counseling prior to filing for divorce. These events occurred in the months prior to her motor vehicle collision. Family medical history was generally unremarkable. Substance use history was denied. Medications at the time of evaluation included Aricept, 5 mg; Zoloft, 50 mg; and salsalate, 1000 mg, b.i.d.

Educational history included 8 years of formal schooling where she reportedly obtained Bs and Cs. Later in her life, she participated in an adult educational program and earned her high school diploma. Vocationally, she had been working as a teacher's aid for the past 15 years, although prior to this position she also worked in janitorial services and as a clerk.

At the time of the evaluation, she reported experiencing difficulties with sleep maintenance, tinnitus, headaches, decreased appetite, occasional blurred vision, dizziness, nausea, and anergia. Cognitively, she felt that her memory was worse since the accident, especially for details of previous conversations and read material. She also complained of bradyphrenia and shaky hand writing. Since the accident, she had experienced dysphoric mood, anhedonia, and irritability. She also was anxious when driving and experienced disturbing dreams, the later of which she attributed to medication side effects (i.e., Zoloft), rather than anxiety symptoms. She reported that she was "sad" that she was not working and very concerned about her perceived memory problems. Although she was recently divorced after 22 years of marriage, she felt that her relationships with friends and other family members was quite good. Functionally, she remained independent in her ability to perform activities of daily living, including managing her medications, finances, personal care, driving, and household chores.

During the feedback session, she brought her mother to the appointment and asked that we share the outcome of the testing with both individuals. At this point, her mother indicated that her daughter's ex-husband was "showing up" at her house without warning and that her daughter had even woken up with him next to her in the bed. The patient reported that these events did not bother her, but her mother contradicted her daughter's response and indicated that her daughter had called her multiple times in tears regarding her ex-husband's behavior. Since beginning Zoloft, however, her emotional distress had lessened somewhat.

Examination Results

Validity of Test Results. As is common in most neuropsychological evaluation, various measures of effort or dissimilation were administered in order to examine engagement in the testing process. As shown in Table 20-1, the patient performed adequately across all cognitive symptom validity measures; however, she displayed a tendency to be overly focused on her somatic complaints and may have exaggerated her symptom presentation on the MMPI-2. Taken together,

her obtained results were likely to be accurate reflections of her cognitive functioning at the time of the evaluation, but impressions regarding her personality and emotional functioning were limited owing to increased probability of symptom promotion.

Intellectual and Cognitive Functioning. As shown in Table 20-2, the patient obtained a WAIS-III Full Scale IQ of 87, which falls in the low-average range traditionally, but compared to persons of similar demographic background was in the average range. Her IQ was consistent with expectations given what was known about her educational and vocational histories and average performances across academic screening measures of single-word reading, spelling, and written arithmetic skills. Her performances across other cognitive domains, including attention-concentration,

Table 20-1. Summary of Effort and Motivation Indicators

California Verbal Learning Test

CVLT Variable	Scores	Millis et al., 2007; Wolfe et al., 2009
LDFR raw score	14	
Total Recall Discrim. standard score	0	
d-prime raw score	3.3	
Recognition Hits raw score	16	
	XB	Probability of Incomplete Effort
3-Variable Model (LDFR, TRD, d')	0.121	0.530213146
Recognition Hits only	−1.33	0.209159365

Green Medical Symptom Validity Test
IR = Pass
DR = Pass
CON = Pass

Minnesota Multiphasic Personality Inventory-2
VRIN T score = 58
TRIN T score = 58 (T)
F T-score = 58
F(B) T score = 58
F(P) T score = 41
Fake Bad Scale raw score = 31
Response Bias Scale raw score = 13 (T score = 80)
L T score = 71
K T score = 50

Reliable Digit Span = 9
Vocabulary SS (Demographically Corrected) = 10

Wisconsin Card Sorting Test-128
Failure to Maintain Set = 0

speed of information processing, visual spatial construction, verbal learning and recall following a delay, and aspects of executive functions such as word generation, novel problem solving, ability to incorporate feedback into decision making, and verbal abstraction skills, were all within the low-average or better ranges. The only exception was on the task of fine motor speed where she displayed impaired performances bilaterally, but she had extremely long fingernails which appeared to impede her performance.

Personality and Emotional Functioning. As shown in Table 20-2, on the MMPI-2, she endorsed items consistent with strong somatization and symptom exaggeration tendencies. With these caveats, emotionally, she also acknowledged experiencing some depressive and anxious symptoms, although not severe in intensity. She also endorsed symptoms of resentment and hostility toward others. Her response pattern indicated that she was unlikely to be overly psychologically minded or insightful. She likely preferred to cope with her difficulties by employing denial, overrationalization, and/or manifesting somatic problems. Interpersonally, the patient was likely to be seen by others as extroverted with a strong need for affection, overly self-controlled, immature, passive, and dependent.

Table 20-2. Summary of Neuropsychological Test Data

Test Name	Standard Score	T-Score
Wechsler Adult Intelligence Test–III		
Full-Scale IQ	87	51
Verbal Comprehension Index	89	54
Perceptual Organizational Index	93	52
Working Memory Index	84	45
Processing Speed Index	93	52
Vocabulary		57
Similarities		51
Arithmetic		41
Digit Span		48
Information		52
Letter-Number Sequencing		52
Picture Completions		52
Digit Symbol		53
Block Design		47
Matrix Reasoning		57
Symbol Search		52
Wide Range Achievement Test–4		
Reading	105	
Spelling	99	
Arithmetic	90	
Test Name	Raw Score	T-Score
Grooved Pegboard Test		
Dominant (right) hand	c91"	27
Nondominant hand	100"	33
Digit Vigilance Test		
Time 417"	42	
Errors 2	64	
Trail-Making Test		
Part A 41"	43	
Part B 114"	41	

(Continued)

Table 20-2. Summary of Neuropsychological Test Data (*Continued*)

Test Name	Raw Score	T-Score
California Verbal Learning Test-II		
Trial 1 5	35	
Trial 5 13	50	
Trials 1–53	48	43
Trial B 6	45	
Short-Delay Free Recall	13	55
Short-Delay Cued Recall	14	55
Long-Delay Free Recall	14	55
Long-Delay Cued Recall	14	50
Recognition Hits	14	35
Discriminability (d')	3.3	50
Intrusions	1	45
Repetitions	2	45
Wisconsin Card-Sorting Test -128		
Categories	6	
Perserative Responses	8	>80
Perserative Errors	8	>80
Minnesota Multiphasic Personality Inventory -2		

Scale	K Corrected T-Scores
1	90
2	79
3	94
4	55
6	52
7	77
8	69
9	65

Discussion

The neuropsychological profile in this case highlights the natural recovery expected from a mild brain injury, but it also reveals the complicated psychological and environmental factors that can influence symptom reporting. Her test results demonstrate good cognitive functioning, with one relatively lower than expected performance on a task requiring fine motor speed. By chance alone, there could be one low score in a larger battery of tests, but in this case the low scores were thought to be most likely related to her excessively long finger nails. Results on the MMPI-2 and data from the clinical interview revealed an individual with strong somatically focused complaints, dysphoric and anxious mood, and probable symptom exaggeration tendencies. Given what is known about the circumstances of her supposed brain injury (i.e., no loss of consciousness, no retrograde amnesia, no sustained posttraumatic confusion, no positive head imaging findings), it is doubtful that she experienced anything greater than a concussion—at worst—at the time of the motor vehicle collision. In such a situation, it is expected that she should experience a rapid and full cognitive recovery within a week to 10 days with 3 months time at the most . Along those lines, no evidence was seen in the test results approximately 2 months after her accident to implicate continued cognitive sequelae status post concussion. Specifically, she performed within the low-average range or better on measures of attention-concentration, speed of information processing, executive functioning, and learning/memory—areas that are commonly impaired in patients who are still recovering from a brain injury.

Her perceived symptom complaints were thought to be accounted for by nonneurological factors, such as her depressed and anxious emotional status, strong somatic focus, and other situational factors, including pending litigation involvement. There were also family dynamics that were contributory factors in this case; for instance, during the feedback session with the patient and mother, the mother seemed to be very overinvolved, stating that she and her daughter were best friends, that she was very involved in her day-to-day activities, and requested contact information from this examiner in case other issues arose. As such, there appeared to be some secondary gain and dependency issues at play between the mother and daughter that could have explained some of the findings noted on the MMPI-2 and the maintained symptom reporting.

Diagnostically, at the time of the evaluation, the patient did not meet formal DSM-IV-TR criteria for postconcussion syndrome (PCS) owing to no objective evidence for deficits in attention-concentration or memory (criteria B) and given that she was only 2 months post-accident (criteria B). Arguably, she also did not meet ICD-10 criteria for PCS because her possible concussion was not "severe enough" to result in a loss of consciousness. Given the concerns about this diagnostic category noted in the introduction of this chapter, this diagnosis was not formally considered anyway. Rather, given her clinical history and objective results garnered from the neuropsychological evaluation, the most appropriate diagnoses were a probable somatoform disorder not otherwise specified (NOS), as the patient manifested her medically unexplained symptoms for less than 6 months, precluding formal diagnosis of an undifferentiated somatoform disorder, and possible depression NOS by history and self-report.

During the feedback session, it was relayed that the patient would likely benefit from education about the following: (1) concussion in terms of duration and expected recovery of common dysfunction (i.e., attention-concentration, speed of information processing, memory), (2) reassurance that on objective testing it appeared that she made a full cognitive recovery, and (3) a simple explanation of how her subjective cognitive complaints were best accounted for by her emotional status (e.g., memory complaints are common in persons with depressed mood) and situation (e.g., recently divorced, with ongoing involvement from ex-husband). A similar educationally based intervention aimed at establishing expectancies of rapid and full cognitive recovery has been shown to reduce the number and duration of subsequent subjective cognitive complaints (i.e., Kashluba et al., 2004; Mittenberg, Tremont, Zielinski, Fichera, & Rayls, 1996).

She was also told that there was no objective evidence seen that would stand in the way of her returning to competitive employment, and that in fact, return to work was most likely going to be helpful in her combating depression, increasing her self-efficacy by feeling that she was a productive person who was contributing to society and her own financial situation, and that it would also help refocus her thoughts from disability to functional independence. She was encouraged to consider participating in short-term psychotherapy to address her emotional distress, to improve coping, while also promoting functional return to activity. To that end, it was thought that she also would likely benefit from an introduction and re-establishment of good sleep hygiene habits. She was advised that her driving apprehension would also diminish in time as she continued to drive (i.e., a naturalistic in vivo exposure intervention), and that if she began to actively avoid driving, her driving anxiety could intensify and persist. Finally, it was recommended that her physiatrist revisit the need for the Aricept prescription, given the fact she was doing so well cognitively.

References

American Psychiatric Association. (2000). *Diagnostic and statistical manual of mental disorder* (4th ed., Text rev.). Washington, DC: Author.

Belanger, H. G., & Vanderploeg, R. D. (2005). The neuropsychological impact of sports-related concussion. *Journal of the International Neuropsychological Society, 11*, 345–357.

Binder, L. M. (2005). Forensic assessment of medically unexplained symptoms. In G. J. Larabee, (Ed.), *Forensic neuropsychology: A scientific approach* (pp. 298–333). New York: Oxford University Press.

Boake, C., McCauley, S. R., Levin, H. S., Pedroza, C., Contant, C.F., Song, J. X., et al. (2005). Diagnostic criteria for post concessional syndrome after mild to moderate traumatic brain injury. *The Journal of Neuropsychiatry and Clinical Neuroscience, 17*, 350–356.

Brolinson, P. G., Manoogian, S., McNeelly, D., Goforth, M., Greenwald, R., & Duma, S. (2006). Analysis of linear head accelerations from collegiate football impacts. *Current Sports Medicine Report, 5,* 23–28.

Carroll, L. J., Cassidy, J. D., Peloso, P. M., Borg, J., von Holst, H., Holm, L., et al. (2004). Prognosis for mild traumatic brain injury: Results of the WHO collaborating centre task force on mild traumatic brain injury. *Journal of Rehabilitation Medicine, 36*(43), 84–105.

Centers for Disease Control and Prevention. (2003). *National Center for Injury Prevention and Control, Centers for Disease Control and Injury Prevention: Report to Congress on mild traumatic brain injury in the United States: Steps to prevent a serious public health problem.* Atlanta, GA. Retrieved October 26, 2008, from: http://www.cdc.gov/ncipc/pub-res/mtbi/report.htm.

Dikmen, S. Machamer, J., Winn, H., & Temkin, N. (1995). Neuropsychological Outcome at 1-Year Post Head Injury. Neuropsychology, 9, 80–90.

Dikmen, S., Machamer, J., & Temkin, N. (2001). Mild head injury: Facts and artifacts. *Journal of Clinical Experimental Neuropsychology, 23,* 729–738.

Dikmen, S., McLean, A., & Temkin, T. (1986). Neuropsychological and psychosocial consequences of minor head injury. *Journal of Neurology, Neurosurgery, and Psychiatry, 49,* 1227–1232.

Holm, L., Cassidy, J. D., Carroll, L. J., & Borg, J. (2005). Summary of the WHO collaborating centre for neurotrauma task force on mild traumatic brain injury. *Journal of Rehabilitation Medicine, 37,* 137–141.

Iverson, G. L. (2005). Outcome in mild traumatic brain injury. *Current Opinion in Psychiatry, 18,* 301–317.

Iverson, G. L., & Lange, R. T. (2003). Examination of "postconcussion-like" symptoms in a healthy sample. *Applied Neuropsychology, 10,* 137–144.

Kashluba, S., Hanks, R. A., Casey, J. E., & Millis, S. R. (2008). Neuropsychologic and functional outcome after complicated mild traumatic brain injury. *Archives of Physical Medicine and Rehabilitation, 89,* 904–911.

Kashluba, S., Paniak, C., Blake, T., Reynolds, S., Toller-Lobe, G., & Nagy, J. (2004). A longitudinal, controlled study of patient complaints following treated mild traumatic brain injury. *Archives of Clinical Neuropsychology, 19,* 805–816.

Levin, H. S., Mattis, S., Ruff, R. M., Eisenberg, H. M., Marshall, L. F., Tabaddor, K., et al. (1987). Neurobehavioral outcome following minor head injury: A three-center study. *Journal of Neurosurgery, 66,* 234–343.

Levine, B., Fujiwara, E., O'Conner, C., Richard, N., Kovacevic, N., Mandic, M., et al. (2006). In vivo characterization of traumatic brain injury neuropathology with structural and functional neuroimaging. *Journal of Neurotrauma, 23,* 1346–1411.

Macciocchi, S. N., Barth, J. T., Alves, W., Rimel, R. W., & Jane, J. A. (1996). Neuropsychological functioning and recovery after mild head injury in collegiate athletes. *Neurosurgery, 39,* 510–514.

McCrea, M. (2008). Biomechanics of TBI. In M. McCrae (Ed.), *Mild traumatic brain injury and postconcussion syndrome* (p. 51). New York: Oxford University Press.

McCrea, M., Guskiewicz, K. M., Marshall, S. W., Barr, W., Randolph, C., Cantu, R. C., et al. (2003). Acute effects and recovery time following concussion in collegiate football players. *Journal of the American Medical Association, 290,* 2556–2563.

Mittenberg, W., Tremont, G., Zielinski, R. E., Fichera, S., & Rayls, K. R. (1996). Cognitive-behavioral prevention of postconcussion syndrome. *Archives of Clinical Neuropsychology, 11,* 139–145.

Rohling, M. L., Meyers, J. E., & Millis, S. R. (2003). Neuropsychological impairment following traumatic brain injury: A dose-response analysis. *The Clinical Neuropsychologist, 17,* 289–302.

Shaw, N. (2002). The neurophysiology of concussion. *Progress in Neurobiology, 67,* 281–344.

Teasdale, G., & Jennett, B. (1974). Assessment of coma and impaired consciousness: A practical scale. *Lancet, 2,* 81–84.

Wang, Y., Chan, R. C. K., & Deng, Y. (2006). Examination of postconcussion symptoms in healthy university students: Relationships to subjective and objective neuropsychological function performance. *Archives of Clinical Neuropsychology, 21,* 339–347.

Wolfe, P., Millis, S.R., Hanks, R.A., Fichtenberg, N., Larabee, G., Sweet, J. (2010). Effort Indicators within the California Verbal Learning Test - II (CVLT-II). *The Clinical Neuropsychologist,* 24 (1), 153–168

Zhang, L., Yang, K. H., & King, A. I. (2004). A proposed injury threshold for mild traumatic brain injury. *Journal of Biomechanical Engineering, 126,* 226–236.

21

Hypoxia after Near Drowning

John T. Beetar

While the human brain does not store oxygen, it requires a constant supply to meet its energy demands (White, Wiegenstein, & Winegar, 1984). When the brain is deprived of oxygen from conditions such as cardiac arrest, carbon monoxide poisoning, obstructive sleep apnea, and near drowning, hypoxic brain injuries can result (Hopkins, Tate, & Bigler, 2005). Necrosis of brain cells is thought to occur when the period of oxygen deprivation exceeds 4–8 minutes (Bigler & Alfano, 1988).

Neuropsychological deficits often result from hypoxia, and they are frequently related to damage to the hippocampus and cerebellum, which are known to be vulnerable to oxygen deprivation. Furthermore, the basal ganglia, watershed cortex, and thalamus also can be areas of insult. Impairments in memory, executive control and behavior, and visuospatial functions often are reported (Caine & Watson, 2000).

When the supply of oxygen is disrupted, a set of cardiovascular adjustments is activated to conserve oxygen for those tissues most sensitive to hypoxia. This reaction is often seen during breath holding while submersed in water. It is referred to as the diving response whereby cardiac output is diminished, secondary to bradycardia. Peripheral vasoconstriction reduces blood flow to a large proportion of the body, including skeletal muscles, so that it is conserved for the heart and brain. It is hypothesized that the diving response explains survival from prolonged submersion (Gooden, 1992) and is

enhanced by both anxiety and cold water (Golden, Tipton, & Scott, 1997). However, there is debate about the effectiveness of bradycardia during submersion in individuals other than infants. Goksor, Rosengren, and Wennergren (2002) argued that the dive reflex declines with increasing age during childhood.

There are approximately 500,000 drownings every year worldwide (Peden, McGee, & Sharma, 2002). In the United States, drowning is second to motor vehicle crashes as a cause of unintentional injury death among children and adolescents (Cohen, Matter, Sinclair, Smith, & Xiang, 2008). Near drowning is defined as survival, at least temporarily, following suffocation by submersion in water (Modell, 1989); it occurs three to five times more often than drowning (Levin, Morriss, Toro, Brink, & Turner, 1993).

Near drowning in cold water is thought to protect the central nervous system for longer periods of time than is usually required to produce cell death. It is theorized that cold water results in rapid loss of body heat. Subsequently, the brain is cooled and metabolism is depressed. Upon recovery, survivors are hypothermic with a reduction of about 7°C or 11°F. In animal studies, a brain temperature of below 29°C to 31°C, or about 85° F, provides increased protection against anoxia. A child's skin surface relative to body weight is larger compared to adults. As such, they lose heat more rapidly and may be protected for periods of longer duration than an adult (Gooden, 1992). Indeed, Samuelson, Nekludov, and Levander (2008) recently reported on two adult survivors of cold water submersions with ongoing neuropsychological deficits. However, in a retrospective study, Suominen et al. (2002) found that children did not have a better outcome than adults despite a higher surface of area to body weight ratio. They concluded that survival and quality of neurological outcome after near drowning is dependent on the duration of submersion rather than the age of the victim.

The Case of A. W.

A. W. was referred for a neuropsychological evaluation by his psychiatrist. At that time, he was 10 years old and lived with his mother, stepfather, and younger half sister. He had not seen his biological father in about 5 years. Family medical history is unremarkable.

A. W. was the 7 pound, 15 ounce product of a gestation complicated by vomiting and the occasional use of alcohol. He was delivered during a head-first vaginal delivery. The neonatal period was notable for jaundice. Developmental milestones reportedly were attained within expected time frames.

Medical/psychiatric history is most significant for aggression toward peers and attention-deficit/hyperactivity disorder (ADHD), diagnosed at about 8 years. Treatment in the form of medication was deferred by A. W.'s family. At 9 years, intellectual testing with the Wechsler Intelligence Scale for Children, Third Edition (WISC-III) revealed average ability given a Verbal IQ (VIQ) of 111, at the 77th percentile, a Performance IQ (PIQ) of 104, at the 61st percentile, and a Full Scale IQ (FSIQ) of 108, at the 70th percentile. Individual subtest scores are listed in Table 21-1.

The subsequent year, A. W. was trialed on Ritalin. However, 2 weeks following the start of medication, he and two other boys fell through the ice of a partially frozen pond. A. W. was submerged for more than 30 minutes. Upon recovery from the water, he presented with fixed and dilated pupils and was taken to the hospital. His body core temperature was 85.1°F. A. W. was in a coma for 12 days, and he required respiratory and cardiovascular support. On hospital day 3, an electroencephalogram (EEG) was abnormal; Dilantin was administered for seizure prophylaxis.

Table 21-1. Test Results

WISC-III Subtests	Subtest Score	WISC-III Subtests	Subtest Score
Information	12	Picture Completion	12
Similarities	12		
Arithmetic	11	Coding	11
Vocabulary	11	Picture Arrangement	11
Comprehension	13		
Digit Span	14	Block Design	12
		Object Assembly	7
		Symbol Search	11
		Mazes	10

On hospital day 8, a computed tomography (CT) scan showed focal hemorrhages, a mild left to right shift, and frontoparietal and occipital hypodensities consistent with a poor prognosis. However, on hospital day 15, A. W. was extubated from the ventilator and began to show rapid improvement in mental status. For example, he could follow simple commands, recognize family members, and speak in complete sentences. He was also emotionally labile. About 3 weeks following the near drowning, A. W. was discharged on Clonidine, Feosol, and Colace. Dilantin had already been discontinued. Screening of intellect at that time revealed average ability. Verbal memory was affected by a primacy effect; nonverbal memory was impacted by inattention. Impaired fine-motor skills reportedly contributed to constructional difficulties. Executive functioning was notable for loss of set.

Following A. W.'s accident, he received tutoring to prepare him for a return to his fifth-grade class, initially on a part-time basis. There had been no premorbid history of retention or special education. When A. W. returned to school, his teacher described him as inattentive, distractible, poorly organized, and forgetful. Poor frustration tolerance often resulted in temper tantrums and hostility.

A. W. was seen twice for neuropsychological evaluations by this writer to assess his recovery from the near drowning. The first assessment occurred about 6 months following the accident; the re-evaluation took place approximately 2 years later. Taken together, observations were notable for slender build. There was no evidence of physical abnormalities; A. W. preferred his right hand. Ability to sustain attention was unremarkable, as were receptive and expressive language skills. During the first assessment session, A. W. was noted to be emotionally labile. In contrast, there was no emotional lability during his second visit.

Examination Results

Given that testing of intellect had been performed a year before the accident, and then rescreened at the time of his discharge, it was not evaluated during the first neuropsychological evaluation. At that time, testing of sensorimotor functions revealed that hand strength and finger tapping speed were below expectations on the right side. Bilateral fine-motor dexterity was deficient. On tasks of tactile perception, A. W. made more errors on the right than on the left. Appreciation of right and left orientation was intact on his own body; however, he reversed right and left on a confronting person.

Assessment of language functions revealed average single-word receptive vocabulary on the Peabody Picture Vocabulary Test (PPVT)–Revised given a scaled score at the 68th percentile. On the Token Test, Part V, ability to follow commands was at the 75th percentile. On the Boston Naming Test, A. W. performed in the low-average range. Word fluency was average to a semantic category, but below average to a phonemic characteristic with perseverative tendencies noted.

Verbal memory on the Rey Auditory Verbal Learning Test (AVLT) was average on all conditions. On the Wide Range Assessment of Memory and Learning (WRAML), sentence repetition was low average, as was story recall. Story recognition memory was within expectations.

On the Hooper Visual Organization Test, A. W. performed in the low-average range. On the Test of Visual-Perceptual Skills (TVPS), visual memory was superior. In contrast, his appreciation of visual-spatial relations, visual form constancy, and visual figure-ground was below expectations.

On measures of visual-motor ability, A. W.'s scores were variable. Specifically, construction on the Beery Visual Motor Integration Test (VMI) was in the average range with evidence of poor planning. His copy of the Rey-Osterrieth Complex Figure (ROCF) was disorganized with an overall below-average score. Delayed recall of the figure was markedly impaired. However, immediate

recall of geometric figures on the Benton Visual Retention Test was within expectations.

Regarding executive functions, A. W. demonstrated the ability to sustain his attention on cancellation tasks. On the Trail Making Test (TMT), he worked within time expectations on both sequencing and switching tasks. With regard to the latter, he failed to correctly alternate the set on two occasions. On the Stroop Color-Word Naming Test, there was no evidence of susceptibility to interference by competing cognitive sets. A. W. performed in the high-average range on the Children's Category Test.

On the Woodcock-Johnson Tests of Achievement–Revised, all basic and applied academic skills were average. Measures of emotional/behavioral functioning revealed anxiety, mood variability, inattention, hyperactivity, impulsivity, and aggression.

Immediately prior to this writer's reevaluation in 1998, A. W.'s local school system re-evaluated his intellect with the WISC-III. He obtained a Verbal IQ of 123, at the 94th percentile, a Performance IQ of 110, at the 75th percentile, and a Full Scale IQ of 118, at the 88th percentile. Academic achievement generally was within expectations except for reading comprehension and written expression. Individual subtest scores for the WISC-III are presented in Table 21-2.

Neuropsychological re-evaluation demonstrated an appreciation of right and left orientation on both self and confronting person. Bilateral strength and dexterity were within expectations.

Assessment of language functions revealed average single-word receptive vocabulary on the PPVT–III given a scaled score at the 70th percentile. On the Token Test, Part V, ability to follow commands was at the 74th percentile.

Table 21-2. Test Results

WISC-III Subtests	Subtest Score	WISC-III Subtests	Subtest Score
Information	13	Picture	15
Similarities	14	Completion	
Arithmetic	16	Coding	9
Vocabulary	12	Picture	13
Comprehension	14	Arrangement	
		Block Design	9
	14	Object Assembly	11

On the Boston Naming Test, A. W. performed in the average range. Word fluency was low average to a semantic category and average to a phonemic characteristic.

Verbal memory on the Rey AVLT ranged from average to high average. On the WRAML, sentence repetition was average, as was story recall. Story recognition memory was within expectations.

On the Hooper Visual Organization Test, A. W. performed in the average range. On measures of visual-motor ability, A. W.'s scores again were variable. Specifically, construction on the VMI was average. His copy of the ROCF was better organized than during the initial evaluation with an overall low-average score. However, delayed recall of the figure again was impaired. Immediate recall of geometric figures on the Benton Visual Retention Test was within expectations.

On measures of executive functioning, A. W. worked slower than expected when required to complete cancellation tasks. On the TMT, he worked within time expectations on both sequencing and switching tasks. On the latter task, there were no errors of set switching. On the Wisconsin Card Sorting Task (WCST), his problem solving was within expectations.

The Case of B. Y.

B. Y. was referred for a neuropsychological evaluation by his psychiatrist. He and A. W. were involved in the same near-drowning accident when B. Y. was 11 years old. At that time, he was living with his mother, older brother, and younger half brother. His father was not involved in his care. Extended family history is notable for diabetes and heart disease on the paternal side.

B. Y. was the 8 pound, 2 ounce product of an uncomplicated gestation. Anesthesia was employed during labor; forceps were used during the vaginal delivery. The neonatal period was unremarkable. Developmental milestones reportedly were attained within expected time frames.

Premorbid educational history was unremarkable. Medical/psychiatric history was significant for ADHD, obsessive-compulsive disorder, and tics. B. Y. was about to start psychostimulant medication when he nearly drowned. His older brother, whom B. Y. attempted to rescue, died in the same accident. B. Y. was submerged for more than 30 minutes. Upon recovery from the water,

his body core temperature was 94°F. B. Y. was comatose for 1 day and suffered posttraumatic amnesia for several weeks. An EEG showed bilateral slowing; however, magnetic resonance imaging (MRI) at the time of discharge, 1 month following the accident, was normal. Regardless, B. Y. had impaired cognition, displayed choreoathetosis, and could not engage in most aspects of self-care. His diagnosis of hypoxic encephalopathy was associated with Parkinson syndrome, consisting of involuntary motor movements that were treated with Amantadine.

Following B. Y.'s discharge, he was admitted first to inpatient and then outpatient rehabilitation. The latter was several years in duration and provided both rehabilitative services and academics. About 1.5 years after the near drowning, B. Y. began a gradual re-entry to his public school. He was placed in a self-contained classroom for most of the day and experienced notable difficulty given poor memory, reduced language comprehension, inattention, and impulsivity. Indeed, the referring psychiatrist reported worsening ADHD symptoms, which were being treated with Ritalin at the time. Compulsions, in the form of picking behaviors, and tics, such as eye blinking and throat clearing, also were present post injury. B. Y. was having difficulty adjusting to the loss of his brother and his own premorbid functioning.

Approximately 1 year after the near drowning, a neuropsychological evaluation was conducted by an outside evaluator. On the WISC-III, B. Y. achieved a Verbal IQ of 75, at the 5th percentile, a Performance IQ of 64, at the 1st percentile, and a Full Scale IQ of 68, at the 2nd percentile. Individual subtest scores are provided in Table 21-3.

Additional measures showed impaired visual scanning, visual-motor skills, and executive functioning. Additionally, postural control was reduced. B. Y. displayed mild coordination deficits. A speech and language evaluation revealed intact expressive vocabulary, but poorer than expected receptive skills. His reading recognition was well below grade-level expectations. Overall impressions were a significant decline in functioning compared to premorbid estimates of generally average ability.

B. Y. was seen by this writer for a neuropsychological evaluation 2 years following his near-drowning injury. At that time, he was

Table 21-3. Test Results

WISC-III Subtests	Subtest Score	WISC-III Subtests	Subtest Score
Information	6	Picture Completion	9
Similarities	9		
Arithmetic	2	Coding	3
Vocabulary	5	Picture Arrangement	1
Comprehension	6		
Digit Span	9	Block Design	2
		Object Assembly	5

Table 21-4. Test Results

WISC-III Subtests	Subtest Score	WISC-III Subtests	Subtest Score
Information	8	Picture Completion	6
Similarities	7		
Arithmetic	5	Coding	3
Vocabulary	6	Picture Arrangement	3
Comprehension	4		
Digit Span	10	Block Design	1
		Object Assembly	4
		Symbol Search	2

11.75 years old. Observations revealed a stocky individual with an awkward gait and involuntary movements of the lower extremities. He was sociable and responsive to humor; rapport was easily established. Conversational speech was difficult to understand given impaired articulation since the accident. B. Y. spoke with a nasal quality; and he often garbled his words. While he was friendly, he could also be oppositional between tasks. B. Y. frequently complained about the duration of testing. Once engaged in an activity, however, he was able to persist with praise and encouragement. He preferred his right hand.

Examination Results

Intelligence testing with the WISC-III yielded a Verbal IQ of 78, at the 7th percentile and a Performance IQ of 60, which is less than the 1st percentile. B. Y.'s Full Scale IQ was 67, at the 1st percentile. In general, results are consistent with those of prior testing. Individual subtest scores are provided in Table 21-4.

With the exception of impaired bilateral tactile discrimination, sensory-perceptual abilities were normal. Hand strength was within expectations on both the right and left hands. However, motor speed and dexterity were impaired, bilaterally. B. Y. also presented with significant overflow movement in the opposite hand and in his face during selected tasks.

Assessment of basic language functions revealed average receptive vocabulary on PPVT-R, given a scaled score at the 37th percentile, and high-average naming on the Expressive One-Word Vocabulary Test (EOWVT) with a scaled score at the 86th percentile. On the Token Test, Part V, B. Y. scored in the low-average range.

Word generation to either a phonemic characteristic or semantic category was impaired at the 1st percentile.

Verbal memory on the Rey AVLT was impaired. B. Y. had no recall of any words on the immediate and delayed recall formats. His recognition memory also was deficient and further spoiled by numerous false-positive responses. On the WRAML, sentence repetition was average. In contrast, story recall was below average. Story recognition memory was low average.

On the Hooper Visual Organization Test, B.Y. performed in the low-average range. On the TVPS, B. Y.'s appreciation of visual figure-ground was average. Otherwise, his other subtest scores on that measure were well below expectations.

Regarding visual-motor ability, construction on the VMI was below average given a standard score of 70, at the 2nd percentile. Immediate recall of geometric figures on the Benton Visual Retention Test also was below expectations.

B. Y.'s ability to sustain his attention on cancellation tasks was below expectations. He became confused during the task and lost his place while scanning. On the TMT, he worked within time expectations and did not make any errors on the sequencing task. However, when required to alternate between cognitive sets, he was slower than expected and made numerous errors. The WCST was discontinued given B. Y.'s significant difficulty with that measure of novel problem solving.

Evaluation of emotional/behavioral functioning revealed inattention, distractibility, impulsivity, withdrawal, and ongoing obsessions and compulsions. B. Y. also had a history of frequent somatic complaints, likely secondary to his prolonged hypoxia.

Table 21-5. Table of Selected Test Results from Neuropsychological Evaluations

	Initial Evaluation: A. W.	Reevaluation: A. W.	Initial Evaluation: B. Y.
Tests			
Motor Functions			
Grooved pegs (preferred)	89" (4th)	67" (55th)	109" (<1st)
(nonpreferred)	127" (<1st)	78" (30th)	106" (<1st)
Finger tapping (preferred)	24.8 (1st)	N/A	32.8 (5th)
(nonpreferred)	32.8 (47th)		26.8 (2nd)
Language Functions			
PPVT-R	107 (68th)	N/A	95 (37th)
PPVT-III	N/A	108 (70th)	N/A
Token Test (Part V)	19 (75th)	19 (74th)	11 (11th)
Boston Naming Test	41 (14th)	48 (34th)	N/A
EOWVT	N/A	N/A	88 (86th)
"F-A-S" word fluency	12 (7th)	29 (48th)	5 (1st)
"Animals" word fluency	14 (27th)	15 (19th)	7 (1st)
Rey AVLT:			
Total Learned	40 (51st)	53 (84th)	25 (4th)
Interference List	5 (61st)	6 (72nd)	4 (39th)
Immediate Recall	10 (72nd)	10 (69th)	0 (1st)
Delayed Recall	7 (43rd)	9 (61st)	0 (1st)
Delayed Recognition	14 (WNL)	15 (WNL)	8 (IMP)
False Positives	2	1	10
WRAML:			
Sentence Repetition	14 (16th)	18 (25th)	20 (37th)
Immediate Story Recall	17 (16th)	33 (75th)	7 (1st)
Delayed Story Recall	17	29	2
Story Recognition	12 (AV)	11 (AV)	8 (LAV)
Visual-Spatial Functions			
Hooper	22 (21st)	26 (54th)	21.5 (16th)
TVPS Perceptual Quotient	92 (30th)	N/A	62 (1st)
VMI	92 (30th)	92 (30th)	70 (2nd)
ROCF:			
Copy	15.5 (6th)	24 (18th)	N/A
Delayed Recall	2 (1st)	11.5 (3rd)	N/A
Executive Functions			
TMT Part A	21" (59th)	18" (59th)	23" (36th)
Part B	53" (50th)	29" (69th)	120" (<1st)
Children's Category Test	12 (89th)	N/A	N/A
WCST Categories	N/A	6	0 (D/C)

Note. Raw scores are provided with the exception of standard scores for the PPVT, VMI, and TVPS. Percentiles or ranges are presented in parentheses.

Discussion

Two boys of approximately the same age, both with premorbid ADHD, unremarkable educational histories, and involvement in the same near-drowning accident, had markedly different neuropsychological outcomes.

On initial neuropsychological evaluation following the accident, A. W. presented with right-sided deficits on tests of sensorimotor functions. He also demonstrated executive dysfunction given occasional loss of set and poor organizational skills. Memory grossly was intact, but impacted by inefficient learning and poor organization of material. Visual perception and construction were variable; the latter also was affected by executive difficulties. Regarding language, receptive skills were intact, while aspects of expressive skills were insecure. Observations and history were notable for emotional lability.

Upon re-evaluation several years later, A. W. had recovered all functioning with the exception of a mild relative weakness in his visual-spatial skills. It was not known whether there had been any premorbid unevenness in that domain or if those discontinuities were due to his brain injury following the near drowning. Observations revealed diminished lability. Medical records revealed that A. W.'s body core temperature had cooled to around 85°F, a temperature thought to be neuroprotective.

In contrast, findings of B. Y.'s neuropsychological testing 2 years following his injuries revealed impairments in numerous areas of functioning. Specifically, overall intellect was below average. He also demonstrated variability in selected language functions, particularly expressive skills, visual-perceptual and visual-motor skills, and executive functioning. Furthermore, B. Y. presented with choreoathetosis and bilateral fine-motor deficits. His medical records indicated that his body core temperature was 94°F upon recovery.

A. W.'s body temperature had cooled to a level thought to be protective of the central nervous system; however, B. Y.'s temperature was only about four degrees colder than normal. While the actual body weights of these boys at the time of their accident are not known, during testing, A. W. was observed to be slender while B. Y. was stocky. Thus, B. Y. may have retained more heat than A. W. because of his build.

There is debate in the literature about the dive reflex during a submersion and subsequent adjustments to conserve oxygen for the brain and heart while blood flow to other organs and muscles is diminished. B. Y. tried to save his brother who drowned. As such, it is hypothesized that the necessary cardiovascular adjustments were not made in B. Y.'s case given the need for blood in his skeletal muscles during his attempted rescue. Taken together, his brain presumably was both insufficiently cooled and perfused with blood. These conditions likely resulted in compromise of brain functioning compared to his premorbid endowment. By contrast, it is reasonable to hypothesize that hypothermia and the dive reflex preserved A. W.'s brain functioning.

References

Bigler, E. D., & Alfano, M. (1988). Anoxic encephalopathy: Neuroradiological and neuropsychological findings. *Archives of Clinical Neuropsychology, 3,* 383–396.

Caine, D., & Watson, J. D. (2000). Neuropsychological and neuropathological sequelae of cerebral anoxia: A critical review. *Journal of the International Neuropsychological Society, 6,* 86–99.

Cohen, R. H., Matter, K. C., Sinclair, S. A., Smith, G. A., & Xiang, H. (2008). Unintentional pediatric submersion-injury-related hospitalizations in the United States, 2003. *Injury Prevention, 14,* 131–135.

Golden, F. C., Tipton, M. J., & Scott, R. C. (1997). Immersion, near-drowning and drowning. *British Journal of Anaesthesia, 79,* 214–225.

Gooden, B. A. (1992). Why some people do not drown: Hypothermia versus the diving response. *The Medical Journal of Australia, 157,* 629–632.

Goksor, E., Rosengren, L., & Wennergren, G. (2002). Bradycardic response during submersion in infant swimming. *Acta Pediatrics, 91,* 307–312.

Hopkins, R. O., Tate, D. F., & Bigler, E. D. (2005). Anoxic versus traumatic brain injury: Amount of tissue loss, not etiology, alters cognitive and emotional function. *Neuropsychology, 19,* 233–242.

Levin, D. L., Morriss, F. C., Toro, L. O., Brink, L. W., & Turner, G. R. (1993). Drowning and near-drowning. *Pediatric Clinics of North America, 40,* 321–336.

Modell, J. H. (1989). Drown versus near-drown: A discussion of definitions. *Critical Care Medicine, 9,* 351–352.

Peden, M., McGee, K., & Sharma, K. (2002). *The injury chart book: A graphical overview of the global burden of injuries.* Geneva, Switzerland: World Health Organization.

Samuelson, H., Nekludov, M., & Levander, M. (2008). Neuropsychological outcome following near-drowning in ice water: Two adult cases. *Journal of the International Neuropsychological Society, 14,* 660–666.

Suominen, P., Baille, C., Korpela, R., Rautanen, S., Ranta, S., & Olkkola, K. T. (2002). Impact of age, submersion time and water temperature on outcome in near drowning. *Resuscitation, 52,* 247–254.

White, B. C., Wiegenstein, J. G., & Winegar, C. D. (1984). Brain ischemic anoxia: Mechanisms of injury. *Journal of the American Medical Association, 251,* 1586–1590.

Part III

Neuropsychiatric Disorders

Neuropsychiatric disorder is a principal reason why an individual may be referred to a clinical neuropsychologist, and there is a long tradition of neuropsychological evaluation and treatment in psychiatric settings. Although the primary presentation is often emotional and behavioral in nature, individuals with neuropsychiatric disorders may also present with identifiable neuropsychological impairment. Such impairment is often related to underlying neurobiological disruption, but it may also be exacerbated by emotional overlay or interaction of the individual and his or her environment. While the scope of neuropsychiatric disorders is broad, and entire books have been dedicated to the topic, the following seven chapters cover a variety of thought disorders.

22

Attention-Deficit/Hyperactivity Disorder and Anxiety Disorder: An Atypical Presentation of a "Typical" Disorder

Kira Armstrong

Attention-deficit/hyperactivity disorder (ADHD) is generally recognized as the most common diagnosis for children leading to a psychiatric or psychological evaluation. Conservative estimates suggest that 4% to 12% of children between the ages of 6 and 18 years may have ADHD, and some reviews found the incidence rate to be as high as 17% (Stefanatos & Baron, 2007). While many clinicians are well grounded in the diagnostic criteria and presentation of a "typical" ADHD child, the majority of children with ADHD have at least one diagnosable comorbid disorder. In fact, Brassett-Harknett and Butler (2007) argue that one is more likely to find a child with ADHD and a comorbidity than to find a child with ADHD alone. Depending on the source, research suggests that 58%–87% of children with ADHD may have at least one comorbid disorder, and up to 20% may meet criteria for three or more comorbid disorders (Stefanatos & Baron, 2007).

Historically, the literature has focused more on children with ADHD and comorbid externalizing disorders. This is due in part to the fact that these disorders are more readily apparent because of their significant impact on the child's parents, teachers, and others. In contrast, as many children with *internalizing* symptomatology do not exhibit disruptive behaviors, their symptoms are easily overlooked and/or misunderstood. Furthermore, many children effectively "hide" their anxiety from parents and teachers, because talking about their fears is anxiety provoking in and of itself.

Consequently, these diagnoses can be missed without specific and targeted inquiry by the clinician (Schatz & Rostain, 2006). Additionally, conducting a cursory review of symptoms may lead clinicians to assume a child's anxiety is merely a "normal feature" of a typical developmental course (Stefanatos & Baron, 2007).

Although internalizing disorders can be less overt, they are nonetheless equally disruptive to a child's adjustment (Stefanatos & Baron, 2007). They are also fairly common in children with ADHD. In fact, several studies suggest that comorbid rates of ADHD and anxiety disorders range from 8% to 50% (Mennin, Biederman, Mick, & Faraone, 2000; Schatz & Rostain, 2006). This finding is especially meaningful, when one is reminded that only 5%–15% of the general population will meet criteria for an anxiety disorder (Schatz & Rostain, 2006). Consequently, a child with ADHD has significantly greater risk for a comorbid anxiety disorder than a child without ADHD.

As neuropsychologists we are, of course, interested in the impact of specific disorders on a child's neurocognitive abilities. Unfortunately, to date there have only been three studies specifically evaluating the cognitive impact of anxiety in children. Furthermore, these studies have varied significantly in their samples, experimental measures, and results. For example, Gunther, Holkamp, Jolles, Herpertz-Dahlmann, and Konrad (2004) demonstrated significant verbal memory difficulties in children with depression but failed to find any cognitive difficulties associated with anxiety. In contrast, Vasa et al. (2007) reported that children with social phobias exhibited deficits in visual memory but not verbal memory. Finally, Toren et al. (2000) reported that anxiety and worry tended to impair performance on tasks of working memory, vocabulary, reading comprehension, mathematics, and problem solving. Their sample also exhibited a rigid adherence to a specific approach to tasks as well as a decreased ability to shift their focus to other tasks or strategies.

There is a somewhat larger literature base regarding the comorbid presentation of children with ADHD and anxiety disorders, although here too the studies are limited. Preliminary findings suggest that children with comorbid ADHD and anxiety may exhibit a different presentation of ADHD symptomatology due to the overlap of their respective disorders. More specifically, many of these children experience significant anxiety associated with perceived judgment, failure, and fears related to reduced competency and performance. Consequently, a child's anxiety may help inhibit impulsive tendencies and hyperactivity, which leads to an ameliorating effect on comorbid conduct disorders. However, studies also suggest that these children may have increased attentional difficulties and exhibit longer reaction times. Furthermore, the combined impact of their ADHD and cautious response style may lead to self-fulfilling prophecies regarding their fears of negative evaluations due to their poor academic performance (Jensen et al., 2001).

The Case of R. G.

R. G. is a 12-year-old boy who was diagnosed with ADHD by his pediatrician in second grade. He has been taking a stimulant since the diagnosis, which has successfully reduced his activity level and led to general improvements in his academic performance. However, it also contributes to notable side effects. For example, R. G. complains of headaches and stomachaches and his parents report lethargy and signs of anhedonia; R. G. does not want to "do anything," including activities he typically enjoys, when he takes his Concerta. When his parents allow him to skip his medication (e.g., on a weekend or during a school vacation), R. G.'s affect brightens

considerably and he becomes more engaged with his friends and family. Furthermore, despite medication management of his ADHD, R. G. continues to exhibit persistent difficulties with working memory, emotional reactivity, and a low tolerance for frustration. Because of these ongoing difficulties, R. G. has participated in two psychological evaluations and one psychiatric evaluation in order to assist with clinical management. Each of these evaluators confirmed R. G.'s ADHD and recommended an increase in stimulant medication. Consequently, at the time of this neuropsychological assessment R. G. was taking 54 mg Concerta as well as 0.1 mg Clonidine to help him sleep at night.

R. G. was born full-term weighing 7 pounds, 12 ounces. His mother's pregnancy was significant for preterm labor at 22 weeks gestation that was delayed by treatment with terbutaline and magnesium sulfate. Perinatal history was uncomplicated and developmental milestones were met within normal limits. Aside from his ADHD, medical history is noncontributory.

Academically, R. G. has never repeated a grade or received special educational services. This neuropsychological evaluation was completed during the summer before sixth grade (which in his district is the first year of middle school). Despite his medication, R. G. frequently forgets to bring homework to school and/or turn it in even when it is in his bag. His folders and materials are also significantly disorganized. When working on homework R. G. becomes extremely frustrated. Sometimes he will become so distressed that he will hit himself with his hand, or lie on the floor crying, "I don't want to do it! I don't want to do it!" At these times he becomes so overwhelmed that he cannot follow or understand simple concepts or homework expectations. R. G. also reports experiencing stomachaches when he is nervous about a test or school activity and when completing homework.

Because of these concerns, R. G. participated in a school-based evaluation several months prior to this neuropsychological assessment. Test results documented an average overall cognitive ability on the WISC-IV with a Full-Scale IQ of 90 (VCI = 87; PRI = 98; WMI = 91; PSI = 97). R. G. demonstrated a relative weakness in his abstract verbal skills on the Similarities subtest, but performance in all other areas was in the low-average to average range. Scaled scores were as follows:

Similarities	6	Block Design	10
Vocabulary	9	Picture Concepts	11
Comprehension	8	Matrix Reasoning	8
Digit Span	9	Coding	9
Letter # Sequencing	8	Symbol Search	10

Within this context, academic skills on the WJ-III were in the low-average to average range, although R. G. demonstrated a consistent weakness on all timed (or "fluency-based") tests. Additionally, auditory working memory was highlighted as a relative weakness. Speech and language testing also documented difficulties with working memory, but all other language based tasks were in the low-average to average range. Based on these findings it was determined that R. G. did not have a learning disorder, and therefore he was deemed ineligible for special educational services.

Although all of R. G.'s previous evaluators had failed to recognize any internalizing symptomatology, it took very little clinical investigation to recognize that R. G. has been experiencing long-standing and significant emotional difficulties. In fact upon questioning, his mother described R. G. as an "extremely anxious boy who is nervous about most new things." Furthermore, he is afraid to go into the family's basement alone, and of riding in elevators. He also worries that if a door shuts (e.g., in a public restroom) he will be unable to open it. He is a perfectionistic child and he can become frustrated if his work is not "just right." R. G. reports having difficulties falling asleep at night because he worries about global warming and other general fears. He also worries that children will laugh at him in social situations and has significant difficulty when he loses at a game.

Socially, although R. G. is actively sought out by children in his neighborhood and at his family's summer home, he does not have any friends at school. He sits alone at lunchtime and has been the target of teasing. Notably, he has a very significant family history of anxiety (including panic attacks) in numerous maternal relatives (family history was otherwise unremarkable), but the relevance of this history had never been addressed in previous evaluations.

Behavioral Observations

R. G. was tested across 3 days. He was on his medications for days 1 and 2, but not for day 3. Across all days of testing R. G. was a likable but very anxious boy. He interacted appropriately with the examiner and was clearly motivated to perform well. He also appeared fairly comfortable with the examiner and the testing process. Nonetheless, R. G. demonstrated a significant reluctance to guess an answer and spent an unusually long amount of time considering responses before answering most open-ended verbal questions. Similarly, he demonstrated notably poor spontaneous recall in the context of extremely strong recognition skills. During the first day of testing R. G. initially engaged in mild "nervous" activity (e.g., picking at his fingers). Over time these behaviors evolved into a more dysregulated style of fidgeting, such as playing with his pencil and wiggling in his seat. Furthermore, on day 3 of testing (when he was not on his medication) R. G. was even more dysregulated, as demonstrated by a tendency to twirl his hair, jiggle his legs, or spin pens. His response style across all three days was slow, methodical, and perfectionistic; however, despite his best efforts R. G. was still prone to impulsive and/or careless errors.

R. G. easily engaged in informal conversation, but he never initiated it. Comprehension was intact, despite R. G.'s tendency toward long latencies for responses. Language expression was appropriate in form and content, aside from occasional word-finding difficulties. Speech was clearly articulated and intelligible. Language pragmatics were intact, and R. G. demonstrated a satisfactory appreciation of paralinguistic features such as gesture, intonation, and facial expression.

R. G. did not demonstrate any unusual physical characteristics. His gait and balance were unremarkable. Graphomotor control was adequate. R. G. preferred his left hand for writing and drawing. He employed a modified tripod grip and produced legible output.

Examination Results

Because the WISC-IV had recently been administered to R. G., his cognitive ability was assessed using the WASI. Consistent with previous testing, his overall cognitive ability was average, with a Full Scale IQ of 107 (around the 70th percentile). His Verbal IQ of 100 was also average (around the 50th percentile), and his Performance IQ of 110 was in the high-average range (around the 75th percentile). T-scores for each subtest were as follows:

| Vocabulary | 48 | Block Design | 58 |
| Similarities | 53 | Matrix Reasoning | 57 |

Outside of the WASI, language skills were vulnerable to difficulties with organized retrieval and fell in the below-average to low-average range. More specifically, phonemic and semantic verbal fluency were below average. In contrast, confrontation naming skills were in the low-average range, as was R. G.'s execution of oral directions. Verbal learning was vulnerable to inattention and anxiety, and fell in the below-average to average range. For example, R. G. reported that he "blanked out" during the immediate and delayed trials of the CMS Stories subtests, which led to a below-average performance. He also demonstrated a significant split in his recall across the two stories. For example on Story 1 he immediately recalled 20 details, but he only recalled 6 details for Story 2 (delayed recall of details was 11 and 3, respectively). However, he accurately identified 27 out of 30 questions on the recognition subtest, leading to an average performance. Furthermore, he demonstrated a clear confidence in his answers to this task (i.e., he was not guessing). R. G.'s initial recall on the CVLT-C was average, as was his total recall across five trials. However, it was noteworthy that he implemented a semantic clustering strategy during the first trial, but then second guessed this strategy and reverted to a less advanced serial recall approach for the remaining four trials. Delayed recall was in the average to high-average range, and recognition was average.

Visual spatial skills were a relative strength for R. G. and fell in the average to above-average range. More specifically, perceptual recognition was average, as were simple visual-motor construction skills. Perceptual matching was in the high-average range. Visual learning and memory were in the average to above-average range. More specifically, R. G.'s ability to learn and recall a number of geometric shapes and their appropriate location was in the average to high-average range. Additionally, immediate facial recognition was in the high-average range, and delayed recognition was above average. Spatial learning and delayed recall were also above average.

Tests of executive functions revealed deficits in working memory (both on and off medication), and organization, as well as variable difficulties in controlling cognitive impulsivity. Divided attention was also impaired when R. G. was not on his medication. More specifically, working memory was impaired on the DKEFS Trail Making Test (Condition 4) even when R. G. was taking his medication. Visual scanning skills were also technically below average on the DKEFS Trail Making Test (Condition 1) because R. G. spent 23 seconds double checking his work before reporting he was done; when scoring the time it actually took him to complete the task, his score was average. R. G.'s working memory off Concerta was impaired and significantly poorer than his digit span score from the WISC-IV (as administered by his school). Divided attention was also impaired (off medication). Finally, R. G. demonstrated marked difficulties with organization on the Rey-Osterrieth Complex Figure. He employed a disjointed and part-oriented approach to copying the design, which led to the production of several errors. R. G. was only able to recall a few isolated details during his immediate and delayed recall drawings of the design. In contrast, abstract reasoning and cognitive flexibility were in the high-average range, and R. G.'s ability to inhibit prepotent responses was average. Finally, on the BRIEF, R. G.'s mother highlighted significant difficulties with initiation and self-monitoring skills (even while on Concerta).

R. G. demonstrated a below-average performance on the Grooved Pegboard with his left, dominant hand (there is a positive family history for sinistrality). However, his approach to this task (and all timed tests) was notably slow, cautious, and methodical; he did not appear to have any actual difficulties with the task itself. Furthermore, rapid graphomotor output was well above the average range on the NEPSY-II Visuomotor Precision subtest.

An academic screener revealed average word recognition and spelling skills. Math skills were in the low-average range because of several careless errors; when given credit for his careless mistakes, R. G.'s performance was average. Reading rate, accuracy, fluency, and comprehension were also average.

R. G. and his mother each completed the CBCL to report on his emotional adjustment. Both respondents endorsed a high number of somatic complaints and sad mood. Additionally, R. G. reported significant difficulties with anxiety and attention. R. G. also completed the MASC and the CDI to further evaluate his mood. His responses to the MASC again revealed significant difficulties with anxiety. In fact, he only responded to two of the items by saying they were "never" a problem for him. His pattern of responses highlights significant symptoms associated with fears of humiliation and rejection, social anxiety, separation/panic symptoms, and performance anxiety. R. G. also endorsed significant feelings of anhedonia and sad mood on the CDI (he denied any suicidal ideation on this measure).

Summary of Findings and Diagnostic Conclusions

Consistent with previous testing, the results from this evaluation indicate that R. G.'s overall cognitive ability (i.e., "IQ") is average. However, he demonstrated difficulties with executive functions such as working memory, divided attention, behavioral regulation, and organization. These problems were evident across all days of testing, although the difficulties were greater when he was not taking his medication. Additionally, R. G. tended to exhibit a relatively slowed approach to tasks driven by an internal need to check for accuracy, perfectionistic tendencies, and heightened anxiety in response to timed tests. These difficulties impacted his performance across all neurocognitive domains. Within this context, basic language skills were in the low-average to average range, although rapid word generation was below average. Verbal learning and spontaneous retrieval were significantly hampered by R. G.'s anxiety and decreased attention, which led to markedly variable performance. More specifically, learning was in the below-average to average range; he performed better when information was repeated. Delayed recall was in the below-average to average range,

and recognition was average (even for material that R. G. was unable to spontaneously recall). Visual-spatial skills, including learning and memory were relative strengths falling in the average to above-average range. Left-sided fine motor speed and dexterity were technically impaired, but R. G.'s slow cautious approach to this task contributed to his slow speed. Rapid graphomotor output and accuracy were average. Academic skills were average. Finally, both R. G. and his mother endorsed symptoms of sadness and anhedonia, and R. G. reported markedly elevated symptoms of anxiety.

As had been documented numerous times by previous evaluators, the results of the neuropsychological assessment again confirmed R. G.'s ADHD diagnosis. More importantly, however, by taking a careful and thorough approach to his overall adjustment and presentation the results also helped to clarify the unexplained source of his ongoing attentional, cognitive, and emotional difficulties. Indeed, although further investigation is warranted, he appears to meet criteria for a generalized anxiety disorder (GAD), according to *DSM-IV* criteria. R. G. also has many symptoms suggestive of social anxiety and phobic tendencies. Furthermore, he appears to be experiencing periods of sadness and anhedonia associated with his anxiety disorder(s), as well as physical side effects from his medication. R. G. did not appear clinically depressed at the time of this evaluation, although it was recommended that his mood be further evaluated by a treating therapist.

Discussion

R. G. had been evaluated by his pediatrician, several psychologists, and a psychiatrist over a 5-year time frame. However, because his ADHD symptoms were so overtly recognizable his ongoing difficulties with attention, emotional reactivity, and decreased frustration tolerance were repeatedly associated with this diagnosis; no one appeared to have investigated whether he might also be experiencing a comorbid psychiatric disorder. R. G. presents an excellent example of what can go wrong when evaluators fail to take a comprehensive biopsychosocial approach to their assessments. In many ways, he should have been an "easy" case. He had a significant family history of anxiety and also demonstrated a performance-based anxiety throughout the neuropsychological assessment. Even upon first meeting R. G. most skilled clinicians should have recognized his nearly palpable anxiety. Unfortunately, the "easy" answer seemed to have eclipsed the other, equally significant etiology underlying R. G.'s difficulties. This led to a poorly developed intervention plan that actually impeded his development and adjustment.

Although R. G. previously had been deemed ineligible for special educational services, the neuropsychological evaluation helped to highlight many specific risk factors that derive from the combined impact of his comorbid anxiety disorder(s) and ADHD. While most educators can recognize the general difficulties that ADHD may have on a child's day-to-day functioning, his anxiety disorder adds another layer to R. G.'s problems. For example, the organizational difficulties inherent in both his ADHD and anxiety disorder contribute to his difficulties with organized retrieval. More specifically, his organization difficulties make it challenging for R. G. to efficiently encode new information and to access it when he needs to share his knowledge with others. Additionally, even when R. G. is able to develop a sound strategy to accomplish a task, he tends to question any approach that is not "approved." Consequently, he second-guesses himself and defaults to a weaker, but better-known strategy (e.g., relying on rote recall rather than semantically clustering information). His anxiety also exacerbates his retrieval difficulties, leading to a tendency to "draw a blank" under timed or other pressured conditions (e.g., tests). His difficulties with organized verbal retrieval and fears of negative social evaluation make it hard for him to share his knowledge during classroom activities and during evaluations. Many children with similar profiles also experience difficulties making inferences if they are unable to "prove" their answer by reviewing text. Finally, R. G.'s perfectionistic tendencies are leading to a markedly slow *performance speed* in the context of an otherwise average *processing speed*. This self-induced slowed response style in turn limits his ability to listen to, remember, and follow multiple step directions, and to complete tasks within an expected time frame. All of these difficulties were expected to become more prominent when R. G. attempts to meet the more

rigorous expectations of middle school in the coming school year.

This evaluation led to several recommendations for clinical and academic management. First, it was suggested that R. G.'s parents meet with their pediatrician to reassess his current medication regimen. While he clearly benefits from Concerta, it will be important for R. G. and his family to work with his health-care providers to find a medication that has less significant side effects. In particular, given his comorbid anxiety disorder, consultation with a psychiatrist was suggested to discuss medication choices other than continuously increasing his stimulant dose. Outpatient psychotherapy services with a cognitive-behavioral emphasis was also recommended as a means to help R. G. learn to better recognize and manage his anxiety symptomatology. Finally, it was recommended that the neuropsychological report be shared with school personnel to re-evaluate his need for special educational services. More specifically, it was suggested that his disabilities were significantly impacting R. G.'s ability to access the curriculum and consequently he required specialized educational assistance. Specific recommendations included consultation with the school counselor to help him apply the skills he would be learning in psychotherapy in the school setting. Of course, this would also require communication with his outpatient therapist. Additionally, it was recommended that R. G. be provided with help designed to support his organizational difficulties that were both "real" (i.e., secondary to his ADHD and associated executive dysfunction) and self-imposed due to his tendency to second-guess his own organizational skills.

The comorbid presentation of anxiety disorders in children with ADHD is poorly understood and often overlooked. However, anxiety can significantly impact the presentation of ADHD symptomatology, and it contributes to numerous problems in its own right. Emphasizing a biopsychosocial approach to a neuropsychological evaluation can help to illuminate problems that may have been overlooked or compartmentalized as being "unrelated" to the child's neurocognitive difficulties by a child's parents, teachers, and health-care personnel. Furthermore, recognizing the complex interaction of these two disorders can help to direct effective interventions in all aspects of the child's life including the child's home functioning, academic performance, and more general clinical management.

References

Brassett-Harknett, A. & Butler, N. (2007). Attention-deficit/hyperactivity disorder: An overview of the etiology and a review of the literature relating to the correlates and lifecourse outcomes for men and women. *Clinical Psychological Review, 27*, 188–210.

Günther, T., Holkamp, H., Jolles, J., Herpertz-Dahlmann, B., & Konrad, K. (2004). Verbal memory and aspects of attentional control in children and adolescents with anxiety disorders or depressive disorders. *Journal of Affective Disorders, 82*, 265–269.

Jensen, P. S., Hinshaw, S. P., Kraemer, H. C., Lenora, N., Newconr, J. H., Abikoff, H. B., et al. (2001). ADHD Comorbidity findings from the MTA study: Comparing comorbid subgroups. *Journal of the American Academy of Child and Adolescent Psychiatry, 40*(2), 147–158.

Mennin, D., Biederman, J., Mick, E., & Faraone, S. V. (2000). Towards defining a meaningful anxiety phenotype for research in ADHD children. *Journal of Attention Disorders, 3*(4), 192–199.

Schatz, D. B., & Rostain, A. L. (2006). ADHD with comorbid anxiety: A review of the current literature. *Journal of Attention Disorders, 10*(2), 141–149.

Stefanatos, G. A., & Baron, I. S. (2007). Attention-deficit/hyperactivity disorder: A neuropsychological perspective towards DSM-V. *Neuropsychological Review, 17*, 5–38.

Toren, P., Sadeh, M., Wolmer, L., Eldar, S., Koren, S., Weizman, R., & Laor, N. (2000). Neurocognitive correlates of anxiety disorders in children: A preliminary report. *Journal of Anxiety Disorders, 14*(3), 239–247.

Vasa, R. A., Roberson-Nay, R., Klein, R. G., Mannuzza, S., Moulton, J. L., Guardino, M., Merikangas, A., Carlino, A. R., & Pine, D. S. (2007). Memory deficits in children with and at risk for anxiety disorders. *Depression and Anxiety, 24*, 85–94.

23

A Case of Somatoform Disorder with Inconsistent Effort

Beth S. Slomine and Ericka L. Wodka

Somatoform disorders are defined as a group of disorders in which there are physical symptoms that suggest a medical condition, although the symptoms cannot be fully explained by a medical condition. To be classified as a somatoform disorder, the symptoms must be causing significant distress and impairment in functioning. The fourth edition of the *Diagnostic and Statistical Manual of Mental Disorders* (*DSM-IV- TR*) describes seven different somatoform disorders (American Psychiatric Association, 2000), each of which will be defined below.

Somatization disorder begins before age 30 years and extends over a period of years and is characterized by a combination of pain, gastrointestinal, sexual, and pseudoneurological symptoms. Because somatization disorder must last for a period of years and must include at least one group of symptoms that is not applicable to young children (sexual symptoms), it is rarely diagnosed in children. *Undifferentiated somatoform disorder* is characterized by unexplained physical complaints lasting 6 months or more. *Conversion disorder* involves unexplained symptoms or deficits affecting voluntary motor or sensory function that suggest a neurological or other medical condition. Psychological factors are judged to be associated with these symptoms. In *pain disorder*, pain is the most significant symptom and psychological factors are judged to play an important role. *Hypochondriasis* is characterized by a preoccupation with the fear of having a serious disease thought to be based on misinterpretation of bodily symptoms. Lastly, *somatoform disorder, not otherwise specified* is used for disorders with somatoform symptoms that do not meet the criteria for a specific disorder.

The prevalence rates for specific *DSM*-defined somatoform disorders vary. Somatization disorder and conversion disorder rates are very low (0.2%–2% and <0.1 to 3%, respectively), whereas pain disorder is more common, occurring in 10%–15% of work-related disability for back pain alone (American Psychiatric Association, 2000). Given the low prevalence rates and the large number of symptoms necessary for diagnosis, the *DSM* criteria, for somatization disorder in particular, have been criticized for being overly restrictive.

Less stringent criteria have been proposed to capture individuals with significant somatizing symptoms (Escobar, Burnam, Karno, Forsythe, & Golding, 1987; Kroenke et al., 1997), which have resulted in higher prevalence rates. These less restrictive criteria are more consistent with how somatization is conceptualized commonly within neuropsychological practice. In neuropsychology, the terms *somatization, somatoform symptoms*, and *somatizing patients* are commonly used interchangeably to describe patients who present with multiple somatic complaints that are medically unexplained and have significant functional impairment or disruption in everyday life (Lamberty, 2008). In children, the concept of somatization is even less clear and, therefore, there is a paucity of literature on identification of these disorders and estimating prevalence in children.

In many cases, the interrelationship between somatizing and medically explained symptoms is also controversial, as a patient's presentation may not necessarily be the result of either somatization or medically explained symptoms but a combination of both. This controversy is particularly clear in the literature regarding mild traumatic brain injury (TBI), where there remains vigorous debate as to physiogenic versus psychogenic nature of postconcussive symptoms (Lee, 2007), especially following mild TBI in children (Yeates & Taylor, 2005).

The American Congress of Rehabilitation Medicine defines a mild TBI as occurring if one of the following is present: any loss of consciousness, any loss of memory for events before and after the incident, any alteration in mental status at the time of the event, or any focal neurologic deficit. Loss of consciousness must be less than 30 minutes, and any period of confusion must be less than 24 hours following the incident (Mild Traumatic Brain Injury Committee of the Head Injury Interdisciplinary Special Interest Group of the American Congress of Rehabilitation Medicine, 1993). After mild TBI, some individuals may develop a constellation of postconcussive symptoms. While there are differences in the classification of postconcussion syndrome between the *DSM-IV TR* and the *International Classification of Diseases, 10th Revision* (*ICD-10*), both classification systems describe a set of symptoms involving somatic, cognitive, and affective functioning (American Psychological Association, 2000; World Health Organization, 1992).

Despite their overall similarities, the *DSM-IV-TR* and *ICD-10* criteria for postconcussion syndrome differ in several important aspects. According to the *DSM-IV-TR* research criteria, postconcussive symptoms must last for at least 3 months after injury, whereas the *ICD-10* only indicates that these symptoms develop within 4 weeks after the incident (without specification pertaining to duration of symptom persistence). The *ICD-10* includes psychological factors (preoccupation with symptoms, fear of brain damage, and adoption of the sick role) in their criteria, whereas the *DSM-IV-TR* requires neuropsychological evidence of cognitive difficulties.

Following mild TBI, symptoms typically resolve over time. For instance, in the adult literature, the vast majority of individuals are symptom free within a month after mild TBI (Lee, 2007). The timing and extent of symptom resolution is less clear in the pediatric literature, and several factors including preinjury vulnerability of the child, family factors, and postinjury changes in brain functioning have been implicated (Yeates & Taylor, 2005).

The Case of Lisa

Referral

At the time of this evaluation, Lisa was a 10-year-old, right-handed girl with a history of chronic headaches and newly developed ataxic gait following two injuries sustained approximately 2 months prior to this evaluation. Lisa was admitted to an inpatient rehabilitation hospital for comprehensive rehabilitation and pain management following the significant limitations her ataxia and headaches had placed on her daily functioning. A neuropsychological evaluation was conducted during this admission.

History of Present Illness

Lisa was in her usual state of good health until she struck her head near the end of a water slide. When she entered the water, her father was there and immediately pulled her up, and she was "hysterical," reportedly crying, screaming, and yelling. There was no reported loss of consciousness or vomiting. Lisa was transported to a local hospital. Initial computed tomography (CT) scan was unremarkable, and she was released from the hospital after about 6–7 hours. Parents report that she "wasn't herself the following day, and was out of it." The new school year began 2 days after this incident, and Lisa attended school the first day. After her first day of school, while completing her homework on a stool at the kitchen counter, Lisa fell backwards and hit her head again. While parents reported that her affect was blunted and she reported that she was in pain, Lisa again did not lose consciousness or vomit. She did not go to the hospital and went to bed early. Parents reported that Lisa's affect was much more blunted after the second incident and that she was reporting much more pain. Lisa went back to school for the next 2 days, but she was sent home on the third day of school due to severe headaches and deterioration of her walking. She went directly to a local county hospital, where she received another CT scan (which was read as normal). After observation she was sent home and remained on bedrest for 1 week. After that week, she returned to school under a modified schedule (dismissed early). However, she only attended school for 1 day, as she complained of increased fatigue and was subsequently admitted to a university medical center. She remained hospitalized for 3 days and was discharged on Imitrex as needed for headache pain. Lisa planned to return to school on the following Monday, but her headaches and inability to walk persisted and instead she returned to the university medical center. During that hospitalization, medication was changed from Imitrex to Elavil in an attempt to address headache pain; she was discharged the same day. Lisa reported that the Elavil decreased the frequency and intensity of her headaches, but that she continued to have daily headaches and difficulty walking. About 1 month after the second incident, Lisa started using a wheelchair to prevent falls.

During a physical therapy evaluation conducted days prior to Lisa's inpatient rehabilitation admission, Lisa was able to walk with one hand held assistance for balance. She was described as having an erratic ataxic-like gait. Her legs often ended up scissoring. During the evaluation, Lisa stated that she could not control her legs. With a posterior walker she was able to walk with supervision. The excursion of her foot placement was narrowed by the containment of her pelvis within the walker, which made her less unsteady.

Family History

At the time of this evaluation, Lisa was living with her parents and brothers (ages 4 and 7 years). Both of her parents completed college; her father was employed as an analyst and her mother owned a business. Family history is significant for anxiety (including panic attacks), mood disorder, migraines, and learning disability; also of note, Lisa's mother sustained a severe TBI about 2 years prior to Lisa's hospital admission and required inpatient hospitalization and rehabilitation for a period of time. At the time of this evaluation, Lisa's mother was back to full activities, including running her own business.

Developmental History

According to her mother, Lisa was born full term, following an uncomplicated pregnancy and delivery. There were no concerns with language or social development; however, mild delay in gross motor development was reported (i.e., Lisa did not walk until she was 18 months of age, and running was always awkward prior to her injuries). There were no reported difficulties with sleep, feeding, or toilet training. Prior to the recent incidents, Lisa had never been hospitalized, and she has never had any surgeries. However, frequent headaches (for which she treated by lying down) predated Lisa's recent injuries. Further, per parent report, Lisa was diagnosed with obsessive-compulsive disorder/anxiety at age 4 years, but she "grew out of it within 6 months of behavioral changes to routine." There is no other history of serious illnesses, neurological problems, or trauma.

At the time of this evaluation, Lisa was in the fifth grade at a public elementary school. Due to the timing of her injuries, Lisa only attended 3 days of school that year, but she had been completing work that her mother brought to the rehabilitation hospital from her teachers. Based on review of available school records, her grades across the four quarters of fourth grade were mostly As and Bs, with two Cs in the first and second quarter of Math; all of her final grades were As and Bs. Of note, parents reported that when Lisa received her first C, she independently signed herself up for tutoring and improved her grade. Lisa missed a total of 5 days of school during the last year. Recent standardized academic achievement testing indicated that Lisa was performing at the 97th to 99th percentile in reading and mathematics, respectively.

Per parent report, Lisa was described as a creative, kind, reflective, helpful, well-mannered, mature, goal-oriented, reliable, and responsible girl. Socially, parents reported that Lisa had many friends and was voted "best friend to have" at school the previous year; Lisa also tutored other children at school. Lisa's weaknesses were described as her disorganization (in planning activities and keeping her room and desk neat).

Parents describe Lisa as being on a "quest for perfection" and that she expects much from herself.

Evaluation and Treatment

Lisa was admitted to an inpatient rehabilitation program 5 weeks after sustaining her second injury. This evaluation was conducted over multiple 30- to 60-minute sessions in a 2-week period during Lisa's admission at an inpatient rehabilitation center. Over the course of her 2.5-week hospitalization, Lisa received daily physical and occupational therapy and worked closely with behavioral psychology for coping and pain management. Psychiatry consultation indicated that Lisa currently met criteria for pain disorder, NOS, with rule out diagnoses of anxiety disorder, conversion disorder, somatization disorder, and parent–child relationship problem. No additional medication was recommended at the time; however, individual and family-based psychotherapy was strongly endorsed.

Behavioral Observations

Lisa generally presented as a friendly, polite, and pleasant girl. Overall, adequate socialization skills were observed during the evaluation, such as using appropriate greetings in response to others saying hello, and attending to individuals speaking to her. Lisa demonstrated an appropriate range of affect during the session. Her underlying affect was typically flat, although she smiled in response to social interaction and positive encouragement. Of note, Lisa never complained of pain or headache during the multiple evaluation sessions.

Lisa was cooperative and appeared to give a good effort throughout the assessment. Specifically, she took her time to think through questions before answering, and there was no evidence of impulsivity or inattention. Of note, when Lisa did not automatically know the response to a question, a distressed look came across her face and she was very hesitant to take a guess (even when encouraged). Additionally, during one session, Lisa was particularly upset at the start of the session, which occurred right after a physically demanding physical therapy session. She was able to calm herself after 10 minutes and participated in the assessment session.

Lisa demonstrated a right-hand preference for printing and drawing, and her pencil grasp during paper-and-pencil tasks was mature. While her writing was neat, her drawing appeared somewhat more ataxic, with poor line quality. Lisa attended to all areas of visual space when scanning a page and generally navigated in her environment without difficulty.

Upon initial evaluation, Lisa's gait was wide-based, unbalanced, and awkward. She was unable to walk a straight path down a hallway and instead weaved unpredictably from side to side. In addition, her arms flailed up and out, disjointed from her steps. While Lisa appeared very unbalanced and ataxic, she never bumped into walls or obstacles and did not fall. Over the course of admission, significant improvements were noted in Lisa's gait. By discharge, she was able to walk independently for short distances, and with bilateral canes or a walker for longer distances. Her physical and occupational therapists reported that her balance was adequate for walking and other more difficult activities (playing lacrosse in the hallway).

Validity

Standardized measures selected for this evaluation are appropriate for Lisa's age, and are considered valid for the purposes of delineating her current neurocognitive strengths and weaknesses. She was not taking any medication for pain that could have affected her cognitive abilities.

Of note, Lisa demonstrated variable performance on measures indicative of her effort. Specifically, she performed within normal limits on a test of visual memory (TOMM), designed to examine effort; however, she demonstrated unusual performance on a measure of verbal memory (CVLT-C). While Lisa was able to learn and recall a list of words adequately for her age, her performance was severely impaired when asked to recognize the words from the list. Furthermore, her performance fell well below age expectations on a simple shape matching task (WISC-IV Symbol Search); while Lisa took her time on this task, 10 items were incorrect and 11 items were correct. Her performance on these measures (as well as the variability in her performance across measures, which will be described later) strongly suggests that Lisa's effort varied throughout the assessment.

Assessment Results

Clinical Interview. Upon admission, Lisa reported that she had two different types of headache pain, which she described as "concussion headaches" and "migraine headaches." She noted that her migraine headaches had decreased significantly prior to admission, but she continued to have "concussion headaches" every 30 minutes (described as a throbbing pain in her head). She reported that one of her doctors told her that she will be "prone to migraines for the rest of her life."

Lisa reported remembering events immediately prior to and following both injuries; therefore, there was no period of retrograde amnesia or posttraumatic amnesia associated with either incident. Neither Lisa nor her parents reported any difficulty with memory or attention or changes in emotional functioning following her injuries.

General Intelligence. Administration of the WISC-IV, a standard measure of general intellectual functioning, revealed high-average verbal (SS = 114, 82nd percentile) and average nonverbal (SS = 106, 66th percentile) problem-solving skills. Due to significant variability in performance across subtests, the Full Scale IQ score is not an accurate estimate of Lisa's abilities. Specifically, while Lisa's performance fell above the 99th percentile on some measures, her performance fell below the 1st percentile on other subtests. However, overall, Lisa demonstrated consistent weakness on measures of working memory (SS = 71, 3rd percentile) and speed of information processing (SS = 62, 1st percentile). Individual subtest scores and overall index scores are listed in Table 23-1.

Visuomotor Integration, Visual Scanning, and Processing Speed. Lisa demonstrated variable performance on visuomotor tasks requiring rapid responding, with greater impairment observed on easier tasks than on harder tasks. For instance, Lisa's performance fell solidly in the average range on a task of graphomotor speed and precision (NEPSY Visuomotor Precision ScS = 10, 50th percentile). However, impaired bilateral fine motor manipulation and planning skills were observed when Lisa was asked to place pegs into appropriate holes across a board (Grooved Pegboard Right [dominant hand] z-score = –8.0, <1st percentile; Left [nondominant hand] z-score = –5.6, <1st percentile). Additionally, when Lisa was asked to quickly draw simple shapes/symbols based on a key, her performance fell in the borderline range (WISC-IV Coding ScS = 5, 5th percentile). Borderline performance was also demonstrated on a task of basic visual scanning (D-KEFS Trail Making Test: Visual Scanning ScS = 5, 5th percentile). Notably, when demands increased slightly, Lisa's performance fell in the average range on tasks of number/letter sequencing (D-KEFS Trail Making Test: Number Sequencing ScS = 8, 25th percentile, Letter Sequencing ScS = 8, 25th percentile).

Lisa's ability to copy a complex geometric design was impaired (RCFT Copy <1st percentile). Her production preserved both the overall gestalt of the figure as well as the details; however, her lines were inaccurate and appeared somewhat ataxic (i.e., were not straight, but "wobbly," did not meet appropriately at corners). Her poor score is reflected in the inaccuracy of her lines and careless errors (e.g., copying an inaccurate number of dots, misplacing the orientation of shapes). Lisa did not hurry through this task, and she made several erasures. Of note, she also repeatedly stated that she is not good at drawing and could only draw cats.

Table 23-1. Test Results

WISC-IV Subtests	Subtest Score (ScS)	WISC-IV Subtests	Subtest Score (ScS)
Similarities	13	Block Design	10
Vocabulary	13	Matrix Reasoning	6
Comprehension	12	Picture Concepts	17
Digit Span	5	Coding	5
Letter Number Sequencing	5	Symbol Search	1

Language. Confrontation naming appeared grossly intact (Boston Naming Test, z-score = 0.5, 69th percentile). Lisa's ability to spontaneously generate as many words as possible that began with a specific letter was within age expectations (D-KEFS Letter Fluency ScS = 8, 25th percentile); semantic fluency also fell in the average range (D-KEFS Category Fluency ScS = 10, 50th percentile).

Memory. Lisa demonstrated variable performance on standardized measures of verbal memory, which was likely impacted by her level of effort. On a list-learning task where Lisa was presented with a list of 15 words, her overall score fell in the high-average range (CVLT-C, Total Score T-Score = 58, 70th percentile). Lisa's initial recall after the first presentation of the list fell in the high-average range (List A, Trial 1 = 8 words, z-score = 1.0, 84th percentile), and her learning curve was low average (z- score = –1.0, 16th percentile). Lisa's performance remained in the average range following a short delay and presentation of a distracter list (Short Delay Free Recall = 8 words, z-score = –0.5, 31st percentile) and following a longer time delay (Long Delay Free Recall = 8 words, z-score = –0.5, 31st percentile). While Lisa was able to spontaneously recall words from the list with average ability, her ability to recognize whether specific words were or were not on the original list (a much easier task) was impaired (Recognition Discriminabiltiy z-score = –3.0, <1st percentile). Of note, Lisa failed to recognize 7 of the 15 correct words (Correct Recognition Hits z-score = –2.5, <1st percentile) and incorrectly identified 6 words that were not on the list (False Positives z-score = 1.5, 93rd percentile), which is very unusual for her age, specifically when considered in the context of her average spontaneous retrieval.

In terms of visual memory, Lisa's ability to reproduce the details of a complex figure after a short and a longer delay (30 minutes) was impaired (RCFT Immediate Recall T-score = 29, <1st percentile; Delayed Recall T-score = 27, <1st percentile). As her copy of the figure was also impaired, it is likely that poor visuoconstructional ability impacted her memory for the figure. In contrast to her performance on measures of verbal memory, Lisa's memory for the design was supported by the recognition trial, as her ability to recognize aspects of the design after a long delay was low average, suggesting adequate encoding of the visual design into memory (Recognition Total Correct T-score = 41, 18th percentile).

Attention and Executive Functioning. Variable performance was also observed on measures of auditory attention. Rote repetition of digits was within the borderline range (WISC-IV Digit Span Forward ScS = 5, 5th percentile, 4 digits forwards), while her ability to repeat strings of digits in reverse order, requiring mental manipulation, was in the low-average range (Digit Span Backward ScS = 7, 16th percentile, 3 digits backwards). Lisa scored in the borderline/low-average range on a simple sustained attention task requiring counting of sounds (TEA-Ch Score! ScS = 6, 9th percentile); however, her performance improved to the average range on a more complex attention task that required dividing her attention (Score DT ScS = 8, 25th percentile).

Lisa's performance on tasks requiring rapid cognitive flexibility, verbal initiation, and verbal inhibition of an automatic response was within to above age expectations (D-KEFS Color-Word Interference Test: Inhibition ScS = 9, 37th percentile, Inhibition/Switching ScS = 11, 63rd percentile; Verbal Fluency: Category Switching ScS = 14, 91st percentile, Switching Accuracy ScS = 12, 75th percentile). Further, she also performed within age expectations on a motor task requiring rapid shifting between two response sets (D-KEFS Trail Making Test: Number-Letter Switching ScS = 9, 37th percentile); given her difficulty with easier motor tasks, her average performance on these more difficult tasks is surprising and again supports her variable effort throughout the assessment.

Lisa's parents rated her behavioral presentation on a standardized questionnaire of everyday executive skills (BRIEF); they were asked to rate Lisa's behavior prior to her recent injuries. Parent report indicated a clinically significant preinjury concern with Lisa's ability to organize her environment. Otherwise, there were no other significant parent-reported preinjury concerns with behavioral/emotional control or metacognitive aspects of executive functioning (e.g., problem solving, working memory, self-monitoring). They also reported no change in these behaviors/skills over the past month and a half.

Behavioral and Emotional. Lisa's parents completed the Behavior Assessment System for Children, Second Edition (BASC-2, PRS-C) based on Lisa's *preinjury* behavioral and emotional functioning. Preinjury, parent report identified clinically significant concern with anxiety (e.g., worries about what parents/teachers/other children think, tries too hard to please others). Otherwise there were no other concerns with either internalizing (e.g., depression, somatization) or externalizing (e.g., aggression, hyperactivity) behavior problems reported by parents. Parents did not report any changes in these behaviors over the past month and a half subsequent to her injuries.

When questioned directly, Lisa denied any current significant mood and behavior symptoms. However, she expressed some concern and worry about her health and being in the hospital (e.g., *Three Wishes Task*: "I wish I could walk," "I wish my cat was here," and "I wish that I could go home"). On projective testing (Family Kinetic Drawing, Sentence Completion), Lisa's overall responses suggested a good relationship with her family (My family is the "best," My mother "is nice," My daddy is "fun"). Nonetheless, other indirect assessment using storytelling about picture cards (Thematic Apperception Test) suggested anxiety surrounding safety/security at home. Specifically, her responses to these cards suggested that she finds significant support in animals and may not view important people in her life as a source of support during difficult times. For example, stories focused around a lone individual who either ran away from home, who was attacked in a home invasion, or who was forced to move away from home. In most of these stories, help was provided only by the protagonist herself or her pets.

Discussion

The current neuropsychological evaluation revealed significant and unusual variability in Lisa's performance on cognitive tasks, inconsistent with any known neurological condition. This variability was attributed to fluctuations in her effort, which had a negative impact on her performance. Specifically, in several instances, Lisa performed much worse on easier tasks relative to more difficult tasks. This is consistent with reports from her inpatient physical and occupational therapists, who noted inconsistent functioning (i.e., difficulty with an easy motor task, while demonstrating the ability to perform a more motorically challenging task, specifically when distracted).

Overall, on measures where effort was thought to be adequate, results suggested typically average to above-average intellectual abilities. Testing also revealed many areas of intact cognitive functioning, including language, response/processing speed, aspects of memory for verbal information, nonverbal memory recognition, and aspects of executive functions (e.g., cognitive flexibility). Lisa more consistently demonstrated difficulty with measures requiring hand-eye coordination and graphomotor speed; however, unusual variability in her performance across such measures was observed, with average performance demonstrated on some measures with increased fine motor demands (as well as increased cognitive demands), and impaired performance observed on other measures with significantly less fine motor demand.

Although Lisa denied significant mood symptoms during clinical interview, projective testing revealed themes of anxiety related to her home, stress related to ineffective coping strategies, and reliance on animals, rather than people for support. Parent report on a standardized measure indicated clinically significant concern with symptoms of anxiety prior to and following Lisa's injuries.

While some of Lisa's physical symptoms (i.e., headaches) may possibly be explained by her recent "concussions" combined with preinjury history of headaches, she does not clearly meet the criteria for having a mild TBI according to the definition of the American Congress of Rehabilitation Medicine (Mild Traumatic Brain Injury Committee of the Head Injury Interdisciplinary Special Interest Group of the American Congress of Rehabilitation Medicine, 1993). Specifically, she had no loss of consciousness or loss of memory surrounding either injury. In addition, the gait disturbance that developed was not consistent with a focal neurologic deficit. On the other hand, given that she was reportedly "out of it" the day after her first injury and had blunted affect following her second injury, it is possible that these changes could be considered an alteration in mental state, as defined by the American Congress of Rehabilitation Medicine criteria.

Importantly, even if she met the criteria for having a mild TBI, the quality and severity of Lisa's gait disturbance, which worsened over time, and variability in performance on cognitive measures cannot be medically explained. Based on the results of this evaluation, these unexplained symptoms were likely related to Lisa's tendency to experience emotional distress (e.g., anxiety) somatically, and consistent with a diagnosis of conversion disorder. Physical problems, such as headache pain and difficulty walking, were thought to be exacerbated when Lisa was under stress, particularly related to her home environment.

While unexplained medical symptoms are commonplace in somatization disorder, in the neuropsychological context, these symptoms can also be conceptualized as poor or inconsistent effort. In forensic evaluations, poor or inconsistent effort is typically attributed to secondary gain, as individuals stand to gain financially from having ongoing symptoms. Therefore, individuals evaluated for forensic purposes who display poor or inconsistent effort are often labeled as malingerers. In clinical settings, determining the underlying reason for poor effort is often more challenging, as secondary gain is not always clear. Moreover, according to the DSM-IV-TR, one of the criteria for conversion disorder is that symptoms are not intentionally produced or feigned, as in factitious disorder or malingering. In Lisa's case, performance was extremely variable and did not improve after multiple prompts and encouragement to try her best. While it is possible that she was volitionally exaggerating her symptoms, there was no clear secondary gain that we could identify.

There are several individual and family characteristics that are associated with somatization symptoms and chronic pain in children. It has been reported that up to one-half of children who experience medically unexplained chronic pain face additional symptoms of mood disorder, specifically anxiety and depression (Stevenson, Simpson, & Bailey, 1988). Several common personality traits have also been identified in children with somatoform disorders, as these children are frequently described as conscientious, obsessive, sensitive, insecure, and anxious, with tendencies towards setting high personal expectations (Garralda, 1996). In addition to individual psychological factors, family factors may be associated with the development of somatization in children. In their review of the psychological models of somatization, Husain, Browne, and Chalder (2007) stress the familial role in the development and maintenance of medically unexplained somatic symptoms, including the effects of the typically high behavioral and academic expectations parents have placed on children who present with somatoform disorders. Additionally, it was noted that family members of children with somatoform disorders have frequently presented with similar conditions and preoccupations with their symptoms.

The individual and family risk factors described above are certainly applicable to Lisa's case. For instance, Lisa's parent ratings described Lisa as having anxiety before and following injury. Parents also qualitatively described Lisa as being on a "quest for perfection" and that she expects much from herself. Lisa's parents are also high-achievers and had placed some degree of pressure upon Lisa, which she likely amplified by placing pressure upon herself. In addition, Lisa's mother also experienced migraines and sustained a significant TBI less that 3 years prior to Lisa's injuries. This constellation of risk factors adds further support to the consistency of Lisa's presentation with a somatoform disorder.

Given that psychological factors are thought to play a major role in the development of somatizing symptoms, careful examination of psychosocial issues is essential when evaluating children thought to have unexplained medical symptoms. The adult literature describing the assessment of somatoform disorders relies heavily upon self-assessment of personality, typically using the Minnesota Multiphasic Personality Inventory (MMPI) and its revision (MMPI-2) to identify patterns of response. For instance, both a "generally elevated profile" and a "Conversion V" (where the Hypocondriasis [HS] and Hysteria [HY] scales are elevated, and the Depression [D] scale is well below all other scales) have been described (Bradley, Prokop, Margolis, & Gentry,

1978; Nordin, Eisemann, & Richter, 2005). In adult samples, these profiles are heavily relied upon to inform diagnosis and treatment. While the MMPI-A is available for adolescents 14 to 18 years old (Butcher et al., 1992), there is no comprehensive measure that considers the role of emotional problems and personality characteristics in the development and maintenance of experienced somatizing symptoms for children and young adolescents.

Self-report measures that examine children's emotional and behavioral functioning are available (e.g., the Behavior Assessment System for Children–Second Edition: BASC-2; Children's Depression Inventory); however, there are several limitations to such measures, including the child's ability to self-monitor and accurately report emotional functioning as well as the potential for underreporting of difficulties due to social desirability influences (Zeman, Klimes-Dougan, Cassano, & Adrian, 2007). Additionally, it has been described that children with somatoform disorders have a tendency for minimizing these emotional difficulties (Kozlowska, 2003). Therefore, standardized parent report and projective measures (e.g., Incomplete Sentences, Thematic Apperception Test) can be a useful means of gaining insight into the child's emotional experience and possible associations with somatoform symptomatology. For instance, Lisa clearly minimized all emotionally related symptoms on interview, while her parents reported clinically significant anxiety, and her own responses to projective measures suggested significant family stress and associated anxiety.

There are a variety of psychological conceptualizations and treatment approaches for children with somatoform disorders ranging from psychoanalytic to behavioral approaches (Lamberty, 2008). Husain and colleagues (2007) reported on the efficacy of cognitive-behavioral therapy and relaxation treatments to address unexplained headache and stomach pain, but they stressed the need for studies with lower attrition rates, as well as those examining treatment for other pain symptoms. In addition, both inpatient and outpatient multidisciplinary programs that include physical therapy, occupational therapy, and psychological treatment have been described in the literature as treatment options for children with somatoform disorders (Palermo & Scher, 2001).

When described in the literature, multidisciplinary treatment programs designed for children with somatoform disorders emphasize the use of positive reinforcement, where healthy behavior is attended to and rewarded, and extinction or withdraw of reinforcement is implemented in response to sick role behaviors (Brazier & Venning, 1997; Eccleston, Malleson, Clinch, Connell, & Courbut, 2005; Garralda, 1996). While childhood somatoform disorders can be addressed with coordinated outpatient treatment, in their case description, Palermo and Scher (2001) document the efficient and cost-effective nature of a well-designed inpatient rehabilitation setting, especially for children with significant functional impairment. With that said, some level of outpatient follow-up subsequent to an inpatient admission is necessary to assist with reintegration and management of potential pitfalls.

While Lisa's functioning was markedly impaired prior to her admission, it should be recognized that despite Lisa's gait disturbance and reported frequent headaches, she functioned adequately throughout the day during this hospitalization with planned ignoring of attention-seeking behaviors (i.e., her gait) along with encouragement and support from the staff for engaging in functional tasks. In addition, reasonable daily functional goals were set by the physical and occupational therapists, so that Lisa could slowly progress her functional skills. Using these strategies, Lisa made daily gains. It was recommended that upon discharge Lisa's family, teachers, and other caregivers provide similar support. In addition, it was recommended that Lisa participate in outpatient psychological therapy to further develop coping and anxiety management skills. Outpatient physical therapy was also recommended to continue to promote functional gains in mobility skills.

Lisa attended a 4-month follow-up rehabilitation outpatient clinic multidisciplinary evaluation. Overall, Lisa was described as doing very well, with decreased intensity and frequency of headaches, with medication taper 6 weeks prior to the appointment. At that time, she was taking Tylenol as needed for headaches. She was discharged from outpatient physical therapy and was able to run "better than ever." The family reported positive implementation of behavioral strategies learned during her inpatient admission. Lisa was reportedly doing well in school, receiving all As and Bs. Her mother reported that she had matured significantly over the past several months and was more open to discussing issues and problems with her family. She was socializing and participating in Girl Scouts.

In conclusion, children with somatoform disorders exhibit a complex set of symptoms that significantly impact daily functioning. Incomplete diagnosis or inadequate treatment can result in significant medical cost, due to the treatment-seeking and chronic nature of the untreated or inappropriately treated disorder. Evaluation and diagnosis of children with somatoform disorders is particularly challenging because many present with a combination of both medically explained and medically unexplained symptoms, and there is often lack of consensus among a child's health-care providers as to the etiology of all of the presenting symptoms. The pediatric neuropsychologist brings an important perspective in understanding such children and providing for their treatment and intervention plans. Neuropsychological assessment is useful in delineating the specific cognitive, emotional, behavioral, personality, and somatic symptoms, understanding these symptoms in relation to brain functioning, and informing treatment planning and promoting functioning within the home, school, and community settings.

References

American Psychiatric Association. *Diagnostic and statistical manual of mental disorders* (4th ed., Text rev.). Arlington, VA: American Psychiatric Association; 2000:760–762.

Bradley, L. A., Prokop, C. K., Margolis, R., & Gentry, W. D. (1978). Multivariate analyses of the MMPI profiles of low back pain patients. *Journal of Behavioral Medicine, 1*, 253–272.

Brazier, D. K., & Venning, H. E. (1997). Conversion disorders in adolescents: A practical approach to rehabilitation. *British Journal of Rheumatology, 36*, 594–598.

Butcher, J. N., Williams, C. L., Graham, J. R., Archer, R. P., Tellgen, A., Ben-Porath, Y. S., & Kaemer, B. (1992). *MMPI-A (Minnesota Multiphasic Personality Inventory-Adolescent): Manual for administration, scoring, and interpretation*. Minneapolis: University of Minnesota Press.

Eccleston, C., Malleson, P. N., Clinch, J., Connell, H., & Sourbut, C. (2003). Chronic pain in adolescents: Evaluation of a programme of interdisciplinary cognitive behavior therapy. *Archive of Disease in Childhood, 88*, 881–885.

Escobar, J. I., Burnam, M. A., Karno, M., Forsythe, A., & Golding, J. M. (1987). Somatization in the community. *Archives of General Psychiatry, 44*, 713–718.

Garralda, M. E. (1996). Somatisation in children. *Journal of Child Psychology and Psychiatry, 37*, 13–33.

Husain, K., Browne, T., & Chalder, T. (2007). A review of psychological models and interventions for medically unexplained somatic symptoms in children. *Child and Adolescent Mental Health, 12*, 2–7.

Kozlowska, K. (2003). Good children presenting with conversion disorder. *Clinical Child Psychology and Psychiatry, 6*, 575–591.

Kroenke, K., Spitzer, R. L., deGruy, F. V., Hahn, S. R., Linzer, M., Williams, J. B., et al., (1997). Multisomatoform disorder: An alternative to undifferentiated somatoform disorder for the somatizing patient in primary care. *Archives of General Psychiatry, 54*, 352–358.

Lamberty, G. J. (2008) Understanding somatization in the practice of clinical neuropyshcology. Oxford Workshop Series. New York: Oxford University Press.

Lee, L. K. (2007) Controversies in the sequelae of pediatric mild traumatic brain injury. *Pediatric Emergency Care, 23*, 580–586.

Mild Traumatic Brain Injury Committee of the Head Injury Interdisciplinary Special Interest Group of the American Congress of Rehabilitation Medicine (1993). Definition of mild traumatic brain injury. *Journal of Head Trauma Rehabilitation, 8*, 86–87.

Nordin, H., Eisemann, M., & Richter, J. (2005). MMPI-2 subgroups in a sample of chronic pain patients. *Scandinavian Journal of Psychology, 46*, 209–216.

Palermo, T. M., & Scher, M. S. (2001). Treatment of functional impairment in severe somatoform pain disorder: A case example. *Journal of Pediatric Psychology, 26*, 429–434.

Stevenson, J., Simpson, J., & Bailey, V. (1988). Research note: Recurrent headaches and stomachaches in preschool children. *Journal of Child Psychology and Psychiatry, 29*, 897–900.

World Health Organizations. The ICD-10 classification of mental and behavioural disorders: Clinical description and diagnostic guidelines. Geneva, Switzerland: 1992.

Yeates, K. O., & Taylor, H. G. (2005). Neurobehavioural outcomes of mild head injury in children and adolescents. *Pediatric Rehabilitation, 8*,(1), 5–16.

Zeman, J., Klimes-Dougan, B., Cassano, M., & Adrian, M. (2007). Measurement issues in emotion research with children and adolescents. *Clinical Psychology: Science and Practice, 14*, 377–401.

24

Obsessive-Compulsive Disorder: A Case Study

Ann C. Marcotte and Miriam T. Goldstein

Obsessive-compulsive disorder (OCD) is a complex neuropsychiatric disorder that falls within the spectrum of anxiety disorders. According to the *DSM-IV TR* (American Psychiatric Association, 2000), OCD is characterized by recurrent, unwanted thoughts, impulses, or images (obsessions) and repetitive, ritualistic, and often covert behaviors that are performed to reduce distress (compulsions). These obsessions are not merely excessive worries about real-life situations; they are thoughts, images, and impulses that come from the mind of the individual with OCD. Individuals with OCD feel compelled to perform the compulsive behavior (e.g., hand washing, checking) or mental act (e.g., praying, counting, repeating words silently) to reduce distress. By definition, the obsessions and/or compulsions associated with OCD are severe enough to be time consuming or to cause considerable impairment in the person's life. In adults, there must be recognition at some point in the course of the disorder that the obsessions and/or compulsions are excessive or unreasonable, while such insight is not needed to reach a diagnosis of OCD in children. The obsessions and compulsions typical of individuals with OCD differ in childhood and adulthood; Geller et al. (2001) provide an excellent review of age of onset symptom differences. Obsessive-compulsive disorder often has a waxing and waning nature, and it is not uncommon for the types of obsessions and compulsions to change over time, and to exacerbate during periods of high stress. In adults, depression, other anxiety disorders, eating disorders, and some personality disorders are commonly comorbid with OCD. In children, OCD can coexist with disruptive behavior disorders, as well as attention-deficit/hyperactivity disorder (ADHD), tic disorders, and learning disorders, with lower rates of coexisting depression reported (American Psychiatric Association, 2000; Geller et al., 2001). Treatments for OCD typically include behavioral strategies, such as event and response prevention that are coupled with cognitive-behavioral therapy (CBT) techniques for anxiety management. Selective serotonin reuptake inhibitor (SSRI) medications have also provided symptom relief for many individuals with OCD. A study of treatment outcomes in children and adolescents with OCD found the most positive treatment effects in those who received both CBT and Zoloft versus Zoloft or CBT alone (Pediatric OCD Treatment Study, 2004).

With regard to possible neurobiological factors associated with this disorder, it is interesting to note that OCD is a psychiatric disorder that can arise in several neurological disorders that affect subcortical-cortical brain regions. Specifically, OCD can emerge in patients with disorders that affect the basal ganglia, such as Parkinson disease, Huntington chorea, Sydenham chorea, and Tourette syndrome. In the past few years, a growing body of research has evolved investigating the biological and neuropsychological underpinnings of OCD. Neuroimaging studies conducted with adults with OCD suggest abnormalities in the orbitofrontal cortex, anterior cingulate cortex, and basal ganglia (e.g., the orbital frontal pathway of the cortico-striatal-thalamo-cortical circuit). In addition, studies have indicated abnormal activation during the resting state in the striatum, orbitofrontal cortex, thalamus, and cingulate gyrus (Chamberlain, Blackwell, Fineberg, Robbins, & Sahakian, 2005; Menzies et al., 2008). Significantly fewer neuroimaging studies have been conducted with children with OCD, and results to date are less conclusive than studies with adults, although some have reported reduced putamen volumes but no changes in frontal lobe regions (Friedlander & Desrocher, 2006).

Given the frontal-subcortical brain structures implicated in OCD, neuropsychological deficits associated with these affected brain regions would not be unexpected. A growing number of neuropsychological studies have explored potential OCD-related cognitive impairments. A review of these studies reveals considerable variability in reported results, which are likely attributable to significant differences between studies with regard to subject characteristics, including the following: age of symptom onset, precise symptom presentation, duration, and severity of symptoms; the presence of comorbid psychiatric (especially other anxiety disorders and depression) or medical diagnoses; medication use at time of study; and other subject variables, such as age and educational level. In particular, the coexistence of depression or ADHD in OCD can cloud neuropsychological testing findings, as each of these psychiatric disorders presents with cognitive features that overlap those often reported in OCD. Another factor that may contribute to variability among study findings includes the measures employed to examine specific neuropsychological constructs. While performances on specific neuropsychological tests have varied across studies, a pattern of neuropsychological deficits in individuals with OCD, nevertheless, has begun to emerge from the literature, and while the majority of studies have investigated the neuropsychological functioning of adults, research conducted with children and adolescents has found similar patterns (Andrés et al., 2007).

The primary neuropsychological deficit identified in individuals with OCD is executive dysfunction, although the specific executive deficits have varied considerably between studies,

possibly as a result of differences in measures employed, methodology, and/or study populations. Mental flexibility and set shifting have commonly been examined using the Wisconsin Card Sort Test (WCST). Several studies have found that individuals with OCD made more errors, completed fewer categories, lost set more often, and had more difficulty learning from feedback than healthy controls, while others found no differences. The Trail Making Test Parts A and B have also been used to examine set shifting in several studies with mixed results. Similarly, on measures of verbal fluency, conflicting findings were obtained, with some studies showing impaired fluency in individuals with OCD and other studies finding no differences. In studies examining planning skills in individuals with OCD using the Tower of Hanoi and the Tower of London tests, the majority found that individuals with OCD did not show deficits in the accuracy of their planning ability and that they reached a similar number of correct solutions as did the controls. In general, while overall performance on set-shifting, verbal fluency, and planning tasks sometimes did not differ from that of healthy controls, the majority of studies found some differences in individuals with OCD, such as increased response latencies, increased rates of perseverative responses, and difficulty utilizing feedback to change behavior. A finding that has been consistent in the research is that individuals with OCD generally demonstrate poorer use of organizational strategies, particularly on visual tasks such as the Rey-Osterrieth Complex Figure Test (Chamberlain et al., 2005; De Geus, Denys, Sitskoorn, & Westenberg, 2007; Greisberg & McKay, 2003; Kuelz, Hohagen, & Voderholzer, 2004; Olley, Malhi, & Sachdev, 2007).

With regard to memory functioning, the majority of studies have found OCD to be associated with weaknesses in visual memory. On the Rey-Osterrieth Complex Figure Test (RCFT), which has been utilized in several studies, individuals with OCD generally performed more poorly than controls on the immediate and delayed recall tasks. However, their reduced performance was often attributed by the investigators to difficulty utilizing effective organizational strategies while initially copying the RCFT, leading to inefficient encoding of the figure, rather than due to a fundamental visual memory deficit (Deckersbach, Otto, Savage, Baer, & Jenike, 2000; Penadés, Catalan, Andrés, Salamero, & Gasto, 2005; Savage et al., 2000). Other studies, however, found that while organizational weaknesses contributed to nonverbal memory difficulties, they did not account for them completely (Shin et al., 2004). Some research that examined OCD patients who did not have depression found no weaknesses in copying or recalling the RCFT (Moritz, Kloss, Jahn, Schick, & Hand, 2003; Simpson et al., 2006). Most studies that assessed verbal working memory, as well as declarative verbal memory, found no deficits in individuals with OCD (Kuelz et al., 2004). However, some studies that examined verbal memory for tasks that require organization of verbal stimuli (such as the California Verbal Learning Test [CVLT]) reported that individuals with OCD performed more poorly than healthy controls (Deckersbach et al., 2005; Savage et al., 2000). There were also some findings that individuals with OCD showed a slightly slower learning curve on the CVLT (De Geus et al., 2007). Differences in performance between individuals with OCD and healthy controls on verbal memory tasks have commonly been associated with depression and inefficient use of organizational strategies.

Research findings generally suggest that basic attention is intact in individuals with OCD (Kuelz et al., 2004). However, some studies found that OCD patients showed a bias in attention processing, as they attended more to stimuli that were relevant to their OCD concerns than they did to neutral stimuli (Chamberlain et al., 2005; Metehan & Flament, 2007). Another study suggested that attention weaknesses might be present in individuals with OCD and may account for findings that individuals with OCD have difficulties maintaining set (De Geus et al., 2007). Other areas of functional deficits that have been implicated in OCD include cognitive processing speed, motor speed, and visual spatial deficits. However, weaknesses in these areas have not been consistently supported by research. Instead, it has been proposed that cognitive and/or motor slowing might be attributable to comorbid depression or medication use, while visual spatial weaknesses might be related to organizational difficulties

rather than perceptual deficits (Kuelz et al., 2004; Simpson et al., 2006).

Another line of research into OCD raises the suggestion that age of onset and duration of symptoms may be related to the permanence of the neurocognitive profile seen in OCD. For example, research on the cognitive response to treatment for OCD has found some differences between adults and children. While some neuropsychological deficits remained in adults even after successful psychopharmacological treatment (Nielen & Den Boer, 2003; Rao, Reddy, Kumar, Kandavel, & Chandrashekar, 2008), neuropsychological functioning in children was reported to improve after such treatment (Andrés, et al., 2008). Due to the briefer duration of the disorder, the neuropsychological deficits in children may not be as lasting as they were in adults. Differences in response to treatment, as well as differing patterns of neuropsychological weaknesses across studies, have raised speculation of differing neurobiology between early- and late-onset OCD (Hwang et al., 2007).

By definition, obsessions and compulsions often lead to functional interference in the life of the individual with OCD. Impairment in social functioning, academic/vocational functioning, and the completion of routine tasks of everyday life are frequently seen in this population and can vary greatly as a function of the specific nature of the obsessions and compulsions. Patients may come to the attention of the clinical neuropsychologist due to concerns about these social or behavioral functioning impairments, as well as due to concern that possible cognitive symptoms may be contributing to problems the patient is encountering meeting with greater success in everyday life at school or work. As obsessions are covert, and many individuals with OCD engage in their compulsive behaviors out of sight of others, OCD may not be the first diagnosis suspected in such cases. Among children and adolescents with OCD, common presenting behaviors can include academic decline, teacher concerns about inattention and work completion, difficulties with the timely completion of homework (sometimes seen with mental blocking and a lot of erasing), considerable time spent getting ready for bed or in the bathroom, and other atypical behaviors. The following case study presents a history of an adolescent patient's behavioral presentation and allows for an exploration of the cognitive profile associated with OCD. This case also highlights some of the challenges that comorbid conditions place on determining whether documented cognitive features seen in testing are specific to this disorder. It also allows for a discussion of ways to address and treat OCD-related symptoms in order to reduce their adverse impact on daily functioning, in this case, with regard to the patient's school performance.

Case Study: C. K.

Background Information

The patient, C. K., was a 15-year-old, right-handed, Caucasian male adolescent referred for a neuropsychological evaluation by his parents to obtain information about his cognitive and learning profiles in order to assist in determining his eligibility to receive accommodations in school. C. K., who had recently completed the eighth grade, presented with a longstanding history of OCD, and he also carried prior diagnoses of ADHD and language arts learning disabilities.

C. K. was the product of a full-term, uncomplicated pregnancy and a Cesarean delivery. He was jaundiced at birth but did not require phototherapy. His neonatal period was otherwise unremarkable. While C. K. achieved early gross motor developmental milestones within the normal time frame, his expressive language acquisition was initially delayed, and he did not speak his first word until 20 months. His subsequent language development, however, was very rapid, and he began speaking in two- to three-word sentences at age 22 months. C. K. showed some mild delays with his fine motor skills and did not learn to tie shoelaces until age 6. C. K. experienced good health and had no history of head injuries, loss of consciousness, or seizures. There was no reported history of learning, attention, or neurological problems in the family, although the family psychiatric history was significant for anxiety and OCD in first-degree relatives.

With regard to educational history, C. K. had attended the same school since kindergarten. He experienced difficulty learning to read and received reading support services at school. He also had initial difficulty acquiring handwriting skills. Since the fourth grade, C. K. received in-school learning support and private tutoring outside of school one to two times a week. At the time of testing, tutoring focused on advancing his higher order reading comprehension and written expression skills. C. K.'s mother also reported that her son's thinking remained concrete and was not as abstract as expected for his age. For a few years, C. K. had been receiving accommodations in school, including extended time on tests due to his very slow work pace and a foreign language course waiver due to language arts learning difficulties. Academically, C. K. was a solid student, often earning "B" marks, and his parents reported that he worked very hard to achieve his grades. Typically, C. K. spent 3–4 hours nightly completing school assignments. He had never posed behavior problems at home or in school and enjoyed very good relationships with family members, teachers, and classmates.

According to his mother, C. K. displayed compulsive and obsessive behaviors beginning at a young age. He did not display unusual problems with separation anxiety. As a preschooler, C. K. would play with electrical devices and seemed obsessed with objects with motors. He never, however, showed a lack of interest in others, and his play skills were otherwise normal. As a youngster, C. K. was also described as hypervigilant of his environment; he continued to remain hypervigilant at the time of referral. During kindergarten, C. K.'s teacher expressed concern about his reduced attention and distractibility, and early learning and handwriting acquisition issues were also reported. C. K. underwent a psychological evaluation at age 6, and results were interpreted as consistent with a presentation of ADHD and language-based learning weaknesses. He subsequently began to receive academic support in school. Medication for ADHD was recommended, and over the ensuing 4 years C. K. was tried on numerous stimulant medications with little positive improvements reported. Toward the end of his fourth grade year, a selective serotonin reuptake inhibitor (SSRI) medication was introduced for the first time to address his obsessive-compulsive symptoms which in conjunction with continued use of a stimulant medication finally provided improvements in C. K.'s presentation. In the years prior to this evaluation, C. K. had never been engaged in a course of therapy. C. K. had displayed fewer compulsive behaviors in school as compared to home over the years; his mother perceived that C. K. worked very hard to contain his obsessions and compulsions during the school day, although they emerged in class during stressful times. During the second grade, C. K. began to engage in compulsive erasing while writing, and his parents grew increasingly aware of his perfectionistic obsessions. Perfectionistic behaviors persisted over the years, although the compulsions C. K. engaged in to reduce his anxiety changed over time. He was reported to work at a very slow pace, which his mother saw as related to ongoing obsessions with perfection. Checking behaviors were intermittently observed at home over the years.

Behavioral Observations

C. K. was on Zoloft and Stratera at the time of testing. He was a friendly and talkative adolescent who was very cooperative and put forth excellent effort on all tasks. Testing C. K. took longer than is typical for young adolescents, in large measure due to his anxiety and OCD-related behaviors. At times, particularly on timed measures, C. K. became noticeably aroused and anxious and would remark that he was "doing a bad job." Throughout testing, C. K. displayed a very slow, deliberate, and cautious work style that adversely affected his performances on timed measures. This very deliberate and slow style was also seen in C. K.'s completion of other tasks. For example, there were often long latencies between the examiner's questions and C. K.'s responses. He took great care and time to organize his thoughts and formulate his answers before responding to questions. He was also quite slow in selecting answers on tests with multiple-choice formats and was noted to carefully examine each option, sometimes more than once, prior to making his selection. His rate of production on tasks with graphomotor output was also quite slow and was affected by his careful and precise work style. When tested on medication, C. K. was not inattentive or distractible. He remained on task and did not require redirection from the examiners. However, his performances on some of the tasks indicated some variable attention to detail. C. K. did not show impulsivity on tasks and sat quietly during testing. C. K.'s spoken language was fluent and free of word-finding problems. His auditory comprehension was intact, although he often asked many questions after instructions to a task had been presented; C. K. seemed to want to be certain that he had understood all of the task parameters and demands prior to commencing the task in order to ensure he would carry it out as requested.

Test Results

The Wechsler Intelligence Scale for Children–Fourth Edition (WISC-IV) was administered to C. K., and his Full Scale IQ was in the average range (FSIQ = 105, 63rd percentile). However, C. K. showed significant variability in his performances across the WISC-IV index scores. His Verbal Comprehension index score (VCI = 106, 66th percentile) was solidly in the average range, as was his Perceptual Reasoning index score (PRI = 96, 45th percentile). On the Working Memory index (WMI = 123, 94th percentile), C. K.'s score fell in the superior range. His Processing Speed index score (PSI = 85, 16th percentile), however, fell within the low-average range and was statistically lower than his other WISC-IV index scores. His subtest performances ranged from the 2nd to the 95th percentile. Within the verbal comprehension domain, C. K.'s scores fell within normal limits (37th–75th percentile), indicating that his verbal reasoning abilities were age-appropriate. C. K. also performed within age expectation on the untimed Matrix Reasoning and Picture Concepts subtests. On the Block Design subtest, he scored at the mean for his age and correctly replicated 12 out of 14 designs, but he earned no bonus points for speed of completion. C. K.'s strongest subtest performances were earned on the Digit Span and Letter Number Sequencing working memory subtests (95th and 84th percentiles respectively). In contrast, on the WISC-IV timed subtests, C. K. achieved lower scores. On the Picture Completion subtest, which requires quick thinking and careful attention to visual detail for good performance, C. K. performed at the 2nd percentile. He gave few incorrect responses on this task, but he did not earn credit on many items because he did not respond within the 20-second time limit. On the Coding subtest, C. K.'s performance fell at the 25th percentile and, while error-free, was slowly executed. On the Symbol Search subtest, C. K. worked slowly and also committed three errors, yielding a performance falling at the 16th percentile.

Academic Achievement

C. K.'s academic achievement was assessed using the Wechsler Individual Achievement Test – Second Edition (WIAT-II) and the Reading Fluency and Math Fluency subtests of the Woodcock-Johnson III Tests of Achievement (WJ-III). C. K.'s reading, decoding, word identification, and spelling skills were well developed, while his reading comprehension was average. He demonstrated solid comprehension for factual information but more emergent skill in answering higher order reading comprehension questions demanding abstraction, inference, and deduction. His reading speed was average on both the WIAT-II and WJ-III; however, he often re-read large portions of the WIAT-II passages prior to answering comprehension questions. C. K. demonstrated some relative weaknesses in his writing skills on the WIAT-II Written Expression subtest. He had difficulty rapidly generating words to fit a semantic cue (Word Fluency = 1st quartile). In addition, in writing an essay, his syntax, word usage, and idea development were simplistic for his age and grade level. His writing was also weak with regard to organization and depth of detail. In contrast, C. K. demonstrated well-developed math skills.

Neuropsychological Testing

C. K.'s language skills were within normal limits, although he displayed anxiety-related mental blocking on the Boston Naming Test, as he was able to retrieve six additional words when provided with phonemic cues. Fine motor speed and dexterity for each hand were well below expectation; C. K. displayed no problems inserting pegs into a pegboard or manipulating the pegs, but he worked at a very slow pace. C. K.'s motor-free

visual-perceptual skills were within age expectations. However, he showed significant weakness on tests involving visual motor integration skills. On the Beery Developmental Test of Visual Motor Integration–5th Edition he performed at the 5th percentile, while his copy of the Rey-Osterreith Complex Figure Test (RCFT) earned a quantitative score falling at the 19th percentile. On both tasks, C. K. showed reduced planning that affected the accuracy of his reproductions. C. K. also showed immature organizational strategy on the RCFT. Rather than initially appreciating the overall design shape and then adding in design details, C. K. drew the complex figure in a fragmented, piecemeal manner. He was also inattentive to some of the details as he copied the design, and he incorrectly placed some of the details in his drawing. When asked to recall the RCFT immediately and after a delay, C. K.'s designs earned scores falling within the low end of average (25th and 29th percentile, respectively), and he showed no loss of information over time. On the WRAML-2 Picture Memory subtest, which did not require him to impose organization, C. K. performed at an average level for his age.

Examination of C. K.'s verbal memory skills revealed them to be intact. However, on the story memory test, C. K.'s spontaneous delayed recall was stronger than his delayed recognition performance, which was examined by having him answer multiple-choice questions; C. K. struggled to make choices on the recognition test and doubted some of his own correct free recall of story elements. C. K.'s verbal learning skills, as measured by the California Verbal Learning Test–Children's Version (CVLT-C), were average, and he retained learned information well over time. His use of semantic clustering for list learning was average. However, C. K. made a significantly high number of intrusions, adding words that were not on the list. It appeared that to reduce his anxiety about forgetting a word, he said words that he thought might possibly have been on the list. The high number of intrusions suggests that he did not monitor his performance well.

C. K. demonstrated significant variability in his executive functioning, with marked problems seen on measures sensitive to mental flexibility and cognitive shifting. He performed in the average range on a simple sequencing task

(Trail Making Test [TMT] Part A), but on a more complex sequencing task that required him to alternate between numbers and letters (TMT Part B), his performance was error free, but his time to completion was very slow (8th percentile). C. K. did not show any difficulty on verbal fluency tasks. However, on the Wisconsin Card Sort Test, C. K. displayed significant weakness. He was only able to complete one out of six card matching sets. Rather than systematically attempting to match the cards along one criteria and then another until a correct match was made, C. K. appeared to make the task more complicated than necessary by attempting to match the cards according to several criteria at the same time. He then appeared to become confused when the examiner's feedback did not match his expectations, and he showed considerable difficulty in shifting set to adapt his performance according to the feedback he received. In addition, he lost set four times, either forgetting or confusing the principle by which he was successfully matching the cards. C. K. performed within normal limits on the Conners' Continuous Performance Test-II, a 14-minute long computerized test of sustained attention, vigilance, concentration, and impulsivity.

Emotional Functioning

As part of the evaluation, C. K. completed a self-rating measure, the Achenbach Youth Self-Report (YSR), about his feelings and behaviors. C. K.'s responses did not yield clinical elevations on any of the problem behavior scales. However, his responses did indicate that he was a worry-prone adolescent. He endorsed that he is sometimes too fearful or anxious and tends to worry a lot. He also reported that he tends to feel the need to be perfect. In addition, C. K. reported engaging in some repetitive behaviors, such as "erasing something when it is okay." He further endorsed some difficulties with attention, reporting that he is sometimes easily distracted and, at times, has trouble concentrating. His pattern of responses did not reveal evidence of depression.

Discussion

C. K.'s neuropsychological profile of strengths and weaknesses was in many ways consistent with the profile of individuals with OCD that has emerged in research. Notably, C. K. showed weaknesses in aspects of executive functioning. He displayed difficulty with self-generated planning and organization, as seen in his use of immature organizational strategies on the RCFT. C. K. also displayed weakness in cognitive mental flexibility and set shifting, which was most vividly seen in his performance on the WCST. Similar to the research on children with OCD, C. K. did not demonstrate deficits in his oral fluency. C. K.'s performances on memory tasks were also consistent with patterns documented in the literature on OCD. His visual and verbal memory skills were intact; however, his performances on the RCFT recall tasks were negatively impacted by his poor organizational skills. C. K. also demonstrated age-appropriate visual spatial skills. However, he did show difficulty on tasks that assessed visual-motor integration (VMI and RCFT), but his poor performances were attributable to reduced attention to detail and poor planning and organization, rather than to innate visual-perceptual weaknesses. As was found in some individuals with OCD, C. K. exhibited considerable cognitive slowing on some tasks, including the Coding and Symbol Search subtests of the WISC-IV, and throughout testing, C. K. displayed a slow, deliberate, and cautious style that affected his performances on timed measures. He also displayed fine motor speed slowness in the absence of fine motor dexterity problems.

At the time of testing, C. K. was on medication for ADHD (Stratterra) and OCD (Zoloft). Unlike the study by Andrés et al. (2008) that found that children and adolescents who underwent psychopharmacological treatment did not continue to show executive dysfunction, C. K. exhibited significant executive functioning deficits. While it was proposed that cognitive deficits associated with OCD might have been reversible for the young participants in the Andrés et al. (2007) study as they had not had the disorder long, C. K. had experienced OCD for several years before he was effectively medicated. His presentation in that respect was more consistent with results of studies that found continuing cognitive deficits in adults with OCD following psychopharmacological intervention.

It was difficult to discern at the time of testing whether C. K.'s cognitive profile was solely attributable to OCD or whether his earlier diagnosis of ADHD could account for some of the executive weaknesses documented. It is also possible that C. K.'s earlier diagnosis of ADHD may have been reached in the absence of consideration of OCD as part of a more complex neuropsychiatric presentation. Obsessive thinking can lend to the appearance of inattention and can also directly affect attention testing results. In this testing, when examined while on medication, C. K. demonstrated no fundamental attention problems. It is possible that he had frank attentional problems independent of OCD that were being improved with the stimulant medication. In the absence of depression, C. K.'s cognitive slowing appeared to be related to his perfectionistic tendencies and his very strong need to be sure of the accuracy of his responses and work product. In evaluating an individual with OCD, it is important to consider the patient's specific obsessions and compulsions, as differing constellations of OCD symptoms may affect neuropsychological testing and daily functioning in varying ways. For example, a preoccupation with perfection, such as constantly checking one's work, can significantly affect the rate at which one can complete work, while an obsession about germs or contamination anxiety likely would not influence work rate.

While the precise etiology(ies) to account for C. K.'s neuropsychological profile remained elusive, what was critical was that the testing provided a clear picture of C. K.'s cognitive, academic, and psychological profile and led to specific treatment recommendations and school accommodations to address his ongoing needs and to improve his functioning. The continued use of medications as part of his treatment was recommended for C. K., as C. K. had made significant gains and was less functionally impaired when on medications. It was further recommended that C. K. be engaged in a course of cognitive-behavioral therapy to further reduce his obsessive thinking and compulsions; he had never been engaged in such treatment, and treatment outcome studies with adolescents have shown the most favorable results when OCD is treated with medication and such therapy. For school, the continued provision of an extended time

accommodation for tests was supported. Given his slow graphomotor output, it was also recommended that C. K. be allowed to use a computer for in-school writing assignments and homework to see if it would make his work completion timelier. Ongoing academic support to further develop C. K.'s inferential reading comprehension and expository writing was also recommended.

References

American Psychiatric Association. (2000). *Diagnostic and statistical manual of mental disorders* (4th ed., Text rev.). Washington, DC: Author.

Andrés, S., Boget, T., Lázaro, L., Penadés, R., Morer, A., Salamero, M., et al. (2007). Neuropsychological performance in children and adolescents with obsessive-compulsive disorder and influence of clinical variables. *Biological Psychiatry, 61*, 946–951.

Andrés, S., Lázaro, L., Salamero, M., Boget, T., Penadés, R., & Castro-Fornieles, J. (2008). Changes in cognitive dysfunction in children and adolescents with obsessive-compulsive disorder after treatment. *Journal of Psychiatric Research, 42*, 507–514.

Chamberlain, S. R., Blackwell, A. D., Fineberg, N. A., Robbins, T. W., & Sahakian, B. J. (2005). The neuropsychology of obsessive-compulsive disorder: the importance of failures in cognitive and behavioural inhibition as candidate endophenotypic markers. *Neuroscience and Biobehavioral Reviews, 29*, 399–419.

Deckersbach, T., Otto, M. W., Savage, C. R., Baer, L., & Jenike, M. A. (2000). The relationship between semantic organization and memory in obsessive-compulsive disorder. *Psychotherapy and Psychosomatics, 69*(2), 101–107.

Deckersbach, T., Savage, C. R., Dougherty, D. D., Bohne, A., Loh, R., Nierenberg, A., et al. (2005). Spontaneous and directed application of verbal learning strategies in bipolar disorder and obsessive-compulsive disorder. *Bipolar Disorders, 7*(2), 166–175.

De Geus, F., Denys, D. A. J. P., Sitskoorn, M. M., & Westenberg, H. G. M. (2007). Attention and cognition in patients with obsessive-compulsive disorder. *Psychiatry and Clinical Neurosciences, 61*, 45–53.

Friedlander, L., & Desrocher, M. (2006). Neuroimaging studies of obsessive-compulsive disorder in adults and children. *Clinical Psychology Review, 26*(1), 32–49.

Geller, D. A., Biederman, J., Faraone, S., Agranat, A., Cradock, K., Hagermoser, L., et al. (2001). Developmental aspects of obsessive-compulsive disorder: Findings on children, adolescents, and adults.

The Journal of Nervous and Mental Disease, 189, 471–477.

Greisberg, S., & McKay, D. (2003). Neuropsychology of obsessive-compulsive disorder: A review and treatment implications. *Clinical Psychology Review, 23,* 95–117.

Hwang, S. H., Kwon, J. S., Shin, Y., Lee, K. J., Kim, Y. Y., & Kim, M. (2007). Neuropsychological profiles of patients with obsessive-compulsive disorder: Early onset versus late onset. *Journal of the International Neuropsychological Society, 13,* 30–37.

Kuelz, A. K., Hogan, F., & Voderholzer, U. (2004). Neuropsychological performance in obsessive-compulsive disorder: A Critical review. *Biological Psychology, 65,* 185–236.

Menzies, L., Chamberlain, S. R., Laird, A. R., Thelen, S. M., Sahakian, B. J., & Bullmore, E. T. (2008). Integrating evidence from neuroimaging and neuropsychological studies of obsessive-compulsive disorder: The orbitofronto-striatal model revisited. *Neuroscience and Biobehavioral Reviews, 32,* 525–549.

Metehan, I., & Flament, M. F. (2007). Neuropsychological profile of childhood-onset obsessive-compulsive disorder. *Turkish Journal of Psychiatry, 18*(4), 293–301.

Moritz, S., Kloss, M., Jahn, H., Schick, M., & Hand, I. (2003). Impact of co-morbid depressive symptoms on non-verbal memory and visuospatial performance in obsessive-compulsive disorder. *Cognitive Neuropschiatry, 8,* 261–272.

Nielen, M. M. A., & Den Boer, J. A. (2003). Neuropsychological performance of OCD patients before and after treatment with fluoxetine: Evidence for persistent cognitive deficits. *Psychological Medicine, 33,* 917–925.

Olley, A., Malhi, G., & Sachdev, P. (2007). Memory and executive functioning in obsessive-compulsive disorder: A selective review. *Journal of Affective Disorders, 104,* 15–23.

Pediatric OCD Treatment Study (POTS) Team. (2004). Cognitive-behavior therapy, sertraline, and their combination for children and adolescents with obsessive-compulsive disorder. *Journal of the American Medical Association, 292*(16), 1969–1976.

Penadés, R., Catalan, R., Andrés, S., Salamero, M., & Gasto, C. (2005). Executive function and non-verbal memory in obsessive-compulsive disorder. *Psychiatry Research, 133*(1), 81–90.

Rao, N. P., Reddy, Y. C. J., Kumar, K. J., Kandavel, T., & Chandrashekar, C. R. (2008). Are neuropsychological deficits trait markers in OCD? *Progress in Neuro-Psychopharmacology and Biological Psychiatry, 32,* 1574–1579.

Savage, C. R., Deckersbach, T., Wilhem, S., Rauch, S. L., Baer, L., Reid, T., et al. (2000). Strategic processing and episodic memory impairment in obsessive compulsive disorder. *Neuropsychology, 14*(1), 141–151.

Shin, M. S., Park, S. J., Kim, M. S., Lee, Y. H., Ha, T. H., & Kwon, J. S. (2004). Deficits of organizational strategy and visual memory in obsessive-compulsive disorder. *Neuropsychology, 18*(4), 665–672.

Simpson, H. B., Rosen W., Huppert, J. D., Lin, S., Foa, E. B., & Liebowitz, M. R. (2006). Are there reliable neuropsychological deficits in obsessive-compulsive disorder? *Journal of Psychiatric Research, 40*(3), 247–257.

25

First-Episode Schizophrenia

Anthony J. Giuliano and Bernice A. Marcopulos

Over the past two decades, there has been increasing attention given to the earliest stages of schizophrenia in an effort to better understand its neuropathology and to differentiate its modal cognitive features from the effects of its treatment, including institutionalization, and other exposures such as comorbid substance dependence. Thus, we chose a case of a young adult with recent-onset schizophrenia rather than an individual in the so-called chronic stage of schizophrenia with multiple episodes of psychosis, hospitalizations, and somatic treatments. We hope that this case presentation will underscore several important considerations in the clinical neuropsychological assessment of persons with schizophrenia (PWS): *(1)* Neurocognitive deficits are widely considered to be a core component of schizophrenia. *(2)* On average, neuropsychological impairment involves multiple domains, is severe to moderately severe compared to healthy age peers, and is relatively independent of clinical symptoms and most drug treatments. *(3)* While the evolution of cognitive deficits remains uncertain, significant cognitive impairment appears to be reliably established by the first episode, and nearly all PWS demonstrate cognitive decline compared with their expected level had they not developed the illness. *(4)* Neuropsychological assessment has clinical value in the management of the illness, precisely because the daily functioning of PWS is most strongly associated with their level of cognitive functioning. Contemporary and developing treatments with medications and/or cognitive remediation or interventions intended to improve cognition may yield functional benefits, and reliable determination of cognitive functioning through clinical neuropsychological assessment may contribute to better outcomes.

Brief Overview of the Neuropsychology of Schizophrenia

Schizophrenia is a complex, heterogeneous lifelong disorder associated with moderate to severe cognitive deficits and substantial functional disability. Cognitive deficits have long been regarded as core features of schizophrenia (Bleuler, 1950; Heinrichs, 2005; Kraepelin, 1950). More recently, cognitive deficits have become the focus of proposals to include cognition within the diagnostic criteria for schizophrenia (Keefe & Fenton, 2007) as well as intervention studies to enhance cognition (Gold, 2004; Green, 2007). The cognitive deficits remain present in treated patients and in those who are no longer symptomatic (Goldberg et al., 2007; Gold, Arndt, Nopoulos, O'Leary, Andreasen, 1999; Keefe, Silva, Perkins, & Lieberman, 1999) and are *not* significantly associated with clinical symptoms, particularly positive symptoms (Bilder et al., 2000). Cognitive deficits in schizophrenia also strongly contribute to functional outcome and quality of life, and their severity is associated with how well PWS engage in or respond to psychosocial rehabilitation, manage in their community, and engage in productive work (Green, 1996; Green, Kern, Braff, & Mintz, 2000; Green, Kern, & Heaton, 2004;

Velligan, Kern, & Gold, 2006; Mohamed, Rosenheck, Swartz, Stroup, Lieberman, & Keefe, 2008).

While there is considerable heterogeneity among the cognitive domains most affected, a modal profile of cognitive performance across domains has been amply documented (Heinrichs & Zakzanis, 1998). Heinrichs and Zakzanis' (1998) meta-analysis of neurocognition in PWS documented that cognitive deficits were present in all domains of cognition assessed, and they ranged from moderate (in motor functions) to very large (in verbal declarative memory). Moreover, this level and pattern of cognitive performance across domains is consistent for recent-onset or first-episode patients, such as in the case presented in this chapter, suggesting that cognitive deficits are reliably present and well established within the phase of early psychosis (Mesholam-Gately, Giuliano, Goff, Faraone, & Seidman, 2009). Mesholam-Gately and colleagues' findings also documented that those in their first episode of schizophrenia are characterized by moderate to severe cognitive deficits that can be viewed as a generalized impairment (Blanchard & Neale, 1994; Dickinson & Harvey, 2009) or as multiple specific "selective" deficits of differential magnitude (Saykin et al., 1994). Deficits were most severe in the domains of verbal memory and processing speed, and least severe in upper extremity motor functioning, though no cognitive function was comparable to age- and gender-matched healthy control subjects.

Clinical neuropsychology is thus a valuable tool in understanding and managing schizophrenia. Neuropsychological assessment of PWS can contribute to differential diagnosis and treatment planning and to elucidate factors affecting recovery and outcome (Marcopulos et al., 2008). For instance, neuropsychological assessment can inform judgments about whether the cognitive deficits are significant enough to impair independent living, competitive employment, and/or educational attainment, and it can help to identify targets for cognitive aids and supports or learning and work accommodations. Neuropsychological assessment can also contribute to decisions about whether (and under what circumstances) the individual has the cognitive capacity to manage his or her own illness effectively and work actively

toward recovery (Kopelowicz, Liberman, Ventura, Zarate, & Mintz, 2005). It can elucidate the influence of coexisting neuropsychological vulnerabilities (e.g., traumatic brain injury, substance abuse/dependence, premorbid learning disabilities) that often complicate the clinical picture and can aid in differential diagnosis (e.g., psychosis due to medical issue vs. primary psychotic disorder). At the individual level, however, neuropsychological assessment cannot reliably differentiate among major mental illnesses such as schizophrenia versus schizoaffective versus bipolar disorders, given the remarkable heterogeneity across individual profiles (Keefe & Fenton, 2007; Schretlen, Cascella, Meyer, Kingery, Testa, Munro, Pulver, Rivkin, Rao, Diaz-Asper, Dickerson, Yolken, & Pearlson, 2007). There is no prototypical neuropsychological testing profile for PWS.

Clinical neuropsychologists can be consulted at any time during the course of the illness. In the case presented here, a neuropsychological assessment was conducted during the first episode of the illness, close to its onset. This case illustrates that cognitive deficits are evident early in the illness and are not simply a secondary effect of psychotic symptoms, such as hallucinations and delusions, or treatment with antipsychotic medications. Identification and treatment of cognitive deficits is essential if functional outcomes for PWS are to be optimized.

Case Presentation

Case History

Mr. Z is a 22-year-old, right-hand-dominant, single Caucasian male who was psychiatrically hospitalized for approximately 1 month during the summer of 2008 for a first episode of psychosis. He is the only child of married parents. His mother completed a masters degree in education and his father completed a masters degree in electrical engineering. Neither parent had a history of psychiatric difficulties. Family history does not include any known first- or second-degree relatives with a primary psychotic disorder. However, Mr. Z's maternal grandmother was described as emotionally flat, socially isolated, and prone to suspiciousness. She was treated with medication for depression but reportedly used it only for brief periods. A cousin was psychiatrically hospitalized while in college for unknown reasons, but she was able to return to school, complete her degree, and work productively in a health-care profession.

Both parents were in their early 30s at the time of his birth, and there were no known obstetric or perinatal complications. Pregnancy and birth history were normative by maternal report. Early developmental history was largely normative, and developmental milestones were achieved at age expectations. Despite repeating kindergarten (reportedly for weaknesses in school "readiness" and social maturity), Mr. Z had always been an above-average student and was attending a competitive college prior to his first psychiatric hospitalization. Mr. Z's only known early risk factors include unspecified diagnoses but possibly related symptoms in one of two second-degree relatives.

Mr. Z's premorbid history includes average social functioning until about the fourth grade, when it started to decline in favor of a focus on his school work and interest in various solitary projects, particularly related to music. By all accounts, he still related adequately to others but his initiation in and time spent in extrafamilial relationships decreased. To an important degree, Mr. Z's intellectual and academic development may have overshadowed his social development. Up until fourth grade, Mr. Z also participated in youth sports such as soccer. In high school, Mr. Z was regarded as academically successful by his teachers and peers. He attended a well-regarded public high school and achieved above-average grades, uniformly in the B+ to A range. His SATs were also above average; he took the "new" SAT in 2005 and achieved a score of 670 on Critical Reading, 650 on Mathematics, and 624 on Writing. His academic performance in college was less positive, though still above average in his freshman year, particularly in his music and math/engineering courses. His early work at a music engineering studio in his sophomore year was also successful.

However, as he explained it, he began to take things "too literally" during his freshman year of college. He also acknowledged considerable alcohol use in this period and missed classes on several occasions due to hangovers. He reported that he sometimes drove drunk, but this scared him and led him to stop drinking toward the end of his freshman year. He also used other drugs in this period. In the year prior to his first episode of psychosis, he used considerable amounts of cannabis regularly and cocaine and hallucinogens episodically (several uses of LSD, ecstasy, and psilocybin).

The onset of Mr. Z's prodrome, or the period before psychosis onset during which he began to show attenuated negative and positive symptoms, is difficult to identify precisely. He reported, however, that around the age of 14, he started to hear "hissing" and "humming" sounds and indistinguishable "chatter" that began low, increased in intensity, and then faded out over periods of seconds to minutes. These experiences occurred intermittently throughout his adolescence, sometimes in periods of stress (e.g., exam times, relationship conflicts, applications and transition to college).

In the year prior to his hospitalization, Mr. Z demonstrated a pattern of escalating adjustment problems in his social and role functioning and symptoms. He reported that his friends began to complain that his drug use was changing his personality. From Mr. Z's perspective, he recalled that he was often a person who "liked and needed to get his point across," but he was having increasing difficulty focusing and finishing his thoughts. He noted that he had a hard time understanding jokes and sarcasm, and by the late fall of his junior year, he could neither convey his thoughts clearly to others nor perform his job in a timely manner. He also reported that he became increasingly withdrawn, irritable, suspicious, and hypervigilant. Within 6–7 months prior to his hospitalization, he began to believe that he was "extraceptive and could read people's minds." He also became focused on religion and apocalyptic views of world conflicts, at one point believing that the world was close to coming to an end and would erupt into nuclear war. He said that the "universe had sent him out the thought that all wars are about religion." He later read a local magazine that published a picture of a "Western" Jesus whom he believed ultimately looked like him, and he thought for a while that he might be Jesus; he later revised this idea in favor of thinking of himself as a prophet. These notions influenced the episodic but strident pressure he placed on his band mates to move away from their hybrid of rock and island music to Christian rock and more Dylan-esque songs about war, peace, and songs that would "instigate peace rallies." He was frequently upset by his band mates' teasing of him in response. He spent many days tearful and frightened, as he felt compelled to change the style of his band's music if in fact he was the "Second Coming." Several other symptoms were notable, including somatic delusions of experiencing "Einstein's Theory of Relativity in my body." His explanation was that he could feel sound speed up and slow down in his body, and that since Einstein believed that speed and motion were relative, he experienced time as really slow, even when not using drugs.

He stopped using cannabis in late winter 2008 as a result of increasing fearfulness and at the urging of his friends. He also quit his job because he had trouble completing job-related tasks. He saw a psychiatrist at that time who recommended a trial of medication. Mr. Z recalled the psychiatrist telling him that his thinking was unclear at times and that he seemed to ramble. During the spring semester, he had increasing difficulty paying attention in class or completing any of his homework, tending to self-care reliably, and he did not finish any of his courses. His parents became concerned about his ongoing "depression" and facilitated his medical withdrawal from school and return home. They also took him to see a different psychiatrist, but again he refused medication. His withdrawal from college and increased support at home appeared to decrease his distress. At that point, he had not told anyone about his psychotic ideas/beliefs, and only acknowledged that he had been depressed and needed some "down" time. At home, he spent much of his time on his computer, surfing Web sites related to his ideas, listening to/downloading music, and playing video games and his instruments, though he reported rarely being able to finish playing an entire song. Socialization included one casual friend who did not attend college and with whom he would play computer games. Days before his next psychiatry appointment in June 2008, EMTs had arrived at a neighbor's home, and he walked down the street to approach one of them. He had been increasingly agitated by his apocalyptic thoughts and notions that he had to do something. He told

the EMTs that he had heard that if he ever needed help, he should tell someone. After 6–7 months of untreated psychosis, he was hospitalized and treated with medication, psychoeducation, and psychosocial therapies for 1 month.

About 2 months after his hospital discharge and 10 months into his illness, Mr. Z was referred by his psychiatrist for his first neuropsychological assessment as part of his participation in a comprehensive early psychosis program. Neuropsychological assessments are commonly requested by treating clinicians in the early psychosis program to document an individual's level and pattern of cognitive functioning, contribute to treatment decision making, and plan for academic and/or work re-engagement. The overarching goals of Mr. Z.'s early psychosis program are earlier detection, diagnosis, and treatment of serious mental illness, with the aim of better outcomes for young people and their families. The program is focused on maintaining a young person's educational and vocational prospects, motivation and self-esteem, peer and family relationships, and physical health and well-being.

The assessment occurred 2 months after discharge from a psychiatric hospital during which he was placed on Abilify (15 mg). As an inpatient, he was prescribed Vistaril for anxiety. At the time of this assessment, he was on medical leave from his university. He was considering the idea of discontinuing his medication, returning to school full time, and returning to his work, which he said he missed. He remained engaged in the early psychosis program, but he had difficulty consistently valuing the benefits of medications and other treatments.

Behavioral Observations

Mr. Z was alert and fully oriented for the two assessment sessions. He was friendly and cooperative, and was anxious to perform well on the assessment. He was very curious about the findings, and he appeared to put forth his best effort on all tasks. As recommended by Marcopulos et al. (2008) and Gorissen, Sanz de la Torre, and Schmand (2005), we made use of an effort measure to index his capacity for sustained mental effort. Mr. Z.'s scores on the Test of Memory Malingering (TOMM) were as follows: Trial 1 = 42, Trial 2 = 49, and Retention = 49, overall indicating adequate task engagement and effort marked by some difficulty initiating set (i.e., early errors on Trial 1). There was no evidence of overt psychosis during the testing itself. He smiled, made conversation, and initiated and responded to humor. Symptom ratings on the Brief Psychiatric Rating Scale (BPRS; Lukoff, Nuechterlein, & Ventura, 1986) at the time of this assessment ranged from 1 to 3 (not present to mild); this is in contrast to retrospective ratings of 6 and 7 (severe range) on items related to suspiciousness, unusual thought content, grandiosity, and hallucinations when he was most symptomatic (early to mid-2008). Thus, he was clinically stable (i.e., psychosis was relatively minimal) at the time of assessment. His processing speed in interpersonal interactions and on problem-solving tasks was somewhat slow and effortful, particularly given his known above-average level of premorbid functioning. Testing was considered a valid

reflection of his current neurocognitive strengths and weaknesses. Test scores are presented in Tables 25-1 through 25-5. Norms used for interpretation were from the test manuals or the Heaton norms, (Heaton, Miller, Taylor, and Grant, 2004).

Test Results

Mr. Z's test performance revealed an interesting pattern of strengths and weaknesses that are common, but not unique, to PWS. Mr. Z's highest scores were on academically based measures such as the Vocabulary and Information subtests of the Wechsler Adult Intelligence Scale (WAIS)-III and Word Attack, Calculation, Letter-Word Identification, and Spelling on the Woodcock-Johnson III Tests of Achievement (see Table 25-1). These scores reflect his history of academic success and interest, particularly in language arts.

Table 25-1. Intelligence and Academic Achievement Test Results

Wechsler Adult Intelligence Scale–III (WAIS-III)

Cognitive Domain/Test	Standard Score/Scaled Score	Percentile Rank	Qualitative Description
Full-Scale IQ	97	42	Average
VCI	112	79	High Average
POI	95	37	Average
WMI	97	42	Average
PSI	86	18	Low Average
Vocabulary	12	75	High Average
Similarities	10	50	Average
Information	15	95	Superior
Comprehension	9	37	Average
Picture Completion	9	37	Average
Block Design	10	50	Average
Matrix Reasoning	9	37	Average
Picture Arrangement	7	16	Low Average
Arithmetic	9	37	Average
Digit Span	9	37	Average
Letter-Number Sequencing	11	63	Average
Digit-Symbol Coding	7	16	Low Average
Symbol Search	8	25	Average
WJ-III			
Letter-Word Identification	125	95	Superior
Word Attack	119	90	High Average
Calculation	112	79	High Average
Spelling	115	84	High Average
Reading Fluency	98	45	Average
Math Fluency	91	27	Average
Passage Comprehension	94	34	Average

VCI, Verbal Comprehension Index; POI, Perceptual-Organization Index; PSI, Processing Speed Index; WMI, Working Memory Index.

Table 25-2. Motor Functioning and Visuospatial Test Results

Motor Functioning

Test	Hand	T Score	Qualitative Description
Finger Tapping	R = 44.8	32	Low
	L = 42	38	Low
Grooved Pegboard	R = 82	27	Very Low
	L = 94	27	Very Low

Visuospatial Functioning

Test	Trial	T-Score	Percentile Rank
Rey Complex Figure	Copy	32	2 to 5
	Immediate	<20	< 1
	Delayed	<20	<1
	Recognition	46	34

The Wide Range Achievement Test-4 Reading subtest, like other word reading measures, was used as an estimate of premorbid intellectual functioning (Griffin, Rivera-Mindt, Rankin, Ritchie, & Scott, 2002); Mr. Z's premorbid intellectual functioning was estimated to fall in the above-average range. Basic word reading (but not reading fluency or comprehension) is believed to be largely unaffected by schizophrenia, and there is strong support for indexing premorbid functioning by level of performance on word reading tests for PWS (Dalby & Williams, 1986; Goldberg et,al., 1990; Kremen et al., 1996). While he appears to have preserved verbal abilities, it is possible that some degree of decline occurred, particularly in verbal abstraction and higher level verbal expressive functions (i.e., WAIS-III Similarities and Comprehension are now at a mid-average level), particularly if Mr. Z's premorbid cognition is indexed by his superior level of

Table 25-3. Learning and Memory Functioning Test Results

CVLT-II

Test	Trial	Raw Score	Standard Score
Standard Form	Trial 1-5	43	42
	(4, 7, 9, 11 and 12)		
	Trial B	4	−1.5
	Short-Delay Free Recall	7	−1.5
	Short-Delay Cued Recall	9	−1.0
	Long-Delay Free Recall	8	−1.5
	Long-Delay Cued Recall	8	−1.5
	Repetitions	12	−1.0
	Recognition	14	0.5
	False Positive	2	
	Forced Choice	16/16	

WMS-III

Subtest	Raw Score	Scaled Score	Percentile Rank	Qualitative Description
Logical Memory I	44	11	63	Average
Logical Memory II	24	10	50	Average
WMS-III Faces I	35	8	25	Average
WMS-III Faces II	33	7	16	Low Average

Table 25-4. Executive Functioning Test Results

Trail-Making Test

Part B	Time = 97 seconds	T = 31	Low

Stroop

Condition	Score	Percentile	Qualitative Description
Word Score	90	18	Average
Color Score	46	1	Low
Color-Word	26	3	Low
Score Interference	9.4	84	Average

D-KEFS

	Raw Score	Scaled Score	Qualitative Description
Verbal Fluency	Letter Fluency = 31	8	Average
	Category Fluency = 35	9	Average
	Category Switching Correct = 11	7	Low Average
	Category Switching Accuracy = 10	8	Average

D-KEFS Proverb Test Total Achievement Score	22	10	Average

Wisconsin Card Sorting Test

	Raw Score	Percentile Rank	Qualitative Description
Categories Achieved	4 (almost 5)	>16	Average
Loss of Set	2		
Percent Perseverative Errors	7.8%	47	Average

single-word reading. This might also be true of his performance on other academic achievement measures, particularly those tapping speed and accuracy. This issue will be discussed later.

Mr. Z completed the Wisconsin Card Sorting test, which emphasizes executive function and has been used extensively in studies of schizophrenia. He performed in the lower end of the average range. His performance on other measures of executive function was variable, and marked by slow processing speed, likely reduced but still average verbal frequency, verbal abstraction, working memory, and set-shifting, and borderline-problem solving efficiency.

Verbal and visual memory and attention are frequently impaired in schizophrenia. In Mr. Z.'s case, performance on measures of learning and

memory varied (Table 25-3). His performance on the WMS-III Logical Memory was average, WMS-III Faces and the CVLT were low average, while performance on the MCCB measures

Table 25-5. MATRICS Consensus Cognitive Battery (MCCB) Domain Scores

Domain	T-Score	Percentile Score
Speed of Processing	28	1.0
Attention/Vigilance	34	5.5
Working Memory	43	24.2
Verbal Learning	33	4.5
Visual Learning	35	6.7
Reasoning and Problem Solving	36	8.1
Social Cognition	64	91.9
Overall Composite	32	3.6

(Table 25-5) was at least mildly impaired. Mr. Z. performed within normative expectations on working memory tasks. His performance on the CPT-IP was low. Difficulties in sustained attention and verbal learning and memory, even if relatively mild as in the case of Mr. Z., are likely to make continuation of his university studies more effortful and challenging.

On motor tests, he performed in the below-average range. Visuoconstructive tasks were impaired (Table 25-2). He produced a poor copy of the Rey-Osterrieth Complex Figure. As is common in PWS (Seidman, Lanca, Kremen, Faraone, & Tsuang, 2003), his approach was fragmented and part-(or detail-)oriented; Mr. Z also appeared to lose his reference point when copying two of the figure's core structural features (including the vertical midline and right vertical line of the central rectangle), resulting in a somewhat disorganized reproduction marked by omission or misplacement of some features. Some research has also shown that copy organization strategy is associated with recall accuracy (Sullivan, Mathalon, Ha, Zipursky, & Pfefferman, 1992).

In addition to more common neuropsychology measures, Mr. Z completed the MATRICS Consensus Cognitive Battery (MCCB; Nuechterlein & Green, 2006). The battery is available commercially and has good normative data. Although it is most commonly used in drug trial studies, it has clinical applications as well and taps a variety of cognitive functions thought to be most affected in schizophrenia. It consists of 10 individually administered tests to measure cognitive performance in seven domains: speed of processing, attention/vigilance, working memory, verbal learning, visual learning, reasoning and problem solving, and social cognition. The test developers conceived four key purposes of the MCCB: as an outcome measure for clinical trials of cognition-enhancing drugs or cognitive remediation, as a sensitive measure of cognitive change in other repeated testing applications, and as a reference point for nonintervention studies of schizophrenia and other severe psychiatric disorders. It is for the latter two purposes that we have included the MCCB in this assessment. His performance on the MCCB reveals deficits across a range of neuropsychological functions compared with the normative sample

(Table 25-5). However, administration and interpretation of MCCB test results is not regarded as a substitute for a comprehensive neuropsychological evaluation. Thus, our battery is augmented with commonly used neuropsychological measures to provide a more comprehensive assessment.

Persons with schizophrenia often have social skills deficits that precede the onset of the disorder (Mueser, 2000), and these may have a wide-ranging impact on their overall functioning and outcome. Social skills deficits are a major focus of intervention strategies for PWS (Tenhula & Bellack, 2008). Cognitive deficits may underlie the difficulties that persons with schizophrenia display in relating effectively to others (Bellack, Sayers, Mueser, & Bennett, 1994; Liberman et al., 1986; Morrison, Bellack, & Mueser, 1988). Within the field of schizophrenia, some researchers have argued that traditional measures of neurocognition leave between 40% and 80% of social functioning unexplained, opening the possibility that social cognition might add relevant explanatory power (Green, Kern, Braff, & Mintz, 2000; Pinkham, Penn, Perkins, & Lieberman, 2003).

While social cognition in schizophrenia can be conceptualized in a variety of ways (e.g., theory of mind, attributional style, facial affect perception; see Penn, Addington, & Pinkham, 2006), the MCCB operationalized the construct with a subtest from the Mayer-Salovey-Caruso Emotional Intelligence Test (MSCEIT; Mayer, Salovey, & Caruso, 2002), and it is this task that was included in this case study battery. The Managing Emotions subtest of the MSCEIT measures how well people perform tasks involving emotions and solving emotional problems, and it requires the patient to (1) rate the effectiveness of alternative actions in achieving a certain result in situations where a person must regulate his/her emotions, and (2) asks the respondent to evaluate how effective different actions would be in achieving an outcome involving other people. In contrast to studies of people both in the early and more chronic stages of schizophrenia that document stable deficits on tasks such as facial affect recognition, Mr. Z performed in the above-average range on the MCCB task of social cognition (Table 25-5). Mr. Z's limited interest in and situation-specific social engagement (i.e., band/music) was evident long before his psychotic symptoms emerged. Nonetheless, one might tentatively conclude that Mr. Z has some intact capacity to use emotions to solve problems (which may be an asset that supports his interest and involvement in music and, despite his psychosis, limited his vulnerability to act out impulsively).

Mr. Z also completed two self-report measures of emotional functioning. On the BAI, (Total Score = 8) which requires the respondent to rate common symptoms of anxiety over the past week, the two most highly endorsed symptoms were inability to relax and fear of losing control. The BDI revealed a mild level of depression (Total Score = 15). Persons with schizophrenia are at risk of developing comorbid depression and have an elevated suicide risk (Palmer, Pankrantz, & Bostwick, 2005).

Discussion

As in most cases of schizophrenia, Mr. Z's disorder had its onset in emerging adulthood (ages 18–25), a transitional stage of life when young adults typically begin to attain independence from their parents and other social and institutional influences, complete educational goals and/or begin to pursue work and/or career goals, and develop intimate relationships (Arnett, 2001). For Mr. Z, this process has been disrupted. One aspect of the illness's toll is reflected in his neuropsychological test performance. Neuropsychological assessment revealed a number of cognitive deficits, primarily in speed of processing, attention and vigilance, verbal and visual memory, psychomotor speed, and executive functioning. While the severity and range of deficits vary widely across patients, deficits in these cognitive domains are fairly common (Savla, Moore & Palmer, 2008). Since at the time of testing his psychopathology symptoms were stable and largely in remission, and he was on a modest dose of a second-generation antipsychotic not usually associated with cognitive problems (Keefe et al., 1999), we concluded that his testing reflected the core deficits manifested by his diagnosis of schizophrenia.

What did neuropsychology add to this case in terms of treatment planning? Cognitive impairment in schizophrenia has been found to be a better predictor of daily functioning and disability than psychotic (positive) symptoms (Green, 1996, 1998; Twamley et al., 2002). Mr. Z's history and presentation are fairly typical and illustrate how cognitive deficits impact employment and academic achievement. Mr. Z's cognitive deficits largely fell within the mild to moderate range of severity, while his premorbid cognitive endowment was above average. Thus, his cognitive difficulties are very apparent to him and are likely to challenge a crucial aspect of his identity as an intellectually talented individual; this aspect of his adjustment will likely require time and support in the context of therapies and recovery to be accommodated. In addition, his cognitive impairments are likely to interfere with, but not prevent him from, achieving some of his educational goals.

In providing a feedback-discussion session, the neuropsychological assessment findings were presented in the context of a vulnerability-stress model to emphasize the point that while his impairments have real-world implications, they were not by themselves able to define his recovery or goal achievement. In addition, Mr. Z was told that his cognitive difficulties, of which he was quite aware, were most likely related to his is overall illness and not a result of his medication treatment. Our hope was to maintain self-esteem and positive expectancies, minimize defeatist performance beliefs (see Grant & Beck, 2008), and enhance his openness to and engagement of treatments such as medication, cognitive adaptations, and practical supports. The neuropsychologist recommended that he consider taking a reduced academic load to minimize stress, work to develop compensations for his cognitive difficulties (e.g., memory and organization aides), and consult with the student disability services center at his university to request support services and accommodations. Becoming aware of the cognitive dysfunction that is part of the schizophrenia symptom complex can help Mr. Z. function in the community and promote recovery (Kopelwicz et al., 2004; Liberman & Kopelowicz, 2005). He was assured that his cognitive symptoms are not likely to get worse, and they may even improve modestly over time (Heaton et al., 2001).

To maximize his recovery and cognition over time, the discussion emphasized the value of health-related behaviors (e.g., sleep, nutrition, exercise), medication adherence in collaboration with a trusted prescribing clinician, openness to and use of cognitive adaptations and supports, avoidance of nonprescribed drugs and alcohol (Kavanaugh, 2008), and gradual return to pleasurable and constructive activities (such as playing music with his bandmates). However, regarding the latter, we also recommended consideration of some education of his bandmates regarding some of Mr. Z's vulnerabilities, and how they might be able to support his recovery; Mr. Z was willing to consider this, but only minimally at the time of our discussion.

The potential future value of vocational supports through a specialized supported employment program was also discussed (Becker, 2008; McGurk & Mueser, 2004). Despite mixed findings to date, it was also recommended that he consider a clinical trial of a computer-based cognitive remediation (e.g., a "brain fitness") program that was being conducted locally by clinical researchers (see Dickinson, Tenhula, Morris, Brown, Peer, Spencer, Li, Gold & Bellack, 2010 and Wykes & Reeder, 2005 for examples and discussion). While appreciating that cognitive remediation may represent more a promissory note than evidence-based treatment, we felt that participation in such a program might address his key concerns directly and support his identity as a cognitively capable individual, as well as facilitate broader treatment engagement.

Lastly, discussion with his parents emphasized noncoercive monitoring and support of health behaviors, psychiatric treatment, and his personal recovery goals. His parents were invited to participate in the early psychosis program's multifamily psychoeducation group therapy (see McFarlane, 2002) to assist them in understanding their son's mental health disorder and support them in constructively participating in his recovery. Meta-analyses have reliably shown that multifamily groups reduce relapse rates, improve social and family functioning, enhance quality of life, and reduce family burden (Kopelowicz, Liberman, & Zarate, 2007). Overall, his and his family's ongoing participation in the early psychosis program, which includes only older adolescents and young adults (16–30 years old) and their families, is geared to provide multimodal services in a developmentally sensitive fashion and is likely to support a positive outcome (Addington, 2007; Lincoln, Wilhelm, & Nestoriuc, 2007).

Mr. Z. is fortunate to reside in a large metropolitan area with several university medical centers with expertise in treating schizophrenia. Mr. Z. was enrolled in a program that included a treatment regimen that represents the "best practices" based on current knowledge of the illness (see Tandon, Keshavan, & Nasrallah, 2008, for a review). The program was designed to intervene early in the illness to mitigate factors that adversely affect outcome, such as frequent relapse of episodes of distressing and disorganizing psychosis, and medical and psychiatric comorbidity (e.g., diabetes, obesity, nicotine and substance abuse, anxiety, and depression). The program also addresses vocational and educational needs, family and peer relationships, and medical-health needs. With proper illness management, treatment and community-based supports, Mr. Z. has good reason to be optimistic. He has a reasonable chance of completing his education, becoming employed, and enjoying a more positive quality of life than is often associated with schizophrenia.

References

Addington, J., (2007). The promise of early intervention. *Early Intervention in Psychiatry*, *1*, 294–307.

Arnett, J. J. (2001). Emerging adulthood: A theory of development from the late teens through the twenties. *American Psychologist*, *55*, 469–480.

Becker, D. R. (2008). Vocational rehabilitation. In K. T. Mueser & D. V. Jeste (Eds.), *Clinical handbook of schizophrenia* (pp. 461–467). New York: Guilford Press.

Bellack, A. S., Sayers, M., Mueser, K. T., & Bennett, M. (1994). An evaluation of social problem solving in schizophrenia. *Journal of Abnormal Psychology*, *103*, 371–378.

Bilder, R. M., Goldman, R. S., Robinson, D., Reiter, G., Bell, L., Bates, J. A., Pappadopulos, E. Willson D. F., Alvir J. M. J., Woerner, M. G., Geisler, S. Kane J. M., & Lieberman J. A. (2000). Neuropsychology of first-episode schizophrenia: Initial characterization and clinical correlates. *American Journal of Psychiatry*, *157*(4), 549–559.

Blanchard, J. J., & Neale, J. M. (1994). The neuropsychological signature of schizophrenia: Generalized or differential deficit? *American Journal of Psychiatry*, *151*(1), 40–48.

Bleuler, E. (1950). *Dementia praecox, or the group of schizophrenias* (J. Zinker, Trans.). New York: International Universities Press.

Dalby, J. T., & Williams, R. (1986). Preserved reading and spelling ability in psychotic disorders. *Psychological Medicine, 27*, 1311–1323.

Dickinson, D., & Harvey, P. D. (2009). Systematic hypotheses for generalized cognitive deficits in schizophrenia: A new take on an old problem. *Schizophrenia Bulletin, 35*, 532–542.

Dickinson, D., Tenhula, W., Morris, S., Brown, C., Peer, J., Spencer, K., Li, L., Gold, J. M., & Bellack, A. S. (2010). A randomized, controlled trial of computer-assisted cognitive remediation for schizophrenia. *American Journal of Psychiatry, 167*, 170–180.

Gold, J. M. (2004). Cognitive deficits as treatment targets in schizophrenia. *Schizophrenia Research, 72*, 21–28.

Gold, S., Arndt, S., Nopoulos, P., O'Leary, D. S., & Andreasen, N. C. (1999). Longitudinal study of cognitive function in first-episode and recent-onset schizophrenia. *American Journal of Psychiatry, 156*, 1342–1348.

Goldberg, T. E., Goldman, R. S., Burdick, K. E., Malhotra, A. K., Lencz, T., Patel, R. C., Woerner, M. G., Schooler, N. R., Kane, J. M., & Robinson, D. G. (2007). Cognitive improvement after treatment with second-generation antipsychotic medications in first-episode schizophrenia: Is it a practice effect? *Archives of General Psychiatry, 64(10)*, 1115–1122.

Goldberg, T. E., Ragland, D., Torrey, E. F., Gold, J. M., Bigelow, L. B., & Weinberger, D. R. (1990). Neuropsychological assessment of monozygotic twins discordant for schizophrenia. *Archives of General Psychiatry, 47*, 1066–1072.

Gorissen, M., Sanz de la Torre, J. C., & Schmand, B. (2005). Effort and cognition in schizophrenia patients. *Schizophrenia Research, 78*, 199–208.

Grant, P. M., & Beck, A. T. (2008). Defeatist beliefs as a mediator of cognitive impairment, negative symptoms, and functioning in schizophrenia. *Schizophrenia Bulletin*, doi:10.1093/schbul/sbn008.

Green, M. F. (1996). What are the functional consequences of neurocognitive deficits in schizophrenia? *American Journal of Psychiatry, 153*, 321–330.

Green, M. F. (1998). *Schizophrenia from a neurocognitive perspective: Probing the impenetrable darkness.* Boston: Allyn and Bacon.

Green, M. F. (2007). Stimulating the development of drug treatments to improve cognition in schizophrenia. *Annual Review of Clinical Psychology, 3*, 159–180.

Green, M. F., Kern, R. S., Braff, D. L., & Mintz, J. (2000). Neurocognitive deficits and functional outcome in schizophrenia: Are we measuring the "right stuff"? *Schizophrenia Bulletin, 26*, 119–136.

Green, M. F., Kern, R. S., & Heaton, R. K. (2004). Longitudinal studies of cognition and functional outcome in schizophrenia: Implications for MATRICS. *Schizophrenia Research, 72*, 41–51.

Griffin, S. L., Rivera Mindt, M., Rankin, E. J., Ritchie, A. J., & Scott, J. G. (2002). Estimating premorbid intelligence: Comparison of traditional and contemporary methods across the intelligence spectrum. *Archives of Clinical Neuropsychology, 17*, 497–507.

Heaton, R. K., Gladsjo, J. A., Palmer, B. W., Kuck, J., Marcotte, T. D., & Jeste, D. V. (2001). Stability and course of neuropsychological deficits in schizophrenia. *Archives of General Psychiatry, 58*, 24–32.

Heaton, R.K., Miller, S.W., Taylor, M.J., & Grant, I. (2004). Revised comprehensive norms for an expanded Halstead-Reitan Battery: Demographically adjusted neuropsychological norms for African American and Caucasian adults. Lutz, FL: PAR.

Heinrichs, R. W. (2005). The primacy of cognition in schizophrenia. *American Psychologist, 60*, 229–242.

Heinrichs, R. W., & Zakzanis, K. K. (1998). Neurocognitive deficit in schizophrenia: A quantitative review of the evidence. *Neuropsychology, 12*, 426–445.

Kavanaugh, D. J. (2008). Management of co-occurring substance use disorders. In K. T. Mueser & D. V. Jeste (Eds.), *Clinical handbook of schizophrenia* (pp. 459–470). New York: Guilford Press.

Keefe, R. S. E., & Fenton, W. S. (2007). How should DSM-V criteria for schizophrenia include cognitive impairment? *Schizophrenia Bulletin, 33*, 912–920.

Keefe, R. S. E., Silva, S. G., Perkins, D. O., & Lieberman, J. A. (1999). The effects of atypical antipsychotic drugs on neurocognitive impairment in schizophrenia: A review and meta-analysis. *Schizophrenia Bulletin, 25*, 201–222.

Kopelowicz, A., Liberman, R. P., Ventura, J., Zarate, R., & Mintz, J. (2005). Cognitive correlates of recovery from schizophrenia. *Psychological Medicine, 35*, 1165–1173.

Kopelowicz, A., Liberman, R. P., & Zarate, R. (2007). Psychosocial treatments for schizophrenia. In P. E. Nathan & J. M. Gorman (Eds.), *Treatments that work* (3rd ed., pp. 243–269). London: Oxford University Press.

Kraeplin, E. (1950). *Dementia praecox and paraphrenia* (J. Zinkin, Trans.). New York: International Universities Press.

Kremen, W. S., Seidman, L. J., Faraone, S. V., Pepple, J. R., Lyons, M. J., & Tsuang, M. T. (1996). The "3 Rs" and neuropsychological function in schizophrenia: An empirical test of the matching fallacy. *Neuropsychology, 10*, 22–31.

Liberman, R. P., & Kopelowicz, A. (2005). Recovery from schizophrenia: A criterion-based definition. In R. O. Ralph & P. W. Corrigan (Eds.), *Recovery in mental illness. Broadening our understanding of wellness* (pp. 101–129). Washington, DC: American Psychological Assocation.

Liberman, R. P., Mueser, K. T., Wallace, C. J., Jacobs, H. E., Eckman, T., & Massel, H. K. (1986). Training skills in the psychiatrically disabled: Learning coping and competence. *Schizophrenia Bulletin, 12,* 631–647.

Lincoln, T. M., Wilhelm, K., & Nestoriuc, Y. (2007). Effectiveness of psychoeducation for relapse, symptoms, knowledge, adherence, and functioning in psychotic disorders: A meta-analysis. *Schizophrenia Research, 96,* 232–245.

Lukoff, D., Nuechterlein, K. H., & Ventura, J. (1986). Manual for the Expanded Brief Psychiatric Rating Scale (BPRS). *Schizophrenia Bulletin, 12,* 594–602.

Marcopulos, B. A., Fujii, D., O'Grady, J., Shaver, G., Manley, J., & Aucone, E. (2008). Providing neuropsychological services for persons with schizophrenia: A review of the literature and prescription for practice. In J. Morgan & J. Ricker (Eds.), *Textbook of clinical neuropsychology* (pp. 743–761). New York: Taylor & Francis.

Mayer, J. D., Salovey, P., & Carouso, D. R. (2002). *Mayer-Salovey-Caruso Emotional Intelligence Test.* Toronto, Ontario: MHS Publishers.

McFarlane, W. R. (Ed.). (2002). *Multifamily groups in the treatment of severe psychiatric disorders.* New York: Guilford Press.

McGurk, S., & Mueser, K. (2004). Cognitive functioning, symptoms, and work in supported employment: A review and heuristic model. *Schizophrenia Research, 70,* 147–173.

Mesholam-Gately, R. I., Giuliano, A. J., Goff, K. P., Faraone, S. V., & Seidman, L. J. (2009). Neurocognition in first-episode schizophrenia: A meta-analytic review. *Neuropsychology, 23,* 315–336.

Mohamed, S., Rosenheck, R., Swartz, M., Stroup, S., Lieberman, J.A., & Keefe, R.S.E. (2008). Relationship of cognition and psychopathology to functional impairment in schizophrenia. *American Journal of Psychiatry, 165,* 978–987.

Morrison, R. L., Bellack, A. S., & Mueser, K. T. (1988). Facial affect recognition deficits and schizophrenia. *Schizophrenia Bulletin, 14,* 67–83.

Mueser, K. T. (2000). Cognitive functioning, social adjustment and long-term outcome in schizophrenia. In T. Sharma & P. Harvey (Eds.), *Cognition in schizophrenia: Impairments, importance and treatment strategies* (pp. 157–177). Oxford, England: Oxford University Press.

Nuechterlien, K. H., & Green, M. F. (2006). *MCCB: MATRICS Consensus Cognitive Battery Manual.* Los Angeles: The Regents of the University of California.

Palmer, B. A., Pankrantz, V. S., & Bostwick, J. M. (2005). The lifetime risk of suicide in schizophrenia: A re-examination. *Archives of General Psychiatry, 62,* 247–253.

Penn, D. L., Addington, J., & Pinkham, A. (2006). Social cognitive impairments. In J. A. Lieberman, T. S. Stroup, & D. O. Perkins (Eds.), *Textbook of schizophrenia* (pp. 261–274). Washington, DC: American Psychiatric Publishing.

Pinkham, A. E., Penn, D. L., Perkins, D. O., & Lieberman, J. A. (2003). Implications for the neural basis of social cognition for the study of schizophrenia. *American Journal of Psychiatry, 160,* 815–824.

Savla, G. N., Moore, D. J., & Palmer, B. W. (2008). Cognitive functioning in schizophrenia. In K. T. Mueser & D. V. Jeste (Eds.), *Clinical handbook of schizophrenia* (pp. 91–99). New York: The Guilford Press.

Saykin, A. J., Shtasel, D. L., Gur, R. E., Kester, D. B., Mozley, L. H., Stafiniak, P., & Gur, R. C. (1994). Neuropsychological deficits in neuroleptic naive patients with first-episode schizophrenia. *Archives of General Psychiatry, 51*(2), 124–131.

Schretlen, D. J., Cascella, N. G., Meyer, S. M., Kingery, L. R., Testa, S. M., Munro, C. A., Pulver, A. E., Rivkin, P., Rao, V. A., Diaz-Asper, C. M., Dickerson, F. B., Yolken, R. H., & Pearlson, G. D. (2007). Neuropsychological functioning in bipolar disorder and schizophrenia. *Biological Psychiatry, 62,* 179-186.

Seidman, L. J., Lanca, M., Kremen, W. S., Faraone, S. V., & Tsuang, M. T. (2003). Organizational and visual memory deficits in schizophrenia and bipolar psychoses using the Rey-Osterrieth Complex Figure: Effects of duration of illness. *Journal of Clinical and Experimental Neuropsychology, 25,* 949–964.

Sullivan, E. V., Mathalon, D. H., Ha, C. N., Zipursky, R. B., & Pfefferman, A. (1992). The contribution of constructional accuracy and organizational strategy to nonverbal recall in schizophrenia and chronic alcoholism. *Biological Psychiatry, 32,* 312–333.

Tandon, R., Keshavan, M. S., & Nasrallah, H. A. (2008). Schizophrenia, "Just the facts": What we know in 2008 Part 1: Overview. *Schizophrenia Research, 100,* 4–19.

Tenhula, W. N., & Bellack, A. S. (2008). Social skills training. In K. T. Mueser & D. V. Jeste (Eds.), *Clinical handbook of schizophrenia* (pp. 240–248). New York: The Guilford Press.

Twamley, E. W., Doshi, R. R., Nayak, G. V., Palmer, B. W., Golshan, S., Heaton, R. K., Patterson, T. L., & Jeste, D. V. (2002). Generalized cognitive impairments, ability to perform everyday tasks, and level of independence in community living situations of older patients with psychosis. *American Journal of Psychiatry, 159*(12), 2013–2020.

Velligan, D. I., Kern, R. S., & Gold, J. M. (2006). Cognitive rehabilitation for schizophrenia and the putative role of motivation and expectancies. *Schizophrenia Bulletin, 32,* 474–485.

Wykes, T., & Reeder, C. (2005). *Cognitive remediation therapy for schizophrenia.* New York: Routledge.

26

Late-Onset Depression versus Dementia

Tracy D. Vannorsdall and David J. Schretlen

Depression and cognitive dysfunction occur together in many diseases and medical conditions, but their co-occurrence raises particularly difficult questions in elderly adults. One of the most common referral questions asked of neuropsychologists who work with elderly adults is whether a patient's memory decline is due to dementia or depression. While such referrals are often couched in terms of an "either/or" question, there are more than two possible answers. One can have depression—or not—and one can have a dementing illness—or not. Some patients have a dementing illness with depression as a symptom. Others develop a "dementia of depression." Furthermore, each condition can distort the other's presentation. For example, depression can lead patients to overestimate their cognitive failures, and dementia can lead observers to misperceive apathy or cognitive slowing as signs of depression. Finally, these complications can change over time. Some patients who develop depression during the early stage of Alzheimer disease (AD) later experience a remission of mood symptoms. Others with AD do not develop depression until later in the illness. Thus, good clinical practice requires the clinician to appreciate complexities that are obscured by the deceptively simple referral question of "dementia versus depression."

Depression is common in older adults. Up to one-third of elderly adults will experience a major depressive episode late in life (Blazer, 2002; Waraich, Goldner, Somers, & Hsu, 2004). Some degree of cognitive dysfunction occurs in 25%–55% of older adults with depression (Butters et al., 2000; Lee, Potter, Wagner, Welsh-Bohmer, & Steffens, 2007; Lockwood, Alexopoulos, Kakuma, & Van Gorp, 2000). The rate of this comorbidity appears to double every 5 years after age 70 (Arve, Tilvis, Lehtonen, Valvanne, & Sairanen, 1999). As a result, there is a sizeable group of older adults for whom the differential diagnosis of depression, dementia/mild cognitive impairment (MCI), or some combination of the two, will be relevant. Distinguishing the cognitive symptoms of depression from those of a dementing illness is crucial for diagnosis and treatment. A thorough clinical history, careful inspection of a patient's neurocognitive profile, and often longitudinal follow-up are essential for accurate diagnostic formulation.

Nearly 50 years ago, Kiloh (1961) coined the term "pseudo-dementia" to describe patients who presented with symptoms of dementia, but whose work-ups revealed no "organic" cause. The term has outlived its usefulness, as it is now widely recognized that individuals with depression can experience genuine cognitive dysfunction without demonstrable neuropathology. Persons with depression perform more poorly than nondepressed controls on cognitive testing (Christensen, Griffiths, Mackinnon, & Jacomb, 1997; Nebes et al., 2003), and elderly individuals with depression can show more severe deficits than younger persons with depression (Dotson, Resnick, & Zonderman, 2008; Gualtieri & Johnson, 2008). The most consistently documented deficits in depressed elderly adults involve psychomotor speed, executive functioning, and new learning/memory (Butters, Bhalla, et al., 2004; Nebes et al., 2000). Thus, the prototypical cognitive deficits resulting from depression resemble those seen in "subcortical-type" dementia (Crowe & Hoogenraad, 2000). There is some evidence that the degree of impairment correlates with depression severity (Boone et al., 1995; Yaffe et al., 1999). In addition, episodic memory might be more impaired in elderly adults with early-onset than late-onset depression (Rapp et al., 2005). However, a recent meta-analysis (Herrmann, Goodwin, & Ebmeier, 2007) found that elderly adults with early- versus late-onset depression showed roughly equivalent deficits in episodic and semantic memory, whereas those with late-onset depression showed more pronounced executive dysfunction and psychomotor slowing.

Whether depressed elderly adults show disproportionate cognitive dysfunction because aging depletes their cognitive reserve, or because any group of elderly adults is likely to include some with undiagnosed dementing illnesses, remains unclear. There is some evidence that new-onset depression in late life can foreshadow the development of dementia (Robert et al., 2003) or be an early symptom of dementia (Chen, Ganguli, Mulsant, & DeKosky, 1999). In some longitudinal studies of adults with MCI, depression is associated with increased rates of conversion to dementia (Modrego & Ferrandez, 2004) and persistent cognitive dysfunction even following resolution of a depressive episode (Lee et al., 2007). However, numerous studies also have shown that any history of depression (including early-onset) is associated with an increased risk of developing dementia in late life (Broe et al., 1990; Green et al., 2003; Jorm, 2001; Speck et al., 1995; Steffens et al., 1997). In fact, one meta-analysis suggested that the more remote the onset of depression the greater the likelihood of developing dementia (Ownby, Crocco, Acevedo, John, & Loewenstein, 2006).

Olin, Katz, Meyers, Schneider, and Lebowitz (2002) outlined clinical characteristics that can differentiate depression from dementia. First, those suffering from a primary affective disorder tend to report more severe cognitive problems than those with dementia (Feehan, Knight, & Partridge, 1991). Individuals with cortical-type dementia syndromes often have less insight into their cognitive dysfunction or may attribute less significance to their cognitive errors. Additionally, the clinical history provided by depressed older adults and their informants frequently suggests a temporal correspondence between the onset of low mood and the complaints of cognitive decline. When depression is primary, the severity of perceived cognitive failures tends to be more tightly coupled with mood fluctuations over time, whereas in early dementia the cognitive symptoms show little relationship to changes in mood. Depressive symptoms in individuals with early dementia also are often less severe and more likely to include social withdrawal and irritability as prominent features (Zubenko et al., 2003). In contrast, depressed individuals who report cognitive problems but do not have primary dementia are more likely to meet criteria for a major depressive episode (Olin et al., 2002).

The pattern of cognitive deficits produced on neuropsychological testing can also help differentiate depression from early dementia. While new learning/memory is usually the first cognitive domain affected by AD, depressed elderly adults often demonstrate more prominent weaknesses on tests of executive functioning and complex attention (Rapp et al., 2005). One hypothesis is that the latter is due, at least in part, to diminished capacity for effortful processing: The more effort a task requires for success, the less well individuals with depression tend to perform on it (Roy-Byrne, Weingartner, Bierer, Thompson, & Post, 1986). Indeed, some evidence suggests that the relationship between depressive symptoms and performance on many cognitive tests is largely mediated by impairments of effortful processing (Butters, Whyte, et al., 2004; Nebes et al., 2000).

When considering performance on tests of learning and memory, both individuals with early AD and those with depression can show poor acquisition and recall. However, those with dementia tend not to benefit from repeated exposure to stimuli, resulting in a flat learning curve, whereas depressed older adults may display inefficient learning on the initial trial, but frequently show greater benefit from repeated exposure (Steffens & Potter, 2008). Additionally, the memory deficits observed in those with early AD tend to be more severe, with more rapid forgetting and notable decrements in delayed recall

(Hart, Kwentus, Hamer, & Taylor, 1987). With recognition cuing, depressed older adults also tend to perform better than their demented peers and they make fewer false-positive errors (Hart et al., 1987; Miller & Lewis, 1977). However, depression may also contribute to increased self-doubt on recognition testing, resulting in a nay-saying bias and false-negative errors (Miller & Lewis, 1977).

Differences in other cognitive domains also can help with differential diagnosis. Patients with early AD are more likely to demonstrate impairments of temporal orientation, naming, praxis, and visuospatial functioning than those with cognitive dysfunction due to primary depression (Crowe & Hoogenraad, 2000; Jones, Tranel, Benton, & Paulsen, 1992).

In some cases, it is simply impossible to differentiate early dementia with depression from the dementia of depression without longitudinal assessment. While dementias due to degenerative diseases worsen over time, progressive cognitive decline is not characteristic of primary depression. However, there is not convincing evidence that effective treatment of major depression leads to substantial improvement in cognitive functioning. Indeed, Nebes et al. (2003) found that even elderly patients with major depression whose mood symptoms responded well to treatment with an antidepressant (paroxetine or nortriptyline) showed no greater improvement over baseline performance in any cognitive domain than untreated healthy controls on five follow-up evaluations taking place over a 12-week period. This and other studies suggest that many of the cognitive deficits shown by elderly adults with primary depression are more trait-like than state-like (Georgotas et al., 1989; Reischies & Neu, 2000). Nevertheless, longitudinal assessment can assist in the differential diagnosis based on whether the patient shows progressive decline over time.

The Case of Ms. S.

Ms. S. is a Caucasian widow who was first referred for a neuropsychological assessment at age 78 by a consulting psychiatrist due to complaints of memory decline over the preceding 8 years. She returned for follow-up testing 3 years later.

The patient's father developed a memory disorder in late life, but she reported no other family history of neuropsychiatric illness. Ms. S. was born and raised in New Jersey, graduated from high school, and left college to marry her first husband. Together they had three children before he died of a heart attack. She remarried at age 47, but her second husband developed dementia. He died of heart disease 1 year after her initial cognitive evaluation. On follow-up, Ms. S. lives alone in an apartment, although she has a full-time housekeeper/cook. She enjoys excellent relationships with her 22 children, grandchildren, and great grandchildren.

Ms. S. has a history of irritable bowel syndrome, hypertension, and aortic artery stenosis for which she underwent an aortic valve replacement. She also has undergone a hysterectomy, hemorrhoidectomy, and cataract removal. Ms. S. fell down three times during the past few years. As a result of these falls, she once fractured her wrist and once struck her head, but she did not lose consciousness. Ms. S. said she deliberately lost 35 pounds in the past few years. She explains that it is not difficult to maintain her current weight because food has little appeal to her; however, she has not continued losing weight, either. She began seeing a psychiatrist shortly before we first examined her. He started her on a selective serotonin reuptake inhibitor (SSRI). She currently is taking medication for hypertension and hypercholesterolemia as well.

Ms. S. reports that she first developed symptoms of depression in her early 70s. She describes persistent sadness, decreased interest in previously enjoyed activities, difficulty concentrating, and forgetfulness. At our initial examination, she reported noticing that her memory had declined over the preceding 1–2 years. Her handwriting seemed sloppier, and she often felt "discombobulated." On follow-up 3 years later, Ms. S. is still bothered by these symptoms, but she denies substantial worsening of them. Nevertheless, having dealt with her late husband's dementia for many years, Ms. S. is worried that her own memory and other cognitive failures might be due to AD.

On both evaluations Ms. S. was nicely dressed, impeccably groomed, alert, and fully oriented in all three spheres. She walked without assistance and displayed no abnormal movements. Her speech was normal in rate, rhythm, volume, and prosody. No word-finding difficulties, para-phasic errors, or other language abnormalities were noted in her discourse. On follow-up she describes her mood as "lethargic" and explains that she finds it difficult to get up and out of the house to do errands or visit others. However, she allows that doing things and seeing others usually lifts her spirits. Her affect is surprisingly bright. She laughs at times but also makes self-denigrating comments about perceived failures during test-ing—at times even as she performs well.

As shown in Table 26-1, on both examina-tions, the patient's single-word reading (NART-R) suggests that her premorbid IQ probably was

Table 26-1. Test Results

Test	2005	Range	2008	Range	Δ
NART-R (est. premorbid IQ)	117	High Average	116	High Average	
WASI (intelligence; age. adj. scores)	121	Superior	120	Superior	
MMSE (global cognitive functioning)	29/30	Normal	29/30	Normal	
GPT (fine manual speed/dexterity)					
Dominant (Right) hand	92"	Average	131"	Low Average	↓
BTA (auditory divided attention)					
Letters raw score	9/10	High Average	7/10	Average	
Trail Making (psychomotor speed)					
Part A	70"	Low Average	66"	Low Average	
Part B	133"	Average	198"	Low Average	↓
Nelson WCST (executive function)					
Category sorts	4/6	Average	2/6	Borderline	↓
Perseverative errors	1	Average	9	Low Average	↓
Boston Naming Test (object naming)	27/30	Average	27/30	Average	
Verbal Fluency (word list generation)					
Letters S & P	25	Average	28	Averae	
Animals and supermarket items	26	Borderline	41	Average	↑
Design Fluency (design generation)					
Novel designs in 4 min	10	Average	13	Average	
Clock Drawing (visual-construction)					
Command	4/5	Normal	5/5	Normal	
Copy	5/5	Normal	4/5	Normal	
Rey CFT (constructional praxis)					
Copy	25/36	Borderline	16.5/36	Abnormal	↓
Recall (5 min delay)	7/36	Low Average	6/36	Low Average	
BVMT-R (verbal learning/memory)					
Immediate recall (trials 1–3)	1, 2, 4	Borderline	4, 4, 8	Average	↑
Delayed recall (20 min)	4/12	Low Average	8/12	Average	↑
Delayed recognition (hits-false-positive errors)	6-0	Average	5-0	Average	
HVLT-R (verbal learning/memory)					
Immediate recall (trials 1-3)	4, 6, 11	Average	6, 8, 10	Average	↑
Delayed recall (20 min)	9/12	Average	10/12	High Average	
Delayed recog. (hits-false pos. errors)	11-0	Average	12-0	High Average	
WMS-III (verbal learning/memory)					
Logical Memory immediate	13	High Average	15	Superior	
Logical Memory delayed	15	Superior	17	Very Superior	
Prospective Memory Test	1 cue	Average	1 cue	Average	

BTA, Brief Test of Attention; BVMT-R, Brief Visuospatial Memory Test–Revised; Rey CFT, Rey-Osterrieth Complex Figure Test; GPT, Grooved Pegboard Test; MMSE, Mini Mental State Examination; NART-R, National Adult Reading Test–Revised; Nelson WCST, modified Nelson Wisconsin Card Sorting Test; HVLT-R, Hopkins Verbal Learning Test–Revised; WASI, Wechsler Abbreviated Scale of Intelligence; WMS-III, Wechsler Memory Scale–III Logical Memory Subtest.

well above average. Consistent with this, she produced a WASI Full Scale IQ score in the superior range. She lost just one point (for drawing intersecting pentagons) on the MMSE dementia screening test, and she was fully oriented to time. Nearly all the patient's other cognitive test performances were well within normal limits on both evaluations.

In examining the pattern of her test performances on both evaluations, Ms. S. showed mild slowing on tests of fine manual speed/dexterity (Grooved Pegboard), and psychomotor speed (Trail Making), with a noticeable decline from her initial evaluation on Part B of the latter test. Declines also were noted on a card-sorting test of executive functioning (mWCST) and the Rey-Osterrieth Complex Figure Test of visual-constructional praxis. Her approach to drawing the latter figure was disorganized. Conversely, compared to her first assessment, Ms. S. showed substantially better performance on selected measures of semantic verbal fluency, learning and delayed recall of simple designs (BVMT-R), and word list learning (HVLT-R). Importantly, her best (i.e., superior) performances were all observed on tests of new learning/memory. She also demonstrated stable and perfectly intact phonemic word fluency, picture naming (BNT), design fluency (DFT), clock drawing, and prospective memory (PMT). In short, testing revealed mildly reduced psychomotor speed, executive functioning, and complex attention, together with impaired visual-constructional praxis, against a background of otherwise intact functioning and unusually good memory.

In addition to cognitive testing, Ms. S. completed four self-report measures both times we examined her, with relatively consistent results. Despite her pleasant demeanor and reasonably bright affect, Ms. S. consistently endorsed numerous symptoms on the Geriatric Depression Scale, suggesting that she continues to experience severe depression. She also produced abnormal scores on several scales of the SCL-90-R psychiatric symptom inventory, reflecting her endorsement of distress related to symptoms of depression, anxiety, and cognitive failures. Compared to testing 3 years ago, Ms. S. also reported needing help to perform more instrumental activities of daily living, such as traveling outside of walking distance, doing housework,

the laundry and handyman work, taking medications as prescribed, and managing her money. Finally, Ms. S. again described herself as an unstable, mildly introverted woman who is more open-minded but much lower in conscientiousness, and about average in agreeableness compared to other women on the NEO Five Factor Inventory (FFI).

Discussion and Conclusions

Ms. S is a hypertensive but otherwise healthy 81-year-old woman. Her premorbid intelligence likely was well above average, if not superior. She has struggled with depression since her early 70s and concern about her memory for 4–5 years. Nearly all of Ms. S.'s cognitive test performances were within normal limits, and most ranged from average to superior. She showed mildly abnormal to low-average performance—and/or declines relative to testing 3 years earlier—on selected measures of psychomotor speed, executive functioning, and divided attention. However, she also showed substantial improvement—and/or unusually good performance—on many other tests, including tests of memory and semantic verbal fluency.

The patient's excellent memory, object naming, and semantic verbal fluency all strongly suggest that Ms. S. does not have AD. However, her reduced psychomotor speed and executive ability point to the presence of a mild cognitive disorder. We suspect that this is due to her persisting depression, possible undiagnosed cerebrovascular changes, or their combination. On our recommendation, Ms. S. underwent a brain magnetic resonance imaging (MRI) scan following our initial examination. It revealed scattered periventricular and subcortical white matter hyperintensities. These occur very frequently in late-onset depression, consistent with the notion of "vascular depression" (Alexopoulos, 2006). Since her last evaluation, Ms. S.'s cerebrovascular risk factors have remained stable over time, and she reports no history of stroke. It is possible that she reports needing more help for instrumental activities of daily living due to functional decline. However, it is also possible that she reports this *because* she hired a full-time housekeeper/cook.

Despite treatment with an antidepressant, Ms. S.'s psychological test results suggest that she continues to suffer from moderately severe major depression. She also continues to show mild, selective cognitive deficits or weakness in domains that are consistent with the neuropsychological dysfunction associated with depression, particularly slowing and executive impairment. The persistence of her affective and cognitive dysfunction in the face of treatment is not uncommon, and evidence suggests that our patient's cognitive deficits might persist even if her depression can be brought under better control. In older depressed adults, fully one-half demonstrate persisting cognitive deficits after their mood symptoms abate (Nebes et al., 2003). That said, neuropsychological evaluation can serve to document an individual patient's areas of residual cognitive strengths and weakness, which can help facilitate development of the most appropriate treatment plan. For instance, some executive functioning deficits associated with depression such as abulia, perseveration, and poor response inhibition are associated both with recurrence of depression (Alexopoulos et al., 2000) and poorer response to an SSRI (Alexopoulos et al., 2005). There is also evidence that in older adults with depression-related executive dysfunction, therapies targeting areas of cognitive weakness, such as problem solving, are associated with reduced remission and improved functional abilities (Alexopoulos, Raue, & Arean, 2003). Taken together, these findings suggest that failing a trial of antidepressant medication is not an effective means of disentangling cognitive dysfunction due to depression from that due to early dementia. Furthermore, it points to the need for greater treatment monitoring and tailoring of interventions in late-onset depression with comorbid cognitive dysfunction.

In summary, objective evidence of cognitive dysfunction frequently accompanies subjective cognitive complaints in older adults with depression. A thorough clinical history and neuropsychological assessment can aid in differentiating cognitive difficulties due to depression from those attributable to early dementia. However, as was seen in our patient, the history and observed deficits on a single evaluation may not provide persuasive evidence to differentiate depression-related dysfunction from very early-stage dementia. Follow-up cognitive assessment allows one to detect declines in cognition occurring over time that would be consistent with a progressive dementia. Alternatively, follow-up assessment may reveal improvements in the deficits observed on an initial evaluation, providing persuasive evidence against a dementia-related etiology and highlighting the need for more aggressive treatment of depression. Furthermore, cognitive dysfunction in older adults with depression may complicate treatment of their mood disorder and may necessitate more comprehensive patient monitoring.

References

Alexopoulos, G. S. (2006). The vascular depression hypothesis: 10 years later. *Biological Psychiatry*, *60*(12), 1304–1305.

Alexopoulos, G. S., Kiosses, D. N., Heo, M., Murphy, C. F., Shanmugham, B., & Gunning-Dixon, F. (2005). Executive dysfunction and the course of geriatric depression. *Biological Psychiatry*, *58*(3), 204–210.

Alexopoulos, G. S., Meyers, B. S., Young, R. C., Kalayam, B., Kakuma, T., Gabrielle, M., et al. (2000). Executive dysfunction and long-term outcomes of geriatric depression. *Archives of General Psychiatry*, *57*(3), 285–290.

Alexopoulos, G. S., Raue, P., & Arean, P. (2003). Problem-solving therapy versus supportive therapy in geriatric major depression with executive dysfunction. *American Journal of Geriatric Psychiatry*, *11*(1), 46–52.

Arve, S., Tilvis, R. S., Lehtonen, A., Valvanne, J., & Sairanen, S. (1999). Coexistence of lowered mood and cognitive impairment of elderly people in five birth cohorts. *Aging (Milano)*, *11*(2), 90–95.

Blazer, D. G. (2002). The prevalence of depressive symptoms. *Journals of Gerontology Series A: Biological Sciences and Medical Sciences*, *57*(3), M150–M151.

Boone, K. B., Lesser, I. M., Miller, B. L., Wohl, M., Berman, N., Lee, A., et al. (1995). Cognitive functioning in older depressed outpatients: Relationship of presence and severity of depression to neuropsychological test scores. *Neuropsychology*, *9*(3), 390–398.

Broe, G. A., Henderson, A. S., Creasey, H., McCusker, E., Korten, A. E., Jorm, A. F., et al. (1990). A case-control study of Alzheimer's disease in Australia. *Neurology*, *40*(11), 1698–1707.

Butters, M. A., Becker, J. T., Nebes, R. D., Zmuda, M. D., Mulsant, B. H., Pollock, B. G., et al. (2000). Changes in cognitive functioning following treatment of late-life depression. *American Journal of Psychiatry*, *157*(12), 1949–1954.

Butters, M. A., Bhalla, R. K., Mulsant, B. H., Mazumdar, S., Houck, P. R., Begley, A. E., et al. (2004). Executive functioning, illness course, and relapse/recurrence in continuation and maintenance treatment of late-life depression: Is there a relationship? *American Journal of Geriatric Psychiatry, 12*(4), 387–394.

Butters, M. A., Whyte, E. M., Nebes, R. D., Begley, A. E., Dew, M. A., Mulsant, B. H., et al. (2004). The nature and determinants of neuropsychological functioning in late-life depression. *Archives of General Psychiatry, 61*(6), 587–595.

Chen, P., Ganguli, M., Mulsant, B. H., & DeKosky, S. T. (1999). The temporal relationship between depressive symptoms and dementia: a community-based prospective study. *Archives of General Psychiatry, 56*(3), 261–266.

Christensen, H., Griffiths, K., Mackinnon, A., & Jacomb, P. (1997). A quantitative review of cognitive deficits in depression and Alzheimer-type dementia. *Journal of the International Neuropsychology Society, 3*(6), 631–651.

Crowe, S. F., & Hoogenraad, K. (2000). Differentiation of dementia of the Alzheimer's type from depression with cognitive impairment on the basis of a cortical versus subcortical pattern of cognitive deficit. *Archives of Clinical Neuropsychology, 15*(1), 9–19.

Dotson, V. M., Resnick, S. M., & Zonderman, A. B. (2008). Differential association of concurrent, base-line, and average depressive symptoms with cognitive decline in older adults. *American Journal of Geriatric Psychiatry, 16*(4), 318–330.

Feehan, M., Knight, R. G., & Partridge, F. M. (1991). Cognitive complaint and test performance in elderly patients suffering depression or dementia. *International Journal of Geriatric Psychiatry, 6*(5), 287–293.

Georgotas, A., McCue, R. E., Reisberg, B., Ferris, S. H., Nagachandran, N., Chang, I., et al. (1989). The effects of mood changes and antidepressants on the cognitive capacity of elderly depressed patients. *International Psychogeriatrics, 1*(2), 135–143.

Green, R. C., Cupples, L. A., Kurz, A., Auerbach, S., Go, R., Sadovnick, D., et al. (2003). Depression as a risk factor for Alzheimer disease: The MIRAGE Study. *Archives of Neurology, 60*(5), 753–759.

Gualtieri, C. T., & Johnson, L. G. (2008). Age-related cognitive decline in patients with mood disorders. *Progress in Neuropsychopharmacology and Biological Psychiatry, 32*(4), 962–967.

Hart, R. P., Kwentus, J. A., Hamer, R. M., & Taylor, J. R. (1987). Selective reminding procedure in depression and dementia. *Psychology and Aging, 2*(2), 111–115.

Herrmann, L. L., Goodwin, G. M., & Ebmeier, K. P. (2007). The cognitive neuropsychology of depression in the elderly. *Psychological Medicine, 37*(12), 1693–1702.

Jones, R. D., Tranel, D., Benton, A., & Paulsen, J. (1992). Differentiating dementia from 'pseudodementia'

early in the clinical course: Utility of neuropsychological tests. *Neuropsychology, 6*(1), 13–21.

Jorm, A. F. (2001). History of depression as a risk factor for dementia: An updated review. *Australia and New Zealand Journal of Psychiatry, 35*(6), 776–781.

Kiloh, L. G. (1961). Pseudodementia. *Acta Psychiatrica Scandinavica, 37*, 336–351.

Lee, J. S., Potter, G. G., Wagner, H. R., Welsh-Bohmer, K. A., & Steffens, D. C. (2007). Persistent mild cognitive impairment in geriatric depression. *International Psychogeriatrics, 19*(1), 125–135.

Lockwood, K. A., Alexopoulos, G. S., Kakuma, T., & Van Gorp, W. G. (2000). Subtypes of cognitive impairment in depressed older adults. *American Journal of Geriatric Psychiatry, 8*(3), 201–208.

Miller, E., & Lewis, P. (1977). Recognition memory in elderly patients with depression and dementia: A signal detection analysis. *Journal of Abnormal Psychology, 86*(1), 84–86.

Modrego, P. J., & Ferrandez, J. (2004). Depression in patients with mild cognitive impairment increases the risk of developing dementia of Alzheimer type: A prospective cohort study. *Archives of Neurology, 61*(8), 1290–1293.

Nebes, R. D., Butters, M. A., Mulsant, B. H., Pollock, B. G., Zmuda, M. D., Houck, P. R., et al. (2000). Decreased working memory and processing speed mediate cognitive impairment in geriatric depression. *Psychological Medicine, 30*(3), 679–691.

Nebes, R. D., Pollock, B. G., Houck, P. R., Butters, M. A., Mulsant, B. H., Zmuda, M. D., et al. (2003). Persistence of cognitive impairment in geriatric patients following antidepressant treatment: A randomized, double-blind clinical trial with nortriptyline and paroxetine. *Journal of Psychiatric Research, 37*(2), 99–108.

Olin, J. T., Katz, I. R., Meyers, B. S., Schneider, L. S., & Lebowitz, B. D. (2002). Provisional diagnostic criteria for depression of Alzheimer disease: Rationale and background. *American Journal of Geriatric Psychiatry, 10*(2), 129–141.

Ownby, R. L., Crocco, E., Acevedo, A., John, V., & Loewenstein, D. (2006). Depression and risk for Alzheimer disease: Systematic review, meta-analysis, and metaregression analysis. *Archives of General Psychiatry, 63*(5), 530–538.

Rapp, M. A., Dahlman, K., Sano, M., Grossman, H. T., Haroutunian, V., & Gorman, J. M. (2005). Neuropsychological differences between late-onset and recurrent geriatric major depression. *American Journal of Psychiatry, 162*(4), 691–698.

Reischies, F. M., & Neu, P. (2000). Comorbidity of mild cognitive disorder and depression—a neuropsychological analysis. *European Archives of Psychiatry and Clinical Neuroscience, 250*(4), 186–193.

Robert, P. H., Schuck, S., Dubois, B., Lepine, J. P., Gallarda, T., Olie, J. P., et al. (2003). Validation of the Short Cognitive Battery (B2C). Value in screening for Alzheimer's disease and depressive disorders in psychiatric practice. *Encephale, 29*(3 Pt. 1), 266–272.

Roy-Byrne, P. P., Weingartner, H., Bierer, L. M., Thompson, K., & Post, R. M. (1986). Effortful and automatic cognitive processes in depression. *Archives of General Psychiatry, 43*(3), 265–267.

Speck, C. E., Kukull, W. A., Brenner, D. E., Bowen, J. D., McCormick, W. C., Teri, L., et al. (1995). History of depression as a risk factor for Alzheimer's disease. *Epidemiology, 6*(4), 366–369.

Steffens, D. C., Plassman, B. L., Helms, M. J., Welsh-Bohmer, K. A., Saunders, A. M., & Breitner, J. C. (1997). A twin study of late-onset depression and apolipoprotein E epsilon 4 as risk factors for Alzheimer's disease. *Biological Psychiatry, 41*(8), 851–856.

Steffens, D. C., & Potter, G. G. (2008). Geriatric depression and cognitive impairment. *Psychological Medicine, 38*(2), 163–175.

Waraich, P., Goldner, E. M., Somers, J. M., & Hsu, L. (2004). Prevalence and incidence studies of mood disorders: A systematic review of the literature. *Canadian Journal of Psychiatry, 49*(2), 124–138.

Yaffe, K., Blackwell, T., Gore, R., Sands, L., Reus, V., & Browner, W. S. (1999). Depressive symptoms and cognitive decline in nondemented elderly women: A prospective study. *Archives of General Psychiatry, 56*(5), 425–430.

Zubenko, G. S., Zubenko, W. N., McPherson, S., Spoor, E., Marin, D. B., Farlow, M. R., et al. (2003). A collaborative study of the emergence and clinical features of the major depressive syndrome of Alzheimer's disease. *American Journal of Psychiatry, 160*(5), 857–866.

27

Release Hallucinations: Uninvited Guests and Phantom Orchestras

Michael Sharland and Thomas A. Hammeke

Declines in visual and auditory acuity commonly occur as symptoms of aging. Unbeknownst to some professionals, hallucinations can accompany these sensory declines outside the context of psychiatric or neurological impairment. These hallucinations are frequently referred to as release hallucinations with the belief that they emanate from a discharge of cells in higher level association areas due to insufficient suppression from afferent stimuli (Fernandez, Lichtshein, & Vieweg, 1997).

Visual hallucinations occurring in the context of impaired vision is also called Charles Bonnet syndrome (Rovner, 2006). The syndrome was coined by George De Morsier, a Swiss physician, in 1967 after Charles Bonnet, a naturalist and philosopher who first described the syndrome in 1760 (Hedges, 2007). Charles Bonnet described the experiences of his 87-year-old grandfather who experienced spontaneous, well-formed visual hallucinations without apparent psychiatric or cognitive deficits (Hedges, 2007). He reported that his grandfather retained his complete faculties and memory and remained independent in his daily activities, but on occasion he saw "figures of men, of women, of birds, of carriages…" that moved, changed size, and appeared and disappeared (Hedges, 2007). His grandfather was able to describe these people, and objects in great detail and noted that the objects never spoke or interacted with him. Charles Bonnet commented that his grandfather had undergone cataract surgery late in life, affecting his visual acuity, and surmised that the cause of these hallucinations

arose in the part of the brain responsible for vision (Hedges, 2007). Of interest, Charles Bonnet himself lost his sight later in life and during his retirement described visual hallucinations characteristic of his eponymous syndrome.

DeMorsier's original definition of Charles Bonnet syndrome (CBS) included visual hallucinations in older individuals without "mental deficiency;" however, later researchers have suggested that reduced visual acuity and brain dysfunction must both be present to diagnose CBS (Fernandez et al., 1997). Pliskin and colleagues (1996) compared 15 CBS patients to age-matched controls and found that the CBS patients exhibited neuropsychological impairment consistent with early dementia.

Prevalence figures for CBS are difficult to accurately ascertain because many patients are hesitant or unwilling to discuss the presence of hallucinations for fear that people will consider them mentally ill or "crazy" (Menon, Rahman, Menon, & Dutton, 2003). Prevalence rate estimations vary from 11% to 15% in visually impaired individuals and 1.8% to 3.5% in psychogeriatric patients over the age of 65 (Menon et al., 2003). CBS syndrome occurs more commonly in elderly individuals with mean ages of incidence between 70 and 80 years of age (Menon et al., 2003). In addition, the disorder is frequently misdiagnosed as psychosis or dementia (Hart, 1997). In one study of 16 patients who consulted their physicians regarding these hallucinations, only one was correctly diagnosed (Teunisse, Cruysberg, Hoefnagels, Verbeek, & Zitman, 1996).

While DeMorsier initially considered CBS a disorder of older men, more recent research has not found a clear sex preference for the disorder.

The content of CBS release hallucinations can vary, but it is most commonly that of a person (Podoll, Osterheider, & Noth, 1989). Faces, geometric designs, objects, and animals have also been described with size varying from miniature to larger than life (Menon et al., 2003). The content of the hallucination is typically well defined, organized, and quite clear and vivid in color (Fernandez et al., 1997). These images may remain stationary, move en bloc, or have dynamic movement (Menon et al., 2003). The hallucination is typically stereotypic or has recurring themes, especially when the hallucination involves movement (Menon et al., 2003). Hallucinations may be more frequently triggered in low-light conditions, and case studies have reported individuals who are able to stop the hallucination by looking away, looking directly at the hallucination, or changing the lighting condition (Menon et al., 2003).

Release hallucinations are not confined to the visual domain. Oliver Sacks described individuals with musical release hallucinations in a recent book (Sacks, 2007). Indeed, authors have suggested that musical hallucinations may have inspired well-known composers such as Haydn, Ravel, and Smetana (Evers & Ellger, 2004). Bedrich Smetana was known to have hearing loss, thought to be due to syphilis, and described his musical hallucinations as a chord in A major and two male voices in G major (Evers & Ellger, 2004).

As with CBS, musical release hallucinations are more common in hearing impaired, elderly individuals, who may also have brain dysfunction (Berrios, 1991). Unlike CBS, it appears that women are more likely to have musical release hallucinations than men (Evers & Ellger, 2004). Overall prevalence rates were reported at 2.5% in a sample of elderly individuals, but it is thought that this may be an underestimation for many of the same reasons as CBS is underreported (Evers & Ellger, 2004).

While musical hallucinations may initially be pleasant, the pleasurable aspects often deteriorate over time, and the music may become too loud or distorted (Brust, 2001) or annoying from continuous repetition. While the musical hallucination is usually constant during waking hours, it can be intermittent. For example, David and Fernandez (2000) report a case of an elderly woman who heard a piano, drums, or full orchestra each evening as she was falling asleep. Typically the hallucinatory experience is attenuated when attention is diverted away from it. Many individuals with musical hallucinations report an ability to change the hallucination by humming or singing a different melody, which then begins a repetitious cycle (Hammeke, McQuillen, & Cohen, 1983). Pathophysiology is considered to be similar to CBS, in that reduced sensory input results in disinhibition of perception-bearing circuits, resulting in the "release" of perceptual traces (Brust, 2001).

Case Sample 1

Ms. Smith is an 89-year-old, right-handed Caucasian woman who was referred by her neurologist for neuropsychological evaluation of her cognitive functioning. She experienced a rapid onset of generalized weakness, confusion, and visual hallucinations 6 months prior to her evaluation. The episode was associated with a bladder infection. Cognitively, she was reportedly functioning rather well prior to this time. However, her daughter reported noticed increasing forgetfulness and word-finding deficits. Her neurologist noted no signs of parkinsonism on neurological examination.

Ms. Smith's visual hallucinations were remarkable for the great detail of the characters and environments involved, repeated occurrence of the same themes (same characters engaging in the same actions over and over again), short duration of the episodes, as well as their more common occurrence in low-light conditions (although they occured also in well-lit conditions, though not as frequently). She initially reported seeing children around her house. A few days later, she reported seeing "parents" with the same children she had seen previously. She stated that these people were not talking. They were all wearing hats and some males' faces were notable for long facial whiskers. She continued to report seeing these same individuals engaged in different kinds of actions inside and outside of her house. They were piling up their personal belongings on her sofa, applying new wallpaper in her living room (the wallpaper was noted to have elaborate patterns), and then taking the wallpaper off. The "kids" showed up in her bathroom and came into her bed. The "parents" would spend their days working outside, and they would show up in the house around lunch and dinner times. Occasionally she would prepare food for these individuals, and she left the television on in the evening for them, expecting that they would turn it off when they went to bed. She noted that she usually saw only the upper body of these individuals and referred to them as "migrant workers." When asked about this, she noted that they were wearing clothing similar to that worn by migrant workers she frequently saw working in the fields when she was a child, close to where she used to live. She had not experienced hallucinations in other sensory modalities (e.g., auditory). In fact, she reported becoming frustrated due to the fact that the individuals she saw in her house never talked or responded to her questions. Ms. Smith reported awareness that the hallucinations were not real, although she responded to them at times as if they were, and she did not find the hallucinations distressing. The hallucinations occurred on a daily basis.

Ms. Smith continued to be mostly independent in basic self-care activities (feeding, dressing, personal hygiene) and in completing simple household tasks (folding newspapers and warming up food in the microwave), although her vision impairment (macular degeneration) interfered with many activities. She needed assistance in instrumental daily activities, such as using household appliances, managing medications, shopping, and handling mail and finances (due to her vision impairment). She denied learning difficulties during schooling. She completed the eighth grade. She worked on the family farm through her working years.

Ms. Smith had a history of colon cancer, macular degeneration, hypertension, hypercholesterolemia, anemia, lumbago, and osteoporosis. No recent changes in her motor functioning were noted by her daughter. Her current medications included Norvasc, Lopressor, tramadol, Tylenol, and Prilosec. Psychiatric history and family psychiatric history are unremarkable. A computed tomography (CT) image of the brain from 10/24/2006 showed no acute abnormalities in the brain. Age-appropriate volume loss was noted, as were white matter signal abnormalities that were thought to represent chronic microvascular ischemia.

Ms. Smith had significant visual impairment due to macular degeneration; therefore, most visually based measures were excluded from the evaluation. She was oriented to person, city, year, and day of the week, but she misreported the day of the month, month, and time of the day, and she did not recall the name of the prior president (she noted that his wife is in the Senate, though). Speech was fluent and free of paraphasic errors, with normal volume and prosody. Occasional word-finding difficulty was noted during casual conversation. Comprehension appeared generally intact during casual conversation. She appeared at times to have hearing difficulty. Mood was euthymic and range of affect was full. Remote memory as assessed by her ability to recall personal historical information appeared adequate. Judgment and insight appeared adequate. Ms. Smith was pleasant and cooperative. She put forth good and consistent effort throughout the evaluation.

Ms. Smith exhibited low average general fund of knowledge and average verbal abstract reasoning skills. She was not able to see enlarged printed words; thus, basic reading skills could not be evaluated.

Immediate and delayed recall of stories was low average for her age. Her recognition of stories was average. Rote learning of a word list was in the impaired range, as was her recall (3/12 words recalled spontaneously). Her recognition of the list was better and in the low average range (11/12 words correctly recognized with two false-positive errors). Confrontation naming could not be reliably and fully assessed due to her vision impairment. She performed in the impaired range on phonemic and semantic verbal fluency tasks. Simple auditory verbal working memory performance was in the low average range (span forward = 5, span backward = 3). Performance on a simple motor inhibition task (go/no-go task) was within normal limits. Ms. Smith endorsed only a few items on a self-report inventory covering common symptoms of depression, indicating no clinically significant depression.

Overall, Ms. Smith showed an abnormal cognitive profile. She showed impairment on tasks of rote verbal learning and retrieval memory, as well as impaired semantic and phonemic fluency performance. However, Ms. Smith presented with cognitive strengths in her performance, including average verbal abstract reasoning, low average remote memory, low average to average verbal recognition memory, and low average verbal working memory. Language comprehension appeared relatively intact during casual conversation. She also followed simple one- to three-step commands, and in general correctly answered questions containing complex ideational materials. Ms. Smith's cognitive profile is consistent with mild dementia, given her impaired performance on select executive functions tasks and memory retrieval difficulty, but relatively well-preserved memory encoding skills (as evidenced by low average to average recognition memory performance). She had impaired daily functioning above and beyond the problems due to her vision impairment, although her impairment seemed to fluctuate with her level of confusion, with better functioning when less confusion is present.

The hallucinations described by Ms. Smith and her daughter were characteristic of release hallucinations associated with vision loss, such as those seen in Charles Bonnet syndrome. In the light of no past psychiatric history, a primary psychiatric etiology for the hallucinations is unlikely. Another possibility is a neurodegenerative condition (such as Lewy-body dementia), where detailed hallucinations also can be seen along with fluctuating cognitive deficits and confusion. The hallucinations did not appear to fluctuate with her mental status, and no parkinsoninsm was noted on her neurological examination, implying that these may represent an independent process (i.e., release hallucinations) from the pathology causing the mental confusion.

Case Sample 2

Ms. Jones is a 75 year-old, right-handed, Caucasian woman who was referred by her neurologist to evaluate a 4-month history of musical hallucinations. Her first experience of hallucinations occurred shortly after a course of antibiotics for a sinus infection. She was awakened from sleep by loud music, which was so vivid that she assumed her neighbors were playing their stereo loudly. She went to find the source of the music.

The music stopped after 1 hour but occurred again the following night and through the subsequent day. Ms. Jones was so bothered by the music that she employed her sister to assist her in locating its source. The frequency of hallucinations increased over the following 3 weeks until they were a constant experience except during sleep, active conversation, or while engaged in effortful mental processing.

Ms. Jones described her hallucinations to include both familiar and unfamiliar melodies. Those songs which she recognized were typically religious hymns or songs from her childhood. The melodies were often played by a single instrument (e.g., guitar) and accompanied by a voice singing baritone. Occasionally, she experienced the songs sung by a choir with full orchestral accompaniment. The melodies were repetitive and increased in intensity when ambient noise levels were low or when she was mentally inactive. She stated that she was able to change the song or alter its speed by mentally replacing the musical passage with another.

Medical history and neurological work-up was unremarkable with the exception of sensorineural hearing loss over the past several years requiring the use of hearing aids. A CT scan of the brain revealed mild diffuse atrophy. Ms. Jones graduated from college and worked as a teacher. At the time of her referral she was retired. She lived alone and was independent in activities of daily living.

Ms. Jones arrived for her appointment on time and unaccompanied. Speech was fluent with normal rate, volume, and tone. Language comprehension was adequate for conversational speech and complex instructions, despite her hearing difficulties. Thought processes were clear and goal directed. Mood and affect were appropriate to the assessment setting. Motivation and effort were adequate.

Ms. Jones performed in the superior range on tests of intellectual abilities (Full Scale IQ = 121, VIQ = 131, PIQ = 106). She performed consistently in the above average range on intellectual subtests with the exception of logical sequential reasoning (i.e., Picture Arrangement), which was in the low average range. Memory abilities were consistent with intellectual abilities and in the superior range. Moreover, she performed in the average to above average range on almost all neuropsychological tasks. Of note, she was impaired on the speech-sounds perception task but performed within normal limits on the seashore rhythm test. Personality testing with the MMPI revealed a valid profile with no elevations on clinical scales.

In sum, Ms. Jones performed in the average to superior range on almost all neuropsychological tests, with the exception of a low average performance on Picture Arrangement and an impaired performance on the Speech-Sounds Perception test. Her neuropsychological profile was essentially normal and not thought to be indicative of mild cognitive impairment, dementia, or a focal neurobehavioral syndrome. It was hypothesized that her hallucinations were caused by her progressive sensorineural hearing loss.

Discussion

The two case reports described earlier illustrate many of the details reported by patients with typical release hallucinations. With the first case report, the patient was an elderly woman with impaired vision who saw repetitive, detailed images of people. These people were similar to individuals she may have interacted with in her childhood and indeed dressed in an outdated style, more consistent with the time period of the patient's youth. They appeared to occur more frequently, but not exclusively during periods of lower ambient light. The detail of the hallucinations was much more vivid than her vision acuity enabled. While the patient exhibited some insight into the unreality of her experiences, she nevertheless attempted to interact with the hallucinations on occasion by making lunch for the people she saw or leaving the television on for them. Neuropsychological testing revealed cognitive deficits consistent with a mild dementia. This neuropsychological profile is consistent with the findings of Pliskin and colleagues (1996).

Differential diagnoses for this patient includes a Lewy body dementia, prolonged delirium, or new-onset psychosis associated with dementia. With Lewy body dementia, one would expect greater fluctuations in cognition and hallucinations as well as Parkinsonian motor symptoms, which were not present during the evaluation. A prolonged delirium is unlikely given her areas of cognitive strength and the absence of a waxing and waning course. While new-onset psychosis associated with dementia is a possibility, the patient only exhibits hallucinations. She did not report frank delusional ideation, mood remains euthymic, and she did not show any other positive symptoms of psychosis. Therefore, the most likely explanation of her hallucinations is a Charles Bonnet syndrome of visual release hallucinations likely due to her macular degeneration. Her underlying mild cognitive deficits may be associated with a diminished capacity in the central nervous system to suppress the release of perceptual memories, thereby lowering the threshold for hallucination onset. Still, as illustrated in the second case report, cognitive deficit does not appear to be a requirement for release hallucination manifestation.

The second case example illustrates musical release hallucinations. In this case an elderly woman presented with new-onset musical hallucinations that began with intermittent frequency but shortly progressed to a constant experience. Like the first case example, this patient also had sensory loss in the modality in which the hallucinations occurred. This patient also experienced repetitive hallucinations of stimuli that were familiar from childhood. The intensity of hallucinations increased in situations of low ambient sensory stimuli and when she was not actively engaged in mental processing. In contrast to the previous case example, this patient was able to alter the nature of her hallucinations by subvocalizing other melodies. In addition, she performed in the average to superior range on almost all neuropsychological measures, and her neurocognitive profile was interpreted as being essentially normal. Finally, she did not report or exhibit any disordered thinking or affective disorder during interview or assessment making a new-onset psychiatric condition unlikely.

Thus, as seen in the second case report, one does not need cognitive dysfunction as a prerequisite to experience release hallucinations. Instead, interruption or degradation of afferent sensory input appears to be the necessary condition for release hallucinations to occur. There are several possible explanations for the observed co-occurrence of release hallucinations and cognitive deficits. Both release hallucinations and cognitive impairment occur at greater frequency in elderly populations; hence, comorbidity may be a result of elevated base rates in the overall population. An alternate possibility is that cognitive deficits, especially those affecting the inhibitory processes of the brain, may result in a lower threshold for hallucination onset with impaired sensory input. Thus, the brain may be less able to suppress the intrinsic perceptual traces that are "released" in the absence of sufficient incoming sensory stimuli.

While these cases illustrate the phenomenon of release hallucinations in the auditory and visual modalities, the phenomenon is know to occur in other modalities as well. For example, phantom limb experiences likely represent a form of release hallucination in the somatic realm in paraplegic patients and patients with limb amputations. The authors also have evaluated a woman with olfactory hallucinations that occurred after resection of the olfactory bulbs in a surgical procedure.

There are no reliable treatments for release hallucinations. Case reports suggest that if one can reverse the sensory loss (i.e., restore vision or hearing to adequate levels), this will result in a cessation of release phenomena (Menon et al., 2003). Conversely, release phenomena tend to ebb as the sensory deficit progresses to a complete loss of sensory input. Thus, individuals who progress to total loss of sight or hearing report a cessation of release phenomena (Evers & Ellger, 2004). Hence, it appears that release hallucinations occur within a certain window of sensory deficit; however, no research has been published to define the window in which release hallucinations can occur. Individuals have reported environmental techniques to minimize release hallucinations. For example, one might use higher wattage light bulbs and avoid low-light conditions to reduce the occurrence of visual hallucinations. Finally, a number of case studies have examined various medications as potential treatments for release phenomena. David and Fernandez (2000) found that the atypical antipsychotic quetiapine was effective in reducing the intensity of musical release hallucinations. In an alternate case report, Lang and colleagues (2007) reported effective treatment of visual hallucinations with venlafaxine, a selective serotonin and noradrenalin reuptake inhibitor.

References

Berrios, G. (1991). Musical hallucinosis: A statistical analysis of 46 cases. *Psychopathology, 24,* 356–360.

Brust, J. (2001). Music and the neurologist: A historical perspective. *Annalls of the New York Academy of Science, 930,* 143–152.

David, R., & Fernandez, H. (2000). Quetiapine for hypnogogic musical release hallucinations. *Journal of Geriatric Psychiatry and Neurology, 13,* 210–211.

Evers, S., & Ellger, T. (2004). The clinical spectrum of musical hallucinations. *Journal of Neurological Sciences, 227,* 55–65.

Fernandez, A., Lichtshein, G., and Vieweg, W. (1997). The Charles Bonnet syndrome: A review. *Journal of Nervous and Mental Disease, 185,* 195–200.

Hammeke, T. A., McQuillen, M. P., & Cohen, B. A. (1983). Musical hallucinations associated with acquired deafness. *Journal of Neurology, Neurosurgery, and Psychiatry, 46,* 570–572.

Hart, J. (1997). Phantom visions: Real enough to touch. *Elder Care, 9,* 30–32.

Hedges, T. (2007). Charles Bonnet, his life, his syndrome. *Survey of Ophthalmology, 52,* 111–114.

Lang, U., Stogowski, D., Schulze, D., Domula, M., Schmidt, E., Gallinat, J., Tugtekin, S., & Felber, W. (2007). Charles Bonnet syndrome: Successful treatment of visual hallucinations due to vision loss with selective serotonin reuptake inhibitors. *Journal of Psychopharmacology, 21,* 553–555.

Menon, G., Rahman, I., Menon, S., & Dutton, G. (2003). Complex visual hallucinations in the visually impaired: The Charles Bonnet syndrome. *Survey of Ophthalmology, 48,* 58–72.

Pliskin, N., Kiolbasa, T., Towle, V., Pankow, L., Ernest, J. T., Noronha, A., & Luchins, D. J. (1996). Charles Bonnet syndrome: An early marker for dementia? *Journal of the American Geriatric Society, 44,* 1055–1061.

Podoll, K., Osterheider, M., & Noth, J. (1989). The Charles Bonnet syndrome. *Fortschritte der Neurologie-Psychiatrie, 57,* 43–60.

Rovner, B. (2006). The Charles Bonnet syndrome: A review of recent research. *Current Opinion in Ophthalmology, 17,* 275–277.

Sacks, O. (2007). *Musicophilia: Tales of music and the brain.* New York: Alfred A Knopf.

Teunisse, R., Cruysberg, J., Hoefnagels, W., Verbeek, A. L., & Zitman, F. G. (1996). Visual hallucinations in psychologically normal people: Charles Bonnet syndrome. *Lancet, 347,* 794–797.

28

Psychogenic Nonepileptic Seizure Disorder: The Case of P. S.

Christopher L. Grote and Maria J. Marquine

Nonepileptic seizures (NESs) are a common presentation in epilepsy clinics. The purpose of this chapter and vignette is to describe some of the common characteristics of such presentations, how neuropsychologists might evaluate patients with known or suspected NESs, and how a recent case in our clinic illustrates some of the challenges associated with such evaluations.

One of the first lessons for a neuropsychologist is that psychological testing cannot reliably differentiate patients with epileptic seizures (ESs) from those with NESs. Instead, the purpose of the neuropsychological consultation should be to identify whether there is sufficient test data and psychosocial data to raise the "index of suspicion" that NESs may be present and to explain at least part of the patient's current presentation. Even in the presence of concordant factors suggesting that a patient's presentation is suggestive of NESs, this in no way eliminates the possibility that ESs may be present. In part, this is because "one cannot prove a negative." The presence of obvious signs of "hysteria" or somaticizing-type behaviors in a patient does not rule out the possibility that ESs were or are occurring. This principle must be remembered by the clinician even in the face of covert or overt pressure from referral sources or other health-care workers for feedback on whether a patient's seizure was "real." Certainly, the seizure-like behavior occurred, but psychological testing and interview cannot absolutely determine the cause of the apparent seizure.

Another caveat regarding the limitation of psychological diagnosis comes from studies showing ESs and NESs can coexist in the same case. There are at least two reasons for this. First, many patients with NESs have been found to have neurological histories, including positive magnetic resonance imaging (MRI) findings or other central nervous system (CNS) diagnoses (Wilkus, Dodrill, & Thompson, 1984). Second, estimates of the coexistence of ESs and NESs range from 10% to 40% (Ramsay, Cohen, & Brown, 1993). The issue of coexistence might be explained, at least in part, by ES patients having knowledge of how a "genuine seizure" appears and then being able to emulate this appearance, perhaps achieving the same gain in having an NES as they might have had with an ES. Some patients with ESs and/or NESs have been able to describe to us some of the "benefits" in having a seizure, regardless of the cause of the seizure-like behavior. These have included financial compensation for having a seizure disorder, attention or sympathy from others, a cathartic release of stress, or being relieved from household or lifestyle obligations and chores. Debates as to whether the pursuit of such benefits are conscious versus unconscious, or intentional versus nonintentional, may be helpful in some cases but counterproductive in others. Instead, the principles of operant conditioning might be recalled to help understand the occurrence of some NES presentations. These state that the likelihood of a particular behavior increases or decreases through positive or negative reinforcement each time the behavior is exhibited. Therefore, an NES may be reinforced through the reactions of others, including family or compensation payers, in reaction to the presence of apparent seizures.

Given the inability of neuropsychologists to reliably differentiate NES from ES patients, is there any point in neurologists seeking out psychological consultations on patients suspected of having NESs? Absolutely! The informed neuropsychologist can be helpful in knowing the common characteristics and test responses of patients with NESs and help develop a treatment plan. While the gold standard of diagnosis of seizures remains video-electroencephalogram (EEG) monitoring, the principle of "you can't prove a negative" also applies here. Although an extended inpatient stay may not result in any definitive ESs being captured on video, the attending neurologist cannot always be confident that such a seizure would not have occurred with a longer period of observation. Therefore, possibly concordant information from the neuropsychologist that motivational or psychological factors do indeed seem to account for at least part of the patient's presentation may be the deciding factor in the neurologist's diagnosis. Such determinations are not insignificant because they may inform the decision as to whether to keep a patient on antiepileptic medications, with their possible side effects, or whether to allow a patient to return to work.

There is no single factor that may cause a clinician to become suspicious about the presence of NESs, but instead there may be a cluster of test scores or psychosocial factors that do. An extensive review of this topic can be found in a review by Bowman and Markand (2005), but a brief summary of some of these findings include female gender and being between the ages of 15 and 35 (Shen, Bowman, & Markand, 1990). Among these patients (young women) in particular but also among all patients with NESs are high rates of reports of having been sexually and/ or physically abused (Bowman, 1993). Bowman and Markand's review (2005) indicates that as many as 85% of patients with NESs report a history of sexual trauma and/or domestic abuse. Obviously, this indicates that the consulting neuropsychologists should skillfully and delicately inquire about such a history. It is not uncommon for patients to "open up" about such events during diagnostic interviews, often for the first time in their lives, about the presence and importance of these traumatic events. Their physicians often have not suspected or asked about traumas, and many patients have not wanted to initiate conversations about such sensitive issues either with their health-care providers, families, or friends. It may be during the course of a sensitively conducted psychological interview that these events come to light. As diagnostically useful as such information may initially seem, the way in which this information is handled must be carefully considered. These issues would include possible duty to report or even duty to warn to authorities, depending on the age of the patient, knowledge of the alleged perpetrator, or the perceived likelihood of further abuses being committed. Another challenge is the disclosure of this information by the neuropsychologists. Should specific events, including identification of the alleged perpetrator, be detailed in verbal or written reports, especially if the reliability of the report is unknown? Finally, there may be a tendency for a rush to judgment that this case indeed must be one of NESs given that the patient just revealed one or many traumatic events that might seem to explain their current presentation. This predisposition must be balanced against the knowledge that there is not always a clear link between a life stressor and a health outcome (Murrell, Norris, & Grote, 1987), and that unfortunately the base rate of some types of trauma is distressingly high. For instance, it has been estimated that some 15%–25% of American girls have been sexually abused by the age of 18 (Leserman, 2005). Just as one would not assume that any one person with a history of sexual abuse has NESs, one should not automatically infer that a referred patient has NESs if she or he reports this abuse.

Other clinical features may help differentiate ESs from NESs (Bowman & Markand, 2005). These include NES patients being *more* likely to have seizure-like episodes: *(1)* only while awake and not from sleep; *(2)* upon suggestion from a health-care worker; *(3)* that are *not* stereotyped, or typical from seizure to seizure; *(4)* that feature forward pelvis thrusting; *(5)* that include emotional displays, including crying; *(6)* in which the eyes are closed; *(7)* with a brief, and not sustained, period of postictal confusion. In addition,

NES patients typically will have normal EEGs during, before, or after the seizure-like event, whereas ES patients of course would show epileptiform activity or slowing on EEG during or after their seizure.

The aforementioned seizure and EEG characteristics would typically be evaluated by a neurologist, as potentially could the abuse and demographic factors, described earlier. Therefore, it is reasonable to ask if there is an advantage to consulting a neuropsychologist on suspected NES cases and whether they can bring in any additional data that would make a difference. Review of the literature suggests that this can be answered in the affirmative for three reasons: effort testing, evaluation of cognition, and personality testing.

Recent studies have shown that a lack of consistent effort on cognitive tests, or exaggerated report of psychiatric, somatic and cognitive symptoms, is surprisingly high among patients presenting for neuropsychological testing (Boone, 2007). This is particularly true among patients who are applying for compensation of some kind, either disability benefits or perhaps through personal injury litigation (Larrabee & Berry, 2007). Thus, it is not surprising that at least one study has emphasized the importance of testing cognitive effort among patients with NESs. Binder, Kindermann, Heaton, and Salinsky (1998) administered a battery of tests, including a measure of cognitive effort, the Portland Digit Recognition Test, to samples of patients with either ESs or NESs. They found that patients with NESs scored significantly lower on the Portland compared to patients with ESs. While there were relatively few NES patients who scored in the "malingering" range on this test, the authors suggested that effort be routinely assessed among patients with NESs.

As previously reviewed, a significant number of patients with NESs show evidence of neurological abnormalities and/or also have had ESs. Therefore, cognitive deficits can also be expected in at least some cases of NESs, as indicated in a review of three different studies (Grote, Smith, & Ruth, 2001). Overall, these studies found that about half of all cognitive test scores obtained by NES patients, or about half of all NES cognitive test protocols, were in the impaired range of

function. Patients with NESs performed more poorly on cognitive tests than did normal controls, but at a level similar to that of patients with ESs only. While these studies did not control for effort on testing, something that should be done in future studies (Heilbronner et al., 2009), it remains that patients with NESs are at risk for cognitive dysfunction because of the likelihood of their having positive neurological symptoms or histories.

The rate of diagnosed psychopathology among patients with NESs has been estimated to range from 43% to 100% (Bowman, 2001). Bowman (2001) notes that depression is the most common psychiatric comorbidity in these patients, occurring in one-third to one-half of patients, probably reflecting the high frequency of past and current life stressors in this population. Anxiety and personality disorders also occur at relatively high rates. Conversion disorder and other types of somatoform disorders are the most commonly made primary diagnosis, and it is not unusual for patients to present with other types of unexplained medical symptoms at other times in their lives. It seems possible that some patients may engage in "symptom substitution." That is, as one type of somaticizing behavior is explained away, they may develop complaints in other parts of the body, such as headaches or back pain.

The primary diagnostic instrument used by neuropsychogists in the evaluation of NES patients has been the MMPI-2. Grote and colleagues (2003) did a retrospective chart study of the MMPIs of ES and NES patients and which type of two-point codes were found. The presence of either a "1-3" or "2-3" code (indicating high scores on the "Hysteria" scale as well as on scales measuring either depression or somatic complaints) had excellent specificity and good sensitivity in differentiating these ES from NES patients. Nearly all of these two-point "1-3"-"2-3" codes were produced by NES patients, but not all NES patients produced these profiles. Similarly, Brown et al. (1991) found that nonepileptic patients showed an increased sensitivity to somatic concerns, as evidenced by a frequent presence of "conversion V" profiles. However, because of the high rate of signs of psychiatric distress among both ES and NES patient groups, neither the MMPI-2 nor any other measures of personality can be exclusively relied on in isolation to make a differential diagnosis.

Case Presentation

We were asked to evaluate patient P. S. at two different times, 6 months apart. At the time of our first encounter with P. S., she was a 36-year-old, single, right-handed, Caucasian female who was referred for inpatient neuropsychological evaluation due to possible psychogenic nonepileptic seizures. A few days prior to our initial evaluation of P. S., she was found by her boyfriend moaning on the floor, with her hands tightly clenched. She had had urinary incontinence and she was unresponsive for several hours and was at least partially disoriented for the next 2 to 3 days. In particular, she was confused about the identity of her boyfriend, being inconsistent in her ability to remember either his name or who he was. An EEG showed diffuse background slowing consistent with "mild encephalopathy," but there was no evidence of epileptiform activity. An MRI of her brain was normal. A number of other medical tests ran through the course of her hospitalization showed no evidence of an organic basis to the patient's presentation. No seizure-like episodes were observed during the course of her inpatient stay.

First Evaluation

On interview with P. S.'s boyfriend and mother, we learned that P. S. had been under significant financial and occupational stress during the months prior to her seizure-like episode. Her boyfriend, who had lived with her for 3 years, had been supporting her financially for a number of months. In addition, she was recently placed on probation at her social work job, because of difficulties in following directions and in performing her duties. Additionally, she had been scheduled to take her licensing exam the day before the seizure that led to her hospital admission. She had failed this exam once before and she had been struggling in studying for it.

P. S.'s family members reported her medical history was unremarkable. However, she had a history of depression dating back to her teenage years, and she had been followed by a psychiatrist and a psychologist for a number of years.

She had no history of suicidal attempts or psychiatric hospitalizations.

On interview with P. S., she was a slender woman, who was appropriately groomed, spoke softly, and appeared frail. She reported that she had a "patchy" memory for the last decade and difficulties remembering day-to-day events. She was uncertain about her reason for hospitalization, did not know for how long she had been hospitalized, and she was unable to provide her current address or describe the apartment she had lived in for 8 years. She knew she was living with her boyfriend but was uncertain for how long.

The patient stated she had some financial concerns prior to her episode, but she denied other current stressors. P. S. described her relationship with her boyfriend as "very good" and had no recollection of an upcoming licensing exam. She described her current mood as "good." She denied any history of suicidal ideation or hallucinations and stated she had never cut herself or otherwise tried to hurt herself. She denied any significant history of substance use.

The patient reported that her parents divorced when she was a child. Both of her parents graduated college and were still in good health. P. S. stated she was sexually abused on one occasion at the age of 9 years by a family friend but denied that this caused her any current difficulties. She reported being an average student throughout high school. After completing 2 years of college, she changed schools because of difficulties with other students. She graduated from a second college with average grades.

Test Results

P. S.'s performance on measures of effort suggested variable effort during the evaluation. She performed within normal limits on one test of effort (Victoria Symptom Validity Test: 23/24 hard items) but failed a second one (Test of Memory Malingering: Trial 1 = 36/50, Trial 2 = 42/50, Retention Trial = 39/50). Thus, her scores on subsequent measures of cognitive ability have to be interpreted with caution.

She had an MMSE score of 24/30. She was oriented to person and place, but she was unable to provide the correct date or day of the week and was unable to recall three words after a short delay.

"Premorbid" intellectual functioning was estimated to be in the average range based on a measure of reading ability (Wechsler Test of Adult Reading: Estimated Full Scale IQ = 103).

She performed quite variably on a screening measure of cognitive ability, with scores ranging from the impaired range on measures of immediate and delayed memory, to the low-average range on measures of language and attention, to the above-average range on a measure of nonverbal ability. Table 28-1 shows the scores from the Repeatable Battery for the Assessment of Neuropsychological Status, both from this and the repeat evaluations.

P. S. also completed the Minnesota Multiphasic Personality Inventory: Second Edition (370-Item Form; MMPI-2). She obtained one significant elevation on the L validity scale (T = 66), which is often observed in individuals who portray themselves in an overly positive manner and who lack insight into the cause of their difficulties. She had significant elevations on two of ten clinical scales (Scale 2: T = 66; Scale 7: T = 66), indicating that she is experiencing clinical significant distress, including symptoms of depression and anxiety.

Based on results from our first neuropsychological evaluation of P. S., we concluded that at least some elements of her presentation were consistent with a somatoform disorder. Although this did not rule out the possibility of an organic basis to her claimed memory impairment, it raised the possibility that psychological factors accounted for at least part of her presentation. We recommended that the patient continue to be followed by her treating psychologist and psychiatrist.

We communicated our findings to the referral physician, who gave the patient and her family feedback about the results of P. S.'s diagnostic work-up during her hospitalization. The patient was discharged to the care of her family a couple of days after our evaluation.

Second Evaluation

Four months later, P. S.'s mother called our clinic for a follow-up evaluation of the patient. P. S.'s mother and sister accompanied her to the evaluation.

On interview with P. S. and her family, P. S. denied having had any additional seizure-like episodes but reported that she continued to have problems in forming new memories, as well as difficulties remembering events of the past year. She reported she had not driven since her hospitalization because she was afraid of doing so. She stated she had not returned to work because she could not remember how to perform her job duties and hence was applying for Social Security disability. She continued to live with her boyfriend, and a family member had been assisting in her daily routine because her family did not think she could function independently.

P. S.'s family reported that they thought her seizure-like episode and subsequent decline in function were likely to be explained by the stressors listed during our first evaluation. As explained above, these included work and financial difficulties, and the stress of studying for the licensing exam. P. S. agreed with her family on this matter. Furthermore, on a separate interview with her alone, she listed another source of stress. She reported that she had been having difficulties in her relationship with her boyfriend for a number of months, and that she had been romantically involved with another man during the 3 months

Table 28-1. P. S.'s Scores on the Repeatable Battery for the Assessment of Neuropsychological Status

Index	First Evaluation		Second Evaluation	
	Index Score	Percentile	Index Score	Percentile
Attention	88	21st	85	16th
Language	85	16th	85	16th
Visuospatial/Constructional	116	86th	84	14th
Immediate Memory	61	<1st	65	1st
Delayed Memory	44	<1st	44	<1st

Note. Form A given first; form B, second.

prior to her seizure-like episode. She had not told anyone about this relationship, in part because he was of a different racial group than her family, and she was quite fearful and certain that her family would disapprove of this relationship both because of the racial issue and because her family was very affectionate with her live-in boyfriend who was continuing to care for her. She continued to secretly see the second boyfriend when she could. She was frustrated in that he reportedly saw the relationship primarily in terms of sexual gratification, while she was hoping that he would "step up" and offer her the chance to move in with him and then financially support her. In the interim, her relationship with her unsuspecting live in-boyfriend had continued to deteriorate. She was not planning on ending the relationship with her boyfriend because she was concerned she would not be able to support herself financially. She stated she did not think her cognitive problems were "brain related" and described them as "overwhelming." She stated she felt "jailed" by her illness and people taking care of her.

As was the case during the previous evaluation, the patient had difficulties relaying aspects of her history, including some dating back to her childhood. P. S.'s mother and sister seemed very concerned about inaccuracies in P. S.'s report of her history, continuously interrupting P. S. during the interview to correct her. Furthermore, they brought typed notes to the evaluation and later mailed others detailing P. S.'s history, and left phone messages with a similar purpose. These inaccuracies, however, were not substantial and for the most part referred to inaccuracies in dates provided by the patient or sequences of events in her distant past.

Test Results

P. S. scored 50 on each of the TOMM trials during this evaluation. However, there were aspects of her performance that suggested inconsistent effort. For example, she provided her correct age at the beginning of the evaluation but later in the day stated she had forgotten how old she was. She was also able to state the current date when signing a Release of Information form but was unable to do so a few minutes

later on formal testing, scoring in the impaired range on a test of orientation (Information and Orientation Wechsler Memory Scale–Third Edition = 8/14). On this test, she was also not oriented to place and could not name the current president.

Repeat testing with the RBANS (alternate form) revealed scores similar to those obtained during the first evaluation (see Table 28-1). She again scored in the impaired range on tests of immediate and delayed memory and in the low-average range across other measures, including nonverbal ability. Her nonverbal ability score dropped significantly from the first to the second evaluation. She also did poorly on a multitrial list learning task, as she recalled 5, 6, 6, and 5 out of 12 words across repeated trials (WMS-III Word List I = 5th percentile). Her performance was notable for a high number of intrusions. After presentation of an interference list, she recalled 1 of 12 words, and after a 25-minute delay she also only provided 1 correct word (Word List II = 9th percentile). Her performance (19/24 correct) on a recognition portion of this test was borderline (Word List II Recognition = 9th percentile).

P. S. was also asked to complete the MMPI-2. She obtained an elevated score on the F scale (T = 75) and on five of the ten clinical scales (Scale 2, 3, 7, 8, 4). Her profile indicated she was experiencing feelings of depression and anxiety, and she was quite focused on her somatic concerns even in the absence of a clear physiological basis for these complaints.

Based on these findings, we concluded that P. S.'s claimed memory problems may be best understood from a psychogenic perspective, in the context of family and interpersonal stressors. We recommended that she continued to be treated by her psychologist and psychiatrist. We also suggested that she might be encouraged to attempt a return to work and resumption of her daily responsibilities of living.

Feedback Session and Follow-Up

A couple of weeks later we gave feedback on our findings to P. S. and her mother and sister. Given that P. S. had reported to us that no one else in her family knew about her affair, we first met with her alone. We told her that we thought the stressors she had relayed to us, including her affair, probably explained at least in part her claimed memory difficulties. She agreed with our explanation and said she would like us to give feedback to her family as well. She asked that we not disclose the affair to them but agreed to us mentioning that there was an extra stressor the family was not aware of. When giving feedback to her family, they seemed receptive to it but were wary about P. S. assuming work and daily living responsibilities. They asked us whether we thought P. S. was going to improve and if so when. We replied that we thought there was a "willful" aspect to her presentation and that P. S. was going to improve when she was ready to be well. P. S. agreed with this during the feedback session.

Approximately a month later we received a letter from P. S.'s job asking us to indicate the date she could return to work and whether there were any restrictions in her doing so. We replied in writing stating that she could return to work immediately because we knew of no certain medical evidence that she was physically ill. Given her claimed symptoms of fatigue and memory difficulties, we recommended that she start working part time and that she was initially restricted from activities regarded as higher risk, such as dispensing medication and driving patients. We emphasized in feedback to the employer that it was difficult to get an accurate assessment of the patient in our evaluations because she had some "personal issues" that affected her effort and the way she presents her concerns or symptoms to others.

We were contacted by P. S.'s referring neurologist 9 months after the feedback session and learned that she had left her boyfriend and was living with her sister. Her memory had improved slightly, but she continued to have difficulties. She had returned to work part time and had not reattempted to take the licensing exam. The status of her disability application was not known.

Discussion

This case seems to be illustrative of patients with NESs in a number of ways. The patient is a young woman with a history of reported sexual abuse in her early years who presented to us and to other health-care professionals with a number of symptoms that could not be easily explained or accounted for. These include her report of being unable to remember many life events of the past decade, a claimed inability to remember most new things presented to her, and a specific but temporary amnesia as to the name and identity of her boyfriend. It was only through extensive interview that it was revealed that she was having an affair with a coworker. Prior to our evaluation, she had not revealed the existence of this relationship to anyone else, in part because of its illicit nature and as her family would object to her dating someone of his racial background. She was frustrated over not being able to share this relationship with anyone, while simultaneously being upset that her affair was not progressing to a more permanent relationship while also fearing that her cuckolded boyfriend would find out what was going on and discontinue his financial support. These events served as the psychosocial context in which she had a reportedly disabling seizure one day before she was scheduled to retake a licensing exam that she had already failed once before.

An EEG had shown some slowing but nothing that could necessarily explain the seizure that had caused her admission. The two neuropsychological evaluations had shown impaired learning and memory scores across time. However, the accuracy of these scores was dubious given her failure on a test of effort during the first exam and her inconsistent response to test questions during the second exam. Her MMPI-2 profiles showed evidence of lack of insight and symptoms of depression and somatization. All of these features are often described in previous studies of NES patients, including EEG abnormalities, poor effort, impaired cognitive abilities, and evidence of psychiatric disturbance.

Bowman and Markand (2005) have written that NESs serve as a distracter or coping mechanism for those patients who cannot deal with their life challenges in more appropriate or healthy ways, probably a useful concept for other somatoform and unexplained illness behaviors. This certainly seems to be true of P. S., who initially claimed not to see any connection between her seizure and contextual life events. At the time of feedback, however, and only in private, she did eventually admit to the relationship between her seizure, claimed memory problems, and life stressors. She, however, did not see any point in telling her treating psychiatrist or therapist about her "secrets," feeling that this was both too embarrassing and that she did not want to face their disapproval for having misled them for so long.

This patient's last-known outcome suggested only partial remission of her symptoms, which also is typical of at least some patients with NESs. These patients often have chronic patterns of maladjusted interpersonal relationships, as well as coexistent mood, anxiety, or dissociative disorders. Therefore, remission of "seizures" may not explain the whole story, as claimed or real cognitive deficits, un- or underemployment, and continuing symptoms of psychopathology may go regardless of seizure status. A review of disparate studies (Bowman & Kanner, 2007) indicated that approximately 45% of NES patients became seizure free, about a third showed significant improvement in seizure frequency, whereas the remainder showed no change in frequency. Patients without a reported history of abuse, and/or those without coexistent psychiatric disorders, were more likely to eventually show a cessation of NESs as compared to those who did have those background characteristics. Unfortunately, it is not clear whether treatment, or what type of treatment, contributes to better outcomes. One study found that neither psychotherapy nor the number of visits predicted outcome (Walczak, 1995). However, it does appear that giving clear and direct feedback about the presence of NESs, and the suspected reasons for its presence, can substantially improve outcome. Another study (Aboukasm, Mahr, Gahry, Thomas, & Barkley, 1998) investigated whether feedback led to changes in NES frequency. None of the patients in the "no feedback" condition became seizure free, whereas over half of those who did receive relevant feedback did become free of their NESs. The authors concluded that diagnostic feedback could be therapeutic in of itself. Whether these patients went on to develop other types of somaticizing type behaviors is not know but might be expected in at least some cases, given the chronicity of some of these patients' difficulties and

their inability to or learn more appropriate ways of dealing with life stressors.

References

Aboukasm, A., Mahr, G., Gahry, B. R., Thomas, A., & Barkley, G. L. (1998). Retrospective analysis of the effects of psychotherapeutic interventions on outcomes of psychogenic nonepileptic seizures. *Epilepsia*, 39, 470–473.

Binder, L. M., Kindermann, S. S., Heaton, R. K., & Salinsky, M. C. (1998). Neuropsychological impairment in patients with nonepileptic seizures. *Archives of Clinical Neuropsychology*, 6, 513–522.

Boone, K. B. (2007). *Assessment of feigned cognitive impairment*. New York: Guilford Press.

Bowman, E. S. (1993). Etiology and clinical course of pseudoseizures. Relationship to trauma, depression and dissociation. *Psychosomatics*, 34, 333–342.

Bowman, E. S. (2001). Psychopathology and outcome in pseudoseizures. In A. B. Etting & A. M. Kanner (Eds.), *Psychiatric issues in epilepsy* (pp. 355–377). Philadelphia: Lippincott Williams & Wilkins.

Bowman, E. S., & Kanner, A. M. (2007). Psychopathology and outcome in psychogenic nonepileptic seizures. In A. B. Ettinger & A. M. Kanner (Eds.), *Psychiatric issues in Epilepsy* (pp. 432–460). Philadelphia: Lippincott Williams & Wilkins.

Bowman, E. S., & Markand, O. (2005). Diagnosis and treatment of pseudoseizures. *Psychiatric Annals*, 35, 306–312.

Brown, M. C., Levin, B. E., Ramsay, R. E., Katz, D.A., & Duchowny, M.S (1991). Characteristics of patients with pseudoseizures. *Journal of Epilepsy*, 4, 225–229.

Grote, C. L., Geary, E., Balabanov, A., Bergen, D., Kanner, A., Palac, S., & Smith, M. (2003). Evidence that the MMPI-2 differentiates patients with epileptic seizures from those with psychogenic nonepileptic seizures. *Journal of the International Neuropsychological Society*, 9, 535.

Grote, C. L., Smith, C. A., & Ruth, A. (2001). Neuropsychological evaluation of the patient with seizures. In A. B. Etting & A. M. Kanner (Eds.), *Psychiatric issues in epilepsy* (pp. 31–44). Philadelphia: Lippincott Williams & Wilkins.

Heilbronner, R. L., Sweet, J. J, Morgan, J. E., Larrabee, G. J., Millis, S. R., & conference participants. (2009). American academy of clinical neuropsychology consensus conference statement on the neuropsychological assessment of effort, response bias, and malingering. *The Clinical Neuropsychologist*, 23, 1093–1129.

Larrabee, G. J., & Berry, D. T. (2007). Diagnostic classification statistics and diagnostic validity of malingering assessment. In G. J. Larrabee (Ed.), *Assessment of malingered neuropsychological deficits* (pp. 14–26). Oxford, England: Oxford University Press.

Leserman, J. (2005). Sexual abuse history: Prevalence, health effects, mediators, and psychological treatment. *Psychosomatic Medicine, 67,* 906–915.

Murrell, S. A., Norris, F. H., & Grote, C. L. (1987). Life events in older adults. In L. H. Cohen (Ed.), *Life events and psychological functioning* (pp. 96–122). Newbury Park, CA: Sage.

Ramsay, R. E., Cohen, A., & Brown, M. C. (1993). Coexisting epilepsy and non-epileptic seizures. In A. J. Rowan & J. R. Gates (Eds.), *Non-epileptic seizures* (1st ed., pp. 47–54). Stoneham, MA: Butterworth-Heineman

Shen, W., Bowman, E. S., & Markand, O. N. Presenting the diagnosis of pseudoseizure. *Neurology, 40,* 756–759.

Walczak, T. S., Papacostas, W., Williams, D.T., Scheuer, M. L., Lebowitz, N., & Notarfrancesco, A. (1995). Outcome after diagnosis of psychogenic nonepileptic seizures. *Epilepsia, 36,* 1131–1137.

Wilkus, R. J., Dodrill, C., & Thompson, P. M. (1984). Intensive EEG monitoring and psychological studies of patients with pseudoepileptic seizures. *Epilepsia, 25,* 100–107.

Part IV

Neurologic/Other Medical Conditions

Acquired cerebral abnormalities are prevalent. Many originate within the central nervous system, but others are the result of non–central nervous system conditions, that is, conditions that originate elsewhere in the body. The 17 chapters in this section explore the effects on the brain of various conditions and diseases that impact cognition, behavior, and emotional adjustment. Some may be devastating to cerebral integrity and life threatening, while for others, contemporary medical treatment may extend life and ameliorate negative neuropsychological effects. The role of the neuropsychologist in such cases involves a balance between assessment and intervention, applied to both the patient and family members.

29

Birth below 500 grams

Jennifer C. Gidley Larson, Ida Sue Baron,
Margot D. Ahronovich, and Mary Iampietro

Neonatal intensive care has progressed consider-ably since its inception in the 1970s, leading to steadily increasing survival rates for those born extremely preterm (<1000 g or <28 weeks gesta-tional age) and for those exceptionally early delivered neonates who are born micropremature (<500 g; Lucey et al., 2004). Medical proce-dures and treatments have advanced sufficiently in the past decade to anticipate the survival of an even greater number of micropremature infants with each subsequent year. However, incidence rates for birth <500 g are not yet routinely reported in the annual National Vital Health Statistics report. Furthermore, physician opin-ions have been variable about whether aggres-sive resuscitation of these borderline viable infants is warranted since these survivors are at substantial risk for lifespan neurodevelopmental and neurocognitive impairment (Hintz et al., 2005; MacDonald, 2002; Schollin, 2005). Thus, greater understanding of how such exceptionally early birth will affect neurodevelopmental and neuropsychological outcomes is needed.

The understandably sparse literature regard-ing birth <500 g is largely due to the infrequency of these children's survival. Most data have been in the form of descriptive case reports, often relying on subjective clinical impressions or general cognitive or neuromotor test results. We found no report of multidomain neuropsy-chological evaluation. These previously pub-lished case reports have been distinctive for their emphasis on the respective micropremature child's remarkably adequate development despite obvious adverse neonatal circumstances. The earliest case report was of a 398 g male born in 1937 at approximately 32 weeks, kept alive in a warm oven and fed drops of brandy mixed with warm water, whose mental and physical condi-tions were judged normal at 12 months (Monro, 1939). In 1950, Fakim reported on a 450 g female, but without cognitive data. Nearly 35 years later, a female born at 25 weeks weighing 440 g was described as exhibiting increased activity and distractibility at 2 years, but no sensorineural, gross motor, or language deficits. Her Bayley Scales of Infant Development mental developmen-tal index (MDI) was 83 (low average) (Pleasure, Dhand, & Kaur, 1984). Moro and Minoli (1991) reported favorable neurodevelopmental out-comes at both 22 months and 47 months for a 450 g female, with the exception of fine motor and visuomotor difficulties (Coccia, Pezzani, Moro, & Minoli, 1992). There have been addi-tional reports of acceptable function for those born at 380 g studied at 20 months (Ginsberg, Goldsmith, & Stedman, 1990), 390 g studied at 24 months corrected age (Amato, 1992), 450 g studied at 12 months (Lelak, Limanowski, & Hager-Malecka, 1973), 460 g (age unreported) (Moro & Minoli, 1991), and for two 480–490 g infants (age unreported) (Corchia, Cossu, & Sanna, 1994). The lowest infant birth weight reported to date was of a female born at 26 weeks 6 days weighing 280 g. Her MDI was 86 (low average) and she had age-appropriate general development and visual-motor perceptual skill at 2 years (Muraskas, Myers, Lambert, &

Anderson, 1992). Follow-up report at 14 years indicated that her national high school examination score fell at the 83rd percentile and her grade point average was 3.7 (on a 4-point scale); no psychosocial problems had emerged (Muraskas, Hasson, & Besinger, 2004).

While these case studies suggest adequate outcomes may be expected in selected circumstances, little has been published for this subset of children regarding school age outcomes, their performance across neuropsychological domains, or their function as a consequence of perinatal morbidities common to micropremature infants. The Vermont Oxford Network, a multisite nonprofit neonatal database, summarized morbidity and mortality data for 4172 infants born weighing 401-500 g between 1996 and 2000 (Lucey et al., 2004). Of 690 infants (17%) who survived to neonatal intensive care unit (NICU) discharge, more were female, the product of singleton birth, small for gestational age (SGA), of greater gestational age (mean 25.3 ± 2 weeks), delivered by Cesarean section, and born to mothers who had received antenatal steroids and prenatal care (Lucey et al., 2004). Most survivors had multiple perinatal morbidities and especially common preterm complications such as patent ductus arteriosus (PDA), retinopathy of prematurity (ROP), and chronic lung disease (CLD) (Lucey et al., 2004). A Canadian study of infants born <500 g (and >20 weeks) from 1983 to 1994 found only 18 of 382 live births (4.7%) survived to NICU discharge. Of these, 13 infants (72.2%) survived to 3 years, including four who had no disability or cerebral palsy (CP) and whose cognitive scores ranged from borderline to average limits, and one who had mild spastic diplegia and functioned within high-average limits (Sauve, Robertson, Etches, Byrne, & Dayer-Zamora, 1998). This wide range of outcomes is consistent with the variability reported in the extremely preterm population. It has been concluded that long-term survival following birth <500 g is likely to be associated with poor growth and development, multiple medical morbidities, and cognitive impairments. None of the aforementioned reports included a sufficiently extensive evaluation to allow for finer discriminations of neuropsychological integrity or dysfunction. Appraisal of neuropsychological strengths and weaknesses has been lacking for these highly at-risk infants, particularly as they mature into the childhood years.

In this chapter, we present the neuropsychological test results obtained on three children born <500 g. These children participated in a study of neuropsychological outcomes at early school age after extremely preterm birth, and their results were considered instructive. Their exceptionally low birth weights (440 g, 480 g, and 482 g) and individual neonatal courses provided a unique opportunity to examine their data from a clinical perspective relative to the extant extremely preterm literature. Each child was assessed within constrained time limits (2 hours) with a test battery designed to measure functions especially susceptible to disruption after preterm birth (see Table 29-1). The history and background of each child is presented, followed by their neuropsychological and behavioral data, and a discussion of their performance similarities and differences.

Case Reports

Demographic and common preterm medical complication characteristics for each child are presented in Table 29-2.

Case 1: N. M.

N. M. was 6 years, 7 months old, right handed, female, and born to college-educated Asian immigrant parents in 1999. She was the product of a Cesarean delivery (singleton, vertex presentation) after a 30-hour labor, born weighing 440 g (<3 percentile) at 24 weeks, and therefore SGA. Apgar scores were 5 at 1 minute and 7 at 5 minutes. The pregnancy was complicated by pregnancy-induced hypertension and pre-eclampsia. Her mother had no previous pregnancies, miscarriages, or fertility consultation, and was 42 years old at delivery; paternal age was 44 years. N. M. was diagnosed with stage 1 ROP, bronchopulmonary dysplasia (BPD), and PDA. She received surfactant therapy, spent 7 days on the oscillator and an additional 20 days on a conventional ventilator, 19 days on nasal continuous positive airway pressure (CPAP), and received corticosteroid (dexamethasone) treatment for 33 days. Cranial ultrasounds revealed normal brain structure. N. M. was discharged from the NICU at 85 days.

Table 29-1. Neuropsychological Measures, Function, and Reported Score by Domain

Domain	Test Instrument	Function	Score Reported
General Intellectual Functioning	DAS General Conceptual Ability (GCA)	General Intellectual Ability (IQ)	Standard Score
	DAS Verbal Cluster	Language/Verbal Reasoning Ability	Standard Score
	DAS Nonverbal Reasoning Cluster	Nonverbal Reasoning Ability	Standard Score
	DAS Spatial Cluster	Spatial/Perceptual Ability	Standard Score
Academic Achievement	DAS Basic Number Skills	Basic Arithmetic	Standard Score
	DAS Spelling	Written Spelling Ability	Standard Score
	DAS Word Reading	Reading Single Words Aloud	Standard Score
Language	DAS Verbal Cluster		Standard Score
	DAS Word Definitions	Word Knowledge	T-Score
	CTOPP Elision	Phonological Awareness	Scaled Score
Nonverbal/ Perceptual	DAS Nonverbal Reasoning Cluster		Standard Score
	DAS Spatial Cluster		Standard Score
	DAS Matrices	Nonverbal Problem Solving and Reasoning	T-Score
	DAS Sequential & Quantitative Reasoning	Numeric Reasoning	T-Score
	DAS Pattern Construction	Visuospatial Ability	T-Score
Motor/ Visuomotor	DAS Speed of Information Processing	Mental Processing Speed	T-Score
	Beery Visual-Motor Integration	Design Copying	Standard Score
	Purdue Pegboard*	Fine Motor Dexterity and Manual Coordination Visuomotor Speed (Time per Target)	T-Score
	TEA-Ch Sky Search Motor Control		Raw Score
	PANESS	Speed of Movements	Z-score
Attention/ Working Memory	WISC-IV Digit Span Forward and Backward	Attention Span and Repetition of Digits	Scaled Score
	Corsi Block-tapping Span†	Spatial Working Memory	T-Score
	TEA-Ch Sky Search	Visual Scanning Accuracy, Scanning Speed	Scaled Score
Executive Functioning	DAS Similarities	Abstract Verbal Reasoning	T-Score
	Phonemic Fluency (FAS)	Letter Fluency	T-Score
	Semantic Fluency (Animals)	Category Fluency	T-Score
	BRIEF Parent Report	Parental Report of Everyday Executive Functioning	T-Score
Learning and Memory	DAS Recall of Designs	Short-term Recall of Visual-Spatial Information	T-Score
	DAS Immediate/Delayed Recall of Objects	Immediate/Delayed Verbal Recall of Visual Information	T-Score
Behavior	BASC-II	Parental Report of Everyday Behavior (Clinical and Adaptive)	T-Score
Parent Perception	PEDS	Parental Report of Child's Learning, Behavior, and Development	Raw Score

*For the Purdue Pegboard Test (Tiffen, 1968), Gardner and Broman (1979) norms were used.

†Corsi Block Span (Corsi, 1972).

BASC-II, Behavior Assessment System for Children: Parent Form (Reynolds & Kamphaus, 1998); BRIEF, Behavioral Rating Inventory of Executive Function: Parent Form (Gioia, Isquith, Guy, & Kenworthy, 2000); C-TOPP, Comprehensive Test of Phonological Processing: Elision Subtest (Wagner, Torgesen, & Rashotte, 1999); DAS, Differential Ability Scales (Elliott, 1990); PANESS, Physical and Neurological Examination of Subtle Signs–Revised (Denckla, 1985); PEDS, Parent's Evaluation of Developmental Status (Glascoe, 2001); TEA-Ch, Test of Everyday Attention in Children: Sky Search Subtest (Manly, Robertson, Anderson, & Nimmo-Smith, 1999); VMI, Beery-Buktenica Developmental Test of Visual-Motor Integration (Beery & Beery, 2004); WISC-IV, Wechsler Intelligence Scales for Children, Fourth edition: Digit Span Subtest (Wechsler, 2003).

Table 29-2. Demographic Information and Presence (+) or Absence (–) of Typical Neonatal Complications

	Case 1: N. M.	Case 2: K. C.	Case 3: M. A.
Birth weight (grams)	440	482	480
Gestational age (weeks)	24	23	26
Age at evaluation	6 yr 7 mo	6 yr 1 mo	6 yr 4 mo
Gender	Female	Male	Female
Ethnicity	Asian	Biracial	Caucasian
Handedness	Right	Left	Right
Sensorineural loss: hearing (H) vision (V)	–	V, H	V
Maternal age (years)	42	36	40
Maternal education (years)	16	16	16
Inborn	+	+	+
Gestational age/weight ratio	SGA	–	SGA
Intrauterine growth retardation	–	–	+
Intraventricular hemorrhage Grade	–	1	–
Hydrocephalus	–	–	–
Retinopathy of prematurity stage	1	2+ or 3	2+ or 3
Periventricular leukomalacia	–	–	–
Bronchopulmonary dysplasia	+	+	+
Confirmed sepsis	–	–	+
Necrotizing enterocolitis	–	–	–
Patent ductus arteriosus	+	+	+
Surfactant therapy	+	+	+
Dexamethasone (no. of days)	33	28	42
Length of Stay (no. of days)	85	117	157

SGA, small for gestational age.

Developmental history for N. M. noted slight delay in acquisition of gross motor function by conventional, uncorrected chronological age. She sat alone at 10 months uncorrected age, stood alone at 16 months uncorrected age, and walked independently at 18 months uncorrected age; however, these accomplishments were age-appropriate when preterm age correction was applied. Fine motor development also developed age-appropriately. At 7 years, her pediatrician noted mild awkwardness and clumsiness but no obvious neurological or musculoskeletal deficits. Hearing and vision were intact. Her parent reported awkward running, skipping, and ball playing compared to her age-matched peers. She had received speech therapy to improve articulation. Her public school first grade special education teacher expressed concern only about this bilingual child's English mastery, especially as English was not spoken in the home. No family medical, neurological, or psychological problems were reported.

Behavioral observations at testing noted that N. M. was engaged, cooperative, and pleasant to work with. She was of average height and weight, without obvious motor problems, but evidenced difficulty with English, particularly with articulation and vocabulary.

Case 2: K. C.

K. C. was 6 years, 1 month old, left handed, biracial, male, and born to college-educated parents in 2001. He was the surviving twin of a Cesarean delivery (vertex presentation) and an otherwise uncomplicated pregnancy, born at 23 weeks weighing 482 grams (3rd percentile). Apgar scores were 1 at 1 minute and 5 at 5 minutes. His mother, who had three previous pregnancies, one miscarriage, and no fertility consultation, was 36 years old at delivery; paternal age was 40 years. K. C. required and responded well to chest compressions in the delivery room. He was diagnosed with stage 3 ROP with plus disease requiring laser surgery, BPD, and PDA. He received surfactant therapy, spent 11 days on the oscillator and an additional 28 days on a ventilator, 29 days on CPAP, and he received corticosteroid (dexamethasone) treatment for 28 days. Cranial ultrasound at 7 days revealed bilateral grade 1 intraventricular hemorrhage (IVH); however, several follow-up scans up to 3 months were normal. K. C. was discharged from the NICU at 117 days with oxygen and a cardiorespiratory monitor. K. C. had surgery for a hernia at 3 months and eye surgery at 7 months. He had a history of febrile seizures, failure to thrive, and difficulty eating (particularly with chewing and swallowing) and sleeping. Left eye blindness and right ear hearing loss were documented. Family history was significant for mood disorder in both parents.

K. C.'s early motor milestones were achieved on time; he had received physical therapy for gross motor and fine motor skills. At testing, his parent reported that he was awkward when running, skipping, and playing ball. K. C. was slow to learn the alphabet, name colors, count, and recognize numbers. He had a history of repetitive behaviors (i.e., hand flapping, playing with air vents, excessive interest in electrical outlets), hyperactivity, inattention, and impulsivity. A second language was spoken occasionally at home. He attended a regular pre-kindergarten class in a private school.

At testing, he was noted to be stubborn, occasionally noncompliant, and he required constant redirection to stay on task. He frequently reported being finished before he actually had completed a task; however, he continued with encouragement although not always with full effort.

Case 3: M. A.

M. A. was 6 years, 4 months old, right handed, Caucasian, female, and born to college-educated parents in 2002. She was born by Cesarean delivery (singleton, vertex presentation) at 26 weeks weighing 480 g (<3rd percentile; SGA). Apgar scores were 5 at 1 minute and 8 at 5 minutes. The pregnancy was complicated by pregnancy-induced hypertension. M. A.'s mother had two previous pregnancies, including one miscarriage, and no fertility consultation. At delivery, maternal age was 40 years and paternal age was 35 years. M. A. received surfactant therapy, spent 6 days on the oscillator and an additional 42 days on a ventilator, 24 days on CPAP, and received corticosteroid (dexamethasone) treatment for

42 days. She was diagnosed with stage 3 ROP with plus disease (requiring laser surgery), confirmed sepsis, BPD, and PDA. Cranial magnetic resonance imaging (MRI) revealed normal brain structure. She was discharged from the NICU at 157 days with an apnea monitor and a gastrostomy tube with continuous feeds. However, 3 days later she was readmitted to a pediatric unit for 1 additional month, due to frequent monitor alarms and feeding tube intolerance. The gastrostomy tube was required until 4.5 years due to poor sucking and chewing. M. A. had eye surgery at 2 months, 26 days, while in the NICU, and ear surgeries for excessive fluid at 2, 3, and 4 years.

M. A.'s gross motor development was severely delayed. She sat alone at 13 months, stood alone at 19 months, and walked at 22 months, uncorrected ages; these milestones were delayed even with preterm age correction. Her parent reported that she was awkward when running, skipping, and playing ball. Physical and occupational therapies were provided from 10 months until 6 years for gross motor skills and balance, and from 6 months up until this evaluation to aid her ability to eat. Additionally, M. A. required speech therapy for vocal cord damage and had delayed speech and language development. Hyperactivity, inattention, and impulsivity were reported, particularly when fatigued. She wore a contact lens in her right eye and bifocal glasses. Hearing was intact. M. A. was beginning first grade in a regular classroom, with special education resource assistance. Father and paternal grandmother had hypothyroidism.

Behavioral observations at testing noted that she was small for her age, soft-spoken (due to vocal cord damage), and she wore corrective eyeglasses. She was fidgety, found it difficult to sit still, and impulsively turned the pages of a stimulus book and grabbed at table-top items. Motor difficulties prevented completion of all motor tasks. While M. A. was slow to warm to the examiner, she appeared interested, attentive, and engaged.

Neuropsychological Evaluation

Each child was administered cognitive and neuropsychological tests while the child's parent completed a developmental history questionnaire and standardized behavioral rating scales. All raw data were converted to standard scores based on age normative data. Ten broad domains were examined: (1) general conceptual ability, (2) academic achievement, (3) language, (4) nonverbal/perceptual, (5) motor/visuomotor, (6) attention span/working memory, (7) executive functioning, (8) learning and memory, (9) behavior, and (10) parent perception. Table 29-1 lists tests by function and domain.

General Cognitive Function

The overall Differential Ability Scale (DAS) general conceptual ability (GCA) scores were below average and ranged minimally, from 76 for N. M. (low, 5th percentile) to 80 for M. A. and 81 for K. C. (below average, 9th and 10th percentiles, respectively). However, each child exhibited variability across summary verbal, nonverbal reasoning, and spatial ability cluster scores. N. M.'s below-average nonverbal reasoning and spatial scores contrasted with a very low verbal score, the latter likely due to this bilingual child's delayed English proficiency. K. C. and M. A. both had average verbal, below-average nonverbal reasoning, and low spatial scores, and both also had a history of severe ROP, a neonatal complication strongly associated with visuospatial and visuoperceptual dysfunction (see Table 29-3).

Academic Achievement

Impressively, DAS academic achievement scores were either consistent with or surpassed expectation based on each child's respective GCA scores. Each obtained average scores for basic

number skills. N. M. and K. C. had below-average word reading but M. A.'s score was elevated into high limits, a clinically significant 40 points higher than her GCA. N. M. and K. C. had their lowest academic scores on spelling (low range), whereas M. A.'s score was within high limits, a clinically significant 41 points above her GCA. M. A.'s performances in particular highlighted that overall expectations should not be based only on summary cognitive scores or pragmatic verbal skill; M. A. was clearly acquiring language related information at age-appropriate limits despite concerns about her expressive language proficiency and a below-average GCA (see Table 29-3).

Language

The DAS verbal cluster scores were derived from performance on subtests assessing word definitions (i.e., word knowledge) and verbal similarities (i.e., verbal reasoning). K. C. and M. A. obtained average scores for word knowledge and verbal reasoning, and also for phonological awareness based on their CTOPP phonological processing (elision subtest) performances. Not surprisingly, N. M.'s scores reflected her weak English proficiency; word knowledge was at the 1st percentile, and phonological awareness and verbal reasoning, which also required verbal expression, fell at the 2nd and 5th percentiles, respectively (see Table 29-4).

Nonverbal/Perceptual

The DAS nonverbal reasoning cluster did not differ significantly from the spatial cluster for

Table 29-3. General Conceptual Ability and Academic Achievement Test Results

| | | | Case 1: N. M. | | Case 2: K. C. | | Case 3: M. A. | |
			Score	Percentile	Score	Percentile	Score	Percentile
DAS Cluster Scores	GCA	SS	76	5	81	10	80	9
Standard Score	Verbal	SS	68	2	94	34	92	30
	Nonverbal Reasoning	SS	84	14	86	18	84	14
	Spatial	SS	86	18	73	4	74	4
DAS Academic	Basic Number Skills	SS	93	32	94	34	102	55
Achievement	Spelling	SS	74	4	76	5	121	92
Standard Score	Word Reading	SS	80	9	89	23	120	91

Table 29-4. Language, Nonverbal/Perceptual, and Motor/Visuomotor Test Results

			Case 1: N. M.		Case 2: K. C.		Case 3: M. A.	
			Score	Percentile	Score	Percentile	Score	Percentile
Language	DAS Verbal Cluster	SS	68	2	94	34	92	30
	DAS Word Definitions	T	27	1	50	50	48	42
	C-Topp Elision	ss	4	2	10	54	11	64
NonVerbal/	DAS NonVerbal							
Perceptual	Cluster	SS	84	14	86	18	84	84
	DAS Spatial Cluster	SS	86	18	73	4	74	4
	DAS Matrices	T	41	19	44	27	50	50
	DAS Seq. & Quan.							
	Reasoning	T	41	19	40	16	32	4
	DAS Pattern							
	Construction	T	41	19	30	2	34	5
Motor/	DAS Speed of Info.							
Visuomotor	Processing	T	41	19	38	12	46	34
	Beery Visual-Motor							
	Integration	SS	91	27	92	30	76	5
	Purdue Pegboard:							
	Dominant Hand	T	21	<1	20	<1	17	<1
	Purdue Pegboard:							
	Nondominant							
	Hand	T	39	14	33	5	29	2
	Purdue Pegboard:							
	Both Hands	T	41	19	22	<1	19	<1
	TEA-Ch Motor							
	Control Time							
	per Target	Raw	3.8	—	5.5	—	2.2	—
	PANESS: Toe-Tap R	Z	−3.2	<1	−7.6	<1	−4.6	<1
	PANESS: Toe-Tap L	Z	−.44	34	−3.6	<1	—	—
	PANESS: Heel-to-							
	Toe R	Z	−.92	18	1.2	86	—	—
	PANESS: Heel-to-							
	Toe L	Z	−2.9	<1	−.19	45	—	—
	PANESS: Hand Pat R	Z	−1.7	5	−1.8	4	−1.5	7
	PANESS: Hand Pat L	Z	−.70	25	−1.5	7	−2.0	2
	PANESS: Hand							
	Pronate/Supinate R	Z	−2.19	1	−1.7	5	−2.7	<1
	PANESS: Hand							
	Pronate/Supinate L	Z	−.60	27	−2.8	<1	—	—
	PANESS: Finger Tap R	Z	.03	53	−1.5	7	.31	61
	PANESS: Finger Tap L	Z	−1.4	8	.95	82	−4.3	<1
	PANESS: Finger							
	Sequence R	Z	−2.75	<1	−2.7	<1	−1.5	7
	PANESS: Finger							
	Sequence L	Z	−4.5	<1	−3.9	<1	−.74	25

any child. Nonverbal problem solving and pictorial reasoning were low average for N. M. (19th percentile), average for K. C. (27th percentile), and average for M. A. (50th percentile). However; N. M., K. C., and M. A. all exhibited less efficient performances on sequential and quantitative (numeric) reasoning, with performance at the 19th, 19th, and 4th percentiles, respectively. K. C. and M. A. had low performance on pattern construction, their scores at the 2nd and 5th percentiles, respectively, whereas N. M.'s score at the 19th percentile was below average (see Table 29-4). K. C. and M. A.'s especially low pattern construction scores may be due to persisting visuomotor and visual perceptual weaknesses related to their history of severe ROP.

Motor/Visuomotor

As commonly reported for extremely preterm children, motor and visuomotor tests highlighted particular weaknesses within this domain. All three children had difficulty on the timed Purdue Pegboard Test of motor dexterity and manual coordination, and all exhibited very low-range dominant hand performance, their scores each <1st percentile. M. A. and K. C. each had low nondominant hand performance, at the 2nd and 5th percentiles, respectively, and N. M.'s below-average nondominant hand performance fell only at the 14th percentile. For coordinated both-hands trials, M. A. and K. C. had very low performance, <1st percentile, and N. M. had below-average performance, at the 22nd percentile. Similarly, the PANESS measure of speeded efficiency of patterned and repetitive bilateral foot, hand, and finger movements found all three children significantly slowed. In particular, they all demonstrated right-sided repetitive foot, repetitive and patterned hand, and finger sequencing slowness. On the DAS speed of information processing subtest, partly dependent on visuomotor function, N. M. and K. C. both obtained below-average scores at the 19th and 12th percentiles, respectively, while M. A. earned an average score at the 34th percentile. Lastly, N. M. and K. C. had average design copying, at the 27th and 30th percentiles, respectively, whereas M. A.'s score was low at the 5th percentile (see Table 29-4).

Attention Span/Working Memory

Consistent with expectations based on the preterm literature, all three children exhibited weakness on tests of focused/selective attention and spatial working memory. Their below-average scores on WISC-IV digit span ranged from the 12th to 16th percentiles. Discrepancy was noted between forward and backward span; although N. M. had low forward span (2nd percentile) and average backward span (39th percentile), K. C. had below-average forward span (16th percentile) but low backward span (2nd percentile), and M. A. had above-average forward span (85th percentile) but low backward span (2nd percentile). All three children exhibited poor spatial working memory on the Corsi block-tapping task, with performances at very low limits and ≤2nd percentile. All three children exhibited low scores on a TEA-Ch sky-search subtest requiring rapid visual scanning, performances ranging from 2nd to 5th percentiles. K. C. and N. M. identified targets slowly, earning low (5th percentile) and very low (<1st percentile) total attention scores, respectively. M. A.'s total attention score was average, at the 30th percentile (see Table 29-5).

Executive Function

Measures of reasoning and verbal fluency revealed variability within and across children. M. A. exhibited average performances for letter fluency (34th percentile), category fluency (25th percentile), and abstract verbal reasoning (25th percentile). K. C. had average abstract verbal reasoning (27th percentile) but low letter fluency (4th percentile) and low category fluency (2nd percentile). N. M. exhibited low abstract verbal reasoning (5th percentile), but average letter fluency and category fluency, both at the 55th percentile. On an experimental, unnormed action-verb fluency test, N. M. produced more verbs (eight) than either M. A. (four) or K. C. (two) (see Table 29-5).

Learning and Memory

N. M.'s ability to immediately recall designs was average (25th percentile), K. C.'s score was below

Table 29-5. Attention/Working Memory, Executive Function, and Learning and Memory Test Results

			Case 1 N. M.		Case 2 K. C.		Case 3 M. A.	
			Score	Percentile	Score	Percentile	Score	Percentile
Attention/	WISC-IV Digit	ss	6	12	7	16	7	16
Working	Span: Total							
Memory	WISC-IV Digit Span: Forward (Span Length)	ss	4 (3)	2	7 (4)	16	13 (6)	85
	WISC-IV Digit Span: Backward (Span Length)	ss	9 (2)	39	5 (2)	5	4 (2)	2
	Corsi Total	T	30 (3)	2	30 (4)	2	27 (4)	1
	Corsi Span (Span Length)	T	30 (3)	2	41 (4)	19	41 (4)	19
	Corsi Basal (Span Length)	T	25 (1)	1	35 (2)	7	35 (2)	7
	TEA-Ch Sky Search Number of Targets	ss	5	5	4	2	5	5
	TEA-Ch Sky Search Time per Target	ss	1	<1	5	5	8	30
	TEA-Ch Search Attention	ss	1	<1	5	5	8	30
Executive	DAS Similarities	T	34	5	44	27	43	25
Function	Phonemic Fluency (FAS)	T	51	55	32	4	46	34
	Semantic Fluency (Animals)	T	51	55	30	2	43	25
	Verb Fluency	Raw	8	—	2	—	4	—
Learning and	DAS Recall of Designs	T	43	25	38	12	36	8
Memory	DAS Immediate Recall of Objects	T	48	42	51	55	51	55
	DAS Delayed Recall of Objects	T	49	45	42	21	40	16

average (12th percentile), and M. A.'s score fell in the low range (8th percentile). Yet all three children had average ability to learn and immediately recall objects presented visually over three learning trials; however, N. M.'s delayed recall of these picture names remained average (45th percentile), while scores for K. C. (21st percentile) and M. A. (16th percentile) were reduced to below-average limits (see Table 29-5).

Behavioral Rating Scales and Parent Perception Report

Behavioral Rating Inventory of Executive Function. Parental report Behavioral Rating Inventory

of Executive Function (BRIEF) scores were within normal limits for N. M., with the exception of elevation into clinically significant limits regarding her planning and organization skills. K. C.'s BRIEF profile indicated difficulty with working memory, planning, and organization, and his general executive composite was elevated into a clinically significant range. M. A.'s BRIEF subtest scores fell consistently within average limits (see Table 29-6).

Behavioral Assessment System for Children-2. Parental report Behavioral Assessment System for Children-2 (BASC-2) composite and subsection scores found N. M.'s internalizing behaviors and behavioral symptoms indexes within the at-risk range due to elevations on aggression, anxiety, and depression, and clinically significant elevations for somatization and atypicality. Functional communication was also at risk. K. C.'s externalizing problems index was elevated to an at-risk range, based on scores for aggression and conduct problems; hyperactivity fell into a clinically significant elevated range. His behavioral

symptoms index was within at-risk limits for withdrawal and there was clinically significant elevation for attention problems. His score for activities of daily living was also within clinically significant limits. M. A.'s scores for withdrawal and leadership fell within an at-risk range, while all other scores fell within normal limits (see Table 29-6).

Table 29-6. Scores for the BRIEF-Preschool, BASC-II, and PEDS

		Case 1: N. M.		Case 2: K. C.		Case 3: M. A.	
		Score	*Percentile*	Score	*Percentile*	Score	*Percentile*
BRIEF	Inhibit	53	*61*	58	*79*	43	*25*
Parent	Shift	64	*92*	63	*91*	45	*32*
Report	Emotional Control	60	*84*	52	*58*	41	*19*
	Behavioral Regulation Index	60	*84*	58	*79*	42	*21*
	Initiate	55	*70*	55	*70*	55	*70*
	Working Memory	57	*77*	70	*98*	57	*77*
	Plan/Organize	69	*97*	65	*94*	46	*34*
	Organization of Material	66	*95*	66	*95*	35	*7*
	Monitor	54	*66*	70	*98*	54	*66*
	Metacognitive Index	63	*91*	67	*96*	49	*45*
	General Executive Composite	63	*91*	65	*94*	46	*34*
BASC-II	**Clinical Scales**						
Parent	Hyperactivity	47	*37*	71	*98*	51	*53*
Report	Aggression	64	*92*	61	*87*	43	*25*
	Conduct Problems	43	*25*	62	*88*	40	*16*
	Anxiety	61	*87*	41	*19*	33	*5*
	Depression	61	*87*	49	*47*	39	*14*
	Somatization	73	*99*	39	*14*	42	*21*
	Atypicality	74	*99*	57	*77*	44	*27*
	Withdrawal	51	*53*	61	*87*	61	*87*
	Attention Problems	56	*73*	70	*98*	50	*50*
	Adaptive Scales						
	Adaptability	46	*34*	51	*53*	55	*70*
	Social Skills	41	*19*	52	*55*	41	*19*
	Leadership	43	*25*	45	*32*	38	*12*
	Activities of Daily Living	47	*37*	26	*1*	54	*66*
	Functional Communication	33	*5*	51	*53*	61	*87*
	Composite Scores						
	Externalizing Problems	52	*58*	67	*96*	44	*27*
	Internalizing Problems	69	*97*	41	*19*	35	*7*
	Behavioral Symptoms Index	62	*88*	65	*94*	47	*39*
	Adaptive Skills	41	*19*	44	*27*	50	*50*
PEDS	Total Score	0	—	0	—	0	—
Parent	Predictive Score	5	—	3	—	2	—
Report	Nonpredictive Score	1	—	0	—	1	—

BASC = Behavioral Assessment System for Children-2; BRIEF=Behavioral Rating Inventory of Executive Function; PEDS = Parent's Evaluation of Developmental Status.

Parent's Evaluation of Developmental Status. Overall, parents expressed great satisfaction with their child's outcomes. M. A.'s parent expressed concern about impulsivity and a short attention span but was satisfied with her daughter's comprehension, speech, vocabulary, motor function, socialization, and learning. N. M.'s parent expressed no concerns other than about her daughter's limited ability to pronounce English words. K. C.'s parent noted his short attention span but was satisfied with his comprehension, speech and vocabulary, motor function, and learning; K. C.'s parent also commented on his overexcitement when socializing with peers and verbal repetitions when frustrated (see Table 29-6).

Discussion

Case reports provide an opportunity for in-depth analysis of extrinsic and intrinsic factors that influence a child's developmental outcome, and they remind us about the importance of maintaining an informed patient-centered focus. They also help us appreciate that when exceptions to "textbook" presentations occur, these singular examples may be especially informative. We found the neuropsychological test results on three early school-aged children who were each born weighing <500 g instructive. Their data reinforced our opinion that neuropsychological function may vary greatly between individuals born micropremature, that gestational age and birth weight are not uniquely predictive, and that expectations for especially negative outcomes after micropremature birth should not be reflexively predicted when one is counseling parents coping with the adverse medical circumstances of their child's exceptionally low birth weight.

The literature has only recently begun to document the likelihood of age-appropriate, average range neurocognition for recently born extremely preterm survivors (Baron, Ahronovich, Erickson, Gidley Larson, & Litman, 2009; Doyle, 2004; Hakansson, Farooqi, Holmgren, Serenius, & Hogberg, 2004; Wilson-Costello et al., 2007). Outcomes for any preterm survivor depend on numerous influential variables that interact synergistically. Antenatal, neonatal, and postnatal medical advances along with improved intensive care practices contributed substantially to the likelihood that these three children would

survive, and their neuropsychological data provide evidence of more optimal outcomes than was expected based on data from micropremature children born in past years. Furthermore, the direct impact of sociodemographic and familial factors on outcome has increasingly been appreciated (Baron, Litman, Ahronovich, & Larson, 2007; Treyvaud et al., 2009). It has become increasingly apparent that favorable variables such as singleton birth, female gender, high parental education, high socioeconomic status, and enriched socioenvironmental conditions contribute to improved neurodevelopmental outcome (Aylward, Pfeiffer, Wright, & Verhulst, 1989; Kesler et al., 2004; Kilbride, Thorstad, & Daily, 2004; Teplin, Burchinal, Johnson-Martin, Humphry, & Kraybill, 1991).

Care center factors are highly relevant but inconsistent across centers (Vohr et al., 2004). Therefore, outcomes emerging from one care center may not generalize sufficiently well to allow for accurate prediction of outcomes for neonates treated elsewhere. A tertiary care NICU within a hospital that has a large volume of high-risk neonates, that encourages physician-coordinated prophylactic care and individualized treatment protocols, and that provides 24-hour in-house coverage by attending neonatalogists has been found to be especially advantageous (Doyle, 2004; Hakansson et al., 2004). Our three children were inborn between 1999 and 2001 at such a hospital; thus, their treatment was initiated immediately and not delayed by need for transport. This NICU also has a documented history of exceptionally low neonatal neurological complications, exemplified by the absence of such complications in our three micropremature children. An absence of neonatal neurological complications has been associated with better outcomes (Baron et al., 2009; Edgin et al., 2008).

Some cautions for reviewing the literature on extremely preterm birth include that those care centers that endorse aggressive resuscitation and intensive interventions for their most at-risk neonates may report poorer outcome data due to their higher volume of seriously ill neonates, and that longitudinal outcome data from studies of preterm children born decades earlier (before many contemporary obstetric and neonatal advances) are often still cited in the current literature and relied on for practice guidelines.

This latter practice remains questionable for newly born neonates. Knowledge of birth cohort year is critical to gauge comparability across studies and the applicability of another center's data to one's own individual patient.

Our three children presented with some typical post-preterm deficits. However, they also demonstrated some unexpected and quite impressive strengths. Neurosensory disability remains a significant problem following early birth (Eichenwald & Stark, 2008), including of hearing and vision (Lorenz, Wooliever, Jetton, & Paneth, 1998). Our child with a history of mild ROP (N. M.) had intact hearing and vision, but the two children that had ROP severe enough to require laser surgery had sensorineural impairments; one (K. C.) had monocular blindness and contralateral unilateral hearing loss, and one (M. A.) had intact hearing but wore corrective eyeglasses.

While none of these three children had severe neonatal or childhood-onset neurological compromise or cerebral palsy, our tests nonetheless detected subtle neuromotor inefficiencies on measures of motor dexterity, manual coordination, and motor and visuomotor processing speed. These highlighted a prevalent weakness associated with extremely preterm birth. Neuromotor morbidities are common in those born <1000 g, occurring in as many as 20%–51% of survivors (Hack et al., 2005; Halsey, Collin, & Anderson, 1993; Holsti, Grunau, & Whitfield, 2002; Whitfield, Grunau, & Holsti, 1997). While major motor impairment (cerebral palsy) occurs in approximately 7%–19% of children born <1000 g (Bracewell & Marlow, 2002; Mikkola et al., 2005; Tommiska et al., 2003), subtle motor impairments are much more common, particularly those of postural control (Arnaud et al., 2007; Leosdottir, Egilson, & Georgsdottir, 2005; Marlow, Hennessy, Bracewell, & Wolke, 2007), movement quality and speed (Marlow et al., 2007), and coordination (Arnaud et al., 2007; Holsti et al., 2002; Leosdottir et al., 2005; Marlow et al., 2007). Despite the knowledge that subtle motor impairments contribute to learning, behavioral, and emotional problems (Denckla, 2005), they are unlikely to be detected in routine pediatric examinations (Arnaud et al., 2007; Burns, O'Callaghan, McDonnell, & Rogers,

2004; Foulder-Hughes & Cooke, 2003; Grunau, Whitfield, & Davis, 2002; Holsti et al., 2002; Whitfield et al., 1997). Additionally, neuromotor evaluation may indicate brain maturational level and aid examination of related neural systems, including those mediating executive function (Denckla, 1974, 2005).

Each of our three children functioned age appropriately on a number of specific measures, including on the DAS. General cognitive and academic achievement test scores have been highly variable among preterm populations but consistently lower for extremely preterm children compared to term-born controls. A meta-analysis found preterm children obtained a mean intelligence quotient (IQ) nearly 11 points below that of term controls (Bhutta, Cleves, Casey, Cradock, & Anand, 2002), and IQ scores range widely but significantly below those of controls across many single-center and multisite studies. While our children had low-average DAS GCA scores (5th to 10th percentiles), each had DAS cluster scores that ranged into low-average or higher limits, and one child's DAS academic achievement scores ranged into superior limits. The educational needs of our three children varied; one child required special education and one of the two enrolled and doing well in regular classes required resource help. Given better than predicted cognitive and academic outcomes, it was of interest that all six parents were college educated and none had a history of learning or neurological problems, underscoring the important influence of cognitive reserve factors (Stern, 2002). These children's performances were especially impressive given their complex medical histories that, while absent neonatal neurological complications, included older maternal age at delivery (36 to 42 years); low 1-minute Apgar scores (1 to 5); perinatal complications, including sepsis, ROP, BPD, PDA; and extended NICU length of stay. The visuoperceptual weaknesses found for K. C. and M. A. are well-documented consequences of their severe ROP (Msall et al., 2004).

Of great interest, each child's parent reported age-appropriate behavioral functioning and expressed overall satisfaction with their child's development. They acknowledged their child's particular weaknesses but judged these as minimal intrusions on an overall satisfactory quality of life. Parental reports consistent with attentional dysfunction were confirmed by speeded visual search and information processing tests, and all had working memory compromise, an early measurable executive function capacity that presages more complex executive functioning later in life (Conklin, Luciana, Hooper, & Yarger, 2007). Furthermore, their profiles were consistent with reports that extremely preterm birth is associated with abnormalities in frontal cortical-subcortical neural pathways and cerebral white matter (Nosarti et al., 2002; Stewart et al., 1999; Woodward, Anderson, Austin, Howard, & Inder, 2006), cortical gray matter (Nosarti et al., 2002; Peterson et al., 2003; Woodward et al., 2006), the cerebellum (Limperopoulos et al., 2007), and in sensorimotor and premotor cortical volume (Peterson et al., 2000).

Our three cases also provided us greater insight regarding likely etiology for some poor test performances, perhaps unrelated to preterm birth. For example, N. M. was being raised in a bilingual home where English was not spoken, a factor likely contributing to her lagging English skills in her first year of formal schooling. Our standardized cognitive measure likely underestimated her true cognitive ability. Yet her relatively intact word retrieval raised interesting questions regarding the interaction between her less capable pragmatic language skills secondary to unfamiliarity with English and her more highly developed word retrieval evidenced on a semantic fluency measure.

In summary, we examined functioning across multiple cognitive, neuropsychological, and behavioral domains and found that each micropremature child demonstrated variable but often acceptable function for his or her chronological age. Although a higher incidence of substantially poor cognitive and neuromotor outcomes after extremely preterm birth is expected, and these children had below-average GCA scores, our three children who were each born <500 g presented a more optimistic neuropsychological profile at early school age than predicted by the existent extremely preterm literature, with respect to academic achievement and behavior. Significant performance variability was evident across these cases, including on discrete neuropsychological measures not yet commonly reported

for such early born children. The combination of factors most predictive of optimal neuropsychological outcome after extremely preterm birth remains to be determined. As noted earlier, and in accord with the Baron Maturational Model of Child Neuropsychological Development (2008), outcome depends on many more factors than birth weight and gestational age. For our three cases, important factors included high maternal educational level (Breslau, Paneth, & Lucia, 2004); an absence of severe neonatal neurological complications; and that these children likely benefitted from specific care center factors, such as 24-hour attending physician care within a tertiary care NICU that routinely has a high volume of profoundly at-risk neonates. Efforts continue to determine the most relevant contributions to optimal outcomes, including for those born at the threshold of viability. Recent studies have enhanced our understanding of how and which medical, neurobiological, socioenvironmental, and care center factors most influence outcomes following preterm birth. This continuing effort to isolate the most contributory factors is expected to lead to even better outcomes for the earliest born infants who, as exemplified by these three micropremature birth cases, may under a specific set of circumstances function at average or better levels, and consistent with regular grade-level expectations. Comprehensive longitudinal neuropsychological evaluation beginning at an early age holds promise for greater understanding about neural system vulnerability in this increasingly prevalent highly at-risk population.

References

Amato, M. (1992). The care of fetal babies: Survival of a 390 g infant. *Acta Paediatrica Supplement*, *382*, 7–9.

Arnaud, C., Daubisse-Marliac, L., White-Koning, M., Pierrat, V., Larroque, B., Grandjean, H., et al. (2007). Prevalence and associated factors of minor neuromotor dysfunctions at age 5 years in prematurely born children: The EPIPAGE Study. *Archives of Pediatric and Adolescent Medicine*, *161*(11), 1053–1061.

Aylward, G. P., Pfeiffer, S. L., Wright, A., & Verhulst, S. J. (1989). Outcome studies of low birth weight infants published in the last decade: A meta-analysis. *Journal of Pediatrics*, *115*(4), 515–520.

Baron, I. S. (2008). Growth and development of pediatric neuropsychology. In J. Morgan & J. Ricker (Eds.), *Textbook of clinical neuropsychology* (pp. 91–104). New York: Psychology Press.

Baron, I. S., Ahronovich, M. D., Erickson, K., Gidley Larson, J. C., & Litman, F. R. (2009). Age-appropriate early school age neurobehavioral outcomes of extremely preterm birth without severe intraventricular hemorrhage: A single center experience. *Early Human Development, 85,* 191–196.

Baron, I. S., Litman, F. R., Ahronovich, M. D., & Larson, J. C. (2007). Neuropsychological outcomes of preterm triplets discordant for birthweight: A case report. *The Clinical Neuropsychologist, 21,* 338–362.

Beery, K. E., & Beery, N. A. (2004). *The Beery-Buktenica Developmental Test of Visual-Motor Integration: Administration, scoring, and teaching manual.* Minneapolis, MN: NCS Pearson, Inc.

Bhutta, A. T., Cleves, M. A., Casey, P. H., Cradock, M. M., & Anand, K. J. (2002). Cognitive and behavioral outcomes of school-aged children who were born preterm: A meta-analysis. *Journal of the American Medical Association, 288*(6), 728–737.

Bracewell, M., & Marlow, N. (2002). Patterns of motor disability in very preterm children. *Mental Retardation and Developmental Disabilities Research Review, 8,* 241–248.

Breslau, N., Paneth, N. S., & Lucia, V. C. (2004). The lingering academic deficits of low birth weight children. *Pediatrics, 114*(4), 1035–1040.

Burns, Y., O'Callaghan, M., McDonnell, B., & Rogers, Y. (2004). Movement and motor development in ELBW infants at 1 year is related to cognitive and motor abilites at 4 years. *Early Human Development, 80,* 19–29.

Coccia, C., Pezzani, M., Moro, G., & Minoli, I. (1992). Management of extremely low-birth-weight infants. *Acta Paediatrica Supplement, 382,* 10–12.

Conklin, H. M., Luciana, M., Hooper, C. J., & Yarger, R. S. (2007). Working memory performance in typically developing children and adolescents: Behavioral evidence of protracted frontal lobe development. *Developmental Neuropsychology, 31*(1), 103–128.

Corchia, C., Cossu, F., & Sanna, M. (1994). How long should we go on reporting single cases of micropremies? *Acta Paediatrica, 83,* 1110.

Corsi, P. M. (1972). Human memory and the medial temporal region of the brain. *Dissertation Abstracts International, 34,* 819.

Denckla, M. B. (1974). Development of motor co-ordination in normal children. *Developmental Medicine and Child Neurology, 16,* 729–741.

Denckla, M. B. (1985). Revised neurological examination for subtle signs. *Psychopharmacology Bulletin., 21*(4), 773–800.

Denckla, M. B. (2005). Why assess motor functions "early and often?" *Mental Retardation and Developmental Disabilities, 11,* 3.

Doyle, L. W. (2004). Changing availability of neonatal intensive care for extremely low birthweight infants in Victoria over two decades. *The Medical Journal of Australia, 181*(3), 136–139.

Edgin, J. O., Inder, T. E., Anderson, P. J., Hood, K. M., Clark, C. A., & Woodward, L. J. (2008). Executive functioning in preschool children born very preterm: Relationship with early white matter pathology. *Journal of the International Neuropsychological Society, 14*(1), 90–101.

Eichenwald, E. C., & Stark, A. R. (2008). Management and outcomes of very low birth weight. *New England Journal of Medicine, 358*(16), 1700–1711.

Elliott, C. D. (1990). *Differential Ability Scales.* San Anontio, TX: The Psychological Corporation.

Fakim, H. (1950). Survival of a 16-oz baby. *British Medical Association Journal, 2,* 445.

Foulder-Hughes, L., & Cooke, R. (2003). Motor, cognitive, and behavioural disorders in children born very preterm. *Developmental Medicine and Child Neurology, 45*(97–103).

Gardner, R. A., & Broman, M. (1979). The Purdue Pegboard: Normative data on 1334 school children. *Journal of Clinical and Child Psychology, 1,* 156–162.

Ginsberg, H., Goldsmith, J., & Stedman, M. (1990). Intact survival and 20-month follow-up of a 380-gram infant. *Journal of Perinatology, 10,* 3.

Gioia, G. A., Isquith, P. K., Guy, S. C., & Kenworthy, L. (2000). *Behavior rating inventory of executive function.* Odessa, FL: Psychological Assessment Resources, Inc.

Glascoe, F. P. (2001). *Parent's Evaluation of Developmental Status (PEDS).* Nashville, TN: Ellsworth & Vandermeer Press.

Grunau, R. E., Whitfield, M. F., & Davis, C. (2002). Pattern of learning disabilities in children with extremely low birth weight and broadly average intelligence. *Archives of Pediatric and Adolescent Medicine, 156,* 615–620.

Hack, M., Taylor, H. G., Drotar, D., Schluchter, M., Cartar, L., Andreias, L., et al. (2005). Chronic conditions, functional limitations, and special health care needs of school-aged children born with extremely low-birth-weight in the 1990s. *Journal of the American Medical Association, 294,* 318–325.

Hakansson, S., Farooqi, A., Holmgren, P. A., Serenius, F., & Hogberg, U. (2004). Proactive management promotes outcome in extremely preterm infants:

A population-based comparison of two perinatal management strategies. *Pediatrics*, *114*, 58–64.

Halsey, C. L., Collin, M. F., & Anderson, C. L. (1993). Extremely low birthweight children and their peers: A comparison of preschool performance. *Pediatrics*, *91*, 807–811.

Hintz, S. R., Poole, W. K., Wright, L. L., Fanaroff, A. A., Kendrick, D. E., Laptook, A. R., et al. (2005). Changes in mortality and morbidities among infants born at less than 25 weeks during the post-surfactant era. *Archives of Disease in Children Fetal Neonatal Edition*, *90*, F128–F133.

Holsti, L., Grunau, R. V. E., & Whitfield, M. (2002). Developmental coordination disorder in extremely low birth weight children at nine years. *Journal of Developmental and Behavioral Pediatrics*, *23*, 9–15.

Kesler, S. R., Ment, L. R., Vohr, B., Pajot, S. K., Schneider, K. C., Katz, K. H., et al. (2004). Volumetric analysis of regional cerebral development in preterm children. *Pediatric Neurology*, *31*, 318–325.

Kilbride, H. W., Thorstad, K., & Daily, D. K. (2004). Preschool outcome of less than 801-gram preterm infants compared with full-term siblings. *Pediatrics*, *113*, 742–747.

Lelak, K., Limanowski, J., & Hager-Malecka, B. (1973). A 1-year-old child whose life was preserved after being born with delivery weight of 450 g. *Ginekologia Polska*, *44*, 435–440.

Leosdottir, T., Egilson, S., & Georgsdottir, I. (2005). Performance of extremely low birthweight children at 5 years of age on the Miller assessment for preschoolers. *Physical and Occupational Therapy in Pediatrics*, *25*, 59–72.

Limperopoulos, C., Bassan, H., Gauvreau, K., Robertson, R. L., Jr., Sullivan, N. R., Benson, C. B., et al. (2007). Does cerebellar injury in premature infants contribute to the high prevalence of long-term cognitive, learning, and behavioral disability in survivors? *Pediatrics*, *120*, 584–593.

Lorenz, J. M., Wooliever, D. E., Jetton, J. R., & Paneth, N. (1998). A quantitative review of mortality and developmental disability in extremely premature newborns. *Archives of Pediatric and Adolescent Medicine*, *152*, 425–435.

Lucey, J. F., Rowan, C. A., Shiono, P., Wilkinson, A. R., Kilpatrick, S., Payne, N. R., et al. (2004). Fetal infants: The fate of 4172 infants with birth weights of 401 to 500 grams—the Vermont Oxford Network experience (1996-2000). *Pediatrics*, *113*(6), 1559–1566.

MacDonald, H. (2002). Perinatal care at the threshold of viability. *Pediatrics*, *110*, 1024–1027.

Manly, T., Robertson, I. H., Anderson, V., & Nimmo-Smith, I. (1999). *The Test of Everyday Attention for Children: Manual*. St. Bury Edmunds, UK: Thames Valley Test Company, LTD.

Marlow, N., Hennessy, E., Bracewell, M., & Wolke, D. (2007). Motor and executive function at 6 years of age after extremely preterm birth. *Pediatrics*, *120*, 793–804.

Mikkola, K., Ritari, N., Tommiska, V., Salokorpi, T., Lehtonen, L., Tammela, O., et al. (2005). Neurodevelopmental outcome at 5 years of age of a national cohort of extremely low birth weight infants who were born in 1996-1997. *Pediatrics*, *116*, 1391–1400.

Monro, J. S. (1939). A premature infant weighing less than one pound at birth who survived and developed normally. *Canadian Medical Association Journal*, *40*, 69–70.

Moro, G., & Minoli, I. (1991). Survival with birth weight of less than 500 grams. *Pediatrics*, *87*, 270–271.

Msall, M. E., Phelps, D. L., Hardy, R. J., Dobson, V., Quinn, G. E., Summers, C. G., et al. (2004). Educational and social competencies at 8 years in children with threshold retinopathy of prematurity in the CRYO-ROP multicenter study. *Pediatrics*, *113*, 790–799.

Muraskas, J. K., Hasson, A., & Besinger, R. E. (2004). A girl with a birth weight of 280 g, now 14 years old. *New England Journal of Medicine*, *351*, 836–837.

Muraskas, J. K., Myers, T. F., Lambert, G. H., & Anderson, C. I. (1992). Intact survival of a 280-g infant: An extreme case of growth retardation with normal cognitive development at two years of age. *Acta Paediatria Supplement*, *382*, 16–20.

Nosarti, C., Al-Asady, M. H., Frangou, S., Stewart, A. L., Rifkin, L., & Murray, R. M. (2002). Adolescents who were born very preterm have decreased brain volumes. *Brain*, *125*(Pt. 7), 1616–1623.

Peterson, B. S., Anderson, A. W., Ehrenkranz, R., Staib, L. H., Tageldin, M., Colson, E., et al. (2003). Regional brain volumes and their later neurodevelopmental correlates in term and preterm infants. *Pediatrics*, *111*(5 Pt. 1), 939–948.

Peterson, B. S., Vohr, B. R., Lawrence, H. S., Cannistraci, C. J., Dolberg, A., Schnieder, K. C., et al. (2000). Regional brain volume abnormalities and long-term cognitive outcome in preterm infants. *Journal of the American Medical Association*, *284*, 1939–1947.

Pleasure, J. R., Dhand, M., & Kaur, M. (1984). What is the lower limit of viability? *American Journal of Diseases of Children*, *138*, 783–785.

Reynolds, C., & Kamphaus, R. W. (1998). *Behavior assessment system for children. Parent rating scale*. Circle Pines, MN: American Guidance Services, Inc.

Sauve, R. S., Robertson, C., Etches, P., Byrne, P. J., & Dayer-Zamora, V. (1998). Before viability: A geographically based outcome study of infants weighing

500 grams or less at birth. *Pediatrics, 101*(3 Pt. 1), 438–445.

Schollin, J. (2005). Viewa on neonatal care of newborns weighing less than 500 grams. *Acta Paediatrica, 94*, 140–142.

Stern, Y. (2002). What is cognitive reserve? Theory and research application of the reserve concept. *Journal of the International Neuropsychological Society, 8*, 448–460.

Stewart, A. L., Rifkin, L., Amess, P. N., Kirkbride, V., Townsend, J. P., Miller, D. H., et al. (1999). Brain structure and neurocognitive and behavioural function in adolescents who were born very preterm. *Lancet, 353*(9165), 1653–1657.

Teplin, S. W., Burchinal, M., Johnson-Martin, N., Humphry, R. A., & Kraybill, E. N. (1991). Neurodevelopmental, health, and growth status at age 6 years of children with birth weights less than 1001 grams. *Journal of Pediatrics, 118*, 768–777.

Tiffen, J. (1968). *Purdue Pegboard: Examiner manual.* Chicago: Science Research Associates.

Tommiska, V., Heinonen, K., Kero, P., Pokela, M. L., Tammela, O., Jarvenpaa, A. L., et al. (2003). A national two year follow up study of extremely low birthweight infants born in 1996-1997. *Archives of Disease in Children Fetal Neonatal Edition, 88*, F29–35.

Treyvaud, K., Anderson, V. A., Howard, K., Bear, M., Hunt, R. W., Doyle, L. W., et al. (2009). Parenting behavior is associated with the early neurobehavioral development of very preterm children. *Pediatrics, 123*, 555–561.

Vohr, B. R., Wright, L. L., Dusick, A. M., Perritt, R., Poole, W. K., Tyson, J. E., et al. (2004). Center differences and outcomes of extremely low birth weight infants. *Pediatrics, 113*, 781–789.

Wagner, R. K., Torgesen, J. K., & Rashotte, C. A. (1999). *Examiner's manual: The Comprehensive Test of Phonological Processing.* Austin, TX: PRO-ED, Inc.

Wechsler, D. (2003). *Manual for the Wechsler Intelligence Scale for Children - 4th edition.* San Antonio, TX: The Psychological Corporation.

Whitfield, M. F., Grunau, R. V., & Holsti, L. (1997). Extremely premature (< or = 800 g) schoolchildren: Multiple areas of hidden disability. *Archives of Disease in Children Fetal Neonatal Edition, 77*, F85–F90.

Wilson-Costello, D., Friedman, H., Minich, N., Siner, B., Taylor, G., Schluchter, M., et al. (2007). Improved neurodevelopmental outcomes for extremely low birth weight infants in 2000-2002. *Pediatrics, 119*, 37–45.

Woodward, L. J., Anderson, P., Austin, N. C., Howard, K., & Inder, T. E. (2006). Neonatal MRI to predict neurodevelopmental outcomes in preterm infants. *New England Journal of Medicine, 355*(7), 685–694.

30

Idiopathic Normal Pressure Hydrocephalus

Lisa D. Ravdin and Heather L. Katzen

Idiopathic normal pressure hydrocephalus (INPH) is a progressive adult-onset disorder historically characterized by gait disturbance, urinary incontinence, and dementia, all observed in the context of enlarged cerebral ventricles. The complete symptom triad was once thought to be necessary for diagnosis; however, it is now recognized that symptoms may become clinically evident at various points along a continuum. The initial presentation of INPH can range from subtle disturbances in one or more of the classic features, to the complete symptom triad representing the more severe end of the spectrum (Relkin, Marmarou, Klinge, Bergsneider, & Black, 2005). Idiopathic normal pressure hydrocephalus can be a diagnostic challenge, particularly since changes in gait, urinary control, and mental status are fairly common in older adults and may result from a variety of other underlying causes.

The incidence and prevalence of INPH have not been well documented; however, it has been suggested that that approximately one-half of a percent of the population over age 65 suffers from INPH-related symptoms (Casmiro et al., 1989; Trenkwalder et al., 1995). Age of onset is most commonly in the sixth and seventh decade of life (Boon, Tans, Delwel, Egeler-Peerdeman, Hanlo, Wurzer, et al. 1997; Mori, 2001), and both men and women are equally affected (Marmarou, Bergsneider, Relkin, Klinge, & Black, 2005). No racial predilection has been described. While the pathophysiology is largely unknown, INPH is thought to be primarily related to a defect or imbalance in cerebrospinal fluid (CSF) production or absorption (Levine, 2008). There are no specific neuropathological criteria for postmortem diagnosis, but discrete abnormalities such as arachnoid fibrosis and dural thickening have been reported (Bech, Waldemar, Gjerris, Klinken, & Juhler, 1999), and postmortem studies have also revealed neuritic plaques and neurofibrillary tangles in a significant number of cases (Silverberg, Mayo, Saul, Rubenstein, & McGuire, 2003). Normal pressure hydrocephalus is distinguishable from other forms of hydrocephalus that occur in neonates and young children.

Characteristic Presenting Features of Idiopathic Normal Pressure Hydrocephalus

Gait Disturbance

Gait disturbance is the most common presenting feature of INPH, followed by cognitive dysfunction and urinary symptoms (Boon, 1997; Krauss et al., 2001; Relkin et al., 2005; Weiner, Constantini, Cohen, & Wisoff, 1995). The gait dysfunction in INPH has been described as "magnetic," "glue-footed," "short-stepped," or "shuffling." Characteristic gait features include reduced stride length, decreased foot-floor clearance, wide-based gait, and diminished counter rotation of the shoulders relative to the opposite hip (Stolze et al., 2000). An abnormality in turning, where patients require multiple small steps to turn in place, is also a distinguishing feature. Gait abnormalities are progressive, and many patients eventually require assistance (i.e., walker or wheelchair) for ambulation. Falls are common and are often the impetus for seeking medical attention (Fisher, 1982; Ravdin et al., 2008).

Urinary Symptoms

Urinary incontinence is the least common symptom and has not been well characterized in INPH. It can be difficult to differentiate from other causes of urinary symptoms in older adults such as bladder dystonia/dysautnomia, urinary tract infections, gynecological abnormalities in women, and prostatism in men (Ahlberg, Norlen, Blomstrand, & Wikkelso, 1988; DuBeau, 1996). Frank incontinence is present in fewer than 50% of cases. More commonly, bladder symptoms of increased urgency and urinary frequency are the presenting symptoms, which left untreated, often evolve into frank incontinence. With this in mind, it is important that the clinician probe beyond incontinence when inquiring about urinary symptoms. Fecal incontinence can develop as the disease advances, but it is relatively rare (Relkin et al., 2005).

Cognitive Deficits

The cognitive profile of INPH is characterized primarily by impairments in attention and memory, executive skills, and visuospatial abilities, a pattern consistent with frontal subcortical dysfunction (Bradley, 2000; Caltagirone, Gainotti, Masullo, & Villa, 1982; Iddon et al., 1999; Klinge, Ruckert, Schuhmann, Dorner et al., 2002; Merten, 1999; Thomsen, Borgesen, Bruhn, & Gjerris, 1986; Vanneste, 2000). Memory problems tend to be attributable to reduced acquisition of material as opposed to the rapid forgetting of information often observed in true amnestic disturbances. Visuospatial difficulties may be reflective of, or exacerbated by, executive dysfunction, which manifests as difficulty conceptualizing, organizing, and planning a response. Reaction time and psychomotor speed are also deficient (Klinge, Ruckert, Schuhmann, Berding et al., 2002). In the early stages, frank dementia is relatively rare; the majority of patients typically present with mild to moderate cognitive dysfunction. Identification of INPH is critically important, as it is one of the few treatable causes of cognitive compromise in older adults.

Neuroimaging in Idiopathic Normal Pressure Hydrocephalus

Ventricular enlargement is often interpreted as consistent with INPH, but it can occur as part of the normal aging process or other neurodegenerative conditions. To establish a diagnosis of INPH, ventriculomegaly should be out of proportion to brain atrophy, as determined by a frontal horn ratio greater than 0.3 on brain imaging (Evans, 1937). The frontal horn ratio, or Evan's index, is calculated by dividing the maximal frontal horn ventricular width by the transverse inner diameter of the skull. Brain imaging must also rule out possible obstructions to CSF flow and other pathologies. Additional imaging findings that are characteristic of INPH include increased callosal angle, enlargement of the temporal horns, and expansion of the third ventricle and doming of the lateral ventricle (Bradley, Jr., 2001; Holodny et al., 1998). In addition to routine structural brain imaging (magnetic resonance imaging [MRI] or computed tomography [CT]), several other techniques have been utilized as potential adjunct measures in the diagnosis of INPH, including quantitative diffusion tensor imaging, positron emission tomography (PET), single-photon emission computed tomography (SPECT), SPECT/acetazolamide challenge, proton magnetic resonance spectroscopy, and nuclear cisternography. Presently, none of these techniques are routinely included in the evaluation of suspected INPH.

Differential Diagnosis

Due to the presenting symptoms and progressive course, INPH is often misdiagnosed as other late-life disorders in which cognition and gait are affected, such as Parkinson's disease, Parkinson plus syndromes, Alzheimer's disease, or cerebrovascular disease. Because of the age of the population at risk, comorbidity is the norm, rather than the exception. Differential diagnosis of INPH from other insidious late life movement disorders is arguably the most challenging to clinicians. In the case of INPH, symptom onset is typically bilateral and progressive. A summary of recent evidence-based diagnostic and management guidelines for INPH are provided in Table 30-1. These practice parameters recognize the heterogeneity of INPH presentations and

Table 30-1. Classification of Idiopathic Normal Pressure Hydrocephalus

Probable INPH

I.   *Clinical Findings*: Presentation must include the following:

    a. Gait/balance disturbance consistent with NPH

    b. Impairment in at least one other domain (cognitive decline, urinary symptoms)

    c. Insidious onset with progression of symptoms over time

    d. Onset after 40 years of age

    e. Symptom duration of at least 3 to 6 months

    f. No antecedent neurological, psychiatric, or general medical condition sufficient to explain the presenting symptoms

II. *Neuroimaging Findings*: CT or MRI showing:

    a. Ventricular enlargement not entirely attributable to cerebral atrophy or congenital enlargement

    b. No macroscopic obstruction to CSF flow

    c. At least one of the following supportive features

       1. Enlargement of the temporal horns of the lateral ventricles not solely related to hippocampal atrophy

       2. Callosal angle >40 degrees

       3. Evidence of altered brain water content, including periventricular signal changes (CT/MRI) not attributable to microvascular ischemic changes or demyelination

       4. An aqueductal or fourth ventricular flow void observed on MRI

III. Physiological Findings: CSF opening pressure in the range of 5–18 mm Hg (or 70–245 mm H2O) as determined by a lumbar puncture or a comparable procedure.

Possible INPH

I.   *Clinical Findings*: Presentation must include the following:

    a. Symptoms of either

       1. Urinary incontinence and/or cognitive impairment in the absence of an observable gait disturbance (or)

       2. Gait disturbance or dementia alone

    b. Symptoms may

       1. Be subacute or indeterminate mode of onset

       2. Follow a nonprogressive or not clearly progressive course

       3. Develop at any age after childhood

       4. Have a duration of less than 3 months or undetermined duration

       5. Follow events such as mild head trauma, remote history of intracerebral hemorrhage, or childhood / adolescent meningitis or other conditions that in the judgment of the clinician are not likely to be causally related

       6. Coexist with other neurological, psychiatric, or general medical disorders but in the judgment of the clinician not be entirely attributable to these conditions

II. *Neuroimaging Findings*: Brain imaging (CT or MRI) showing ventricular enlargement consistent with hydrocephalus but associated with either

    a. Evidence of cerebral atrophy sufficient to potentially explain ventricular size (or)

    b. Structural lesions that may influence ventricular size

III. *Physiological Findings*: No opening pressure measurement available or pressure outside the range required for probable INPH

Unlikely INPH

1. No evidence of ventriculomegaly

2. Signs of increased intracranial pressure such as papilledema

3. No component of the clinical triad of INPH is present

4. Symptoms fully explained by other causes (e.g., spinal stenosis)

Note. Details regarding the specific gait, cognitive, and urinary symptoms necessary for the diagnosis are reviewed in detailed elsewhere (Relkin et al., 2005).

CSF, cerebrospinal fluid; CT, computed tomography; INPH, idiopathic normal pressure hydrocephalus; MRI, magnetic resonance imaging.

recommend a classification scheme that groups patients into "probable," "possible," and "unlikely," depending on the presence of characteristic symptoms (Relkin et al., 2005).

Treatment and Prognostic Procedures in Idiopathic Normal Pressure Hydrocephalus

Patients with INPH can be treated by placement of a ventricular shunt that diverts CSF out of the cerebral ventricles. Many patients realize complete and lasting symptom remission following this relatively straightforward neurosurgical procedure; however, overall, response rates vary widely, with estimates from 30% to 96% (Klinge, Marmarou, Bergsneider, Relkin, & Black, 2005). There is also a high degree of morbidity associated with shunt placement (Vanneste, Augustijn, Dirven, Tan, & Goedhart, 1992), including permanent neurological deficits, intracerebral hemorrhage, subdural hemorrhage, meningeal infection, as well as death (Hebb & Cusimano, 2001; Meier, Konig, & Miethke, 2004; Vanneste et al., 1992). Gait is the symptom most likely to improve (Hebb & Cusimano, 2001); however, changes in cognitive function and urinary incontinence have also been documented (Chang, Agarwal, Williams, Rigamonti, & Hillis, 2006; Iddon et al., 1999; Klinge et al., 2005; Raftopoulos et al., 1994; Thomsen et al., 1986). In recent years, shunt technology has advanced with the advent of programmable valves that allow shunt settings to be changed noninvasively, permitting greater optimization of shunt function in correlation with patient symptoms. The potential benefit is that these devices may minimize the need for re-operation and can help reverse adverse outcomes when they occur; however, this has not been systematically studied.

Cerebrospinal fluid drainage procedures, such as the tap test (TT) or external lumbar drainage, are procedures used in an effort to identify good surgical candidates for shunt placement. Clinical improvement following TT with removal of 50 cc of CSF has been shown to have a positive predictive value of 73%–100% (Marmarou, Young et al., 2005). External lumbar drainage (ELD), a procedure in which greater amounts of CSF (100–600 cc) are drained over an extended 24–72-hour period, has been shown to have

better prognostic value with a sensitivity of 50%–100%, a specificity of 60%–100%, and a positive predictive value of 80%–100% (Marmarou, Young et al., 2005; Williams, Razumovsky, & Hanley, 1998). Given that ELD requires hospitalization, is somewhat more invasive, and can be associated with a number of complications such as infection, it is currently done at a limited number of centers, and in some cases is only employed when there is a strong suspicion of INPH despite a negative tap test. In addition to drainage procedures, there are CSF dynamic tests that can be conducted to improve diagnostic accuracy. Cerebrospinal fluid outflow resistance measured via an infusion test, in which change in pressure is determined following injection of several small boluses of saline into the CSF space during a spinal tap, has been shown to improve the sensitivity (57%–100%) and positive predictive value (75%–92%) of the CSF TT (Marmarou, Young et al., 2005). However, these tests require specialized laboratories for proper performance and are not currently available at many centers.

Methods for selecting shunt candidates vary widely between centers, with little consensus regarding the best means to assess response following one of the diagnostic procedures outlined earlier. Clearly, an objective assessment of both gait and cognition is preferable; however, standard of care often consists of the physician's subjective impression of gait change following a diagnostic procedure such as TT or ELD. Neuropsychologists, given their use of behavioral observation in the context of objective standardized assessments, have a specialized skill set that can be of great value in determining responsiveness to diagnostic procedures for NPH, as well as identifying those who may not otherwise be good candidates for shunt surgery (i.e., comorbid dementia, depression, etc). In additional, standardized postsurgical neuropsychological examinations may be useful in providing feedback regarding the extent of improvement following shunt placement.

The Case of W. G.

Background and Referral

W. G. initially presented to a neurologist with complaints of memory problems at the age of 73.

The neurologic exam was remarkable for reduced mental status (mainly attention), decreased naso-labial fold on the left, and mirror movements when performing rapid alternating movements with the right hand. The patient had difficulty with tandem gait, but balance and other aspects of gait were otherwise intact. The neurologist's impression was that the findings were consistent with a frontal systems disturbance most sugges-tive of cerebrovascular disease, but other etiolo-gies needed to be ruled out. An MRI revealed minimal bilateral periventricular white matter changes and enlargement of the lateral ventricles; the image was interpreted as suspicious for nor-mal-pressure hydrocephalus. The patient was referred for a cognitive evaluation to another neuropsychologist where the results found high-average performance across the majority of cognitive domains, with relative weaknesses in organizing and acquiring new information. The exam was interpreted as consistent with mild executive dysfunction. Given the absence of significant balance, gait, and incontinence prob-lems at that time, no further work-up for hydro-cephalus was undertaken. Interval re-examination was advised.

Over the next 3 years, W. G. was followed by the neurologist, and no significant change in his gait was documented. A follow-up neuropsychologi-cal exam conducted by the same neuropsycholo-gist was remarkable for reduced performance on tasks of psychomotor speed and timed sequenc-ing. The working diagnosis was cerebrovascular disease with possible hydrocephalus. Since no change in gait was observed, no further work-up for hydrocephalus was undertaken at that time.

One year later, the patient returned for neuro-logic follow-up exam with complaints of increased unsteadiness and periods of confusion. The neu-rologic exam was remarkable for increasing imbalance as well as reports of three episodes of incontinence. Although the patient had under-gone radical prostatectomy in the remote past, the patient had not experienced any episodes of incontinence until this time. Repeat neuroimag-ing did not indicate any interval change in com-parison to prior scans; ventriculomegaly persisted but appeared stable. Given the change in gait and new episodes of incontinence, the neurologist decided to perform additional diagnostic work-up for NPH. At that time, the patient was referred to

our clinical program for an evaluation of cogni-tion and gait pre and post tap test.

Age of the patient at the time of the referral to our service was 77 years old. In addition to the history described earlier, medical history was remarkable for borderline diabetes (managed by diet), bilateral cataracts, and radical prostatec-tomy (age 71). Family medical history was nota-ble for lung cancer and alcohol dependency in his mother; colon cancer, gout, cerebrovascular disease, and severe depression in his father. The patient's sister was also deceased following a stroke. Psychiatric history was remarkable for periods of anxiety and participation in psycho-therapy at times throughout his adult life.

Social History

The patient obtained a bachelor's degree from an Ivy League university. After working as a writer for many years, he later returned to school for a master's degree in social work. He reported drinking alcohol socially; alcohol dependence was denied. He acknowledged a remote history of tobacco use.

Results of Pre- and Post-Tap Exam

On exam, the patient was fully alert and ori-ented. Spontaneous speech was fluent and infor-mative. There was no evidence of significant word-finding difficulties, paraphasias, or gram-matical errors. Affect was appropriate to situa-tion with a mildly depressed mood. Formal neuropsychological assessment revealed frontal systems dysfunction, which manifested as reduced initiation, decreased acquisition of new material, and deficits on higher level complex attentional tasks. Psychomotor slowing and reduced response speed were observed through-out the exam. The patient endorsed signs and symptoms associated with a mild depression on a self-report measure. In comparison to the neu-ropsychological exam conducted 2 years prior, moderate declines were noted on tests depen-dent on the integrity of executive functions and psychomotor speed.

Approximately 3 hours following the 50 cc tap test, select cognitive measures were readmin-istered, using alternate forms when available. Post-tap testing revealed improved scores on measures of psychomotor speed and manual dexterity. Qualitative improvements were observed as well. Despite inability to complete an alternating sequencing test (Trails B), the patient demonstrated improved mental sequencing and increased response speed. Both simple and more complex motor speed showed clinically significant post-tap improvements. Basic attention continued to be a strength post tap. Measures of complex attention and executive function were unchanged compared to the pre-tap baseline. During a repeat

gait evaluation, the patient demonstrated improved balance and intact retropulsion. Scores on a standardized gait scale improved from pre-tap, as he walked 10 meters in 10 seconds (9 steps) as compared to baseline in which he walked 10 meters in 12 seconds (14 steps). Results of the pre- and post-tap examination are presented in Table 30-2. Collectively, the cognitive and gait evaluation were interpreted as a positive test response. The patient was referred to a neurosurgeon and subsequently underwent VP shunt placement.

Table 30-2. Neuropsychological Test Performance of W. G.

Test Administered	Pre tap	Post tap	One Year post Shunt
Modified Mental Status Exam	26	23	29
Modified Mini Mental (3MS)	86	81	96
DRS	123	NA	135
Attention	37		36
I/P	28		33
Construction	6		6
Conceptualization	35		39
Memory	17		21
Boston Naming Test	49/60	NA	54/60
WAIS-III-Digit Span	13	12	14
No. F	6	6	6
No. B	4	4	4
Scaled score	9	8	9
Symbol Digit	14	17	23
Verbal Fluency			
FAS	12	discontinued	15
Animals	4	11	13
Hopkins Verbal Learning Test-Revised			
Trial 1	1	4	5
Trial 2	4	4	5
Trial 3	4	4	4
Delayed Recall	0	0	0
Cued Recall	1	0	6
Recognition	7	8	12
False positives	4	6	2
Trail-Making Test			
A	118"	82"	45"
B	discontinued	discontinued	185"
Grooved Pegboard			
Right	172"	121"	107"
Left	164"	158"	118"
Line Tracing Test	130"	86"	91"
Serial Dotting Test	70"	73"	63"
Clock Drawing Test	7	NA	10
Gait Scale	8	6	4

Post Shunt

Two weeks post shunt, the neurosurgeon's note indicated that the immediate postoperative period was remarkable for cognitive worsening, but recovery was otherwise uncomplicated. The patient was observed to have improved gait and a mildly depressed affect with mild anxiety. By 1 month post shunt, cognition was improved relative to the early postoperative period but had not returned to baseline. Three months post shunt, the neurologist's note indicated that the patient was more alert and focused; he was observed to be in good spirits and more energetic. His surgical wounds were well healed. Gait was much improved although still "a bit deliberate."

Repeat neuropsychological assessment was conducted 1 year following shunt surgery. The patient reported he did not notice any further decline since his surgery. His mood was reported as good. Results of the post-shunt exam are provided in Table 30-2. On exam, the patient was fully alert and oriented. Overall, he was pleasant and cooperative with testing, but he had periods where he became somewhat disengaged secondary to apparent fatigue. As a result, effort was somewhat inconsistent and, at times, suboptimal. The patient and his wife reported that he had experienced increased independence in activities of daily living, and he had assumed many of the responsibilities for conducting daily errands due to his wife's declining health. The post-shunt exam was remarkable for improvement in gait and cognition, most notably improved balance and psychomotor speed. A significant improvement from initial pre-tap evaluation was observed on a measure of overall generalized cognitive functioning. Detailed testing revealed improvement in confrontation naming, word list learning and recall, semantic fluency, and several measures of motor and psychomotor speed. Despite overall improvement from baseline pre-shunt assessment, mild to moderate executive dysfunction persisted.

Discussion

This is a case of a 77-year-old gentleman who presented with subtle gait changes and mild executive dysfunction. Over a 4-year period, worsening of gait disturbance, progression of cognitive decline, and development of urinary symptoms led to a comprehensive work up for INPH. Following a positive tap test, the patient underwent shunt placement, with subsequent improvement in gait and some aspects of cognitive function maintained at 1 year follow-up. This case illustrates that the symptoms associated with INPH present along a continuum and may evolve over a period of several years. Here, cognitive dysfunction preceded changes in gait and urinary functions. Although a gait disturbance is often the presenting symptom, it is important to remember that some of the earliest descriptions of the disorder included those with only cognitive symptoms early on (Adams, Fisher, Hakim, Ojemann, & Sweet, 1965; Hakim & Adams, 1965). While the diagnosis was not made in this case until the gait symptoms progressed, it is likely that the subtle executive dysfunction observed at the time of the initial neuropsychological evaluation may have been the earliest manifestation of INPH in this patient.

Neuropsychological findings over the 4-year period showed progressive frontal systems functions. Neuroimaging was repeated several times over the years, yet there were no apparent changes in the degree of ventricular enlargement. Despite the absence of radiographic change, progression of cognitive decline and worsening of gait were identified on objective testing, highlighting the contribution of the neuropsychological exam for the diagnosis of INPH. The neuropsychological exam was also valuable in providing information regarding shunt candidacy by quantifying a positive tap test response. Standard of care for determination of tap test response is typically a physician's perception or the family's report of a change in gait; it is rarely evaluated objectively. At our center, we utilize a formal measure adapted from the Dutch hydrocephalus study (Boon, 1997), which is a timed assessment that also rates aspects of gait typically affected in INPH. This scale was described in detail in a recent study examining which aspects of gait were most responsive to the tap test (Ravdin et al., 2008). The scale is not without limitations, and qualitative improvements in gait may be missed by using this scale in isolation. In this case, only a subtle gait change was observed post tap test. It was the improvement in several aspects of information processing speed and executive functions observed on the neuropsychological exam that provided substantive evidence of tap test response. We have found that measures of upper extremity motor speed are helpful predictors in determining tap test responsiveness, particularly in cases where mild changes in gait are difficult to identify on clinical exam (Tsakanikas, Katzen, Ravdin, & Relkin, 2009).

Identifying INPH in older adults is confounded by the high frequency of age-associated changes in gait and balance, mental status, and urinary symptoms that may be present in this population for a variety of different reasons. This gentleman had a history of radical prostectomy; however, his urinary symptoms were interpreted to be unrelated since they occurred many years following the procedure, after a lengthy period of time without any urinary disturbance. The initial working diagnosis for this patient was cerebrovascular disease. The early symptoms of subtle gait disturbance with some mild executive dysfunction could be fully explained by microvascular disease, which was evident on the MRI scan. The clear progression of the dysexecutive syndrome in conjunction with the worsening of gait and new bladder symptoms prompted the further work-up for INPH. The post-tap changes on the standardized neuropsychological exam were critical to the diagnosis and the decision to proceed with shunt.

A common presentation of INPH, as well as many other cognitive disorders in older adults, is that the individual (or family member) reports "memory problems." Cognitive decline is often perceived as and reported as a "memory problem," when in fact, other aspects of cognition are affected. In this case, the difficulties were perceived as memory changes, even though cognitive compromise had more to do with reduced acquisition of material rather than impaired retention. Memory complaints may also be the presenting symptom for visual spatial deficits (reports of difficulty finding their way around familiar places) or language impairment (reports of forgetting names or trouble recalling other words). The astute clinician needs to probe further on clinical interview, obtain corroborating information when available, and perform a detailed assessment to determine the objective nature of the complaints.

Neurobehavioral manifestations of INPH have been described, with depression as perhaps the most commonly occurring symptom.

Patients may also simply *appear* depressed secondary to motor slowing and reduced information processing speed. Post-shunt depression as observed in this gentleman is relatively common in the early postoperative period. Often times, although the patient may demonstrate significant improvements in cognitive functioning post shunt, they may not return to their baseline level of functioning. In this patient, there was the expectation that he would be able to return to driving and work, and his inability to do these things, despite an overall improvement, may have contributed to his persistent mood disturbance.

Idiopathic normal pressure hydrocephalus is often referred to as a "reversible" dementia. Although significant improvement can be realized post shunt, the extent of improvement can be variable, and some degree of cognitive dysfunction may persist. A positive prognosis for shunt response is generally associated with lack of comorbidities, younger age, independence in activities of daily living, shorter duration of symptoms, and mild cognitive decline. Further, a cognitive profile of isolated frontal systems dysfunction, as opposed to signs suggestive of other cortical involvement (i.e., aphasia), is typically associated with better outcome. The case presented here highlights how a formal neuropsychological evaluation can play a key role in both diagnosis and treatment planning of individuals with suspected INPH.

References

Adams, R. D., Fisher, C. M., Hakim, S., Ojemann, R. G., & Sweet, W. H. (1965). Symptomatic occult hydrocephalus with "normal" cerebrospinal-fluid pressure. A treatable syndrome. *New England Journal of Medicine, 273*, 117–126.

Ahlberg, J., Norlen, L., Blomstrand, C., & Wikkelso, C. (1988). Outcome of shunt operation on urinary incontinence in normal pressure hydrocephalus predicted by lumbar puncture. *Journal of Neurology, Neurosurgery and Psychiatry, 51*(1), 105–108.

Bech, R. A., Waldemar, G., Gjerris, F., Klinken, L., & Juhler, M. (1999). Shunting effects in patients with idiopathic normal pressure hydrocephalus; Correlation with cerebral and leptomeningeal biopsy findings. *Acta Neurochirurgica, 141*(6), 633–639.

Boon, A., Tans, J. T., Delwel, E. J., Egeler-Peerdeman, S.M., Hanlo, P.W., Wurzer, J.A.L, et al. (1997).

Dutch normal-pressure hydrocephalus study: Baseline characteristics with emphasis on clinical findings. *European Journal of Neurology, 4*, 39–47.

Bradley, W. G. (2000). Normal pressure hydrocephalus: New concepts on etiology and diagnosis. *American Journal of Neuroradiology, 21*(9), 1586–1590.

Bradley, W. G., Jr. (2001). Diagnostic tools in hydrocephalus. *Neurosurgery Clinics of North America, 12*(4), 661–684, viii.

Caltagirone, C., Gainotti, G., Masullo, C., & Villa, G. (1982). Neurophysiological study of normal pressure hydrocephalus. *Acta Psychiatrica Scandinavia, 65*(2), 93–100.

Casmiro, M., D'Alessandro, R., Cacciatore, F. M., Daidone, R., Calbucci, F., & Lugaresi, E. (1989). Risk factors for the syndrome of ventricular enlargement with gait apraxia (idiopathic normal pressure hydrocephalus): A case-control study. *Journal of Neurology, Neurosurgery and Psychiatry, 52*(7), 847–852.

Chang, S., Agarwal, S., Williams, M. A., Rigamonti, D., & Hillis, A. E. (2006). Demographic factors influence cognitive recovery after shunt for normal-pressure hydrocephalus. *Neurologist, 12*(1), 39–42.

DuBeau, C. (1996). Interpreting the effect of common medical conditions on voiding dysfunction in the elderly. *Urologic Clinics of North America, 23*(1), 11–18.

Evans, W. A. (1942). An encephalographic ratio for estimating ventricular enlargement and cerebral atrophy. *Archives of Neurology and Psychiatry, 47*, 931–937.

Fisher, C. M. (1982). Hydrocephalus as a cause of disturbances of gait in the elderly. *Neurology, 32*(12), 1358–1363.

Hakim, S., & Adams, R. D. (1965). The special clinical problem of symptomatic hydrocephalus with normal cerebrospinal fluid pressure. Observations on cerebrospinal fluid hydrodynamics. *Journal of the Neurological Sciences, 2*(4), 307–327.

Hebb, A. O., & Cusimano, M. D. (2001). Idiopathic normal pressure hydrocephalus: A systematic review of diagnosis and outcome. *Neurosurgery, 49*(5), 1166–1184.

Holodny, A. I., Waxman, R., George, A. E., Rusinek, H., Kalnin, A. J., & de Leon, M. (1998). MR differential diagnosis of normal-pressure hydrocephalus and Alzheimer disease: Significance of perihippocampal fissures. *American Journal of Neuroradiology, 19*(5), 813–819.

Iddon, J. L., Pickard, J. D., Cross, J. J., Griffiths, P. D., Czosnyka, M., & Sahakian, B. J. (1999). Specific patterns of cognitive impairment in patients with idiopathic normal pressure hydrocephalus and Alzheimer's disease: A pilot study. *Journal of Neurology, Neurosurgery and Psychiatry, 67*(6), 723–732.

Klinge, P., Marmarou, A., Bergsneider, M., Relkin, N., & Black, P. M. (2005). Outcome of shunting in idiopathic normal-pressure hydrocephalus and the value of outcome assessment in shunted patients. *Neurosurgery, 57*(Suppl. 3), S40–S52.

Klinge, P., Ruckert, N., Schuhmann, M., Berding, G., Brinker, T., Knapp, W. H., et al. (2002). Neuropsychological sequels to changes in global cerebral blood flow and cerebrovascular reserve capacity after shunt treatment in chronic hydrocephalus: A quantitative PET-study. *Acta Neurochirurgica Supplementum, 81*, 55–57.

Klinge, P., Ruckert, N., Schuhmann, M., Dorner, L., Brinker, T., & Samii, M. (2002). Neuropsychological testing to improve surgical management of patients with chronic hydrocephalus after shunt treatment. *Acta Neurochirurgica Supplementum, 81*, 51–53.

Krauss, J. K., Faist, M., Schubert, M., Borremans, J. J., Lucking, C. H., & Berger, W. (2001). Evaluation of gait in normal pressure hydrocephalus before and after shunting. *Advanced Neurology, 87*, 301–310.

Levine, D. N. (2008). Intracranial pressure and ventricular expansion in hydrocephalus: Have we been asking the wrong question? *Journal of the Neurological Sciences, 269*(1–2), 1–11.

Marmarou, A., Bergsneider, M., Relkin, N., Klinge, P., & Black, P. M. (2005). Development of guidelines for idiopathic normal-pressure hydrocephalus: Introduction. *Neurosurgery, 57*(Suppl. 3), S1–S3.

Marmarou, A., Young, H. F., Aygok, G. A., Sawauchi, S., Tsuji, O., Yamamoto, T., et al. (2005). Diagnosis and management of idiopathic normal-pressure hydrocephalus: A prospective study in 151 patients. *Journal of Neurosurgery, 102*(6), 987–997.

Meier, U., Konig, A., & Miethke, C. (2004). Predictors of outcome in patients with normal-pressure hydrocephalus. *European Neurology, 51*(2), 59–67.

Merten, T. (1999). Neuropsychologie des Normaldruckhydrozephalus. *Nervenarzt, 70*(6), 496–503.

Mori, K. (2001). Management of idiopathic normal-pressure hydrocephalus: A multi-institutional study conducted in Japan. *Journal of Neurosurgery, 95*(6), 970–973.

Raftopoulos, C., Deleval, J., Chaskis, C., Leonard, A., Cantraine, F., Desmyttere, F., et al. (1994). Cognitive recovery in idiopathic normal pressure hydrocephalus: A prospective study. *Neurosurgery, 35*(3), 397–404.

Ravdin, L. D., Katzen, H. L., Jackson, A. E., Tsakanikas, D., Assuras, S., & Relkin, N. R. (2008). Features of gait most responsive to tap test in normal pressure hydrocephalus. *Clinical Neurology and Neurosurgery, 110*(5), 455–461.

Relkin, N., Marmarou, A., Klinge, P., Bergsneider, M., & Black, P. M. (2005). Diagnosing idiopathic normal-pressure hydrocephalus. *Neurosurgery*, 57(Suppl. 3), S4–S16.

Silverberg, G. D., Mayo, M., Saul, T., Rubenstein, E., & McGuire, D. (2003). Alzheimer's disease, normal-pressure hydrocephalus, and senescent changes in CSF circulatory physiology: A hypothesis. *Lancet Neurol*, 2(8), 506–511.

Stolze, H., Kuhtz-Buschbeck, J. P., Drucke, H., Johnk, K., Diercks, C., Palmie, S., et al. (2000). Gait analysis in idiopathic normal pressure hydrocephalus–which parameters respond to the CSF tap test? *Clinical Neurophysiology*, 111(9), 1678–1686.

Thomsen, A. M., Borgesen, S. E., Bruhn, P., & Gjerris, F. (1986). Prognosis of dementia in normal-pressure hydrocephalus after a shunt operation. *Annals of Neurology*, 20(3), 304–310.

Trenkwalder, C., Schwarz, J., Gebhard, J., Ruland, D., Trenkwalder, P., Hense, H. W., et al. (1995). Starnberg trial on epidemiology of Parkinsonism and hypertension in the elderly. Prevalence of Parkinson's disease and related disorders assessed by a door-to-door survey of inhabitants older than 65 years. *Archives of Neurology*, 52(10), 1017–1022.

Tsakanikas, D., Katzen, H.L., Ravdin, L.D., & Relkin, N.R. (2009). Upper extremity motor measures of tap test response in normal pressure hydrocephalus, *Clinical Neurology and Neurosurgery*, Nov: 111 (9): 752-7.

Vanneste, J. A. (2000). Diagnosis and management of normal-pressure hydrocephalus. *Journal of Neurology*, 247(1), 5–14.

Vanneste, J., Augustijn, P., Dirven, C., Tan, W. F., & Goedhart, Z. D. (1992). Shunting normal-pressure hydrocephalus: do the benefits outweigh the risks? A multicenter study and literature review. *Neurology*, 42(1), 54–59.

Weiner, H. L., Constantini, S., Cohen, H., & Wisoff, J. H. (1995). Current treatment of normal-pressure hydrocephalus: Comparison of flow- regulated and differential-pressure shunt valves. *Neurosurgery*, 37(5), 877–884.

Williams, M. A., Razumovsky, A. Y., & Hanley, D. F. (1998). Comparison of Pcsf monitoring and controlled CSF drainage diagnose normal pressure hydrocephalus. *Acta Neurochirurgica Supplementum*, 71, 328–330.

31

A Case of Childhood Lead Poisoning

Marsha J. Nortz and M. Douglas Ris

Lead is the most abundant heavy metal in the earth's crust. Since antiquity, it has been used to sweeten wine, as medicine, for lead type, in plumbing, in ceramics, and in make-up. Humans have long been aware of the toxic properties of lead, yet we have paradoxically found ingenious ways to increase rather than decrease lead use and exposure. Indeed, the industrial revolution resulted in a tremendous increase in human exposure to lead. It was not until the elimination of lead in gasoline and paint in the United States that population lead exposure decreased dramatically.

Current Exposure Levels in the United States

Screening data from the late 1960s and early 1970s showed that 20%–40% of children had blood lead (PbB) $\geq$ 40 µg/dL (Bernard & McGeehin, 2003). The Third National Health and Nutrition Examination Survey (NHANES III) Phase 1 data (1988–1991) showed a decline to a mean of 3.6 µg/dL for children between 1 and 5 years of age, and NHANES III Phase 2 (1991–1994) showed a further decline to 2.7 µg/dL.

Despite these data evidencing overall declines, higher exposures continue in subpopulations. While the overall prevalence of PbB $\geq$ 5 µg/dL is 25% (most <10 µg/dL), there are huge disparities across ethnic groups. For non-Hispanic black children this rate was 46.8%; for Hispanic children it was 27.9%; and for non-Hispanic white children it was 18.7%. Overall, non-Hispanic black children are seven times more likely than non-Hispanic white children to have PbB in the 10–20 µg/dL range, data that have disturbing social justice implications given evidence of developmental risks at even lower levels of exposure than these (Dilworth-Bart & Moore, 2006). Lanphear et al. (2005) pooled data from seven large international studies and found adverse effects of lead levels below 10 µg/dL on the intelligence quotient (IQ). Moreover, the dose–response curve was steeper below this level than above it. This calls into question whether, from a public health standpoint, any level of exposure is without risk.

As of 1991, the Centers for Disease Control and Prevention (CDC) action level declined from PbB levels of 60 µg/dL to 10 µg/dL. Recommendations for pediatric practice are that PbB levels in the 10–20 µg/dL range be monitored every 3 to 4 months, with concomitant efforts to decrease exposure and insure sufficient dietary intake of calcium and iron. PbB levels over 20–44 µg/dL are monitored more frequently, and, while oral chelation can be considered, it is not recommended by the American Academy of Pediatrics until PbB levels reach the 45–69 µg/dL range. PbB levels >69 µg/dL are rare and, when they occur, are considered a medical emergency usually resulting in obvious encephalopathy.

Modern Era of Lead Research

In 1979 Herbert N. Needleman published a landmark study in the *New England Journal of Medicine* showing a relationship between dentine lead levels in deciduous teeth and IQ (Needleman et al., 1979). Soon after, several international prospective longitudinal studies (Boston [Bellinger, Stiles, & Needleman, 1992], Cincinnati [Dietrich, Succop, Berger, Hammond, & Bornschein, 1991], Kosovo [Wasserman et al., 1997], and Port Pirie [Baghurst et al., 1992]) were launched. These studies represented a scope and level of scientific rigor previously unparalleled in research on lead effects. Over three decades, these and other studies produced a wealth of data indicating the following: *(1)* long-term effects of lead on intelligence are measurable; *(2)* these effects appear to be more related to post- rather than prenatal exposure; *(3)* there is no distinct "behavioral signature" of lead; *(4)* effect size falls in the range of .25 IQ points per μg/dL increase in blood lead (PbB).

Despite the convergence of data leading to these conclusions in the literature, a discussion of the neurobehavioral effects of lead would not be complete without due mention of the related controversy. Claire Ernhart has been the most persistent in pointing out troublesome inconsistencies across studies: "In view of the methodological limitations we may never be able to say with certainty that low-level lead exposure has adverse effects…if there is an effect…it is small" (Ernhart, 1995, p. 231). Bellinger has countered that complete uniformity of findings is not to be expected and that scientists must consider the role of *effect modification*

(Bellinger, 2000). It has been further asserted by Ris (2003) that modeling lead effects on development will likely require conceptions of causality that are more complex, such as Gottlieb's notion of "probabilistic epigenesis," which proposes that bidirectional genetic, neural, behavioral, and environmental factors have an overall *probabilistic* effect over the course of development (Gottlieb, 1992).

The small effect sizes found in developmental lead research have also been questioned on the basis that fractions of an IQ point are nonsensical (Kaufman, 2001). Yet, from a population perspective, small effects can have significant impact on human health, whether it be small changes in ultraviolet light influencing rates of skin cancer or, as pointed out by Nation and Gleaves (2001), small changes in adiposity affecting rates of heart disease and Type II diabetes.

Biologic Plausibility

One of the criteria for establishing a causal relationship is biologic plausibility, that is, there has to be some reasonable biological mechanism by which the toxicant can exert the putative effect (Hill, 1965). While specific mechanisms of action in humans are still being investigated, enough is known about the physiologic effects of lead on the body and nervous system to draw a plausible connection (Figure 31-1). Many of these effects

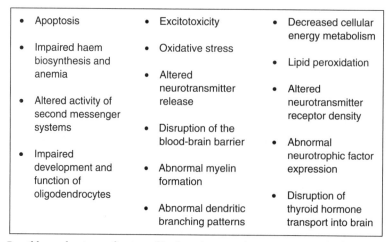

- Apoptosis

- Impaired haem biosynthesis and anemia

- Altered activity of second messenger systems

- Impaired development and function of oligodendrocytes

- Excitotoxicity

- Oxidative stress

- Altered neurotransmitter release

- Disruption of the blood-brain barrier

- Abnormal myelin formation

- Abnormal dendritic branching patterns

- Decreased cellular energy metabolism

- Lipid peroxidation

- Altered neurotransmitter receptor density

- Abnormal neurotrophic factor expression

- Disruption of thyroid hormone transport into brain

Figure 31-1. Possible mechanisms of action of lead on the central nervous system (Lidsky & Schneider, 2003).

are associated with the chemical similarity of lead to calcium and the competition in physiologic pathways between the two.

Modern imaging methodologies have been used to investigate the biological effect of lead on brain structure and function. Stewart et al. (2006) has shown an association between cumulative lead dose in industrial exposure and structural lesions on magnetic resonance imaging (MRI). Yuan et al. (2006) reported a relationship between early lead exposure and atypical activation patterns on functional magnetic resonance imaging (fMRI). In an overlapping sample, Cecil et al. (2008) have shown an inverse relationship between brain volume measures and early exposure to lead.

One can also consider the evolutionary plausibility of adverse developmental effects of lead. Given the ubiquity of lead in the earth's crust, how plausible is it that humans would be so highly vulnerable to this toxicant, particularly at the low levels (<10 µg/dL) cited earlier? Would not humans have evolved mechanisms to mitigate the deleterious effects of lead? Yet we know from prehistoric human remains and samples taken from the polar ice cap that levels of lead in the environment during human evolution were exquisitely low (Flegal & Smith, 1992), obviating the need to evolve a defense against this substance that has no known biologic purpose. Thus, even the lower exposure levels today are many times greater than those to which our prehistoric ancestors were exposed.

Neurobehavioral Phenotype of Lead

Diverse effects of lead on the development of children have been reported, including effects on executive, visuospatial, motor, language, and other functions (Canfield, Kreher, Cornwell, & Henderson, 2003; Coscia, Ris, Succop, & Dietrich, 2003; Lidsky & Schneider, 2006). The most commonly reported outcome index has been IQ, with exposure increase from 10–20 µg/dL being associated with a 2–3 point "loss" in IQ (Schwartz, 1994). This literature does not indicate a distinct "lead phenotype" or "behavioral signature." Rather, degree and nature of effects are likely moderated by a host of subject factors (e.g., age) and ecological factors (e.g.,

exposure type and patterns). Nevertheless, certain deficits may be seen at higher rates in lead-exposed children, but they may not necessarily be present in the majority of such children nor specific to lead exposure.

While most of the research on the developmental effects of lead has focused on effects on cognition (most commonly IQ), there has long been recognition that effects can also be seen on behavioral measures (Byers & Lord, 1943). More recently, this includes the Philadelphia Collaborative Perinatal Project Survey (Denno, 1990), in which the strongest predictor of criminality was a history of lead exposure. Furthermore, studies have shown that adjudicated delinquents have significantly higher bone lead than controls (Needleman, Mcfarland, Ness, Fienberg, & Tobin, 2002), and the connection between early lead exposure and later risk of criminal behavior remains after correction for potential confounding variables (Wright et al., 2008). Historical records have reflected a connection between rates of both unwed pregnancy and violent crime and lead production in the United States and in other countries (Nevin, 2000, 2007). Elevations on certain scales of the Child Behavior Checklist are significantly associated with PbB (Needleman, Riess, Tobin, Biesecker, & Greenhouse, 1996).

The Case of A. M.

A. M. was a 14-year-old, Caucasian female who was the product of a pregnancy and birth history that was unremarkable with the exception of maternal tobacco use unassociated with prematurity or low birth weight. Early medical history was remarkable for an elevated lead level of 41 µg/dL documented at age 14 months secondary to residential exposure. No oral chelation was recommended, but residential lead abatement was ordered by the State Department of Health. Lead levels thereafter declined but remained mildly above recommended levels through age 4 years (Figure 31-2). Medical history was otherwise remarkable for mild anemia, and medical records indicated poor compliance with iron supplementation due to undesirable side effects.

Despite developmental risk in the context of lead exposure, A. M.'s developmental milestones were reportedly met within normal timeframes.

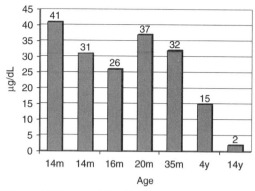

Figure 31-2. A. M.'s lead levels over time (m = months; y = years)

Family interview identified no academic concerns during preschool through the first grade, but subsequent onset of academic difficulties led to repetition of the second grade. Grades were thereafter below average throughout A. M.'s elementary school education. No formal interventions were implemented within the school setting, but A. M. did attend summer school during several summer breaks.

At the time of this evaluation, A. M. was completing the eighth grade in a public school setting. Family report and academic records documented grades that were below average to failing, and particular concerns were documented in reading and writing. Parents had recently completed paperwork to initiate a school-based evaluation to determine eligibility for services. A. M.'s more recent school history was remarkable for frequent school absences due to anemia-related lethargy and other illnesses. Parents also suspected low motivation toward school as a contributor to these absences. A. M. herself reported a significant amount of peer teasing in the school setting.

A. M.'s mental health history was remarkable for diagnosed depression and associated suicidal gestures. Ongoing concerns of lethargy, moodiness, and sadness were reported by the family. A. M. had briefly participated in psychotherapy for approximately 3–4 months prior to this evaluation, but therapy was discontinued by family due to limited rapport with the treating professional.

A. M. lived with her biological parents and younger sister (age 13). Parents each completed high school. A. M.'s father was employed as a laborer, and her mother was a homemaker at the time of this evaluation. There is no known family history of learning disability or other developmental disorder. In fact, A. M.'s sister was maintaining above-average grades. Family history was significant for depression and bipolar disorder.

Examination Results

A. M.'s clinical evaluation was requested to delineate her neuropsychological strengths and weaknesses, as well as to assist in appropriate intervention planning. This evaluation was not performed for forensic purposes or to directly address questions of causality, as can often be the case for neuropsychological referrals following childhood lead exposure. Since there is no distinct behavioral phenotype of childhood lead exposure, a broad battery of neuropsychological tests was designed with the goals of assessing areas at known risk following lead exposure, areas considered at risk given A. M.'s personal history, and screening remaining domains to ensure a complete assessment to address the referral questions. Test scores are reported in Tables 31-1, 31-2, and 31-3.

A. M. presented as a shy young lady. Affect remained restricted in range throughout the full-day testing session. She did not typically initiate conversation, but she responded appropriately

Table 31-1. Intelligence and Academic Achievement Scores Based upon Age for A. M.

Test	Standard Score (mean = 100, SD = 15)
WISC-IV	
Verbal Comprehension Index	85
Perceptual Reasoning Index	96
Working Memory Index	88
Processing Speed Index	100
Full Scale IQ	89
WIAT-II	
Word Reading	79 (84)
Spelling	89 (87)
Numerical Operations	94 (93)

Note. Grade-based scores are provided in parentheses for academic skill areas.

WIAT-II, Wechsler Individual Achievement Test–II; WISC-IV, Wechsler Intelligence Scale for Children–IV.

Table 31-2. Additional Neuropsychological Test Scores for A. M.

Test	Standard Score (mean = 100, SD = 15)
Rey-Osterreith Complex Figure Test	
Copy	77–81 range
Immediate Recall	93
Delayed Recall	97
Recognition Total Correct	93
Children's Memory Scale	
Stories Immediate Recall	95
Stories Delayed Recall	95
Stories Recognition Memory	85
Word Lists Learning	95
Word Lists Delayed Recall	105
Word Lists Recognition Memory	100
Delis-Kaplan Executive Function System Trail-Making Test	
Visual Scanning	90
Number Sequencing	90
Letter Sequencing	95
Number Letter Switching	100
Motor Speed	110
Delis-Kaplan Executive Function System Color Word Interference	
Color Naming	85
Word Reading	80
Inhibition	90
Inhibition/Switching	110
Delis-Kaplan Executive Function System Letter Fluency	120
Wisconsin Card Sorting Test	
Total Errors	69
Perseverative Responses	100
Perseverative Errors	98
Nonperseverative Errors	57
Grooved Pegboard	
Dominant (Right) Hand	87
Nondominant Hand	116

to the questions posed by the examiner. Her expressive and receptive language appeared age-appropriate during conversational interactions. A. M. was cooperative and appeared to exert appropriate effort throughout the testing session. However, she appeared to lack confidence and required encouragement to take guesses and persevere in the face of challenge. A. M. also appeared to have mild difficulty with focused and sustained attention at the end of the morning testing session as well as again in the afternoon session following a lunch break. No motor abnormalities were noted upon gross observation.

Overall, the test results were considered to be valid.

With respect to intellectual and academic functioning, A. M. generally performed in the low-average to average range. Her pattern of intellectual functioning was remarkable for a relative strength on component measures of visual scanning/psychomotor speed. Academic achievement was generally commensurate with intellectual functioning, though age-based word reading skills were in the borderline normative range. Due to A. M.'s history of grade retention, however, grade-based scores were calculated and were notable for

Table 31-3. Parent and Teacher Ratings of A. M.'s Daily Functioning on Behavioral Inventories.

Behavioral Inventory	Parent Standard Score (mean = 100, SD = 15)	Teacher Standard Score (mean = 100, SD = 15)
BASC-2		
Hyperactivity	94	109
Aggression	108	98
Conduct Problems	112	108
Anxiety	100	88
Depression	119	88
Somatization	112	121
Atypicality	119	96
Withdrawal	121	85
Attention Problems	106	121
Learning Problems	N/A	110
Social Skills	138	111
Leadership	124	121
Study Skills	N/A	117
BRIEF		
Inhibit	116	115
Shift	128	100
Emotional Control	134	108
Initiate	98	127
Working Memory	132	136
Plan/Organize	96	137
Organization of Materials	96	113
Monitor	110	108

Note. Higher standard scores indicate greater clinical symptomatology.

BASC-2, Behavior Assessment System for Children-2; BRIEF, Behavior Rating Inventory of Executive Function.

low-average performance in reading and spelling, consistent with her related difficulty in speeded naming of colors and words on the Delis-Kaplan Executive Function System (D-KEFS). Despite her eighth grade placement at the time of evaluation, reading and spelling grade equivalencies were around the mid-fifth to sixth grade level.

Broader neuropsychological functioning was largely consistent with A. M.'s intellectual functioning. Specifically, her performance was average to low average across measures of verbal and visual reasoning, verbal and visual learning and memory, working memory, and visual scanning/sequencing. A. M.'s expressive verbal fluency was an area of significant strength for her age and overall neuropsychological profile.

Although A. M.'s performance on a measure of complex visuospatial construction requiring her to copy a complex geometric figure (Rey-Osterrieth Complex Figure Test) was mildly impaired compared to test norms, qualitative inspection of her performance identified no significant visuospatial distortion but rather mild visuomotor imprecision of detail placement that led to score reductions. Interestingly, although fine motor dexterity and speed were intact bilaterally, she did not demonstrate the expected degree of dominant hand advantage on a grooved pegboard task, and performance on this task was also remarkable for one peg drop with each hand.

A. M. demonstrated her most significant area of neuropsychological impairment on tasks assessing the executive functions of problem solving and concept formation. Parent and teacher ratings of A. M.'s everyday executive functioning on the Behavior Rating Inventory of Executive Function (BRIEF) provided corroborating evidence of weaknesses in executive functioning. That is, both raters endorsed clinically significant concerns regarding everyday working memory skills. Teacher's ratings provided evidence of additional metacognitive impairments in planning, strategizing, and self-initiation as well as related but mild symptoms of inattention through her ratings on the Behavior Assessment System for Children-2 (BASC-2).

A. M.'s mood regulation and depression were additional areas of clinical concern identified in the course of her evaluation. Parent ratings identified clinically significant concerns regarding emotional control and cognitive/behavioral flexibility. Similarly, parent ratings on the BASC-2 reflected mild concerns of mood dysregulation, whereas teacher ratings identified no mood concerns other than mild somatization. A. M. herself, however, rated clinically significant levels of overall depression on the Children's Depression Inventory (Standard Score = 154). Specifically, she endorsed items reflecting significant negativity, low self-esteem, and interpersonal problems. She also endorsed suicidal thoughts that, upon further interview, were determined to be without associated plan or current intent to harm herself.

Discussion

Although A. M.'s evaluation clearly identified neurocognitive and emotional concerns in need of intervention, it was not possible to definitively state that her deficits were conclusively and exclusively related to her early lead exposure. Certainly, A. M.'s peak levels of exposure at and around age 2 years were above both the CDC cutoff and the level at which developmental risk has been demonstrated in the literature. However, as argued by Hebben (2001), the neuropsychologist must avoid the logical fallacy of causally relating one event to a preceding event based solely upon their temporal relationship. Because the lead literature has yet to demonstrate a clear, behavioral phenotype of low-level lead exposure, a linear dose–response relationship, or a consistent effect of timing of low-level lead exposure on IQ, neuropsychologists must be cautious about drawing such a conclusion in their clinical work. The need for caution is further highlighted by the small amount of variance in cognitive outcome (i.e., IQ) accounted for by lead exposure relative to that accounted for by covariates such as heritability, parenting, and social factors.

For A. M., we concluded that her history of lead exposure was one risk factor for the areas of neurocognitive impairment and academic difficulty reflected in her evaluation. Her overall intellectual functioning was mildly below population norms, and her family history, including the strong performance of her sister in the same educational system, is suggestive of functioning closer to the population mean rather than functioning that is largely low average. The fact that her greatest neurocognitive risk was in the area of executive functioning is certainly consistent with a model of specific brain insult, in that complex skills such as these are particularly sensitive to more subtle insult. However, several other factors were also believed to impact A. M.'s functioning over time, consistent with the concept of "probabilistic epigenesis." These factors included her significant depression, poor motivation and lethargy, history of school absenteeism, and lack of educational interventions for her early academic problems. Her mood disorder itself was likely multidetermined in the context of her family history of mood disorder but also the secondary impact of her academic and social difficulties.

Recommendations were formulated to address the multiple areas of risk identified. Most urgently, A. M. and her family were referred for psychotherapy services to address her mood disorder, with services to address both her emotional coping as well as risk management of suicidal ideation. Family education regarding risk management was provided, as was a safety plan. Additional instruction in behavioral management strategies to facilitate school attendance and motivation as well as adherence to anemia treatments was offered. Monitoring for the emergence of externalizing behavior problems was recommended, as A. M.'s combination of lead exposure, academic and broader neurocognitive risks, depression, and social risks were considered to place her at higher risk for such concerns.

Academically, educational interventions were discussed, including recommendations for implementation of an Individual Education Program (IEP) given her academic performance that fell below grade level and additional risks associated with her executive dysfunction and depression. Given the mild level of impairment, regular education instruction was considered appropriate, supplemented with "pull out" intervention and additional accommodations for language arts and organizational skills.

Summary

Overall, the large body of research in the area of childhood lead exposure provides a rich scientific context upon which clinicians can and should draw. However, extrapolation from research studying large groups to individual patients can be problematic, particularly with exposures at the lower end of the scale and smaller effect sizes, and in the context of other developmental risk factors (e.g., poverty). Scientific findings must be combined with clinical acumen to address such questions.

References

Baghurst, P. A., McMichael, A. J., Wigg, N. R., Vimpani, G. V., Robertson, E. F., Roberts, R. J., et al. (1992). Environmental exposure to lead and children's intelligence at the age of seven years. The Port Pirie Cohort Study. *New England Journal of Medicine, 327*(18), 1279–1284.

Bellinger, D. C. (2000). Effect modification in epidemiologic studies of low-level neurotoxicant exposures and health outcomes. *Neurotoxicology Teratology, 22*(1), 133–140.

Bellinger, D., Stiles, K., & Needleman, H. (1992). Low-level lead exposure, intelligence, and academic achievement: A long-term follow-up study. *Pediatrics, 90*, 855–861.

Bernard, S. M., & McGeehin, M. A. (2003). Prevalence of blood lead levels ≥ 5 μg/dL among US children 1 to 5 years of age and socioeconomic and demographic factors associated with blood lead levels 5 to 10 μg/dL, Third National Health and Nutrition Examination Survey, 1988-1994. *Pediatrics, 112*, 1308–1313.

Byers, R. K., & Lord, E. E. (1943). Late effects of lead poisoning on mental development. *American Journal of Diseases of Children, 66*, 471–494.

Canfield, R. L., Kreher, D. A., Cornwell, C., & Henderson, C. R. (2003). Low level lead exposure, executive functioning, and learning in early childhood. *Child Neuropsychology, 9*, 35–53.

Cecil, K. M., Brubaker, C. J., Adler, C. M., Dietrich, K. M., Altaye, M., Egelhoff, J. C., Wessel, S., Elangovan, I., Hornung, R., Jarvis, K. & Lanphear, B. P. (2008). Decreased brain volume in adults with childhood lead exposure. *PLoS Medicine, 5*, 0741–0750.

Coscia, J. M., Ris, M. D., Succop, P. A., & Dietrich, K. N., (2003). Cognitive development of lead exposed children from ages 6 to 15 years: An application of growth curve analysis. *Child Neuropsychology, 9*, 10–21.

Denno, D. (1990). *Biology and violence: From birth to adulthood.* New York: Cambridge University Press.

Dietrich, K. N, Succop, P. A., Berger, O., Hammond, P. B., & Bornschein, R. L. (1991). Lead exposure and the cognitive development of urban preschool children: The Lead Study cohort at age 4 years. *Neurotoxicology and Teratology, 13*, 203–211.

Dilworth-Bart, J., & Moore, C. F. (2006). Mercy mercy me: Social injustice and the prevention of environmental pollutant exposures among ethnic minority and poor children. *Child Development, 77*, 247–265.

Ernhart, C. B. (1995). Inconsistencies in the lead-effects literature exist and cannot be explained by "effect modification." *Neurotoxicology Teratology, 17*, 227–233; 249–251.

Flegal, A. R., & Smith, D. R. (1992). Lead levels in pre-industrial humans. *New England Journal of Medicine, 326*, 1293–1294.

Gottlieb, G. (1992). *Individual development and evolution: The genesis of novel behavior.* New York: Oxford University Press.

Hebben, N. (2001). Low lead levels and neuropsychological assessment: Let us not be misled. *Archives of Clinical Neuropsychology, 16*, 353–357.

Hill, A. B. (1965). Environment and disease: Association or causation? *Proceedings of the Royal Society of Medicine, 58*, 295–300.

Kaufman, A. S. (2001). Do low levels of lead produce IQ loss in children? A careful examination of the literature. *Archives of Clinical Neuropsychology, 16*, 303–341.

Lanphear, B. P., Hornung, R., Khoury, J., Yolton, K., Baghurst, P., Bellinger, D. C., et al. (2005). Low environmental lead exposure and children's intellectual function: An international pooled analysis. *Environmental Health Perspective, 113*, 894–899.

Lidsky, T. I., & Schneider, J. S. (2006). Adverse effects of childhood lead poisoning: The clinical neuropsychological perspective. *Environment Research, 100*, 284–293.

Nation, J. R., & Gleaves, D. H. (2001). Low-level lead exposure and intelligence in children. *Archives of Clinical Neuropsychology, 16*, 375–388.

Needleman, H. L., Gunnoe, C., Leviton, A., Reed, R., Peresie, H., Maher, C., et al. (1979). Deficits in psychologic and classroom performance of children with elevated dentine lead levels. *New England Journal of Medicine, 300*, 689–695.

Needleman, H. L., Mcfarland, C., Ness, R. B., Fienberg, S. E., & Tobin, M. J. (2002). Bone lead levels in adjudicated delinquents: A case-control study. *Neurotoxicology and Teratology, 24*, 711–717.

Needleman, H. L., Riess, J. A., Tobin, M. J., Biesecker, G. E., & Greenhouse, J. B. (1996). Bone lead levels and delinquent behavior. *Journal of the American Medical Association*, *275*, 363–369.

Nevin, R. (2000). How lead exposure relates to temporal changes in IQ, violent crime, and unwed pregnancy. *Environmental Research*, *83*, 1–22.

Nevin, R. (2007). Understanding international crime trends: The legacy of preschool lead exposure. *Environmental Research*, *104*, 315–336.

Ris, M. D. (2003). Casual inference in lead research: Introduction to the special section on the neurobehavioral effects of environment lead. *Child Neuropsychology*, *9*, 1–9.

Schwartz, J. (1994). Low-level lead exposure and children's IQ: A meta-analysis and search for a threshold. *Environmental Research*, *65*, 42–55.

Stewart, W. F., Schwartz, B. S., Davatzikos, C., Shen, D., Liu, D., Wu, X., et al. (2006). Past adult lead exposure is linked to neurodegeneration measured by brain MRI. *Neurology*, *66*, 1476–1484.

Wasserman, G. A., Liu, X., Lolacono, N. J., Factor-Litvak, P., Kline, J. K., Popovac, D., et al. (1997). Lead exposure and intelligence in 7-year old children: The Yugoslavia Prospective Study. *Environmental Health Perspectives*, *105*, 956–962.

Wright, J. P., Dietrich, K. N., Ris, M. D., Hornung, R. W., Wessel, S. D., Lanphear, B. P., Ho, M., & Rae, M. N. (2008). Association of prenatal and childhood blood lead concentrations with criminal arrests in early adulthood. *PLoS Medicine*, *5*, 0001–0008.

Yuan, W., Holland, S. K., Cecil, K. M., Dietrich, K. N., Wessel, S. D., Altaye, M., Hornung, R. W., Ris, M. D., Egelhoff, J. C., & Lanphear, B. P. (2006). The impact of early childhood lead exposure on brain organization: A functional magnetic resonance imaging study of language function. *Pediatrics*, *118*, 971–977.

32

Neurobehavioral and Neurodevelopmental Sequelae Associated with Congenital Cytomegalovirus Infection

Helen A. Steigmeyer and Antolin M. Llorente

Cytomegalovirus (CMV) is the leading cause of congenital (vertical) infection in newborns, occurring in approximately 0.5% to 1% of neonates in the United States each year (Noyola et al., 2000; Ross, Dollard, Victor, Sumartojo, & Cannon, 2006). Cytomegalovirus is the most ubiquitous member of the Herpesviridae virus family and is related to other well-known viruses such as varicella (chicken pox) and mononucleosis (Santos de Barona, 1998).

Epidemiology

Cytomegalovirus is present throughout diverse regions of the world; however, the virus is increasingly prevalent in lower socioeconomic areas within underdeveloped and developed nations (Centers for Disease Control and Prevention, 2006). It is estimated that 1 in 150 infants are born with congenital CMV infection each year in the United States. Although the majority of infected neonates are asymptomatic, approximately 1 in 750 children will be symptomatic and affected by significant long-term disability. An estimated 8000 children per year infected with CMV are born with or proceed to develop permanent sequelae, including mental retardation, vision loss, sensorineural hearing loss (SNHL), microcephaly, motor disabilities, cardiac anomalies, and seizures (Castillo, Voigt, Demmler, & Llorente, unpublished manuscript; Cannon & Davis, 2005). Other common symptoms include jaundice, liver-spleen infections, pneumonia, chorioretinitis, mononucleosis,

petechiae, and fetal growth retardation. In addition, and very salient to this chapter, is the fact that asymptomatic CMV is not necessarily "silent" in its presentation, and approximately 90% of infants with *asymptomatic* CMV are at risk for developing progressive or delayed symptoms, most commonly manifesting as vision or hearing loss (Noyola et al., 2000).

Basic Virology of Congenital Cytomegalovirus Infection

The origins of CMV remain uncertain, but the virus has exhibited transmission and shedding through bodily fluids for extended periods of time (Noyola et al., 2001). The kidneys and salivary glands are affected by CMV, enabling detection of the virus via urine and saliva specimens, in addition to viral cultures (Demmler, 1991; Noyola et al., 2000). Excretion of the virus indicates that CMV has the capability to replicate in the host for prolonged periods, remain latent, or reactivate at a later period (Noyola et al., 2000). CMV reinfection may also occur with a new strain of the virus. The prolonged periods of virus excretion documented in the literature have been found in both symptomatic and asymptomatic children and, in some instances, for years after initial infection.

Early detection of fetal CMV infection allows mothers the option of pregnancy termination or fetal treatment with antiviral chemotherapy (Lazzarotto, Varani, Gabrielle, Spezzacatena, & Landini, 1999). Diagnosis of fetal CMV during the gestational period has improved with developments in anticytomegalovirus (anti-CMV) IgM detection. After initial screening identifying IgM-positive women, carriers with primary infection should be identified. One possibility includes microneutralization assay 15 weeks or beyond the point of infection. The absence of neutralizing antibodies indicates a recent primary infection. Antibody avidity may be used up to 18–20 weeks after symptoms first occur in a mother with a functional immune system. Low IgG avidity for the antigen is evident in the weeks following infection and has demonstrated high reliability and sensitivity. Immunoblotting uses IgM detection to determine mothers at risk of transmitting the virus to their fetus.

Amniocentesis is used in cases of maternal primary infection or viremia to assess the status of the fetus (Lazzarotto, Varani, Gabrielle, Spezzacatena, & Landini, 1999). Diagnostic tests are most accurate between 21 and 23 weeks, as the amniotic fluid provides the best likelihood of virus detection later in the gestational period. Despite the advances in diagnostic assays, fetal CMV infection does not indicate outcome.

Neurological Consequences of Congenital Cytomegalovirus Infection

The prognosis of children infected with congenital CMV is variable and often relates to the extent of infection at birth (Castillo et al., unpublished manuscript). The time of infection during gestation has been shown to be an indicator of future neurological outcome (Mejaski-Bosnjak, 2008). Early CMV infection, prior to 18 weeks of gestation, often indicates a poor neurodevelopmental prognosis. A later onset occurring in the third trimester tends to result in more variable outcomes. The most severe manifestations of CMV are more likely to occur in primary maternal infection of the virus, rather than recurrent infection during pregnancy (Dobbins & Adler, 1994; Kenneson & Cannon, 2007).

Serious complications and mortality may result from infection in immunocompromised children with symptomatic CMV (Santos de Barona, 1998). *Symptomatic* children who display clinically apparent effects of the virus (i.e., microcephaly, jaundice, or chorioretinitis) may subsequently develop serious central nervous system (CNS) sequelae, such as CMV-related encephalopathy. Barkovich and Lindan (1994) utilized imaging analysis to identify indicators of significant brain injury in congenital CMV infection that include vasculitis with ischemia, necrotic inflammation, gliosis, and calcification. *Asymptomatic* children may develop sequelae as they continue to grow, however, although present in some cases, CNS damage does not commonly occur.

Neurodevelopmental Findings in Congenital Cytomegalovirus

Microcephaly, chorioretinitis, and neurologic abnormalities at birth have been associated with a poor neurodevelopmental outcome(Noyola et al., 2001). Noyola and colleagues determined that the most specific predictor of poor cognitive outcome in children with symptomatic congenital CMV was the presence of microcephaly at birth (adjusted for gestational age and weight). In contrast, subtle brain abnormalities detected by computed tomography (CT), including white matter abnormalities and single punctate calcifications, were not indicative of a poor neurodevelopmental outcome. Normal head CT scans in addition to proportional head circumference were almost universally indicative of intellectual functioning greater than an intellectual quotient/developmental quotient (IQ/DQ) of 70. Symptomatic children demonstrate a risk for developing sequelae, including ataxia, clumsiness, hyperactivity, hypotonia, mental retardation, reduced pain sensation, SNHL, severe motor deficit, visual problems, and other neurodevelopmental and neurobehavioral problems (Mejaski-Bosnjak, 2008).

Noyola and colleagues found that growth, intellectual function, and development were not significantly affected among a sample of children with prolonged CMV excretion. Other studies have supported this finding, concluding that the intellectual and behavioral functioning of children with asymptomatic CMV is similar to that of controls (i.e., Connolly, Jerger, Williamson, Smith, & Demmler, 1992). Temple, Pass, and Boll (2000) expanded upon measures of intelligence to compare multiple facets of neuropsychological functioning in children with asymptomatic CMV and children without the virus. No significant discrepancies were found between the groups on measures of problem solving, memory, motor speed, tactile-perceptual skills, and visual-motor skills. From a longitudinal perspective, a study of two twin sets, each containing one sibling with asymptomatic CMV infection and the other with no indication of the virus, evidenced no apparent effects of CMV on cognitive, academic, language, or executive functioning (Castillo et al., unpublished manuscript).

In contrast to these findings, a longitudinal study of children with asymptomatic CMV in the Qinba mountain area of China found a significant difference in their intellectual development compared to children without the virus (Zhang et al., 2007). The DQ of children 18 to 36 months of age was significantly lower for those with asymptomatic CMV. The Full-Scale IQ (FSIQ) and Verbal IQ (VIQ) of children 48 to 72 months were significantly lower for those infected with the virus than controls. The greatest disparity was found among the verbal reasoning scores of the two groups, with those infected with CMV functioning at a significantly lower level.

The long-term progression of CMV necessitates continuous monitoring of possible neuropsychological sequelae that may not present until critical developmental periods (Kylat, Kelly, & Ford-Jones, 2006). For example, neurological symptoms may improve, but the virus may contribute to dyslexia, other learning disorders, attention problems, and additional cognitive difficulties.

In addition to overall intellect, other functional areas have been shown to be impacted by CMV infection, including auditory and visual processing. Cytomegalovirus is a prominent cause of SNHL, the most common symptom of both symptomatic and asymptomatic infection (Mejaski-Bosnjak, 2008). Studies comparing asymptomatic children infected with congenital CMV to controls present an increased likelihood of sensorineural hearing loss and higher order auditory processing difficulties among the infected individuals (Connolly et al., 1992; Williamson, Demmler, Percy, & Catlin, 1992). Impaired visual processing is another frequent symptom of CMV infection that is seen more commonly in symptomatic infants (Mejaski-Bosnjak, 2008).

Treatment

No consistent and reliable vaccines or treatment for CMV have been established for regular use (Centers for Disease Control and Prevention, 2006). Areas of current research for a vaccine include recombinant Towne strains, gB glycoprotein, Vactor, and DNA vaccines (Kylat et al., 2006). Antiviral drugs, such as ganciclovir, may aid symptoms such as hearing loss but also present the risk of harmful side effects. Noyola and colleagues (2000) noted that antiviral treatment with ganciclovir may only suppress viral replication during therapy. This was signified by the temporary decrease in viral shedding, but no difference in the overall duration of viral replication when compared to untreated children in the study.

Review of available case reports, uncontrolled studies, and randomized studies of ganciclovir treatment indicated that a particular group of CMV patients are most likely to attain benefits from antiviral therapy (Smets et al., 2006). The results suggest that symptomatic infants with growth retardation, petechiae, or CNS sequelae will likely experience improvements or the prevention of hearing loss. However, potential risks associated with ganciclovir treatment include neutropenia or other hematological abnormalities, catheter infection or malfunction, or possible toxicity similar to the results of animal studies that demonstrated carcinogenic effects and gonadal harm. Long-term follow-up of symptom progression, monitoring of dosage, and attention to toxicity levels are necessary for patients receiving treatment.

The sole randomized, controlled study in the previously stated review revealed that 6 weeks of ganciclovir treatment prevented hearing deterioration for a period of 6 months in symptomatic infants with CNS manifestations of the virus (Kimberlin et al., 2003). In this study, approximately two-thirds of the infants experienced neutropenia as the most significant adverse outcome; however, the negative effects of long-term therapy were not evaluated.

Cannon and Davis (2005) call attention to preventative factors. Emphasis is placed on the importance of hygienic practices, such as hand washing, to aid in the avoidance of maternal infection and transmission of the virus during pregnancy. Promotion of such practices has significant potential benefit for women who are pregnant, or those planning to become pregnant, while in contact with other young children. The significant prevalence of a uniform virus strain within daycare centers suggests CMV is transmitted at high rates among children in such facilities (Dobbins & Adler, 1994). Viral strains may be spread through bodily fluids by means of daycare workers, contaminated toys, or by children themselves. Dobbins and Adler (1994) found CMV to be most common in children 13 to 24 months of age, while children over 3 years of age appeared to cease spreading the virus.

In conclusion, the progressive and variable course of CMV can involve serious neurological and neuropsychological outcomes, reinforcing the need for children to receive continuous follow-up that involves the most comprehensive assessment possible (Kylat et al., 2006).

Case Study: Aron Patient

Identifying Information and Reason for Referral

Aron Patient is a 9-year-old, right-handed, Caucasian male. He presently attends the fourth grade at a private school. He was referred for a neuropsychological evaluation as a result of recently discovered mild, bilateral sensorineural hearing loss (<40 db) with reported consequences in social development within an overall backdrop of a diagnosis of congenital "asymptomatic cytomegalovirus." The current evaluation was requested by his pediatric specialist (Infectious Diseases) to rule out a receptive language disorder. In addition, he was referred to develop appropriate recommendations for intervention. Aron currently does not receive psychotropic medication.

Presenting Problem and Relevant History

According to his mother, Aron reportedly was recently diagnosed with mild, bilateral sensorineural hearing loss. She noted that she had been told that he was shedding "CMV virus shortly after birth," but all subsequent pediatric check-ups eventually led to a diagnosis of "asymptomatic CMV." During his "pediatric visit 6 years ago," she was told not to worry since "silent" (asymptomatic) CMV usually did not lead to problems, but that he would have to be monitored in the future. Earlier this year, Aron began to exhibit difficulty following through on commands. He was subsequently examined by a clinician in the community, and he was diagnosed with attention-deficit/hyperactivity disorder (ADHD) (Predominantly Inattentive Type). He was placed on stimulant medication at that time, yet this intervention did not curtail his problems. His mother noted that "although he smiled and nodded a lot," as if he had understood what he was told, "his listening comprehension was not what it used to be." She then took him to a nearby pediatric hospital where she learned that her child had originally been diagnosed with "asymptomatic" congenital CMV, and he was referred for a thorough pediatric evaluation that led to referrals to infectious diseases and audiology. Hearing tests discovered the presence of mild, bilateral sensorineural hearing loss, as noted earlier. The mother further noted that it appears as if Aron's difficulties are not related to his "intelligence," but rather to difficulties understanding language. When asked about course, the mother indicated that his difficulties have increased over time culminating in his current status. She was not able to pinpoint the specific onset of his difficulties, but she noted that "his real problems" became evident this year. She finally noted that his difficulties impacted his self-esteem and that he has expressed that he is "not smart" on several occasions to her and to one of his teachers. His mother also has noted a newly developed reticence to make new friendships in school and in his neighborhood. Aron has no sleep difficulties. His appetite is normal. Episodes of enuresis or encopresis were not reported. His vision had been checked and was found to be within normal limits.

Aron was the product of Ms. Patient's fifth pregnancy; she never experienced a miscarriage. Her pregnancy with Aron was unremarkable, and she denied the use of alcohol, tobacco products, or controlled substances during the pregnancy.

Labor was spontaneous and delivery occurred 1.5 weeks preterm via normal vertex procedures without complications. Aron weighed 8 pounds at birth and had no perinatal difficulties. Aron was reportedly a very pleasant baby after he was brought home. He did not experience feeding or sleeping problems, and he exhibited a good temperament. According to his mother, he did not exhibit any speech delays; he spoke single words at 11 months and telegraphic speech at 14 months. His recent language difficulties involved only receptive language. He does not receive tutoring or speech-language therapy. Motor skills and all other developmental aspects appeared to be spared. Aron walked independently by 11 months and rode a bike with training wheels at 14 months. With regard to medical illnesses, Aron suffered from mild ear infections treated with antibiotics, and without the need for tube placement. He underwent hearing aid placement 1 week before this evaluation. There was no history of head injury with LOC, hospitalization, or psychosocial stressors. Family medical history is significant for births defects (one maternal aunt) and unremarkable for psychiatric or neurologic disease. From a psychosocial standpoint, Aron's parents have been married for 16 years, without marital problems. A review of medical records revealed laboratory tests that were normal except for "minimal but continued urinary CMV shedding."

Behavioral Observations

Aron was brought to Mt. Washington Hospital for examination by his mother. He appeared to be his stated age and was appropriately dressed and groomed for his evaluation. Aron's spontaneous speech, prosody, and rate of speech were within normal limits, without evidence of dysarthria. The content of his speech was coherent. He informally exhibited mild receptive language problems verified through his inability to follow through correctly on three-step commands, and instructions to complex tests had to be repeated on several occasions. He was friendly towards the examiner throughout the assessment process. Aron's cooperation and attention were appropriate. He exhibited mild squirming but no fidgeting or impulsivity, and his behavior never required the use of redirection. It should also be noted that during the first day of evaluation, Aron had a mild spontaneous nose bleed and had frequently experienced such episodes in the past. These have reportedly diminished in frequency and severity over the years (this was his first episode this year). Correlates of seizures were not noted. Consistent with hospital policy, the presence of pain was assessed with unremarkable findings. Aron's motivation appeared appropriate. He exhibited significant commitment to the testing process and always appeared to be producing his best performance. For these reasons, the results of this examination were considered to be a valid measurement of his current abilities.

The following procedures and tests were administered (in order of administration): Day 1: Hand Preference Demonstration Test; Grooved Pegboard Test; The Children's Auditory Verbal Learning Test–Second Edition (CAVLT-2); Judgment of Line Orientation (JLO); Children's Depression Inventory (CDI); Developmental Test of Visual-Motor Integration (VMI); Behavior Assessment Scale for Children (BASC-2) Self- and Parent Scale; Attention Rating Scale–IV Edition, Home Version; Children's Color Trail Test 1 and 2 (CCTT 1, CCTT 2); Day 2: Wechsler Abbreviated Scale of Intelligence (WASI); NEPSY (selected subtests as noted); Children's Memory Scale (CMS)-Dot Locations, Numbers and Stories only; Rey-Osterrieth Complex Figure (ROCF) (Copy and 30-Minute Delay); Behavior Rating Inventory of Executive Functioning (BRIEF)–Teacher Version and Parent Version.

General Intelligence

Aron's performance revealed an overall intellectual score in the average range. His Full Scale IQ score of 97, (42nd percentile), Verbal IQ score of 93 (32nd percentile), and Performance IQ score of 101 (53rd percentile) all fell within the average range. The eight-point discrepancy between VIQ and PIQ scores is statistically significant ($p < .15$), but the magnitude of this score differential was observed in over 25% of the individuals comprising the WASI standardization sample; therefore, this difference most likely is not clinically significant. With regard to the verbal reasoning skills, he obtained scores within the average range on a subtest assessing word knowledge (Vocabulary) and on a subtest assessing his ability to determine similarities between objects or concepts (Similarities). With regard to visual reasoning skills, he obtained a score within the high-average range on a subtest requiring him to reproduce designs using blocks (Block Design) and within the average range on a test requiring the solution of matrices (Matrix Reasoning).

Attention/Concentration and Executive Function

Aron was administered selected tasks from the CMS in an attempt to assess auditory attention. He obtained a score in the average range (37th percentile) on the digit repetition subtest. On a procedure assessing visual attention (CCTT 1 and CCTT 2), Aron's performance times fell within the average range at the 54th and 38th percentiles, respectively. His numbers of errors also fell within the average range, similar to his interference score (>16th percentile). On the BRIEF, all executive function subscales fell within expected limits for his chronological age, according to maternal report. No impairments of working memory, planning, or organizational difficulties were noted.

Language

Aron's performance on language measures was variable. He performed within the average range (50th percentile) on a task that required sentence formulation in response to a picture stimulus. He performed within the average range (37th percentile) when he had to produce words within specific categories on the NEPSY, Verbal Fluency subtest. On a task that required him to understand and follow instruction (CELF-4 Concepts and Directions), his scores fell within in the average range (37th percentile). He performed within the high-average range (84th percentile) on a NEPSY subtest assessing emerging phonological processing. Aron also scored within the high-average range on a task that measured his knowledge of grammatical rules in a sentence–completion task (CELF-4 Word Structure, 75th percentile).

Visual Processing

Aron performed within the high-average range (84th percentile) on a test of visuo-construction and perceptual organization (WASI Block Design). He also obtained a score in the average range (45th percentile) on the VMI measure assessing visuomotor skills requiring that he copy geometric designs of increasing complexity. His score on a motor-free visual perceptual task assessing his ability to determine the angular distance between lines (Judgment of Line Orientation) fell within the average range (62nd percentile). Aron obtained a score in the average range (34th percentile) on a more difficult visual-motor task (Rey-Osterrieth Complex Figure) requiring significant organization and planning.

Verbal Learning and Memory

Aron obtained a score within average limits on all indices of the CAVLT-2, including immediate memory span (79th percentile), level of learning (82nd percentile), immediate recall (25th percentile), and delayed recall (42nd percentile). His score on a recognition memory task fell within average limits (>16th percentile). Aron's performances fell within average limits on the CMS task assessing Aron's immediate recall (37th percentile) and long-delay recall of stories (50th percentile), and recognition memory after a 30-minute delay (25th percentile).

Visual Learning and Memory

Aron's score on the 30-minute delayed portion of the Rey-Osterrieth Complex Figure test was average (32nd percentile); he was able to recall about 80% of the figure initially learned. This performance was consistent with his average performance on the CMS Dot Location visual memory learning score and recall (63rd percentile).

Lateral Dominance and Fine Motor Skill

Aron obtained a score of 27/27 on the Hand Preference Demonstration Test, suggesting right-hand dominance on a test of manual dexterity. Aron performed within average limits on the Grooved Pegboard Test for both his dominant (73 sec; 74th percentile) and nondominant (90 sec; 45th percentile) hands; he obtained a nonsignificant raw score lateralizing difference of 19%.

Behavioral and Emotional Functioning

Aron and his mother both completed Behavior Assessment System for Children–2 questionnaires, and no statistically significant elevation emerged on any scale. Aron's scores were well within average limits on the Children's Depression Inventory.

Summary and Clinical Impressions

Aron Patient is a 9-year-old, right-handed, Caucasian male in the fourth grade. He was referred for a neuropsychological evaluation as a result of recently discovered mild, bilateral sensorineural hearing loss (<40 db), mild academic difficulties possibly related to a receptive language disorder, and concern about his social development, and with a diagnosis of congenital asymptomatic cytomegalovirus.

Aron's overall performance on a standardized intellectual measure fell in the average range of functioning. The discrepancy between his VIQ and PIQ scores was found to be statistically significant, but small in magnitude and seen in a large proportion of children comprising the WASI standardization sample. Therefore, the split is not considered clinically significant, and both skills appear to be developing at an even rate at this time.

With regard to neuropsychological functioning, the present results revealed findings within normal limits on all domains of functioning, including auditory and visual attention and concentration, visual processing and perceptual organization, rote and contextual visual and auditory learning and memory skills, and fine motor skills. In addition, his profile revealed scores within normal limits on measures of executive skills. With regard to language skills, as a rule-out for receptive language was requested, these skills were assessed with greater degree of depth and breadth. Nevertheless, his scores in this domain fell within normal limits, including receptive and expressive skills, verbal fluency, and phonemic processing. Clearly, his scores in this domain permit a rule-out of a receptive language disorder at this time and point to his hearing difficulties for the "problems" in receptive language he reportedly has

recently experienced. The present findings are consistent with his history of CMV, in that asymptomatic congenital CMV does not always remain "silent" in a proportion of children, approximately 10%–12% of whom go on to develop sensorineural hearing losses (Noyola et al., 2001). If not appropriately detected and diagnosed, but particularly if left untreated, unlike this case, children with asymptomatic CMV with sequelae are capable of developing greater difficulties, including language disorders. From a brain–behavior relationship standpoint, such effects (sensorineural hearing loss) are the result of the impact of CMV on cranial nerves, particularly cranial nerve VIII, and the indirect effects of such hearing losses on language functions. However, although hearing losses are evident in this patient, his profile does not currently support the presence of a receptive language disorder.

Despite parental report of Aron's socialization difficulties, the current results did *not* reveal the presence of significant emotional or behavioral problems. However, in conjunction with his history of asymptomatic CMV, his development of socialization skills warrants continued attention. Placement in a brief, focused social skills training program was recommended. At the same time, it is considered likely that his social contacts will increase appreciably, as he has been fitted with hearing aids.

Aron has several factors working for him. He has a loving and concerned support system consisting of his family and teachers. His estimated cognitive abilities appear to be intact and his neuropsychological profile is within normal limits across all domains, suggesting the potential for more adaptive levels of functioning despite his recently diagnosed hearing loss and reported social difficulties. In addition, Aron responds well to reward systems, and coupled with the aforementioned factors, his positive responses should serve him well in the future if given the appropriate assistance. Toward that end, the following recommendations were offered:

General Recommendations
- Given the history of hearing loss, and the progressive nature of hearing loss in patients with CMV, hearing tests should be conducted

regularly to determine whether further hearing loss has occurred and to address in a timely manner such hearing losses though the use of adaptive methods (e.g., new or reprogrammed hearing aids).

- Aron's teachers and parent should be alert to the emergence of any further academic difficulties so that he may continue to receive needed individual tutoring.
- Aron would benefit from social skills training, and referral is made to the XXX Clinical Centers.
- Reevaluation should be considered in approximately 1 year.
- His parents and teachers may find the following references helpful:

   http://www.ninds.nih.gov/disorders/ cytomegalic/cytomegalic.htm.

   Kelly, M. L. (1990). *School-home notes*: *Promoting children's classroom success.* New York: Guilford Press.

Recommendations for the School

- Students with hearing deficits often learn and perform better in classrooms that have four walls rather than an open classroom arrangement that provides too many visual and auditory distractors throughout the school day.
- Aron's desk should be situated near the teacher (for prompting and redirection). Seat location in the front of the classroom, near the chalkboard, and close to the instructional area will be helpful. The most academically demanding tasks should be scheduled in the morning.
- Placement in a classroom with a small student to teacher ratio should additionally enable his teacher to provide an increased amount of direction, feedback, and positive reinforcement.
- It is recommended that Aron be provided with increased supportive supervision and assistance in understanding instructions when taking standardized tests, and that rest breaks be offered when possible during standardized examinations.
- Aron should function more adaptively when he can anticipate when he must concentrate. A visual representation of the day's schedule will be useful along with an emphasis on visual cues to help him internalize classroom routine. Stimulating and engaging activities, a varied instructional program, and activities and lessons that emphasize hands-on experience are likely to be of greater interest.

- Criterion-based learning should be supplemented with assignments made as a function of how well he has learned a concept.
- Aron will benefit from directions given one step at a time. Aron should establish eye scontact when receiving direction/instruction to enhance understanding and follow-through. Having him paraphrase what the teacher has said may aid his comprehension and enable him to check whether he has understood the directions accurately. Changes in the instructor's voice level and variation in word-pacing may also better sustain Aron's attention.
- A combination of verbal directions with illustrations or other visual stimuli—a multimodality approach—should be attempted.
- A prearranged cueing system with the teacher can be arranged, in which the teacher gives a visual signal (touching the ear) or verbal phrase ("Remember, I'm looking for good listeners") when a targeted inappropriate behavior occurs. The cue can remind the student to correct behavior without direct confrontation or loss of self-esteem. It can involve the classroom teacher or any support personnel available to Aron.
- Aron should be permitted to use assistive technology as needed to enhance his ability to hear classroom lectures and instructions.

Recommendations for the Home

- The use of established routines in the home has been found to be beneficial for children with difficulties similar to those displayed by Aron.
- Parents of a child with hearing loss may benefit from enrollment in an *applied* parenting skill class.
- Aron's parents may want to implement a schedule to help him plan, become more organized, and improve his memory. For example, Aron and his parents may develop his memory skills by learning memory strategies such as "chunking."

Appendix: Assessment Data

Cognitive Functioning

Wechsler Abbreviated Scale of Intelligence (WASI).

Composite Scales	Standard Score	Confidence Intervals (90%)
Verbal IQ Score	93	87–100
Performance IQ Score	101	95–107
Full Scale IQ Score	97	92–102

Verbal Subtests	Scaled Score	Percentile	Performance Subtests	Scaled Score	Percentile
Similarities	9	37th	Block Design	13	84th
Vocabulary	8	25th	Matrix Reasoning	8	25th

Attentional and Executive Functioning

Behavioral Rating Inventory of Executive Function (BRIEF).

BRIEF Scales	Parent Rating T-Score	Teacher Rating T-Score
Inhibit	55	54
Shift	54	54
Emotional Control	54	60
Initiate	59	58
Working Memory	60	58
Plan/Organize	50	54
Organization of Material	49	50
Monitor	56	55

Children's Color Trails Test (CCTT).

CCTT Measure	Percentile
CCTT-1 Time	54th
CCTT-2 Time	38th
Interference	>16th

Visual-Perceptual/Visual-Motor Skills

Beery-Buktenica Test of Visual-Motor Integration (VMI).

VMI Standard Score
98

Judgment of Line Orientation (JLO).

JLO Z-Score	Percentile
+0.30	62nd

Rey-Osterrieth Complex Figure Test (RCFT)

Trial	Percentile
Copy	34th

Fine Motor Skills

Grooved Pegboard Test (GPT).

Pegboard Trials	Seconds	Percentile
Dominant Hand (Right)	73	74th
Nondominant Hand (Left)	90	45th

Learning and Memory

Children's Memory Scale (CMS).

Subtest	Scaled Score
Stories Immediate	9
Stories Delayed	10
Stories Delayed Recognition	8
Dot Locations Learning	9
Dot Locations Recall	11
Numbers	9

Rey-Osterrieth Complex Figure Test (RCFT).

Trial	Percentile
30 Minute Recall	32nd

Children's Auditory Verbal Learning Test–Second Edition (CALVT-II).

Measure	Percentile
Level of Learning	82nd
Immediate Memory Span	7th
Immediate Recall	25th
Delayed Recall	42nd
Recognition	16th

Language Skills

Clinical Evaluation of Language Fundamentals–Fourth Edition (CELF-4).

A Developmental Neuropsychological Assessment–Second Edition (NEPSY-II).

Measure	Scaled Score
CELF-4 Word Structure	12
CELF-4 Concepts & Following Directions	9
CELF-4 Formulated Sentences	10
NEPSY-II Speed Naming	9

Phonological Processing

A Developmental Neuropsychological Assessment–Second Edition (NEPSY-II).

Measure	Scaled Score
Phonological Processing	13

Behavioral/Emotional Functioning

Behavior Assessment System for Children (BASC). (Please note that on this measure, a score over 70 is considered an area of concern, while scores of 60 and above indicate "at risk" areas.)

BASC Scales	Mother Rating T-Score	Self Rating T-Score
Hyperactivity	50	
Aggression	55	
Conduct Problems	52	
Anxiety	48	38
Depression	50	39
Somatization	53	
Atypicality	60	54
Withdrawal	50	
Attention Problems	60	
Attitude toward School		43
Attitude toward Teachers		48
Locus of Control		43
Social Stress		43
Sense of Inadequacy		51

Children's Depression Inventory (CDI).

CDI Measure	T-Score
Total CDI Score	42
Negative Mood	42
Interpersonal Problems	50
Ineffectiveness	38
Anhedonia	35
Negative Self-Esteem	42

References

Barkovich, A. J., & Lindan, C. E. (1994). Congenital cytomegalovirus infection of the brain: Imaging analysis and embryonic consideration. *American Journal of Neuroradiology, 15*, 703–715.

Cannon, M. J., & Davis, K. F. (2005). Washing our hands of the congenital cytomegalovirus disease epidemic. *BMC Public Health, 5*, Article 70. Retrieved August 27, 2008, from http://www.biomedcentral.com/1471-2458/5/70

Castillo, C. L., Voigt, R. G., Demmler, G., & Llorente, A. M. (unpublished manuscript). Congenital cytomegalovirus infection: a longitudinal pediatric, twin case study examining neurocognitive and neurobehavioral correlates.

Centers for Disease Control and Prevention. (2006). *Cytomegalovirus (CMV)*. Retrieved February 12, 2010, from http://www.cdc.gov/cmv/index.htm

Connolly, P. K., Jerger, S., Williamson, W. D., Smith, R. J., & Demmler, G. (1992). Evaluation of higher-level auditory function in children with asymptomatic congenital cytomegalovirus infection. *The American Journal of Otology, 13*(2), 185–193.

Demmler G. (1991). Summary of a workshop on surveillance for congenital cytomegalovirus disease. *Review of Infectious Diseases, 13*, 315.

Dobbins, J., & Adler, S. (1994). The risks and benefits of cytomegalovirus transmission in child day care. *Pediatrics, 94*(6), 1016.

Kenneson, A., & Cannon, M. J. (2007). Review and meta-analysis of the epidemiology of congenital cytomegalovirus (CMV) infection. *Reviews in Medical Virology, 17*(4), 253–276.

Kimberlin, D. W., Lin, C., Sánchez, P. J., Demmler, G. J., Dankner, W., Shelton, M., et al. (2003). Effect of ganciclovir therapy on hearing in symptomatic congenital cytomegalovirus disease involving the central nervous system: A randomized, controlled trial. *The Journal of Pediatrics, 143*, 16–25.

Kylat, R., Kelly, E., & Ford-Jones, E. (2006). Clinical findings and adverse outcome in neonates with symptomatic congenital cytomegalovirus (SCCMV) infection. *European Journal of Pediatrics, 165*(11), 773–778.

Lazzarotto, T., Varani, S., Gabrielli, L., Spezzacatena, P., & Landini, M. (1999). New advances in the diagnosis of congenital cytomegalovirus infection. *Intervirology, 42*, 390–397.

Mejaski-Bosnjak, V. (2008). Congenital CMV infection: A common cause of childhood disability. *Developmental Medicine and Child Neurology, 50*(6), 403.

Noyola, D. E., Demmler, G. J., Williamson, W. D., Griesser C., Sellers, S., Llorente, A., et al. (2000). Cytomegalovirus urinary excretion and long term outcome in children with congenital cytomegalovirus infection. *The Pediatric Infectious Disease Journal, 19*(6), 505–510.

Noyola, D. E., Demmler, G. J., Nelson, C. T., Griesser, C., Williamson, W. D., Atkins, J. T., et al. (2001). Early predictors of neurodevelopmental outcome in symptomatic congenital cytomegalovirus infection. *The Journal of Pediatrics, 138*(3), 325–331.

Ross, D., Dollard, S., Victor, M., Sumartojo, E., & Cannon, M. (2006). The epidemiology and prevention of congenital cytomegalovirus infection and disease: Activities of the Centers for Disease Control and Prevention Workgroup. *Journal of Women's Health (15409996), 15*(3), 224–229.

Santos de Barona, M. (1998). Cytomegalovirus. In L. Phelps (Ed.), *Health-related disorders in children and adolescents: A guidebook for understanding and educating* (pp. 213–218). Washington, DC: American Psychological Association.

Smets, K., Coen, K. D., Dhooge, I., Standaert, L., Laroche, S., Mahieu, L., et al. (2006). Selecting neonates with congenital cytomegalovirus infection for ganciclovir therapy. *European Journal of Pediatrics, 165*(12), 885–890.

Temple, R., Pass, R., & Boll, T. (2000). Neuropsychological functioning in patients with asymptomatic congenital cytomegalovirus infection. *Journal of Developmental and Behavioral Pediatrics, 21*(6), 417–422.

Williamson, W. D., Demmler, G. J., Percy, A. K., & Catlin, F. I. (1992). Progressive hearing loss in infants with asymptomatic congenital cytomegalovirus infection. *Pediatrics, 90*(6), 862–866.

Zhang, X., Li, F., Yu, X., Shi, X., Shi, J., & Zhang, J. (2007). Physical and intellectual development in children with asymptomatic congenital cytomegalovirus infection: A longitudinal cohort study in Qinba mountain area, China. *Journal of Clinical Virology, 40*(3), 180–185.

33

Language-Dominant Neocortical Temporal Lobe Epilepsy

Deborah Cahn-Weiner

Epilepsy surgery is an effective treatment for patients with temporal lobe epilepsy (TLE). Patients who are identified as being good candidates for epilepsy surgery are predicted to have a very high chance of achieving seizure freedom after undergoing anterior temporal lobe resection. Factors that identify a patient as being a good candidate include younger age at time of surgery, magnetic resonance imaging (MRI)-documented evidence of ipsilateral mesial temporal sclerosis (MTS), unilateral temporal abnormalities on fluorodeoxyglucose (FDG)-positron emission tomography (PET), and absence of tonic-clonic seizures (Uijl et al., 2008). While such patients may enjoy a significant reduction or cessation in seizures, many experience some decline in memory functioning after surgery. Another group of patients who also have temporal lobe epilepsy carry even greater burden of risk with regard to memory outcome. A substantial number of patients show no MRI abnormalities; this group has been referred to as "cryptogenic," or MRI-negative temporal lobe epilepsy. Possible sources of the seizure focus in these patients include subtle MTS not readily identifiable on MRI, other medial temporal lobe pathology including microdysgenesis, or temporal neocortical pathology such as cortical dysplasia. The challenge in these cases is determining the specific target for resection and reducing the impact on eloquent and functional brain structures. Such patients have been reported to have worse surgical outcomes in terms of seizure

reduction relative to patients with an identifiable lesion (Cohen-Gadol et al., 2005).

A number of neuropsychological differences have been identified when mesial temporal lobe epilepsy (MTLE) and MRI-negative TLE groups are compared. At baseline, patients with lateralized MTLE evidence material-specific memory deficits, show greater impairments on other cognitive measures, and show greater memory asymmetry on Wada memory testing as compared to patients with non-MTLE. Postoperatively, language-dominant non-MTLE patients show greater cognitive impairments than MTLE patients, including significant decline in verbal memory, confrontation naming, and verbal comprehension skills. Additionally, the decline in verbal memory observed in this patient group appears to occur regardless of seizure outcome (Seidenberg et al., 1998).

The negative impact of medically intractable seizures on quality of life is well documented. Many patients who are at risk for less than optimal seizure outcome or poor memory outcome may still pursue epilepsy surgery because of the social, occupational, and medical challenges they face. The neuropsychologist plays an important role in the preoperative evaluation of epilepsy patients who are surgical candidates. In addition to providing baseline neuropsychological testing, the neuropsychologist assists with the Wada evaluation and informs both the surgical team and the patient about possible risks to cognitive function. In patients with MRI-negative TLE, presentation of the risks and benefits is a sensitive and difficult task.

The Case of Ms. T.

Ms. T. is a 31-year-old, right-handed, single Caucasian woman with a 10-year history of medically refractory complex partial seizures. She was referred for a neuropsychological evaluation to assess her risk for postoperative cognitive complications and to provide baseline neuropsychological test results as part of her presurgical workup in a University Epilepsy Center.

Ms. T. began experiencing seizures at the age of 21. She underwent numerous trials of antiepileptic drugs, but her seizures remained refractory to medication. She reported two different seizure types. The first is a complex partial seizure characterized by an initial feeling of déjà vu followed by inability to speak and staring. These episodes typically last less than 2 minutes. She reported having this type of seizure approximately two to three times per week. Her second seizure type is a generalized tonic clonic seizure. These events occur much less frequently, approximately once or twice a year. Her current medications include Lamotragine (450 mg bid) and Levetiracetam (4000 mg bid). Neurologic exam to date has been negative. She was admitted to the video electroencephalogram (EEG) monitoring unit for 6 days. During this monitoring, she experienced four events; three of these were secondarily generalized seizures. Ictal EEG recordings revealed left posterior temporal onset. Interictally, there were frequent bursts of spike-and-wave discharges over the left posterior temporal area.

A brain MRI performed on the patient showed no focal anatomic abnormality or signal abnormality in the left temporal region. Magnetic source imaging did not show any abnormal spikes in the left temporal lobe region. A brain PET scan showed no specific focus of hypometabolism to suggest a seizure focus. Ms. T. underwent intracarotid amobarbital (Wada) testing. She exhibited significant aphasic symptoms with the left injection. Memory performance with the left injection revealed strong memory for the contralateral, right hemisphere (11/12). With the right injection, there was no evidence of aphasia and memory was again very good (11/12) for the contralateral left hemisphere.

Ms. T. reported that she has experienced some word-finding difficulties that have made her feel uncomfortable in social situations. Additionally, she reported having memory dysfunction and finds that she has to write things down or she will forget them. The patient indicated that these problems have been relatively stable over the past several years, but they represent a decline from her previous level of functioning prior to the onset of epilepsy 10 years ago.

Other medical history is noncontributory. There is no history of meningitis, encephalitis, febrile seizures, or head injury. There is no family history of seizure disorder. She denied history of tobacco, alcohol, or illicit drug use. She endorsed increased anxiety and depression recently and attributed these feelings to her frequent seizures and possible impending surgery. She has never been prescribed an antidepressant, and there is no history of suicidal ideation or past psychiatric hospitalization. There is no family history of psychiatric illness.

Ms. T. reported a happy childhood, no significant childhood medical problems, and no history of developmental delay. She performed well in school, with no apparent learning difficulties, and graduated from a 4-year university with excellent grades. She currently works full time in a sales position. She has not been driving for the past 6 months.

Examination Results

General Behavior. Ms. T. was oriented to person, place, day of the week, date, year, and month. Her speech was fluent, prosodic, and of normal rate, rhythm, and tone. No significant word-finding difficulties were noted in conversational speech, but they were apparent on formal language assessment. She was easily engaged in conversation and made very good eye contact. Thought processes were logical. Her recent and remote personal memory appeared grossly intact. Her affect was appropriate to the situation and mood was considered to be euthymic. She was very pleasant to work with and was forthcoming with information. Her cooperation and effort were very high. The results of this evaluation are therefore believed to be a valid estimation of her current level of neurocognitive functioning. Neuropsychological test results are presented in Table 33-1.

Table 33-1. Neuropsychological Assessment Test Results

Test	Index	Percentile
Intellectual Ability		
WAIS-III		
Full Scale IQ (FSIQ)	(115)	84
Verbal IQ	(112)	79
Performance IQ	(117)	87
Verbal Comprehension Index (VCI)	(112)	79
Perceptual Organization (POI)	(107)	68
Working Memory Index (WMI)	(104)	61
Processing Speed (PSI)	(117)	87

	Raw	Percentile
Verbal Subtests		
Vocabulary	59	95
Similarities	26	63
Arithmetic	15	63
Digit Span	19	63
Information	17	63
Comprehension	26	84
Letter-Number Sequencing	11	50
Performance Subtests		
Picture Completion	22	75
Digit Symbol-Coding	108	98
Block Design	35	37
Matrix Reasoning	21	84
Symbol Search	34	50
Memory Functioning		
Wechsler Memory Scale- III		
Information and Orientation	14	67
Auditory Memory		
Logical Memory I	52	84
Logical Memory II	33	84
Verbal Paired Associates I	32	98
Verbal Paired Associates II	8	84
Auditory Recognition - Delayed	52	75
Visual Memory		
Visual Reproduction I	85	37
Visual Reproduction II	61	37
Visual Reproduction Recog.	48	91
Faces I Recognition	42	75
Faces II Recognition	45	95
California Verbal Learning Test - II		
Trials 1-5	65	90
Trial B	5	16
Short Delay Free Recall	15	84
Short Delay Cued Recall	15	84
Long Delay Free Recall	16	93
Long Delay Cued Recall	16	84
Total Recognition Discriminability	4	84
Rey-Osterrieth Complex Figure Test		
Delayed Recall	13	27

(*Continued*)

Table 33-1. Neuropsychological Assessment Test Results (*Continued*)

Test	Index	Percentile
Language Functioning		
Boston Naming Test	51	4
Auditory Naming Test	48	4
Visuospatial Functions		
Judgment of Line Orientation	24	40
Rey-Osterrieth Complex Figure (copy)	29	21
Attention/Executive Functioning		
Wechsler Memory Scale - III		
Spatial Span	20	84
Mental Control	29	63
D-KEFS		
Trail Making Test (seconds)		
Visual Scanning	14	84
Number Sequencing	16	91
Letter Sequencing	25	75
Number-Letter Switching	50	75
Motor Speed	13	84
Verbal Fluency		
Letter Fluency - Total correct	49	84
Category Fluency-Total Correct	38	37
Design Fluency		
Filled Dots: Total Correct	13	84
Empty Dots: Total Correct	14	84
Switching: Total Correct	12	91
Design Fluency Total Correct	40	95
Color Word Interference Test		
Color Naming	17	95
Word Reading	15	91
Inhibition	33	95
Inhibition/Switching	38	91
Wisconsin Card Sorting Test		
Categories	6	>16
Errors	9	58
Perseverative Responses	4	61
Failure to Maintain Set	0	>16
Motor Functioning		
Finger Tapping		
Dominant Hand	37.2	4
Nondominant Hand	33.9	4
Grooved Pegboard (seconds)		
Dominant Hand	65	12
Nondominant Hand	81	2
Mood/Personality		
Beck Depression Inventory - II	28	mod-severe
QOLIE-89 Overall Score	53	16

Intellectual Functions. Overall intellectual functioning was in the high-average range (FSIQ = 115, 84th percentile). Analysis of Index Scores indicated that her verbal comprehension (i.e., vocabulary, verbal abstraction, and general fund of information) was in the high-average range (Verbal Comprehension Index = 112, 79th percentile). Her visuospatial problem solving skills (i.e., visual analysis, construction, and nonverbal fluid reasoning) were average (Perceptual Organization Index = 107, 68th percentile). This degree of discrepancy was not statistically significant and occurs in approximately 66% of standardization sample of the WAIS-III. Working memory skills were average (Working Memory Index = 104, 61st percentile), while processing speed (Processing Speed Index = 117, 87th percentile) was high average. Among the AIS-III Index Scores, only the Working Memory Index and Processing Speed Index differed significantly.

Within the verbal scale, word knowledge (Vocabulary) was a relative strength (95th percentile). All other verbal subscale performances ranged from 50th to 84th percentile. In terms of performance skills, there was somewhat more variability, with scores ranging from 37th to 84th percentile. Psychomotor speed (Digit Symbol-Coding) was a relative strength (98th percentile).

Memory Functions. Ms. T. displayed average to above-average memory performance across several memory tests administered. Verbal learning and memory skills were generally above average. Her learning and recall of short-story paragraphs (Logical Memory, WMS-III) was above average, and she showed average retention of the information across a 30-minute delay. Similarly, on a test requiring her to learn word pairs (Verbal Paired Associates, WMS-III), she showed high-average learning and retention across a 30-minute delay. Recognition discriminability was high average on the WMS-III verbal memory tests. On the CVLT-II, Ms. T. displayed superior skills in learning a word list across five trials. She showed below-average skills on learning a second, interfering list, suggesting some susceptibility to proactive interference. Her immediate and delayed recall of the original list were above average and superior, respectively. Recognition discriminability on the CVLT-II was also above average.

In the nonverbal, spatial domain, Ms. T. showed average learning and retention of simple geometric figures (Visual Reproduction, WMS-III). Her recognition discriminability was superior. Immediate and delayed face recognition (Faces, WMS-III) were high average and superior, respectively. Delayed recall of a complex geometric figure (ROCF) was average for her age.

Language Functions. Naming skills were assessed with both visual naming (BNT) and auditory naming (Auditory Naming Test) tasks. Visual naming was found to be mildly to moderately impaired for her age and education (51/60, 4th percentile). Examination of her performance indicates that she benefited from phonemic cueing approximately 50% of the time. Auditory naming (48/50; 4th percentile) performance was also impaired relative to individuals with similar educational background. Her performance on verbal fluency tasks indicates above-average skills for phonemic fluency (84th percentile) and average performance for category fluency (50th percentile). Reading skills were also assessed, and she displayed post–high-school-level abilities (73rd percentile), consistent with her educational background. Reading speed, as assessed by the D-KEFS Word Reading subtest, was superior (91st percentile). Performance on verbal subtests of the WAIS-III demonstrated superior word knowledge, above-average social reasoning, and average abstract verbal reasoning and knowledge typically acquired in school.

Spatial Functions. Basic visuoperception, as assessed by her ability to make accurate line angle judgments (JLOT) was average (40th percentile). Her copy of a complex geometric figure (ROCF) was slightly below average for her age (21st percentile). Although she accurately reproduced the overall gestalt, she showed a tendency to rush and as such the placement of internal details was imprecise. Her performance on WAIS-III subtests demonstrated above-average nonverbal reasoning skills, high-average attention to detail, and average perceptual organization skills.

Attention/Executive Functions. Basic auditory attention was average (63rd percentile), with eight digits repeated forward and six digits repeated backward. Spatial attention was above average (84th percentile) with seven blocks tapped forward and seven tapped backward. Mental control, as assessed by the WMS-III, was average for her age (63rd percentile). Mental computation skills were found to be in the average range (63rd percentile) on the Arithmetic subtest of the WAIS-III. On a test of working memory (Letter Number Sequencing, WAIS-III), she displayed average abilities (50th percentile).

Executive functioning skills were found to fall in the above-average to superior range. On the Trail Making Test (D-KEFS), Ms. T. displayed generally above-average skills on simple and complex sequencing tests. Her ability to generate novel designs (Design Fluency) was also above average across simple and more complex conditions. She showed no evidence of disinhibition or difficulty switching sets on the Color Word Interference Test. Ms. T. completed 6/6 card sorts on the WCST and made an average number of errors on this test. Overall, attentional skills and executive functioning were found to be generally average to above average with no evidence of deficits noted.

Motor Dexterity and Speed. On two tests of simple motor speed and dexterity (Finger Tapping, Grooved Pegboard), Ms. T. displayed mildly to moderately impaired skills, but there was no evidence of lateralized impairment. In contrast, her performance on tests of psychomotor speed was more variable, with a superior performance on Digit Symbol-Coding (98th percentile) and an average performance on Symbol Search (50th percentile), both from the WAIS-III.

Mood/Personality. Ms. T.'s affect was generally positive and appropriate to context. During the clinical interview she admitted to feelings of anxiety and depression related to her seizures and impending surgery. A self-report measure of syndromal depression (BDI-II) revealed moderate to severe depressive symptoms currently. She endorsed feelings of sadness, pessimism, loss of pleasure, self-dislike, self-criticalness, increased crying, agitation, loss of interest, indecisiveness, loss of energy, decreased sleep, irritability, decreased appetite, poor concentration, and fatigue. She denied suicidal ideation.

On the QOLIE-89, a quality-of-life inventory designed for patients with epilepsy, Ms. T.'s responses suggested a poorer quality of life than the average person with epilepsy. Her overall score was one standard deviation below average, and her responses to individual subtest scale items suggested prominent quality-of-life problems in role limitations (emotional), energy/fatigue, emotional well-being, health discouragement, worry about seizures, and medication effects.

On the PAI, Ms. T. generated a valid profile. There were significant elevations (T > 70) on three clinical scales: Somatic Complaints (T = 74), Anxiety (T = 71), and Depression (T = 75). All other clinical scales were within normal limits. Her profile indicates that she experiences significant concerns about her physical functioning and likely sees her life as disrupted by a number of physical problems. In addition to leaving her feeling unhappy and discouraged about her future, these problems have also likely affected her performance in social roles, and her lack of success in this area serves as an additional source of stress. She endorsed a variety of minor physical symptoms as well as vague complaints of ill health and fatigue. Ms. T. endorsed a number of items consistent with significant depressive symptoms. While she does not experience physiological signs of depression, she reports feelings of sadness, loss of interest in normal activities, and loss of sense of pleasure in activities that were previously enjoyed. Ms. T.'s profile is also suggestive of a moderate level of anxiety. Her responses indicate that worrying likely interferes with her ability to concentrate. Similar to her depressive feelings, she endorsed few physical signs of tension and stress. There were no significant problems noted in the following areas: unusual thoughts or peculiar experiences, antisocial behavior, problems with empathy, undue suspiciousness, unusually elevated mood or activity, or problematic behaviors to manage anxiety. Finally, Ms. T. denied significant problems with alcohol or drug abuse or dependence.

The diagnostic possibilities generated by the configuration of PAI scale scores include on Axis I: Major Depressive Disorder vs. Dysthymic Disorder. This diagnosis is consistent with her report of symptoms both on the BDI-II and during the clinical interview. Rule-out Personality

Disorder NOS was suggested by the PAI profile for Axis II. Although the PAI profile generated an additional Axis I rule out of Somatization Disorder/Undifferentiated Somatoform Disorder, similar symptoms in these disorders could be attributable to her epilepsy.

Discussion

The results of this assessment indicate that Ms. T. is currently functioning quite well from a cognitive standpoint. Most of her test scores fell in the average to above-average range, and she showed above-average intellectual functioning overall. Ms. T. did not display signs of mesial temporal lobe dysfunction, as her memory skills, including learning, retention, recall, and recognition were quite good on all memory tests administered, regardless of format (e.g., verbal vs. visual). Her performance in other cognitive domains also revealed strong scores on tests of executive functioning, spatial ability, and attention. The exception to this pattern is with regard to her language functions, particularly her scores on auditory and visual naming, which were both significantly impaired for her age and education. In contrast, she performed well on other tests of language, including abstract reasoning, word knowledge, and reading. The finding of a circumscribed deficit in naming is likely related to a structural or functional abnormality in the left temporal lobe, as documented by the video EEG results showing a left temporal lobe seizure origin. Together with the finding of strong memory skills, her neuropsychological test performance suggests dysfunction not in the mesial temporal lobe, but rather in neighboring neocortical structures that are specialized in naming.

The results of this evaluation raise a number of concerns regarding risk for postoperative cognitive complications. With regard to memory, Ms. T. possesses many of the risk factors for postoperative verbal memory decline, including planned surgery in the language dominant hemisphere, absence of MRI findings of mesial temporal sclerosis, good baseline verbal memory performance, and intact memory bilaterally on the Wada test. The neuropsychologist's role to inform both the neurosurgical team and the patient about the relative risks was extremely important.

Following completion of this evaluation and consultation with the Epilepsy Center neurosurgical team, recommendation was made for invasive monitoring with a subdural grid and depth electrodes to better localize her seizure focus. During this monitoring period, extensive language mapping was planned to reduce the risk for further postoperative language problems. Given the risks outlined earlier for possible language and memory decline following surgery, a frank discussion with this patient regarding these risk factors was also planned. Given her high level of cognitive function, she was expected to be able to weigh the risks and benefits adequately. Given the patient's current report of depressive symptoms, she was encouraged by the neuropsychologist to undergo a psychiatric evaluation to determine whether pharmacologic intervention and/or psychotherapy would be beneficial. Finally, repeat neuropsychological assessment 1 year post surgery was recommended.

Ms. T. did undergo invasive monitoring that identified her seizure focus as the left inferior temporal lobe. She subsequently underwent resection of the left inferior temporal lobe; pathology revealed cortical dysplasia. She will be closely monitored by the Epilepsy Center team with repeat neuropsychological assessment during her recovery.

References

Cohen-Gadol, A. A., Bradley, C. C., Williamson, A., Kim, J. H., Westerveld, M., Duckrow, R. B., & Spencer, D. D. (2005). Normal magnetic resonance imaging and medial temporal lobe epilepsy: The clinical syndrome of paradoxical temporal lobe epilepsy. *Journal of Neurosurgery, 102,* 902–909.

Seidenberg, M., Hermann, B., Wyler, A. R., Davies, K., Dohan, F. C., & Leveroni, C. (1998). Neuropsychological outcome following anterior temporal lobectomy in patients with and without the syndrome of mesial temporal lobe epilepsy. *Neuropsychology, 12,* 303–316.

Uijl, S. G., Leijten, F. S., Arends, J. B., Parra, J., van Huffelen, A. C., & Moons K. G. (2008). Prognosis after temporal lobe epilepsy surgery: The value of combining predictors. *Epilepsia, 49*(8), 1317–1323.

34

Language Dominant Mesial Temporal Lobe Epilepsy

William J. McMullen

Temporal lobectomy is a proven and well-accepted method of treatment for medically refractory focal epilepsy (Wiebe, Blume, Girvin, & Eliasziw, 2001). Together with video-electroencephalogram (EEG) monitoring and magnetic resonance imaging (MRI), neuropsychological evaluation has become a key component of the presurgical evaluation of patients with medically intractable epilepsy. Results of neuropsychological evaluation can be used to educate patients and families regarding cognitive difficulties, document when cognitive difficulties are contributing to significant functional impairment in the social or occupational arenas for legal purposes, and assist the treatment team in evaluating the potential risks and benefits of surgery for resection of the epileptogenic focus.

In evaluating these risks and benefits the primary issues that the treatment team needs to address are the likelihood of a dramatic reduction or elimination of seizures post surgery, and the likelihood of cognitive decline following surgery. A recent study documented how quality of life following temporal lobectomy relates primarily to seizure outcome and presence of memory decline (Langfit et al., 2007). Individuals who were seizure free following surgery reported improved quality of life even if they experienced memory decline. Those who were not seizure free following surgery and who experienced decline in memory reported worsened quality of life.

Factors that have been shown to predict seizure outcome following temporal lobe resection for treatment of medically refractory mesial temporal

lobe epilepsy (TLE) include presence of MRI abnormalities (e.g. atrophy, increased T2 signal) in the surgical mesial temporal lobe (Berkovic et al., 1995; Garcia, Laxer, Barbaro, & Dillon, 1994), absence of generalized tonic clonic seizures (Spencer et al., 2005), extent of resection (Wyler, Hermann, & Somes, 1995), and Wada memory asymmetry (Lee et al., 2003; Perrine et al., 1995; Sabsevitz, Swanson, Morris, Mueller, & Seidenberg, 2001). The Wada memory asymmetry score is defined as the difference between the memory scores achieved by each hemisphere. A favorable score would reflect that the nonepileptogenic mesial temporal lobe performs better on Wada memory testing than the epileptogenic mesial temporal lobe.

Factors that have been shown to predict cognitive outcome include side of surgery (Chelune, Naugle, Luders, & Awad, 1991; Clusmann et al., 2002; Hermann, Seidenberg, Haltiner, & Wyler, 1995), age at onset of seizures (Hermann et al., 1995), preoperative neuropsychological performance (Chelune et al., 1991; Clusmann et al., 2002; Hermann et al., 1995), and Wada memory asymmetry score (Lee et al., 2003; Sabsevitz et al., 2001). Findings have generally demonstrated that in language dominant (usually left) anterior temporal lobectomy (ATL) patients, the better the preoperative verbal memory, the greater the risk for postoperative verbal memory decline. Findings have additionally suggested that in these patients, the better the preoperative confrontation naming skill, the greater the risk for postoperative decline in naming.

From the above it can be argued that the more likely it is that seizure onsets are restricted to a single, functionally inadequate, mesial temporal lobe the more likely that removal of that mesial temporal lobe will result in elimination or dramatic reduction in seizures and the less likely it is that cognitive performance will deteriorate. In contrast, removal of a functionally adequate mesial temporal lobe is more likely to contribute to cognitive decline, and individuals with characteristics suggesting functionally adequate tissue (no MRI abnormality, reversed Wada asymmetry, good preoperative neuropsychological performance) are known to have a lower rate of good seizure outcome.

Neuropsychological testing and Wada testing therefore provide information that is key to predicting risk for cognitive decline following surgery, and that, along with other important data, helps to inform the prediction regarding seizure outcome. The integration of neuropsychological and Wada testing data in the service of these goals is illustrated in the following case.

The Case of A. S.

A. S. is a 49-year-old, right-handed, divorced white female with a history of epilepsy dating to age 39. She continued to experience seizures despite escalating doses of multiple antiepileptic medications. She was referred at the age of 46 for neuropsychological evaluation as part of her comprehensive presurgical work up. She then underwent left anterior temporal lobectomy with cortical language mapping 4 months following neuropsychological evaluation, and she has since undergone postoperative neuropsychological assessment at 14 months and 34 months post surgery.

A. S. reported that she was having slightly less than one seizure per month at the time of initial evaluation. She noted that the frequency of her seizures was escalating year over year. Most of her seizures were described as generalized tonic clonic convulsions. She also reported episodes during which she did not lose consciousness, but she became unable to respond to others around her and she had trouble understanding them. When asked about her cognitive symptoms, she reported that she believed that her verbal memory had been worsening over the prior 10 years.

She felt that her mathematics skills had also worsened and that she had increasing problems with auditory comprehension. She also reported a long history of depression. Medications at the time of initial evaluation included Lamictal, Lexapro, Dilantin, and aspirin.

A. S. reported that she is the product of a normal pregnancy, labor, and delivery. She denied history of meningitis and encephalitis. She denied history of learning disorder or attention deficit as a child and stated that she completed 14 years of formal education.

Medical history was reported to include motor vehicle accident in the late teen years during which A. S. reports that she did *not* lose consciousness. She reported that she was the unrestrained passenger in a car that struck a parked car at 20 mph. She reported that her face struck the windshield and that following the accident she experienced problems with her memory that were sufficient to cause her problems at work. She gradually recovered over a 1-year period, but she was unsure at the time of evaluation whether her memory had ever fully recovered.

A. S. reported that she had never used tobacco products and that she had ceased alcohol consumption following onset of seizure disorder. She denied family history of neurological disorder, including epilepsy. She reported that many of her relatives have experienced clinically significant depression.

Neurological evaluation was normal. MRI demonstrated left hippocampal atrophy and EEG demonstrated well-localized left temporal seizure onsets. A. S. underwent the intracarotid amobarbital procedure (IAP) or Wada test. Results found that the left hemisphere was dominant for language with prominent aphasia produced by injection of 120 mg of amobarbital into the left internal carotid artery. Memory was 10/12 with left injection and 10/12 with right injection (Memory asymmetry score = 0).

Preoperative Examination Results

Behavior Observations. A. S. was seen at bedside during her inpatient video-EEG monitoring stay. She was alert and oriented times three. She wore glasses and stated that her hearing was fine. She ambulated independently without obvious evidence of movement abnormality. Affect was broad and appropriate to content with mood described as euthymic. Suicidal and homicidal ideation/plan/intent were denied. Speech was clear and spontaneous and of normal volume, tone, and rate.

General Level of Intellectual Ability. A. S. was administered the Wechsler Adult Intelligence Scale III, on which her performance placed her within the average range (FSIQ = 104; 61st percentile). Verbal and nonverbal scales were comparable (VIQ = 104; PIQ = 104).

Inspection of index scores found that perceptual organization was at the upper end of the average range (PO index = 109; 73rd percentile). Verbal comprehension was at the mid-average range (VC index = 101; 53rd percentile). Working memory was at the mid-average range (WM index = 99; 47th percentile), while processing speed was at the low end of the average range (PS index = 93; 32nd percentile). Statistical analysis of inter-index discrepancies suggested that processing speed was significantly weaker than perceptual organization skills.

Examination of intersubtest variability found that, within the verbal scale, performance on a measure of mental arithmetic was a significant weakness (Arithmetic = 9th percentile) while performances on measures of digit repetition and social judgment were significant strengths (Digit Span = 91st percentile; Comprehension = 91st percentile). Within the nonverbal scale, performance on a measure of processing speed was a significant weakness (Digit Symbol-Coding = 16th percentile), while performance on a measure of visual reasoning was a significant strength (Matrix Reasoning = 84th percentile). There was no other significant intersubtest variability noted within either scale.

Achievement. A. S. was administered a screening measure of academic achievement in reading recognition, spelling, and arithmetic (Wide Range Achievement Test III). On this measure, her performance resulted in average scores for reading recognition (SS = 102) and spelling (SS = 95) and a low-average score for arithmetic (SS = 84).

Attention. Auditory attention and concentration skills were noted to be average to strong on the WAISIII (Digit Span = 91st percentile; Letter Number Sequencing = 50th percentile). Visual attention and concentration were average on the Picture Completion subtest of the WAISIII (50th percentile) and average on the spatial span subtest of the WMSIII (63rd percentile).

Processing Speed. Processing speed was low average to average on the WAISIII (Digit Symbol Coding = 16th percentile; Symbol Search = 63rd percentile). Processing speed associated with language (Stroop Word Reading and Color Naming) was notably weak (Word Reading Speed = 25th percentile; Color Naming Speed = 19th percentile).

Language. Confrontation naming was intact on the Boston Naming Test (57 Points; 46th percentile). Repetition was slightly weak, but not impaired, on a phrase repetition task (14/16). Verbal fluency was mixed; with generation of words to phonetic cue at the mid-average range (FAS = 45 words; 46th percentile), and generation of words to semantic cue at the borderline range (Animal Naming = 16 words; 8th percentile). Comprehension was adequate for task demands.

Visual Spatial Skill. Basic attention to visual detail was intact as noted earlier. Performance on the Block Design subtest of the WAISIII placed A. S. at the 75th percentile and suggested intact basic visual form discrimination, pattern recognition, visual organization, and visual motor integration. Performance on the Matrix Reasoning subtest placed A. S. at the 84th percentile and suggested intact visual reasoning skill as well. Visual sequencing was also intact on the picture arrangement subtest of the WAISIII (PA = 63rd percentile).

Memory. Memory was evaluated in both auditory and visual modalities using the Wechsler Memory Scale III. Auditory memory was found to be very poor (Auditory Immediate and Delayed Memory Scaled Scores both = 77), while visual memory was exceptionally strong (Visual Immediate Memory SS = 121; Visual Delayed Memory SS = 129). Statistical analysis of inter-index discrepancies found that auditory memory was significantly weaker than visual memory at both immediate and delayed recall.

Auditory memory was also found to be significantly weaker than expectations based on performance IQ. A. S. did not benefit substantially from cueing on auditory memory tasks, suggesting that her difficulty with memory was related not only to poor retrieval, but to impaired encoding and storage of verbal material as well.

Executive Functioning. Initiation skills were evaluated in both verbal and nonverbal modalities using tests of fluency. Performance on a test of verbal fluency was at the mid-average range on the FAS test (46th percentile), suggesting average verbal initiation skills. Nonverbal fluency was at the average range on the Ruff Figural Fluency Test (43rd percentile), suggesting average nonverbal initiation as well.

On the Stroop Test, A. S. was somewhat slow across reading and naming trials. However, her score on the interference index was at the average range. No problem with response inhibition per se was therefore suggested by her performance on this measure.

On the Wisconsin Card Sorting Test, a measure requiring good concept formation, self-monitoring, and problem-solving skills for successful performance, A. S. scored quite well overall. She earned all six categories, made only 12 errors (63rd percentile), six of which were perseverative (63rd percentile). She did, however, lose set twice (borderline to low average), suggesting some difficulty with sustaining attention.

Motor Functioning. A. S. was administered the Grooved Pegboard Test to evaluate fine motor coordination and speed. Her performance resulted in average scores for both right (58th percentile) and left (42nd percentile) hands. No significant or lateralizing problem was therefore identified in fine motor coordination.

Emotional Status. A. S. was administered the Personality Assessment Inventory, a standardized self-report personality questionnaire. Her responses to the validity scale items suggested that she produced a valid profile. Her responses to the clinical scale items resulted in a significant scale elevation on the DEP scale (T = 73). She reported a number of difficulties consistent with a significant depressive experience. She admitted openly to feelings of sadness, a loss of interest in normal activities, and a loss of sense of pleasure in things that were previously enjoyed. However, there were relatively few physiological signs of depression. There were no significant reports of suicidal ideation or anger management problems. A. S. also reported some concerns about physical functioning and health matters in general. Her responses suggested that others may see her as fairly impulsive and prone to behaviors likely to be self-harmful or self-destructive. Her interpersonal style appeared best characterized as self-effacing and lacking confidence in social interactions.

Rating Scales. A. S. was administered the Quality of Life in Epilepsy-89, an inventory that compares the individual with other individuals diagnosed with epilepsy in terms of self-reported quality of life. She neglected to complete items 3 through 13 and therefore the physical function scale and the overall score could not be computed. Her responses to the inventory resulted in significantly low ratings for scales measuring health perceptions, impact of epilepsy on work/driving/social functioning, and medication effects. Several additional areas were rated as low average in comparison to others with epilepsy, including overall quality of life, physical role limitations, attention and concentration, health discouragement, seizure worry, memory, social support and social isolation.

Postoperative Examination Results

A. S. was evaluated twice following surgery; at 14 and 34 months post surgery. She has been seizure free since surgery. At the first postoperative assessment she reported problems with memory and word finding, but by the second postoperative evaluation she noted that these issues had improved. She remained depressed at both time points but attributed this to significant social issues that were unrelated to her epilepsy.

Intellectual testing found an initial decline in verbal and nonverbal IQ postoperatively (VIQ = 95; PIQ = 97). At 34 months verbal IQ remained at the average range (VIQ = 97), but performance IQ had risen to high average (PIQ = 116). Verbal comprehension was average at both postoperative time points, but perceptual organization showed significant change; dropping to a standard score of 99 initially, and then rising to a scaled score of 123 at 34 months post. Working memory and processing speed were relatively stable and consistent from pre- to post-surgery.

Confrontation naming initially declined on the Boston Naming Test to 49 points (4th percentile; mild impairment) from the average range. At 34 months naming had improved to 54 pts (18th percentile; low average). Word generation to phonetic cue was stable at 14 months (62nd percentile) but improved at 34 months (92nd percentile). Animal naming declined initially (<1st percentile) but then recovered to the average range at 34 months (31st percentile). Repetition remained intact throughout.

Visual spatial skills initially declined somewhat following surgery, but at 34 months, scores had improved significantly so that they exceeded preoperative levels.

Memory performance on the Wechsler Memory Scale III demonstrated stable (and very poor) verbal memory following surgery at 14 months (Auditory Immediate Memory =74; Auditory Delayed Memory =71). At 34 months verbal memory improved to the low-average range (Immediate and Delayed Memory both SS = 89). Visual memory, perhaps surprisingly, declined significantly at 14 months following surgery; from the superior range to the average range (Visual Immediate Memory = 105; Visual Delayed Memory = 97). At 34 months visual memory improved to the high-average range for immediate memory (SS = 112), and remained at the average range for delayed visual memory (SS = 103).

Executive functioning demonstrated improvement in verbal and nonverbal initiation by 34 months. Stroop test performance was stable. Performance on the Wisconsin Card Sorting Test was intact at all assessments. Fine motor coordination was intact at follow-up.

Overall quality of life on the QUOLIE-89 was average with some problems reported with attention and emotional functioning. As noted above, a depression was present that was reported to be unrelated to health issues.

Discussion

This case presents an interesting mix of factors in an individual with left temporal lobe epilepsy.

The patient's seizure disorder was late onset, she showed intact function bilaterally on the Wada test, and she showed intact confrontation naming prior to surgery. All of these factors would suggest risk of decline in cognition (verbal memory and language skill) and some risk for poor seizure outcome. In contrast, she was known to have hippocampal atrophy on the left, and she was noted to have had very localized left temporal lobe onsets. These latter factors would argue that she was likely to have a good seizure outcome. The Wada test demonstrated intact function bilaterally, but the memory asymmetry score, though not in the favored direction, was not in the unfavorable direction (Score = 0).

Neuropsychological testing suggested very poor verbal memory and very strong visual memory. This pattern was consistent with the known left-temporal lobe onsets and would not suggest likely verbal memory decline following left ATL. Confrontation naming, in contrast, was strong and thus raised the possibility that word-finding skill might decline following surgery. Semantic verbal fluency was significantly weak at the preoperative evaluation, but not frankly impaired.

Taking all of these data into account, it was felt that A. S. was at some risk for decline in both language and verbal memory following surgery (though the level of risk for memory decline was difficult to quantify given conflicting Wada and neuropsychological memory results). Her risk of postoperative seizures was felt by the treatment team to be low given the MRI and EEG results.

Postoperative testing confirmed an initial decline in semantic verbal fluency and confrontation naming skill that improved by the retesting at 34 months. Verbal memory was unchanged initially and then later improved to the low-average range. Visual spatial functions improved significantly by the second postoperative assessment and executive functioning was stable or improved. Surprisingly, visual memory declined significantly following surgery and has not fully recovered to the level achieved preoperatively. While weaker than prior to surgery, visual memory is clearly functional (average to high average) and the patient reports being satisfied with surgery and reports improved overall quality of life, though unrelated social issues have continued to contribute to mood disturbance. As noted

Table 34-1. Comparison between preoperative (left temporal lobectomy), postoperative 1, and postoperative 2 evaluation scaled scores (or raw scores as indicated) and percentiles for patient A.S.

TEST/AREA	MEASURE	2004 Scaled Score	2006 Scaled Score	2007 Scaled Score	2007 Percentile
WAIS-III	Vocabulary	10	10	11	63
	Similarities	12	11	11	63
	Arithmetic	6	4	4	2
	Digit Span	14	14	12	75
	Information	9	8	10	50
	Comprehension	14	9	10	50
	Letter-Number Seq	10	8	11	63
	Picture Completion	10	8	14	91
	Digit Symbol-Coding	7	6	8	25
	Block Design	12	12	16	98
	Matrix Reasoning	13	10	11	63
	Picture Arrangement	11	12	13	84
	Symbol Search	11	11	11	63
WRAT-III	Reading	102	102	100	50
	Spelling	95	98	105	63
	Math	84	87	92	30
WMS-III	Auditory Immediate	77	74	89	23
	Auditory Delayed	77	71	89	23
	Auditory Recognition	75	75	70	2
	Visual Immediate	121	105	112	79
	Visual Delayed	129	97	103	58
	General Memory	93	78	87	19
	Working Memory	102	93	108	70
Language	Boston Naming	57	49	54	18
	COWAT (FAS)	45	49	60	92
	Animal Naming	16	12	20	31
	Phrase Repetition	14/16	16/16	16/16	N/A
Executive	COWAT (FAS)	45	49	60	92
	Ruff Figural Designs	91	104	110	75
	Ruff Persev Ratio	0.1209	0.1827	0.0909	77
	Golden Stroop Words	107	97	108	66
	Golden Stroop Color	67	62	69	24
	Golden Color-Word	38	38	40	50
	Interference Index	-0.30	0.00	-0.20	42
	Wisconsin Categories	6	6	6	>16
	Wisconsin Errors	12	20	11	66
	Wisconsin PE	6	9	5	68
	Wisconsin Set Loss	2	1	0	>16
Motor Skill	GP Dominant	60	87	51	97
	GP Nondominant	71	80	62	82

earlier, she has remained seizure free nearly 4 years post temporal lobectomy.

Epilepsy is a common neurological disorder and medically refractory temporal lobe epilepsy often impacts negatively on quality of life, social and occupational function, driving, and independence. Uncontrolled epilepsy also carries with it the potential for cognitive decline over time as well as the risk of sudden unexpected death in epilepsy (SUDEP). Surgery to remove the epileptogenic focus is an effective treatment in localization-related focal epilepsies in properly selected patients. The neuropsychologist can play an important role as part of the epilepsy treatment team by helping to assess the level of cognitive risk posed by a suggested surgical intervention, as well as by assisting in identifying whether the patient is in a group of patients who are likely to experience a dramatic reduction or elimination of seizures following surgery. Because new nonresective treatment options are potentially on the horizon for individuals classified as high risk for cognitive decline following surgery (e.g., responsive neurostimulation, deep brain stimulation), it will likely be ever more important for neuropsychologists to assist in informing the treatment team, and educating potential surgical candidates, regarding the risks and potential benefits of resective surgery to treat refractory epilepsy.

References

Berkovic, S., McIntosh, A., Kalnins, R., Jackson, G., Fabinyi, G., Brazenor, G., Bladin, P., & Hopper, J. (1995). Preoperative MRI predicts outcome of temporal lobectomy: An actuarial analysis. *Neurology*, 45, 1358–1363.

Chelune, G., Naugle, R., Luders, H., & Awad, I., (1991). Prediction of cognitive change as a function of preoperative ability status among temporal lobectomy patients seen at 6-month follow-up. *Neurology*, 41(3), 399–404.

Clusmann, H., Schramm, J., Kral, T., Helmstaedter, C., Ostertun, B., Fimmers, R., Haun, D., & Elger, C. (2002). Prognostic factors and outcome after different types of resection for temporal lobe epilepsy. *Journal of Neurosurgery*, 97, 1131–1141.

Garcia, P., Laxer, K., Barbaro, N., & Dillon, W. (1994). Prognostic value of qualitative magnetic resonance imaging hippocampal abnormalities in patients undergoing temporal lobectomy for medically refractory seizures. *Epilepsia*, 35(3), 520–524.

Hermann, B., Seidenberg, M., Haltiner, A., & Wyler, A. (1995). Relationship of age at onset, chronological age, and adequace of preoperative performance to verbal memory change after anterior temporal lobectomy. *Epilepsia*, 36(2), 137–145.

Langfitt., J., Westerveld, M., Hamberger, M., Walczak, T., Cicchetti, D., Berg, A., Vickrey, B., Barr, W., Sperling, M., Masur, D., & Spencer, S. (2007). Worsening of quality of life after epilepsy surgery; effects of seizures and memory decline. *Neurology*, 68, 1988–1994.

Lee, G., Park, Y., Westerveld, M., Hempel, A., Blackburn, L., & Loring, D. (2003). Wada memory performance predicts seizure outcome after epilepsy surgery in children. *Epilepsia*, 44(7), 936–943.

Perrine, K., Westerveld, M., Sass, K., Devinsky, O., Dogali, M., Spencer, D., Luciano, D., & Nelson, P. (1995). Wada memory disparities predict seizure laterality and postoperative seizure control. *Epilepsia*, 36(9), 851–856.

Sabsevitz, D., Swanson, S., Morris, G., Mueller, W., & Seidenberg, M. (2001). Memory outcome after left anterior temporal lobectomy in patients with expected and reversed Wada memory asymmetry scores. *Epilepsia*, 42(11), 1408–1415.

Spencer, S., Berg, A., Vickrey, B., Sperling, M., Bazil, C., Shinnar, S., Langfitt, J., Walczak, T., & Pacia, S. (2005). Predicting long-term seizure outcome after resective epilepsy surgery; the multi-center study. *Neurology*, 65, 912–918.

Wiebe, S., Blume, W., Girvin, J., & Eliasziw, M. (2001). A randomized, controlled trial of surgery for temporal-lobe epilepsy. *New England Journal of Medicine*, 345(5), 311–318.

Wyler, A., Hermann, B., & Somes, G. (1995). Extent of medial temporal resection on outcome from anterior temporal lobectomy: A randomized prospective study. *Neurosurgery*, 37(5), 982–991.

35

Motor and Cognitive Characteristics in a Case of Static Encephalopathy

David E. Tupper

Chronic neurodevelopmental disorders seen by pediatric neuropsychologists are often divided into progressive, paroxysmal, and/or static conditions. Progressive childhood neurological disorders can involve genetic or neoplastic etiologies, and they may engender a great deal of urgent clinical attention to help identify concerns as soon as possible, so that the child's life may be extended or the disorder cured. Paroxysmal disorders such as seizures/epilepsy, and episodic disorders of movement or awareness, often benefit from focused neurological assessment and intervention to identify and treat their source, and thus, to optimize their outcome. Static neurological disorders, in contrast, such as cerebral palsy or a specific learning disability, represent a category of childhood chronic disorder that may receive less urgent neurological or pediatric interest but deserve neuropsychological assessment and intervention.

Static encephalopathy is a term used to indicate the fairly common lifelong morbidity from a single or limited neurological etiology suffered in early brain development (Tomlin & St. Clair Forbes, 1995). It is a very general term and the etiologies of static encephalopathy are potentially quite varied. The more common conditions include traumatic brain injury in early life, perinatal hypoxic/ischemic encephalopathy in premature and low-birth-weight infants, perinatal asphyxia, fetal alcohol exposure, and pediatric stroke (see Pellock & Myer, 1992). Other less common etiologies for static encephalopathy include infections (encephalitis or meningitis), human immunodeficiency virus (HIV)-associated encephalopathy of childhood, carbon monoxide poisoning, or radiation necrosis, among many possibilities (Trescher & Johnston, 1992). Sometimes the etiology is inferred based on only indirect evidence of a specific cerebral insult. Any functions of the brain may be affected in varying combinations in a static encephalopathy, depending on the type, localization, timing, and degree of pathology.

Children with static encephalopathy are characterized by continued acquisition of skills at rates below expected levels of normal development but commensurate with their overall level of functioning (Taylor, 1959). The delays typically observed longitudinally in these children remain relatively stable over time compared to initial levels of functioning, although the overall outcome can be quite varied. The gradual decline, or lack of gains, in development observed in other, more progressive encephalopathies is not seen in children with static encephalopathy. However, there may be symptomatic progression, or progression of some of the behavioral and cognitive difficulties, in many children with static encephalopathy as they grow older because they are presented with increasingly complex developmental demands (Dennis, 2000; Goldstein, 2004; Nelson, 2005). The interaction between a chronic brain dysfunction, the developing brain, and the environment adds variation to possible outcomes.

Closely associated with the concept of static encephalopathy is the category of cerebral palsy.

Cerebral palsy is an umbrella term used to refer to a group of nonprogressive disorders of movement and posture that result from a lesion of the immature brain. Cerebral palsy was first described in the early 1800s and investigated formally by William John Little in 1861, who thought it was related specifically to perinatal asphyxia during difficult birth deliveries. Cerebral palsy is the most common cause of physical disability in childhood (Warschausky, 2006), and it reflects a range of conditions resulting from a variety of prenatal, perinatal, and postnatal etiologies. Cerebral palsy is actually one of the static encephalopathies that are characterized by motor deficits with onset in early infancy. While the defining features of cerebral palsy emphasize motor impairment, there are usually other associated limitations in orthopedic and muscular function, visual and perceptual capabilities, cognitive processing, and neurological and emotional function. The prevalence of cerebral palsy is thought to be approximately 2–4 per 1000 children, or about 1 in 500 live births, and the severity of impairment ranges from subtle motor difficulties and clumsiness to involvement of the whole body.

The diagnosis of cerebral palsy is typically made when a child fails to meet motor developmental milestones (Blondis, 1996). The most important diagnostic consideration is that there is no evidence of progressive disease, and neurologists frequently try to rule out a number of genetic, degenerative, or inherited metabolic disorders before identifying cerebral palsy in a child. Neurological and developmental evaluations emphasizing history and physical examination, as well as laboratory screening tests, neuroimaging, electrophysiological tests, and neuropsychological evaluation can provide information to support the diagnosis. According to Blondis (2004), cerebral palsy can be classified according to its clinical motor presentation (extent of tone, spasticity, or movement abnormality demonstrated), the cerebral pathophysiology involved (pyramidal vs. extrapyramidal involvement; traumatic, hypoxic-ischemic, or other etiology), or topographically (diplegia, hemiplegia, triplegia, quadriplegia). Clinically, children with cerebral palsy demonstrate a variety of neuromotor and neuropsychological characteristics that result in functional disability, such as muscle tone abnormalities, muscle weakness, loss of selective movements, and altered patterns of muscle activation. Deficits are often more pronounced in fine motor than in gross motor activities, and problems with motor learning are also seen. In addition to the motor dysfunction, persons with cerebral palsy often suffer from deficits in sensation, perception, learning, emotion, and interpersonal relationships.

Outcomes for individuals with cerebral palsy (and static encephalopathy) are quite varied, given the heterogeneity of functioning seen. Often a continuum of central nervous system dysfunction is seen, with mental retardation present in as much as 60% of children with cerebral palsy (Badawi et al., 2005; Madge et al., 1993). Children with seizures also have a poorer long-term prognosis, and feeding and swallowing problems often affect physical growth. Spasticity and other orthopedic problems lead to decreased functional capabilities. Neuropsychologically, it is difficult to make clear generalizations about the relationship between cerebral palsy and cognitive functioning (Burns & Van Winkle, 2006). A range of IQs has been documented in a number of studies, and any intellectual deficits are likely to be either general or specific in a particular case, depending upon particular aspects of the original static lesion. Relatively few studies of specific neurocognitive deficits have been performed in children with cerebral palsy or static encephalopathy (Fennell & Dikel, 2001). Children with spastic diplegia often show visuoperceptual impairments, and these are thought to be a function of sensory and motoric abnormalities as much as visuospatial function. Hemiplegic cerebral palsy often leads to neuropsychological effects consistent with lateralized early life lesions, dependent upon the hemisphere involved (see Tupper, 2007). In the long term, some children with cerebral palsy who show characteristics of a nonverbal learning disability may demonstrate problems in adaptive behavior and personality adjustment (Del Dotto, Fisk, McFadden, & Rourke, 1991).

In child neuropsychology, there are other differential diagnostic possibilities that need to be considered in evaluating children with motor dysfunction or unexplained clumsiness (Bagnato & Campbell, 1992; Fox & Lent, 1996). Prominent among them is *developmental coordination disorder* (DCD), a term that is used to differentiate children with idiopathic motor problems from children who are suspected of showing some type of early life cerebral insult leading to an acquired static encephalopathy (i.e., mild cerebral palsy). According to the *DSM-IV* (American Psychiatric Association [APA], 2000), children with DCD demonstrate motor performances substantially below expectation given their chronological age and measured intelligence, and the motor disturbance must interfere with academic achievement or activities of daily living. Since it is considered a developmental disorder, the term *DCD* is not applied if cerebral palsy or another neuromuscular or medical condition is present. Nevertheless, the differentiation of a subtle acquired motor disorder from a developmental coordination disorder is not always easy or readily apparent (Deuel, 2002). The absence of evidence of an early-life cerebral lesion is often used in the discrimination of a mild form of cerebral palsy from a developmental coordination disorder, but many children with cerebral palsy do not have definitive lesions on imaging or abnormal neurological findings. Hence, the profile of neuropsychological results in an assessment may provide the needed information to help identify an acquired pattern of motor and associated abnormalities from one where motor function is delayed.

Case Study: S. E.

S. E. was a 15-year, 7-month-old, right-handed male when seen for neuropsychological evaluation. He was referred by a local pediatrician who specializes in developmental pediatrics, based on a desire to gain a better understanding of his cognitive profile to assist with long-term planning for his developmental needs. The pediatrician had followed S. E. for about 12 years, after S. E. was first identified with delays in his speech/language acquisition, motor functioning, and coordination.

History

S. E. was born full term after a long labor with no obvious delivery complications, and with a birth weight of 7 lb, 15 oz. Meconium staining was present at birth, suggestive of fetal distress and/or low oxygenation, but his Apgar scores were acceptable at 7 at 1 minute and 9 at 5 minutes. His nursing and later feeding were described as slightly delayed during infancy, and he only began walking at about 18 months of age; S. E. was described as having "toe-walked" through

the preschool ages. He was a large infant whose growth slowed in his first few years, to the average to low-normal range. His speech development was similarly delayed, with S. E. only using short sentences by the time he was 3 years old, and with reportedly better understanding than expression of language at that time. S. E.'s delays in speech and motor skills became more apparent at about age 3, when he began receiving early childhood education services to help support his developmental progress.

At age 5 years, 10 months, because of persisting concerns about these developmental delays, his pediatrician sent S. E. for a more extensive neurodevelopmental evaluation that included several components. He was then in kindergarten and was described as small for his age, as well as socially immature. S. E. was found to be 2 standard deviations below the mean height for his age, with average weight, but with small head size (one standard deviation below the mean). Audiological assessment showed mild conductive hearing loss, an evaluation by an otolaryngologist noted mild midface underdevelopment, and no pulmonary issues were noted. Neurologically, S. E. had stable but abnormal neurological findings, including low muscle tone in his upper limbs, high muscle tone in his lower limbs, and proximal muscle weakness. He was described as having spastic quadriparesis, and impaired coordination and motor planning. Language assessment found normal recognition vocabulary and basic communication but delays in understanding concepts and lengthy information. Intellectual assessment (using the WPPSI-R) documented a Full-Scale IQ of 78, Verbal IQ of 86, and Performance IQ of 73. Denver Developmental Screening test results demonstrated developmental delays in fine and gross motor development as well as personal-social development. The overall neurodevelopmental diagnosis was of mild cerebral palsy due to static encephalopathy.

S. E. had a number of subsequent medical and psychological assessments during childhood and early adolescence. During a 3-year follow-up assessment, at about 8 years of age, S. E. had an electroencephalogram (EEG) following a fall off a bicycle related to an apparent fainting spell. The EEG showed anterior left quadrant spikes during wakefulness, thought to be evidence of potential epileptogenic dysfunction in the left frontotemporal region. However, S. E. has never been noted to demonstrate seizures, has never been placed on antiepileptic medication, and had no subsequent syncopal episodes. Additionally, brain magnetic resonance imaging (MRI) at that time was reported to be normal. Because of his previously described mild dysmorphic features, he also underwent chromosomal analysis and fragile X DNA testing, which was described as within normal limits; the pediatrician thought that his appearance suggested a syndrome, but none was identified. He was found at age 8–9 years to have a growth hormone deficiency and was treated with growth hormones for several years, with a good spurt in his growth associated with this treatment. No major changes in S. E.'s clinical neurological status occurred, and he continued to be diagnosed with mild cerebral palsy based on his persisting motor difficulties. Educationally, S. E. was in mostly regular classes at school, although he had an individualized educational plan (IEP) developed under the "physical and other health impaired" classification to provide him partial (1 hour/day of resource room assistance) special educational support.

At about 9 years of age, S. E.'s family described him as being somewhat depressed, and they had concerns about his self-esteem. This led to a limited mental health and pediatric assessment. These concerns reportedly stemmed from comments that S. E. made, such as calling himself "stupid" and saying that other children called him "retarded." Schoolwork was also described as becoming more difficult, as he had entered fourth grade, and he was more frustrated with the increased complexity of the academic curriculum; increased "hyperactive" behavior was described at school. He underwent a limited assessment of his academic and attentional skills at that time and was noted to perform better on verbal than nonverbal tasks, to have problems with multistep tasks, and to show possible learning difficulties. He was diagnosed with attention-deficit/hyperactivity disorder (ADHD), and Ritalin was prescribed with good benefit. School services were increased, and he began receiving adaptive physical education along with limited special education, occupational therapy, and physical therapy. Aside from these changes, it is unclear whether any additional mental health services were provided, although a subsequent pediatric note described developmental immaturity in self-care and social emotional skills,

apparently documented on a Vineland Adaptive Behavior Scales inventory.

S. E. maintained effective functioning for several years with his ongoing developmental pediatric care, medication, and special educational and supportive services. When seen in neurodevelopmental follow-up at age 14-½ years, he was described as showing good growth velocity, had continued good benefit from Ritalin, and no major medical issues had emerged. He was judged to possibly be showing a plateau in his mental skills, because of his "static encephalopathy," and more detailed cognitive assessment was considered. S. E. had a repeat Vineland Adaptive Behavior Scales assessment at age 14 years, 9 months, as part of a very limited psychological assessment. He was found to demonstrate limited adaptive behavioral skills overall, with particularly reduced socialization (standard score = 58), daily living skills (standard score = 55), and motor skills (standard score = 56) compared to only moderately low communication (standard score = 70). Recommendations were made for his pediatrician to work closely with S. E.'s mother and school regarding his developmental needs, and to obtain a more detailed neuropsychological evaluation.

Neuropsychological Evaluation

The county developmental disabilities worker involved with S. E. thought that it might be beneficial to request a neuropsychological evaluation, based on the previous psychologist's recommendation. S. E.'s pediatrician agreed and the evaluation was conducted when S. E. was age 15 years, 7 months. S. E. was accompanied to the appointment by his mother, and she participated in an interview and completed several forms. S. E. was observed to be somewhat small and thin for his age, with subtle dysmorphic features, including large ears and a large mouth. He was well dressed and neatly groomed. He had mild misarticulation errors and subtle dysarthria, but these were not impairing and he had otherwise functional communication skills. S. E.'s motor speed was slow and his movements were awkward and labored at times; he also tended to keep his head close to the paper when working on pencil-and-paper tasks. No obvious chorea was noted, and gait was broadly within normal limits. He demonstrated a full range of affect, and his mood was generally euthymic. S. E. reported that he was referred because of his ADHD, and that his medication helped him concentrate on classwork; otherwise he would be "hyper," have high energy, and he would move around a lot. S. E. reported that his problems in school were primarily in math, referring to his Algebra class. In separate interview, S. E.'s mother reported that he was diagnosed at about age 5 years with "mild CP," and that while developmental delays were noted prior to 5 years he had not received a diagnosis. She reported that he had scattered skills, and that his cognitive discrepancies were more notable now that he is older. She noted that his math skills were his weakest, and that even "basic skills" like multiplication and division were difficult. She said that S. E. tended to be drawn to younger children in his social interactions, acted younger behaviorally, and generally did not enjoy socializing with same-age peers.

At the time of this evaluation, S. E. was in 10th grade at a local high school and was primarily mainstreamed in regular education classes, with approximately 1 hour/day of special education assistance. He received assistance in homework strategy, for example, "pacing" himself, and organizational skills, in his special education class. His IEP had been recently updated under the physical and other health impaired classification. He was doing fairly well in language-based classes, such as English and Social Studies, but struggled most in math. Overall, he was a B honor roll student. S. E. resided at home with his mother and younger sister. His parents were divorced when he was young, but his father remained involved in his upbringing and he stayed with his father on weekends. S. E.'s mother had a college education and worked full time in an educational setting. His father had a high school education and worked as a driver. Relevant family history included that his sister had been diagnosed with childhood-onset bipolar disorder and was subject to stormy and volatile behavior. She got along adequately with S. E., but she had lived for a brief time outside of the family home.

S. E. was administered a comprehensive neuropsychological assessment battery, tailored to his age and the referral questions. Thus, he completed measures of general cognitive and intellectual functioning, academic skills, attention and concentration, learning and memory, motor skills, and conceptual and executive skills. In addition, S. E. and his mother completed objective behavioral and psychological inventories about his functioning. S. E. was cooperative and appeared to demonstrate appropriate effort for the evaluation, so the results were judged to be reasonably reliable and valid indicators of his capabilities. He stated that he had taken his stimulant medication (Concerta) before the appointment, and he was attentive throughout the evaluation. According to parent report, this was the only neuropsychological evaluation that S. E. had ever completed, although he had previously participated in a number of psychological, educational, and developmental assessments.

Table 35-1 provides details of the overall neuropsychological evaluation findings for S. E. As can be seen, the Wechsler Abbreviated Scale of Intelligence (WASI) was used to obtain a general estimate of intellectual functioning and, additionally, the Das-Naglieri Cognitive Assessment System (CAS) was administered as another measure of overall cognitive functioning, one which tapped more specific cognitive processes. On the WASI, S. E. received low-average to borderline intellectual scores, which were similar in pattern to previous test results, but several points higher. This likely was indicative of differences in test instruments used over the years. S. E. showed statistically higher (.05 significance level) verbal intellectual skills, especially verbal vocabulary, than nonverbal or visually based intellectual skills. His lowest score was on the Block Design subtest, a measure of visuo-constructional skills. On the CAS, S. E. showed slightly lower scores than on the WASI, which ranged from low-average to the borderline range. His CAS Full Scale score of 68 was at the 1.6th percentile and clearly lower than his WASI FSIQ of 81, which was at the 10th percentile. Interestingly, S. E. demonstrated moderate variability on specific CAS scales, although none of them were statistically different from one another. He received standard scores of 77 for Planning, 74 for Simultaneous cognitive processing, 82 for Attention, and 71 for Successive cognitive processing. Within CAS scales, S. E. demonstrated a pattern of strengths and weaknesses, that is, strength on the Word Series subtest and weakness on the Nonverbal Matrices and Sentence Questions subtests.

Interestingly, academic skills assessed with the Wide Range Achievement Test–Third edition

Table 35-1. Neuropsychological Evaluation Results for Case S. E., Age 15 Years, 7 Months*

	Standard, Scaled, or z Score	Percentile
General Cognitive/Intellectual Skills		
Wechsler Abbreviated Scale of Intelligence (WASI)		
Full Scale IQ	81	10th percentile
Verbal IQ	88	21st percentile
Vocabulary	9	
Similarities	6	
Performance IQ	77	6th percentile
Block Design	4	
Matrix Reasoning	7	
Das-Naglieri Cognitive Assessment System (CAS)		
Full Scale score	68	1.6th percentile
Planning Scale	77	6th percentile
Matching Numbers	7	
Planned Codes	6	
Planned Connections	6	
Simultaneous Processing Scale	74	4th percentile
Nonverbal Matrices	4 (weakness)	
Visual Spatial Relations	8	
Figure Memory	6	
Attention Scale	82	12th percentile
Expressive Attention	7	
Number Detection	8	
Receptive Attention	6	
Successive Processing Scale	71	3rd percentile
Word Series	8 (strength)	
Sentence Repetition	6	
Sentence Questions	2 (weakness)	
Academic Skills		
Wide Range Achievement Test (3rd edition)		
Reading (word recognition)	84	14th percentile
Spelling	90	25th percentile
Arithmetic	88	21st percentile
Attention		
WISC-III Digit Span subtest		
4 digits forward, 3 digits backward	3	
Connors' Continuous Performance Test-II		
55.8% clinical confidence index; only subscore that is atypical is Hit SE Block Change		
Language		
DKEFS Verbal Fluency subtest		
Letter Fluency	8	
Category Fluency	12	
Category Switching		
Total correct responses	14	
Total switching accuracy	16	
Memory		
Wide Range Assessment of Memory and Learning (WRAML)		
Design Memory subtest	5	

(Continued)

Table 35-1. Neuropsychological Evaluation Results for Case S. E., Age 15 Years, 7 Months (*Continued*)

Standard, Scaled, or z Score			Percentile
California Verbal Learning Test for *Children (CVLT-C)*			
Trials 1–5	T = 49		
Short delay free recall	−1.0		
Short delay cued recall	−0.5		
Long delay free recall	−0.5		
Long delay cued recall	−1.5		
Recognition hits	0.0		
Recognition false positives	+3.0		
Rey Complex Figure and Recognition Trial			
Immediate recall	raw score = 9.5, T = 23		
Delayed recall	raw score = 5.5, T < 20		
Recognition total	raw score = 18, T = 33		
Motor/Visuo-motor Skills			
Finger Tapping Test	Right hand	mean of 24.4 taps/10 seconds	
	Left hand	mean of 22.4 taps/10 seconds	
Purdue Pegboard	Right hand	12.0 (raw score)	<10th percentile
(pegs placed)	Left hand	10.5 (raw score)	<10th percentile
	Both hands	8 (pairs)	<10th percentile
Beery Test of Visual-Motor Integration	71		3rd percentile
Rey Complex Figure and Recognition Trial			
Copy	raw score = 17		<1st percentile
Executive Functioning			
D-KEFS Tower	Achievement score = 11		
Wisconsin Card Sorting Test (WCST)			
3 categories achieved (6–10th percentile)			
56 errors (SS = 79)			
25 perseverative errors (SS = 83)			
33 perseverative responses (SS = 80)			
2 failures to maintain set (>16th percentile)			

Behavioral/Emotional Ratings

Achenbach Child Behavior Checklist (CBCL)—completed by mother; elevated internalizing problems (withdrawal, anxious/depressed, social problems, attention problems)

Achenbach Youth Self Report (YSR)—completed by S.E.; no clinically significant problems endorsed

Behavior Rating Inventory of Executive Functions (BRIEF)—parent profile, completed by mother; elevations on most scales, especially shifting, initiation, working memory

*Standard or scaled scores are provided, except as noted.

(WRAT-3) were slightly higher than his intellectual/general cognitive skills, with scores ranging from low average to average, although they were below grade level (reflecting mostly fifth to sixth grade equivalent performances). S. E.'s single-word reading and spelling skills earned standard scores of 84 and 90, respectively, and errors were phonetically accurate. Arithmetic was at a similar level, with a standard score of 88. S. E. demonstrated weaknesses in working with common fractions, and he ultimately did not solve any algebraic equations.

S. E.'s attention and concentration were assessed with several measures. As noted earlier, he demonstrated low-average attentional capabilities on the CAS Attention scale, with no statistical strengths or weaknesses demonstrated. Immediate auditory attention as assessed on the WISC-III Digit Span subtest was moderately impaired; he repeated four digits forward and three digits backward, a performance that was below normal for his age. Sustained attentional skills, as assessed on the Connor's Continuous Performance Test-II, were consistent with an

ADHD sample. He demonstrated a borderline level of clinical significance, poor vigilance, and less consistent responding over the duration of the task.

Expressive language skills were assessed with the Delis-Kaplan Executive Function System (D-KEFS) Verbal Fluency subtest. S. E. performed fairly well. He showed low-average phonemic fluency, high-average category fluency, and performed within high-average limits for category switching. He showed somewhat variable performances on the verbal/language subtests of the WASI and CAS. As noted, he was average on the WASI Vocabulary subtest and he had borderline verbal reasoning on the WASI Similarities subtest. On the CAS Successive processing scale, which is highly verbal, he demonstrated relative strength repeating series of words of varying lengths, demonstrated borderline capability repeating sentences, but showed a clear weakness on the Sentence Questions subtest, which requires grammatical understanding of complex, noncontextual sentences.

Learning and memory capabilities were assessed in both the verbal and visual/figural domains. On the California Verbal Learning Test for Children (CVLT-C), a measure of verbal learning and memory, his performance fell within normal limits. He demonstrated an average learning curve over repeated presentations of a word list, and he showed low-average to average immediate and delayed recall of the word list, with slight confusion on delayed cued recall and recognition. Thus, he was able to encode novel verbal information and recall this information, but he had difficulty correctly discriminating the words he had learned from closely associated words or interfering stimuli. Visual/figural memory was assessed using the Wide Range Assessment of Memory and Learning (WRAML) Design Memory subtest and the Rey-Osterrieth Complex Figure (ROCF). Immediate memory for more simple Design Memory visual stimuli was borderline to mildly impaired. S. E. showed significant nonverbal memory difficulty on the more difficult Rey figure memory trials (see also Figure 35-1B and 35-1C). S. E. demonstrated a notably impaired initial copy production of the figure, and recall performances below the first percentile that only improved slightly (to the 4th percentile) on a multiple-choice recognition trial. Hence, S. E. demonstrated better recall for verbal than nonverbal stimuli, although his visual memory difficulties were likely compounded by poor organizational skills on visuoconstructional/ visuomotor tasks (see later discussion).

S. E. showed variable and mostly poor basic motor performances. Simple finger speed on the Finger Tapping test was impaired bilaterally, but with slight dominant (right) hand performance superiority as expected. Fine motor dexterity was assessed with the Purdue Pegboard and was also significantly impaired bilaterally, with scores below the 10th percentile but also with a slight dominant hand performance superiority. Dexterity on the both hands (bilateral) trial was also limited. With regard to visuomotor performances, S. E. demonstrated reduced visuomotor or drawing skill on the Beery-Buktenica Test of Visual-Motor Integration. His performance was well below age expectations, at about the 8-year-old level. As described previously, when presented with even more complex visual stimuli such as the ROCF, S. E. showed severe constructional and organizational difficulties. His score fell at the 1st percentile, but most importantly, he showed notable distortion of the figure in his reproduction (see Figure 35-1A).

Conceptual and executive skills were also assessed. S. E. demonstrated low-average simple planning capabilities on the CAS Planning scale, which was a relative (but nonstatistical) strength among cognitive processing skills assessed by that measure. Another relative strength in planning was noted on the D-KEFS Tower subtest; S. E. received an average score. Reasoning skills, as measured with the WASI Similarities and Matrix Reasoning subtests, were in the borderline range. Slightly lower nonverbal reasoning skills were noted on the CAS Nonverbal Matrices subtest. On the Wisconsin Card Sorting Test, a measure of concept formation and the ability to utilize external feedback, S. E. again demonstrated borderline skills that were fairly consistent with current intellectual expectations. He attained three of six conceptual categories and showed a mild perseverative response tendency, suggesting mild rigidity in his thought processes and difficulty in complex problem-solving skills.

Finally, S. E. and his mother completed objective behavioral and psychological inventories.

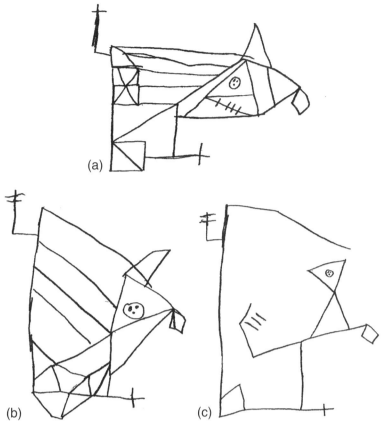

Figure 35-1. Reproduction of the Rey-Osterreith Complex Figure by S. E. (*a*) Copy, (*b*) 3-minute immediate recall, and (*c*) 30-minute delayed recall.

Unfortunately, teacher report forms were sent but not returned. S. E. completed the Achenbach Youth Self-Report Form, and his responses yielded no clinically significant endorsements. Notably, he did write in that he "used to" have concerns about inattention and impulsivity on those items, but he did not rate these as significant. In the personal interview, S. E. denied problems in general, saying that he does well in school, and that his ADHD symptoms are controlled with medication. Maternal endorsements on the Achenbach Child Behavior Checklist resulted in clinically significant elevations on the internalizing problems scales, with increased concern about withdrawal, anxious/depressed, and social interaction characteristics as well as attentional problems. Maternal endorsements on the Behavior Rating Inventory of Executive Function (BRIEF) reflected increased concerns on both the Behavioral Regulation Index and Metacognition Index, with difficulties shifting,

inhibiting, and monitoring behavior reported, as well as problems with initiation, planning, and working memory.

Overall, S. E.'s neuropsychological evaluation documented a general level of cognitive functioning mostly in the borderline to low-average range, with moderate variability, and a clear profile of relative strengths and weaknesses. Strengths were noted in academic skills, and many areas of verbal functioning, including verbal memory, verbal fluency, and vocabulary. He also had strengths with regard to his planning capabilities. Weaknesses were seen particularly in motor speed, coordination, and geometric copying, and he had poor visuospatial organization and constructional functioning. Nonverbal memory, nonverbal reasoning, sustained attention, and complex verbal processing were also identified as relative weaknesses. Notably, S. E.'s variable memory capabilities included better verbal than visual/nonverbal memory. S. E. also demonstrated an internalizing profile with anxious and depressive tendencies, and problems in age-appropriate social interactions.

Diagnostically, S. E.'s neuropsychological findings were interpreted to be consistent with his past diagnosis of ADHD (combined type), as he met major diagnostic criteria (although complete informant information was not currently available to confirm the diagnosis). His overall level of cognitive functioning did not indicate developmental cognitive impairment (i.e., mental deficiency), but he showed borderline to low-average intellectual capabilities, in general. His profile of functioning presented many similarities to a nonverbal learning disability, and therefore, a rule-out diagnosis of Learning Disorder NOS was suggested, although he demonstrated limited academic deficiencies in his current educational setting. Most notably, a diagnosis of Motor Skills Disorder was appropriate to reflect his severe difficulties in motor and visuomotor functioning. It was suggested the he receive further evaluation for an additional Disorder of Written Expression diagnosis. S. E.'s diagnoses were thought to be consistent with his earlier developmental history of static encephalopathy, mild cerebral palsy, and growth hormone deficiency. It was also noted that his lower adaptive functioning (as reported in previous assessments) may be a function of his unique combination of deficits that when taken together, may result in greater functional impairment than indicated by the magnitude of the individual difficulties alone.

A number of recommendations were therefore provided for S. E., including the obvious need for continued academic support services to help him maintain his basic academic skills, consultation with an occupational therapist about his continued difficulties in writing and drawing, consideration of group psychotherapy to address his social skills, a vision screening because of his tendency to keep his head very close to the paper on pencil-and-paper tasks, and continued monitoring of his attentional and emotional functioning and needs. A feedback session to provide the results and recommendations to S. E. and his mother was held, and copies of his report were provided to his mother, and, with her permission, to his pediatrician and developmental disabilities worker.

Comments

As with many similar cases, there was no clear, well-documented etiology for S. E.'s neuropsychological deficiencies. A pediatric neuropsychological assessment that considered quantitative and qualitative findings within a developmental context was beneficial to understanding his uniquely personal pattern of strengths and weaknesses (see Baron, 2004; Bernstein & Waber, 2003). Historically, S. E. had consistently demonstrated delays in motor functioning in particular, with neuromotor abnormalities also present. Thus, he was given the presumed diagnosis of cerebral palsy resulting from a suspected static encephalopathy. A diagnosis of developmental coordination disorder or consideration that it was an idiopathic condition was not thought to best represent the nature of his disorder, and the neuropsychological findings also indicated other deficits in functioning. S. E. clearly showed motor dysfunction during his neuropsychological evaluation, although a number of other neurocognitive deficits were also seen. In particular, S. E. showed a slight dissociation between his better crystallized intellectual skills, as documented on the WASI, and his lower overall cognitive processing capabilities, as seen on the CAS. The CAS, in fact, was designed to detect inefficiencies in various types of cognitive processing that are not as easily identified on traditional intellectual measures, and may have been the more sensitive cognitive measure in this case (Naglieri, 2001). S. E. showed evidence of broad-based cognitive and motor dysfunction consistent with a static encephalopathy.

The motor system works as an integrated unit in concert with other brain systems, with many neural parts, systems, and processes functioning simultaneously at any one time. Many different brain diseases and developmental disorders can therefore give rise to deficits of movement and coordination. In addition, it is very common for disorders that affect motor functioning to also affect other functional domains assessed in neuropsychology. Thus, although a primary motor dysfunction may be prominent in an individual, there is a high likelihood that other related neuropsychological deficits will be apparent (Atkinson & Nardini, 2008). Case S. E. represents an example of an individual who showed interrelated developmental delays and abnormalities across several neuropsychological domains, but with most dramatic motor and attentional/processing difficulties.

References

American Psychiatric Association (APA). (2000). *Diagnostic and statistical manual of mental disorders* (4th ed., Text rev.). Washington, DC: Author.

Atkinson, J., & Nardini, M. (2008). The neuropsychology of visuospatial and visuomotor development. In J. Reed & J. Warner-Rogers (Eds.), *Child neuropsychology: Concepts, theory, and practice* (pp. 183–217). Malden, MA: Wiley-Blackwell.

Badawi, N., Felix, J. F., Kurinczuk, J. J., Dixon, G., Watson, L., Keogh, J. M., Valentine, J., & Stanley, F. J. (2005). Cerebral palsy following term newborn encephalopathy: A population-based study. *Developmental Medicine and Child Neurology, 47*, 293–298.

Bagnato, S. J., & Campbell, T. F. (1992). Comprehensive neurodevelopmental evaluation of children with brain insults. In G. Miller & J. C. Ramer (Eds.), *Static encephalopathies of infancy and childhood* (pp. 27–44). New York: Raven Press.

Baron, I. S. (2004). *Neuropsychological evaluation of the child*. New York: Oxford University Press.

Bernstein, J. H., & Waber, D. P. (2003). Pediatric neuropsychological assessment. In T. E. Feinberg & M. J. Farah (Eds.), *Behavioral neurology and neuropsychology* (2nd ed., pp. 773–781). New York: McGraw-Hill.

Blondis, T. A. (1996). The spectrum of mild neuromotor disabilities. In A. J. Capute & P. A. Accardo (Eds.), *Developmental disabilities in infancy and childhood, Vol. II: The spectrum of developmental disabilities* (2nd ed., pp. 199–208). Baltimore: Paul H. Brookes.

Blondis, T. A. (2004). Neurodevelopmental motor disorders: Cerebral palsy and neuromuscular diseases. In D. Dewey & D. E. Tupper (Eds.), *Developmental motor disorders: A neuropsychological perspective* (pp. 113–136). New York: Guilford.

Burns, T. G., & Van Winkle, A. (2006). Cerebral palsy: Recognizing early neurodevelopmental factors that influence outcome in the school age child. *Newsletter 40 (APA), 24*(1), 13–27.

Del Dotto, J. E., Fisk, J. L., McFadden, G. T., & Rourke, B. P. (1991). Developmental analysis of children/adolescents with nonverbal learning disabilities: Long-term impact on personality adjustment and patterns of adaptive behavior. In B. P. Rourke (Ed.), *Neuropsychological validation of learning disability subtypes* (pp. 293–308). New York: Guilford.

Dennis, M. (2000). Childhood medical disorders and cognitive impairment: Biological risk, time, development, and reserve. In K. O. Yeates, M. D. Ris, & H. G. Taylor (Eds.), *Pediatric neuropsychology: Research, theory, and practice* (pp. 3–22). New York: Guilford.

Deuel, R. K. (2002). Motor soft signs and development. In S. J. Segalowitz & I. Rapin (Eds.), *Handbook of neuropsychology: Vol. 8, Child neuropsychology, part I* (2nd ed., pp. 367–383). Amsterdam, Netherlands: Elsevier.

Fennell, E. B., & Dikel, T. N. (2001). Cognitive and neuropsychological functioning in children with cerebral palsy. *Journal of Child Neurology, 16*(1), 58–63.

Fox, A. M., & Lent, B. (1996). Clumsy children: Primer on developmental coordination disorder. *Canadian Family Physician, 42*, 1965–1971.

Goldstein, G. W. (2004). Static encephalopathies become dynamic. *Current Opinion in Neurology, 17*, 93–94.

Madge, N., Diamond, J., Miller, D., Ross, E., McManus, C., Wadsworth, J., Yule, W., & Frost, B. (1993). *The National Childhood Encephalopathy Study: A 10-Year Follow-Up*. London: MacKeith Press.

Naglieri, J. A. (2001). Using the Cognitive Assessment System (CAS) with learning-disabled children. In A. S. Kaufman & N. L. Kaufman (Eds.), *Specific learning disabilities and difficulties in children and adolescents: Psychological assessment and evaluation* (pp. 141–177). Cambridge, England: Cambridge University Press.

Nelson, K. B. (2005). Neonatal encephalopathy: Etiology and outcome. *Developmental Medicine and Child Neurology, 47*, 292.

Pellock, J. M., & Myer, E. C. (1992). Static encephalopathy and related disorders. In D. M. Kaufman, G. E. Solomon, & C. R. Pfeffer (Eds.), *Child and adolescent neurology for psychiatrists* (pp. 195–206). Baltimore: Williams & Wilkins.

Taylor, E. M. (1959). *Psychological appraisal of children with cerebral defects*. Cambridge, MA: Harvard University Press.

Tomlin, P. I., & St. Clair Forbes, W. (1995). The static encephalopathies. In R. W. Newton (Ed.), *Color atlas of pediatric neurology* (pp. 203–215). London: Mosby-Wolfe.

Trescher, W. H., & Johnston, M. V. (1992). Neurobiology of static encephalopathies. In G. Miller & J. C. Ramer (Eds.), *Static encephalopathies of infancy and childhood* (pp. 219–234). New York: Raven Press.

Tupper, D. E. (2007). Management of children with disorders of motor control and coordination. In S. J. Hunter & J. Donders (Eds.), *Pediatric neuropsychological intervention: A critical review of science & practice* (pp. 338–365). Cambridge, England: Cambridge University Press.

Warschausky, S. (2006). Physical impairments and disability. In J. E. Farmer, J. Donders, & S. Warschausky (Eds.), *Treating neurodevelopmental disabilities: Clinical research and practice* (pp. 81–97). New York: Guilford.

36

Juvenile Pilocytic Astrocytoma: Postresection Amnesia in a College Student

Benjamin L. Johnson-Markve and Gregory P. Lee

Juvenile pilocytic astrocytoma is among the most common astrocytic brain tumors found in children and young adults. These tumors comprise approximately 85% of cerebellar astrocytomas and 60% of optic gliomas, and they affect both sexes equally (Allen, 2000). Although pilocytic astrocytomas most often arise within the cerebellum, they are also found in the diencephalon, most commonly in the optic chiasm, hypothalamus, thalamus, and related third ventricular structures. Optic pathway/hypothalamic astrocytomas typically develop from a slower growing, low-grade form of juvenile pilocytic (i.e., composed of fiber-shaped cells) astrocytoma, while thalamic pilocytic astrocytomas tend to be more aggressive and invasive tumors. Although low-grade astrocytomas are common in the cerebellum and cerebral cortex, it is more rare for these tumors to arise in the diencephalon, accounting for only about 5% of cases. Within the diencephalon, most low-grade pilocytic astrocytomas develop in the optic nerves and optic chiasm (~4%), while only about 1% of are located in the hypothalamus and thalamus (Hjalmars, Kulldorff, Wahlqvist, & Lannering, 1999).

Symptoms of Pilocytic Astrocytoma

The case reported in this chapter is one of those rare instances in which a pilocytic astrocytoma developed adjacent to the optic pathways and hypothalamus extending into the anterior portion of the third ventricle. Depending upon the site of lesion and direction of growth, optic pathway/hypothalamic pilocytic astrocytomas may present with visual, endocrine, or neurological signs and symptoms. Visual signs may include impaired acuity, visual field defects, or nystagmus. Endocrine signs often include diabetes insipidus, short stature, precocious puberty, and after onset of puberty, amenorrhea. As the tumor continues to grow, signs of increased intracranial pressure due to mass effect typically develop, such as headache, nausea, vomiting, inattention, lethargy, irritability, ataxic gait, and diplopia.

These diencephalic tumors are often diagnosed only after they have grown quite large if they do not involve the optic chiasm or nerve. Hydrocephalus frequently develops when the mass fills the third ventricle. Large diencephalic pilocytic tumors, or their cystic components, may expand to impinge upon the nearby frontal and temporal lobes. Juvenile pilocytic astrocytomas have been associated with Von Recklinghausen disease, more commonly called neurofibromatosis, type 1—especially those tumors arising in the optic pathways. Neurofibromatosis, type 1, is an autosomal dominant disorder characterized by the emergence of tumors (usually benign) and changes in skin pigmentation. Between 20% and 30% of children with optic pathway/hypothalamic gliomas have neurofibromatosis, type 1 (Janss, Grundy, Cnaan, Savino, & Packer, 1995).

Prognosis of Pilocytic Astrocytoma

Overall, juvenile pilocytic astrocytomas have an excellent prognosis with a 10-year survival rate between 85% and 90% in those cases where complete tumor resection was possible, especially when located in the posterior fossa (Allen, 2000). There is, however, considerable morbidity and mortality associated with these tumors when they arise in the diencephalon; probably owing to their relative inaccessibility to surgical treatment and the complications that may follow surgery in this deep region of brain. In addition, juvenile pilocytic astrocytomas show more aggressive growth and more frequent recurrence after subtotal resection in patients younger than 5 years and older than 20 years (Alshail, Rutka, Becker, & Hoffman, 1997).

Treatment of Pilocytic Astrocytoma

Treatment recommendations for chiasmatic/hypothalamic pilocytic astrocytoma are fairly consistent across cancer centers (Allen, 2000; Alshail et al., 1997). Conservative treatment, consisting of shunting for hydrocephalus and medical therapy for endocrine dysfunction, is suggested for patients without neurologic dysfunction and slow tumor growth. In patients with progressive visual loss, neurologic dysfunction, and magnetic resonance imaging (MRI)-confirmed tumor growth, a gross subtotal surgical resection of the tumor via a transcallosal approach is undertaken to relieve the hydrocephalus and symptoms of hypothalamic and pituitary dysfunction. In those patients who continue to show disease progression after surgical resection, chemotherapy or radiation therapy is initiated. If chemotherapy is initiated first but proves ineffective in stabilizing progression of the disease, radiation therapy will typically follow, especially in patients over the age of 5 years (Alshail et al., 1997).

The Case of C. S.

Six months prior to the neuropsychological examination, C. S. was an apparently healthy normal 22-year-old, right-handed female, who was a senior at a large university in the southeast United States majoring in journalism. Her academic abilities were generally above average (GPA = 3.5–4.0), although she reported a long-standing weakness in mathematics. At the beginning of the final semester of her senior year, C. S. experienced a few days of flu-like symptoms including fatigue, headache, and somnolence. She went to the student health clinic and was given a prescription for headache relief, which was not effective. The flu-like symptoms persisted over the course of 6 days and progressively worsened to the point where others began to notice disorientation and confusion that prompted a visit to the emergency room.

Medical Evaluation

Upon initial evaluation, C. S. was awake, alert, and mildly disoriented to time with a Glasgow Coma Scale of 14. Neurological exam revealed no sensory or motor impairment, normal reflexes, and normal cranial nerve exam but mild symptoms of possible increased intracranial pressure were observed, including headache, nausea, somnolence, and inattention. Mental status testing revealed partial disorientation and calculation difficulties on serial 7's resulting in a Folstein Mini Mental Status Examination score of 27/30. There were no reported seizures.

A brain MRI at that time revealed a large mass lesion embedded within the anterior septum pellucidum adjacent to the interventricular foramen of Monro with extension into the third ventricle and hypothalamic region with evidence of both calcification and hemorrhage within the tumor mass. Differential diagnosis of the tumor included ependymoma and oligodendroglioma.

Surgery

Two days later, C. S. underwent a right frontal craniotomy for a gross total resection of the large third ventricular tumor. The resection was performed via a transcallosal approach and utilized microscopic tumor dissection. An approximately 2 cm corpus callosotomy was performed in the midline, and the fornices were split to allow entrance to the tumor site through the roof of the third ventricle. Abnormal hemorrhagic tissue was also taken from the lateral wall of the third ventricle, anteriorly at the lamina terminalis, and from the posterior curve of the A2 segments of the anterior cerebral arteries bilaterally. An external ventricular drain (EVD) was placed in the third ventricle through the area of the callosotomy for relief of mild hydrocephalus.

Surgical pathology indicated the resected mass was a mildly invasive WHO Grade I pilocytic astrocytoma with high-grade features. Postoperatively, C. S. developed endocrine dysfunction including diabetes insipidus and panhypopituitarism with hypothyroidism and hypocortisolism thought to be caused by involvement of the pituitary gland and hypothalamic afferents in the tumor resection. She was prescribed desmopressin acetate (DDAVP), a synthetic analogue of the pituitary hormone vasopression, synthroid, prednisone, and prilosec. Repeat MRI the day after surgery revealed significant debulking of the anterior diencephalic mass with minimal residual abnormal enhancing tissue within the cistern of the lamina terminalis. A vertical corticotomy defect was also seen in the midfrontal region extending through the midline with a partial anterior corpus callosotomy (see Figure 36-1).

Following her 9-day hospitalization and acute recovery, C. S. was discharged to an inpatient

rehabilitation facility that included physical, occupational, and speech therapies to enhance physical strength, coordination, endurance, and cognitive recovery.

Complaints

Six months after tumor resection, C. S. reported persisting problems with memory, slowing of response to questions, and reduced thinking efficiency. Memory complaints included difficulties recalling parts of conversations, appointments, events from earlier in the day and forgetting what she had read within a brief period of time. The family also complained she had significant difficulties remembering day-to-day events. For example, she could not recall the rides and other aspects of a recent trip to Disney World and would often mix up the order and timing of events. She would also sometimes be able to remember something, but be unable to recall where, when, or how she acquired the information (source amnesia). Providing structure or giving cues enhanced C. S.'s ability to recall recently learned material and past events.

Although C. S. denied any significant personality alterations after surgery, her parents noted marked changes in her personality and behavioral functioning. She had become more complacent with decreased drive, abulia, and apathy. They described her affective expression as being significantly "muted" stating, "She's just not the same bubbly person we used to know."

Neurological examination was essentially normal at the time of neuropsychological examination, although there was some mild clumsiness and incoordination of the left hand. C. S. continued to show neurovegetative and endocrine symptoms caused by disruption of hypothalamic/pituitary gland functions, including fatigue, hypersomnolence, diminished libido, amenorrhea, weight gain, hypothyroidism, and diabetes insipidus. These cognitive, personality, and vegetative changes raised concerns about her ability to live independently; therefore, she moved in with relatives to ameliorate these concerns and to provide her support and structure to assist with organizational strategies. She had only one semester left to finish college and planned to complete the requirements for her degree in the semester beginning 2 weeks after neuropsychological examination.

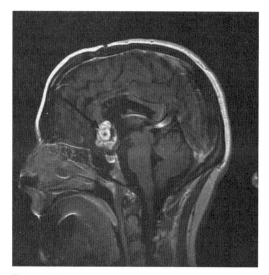

Figure 36-1. Sagittal T1 fluid-attenuated inversion recovery (FLAIR) magnetic resonance imaging scan showing anterior corpus callosotomy and tumor in the anterior third ventricular/hypothalamic region.

Neuropsychological Examination Results

Intellectual Functions

C. S. was administered the Wechsler Adult Intelligence Scale–Third Edition (WAIS-III), and she obtained a Verbal IQ of 111 and a Performance IQ of 119. Processing Speed Index was unexpectedly high, in the superior range (PSI = 128), but otherwise there was little disparity across subtests; most falling within the average to high-average range. Neuropsychological test results are presented in Table 36-1.

Speech and Language

Spontaneous speech was fluent, prosodic, normally articulated, and without paraphasic errors. There was no evidence of perseveration, circumlocution, or echolalia. On the Multilingual Aphasia Examination (MAE), visual naming and sentence repetition were normal, as was the understanding and execution of complex Token Test commands. There was a weakness, however, in associative word (phonemic) fluency. Oral word reading and written spelling on the Wide Range Achievement Test (WRAT-3) were in the normal range.

Attention and Concentration

Performance on all measures of attention-concentration and freedom from distractibility were also in the normal range. C. S. obtained a score of 109 on the WAIS-III Working Memory Index, and attention-concentration subtests from the

Table 36-1. Neuropsychological Test Results in a Case of Juvenile Pilocytic Astrocytoma

Intellectual Functions

Wechsler Adult Intelligence Scales–III	
Full-Scale IQ	= 115 (84th percentile)
Verbal IQ	= 111 (77th percentile)
Verbal Comprehension Index	= 110 (75th percentile)
Vocabulary	= 14 (91st percentile)
Similarities	= 11 (63rd percentile)
Information	= 11 (63rd percentile)
Working Memory Index	= 109 (73rd percentile)
Arithmetic	= 11 (63rd percentile)
Digit Span	= 13 (84th percentile)
Letter-Number Sequencing	= 11 (63rd percentile)
Performance IQ	= 119 (90th percentile)
Perceptual Organizational Index	= 107 (68th percentile)
Picture Completion	= 13 (84th percentile)
Block Design	= 10 (50th percentile)
Matrix Reasoning	= 11 (63rd percentile)
Processing Speed Index	= 128 (97th percentile)
Digit Symbol Coding	= 14 (91st percentile)
Symbol Search	= 16 (98th percentile)
Language Functions	
Multilingual Aphasia Examination	
Visual Naming	= 56/60 (64th percentile)
Controlled Oral Word Association	= 28 (17th percentile)
Token Test	= 43/44 (67th percentile)
Sentence repetition	= 13/14 (65th percentile)
WRAT-3–Reading	= 103 (58th percentile)
WRAT-3–Spelling	= 110 (75th percentile)

(Continued)

Table 36-1. Neuropsychological Test Results in a Case of Juvenile Pilocytic Astrocytoma *(Continued)*

Attention/Concentration Functions

WAIS-III–Working Memory Index	= 109 (73rd percentile)
Digits Forward	= 7 (56th percentile)
Digits Backward	= 5 (47th percentile)
Wechsler Memory Scale-III	
Spatial Span	= 14 (91st percentile)
Mental Control	= 10 (50th percentile)
Trail Making Test–A	= 17" (88th percentile)
Trail Making Test–B	= 69" (17th percentile)

Verbal Learning and Memory Functions

Wechsler Memory Scale-III	
General Memory Index	= 86 (18th percentile)
Auditory Immediate Index	= 117 (87th percentile)
Logical Memory I	= 14 (91st percentile)
Verbal Paired Associates I	= 12 (75th percentile)
Auditory Delayed Index	= 80 (9th percentile)
Logical Memory II	= 2 (1st percentile)
Verbal Paired Associates II	= 4 (2nd percentile)
Auditory Recognition Delayed Index	= 110 (75th percentile)

California Verbal Learning Test-II

Total Trials 1–5 (8,7,9,10,9)	= 43 (9th percentile)
Trial 1	= 8 (50th percentile)
Trial 5	= 9 (<1st percentile)
List B	= 8 (50th percentile)
Short-Delay Free Recall	= 6 (1st percentile)
Short-Delay Cued Recall	= 6 (1st percentile)
Long-Delay Free Recall	= 3 (<1st percentile)
Long-Delay Cued Recall	= 5 (<1st percentile)
Recognition Hits	= 9 (<1st percentile)
Total False Positives	= 4 (6th percentile)

Nonverbal Learning and Memory Functions

Wechsler Memory Scale-III	
Visual Immediate Index	= 84 (14th percentile)
Faces I	= 9 (37th percentile)
Family Pictures I	= 6 (9th percentile)
Visual Delayed Index	= 62 (1st percentile)
Faces II	= 3 (1st percentile)
Family Pictures II	= 5 (5th percentile)
Visual Reproduction I	= 9 (37th percentile)
Visual Reproduction II	= 2 (1st percentile)
Rey-Osterrieth Complex Figure	
Immediate Recall	= 15.5 (1st percentile)
Delayed Recall	= 13 (<1st percentile)
Recognition Total Correct	= 19 (4th percentile)

Visuospatial/Perceptual Functions

Facial Recognition Test	= 48/54 (76th percentile)
Rey Complex Figure, Copy	= 35/36 (>16th percentile)
Judgment of Line Orientation	= 26/30 (56th percentile)

Table 36-1. Neuropsychological Test Results in a Case of Juvenile Pilocytic Astrocytoma (*Continued*)

Executive/Motor Functions

Wisconsin Card-Sorting Test

Categories	= 6 (>16th percentile)
% Perseverative Responses	= 7 (73rd percentile)
% Perseverative Errors	= 7 (73rd percentile)
Trials to 1st Category	= 11 (>16th percentile)
Failure to Maintain Set	= 0 (<16th percentile)
WISC-III Mazes	= 10 (50th percentile)
Controlled Oral Word Association (MAE)	= 28 (17th percentile)

Delis-Kaplan Executive Functions

Design Fluency

Condition 1	= 11 (63rd percentile)
Condition 2	= 10 (50th percentile)
Condition 3	= 11 (63rd percentile)
Set Loss Designs	= 14 (91st percentile)
Repeated Designs	= 13 (84th percentile)

Sorting Test

Condition 1	= 11 (63rd percentile)
Condition 2	= 11 (63rd percentile)

Grooved Pegboard

Dominant (right) hand	= 58" (47th percentile)
Nondominant (left) hand	= 77" (4th percentile)

Frontal Systems Behavior Scale (T scores)

	Before	Present
Self-Rating		
Apathy	30	34
Disinhibition	34	36
Executive Dysfunction	42	34
Total	35	34
Family Rating		
Apathy	44	48
Disinhibition	45	35
Executive Dysfunction	46	49
Total	44	43

Personality Functioning

Minnesota Multiphasic Personality Inventory–2

L	57
F	44
K	67
1	46
2	42
3	49
4	49
5	55
6	48
7	51
8	52
9	56
0	32

Note. Standard and raw scores and percentile ranks were derived from normative tables.

Wechsler Memory Scales (WMS-III) were mostly in the average range, although Spatial Span was in the superior range. There was a disparity between Trails A and Trails B performance; Trails A performance was high normal (88th percentile) while Trails B was low normal (17th percentile).

Verbal Learning and Memory

Assessment of new verbal learning and memory generally revealed normal immediate memory, but moderate impairments in learning and severe impairments in delayed recall, although there were some inconsistencies across memory tests. Delayed recall usually improved when using a recognition format. On the WMS-III, the patient's overall General Memory Index was 86, which was below expectations based upon IQ, and clearly suggested some form of memory disorder.

There was a flat learning curve on California Verbal Learning Test (CVLT-II) as revealed by a normal score on Trial 1 (raw score = 8; 50th percentile) but a severely defective score by Trial 5 (raw score = 9; <1st percentile). Immediate recall was normal on all three verbal memory measures (story recall, paired associates, word list learning), reflecting preserved working memory (attention span) skills in contrast to severely impaired delayed recall for story memory (Logical Memory II) and paired associates (Verbal Paired Associates II) as well as short- and long-term delayed recall for the CVLT word list. Cueing clearly improved performance on the recognition trial for the WMS-III while improvement on the CVLT was equivocal: there was a three-fold increase (from three to nine items) during recognition, but there were also four false positives.

Nonverbal Learning and Memory

Assessment of new visual-spatial learning and memory revealed impairments across all nonverbal memory tests. Specifically, there were mild to severe deficits in delayed recall for faces, family pictures, and drawn geometric figures (Visual Reproduction II) on the WMS-III as well as for the Rey-Osterrieth Complex Figure. The Rey-Osterrieth copy trial was normal (raw score = 35/36), but performance was poor on the immediate recall trial (score = 15.5/36, 1st percentile)

and severely impaired on the delayed recall trial (score = 13/36, <1st percentile).

In contrast, immediate recall of visual-spatial information was in the low-average range, which was poorer than immediate verbal recall, on the WMS-III, but considerably superior to the deficient delayed recall for both verbal and non-verbal materials. Consistent with performance on the verbal recognition memory trials, C. S.'s delayed recall for the Rey-Osterrieth figure improved considerably with cueing (ROCF Recognition Total Correct = 19/36, 8th percentile).

Summarizing, both verbal and visual-spatial memory declined significantly from immediate to delayed recall, and delayed recall was significantly aided when using a recognition format. These defective verbal and visual-spatial memory test results unambiguously confirmed the presence of a severe global (i.e., material nonspecific) memory disorder.

Visuoperception and Spatial Reasoning

Evaluation of visual-spatial, visuoconstructional, and visuoperceptual abilities revealed normal functions across these domains. On the WAIS-III, the Perceptual Organization Index was in the average range (SS = 107), and ability to judge the spatial orientation of lines was in the normal range. Normal constructional abilities were revealed through an excellent copy of the Rey-Osterrieth complex figure. Qualitatively, there was good organization and planning in the patient's Rey-Osterrieth figure. Visuoperception for the discrimination of unfamiliar faces was in the high-average range.

Executive Functions

Executive cognitive functions were normal across most measures. On the Wisconsin Card Sorting Test, C. S. demonstrated a preserved capacity to generate hypotheses, test these hypotheses, and modify performance based upon feedback. She did not display any tendency toward perseveration on this task. Visual planning, measured by the WISC-III Mazes subtest, was also in the normal range. Rapid production of unique figural designs on the Delis-Kaplan Executive Function System (D-KEFS) Design Fluency subtest was normal for all conditions with no inclination toward perseveration. The D-KEFS Sorting Test, which attempted to assess concept formation and initiation of problem-solving behavior, was also in the normal range. The only equivocal measure was a low-normal performance on verbal fluency (MAE Controlled Oral Word Association).

Motor

Although the patient generally showed fluid and purposeful movements of the hands without noticeable tremor or obvious apraxia, there was some subtle clumsiness and incoordination of the left hand during bimanual tasks. This was also seen on Grooved Pegboard where performance was normal with the dominant (right) hand but mildly impaired with the nondominant (left) hand. Performance on graphomotor alternation tasks, measured by drawing Luria figures, was within normal limits. Balance and gait were normal.

Personality–Emotional Functioning

Emotional and behavioral problems associated with frontal lobe dysfunction were assessed using self- and family-report measures from the Frontal Systems Behavior Scale (FrSBe). Both C. S. and her mother reported an absence of significant apathy, disinhibition, or executive dysfunction; however, during the interview her mother did describe notable signs of abulia, including lack of initiative and reduced drive.

Personality assessment using the Minnesota Multiphasic Personality Inventory (MMPI-2) revealed a validity profile consistent with a marked tendency to be defensive and to present oneself in a very favorable light, thus possibly lowering the clinical profile in certain respects. The clinical scales were nevertheless normal. Individuals who obtain similar validity scale profiles often exhibit a lack of insight and tend to minimize or overlook faults in themselves and their circumstances. Nevertheless, there was no strong evidence of any significant mood disorder or other form of psychopathology.

Case Formulation

Neuropsychological evaluation was conducted 6 months following debulking of a pilocytic

astrocytoma in the region of the lamina terminalis and anterior portion of the third ventricle (see Figure 36-2), just adjacent to the hypothalamus. In addition there were also surgical defects involving the medial frontal region and anterior corpus callosum.

Even a casual review of the test results demonstrates that C. S. has a relatively selective impairment of verbal and nonverbal new learning and memory that meets criteria for a neurobehavioral diagnosis of amnesia. The patient's severe global amnesia is supported by history (e.g., difficulty remembering the specifics of past events), family complaints (e.g., forgetting day-to-day events, mixing up the order of events), and by examiner observations during testing (e.g., could not recall parking place, got lost returning to exam room from restroom).

Some signs accompanying the amnesia in this case (e.g., deficits in temporal order judgment, source amnesia, and enhanced recall with cueing), in conjunction with the apparent location of lesion (i.e., diencephalon/peri-third ventricular region), suggests the type of memory disorder most closely resembles a diencephalic or basal forebrain amnesia (Bauer, Grande, & Valenstein, 2003). On the other hand, the absence of retrograde amnesia, lack of confabulation, and rapid forgetting rate are more suggestive of

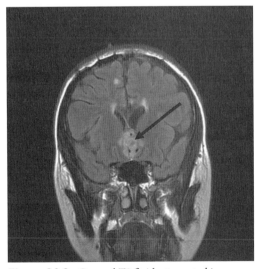

Figure 36-2. Coronal T2 fluid-attenuated inversion recovery (FLAIR) magnetic resonance imaging showing tumor in the anterior third ventricular/hypothalamic region and absent corpus callosum.

a bihippocampal form of amnesia. The large surgical lesion near the lamina terminals may have caused disruption of some basal forebrain nuclei and/or their connections (e.g., septal nuclei, diagonal band of Broca, substantia innominata), which project to the hippocampus. To our knowledge, however, both hippocampi were intact, and the fornices were not severed from their hippocampal inputs or outflow to the mammillary bodies despite having had their commissural fibers spilt. The combination of these anatomical considerations and behavioral features of the memory disorder in this case suggest the amnesia might best be characterized as a mixed amnesia comprised of elements commonly seen in the diencephalic, basal forebrain, and bitemporal types of amnesia.

In addition to the severe memory disorder, the patient showed remnants of a probable left-hand callosal apraxia that first emerged as left-handed clumsiness and akinesia, without alien hand phenomenon, immediately following surgery and has gradually improved with time. During the neuropsychological examination, this was primarily seen in reduced dexterity and speed of the left hand on the Grooved Pegboard test as well a by observations of mild incoordination of the left hand during bimanual tasks, such as Block Design. As with many so-called split brain symptoms following partial callosotomy, this would be expected to improve to the point of clinical insignificance or completely resolve in the near future.

The other major neurobehavioral consequence of the patient's tumor and subsequent surgical debulking was the subtle personality changes consisting of reduced initiative and drive with mild apathy and abulia (i.e., loss of will). The patient's poor insight into the severity of her memory disorder may also be related to these changes, although anosognosia and/or psychological denial are other plausible explanations. These subtle behavioral changes are consistent with the MRI-confirmed surgical damage to the medial frontal lobes causing apparent dysfunction of the anterior cingulate-mesial frontal lobe circuitry.

These frontal lobe behavioral changes are difficult to capture on cognitive testing, so rating scales, such as the Behavior Rating Inventory of Executive Function (BRIEF) and Frontal Systems Behavior Scale (FrSBe), have been developed to evaluate these more subtle behavioral changes. Unfortunately, neither the patient nor her mother rated C. S. as being more apathetic on the FrSBe, although both felt this was a problem acknowledged in separate interviews. After consideration of these factors, it was concluded the patient likely had some mildly reduced initiative and drive. However, given the severity of her amnesia, these mild behavioral changes were considered to be a less important consequence of surgery.

The patient and her family were determined that she at least attempt to complete the last semester required to obtain her undergraduate degree. Cognitive strengths and weakness revealed by neuropsychological testing were reviewed with the patient and her family and suggestions for coping and compensation were discussed. In general, patients with similar memory disorders are helped by providing support and structure. Frequent repetition and review of the material to be learned should also be a useful strategy. Finally, the use of external memory aids and cues should assist with encoding as well as recall. C. S. was referred to the academic support program at her university and a plan for assistance and special accommodations for the upcoming semester was developed. Somewhat unexpectedly to the neuropsychologist (considering the severity of the memory disorder), the patient passed the two final courses required for graduation and received her undergraduate degree. By way of explanation, both courses were graded on the basis of turning in regular assignments and writing term papers. No mid-term or final examinations were required.

Case Follow-Up

After graduation from college, the patient moved back home to live with her family. She was employed full time as a receptionist at a financial institution. One year after surgery, MRI indicated a small tumor recurrence, which was treated with gamma knife irradiation. Follow-up evaluation 6 months later once again revealed probable tumor progression, and she was subsequently treated with fractionated radiation (60 Gy to tumor bed area) using proton beams to minimize the chance of toxicity due to the sensitive location of the tumor in the vicinity of the anterior third ventricle next to the optic tracts and hypothalamus.

Since the radiation therapy, C. S. has been medically and neurologically stable. There have been no visual complaints, sensory or motor impairments, or cranial nerve defects. Other than the persistent cognitive deficits involving new learning and memory and subtle personality changes, there are no persistent neurological impairments. The patient continues regular follow-up and treatment with her endocrinologist for the diabetes insipidus and hypothyroidism secondary to the hypopituitarism, and she undergoes serial brain MRI and neurologic examination approximately every 2 months to check for tumor recurrence.

References

Allen, J. C. (2000). Initial management of children with hypothalamic and thalamic tumors and the modifying role of neurofibromatosis-1. *Pediatric Neurosurgery, 32,* 154–162.

Alshail, E., Rutka, J. T., Becker, L. E., & Hoffman, H. J. (1997). Optic chiasmatic-hypothalamic gliomas. *Brain Pathology, 7,* 799–806.

Bauer, R. M., Grande, L., & Valenstein, E. (2003). Amnesic disorders. In K. M. Heilman & E. Valenstein (Eds.), *Clinical neuropsychology* (4th ed., pp. 495–573). New York: Oxford University Press.

Hjalmars, U., Kulldorff, M., Wahlqvist, Y., & Lannering, B. (1999). Increased incidence rates but no space-time clustering of childhood astrocytoma in Sweden, 1973-1992: A population-based study of pediatric brain tumors. *Cancer, 85,* 2077–2090.

Janss, A., Grundy, R., Cnaan, A., Savino, P., & Packer, R. (1995). Optic pathway and hypothalamic/chiasmatic gliomas in children younger than 5 years with a 6-year follow-up. *Cancer, 75,* 1051–1059.

37

Cerebral Neoplasm: Glioblastoma Multiforme

Robert E. Hanlon, Martin D. Oliveira, and James P. Chandler

Intrinsic tumors of the central nervous system (CNS) are considered uncommon—17,000 to 20,000 annually (DeMonte, 2007)—relative to other life-threatening conditions, with primary brain tumors accounting for 2% of all malignant diseases (Stupp et al., 2002). However, the often dismal outcome involving nearly 13,000 deaths per year in the United States (Reis et al., 2001) despite medical and surgical advances and technological improvements make tumors of the CNS a prominent focus in oncology (DeMonte, 2007). Of the estimated 18,000 new cases diagnosed annually, progression of the disease results in death in two-thirds of patients and significant functional impairment in those who survive (DeMonte, 2007). The etiology of brain tumors is not thoroughly understood because contributing genetic and environmental factors have not been conclusively determined (DeMonte, 2007; Wrensch, Minn, Chew, Bondy, & Berger, 2002). Yet descriptive epidemiological research has outlined valuable criteria, including incidence rates and outcome variables (DeMonte, 2007).

In 2007, the American Cancer Society estimated that 20,500 people in the United States would be diagnosed with a malignant tumor of the brain or spinal cord (11,170 in men and 9330 in woman), and approximately 12,740 people (7150 men and 5590 women) would die from their disease during the same year. Brain tumors rank tenth in the order of cancer-related deaths among woman. Among woman from age 20 to 39, brain tumors are the fifth leading cause of cancer deaths. Among persons under the age of 20,

regardless of gender, tumors of the brain are considered the most common solid tumor, as well as the second leading cause of cancer-related deaths (Jemal et al., 2005).

Diffuse and infiltrative gliomas constitute 40% of all primary and 78% of all malignant CNS neoplasms, making these tumors the most common among other histological variants. More than 80% of these cases are classified as grade III or IV, based on diagnostic criteria from the World Health Organization (WHO), which is currently the most widely used classification system (Batchelor, 2005; Miller & Perry, 2007). The grade IV astrocytoma (AA), also commonly referred to as glioblastoma multiforme or glioblastoma (GBM), is one of the most prevalent histologies among adults (Burger, Vogel, Green, & Strike, 1985; Kleihues, Burger, & Scheithauer, 1993), accounting for 50.7% of all malignant gliomas (Central Brain Tumor Registry of the U.S. [CBTRUS], 2005). Glioblastomas are differentiated based on WHO specifications assessing microvascular proliferation (MVP), encompassing features such as endothelial hypertrophy, endothelial hyperplasia, glomeruloid vessels, and/or necrosis (Miller & Perry, 2007).

Mallory is credited with coining the term *glioblastoma multiforme* in 1914, which was further established in the field of neuro-oncology by Percival Bailey and Harvey Cushing in 1926 (Bailey, 1926). The term *multiforme* was initially applied in reference to the variation in histological makeup between tumor cases and within specific tumors. Thus, an existing GBM may be comprised of varying cellular features, giving it a specific clinical designation. Based on the current WHO classification system, three forms of GBM pathology are diagnostically applied, including conventional GBM, giant cell GBM, and gliosarcoma (Miller & Perry, 2007). Radiographic appearance can reveal edema along with mass effect potentially causing midline shift and herniation (DeAngelis, 2001). In addition, a distinguishing radiographic feature viewed with GBM involves varying ring-like enhancement reflecting MVP (DeAngelis, 2001). Although the tumor often appears to have a distinct encapsulating border on neuroimaging, surgical intervention reveals that the pathology is widely infiltrated (DeAngelis, 2001).

The histopathological occurrence of GBM is maximized between the sixth and eighth decades of life and is thus more prevalent in the elderly population 65 years of age and older. Glioblastoma cases have increased across absolute and age-adjusted incidence (Greig, Ries, Yancik, & Rapoport, 1990; Hess, Broglio, & Bondy, 2004), and the typically poor prognosis has remained relatively constant with minimal improvement over the past 30 years (Barnholtz-Sloan, Sloan, & Schwartz, 2003). Survival rates of 10 years or longer have been reported, although such cases are rare, as documented by Sabel, Reifenberger, Weber, Reifenberger, and Schmitt (2001), who found only 30 published cases between the years of 1990 and 2001. As such, GBM is a life-threatening condition that continues to result in a median survival of approximately 1 year (Daumas-Duport, Scheithauer, O'Fallon, & Kelly, 1988; Galanis & Buckner, 2000), which is often determined by the patient's age (Stupp et al., 2002). The 2-year survival rate is roughly 30% for affected patients under the age of 45 and less than 2% for patients 75 years and older (DeMonte, 2007). The 5-year survival rate for those affected over the age of 45 is only 2% or less (American Cancer Society [ACS], 2006). Other GBM prognostic indicators include presence of necrosis, proliferation, genetic alterations, and degree of surgical resection (Chandler, Prados, Malec, & Wilson, 1993; Schmidt et al., 2002; Scott et al., 1999).

The standard treatment of malignant gliomas typically involves maximal surgical resection followed by radiotherapy (RT), as well as concomitant or adjuvant chemotherapy if clinically indicated (Kristiansen et al., 1981; Walker et al., 1978). The benefit of RT has been accepted since the 1970s based on documented positive results (Kristiansen et al., 1981; Walker et al., 1978; Walker et al., 1980). Historically, chemotherapy has been clinically limited due to probable mechanisms preventing sufficient infiltration of the blood–brain barrier (Stupp et al., 2002). Substantial data provided by the British Medical Research Council (2001) suggested that adjuvant procarbazine, lomustine, and vincristine chemotherapy did not prolong survival rates of patients with AA or GBM, noting an average survival of only 10 months.

However, the novel alkylating agent, Temozolomide (TMZ), has demonstrated efficacy in CNS malignancies (Gilbert et al., 2002; Nicholson et al., 1998; Yung et al., 2000), including recurrent gliomas (Newlands, Stevens, Wedge, Wheelhouse, & Brock, 1997; Reid, Stevens, Rubin, & Ames, 1997; Stupp, Gander, Leyvraz, & Newlands, 2001). Similar benefits were also demonstrated in an extensive randomized phase II trial comparing TMZ to procarbazine (Yung et al., 2000), in which 21% of patients treated with the novel alkylating agent had a 6-month survival rate without progression of tumor, and only 8% achieved the same results with procarbazine. All participants in the clinical trial received a controlled dose in the range of 150 to 200 mg/m2/d for 5 days on a 28-day cycle. Treatment is well tolerated with grade 3 and 4 thrombocytopenia and neutropenia affecting less than 10% of those treated with TMZ in general clinical practice (Stupp et al., 2002). Quick absorption results in close to 100% bioavailability following oral administration (Newlands et al., 1992), and as such, TMZ effectively penetrates the blood–brain barrier with an estimated plasma-CSF ratio in the range of 30% to 40% (Marzolini et al., 1998). Although this agent has been reported to be less beneficial for those with relapsed or progressive GBMs (Brada et al., 2001; Yung et al., 2000), treatment with TMZ has been successfully utilized in challenging cases, involving repeated surgeries as demonstrated in a recent study that extended survival times from an estimated 9-month period, to an average of 15.1 months (Terasaki et al., 2007). Clinical data have also suggested probable synergistic effects when TMZ is combined with RT, and consistent administration on a daily basis has been shown to be safe and effective in prolonging the lives of individuals diagnosed with GBM (Stupp et al., 2002).

Naturally, one common effect of a space-occupying infiltrative cerebral mass, such as a GBM, is neurocognitive dysfunction, which may result from the neoplastic pathology, reactive emotional distress, secondary seizure activity, and the resultant effect of surgical resection, antiepileptic medication, corticosteroids, and RT combined with frequently administered chemotherapy. Additional factors include local or diffuse tumor reoccurrence, leptomeningeal metastasis, and/or metabolic alterations. Given the multifactorial implications, both primary and secondary, cognitive dysfunction is commonly due to a combination of the aforementioned variables (Taphoorn & Klein, 2004).

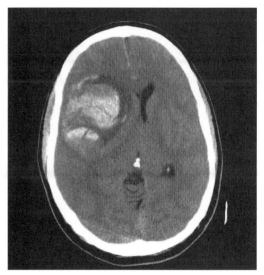

Figure 37-1. Preoperative axial computed tomography scan demonstrating large right frontal hemorrhagic tumor with mass effect and midline shift.

Cases

Case Report 1

Mr. X was a 44-year-old, right-handed male. He completed 18 years of formal education, including a BA and an MBA. Prior to his initial tumor workup, he was employed as a corporate banker for 21 years. Medical/surgical history was remarkable for migraine headaches. He had no history of head trauma or concussion and no history of psychological disorder or psychiatric treatment. He smoked 4–5 cigarettes per day but denied the use of alcohol or illegal drugs. Psychosocial stressors involved searching for employment.

He was in his usual state of reasonable health until October 2003, at which point he suffered a generalized seizure. A computed tomography (CT) scan of the brain revealed a large right frontal lobar hemorrhage with mass effect, as well as right to left midline shift prompting an emergent right frontotemporoparietal craniotomy and resection of a primary high-grade hemorrhagic tumor (see Figure 37-1). Follow-up magnetic resonance imaging (MRI) of the brain in November 2003 revealed nodular enhancement along the margins of the resection cavity consistent with residual tumor, as well as a small infarct in

the left thalamus. At that time, he underwent a second resection of a recurrent high-grade GBM and sustained postoperative complications, including meningitis. He subsequently underwent a 6-week course of RT followed by chemotherapy.

He underwent an initial neuropsychological evaluation at that time. Subjective complaints included memory difficulty, decreased concentration, fatigue, decreased sense of taste, periodic seizures, and depression. He presented as alert, responsive, and oriented to person, place, time, and reason for evaluation. He ambulated independently with normal gait, and sitting posture was symmetric. Dominant right-handed graphomotor functions were intact for paper-and-pencil tasks. Spontaneous speech was fluent and articulate, with normal rate, tone, and volume. Affect was responsive and he revealed full affective range with consistent neutral mood. Thought processes were logical, linear, and goal directed. Frustration tolerance was well preserved, based on his engagement and perseverance on a series of cognitively demanding tasks. Self-regulation behavior was characterized by normal initiation, persistence, and termination of responses. Objective neuropsychological assessment revealed the remarkable preservation of basic neurocognitive functions, with the exception of mildly diminished visuospatial processes, and mildly decreased rate of visual information processing consistent with a right frontal mass.

An MRI in June 2004 redemonstrated interval increase in nodular enhancement around the resection cavity, as well as retraction of the frontal horn of the right lateral ventricle, suggestive of combined radiation necrosis and recurrent GBM. A positron emission tomography (PET) scan of the brain in July 2004 revealed diffuse hypometabolism in the right frontal lobe, and an MRI in July 2004 confirmed continued medial extension of a recurrent GBM. As a result, the patient underwent another right frontal craniotomy and resection of recurrent GBM. A postoperative MRI in November 2004 revealed diminished enhancement around the resection cavity.

Two months later, a follow-up neuropsychological evaluation was conducted to objectively

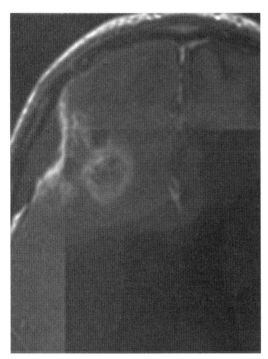

Figure 37-2. A positron emission tomography scan obtained after two resections demonstrating hypometabolism in the right frontal lobe indicative of recurrent glioblastoma multiforme.

assess interval change. Subjective complaints included memory difficulty, decreased concentration, organizational difficulties, decreased decision-making capacity, sleep disturbance, decreased appetite, and anxiety. He also reported worrying about securing employment. His wife had reportedly observed significant personality changes. Upon neuropsychological reassessment, he continued to reveal the preservation of basic neurocognitive functions, including anterograde memory, language, and visuoperceptual processes. However, he revealed significant executive dysfunction not previously demonstrated, involving deficient concept formation and decision-making capacity. Attentional functions remained mildly deficient but unchanged relative to his status at the time of the initial evaluation. Visual-nonverbal memory functions remained within normal limits, but they were notably decreased relative to verbal memory functions. In addition to a mild neurocognitive decline, he also revealed amplified emotional distress, involving increased depressive symptomatology, anxiety, and worry about the future consistent with his diagnosis and prognosis. No significant personality pathology was evident.

In summary, Mr. X continued to demonstrate relative preservation of neurocognitive functions, with the exception of mild but significant executive dysfunction, attentional disturbance, and mildly deficient visuospatial processing. It is likely that his reported organizational and decision-making difficulties were due to his executive dysfunction, and clearly his executive/attentional dysfunction was consistent with a right frontal GBM post three surgical resections. Mr. X died 5 years after his initial diagnosis. Neuropsychological data are shown in Table 37-1.

Case Report

Ms. Z was a 53-year-old, single, right-handed female without children who lived alone. She completed 18 years of education and was employed as an administrator at a law firm. Past medical history was notable for a breast cyst only. She denied the use of tobacco and reported drinking 3–4 alcoholic beverages per week. She was in her usual state of reasonable health until February 2002, when she began to develop

Table 37-1. Neuropsychological Test Results

Test	Standard Score (time 1)	Standard Score (time 2)
Wechsler Test of Adult Reading Estimated Full-Scale IQ	123 (94th percentile)	...
Wide Range Achievement Test–III Reading	SS = 111	...
Wechsler Abbreviated Scale of Intelligence		
Full Scale IQ	108 (70th percentile)	...
Verbal IQ	118 (88th percentile)	...
Performance IQ	97 (42nd percentile)	...
Vocabulary	$T = 65$	...
Block Design	$T = 47$	...
Similarities	$T = 57$	...
Matrix Reasoning	$T = 50$	...
Wechsler Memory Scale–III		
Information and Orientation	14/14	14/14
Logical Memory I	SS = 14	SS = 13
Logical Memory II	SS = 15	SS = 15
Face Recognition I	SS = 9	SS = 9
Face Recognition II	SS = 10	SS = 9
Verbal Paired Associates I	...	SS = 16
Verbal Paired Associates II	...	SS = 13
Family Pictures I	...	SS = 9
Family Pictures II	...	SS = 11
Letter-Number Sequencing	SS = 10	SS = 9
Digit Span	SS = 8	SS = 7
Trail-Making Test		
Part A	$T = 42$	$T = 42$
Part B	$T = 50$	$T = 67$
Controlled Oral Word Association Test	76th percentile	95th percentile
Boston Naming Test	$z = 0.6$	$z = 0.6$
Judgment of Line Orientation Test	40th percentile	56th percentile
Stroop Color-Word Test		
Word Score	$T = 55$	$T = 54$
Color Score	$T = 51$	...
Color-Word	$T = 57$	$T = 65$
Wisconsin Card-Sorting Test		
Categories Completed	4	...
Total Errors	42 (5th percentile)	...
Perseverative Responses	19 (10 percentile)	...
Grooved Pegboard Test		
Dominant	$T = 45$	$T = 54$
Nondominant	$T = 47$	$T = 60$
Beck Depression Inventory-2	12	24

... not administered at evaluation time point.

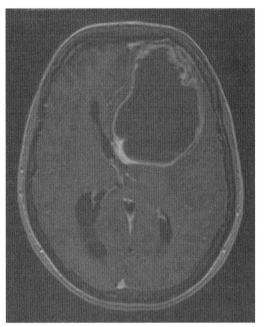

Figure 37-3. Preoperative axial magnetic resonance image demonstrating a large necrotic tumor in the left frontal lobe.

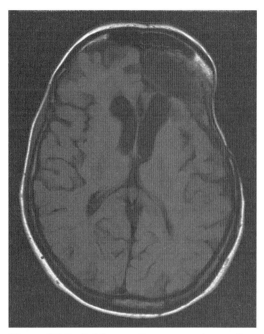

Figure 37-5. Axial magnetic resonance image after three previous resections demonstrating progression of edema.

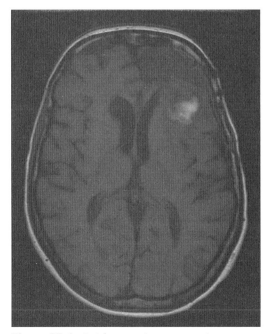

Figure 37-4. Axial magnetic resonance image obtained after initial resection of the mass, demonstrating enhancement in the left frontal area and hemorrhage in the tumor cavity.

expressive language difficulties. An MRI of the brain in April 2002 revealed a large necrotic tumor in the left frontal lobe, prompting a left frontal craniotomy and resection of the mass in April 2002. Pathological analysis confirmed a GBM, and she underwent a second craniotomy and resection of residual mass in May 2002.

An initial brief neuropsychological evaluation in June 2002 revealed mildly deficient generative fluency combined with the general preservation of all other basic neurocognitive functions. In August 2004, neuroimaging studies revealed enhancement in the left frontal area and hemorrhage in the tumor cavity. As a result, she underwent a left frontal craniotomy, resection, and evacuation of the hematoma. She subsequently underwent skull surgery on the cranial flap. A follow-up neuropsychological evaluation in November 2004 revealed multiple neurocognitive deficits and significant cognitive decline, relative to her status in June 2002. At that time, she manifested significant attentional disturbance, defective generative fluency, mild dysnomia, executive dysfunction, and defective verbal memory functions, which were compounded by dysnomia.

Magnetic resonance imaging of the brain in January 2006 revealed no significant change in the left frontal enhancement. However, at about that time, she reported multiple falls from standing with brief loss of consciousness on two occasions. Despite increasing memory instability and pressure from her friends, she continued to live alone. A follow-up neuropsychological evaluation in February 2006 revealed further neurocognitive decline, relative to her status in November 2004. She manifested defective generative fluency, attentional dysfunction, executive dysfunction, and worsening verbal memory dysfunction, which was compounded by her word-finding difficulty. Her mood was stable and she revealed no evidence of significant or disabling psychopathology.

She was readmitted in May 2006, due to tumor regrowth and expansion, combined with her documented cognitive decline. An MRI of the brain in May 2006 revealed progression of edema from the frontal lobe into the anterior left parietal lobe, and into the external capsule and posterior limb of the internal capsule on the left. Compared to the study in January 2006, there was significant increase in the size of the two nodular enhancing lesions located within the corona radiate, a new lesion with abnormal enhancement connected to the large corona radiate lesion located in the region of the posterior limb of the left internal capsule, and an increase in mass effect.

In light of her condition, a follow-up inpatient neuropsychological consultation was requested to objectively assess interval change and to determine her capacity to make independent and informed decisions regarding her discharge

Table 37-2. Neuropsychological Test Results

Test	Standard Score (time 1)	Standard Score (time 2)	Standard Score (time 3)	Standard Score (time 4)
Wechsler Test of Adult Reading				
Estimated Full-Scale IQ	...	116 (86th percentile)	...	...
Wide Range Achievement Test–III				
Reading	SS = 109	SS = 111	...	...
Repeatable Battery for the Assessment of Neuropsychological Status				
Immediate Memory		SS = 69	SS = 78	SS = 57
Visuospatial/Constructional	SS = 100	SS = 100	SS = 100	SS = 84
Language	SS = 94	SS = 90	SS = 82	SS = 60
Attention	SS = 106	SS = 85	SS = 91	
Delayed Memory	SS = 105	SS = 56	SS = 60	SS = 91
Total Scale		SS = 75	SS = 78	
Trail Making Test				
Part A	...	$T = 43$	$T = 31$	$T = 9$
Part B	...	$T = 27$	$T = 28$	DC
Controlled Oral Word Association	<1st percentile	<1st percentile	<1st percentile	<1st percentile
Boston Naming Test	$z = -0.4$	$z = -1.7$	$z = -0.8$	$z = -4.5$
Stroop Color-Word Test				
Word Score	...	$T = 47$	$T = 50$	...
Color Score	...	$T = 49$	$T = 49$	...
Color-Word	...	$T = 47$	$T = 38$	...
Beck Depression Inventory–2	...	6	...	...

..., Not administered at evaluation time point; DC, discontinued; SS, standard score.

plans, independent living, and employment. On objective neuropsychological assessment, she revealed a mild to moderate decline in cognitive functioning, relative to her status in February 2006. She revealed moderate to severely reduced language functions, characterized by moderate dysnomia and moderately dysfluent, perserverative, and circumlocutory speech. She also manifested severely defective attentional capacity, mild executive dysfunction, and mildly defective anterograde memory functions, all of which were impacted by her aphasia. Overall, her decreased neurocognitive state relative to her status on February 2006 was consistent with combined effects of recurrent growth of her left frontal GBM, and serial craniotomies and resections. Considering her overall neurocognitive status, she was deemed not capable of making independent and informed decisions regarding her discharge plans, independent living, and employment. As such, placement in a supervised setting was recommended in order to insure her safety. Given her cognitive limitations, consideration of employment discontinuation and disability funding was also recommended. She died in a hospice 5 years after onset.

Discussion

As demonstrated with the two cases presented, patients affected with brain neoplasms such as GBM may exhibit varying neurocognitive deficits depending on multiple variables, including the original topography tumor site. Mr. X initially presented with mild visuoperceptual deficits consistent with a right frontal mass, while Ms. Z's initial neuropsychological profile was limited to language/attention-based difficulty attributable to a left frontal mass. Further neuropsychological implications stemming from subsequent treatment effects, as evidenced in both Mr. X and Ms. Z, are typically reflective of frontal-subcortical white matter dysfunction (Archibald et al., 1994; Grant, Slattery, Gregor, & Whittle, 1994; Scheibel, Meyers, & Levin, 1996). Overall, resulting neurocognitive profiles may be characterized by reduced attentional capacity, executive dysfunction, reduced processing speed, language deficiency, impaired visuoperceptual abilities, and anterograde memory

disturbance with or without retentive memory impairment (Ammirati, Vick, Liao, Ciric, & Mikhael, 1987; Scheibel et al., 1996). Such neurocognitive deficits have been documented across several studies assessing affected patients considered long-term survivors (Archibald et al., 1994; Gregor et al., 1996; Imperato, Paleologos, & Vick, 1990; Scott et al., 1999). As resilient patients such as Mr. X and Ms. Z continue to counter the historical survival rates, disability secondary to evolving neurocognitive impairment becomes a life-altering factor.

Multiple measures incorporated across various brain cancer treatment trials provide a more thorough clinical picture than the often exclusive markers of survival time and progression-free survival. One study correlating tumor-related neurocognitive changes with MRI proposes that cognitive changes are evident approximately 1 month prior to neuroimaging of actual tumor reoccurrence (Meyers, Hess, Yung, & Levin, 2000). These results indicate that neuropsychological assessment can assist in optimizing patient care by providing preliminary data that may warn of developing pathology, and by clarifying the benefits and risks of probable treatment reinstatement (Meyers et al., 2000). A comprehensive patient profile that includes neurocognitive data, combined with the more widely used assessments of quality of life and activities of daily living can also be more informative when educating the patient and his or her family members about the course of illness and treatment.

Caregivers are often the most affected by the patient's decline in cognitive capacity. Increased demands are reflected in the level of care needed with further progression of the aforementioned neurocognitive functions. Caregivers are thus not only required to alter their lifestyles to meet these demands, but they are also faced with the emotional challenge of caring for a loved one whose declining neurocognitive capacity, as well as changes in personality, transforms the previously independent individual once familiar to them. Disability funding and rehabilitation when possible are potential resources that can be of assistance. The clinical investigation of progressing neurocognitive implications allows for focused informed decisions that can ultimately enhance the quality of life for patients and their caregivers (Hahn et al., 2003).

In sum, the atypical long-term survival of the two patients presented suggests that despite the current 12-month median survival rate (Fine, 1994; Forsyth & Cairncross, 1995), GBM is a manageable form of cancer that can eventually translate into greater survival times. As such, neuropsychology is an essential component that should be included in all prospective treatment outcome studies, as well as ongoing investigations assessing quality of life and activities of daily living (Gregor et al., 1996). Systematic objective data collection serves to ameliorate baseline tumor implications and subsequent treatment effects, inform appropriate reintervention strategies, and clarify after care and rehabilitation needs for long-term survivors.

References

American Cancer Society (ACS). (2006). *Cancer facts and figures–2006*. Atlanta, GA: Author.

Ammirati, M., Vick, N., Liao, Y. L., Ciric, I., & Mikhael, M. (1987). Effect of the extent of surgical resection on survival and quality of life in patients with supratentorial glioblastomas and anaplastic astrocytomas. *Neurosurgery, 21*(2), 201–206.

Archibald, Y. M., Lunn, D., Ruttan, L. A., Macdonald, D. R., Del Maestro, R. F., Barr, H. W., et al. (1994). Cognitive functioning in long-term survivors of high-grade glioma. *Journal of Neurosurgery, 80*(2), 247–253.

Bailey, P., Cushing, H. (1926). *A classification of the tumors of the glioma group on the histogenic basis with a correlated study of prognosis*. Philadelphia: JB Lippincott Co.

Barnholtz-Sloan, J. S., Sloan, A. E., & Schwartz, A. G. (2003). Relative survival rates and patterns of diagnosis analyzed by time period for individuals with primary malignant brain tumor, 1973-1997. *Journal of Neurosurgery, 99*(3), 458–466.

Batchelor, T. D., & Hunter, D. J. (2005). Epidemiology, pathology, and imaging of brain tumors. In M. Peter & J. S. L. Black. (Eds.), *Cancer of the nervous system* (2nd ed., pp. 1–13). Philadelphia: Lippincott Williams & Wilkins.

Brada, M., Hoang-Xuan, K., Rampling, R., Dietrich, P. Y., Dirix, L. Y., Macdonald, D., et al. (2001). Multicenter phase II trial of temozolomide in patients with glioblastoma multiforme at first relapse. *Annals of Oncology, 12*(2), 259–266.

Burger, P. C., Vogel, F. S., Green, S. B., & Strike, T. A. (1985). Glioblastoma multiforme and anaplastic astrocytoma: Pathologic criteria and prognostic implications. *Cancer, 56*(5), 1106–1111.

Central Brain Tumor Registry of the United States (CBTRUS). (2005). *Statistical report: Primary brain tumors in the United States, 1998-2002*. Hinsdale, IL: Author.

Chandler, K. L., Prados, M. D., Malec, M., & Wilson, C. B. (1993). Long-term survival in patients with glioblastoma multiforme. *Neurosurgery, 32*(5), 716–720.

Daumas-Duport, C., Scheithauer, B., O'Fallon, J., & Kelly, P. (1988). Grading of astrocytomas. A simple and reproducible method. *Cancer, 62*(10), 2152–2165.

DeAngelis, L. M. (2001). Brain tumors. *New England Journal of Medicine, 344*(2), 114–123.

DeMonte, F., Gilbert, M., Mahajan, A., & McCutcheon, I. (2007). *Tumors of the brain and spine*. New York: Springer Science+Business Media, LLC.

Fine, H. A. (1994). The basis for current treatment recommendations for malignant gliomas. *Journal of Neurooncology, 20*(2), 111–120.

Forsyth, P. A., & Cairncross, J. G. (1995). Treatment of malignant glioma in adults. *Current Opinion in Neurology, 8*(6), 414–418.

Galanis, E., & Buckner, J. (2000). Chemotherapy for high-grade gliomas. *British Journal of Cancer, 82*(8), 1371–1380.

Gilbert, M. R., Friedman, H. S., Kuttesch, J. F., Prados, M. D., Olson, J. J., Reaman, G. H., et al. (2002). A phase II study of temozolomide in patients with newly diagnosed supratentorial malignant glioma before radiation therapy. *Neuro-Oncology, 4*(4), 261–267.

Grant, R., Slattery, J., Gregor, A., & Whittle, I. R. (1994). Recording neurological impairment in clinical trials of glioma. *Journal of Neurooncology, 19*(1), 37–49.

Gregor, A., Cull, A., Traynor, E., Stewart, M., Lander, F., & Love, S. (1996). Neuropsychometric evaluation of long-term survivors of adult brain tumours: Relationship with tumour and treatment parameters. *Radiotherapy and Oncology, 41*(1), 55–59.

Greig, N. H., Ries, L. G., Yancik, R., & Rapoport, S. I. (1990). Increasing annual incidence of primary malignant brain tumors in the elderly. *Journal of the National Cancer Institue, 82*(20), 1621–1624.

Hahn, C. A., Dunn, R. H., Logue, P. E., King, J. H., Edwards, C. L., & Halperin, E. C. (2003). Prospective study of neuropsychologic testing and quality-of-life assessment of adults with primary malignant brain tumors. *International Journal of Radiation Oncology Biology Physics, 55*(4), 992–999.

Hess, K. R., Broglio, K. R., & Bondy, M. L. (2004). Adult glioma incidence trends in the United States, 1977-2000. *Cancer, 101*(10), 2293–2299.

Imperato, J. P., Paleologos, N. A., & Vick, N. A. (1990). Effects of treatment on long-term survivors with malignant astrocytomas. *Annals of Neurology, 28*(6), 818–822.

Jemal, A., Murray, T., Ward, E., Samuels, A., Tiwari, R. C., Ghafoor, A., et al. (2005). Cancer statistics, 2005. *CA: A Cancer Journal for Clinicians, 55*(1), 10–30.

Kleihues, P., Burger, P. C., & Scheithauer, B. W. (1993). The new WHO classification of brain tumours. *Brain Pathology, 3*(3), 255–268.

Kristiansen, K., Hagen, S., Kollevold, T., Torvik, A., Holme, I., Nesbakken, R., et al. (1981). Combined modality therapy of operated astrocytomas grade III and IV. Confirmation of the value of postoperative irradiation and lack of potentiation of bleomycin on survival time: A prospective multicenter trial of the Scandinavian Glioblastoma Study Group. *Cancer, 47*(4), 649–652.

Marzolini, C., Decosterd, L. A., Shen, F., Gander, M., Leyvraz, S., Bauer, J., et al. (1998). Pharmacokinetics of temozolomide in association with fotemustine in malignant melanoma and malignant glioma patients: Comparison of oral, intravenous, and hepatic intra-arterial administration. *Cancer Chemotherapy & Pharmacology, 42*(6), 433–440.

Meyers, C. A., Hess, K. R., Yung, W. K., & Levin, V. A. (2000). Cognitive function as a predictor of survival in patients with recurrent malignant glioma. *Journal of Clinical Oncology, 18*(3), 646–650.

Miller, C. R., & Perry, A. (2007). Glioblastoma. *Archives of Pathology and Laboratory Medicine, 131*(3), 397–406.

Newlands, E. S., Blackledge, G. R., Slack, J. A., Rustin, G. J., Smith, D. B., Stuart, N. S., et al. (1992). Phase I trial of temozolomide (CCRG 81045: M&B 39831: NSC 362856). *British Journal of Cancer, 65*(2), 287–291.

Newlands, E. S., Stevens, M. F., Wedge, S. R., Wheelhouse, R. T., & Brock, C. (1997). Temozolomide: A review of its discovery, chemical properties, preclinical development and clinical trials. *Cancer Treatment Reviews, 23*(1), 35–61.

Nicholson, H. S., Krailo, M., Ames, M. M., Seibel, N. L., Reid, J. M., Liu-Mares, W., et al. (1998). Phase I study of temozolomide in children and adolescents with recurrent solid tumors: A report from the Children's Cancer Group. *Journal of Clinical Oncology, 16*(9), 3037–3043.

Reid, J. M., Stevens, D. C., Rubin, J., & Ames, M. M. (1997). Pharmacokinetics of 3-methyl-(triazen-1-yl) imidazole-4-carboximide following administration of temozolomide to patients with advanced cancer. *Clinical Cancer Research, 3*(12 Pt. 1), 2393–2398.

Reis, L. A. G., Esiner, M. P., Kosary, C. L., Hankey, B. F., Miller, B. A., Clegg, L., & Edwards, B. K. (Eds). (2001). *SEER Cancer Statistics, 1973-1998.* Bethesda, MD: National Cancer Institute.

Sabel, M., Reifenberger, J., Weber, R. G., Reifenberger, G., & Schmitt, H. P. (2001). Long-term survival of a patient with giant cell glioblastoma. Case report. *Journal of Neurosurgery, 94*(4), 605–611.

Scheibel, R. S., Meyers, C. A., & Levin, V. A. (1996). Cognitive dysfunction following surgery for intracerebral glioma: influence of histopathology, lesion location, and treatment. *Journal of Neurooncology, 30*(1), 61–69.

Schmidt, M. C., Antweiler, S., Urban, N., Mueller, W., Kuklik, A., Meyer-Puttlitz, B., et al. (2002). Impact of genotype and morphology on the prognosis of glioblastoma. *Journal of Neuropathology and Experimental Neurology, 61*(4), 321–328.

Scott, J. N., Rewcastle, N. B., Brasher, P. M., Fulton, D., MacKinnon, J. A., Hamilton, M., et al. (1999). Which glioblastoma multiforme patient will become a long-term survivor? A population-based study. *Annals Neurology, 46*(2), 183–188.

Stupp, R., Dietrich, P. Y., Ostermann Kraljevic, S., Pica, A., Maillard, I., Maeder, P., et al. (2002). Promising survival for patients with newly diagnosed glioblastoma multiforme treated with concomitant radiation plus temozolomide followed by adjuvant temozolomide. *Journal of Clinical Oncology, 20*(5), 1375–1382.

Stupp, R., Gander, M., Leyvraz, S., & Newlands, E. (2001). Current and future developments in the use of temozolomide for the treatment of brain tumours. *Lancet Oncol, 2*(9), 552–560.

Taphoorn, M. J., & Klein, M. (2004). Cognitive deficits in adult patients with brain tumours. *Lancet Neurology, 3*(3), 159–168.

Terasaki, M., Ogo, E., Fukushima, S., Sakata, K., Miyagi, N., Abe, T., et al. (2007). Impact of combination therapy with repeat surgery and temozolomide for recurrent or progressive glioblastoma multiforme: A prospective trial. *Surgical Neurology, 68*(3), 250–254.

Walker, M. D., Alexander, E., Jr., Hunt, W. E., MacCarty, C. S., Mahaley, M. S., Jr., Mealey, J., Jr., et al. (1978). Evaluation of BCNU and/or radiotherapy in the treatment of anaplastic gliomas. A cooperative clinical trial. *Journal of Neurosurgery, 49*(3), 333–343.

Walker, M. D., Green, S. B., Byar, D. P., Alexander, E., Jr., Batzdorf, U., Brooks, W. H., et al. (1980). Randomized comparisons of radiotherapy and nitrosoureas for the treatment of malignant glioma after surgery. *New England Journal of Medicine*, *303*(23), 1323–1329.

Wrensch, M., Minn, Y., Chew, T., Bondy, M., & Berger, M. S. (2002). Epidemiology of primary brain tumors: Current concepts and review of the literature. *Neuro-Oncology*, *4*(4), 278–299.

Yung, W. K., Albright, R. E., Olson, J., Fredericks, R., Fink, K., Prados, M. D., et al. (2000). A phase II study of temozolomide vs. procarbazine in patients with glioblastoma multiforme at first relapse. *British Journal of Cancer*, *83*(5), 588–593.

38

A Case of Acute Lymphocytic Leukemia

Robert Butler

Acute lymphoblastic leukemia (ALL) is the most common malignancy in childhood/adolescence. Of all children diagnosed with cancer, approximately 12,000 per year, ALL accounts for 40%–50% of these patients (Ries et al., 2007). In the 1950s and 1960s, the diagnosis of ALL was associated with almost uniform mortality. In the twenty-first century, approximately 90% of these individuals obtain extended disease-free survival and are considered cured of their cancer. It is generally accepted that the primary reason for this dramatic change in prognosis is a function of the introduction of central nervous system (CNS) prophylaxis (Janzen & Spiegler, 2008). Systemic chemotherapy, at the doses administered for ALL, does not typically cross the blood–brain barrier, and any CNS treatment impact was mild and indirect. Prior to the institution of CNS prophylaxis, children typically returned to oncology clinics having suffered a relapse of their disease in the CNS or other regions. Oncologists realized that an intervention needed to be directly applied to the CNS. Initially, direct treatment to the brain in order to eliminate cancerous cells involved whole-brain, cranial-spinal irradiation. It is well documented that cranial irradiation therapy (CRT) was, and remains, associated with significant neurocognitive deficits in most children/adolescents (Eisner, 2004; Mulhern & Butler, 2004, 2006).

Considerable knowledge has been accumulated regarding the effects of CRT in the pediatric population. Of note, deficits in sustained attention, working memory, information processing speed, and nondominant hemisphere deficits are widely acknowledged and vary according to risk factors such as age at diagnosis, dose of treatment, and gender (Mulhern & Butler, 2004). For unknown reasons, females appear to be more susceptible to the effects of CRT. In an attempt to increase our knowledge of risk factors, attention is being increasingly directed toward possible genetic markers.

As the accumulation of literature clearly indicated the neurocognitive toxicity of irradiation as a CNS prophylaxis, pediatric oncologists took a bold move, replacing CRT with intrathecal injections of chemotherapy, most commonly methotrexate. On a very positive note, evidence suggests that this advance did decrease resultant late neuropsychological and behavioral effects in the ALL population with preserved disease-free survival rates. Nevertheless, individuals who receive intrathecal methatrexate (IT-MTX) can still experience neurocognitive deficits because, as with CRT, IT-MTX results in white matter damage (Moleski, 2000). Risk factors are identical between the two prophylactic preventions.

Standard risk ALL, most commonly treated with the prophylaxis of IT-MTX, can result in neurocognitive involvement that has a significant impact on school performance. Most commonly, learning of mathematics is particularly influenced, likely due to the fact that arithmetic is very demanding of attentional abilities and also affected by nondominant hemisphere deficits. While language-related functions tend to be preserved in many children, this is not necessarily the case if risk factors such as elevated dose, young age at treatment, and female gender are present.

The Case of X. Y.

X. Y. was an 8-year-old, right-handed male who was attending the second grade in the public school system at the time of his referral for an assessment of neurocognitive and behavioral functioning. He was seen 5 years post his initial diagnosis of ALL. He received IT-MTX, but no CRT. Over the course of his treatment protocol, which lasted slightly under 3 years, there were no significant medical complications, such as seizures related to chemotherapy administration. Based on review of medical records and an interview with the patient's mother, the mother's pregnancy and delivery were without complications and developmental milestones had been met at either appropriate or advanced time periods. There was no other history of significant medical illness. X. Y. had no history of traumatic brain injury or any prediagnosis complications.

X. Y.'s mother had completed 18 years of education and was employed as a teacher. His father completed 13 years of education and worked in the area of supervision within a product development company. The parents were married. The patient had two siblings, a 4-year-old brother and a 2-year-old sister, who were all developing without incident.

X. Y. did not receive special services such as 504 considerations or an individualized education plan (IEP) through the school system. He is being raised bilingually by choice, and he attends dual language classes in English and Spanish. Following cessation of treatment, the patient did continue to experience chronic headache pain. Of note, his headaches are typically most apparent following the cessation of a school day. They are considered mild to moderate in intensity, and they do not unduly influence his ability to be involved in extracurricular activities, including sports. At the time of his evaluation he was not taking any prescribed medication, but he was benefiting from over-the-counter pain relief treatments.

The patient's mother brought her son in for the neuropsychological evaluation. Her primary concerns related to the fact that X. Y. appeared to fatigue over the course of a school day, and that she believes that he may tend to "tune things out"

cognitively. There were concerns regarding lapses in attention. Overall, the patient performs well in school, but the mother was becoming concerned over possible late effects from his ALL treatment, particularly as schooling was becoming increasingly demanding. X. Y. was described as somewhat of a perfectionist, and one who can become frustrated if task mastery does not occur quickly. Overall, she did not note highly significant changes in his cognitive status associated with treatment, but this comes with the caveat that he was diagnosed and treated at a very early age, prior to school enrollment. Behaviorally, she described her son as "kind of a nervous guy."

The patient's sleep was described as adequate, but he did experience nightmares that occur approximately two times per week. Thematic content was not related to medical events, but it did appear to consistently involve being attacked by "monsters and stuff." He typically obtains 10 hours of rest per evening. Appetite and nutrition were described as quite adequate. Energy is extremely sufficient on non-school days and adequate over the course of schooling, but, as identified earlier, he does tend to fatigue and experience headache, perhaps secondary to the stress of involvement in the classroom. Overall, X. Y. is considered a happy child. He socializes well, and teachers enjoy his presence in class. There was no evidence of a significant behavioral disturbance or management issues.

Over the course of the current evaluation, the patient was well motivated and demonstrated good attention and concentration. He did become perplexed and frustrated when tasks were difficult, as evidenced by verbal expressions of confusion, and increased motor activity such as extraneous movements and shifting in his chair, but he did maintain task involvement. There was a mild degree of self-distraction, but no evidence of impulsivity or environmental dependency. It was felt that a valid assessment of current neuropsychological functioning had been obtained.

Examination Results

Intelligence

X. Y. was administered the Wechsler Abbreviated Scale of Intelligence (WASI) and earned a verbal I.Q. of 119, a performance I.Q. of 125, and

Table 38-1.

Subtest	Scaled Score
Vocabulary	13
Block Design	15
Similarities	14
Matrix Reasoning	13

a full-scale I.Q. of 125. Intellectual functioning placed within the upper limits of the normal to superior functioning ranges. Individual subtest scores are presented in Table 38-1.

Interestingly, while the patient's performance on the Block Design subtest was characterized by significantly advanced nonverbal reasoning development, the patient received very few processing speed–related bonus points. Thus, even his excellent score is considered to be somewhat of an underestimate due to possible reduced information processing efficacy. In support of this, he completed the Coding subtest of the Wechsler Intelligence Scale for Children–Fourth edition (WISC-IV) and received a scaled score of 6, which suggests mild delays in psychomotor speed. Focused attention, as assessed with the Digit Span subtest from the WISC-IV, placed within the low-normal to borderline range. He received a scaled score of 7, and he recalled four digits forward and four digits backward. Fund of general knowledge was age appropriate, and his Information scaled score was 11.

Attention

Attentional abilities for verbal material and auditory processing, as assessed with the Sentence Memory subtest from the Wide Range Assessment of Memory and Learning (WRAML), were age appropriate and his scaled score was 10. The patient's performance on the Connors Continuous Performance Test–II (CPT-II) resulted in a clinical confidence index of 75%. He made numerous errors of omission (96th percentile), and his performance was extremely variable over the course of the procedure (94th percentile). Thus, there was highly significant evidence of difficulty with the maintenance of attention under conditions of vigilance. There was no evidence of impulsive responding tendencies, and the number of commission errors was age appropriate.

Memory/Learning

Verbal and nonverbal memory were assessed with the Stories and Faces subtests from the Children's Memory Scale (CMS). Immediate recall for verbal material was within the borderline range (scaled score = 7). He, nevertheless, retained 100% of the material at one-half hour delay (scaled score = 7). Immediate and delayed recall for nonverbal material, as assessed with the Faces subtest, was moderately impaired on initial recall (scaled score = 5), but performance improved at one-half hour delay (scaled score = 8), resulting in 113% retention. This may be reflective of processing speed difficulty. X. Y. was administered the Memory Card test from the Colorado Assessment Tests (CAT). This is a nonverbal task that measures learning over two successive presentations following an initial exposure. He exhibited a positive, accelerated learning curve.

Language

On the Boston Naming Test, a measure of confrontational anomia, he earned an age-appropriate raw score of 42. Four objects were identified following a phonemic cue, which is within the normal range for his age. On brief screening with the short form of the Token Test, language comprehension was intact.

Visual/Spatial–Constructional

Spatial awareness was assessed with the Judgment of Line Orientation Test, and his performance was age appropriate. Similarly, he earned a score well within the normal range on the Hooper Visual Organization Test. His performance on the Visual-Motor Integration Measure resulted in a standard score of 95.

Mental Flexibility

While there was earlier evidence of difficulty in processing speed, X. Y. performed well on the Trail Making A & B Tests. He was administered the Wisconsin Card Sorting Test, a measure of flexible problem solving, and completed all six categories. There were only seven preservative responses, two other responses, and there were no instances of a failure to maintain set. Thus, consistent with his advanced intellectual development, under problem-solving conditions he benefitted extremely well from feedback on his own performance, exhibited no evidence of preservative tendencies, nor was he susceptible to distraction.

Achievement

Academic achievement was assessed with the Wide Range Achievement Test–Fourth Edition (WRAT-IV). He earned a Word Reading standard score of 128, a Sentence Comprehension standard score of 114, a Spelling standard score of 116, and a Math Computation standard score of 95. Language skills are clearly grade advanced and consistent with measured intelligence. Arithmetic computation, on the other hand, is a relative weakness, and, even though age appropriate, a qualitative analysis of his performance suggested errors in computation that were likely influenced by inattention.

Personality

X. Y.'s mother completed both the Behavioral Assessment System for Children–Second Edition–Parent Rating (BASC-II-PR) and the Parenting Stress Index (PSI). Her responses to the BASC-II-PR resulted in a valid profile. The patient did receive a clinically significant elevation on the Anxiety Scale. Adaptive functioning was rated as advanced in all areas. Item analysis indicated that X. Y. tends to worry on a regular basis and is excessively concerned about what his teachers will think regarding his performance. He was described as a serious child, and items were endorsed that indicate he has excessive fears and is very preoccupied over making mistakes and what others think of him in this regard. Responses to the PSI indicate that the parent–child relationship is likely to be characterized by excellent emotional health, and both can be expected to be well adjusted to their respective roles. The family system appears to be intact based on her responses, and life stress is manageable at this time.

X. Y. completed the Self-Report version of the BASC-II, and the resultant profile was valid.

There were no clinically significant elevations. He does not view himself as having issues with worry, fears, and anxiousness at a level consistent with the mother's summary and perceptions.

Discussion

On a very positive note, this young man enjoys considerable neuropsychological strengths, even with the highly significant risk factors of diagnosis of, and treatment for, ALL at a very young age. This evaluation followed his CNS prophylactic treatment and also systemic chemotherapy, which we are beginning to understand may not be as benign to the CNS as previously thought. More specifically, intellectual development was in the bright normal to superior range, and nondominant hemisphere functions were generally intact. It may be significant, however, that his nonverbal memory was somewhat more fragile than his verbal memory. His problem-solving approach was quite advanced for his age and consistent with his intelligence. Also, basic language functions, and related academic achievement, were significantly grade advanced.

There were several areas of concern. Most prominently, deficits in the maintenance of attention under conditions of vigilance were present. X. Y. manifested difficulty in maintaining attention over time, and he also exhibited impairment in response consistency. He was not, however, impulsive in his reactions. This is quite consistent with the profile of neuropsychological involvement following ALL treatment protocols. The qualitative nature of dysfunction in this population is quite different from what teachers are most likely to experience, commonly attention-deficit/hyperactivity disorder (ADHD). Of note, subtle attentional difficulties may not be apparent given that children appear to be maintaining attention, are cooperative, and are not impulsive. In the case of X. Y., while grade appropriate, his arithmetic performance is beginning to show evidence of declines. This may be likely due to the fact that arithmetic is demanding of the attentional system. Furthermore, his information processing efficacy was mildly delayed, which is not uncommon following a CNS insult in childhood. In sum, X. Y. is experiencing delays in processing speed that are variable and also difficulties in the maintenance of vigilance attention. However, he does not present with symptoms that would be consistent with a diagnosis of ADHD and is likely to be perceived by his teachers as extremely intelligent. Thus, while in need of an intervention for these issues, he certainly would not meet educational based guidelines for a learning disability.

The current evaluation provides evidence of some subtle, but perhaps significant involvement in terms of psychological factors contributing to the patient's clinical presentation, such as increased anxiety and worrying, particularly in regard to school performance. The neuropsychological evaluation is clearly directing us toward specific interventions in order to assist this young man's continued success in school, particularly given the fact that he is only now just about to complete the second grade.

Recommendations include 504 considerations to address mild processing speed difficulties and attentional problems. These considerations should include increased time for testing and homework assignments, in addition to factors such as preferential seating at the front of the class. The parents were advised as to the potential benefits of a stimulant medication, a treatment modality that has been shown to be potentially beneficial with children treated for a pediatric malignancy (Mulhern et al., 2004). Furthermore, the patient is also an excellent candidate for a cognitive remediation program (Butler et al., 2008). If he becomes involved in this intervention, he would also receive treatment directed toward stress management and anxiety within a cognitive-behavioral framework. Even without attendance in brain injury rehabilitation, this intervention is recommended because of the possibility that he fatigues over the school day because of its demands on his deficient abilities.

Central nervous system involvements following prophylactic treatments associated with leukemia are quite different in their vector of damage when compared to other sources of brain damage in childhood, such as traumatic brain injury and epilepsy. Acute lymphoblastic leukemia–related prophylactic treatments tend to result in delayed, slow, and progressive insidious declines in functioning over time. These are complicated by the fact that the damage has occurred in a developing brain, and the concept of spontaneous recovery is not necessarily appropriate within the ALL population. On a very positive note, the decline in using CRT as a first-line CNS prophylaxis has resulted in decreased neurocognitive deficits in survivors of childhood ALL. Nevertheless, many patients continue to experience CNS toxicity that impacts their quality of life.

As noted in the background section, X. Y. is well positioned for success. From an oncology standpoint, he has received a CNS prophylactic regimen that typically results in less neuropsychological involvement. Additionally, neuropsychological research and clinical evaluations have progressed considerably, and we not only understand many of the likely deficits but are now able to recommend treatment protocols. Ongoing research is directed toward further improving our ability to effectively intervene in this population and also applying our results to other areas of pediatric brain injury.

References

Butler, R.W., Copeland, D. R., Fairclough, D. L., Mulhern, R. K., Katz, E. R., Kazak, A. E., Noll, R. B., Patel, S. K., & Sahler, O. J. (2008). A multicenter, randomized clinical trial of a cognitive remediation program for childhood survivors of a pediatric malignancy. *Journal of Consulting and Clinical Psychology, 76,* 367–378.

Eisner, C. (2004). Neurocognitive sequelae of childhood cancers and their treatment. *Pediatric Rehabilitation, 7,* 1–16.

Janzen, L. A., & Spiegler, B. J. (2008). Neurodevelopment sequelae of pediatric acute lymphoblastic leukemia and its treatment. *Developmental Disabilities Research Reviews, 14,* 185–195.

Moleski, M. (2000). Neuropsychological, neuroanatomical, and neurophysiological consequences of CNS chemotherapy for acute lymphoblastic anemia. *Archives Clinical Neuropsychology, 5,* 603–630.

Mulhern, R. K., & Butler, R. W. (2004). Neurocognitive sequelae of childhood cancers and their treatment. *Pediatric Rehabilitation, 7,* 1–14.

Mulhern, R. K., & Butler, R. W. (2006). Neuropsychological late effects. In R. T. Brown (Ed.), *Comprehensive handbook of childhood cancer and sickle cell disease: A biopsychosocial approach* (pp. 262–278). New York: Oxford University Press.

Mulhern, R. K., Khan, R. B., Kaplan S., Helton, S., Christensen, R., Bonner, M., Brown, R., Xiong, X., Wu, S., Gururangan, S., & Reddick, W. E. (2004). Short-term efficacy of methylphenidate: A randomized, double-blind, placebo-controlled trial among survivors of childhood cancer. *Journal of Clinical Oncology, 22,* 4795–4803.

Ries, L. A. G., Melbert, D., Krapcho, M., Stinchcomb, D. G., Howlader, N., Horner, M. J., Mariotto, A., Miller, B. A., Feuer, E. J., Altekruse, S. F., Lewis, D. R., Clegg, L., Eisner M. P., Reichman, M., & Edwards, B. K. (Eds.). (2007). *SEER cancer statistics review, 1975-2005, National Cancer Institute.* Bethesda, MD. Retrieved February 13, 2010, from http://seer.cancer.gov/csr/1975_2005/results_merged/topic_survival_by_year_dx.pdf.

39

Detecting Deficits in High-Functioning Patients

Bradley N. Axelrod

One of the more difficult activities for neuropsychologists is to provide bad news to patients and their families. Obviously, being prepared to tell individuals that they have a progressive dementia or will not recover cognitively from a stroke that has occurred is a difficult task. Despite the frequency of providing such difficult information to our patients, there is often little training provided to do so.

Likewise, most neuropsychology training programs do not discuss another challenging event, such as evaluating an individual who is most similar to the psychologist. We are surely aware that if a friend or family member were to be referred for evaluation, they would be referred out to another clinician. However, in some situations, the examinee might be of a close enough background, age, or profession to the psychologist that we might identify with the patient.

The individual discussed in this chapter is of interest for a number of reasons. First, he is a clinical psychologist who has familiarity with the profession and many of the principles included in test construction and administration. Walking the balance of administering tasks that he had no knowledge of while still providing a thorough evaluation was an initial challenge; this required an in-depth conversation before the measures were initially selected. Second, the individual's level of impairment required a careful follow-up session in which the specifics regarding his inability to return to active employment as a psychologist were discussed. Although this would be a difficult task under the best of

conditions, providing this type of feedback to a learned colleague was unusually sensitive. Finally, the clinical presentation of this patient is of interest by highlighting cognitive disruption resulting from radiation therapy. Thus, while evaluating the history, cognition, and emotional presentation of this individual, also consider your own reaction to evaluating someone whose background is not dissimilar from your own.

Background Information

At the time of referral, Dr. Smith was 55 years old. He was referred by his neurologist for an evaluation of both cognitive and emotional functioning. He was raised in an urban setting and obtained grades in the A/B range throughout much of his academic history. He served in the Army for 2 years, beginning in 1968. While serving in Vietnam, he was exposed to Agent Orange, a defoliant subsequently found to be associated with high rates of carcinomas in soldiers who used it. Following completion of his college degree, Dr. Smith obtained his Ph.D. in clinical psychology from a state university. He then obtained a position in a Midwestern state college teaching introduction to psychology, psychological research, research methods, experimental psychology, and biological psychology, among other classes. Dr. Smith indicated that his preferred class to teach was experimental psychology because he would hold it like a journal club. The students read relevant articles in psychology. In the course, Dr. Smith would point out weaknesses in the study design, major conclusions, and implications of the manuscripts.

Medical History

Dr. Smith's medical history began with the diagnosis of Burkitt lymphoma in 1988, 15 years prior to the evaluation with me. The onset of the lymphoma was considered related to Dr. Smith's exposure to Agent Orange. He underwent chemotherapy and whole-brain radiation therapy in the late 1980s. He required a 2-year leave of absence from work for treatment and convalescence. After the 2 years, he returned to his university position, taking up his full course load and academic duties.

In an unrelated incident, Dr. Smith was a driver of a vehicle that was rear-ended while on an expressway. His car went off the road and fell into a nearby body of water. He struck his head against the windshield with enough force that it shattered the glass. Dr. Smith did not believe that he lost consciousness. As the vehicle was sinking, he was able to get his family out of the car. He denied any cognitive or emotional changes after that event.

Beginning 10 years following radiation therapy, Dr. Smith noted difficulty in preparing his lectures for class. In addition, he would try to read journal articles but would fail to comprehend the entire content contained within. He began reading and teaching from easier journals. He related that he had found it increasingly difficulty to analyze information from the professional literature without someone else having first offered a synthesis of the data. Dr. Smith's wife noticed that he was increasingly distressed when he prepared lectures. He noticed that it also took a longer time to prepare the same material, making him even more anxious when doing so.

Eventually, Dr. Smith was referred to a neurologist who performed an initial evaluation 2 years after the symptoms began. In her report, she noted complaints of forgetfulness, misplacing objects, repeating conversations, and dysnomia as reported by Dr. Smith and his wife. He reported that his mood was variable, often associated with feeling grateful for having beaten lymphoma but also feeling overwhelmed and easily frustrated when trying to prepare for classes or write professional papers. He slept

6 hours at night, no change from before. He denied any changes in his weight or appetite. The neurological evaluation found Dr. Smith to have good insight and attention, with mildly impaired executive functions. His affect was appropriate. Diagnostically, it was thought that Dr. Smith likely suffered from delayed demyelination, which might also lead to a degenerative cognitive disorder. Dr. Smith was started on Aricept to minimize the ongoing cognitive decline.

Upon neurological reevaluation 1 year later, Dr. Smith's presentation appeared slightly improved in comparison to the initial assessment, although it was still impaired relative to age and education peers. For example, he had previously been able to recite six digits forward and none backward, but 1 year later he produced seven digits forward and five digits backward. No additional cognitive assessment was available for review.

Clinical Interview

Dr. Smith was referred for a neuropsychological evaluation at the request of the neurologist to obtain a more objective and standardized assessment of Dr. Smith's cognition. He attended the appointment accompanied by his wife who remained present during the interview, but not the face-to-face testing. The background information obtained from Dr. Smith and his wife was consistent with the information presented earlier.

A conversation was held with Dr. Smith to discuss the neuropsychological tests with which he might be familiar. While not a neuropsychologist, he had familiarity with issues relating to test construction and test development. The list of tests that were considered to be used for the assessment was shown to him to ensure that he was not intimately familiar with the test items or even the procedures involved in the tasks to be administered.

Behavioral Observations

Dr. Smith was cooperative and compliant throughout the interview and evaluation. He responded to interview questions with responses that were coherent and goal directed. His speech was of normal rate, articulation, volume, and prosody.

He presented with good hygiene, wearing a sport shirt and jacket. Rapport was easily established with Dr. Smith, as he was friendly and fully cooperative with the assessment process.

During the evaluation, Dr. Smith had no difficulty understanding task instructions and demonstrated good stamina across the evaluation. He was aware of failed performance, becoming frustrated when met with failure. Dr. Smith demonstrated a normal range of affect. His mood was affable and otherwise unremarkable.

Tests Administered

Wechsler Adult Intelligence Scale–III (WAIS-3)
Peabody Picture Vocabulary Test–III (PPVT-3)
North American Adult Reading Test (NAART)
Wide Range Achievement Test–III (WRAT-3)
Wechsler Memory Scale–III (WMS-3)
Rey Auditory Verbal Learning Test
Rey Complex Figure Test
Trail-Making Test
Controlled Oral Word Association Test
Category Exemplar Examination
Wisconsin Card Sorting Test (WCST)
Finger Oscillation Test
Grip Strength Test
Grooved Pegboard Test
Minnesota Multiphasic Personality Inventory–II (MMPI-2)

Test Results

Cognitive Functioning

A summary of the quantitative test findings appears in Table 39-1. The narrative for this report follows.

At the time of assessment, Dr. Smith's current level of intellectual functioning fell in the superior range (FSIQ = 126; 96th percentile). He demonstrated relatively lower performance (PIQ = 117) abilities in comparison to his verbal (VIQ = 128) skills. His performance on these tasks was consistent with estimates of intellectual functioning based on performance from a complex reading test and based on demographic information. His performance on the index scores likewise revealed higher verbal comprehension skills (SS = 126) relative to his perceptual organizational (SS = 114) and working memory (SS = 117) skills. He demonstrated relative

weaknesses on Letter-Number Sequencing and Matrix Reasoning, with scores on the other subtests all falling in the high-average to superior range. Performance on a supplemental measure of verbal functioning also fell in the high-average range (SS = 112), consistent with his WAIS-III performance.

Achievement testing revealed average performance on tasks of sight reading (SS = 107), spelling (SS = 107), and arithmetic computation (SS = 102) skills. These scores all fell close to the ceiling of the WRAT-3 for each of the subtests.

Memory functioning, as assessed by the Wechsler Memory Scale-III, revealed borderline deficient performance for previously learned material (SS = 73), significantly worse than his performance on the WAIS-III. His performance following a 30-minute delay was comparable (SS = 69), again deficient relative to his current level of intellectual functioning. On a more complex test of verbal list learning (Rey Auditory Verbal Learning Test), Dr. Smith demonstrated no improvement in learning, even after being given the same list of 15 words five times. He initially recalled four (SS = 79) of the 15 words, still recalling only four words (SS < 55) after the list had been read to him five times. He recalled one of the words after a brief delay (SS < 55) and none 30 minutes later (SS < 55). In contrast to his deficient verbal memory, performance on a complex visual memory test fell in the average range after both brief (SS = 108) and 30-minute (SS = 109) delays. Recognition memory was significantly lower (SS = 88), in part because of a negative response bias. In other words, Dr. Smith was more likely to not respond to an item for fear that he might include a distracter (false-positive errors = 0). However, he obtained 7 of 12 hits when identifying words that had actually been presented. Although less impaired than verbal memory, his performance still represents deficient memory in comparison to his intellectual abilities. Overall, Dr. Smith demonstrated deficient memory performance, with worse performance on tasks of verbal memory.

Dr. Smith's performance on tests of cognitive flexibility ranged from the average range to the superior range. He performed in the superior range on a connect-the-dots test of psychomotor speed (Trail Making Test–A). When the task was

Table 39-1. Summary Table of Neuropsychological Test Data

PREMORBID INTELLECTUAL FUNCTIONING
North American Adult Reading Test   113
Peabody Picture Vocabulary Test–III   112

INTELLECTUAL FUNCTIONING
Wechsler Adult Intelligence Scale–III

FSIQ	126
VIQ	128
PIQ	117
VCI	126
POI	114
WMI	117
Similarities	15
Vocabulary	15
Arithmetic	14
Digit Span	14
Information	14
Letter-Number Sequencing	11
Picture Completion	13
Digit Symbol	13
Block Design	13
Matrix Reasoning	11

ACADEMIC ACHIEVEMENT
Wide Range Achievement Test–3 (WRAT-III)

Reading	107
Spelling	107
Math	102

MEMORY (Standard Scores)
Wechsler Memory–III

Immediate Memory	73
General Memory	69
Auditory Recognition	65

Rey Auditory Verbal Learning Test

Trial 1	79
Trial 5	<55
Total 1 to 5	<55
Recall (immediate)	<55
Delayed memory	<55

Rey Complex Figure Test

Immediate	108
Delayed	109
Recognition Memory	88

EXECUTIVE FUNCTIONING (Standard Scores)
Trail-Making Test

TMT-A	117 (19 sec)
TMT-B	97 (58 sec)
Word Generation (COWAT)	107 (45 words)
Animals & Fruits/Vegetables	115 (46 words)

Wisconsin Card-Sorting Test (demographic correction)

% Conceptual Responses	111
Preservative Responses	101
Perseverative Errors	102

MOTOR TESTS (T-scores)

Finger tapping-dominant	57
Finger tapping-nondominant	41
Grip Strength-dominant	59
Grip Strength -nondominant	54
Grooved pegs-dominant	40
Grooved pegs-nondominant	45

MINNESOTA MULTIPHASIC PERSONALITY
   INVENTORY-II

Scale	T-score
L	52
F	45
K	68
1	64
2	50
3	66
4	69
5	42
6	53
7	59
8	65
9	51
0	39

made more complex (Trail Making Test–B), shifting between numbers and letters, his performance dropped to the average range. Dr. Smith demonstrated intact performance on verbal fluency tasks when either phonemic (i.e., words beginning with a specific letter) or semantic (e.g., animal names) limitations were made. Finally, his performance on the WCST, a problem-solving test of hypothesis generation, modification, and revision, fell in the superior range. Dr. Smith understood the task and was able to consistently benefit from feedback by the examiner. He completed all six categories on the WCST within 70 response cards.

Dr. Smith completed tasks of motor functioning. Intact performance was observed, bilaterally, on measures of finger dexterity, fine motor speed, and grip strength, relative to age, gender, and education peers.

Emotional Functioning

Dr. Smith completed the MMPI-2 (MMPI-2 Welsh code: 4381-7692/5:0# K-L/F), a standardized assessment of emotional functioning, as part of his evaluation. Inspection of the validity scales reveals an individual who has poor insight into his own psychological difficulties, evades discussions about psychological difficulties, and may overcompensate for feeling inadequate.

Evaluation of the secondary validity scales confirms an underreporting of psychological symptoms. The difference score between his F (raw score = 3) and K (raw score = 24) scales falls at −21. According to Greene (1991), this level of defensiveness is greater than that observed in 99.9% of all males and 99.9% of all psychiatric patients. His Superlative Self-Presentation was his highest score (T-score = 65). Similarly, he endorsed 16 of the Lachar-Wrobel critical items, also indicative of an underreporting of emotional difficulties. The difference between the Weiner-Harmon Subtle and Obvious scales falls at a level (total difference score = −55) that again demonstrated minimization of psychological symptoms.

On the restructured clinical scales, he denied any symptoms included in the Demoralization scale (RCd). His highest elevation throughout the entire MMPI-2 was on the Superlative Self-Presentation scale.

The extreme minimization of psychological symptoms made the interpretation of clinical items meaningless. Any information outside of recognizing that his presentation was an attempt to make him appear less distraught than was truly the case would be conjecture.

Findings

Dr. Smith's current performance on measures of intellectual functioning falls in the high-average to superior range. His verbal abilities are comparable to nonverbal abilities. He similarly presents with superior performance on measures of executive functioning. Achievement testing was slightly lower, in the average range, as was Dr. Smith's performance on motor tasks. In contrast to intact performance in the aforementioned areas, Dr. Smith's performance on memory tasks fell in the impaired range. Dr. Smith's performance on the memory measures revealed greater impairment on tasks of verbal memory than on those tapping nonverbal memory.

From an emotional point of view, Dr. Smith's presentation is consistent with one who is well educated and attempts to present himself in an overly positive light. He minimized any psychological stressors, preferring to assume that he can cope with such concerns independently.

In summary, Dr. Smith's cognitive presentation is consistent with the deficits observed by his neurologist. Specifically, isolated cognitive impairment in memory functioning is observed. A possible progressive lateralized dementia should be considered.

In terms of potential limitations, Dr. Smith's ability to return to full-time employment as a college professor is compromised because of his severe memory disability. Although he would be able to have a conversation about information for which he already has knowledge, Dr. Smith's ability to incorporate and integrate new information is clearly abnormal.

Recommendations

There is a common saying that physicians make the worst patients. The same might also be said about psychologists. What recommendations would you make to a psychologist who has cognitive difficulties and adamantly refuses to report any emotional symptoms related to his current state? A recommendation for psychotherapy might be indicated for an individual who wishes to address issues relating to unemployability and its effect on self-esteem, finances, and social support. However, in a psychologist who is so resistant to acknowledging the potential implications of his cognitive condition, any treatment attempts would be thwarted. In such a circumstance, it is the responsibility of the practicing psychologist to work with the patient-psychologist as one would with any learned client. Although not needing to explain the intricacies of psychotherapy, one instead must open the door for the patient-psychologist so that if affective reactions were to crop up in the future, an individual who can provide treatment is already in place.

Neuropsychologists have the opportunity to evaluate individuals presenting with severe cognitive ailments, mild abnormalities, psychiatric conditions, and fabricated deficits. The individual presented in this chapter had true verbal memory deficits. Not only is it difficult to assess "bad news" for individuals as young as Mr. Smith, but the difficulty was compounded by knowing that he was a psychologist who was not very dissimilar from the evaluating clinician.

40

Neuropsychological Effects of Surgical Resection of a Colloid Cyst: A Case Presentation

Aaron C. Malina

Colloid cysts are benign intraventricular tumors. They were first described by Wallman in 1858 and successfully resected by Dandy in 1921 (Chin, 2008). Colloid cysts account for 0.3%–2.0% of intracranial tumors and about 15%–20% of intraventricular masses. They are the most common tumors found in the third ventricle. Colloid cysts are spheroid lesions, typically located in the anterosuperior third ventricle, between the columns of the fornix. They are usually attached to the roof of the third ventricle and sometimes to the choroid plexus, occurring rarely in other locations. Size can vary, but colloid cysts are typically a few millimeters to about 4 cm in diameter. They are problematic because of their location, as they can obstruct the Foramen of Monro, causing obstructive hydrocephalus. The cysts are felt to be developmental, but they are slow growing and the clinical presentation is usually in the third to fifth decade of life. Gender ratio varies across studies from equivocal to 2:1 male to female. There is no known genetic relationship or racial predilection (Amy & Walker, 2003; Spears, 2004; Urso, Ross, Parker, Patrizi, & Stewart, 1998).

Colloid cysts are composed of periodic acid-Schiff-positive amorphous material, necrotic leukocytes, and cholesterol clefts, and they increase in size by accumulation of secreted fluid of the epithelial lining or its breakdown (Amy & Walker, 2003; Motoyama, Hashimoto, Ishida, & Iida, 2002). Colloid cysts typically occur sporadically. The etiology of colloid cysts is debated, but they are generally believed to be

congenital. Hypothesized sources include the paraphysis, choroid plexus, ependyma, primitive neuroectoderm, or endodermal tissue (Akins, Roberts, Coxe, & Kaufman, 1996; Chin, 2008).

The discovery of colloid cysts is typically incidental or after causing an acute obstructive hydrocephalus (Beems, Menovksy, & Lammens, 2006). Clinical presentation varies, and the cyst can be asymptomatic, especially when smaller. Symptoms are generally due to hydrocephalus and increased intracranial pressure, with headache as the most common presenting complaint. Intracystic hemorrhage is rare. The headache can be nonlocalized, but bifrontal, frontal-parietal, or frontal-occipital presentations are common. The "classic" presentation is often reported to be paroxysmal headache associated with change in head position, but, in reality, this is actually quite rare. Other symptoms can include nausea and/or vomiting, vision changes, gait changes, cognitive, psychiatric, and/or behavioral changes. Seizures or sudden death can occur in up to 10% of cases (Akins et al., 1996; Morita & Kelly, 1993; Motoyama et al., 2002; Spears, 2004).

Relatively accurate diagnosis of colloid cysts can be made with computed tomography (CT) and magnetic resonance imaging (MRI) (Hamlat, Casallo-Quiliano, Saikali, Adn, & Brassier, 2004). Radiologically, colloid cysts appear as hyperdense in about two-thirds of cases and isodense in one-third on CT. On MRI, the appearance is variable, but generally hyperintense on T1-weighted images and hypointense on T2-weighted images.

Rim enhancement is commonly seen with contrast (Sener, 2007; Urso et al., 1998). Imaging characteristics vary with the cysts' cholesterol and protein contents (Amy & Walker, 2003).

Management of colloid cysts varies depending on symptom presentation and can range from observation, shunting, sterotactic aspiration, or microsurgical partial or total resection (Amy & Walker, 2003; Parwani, Fatani, Burger, Erozan, & Ali, 2002). Aspiration alone is often inadequate due to a high degree of recurrence, which can be as high as 30% to 80% (Bergsneider, 2007; Grondin, Hader, MacRae, & Hamilton, 2007). Hydrocephalus is the primary indication for surgery. Depending on the cyst, surgical approaches can be endoscopic, transcortical-transventricular, or transcollosal-interforniceal. With an endoscopic approach, the cyst is aspirated, as much of the cyst as possible is removed, and the remainder is cauterized. The goal of treatment is to remove the cerebrospinal fluid (CSF) obstruction, normalize intracranial pressure, and remove the lesion. The most important factor in outcome is early diagnosis and surgical intervention (Amy & Walker, 2003; Chin, 2008; Urso et al., 1998).

Third ventricle tumors, such as colloid cysts, and their surgical removal can cause significant cognitive dysfunction. Cognitive changes can result from both direct cyst effects as well as from treatment. As a result, neuropsychological outcome is relevant to treatment planning for patients with colloid cysts (Friedman, Meyers, & Sawaya, 2003). The region of the brain where the cysts occur is rich in structures and connections that are associated with cognitive functioning, including the mamillary bodies, fornix, thalamic nuclei, septal nuclei, and the mammillothalamic tract (Brand et al., 2004; Moudgil, Azzouz, Abdulkader, Haut, & Gutmann, 2000). The fornix is a major efferent pathway connecting the hippocampus and other limbic and diencephalic structures. Cognitive deficits, particularly memory impairment, are not an unusual postoperative complication and deficits can range in severity from mild to severe (Desai, Nadkarni, Muzumdar, & Goel, 2002; Friedman et al., 2003). Fornix damage is sufficient to induce amnesia. There is variability across studies with some patients making a full recovery postoperatively without cognitive complications, while others are left with significant cognitive residuals (Aggleton

et al., 2000; Mougdil et al., 2000; Poreh et al., 2006). The structures around the third ventricle also have connections with limbic and frontal areas, which can lead to behavioral changes postoperatively (Brand et al., 2007). Preoperative evaluation is useful to assess for presurgical versus postoperative changes (Aggleton et al., 2000; Moorthy, Vinolia, Tharyan, & Rajshekhar, 2006). However, because the onset of symptoms can be acute and severe, preoperative testing may, in some cases, not be practical or possible.

Case Presentation

The patient is a 47-year-old, right-handed, Caucasian male who had been having headaches for a few months, which his primary care physician believed were due to sinusitis. He also had esophageal reflux and underwent an upper endoscopy with twilight sedation. On the morning of the endoscopy, the patient awoke with a headache. After he came out of sedation, the headache worsened and he developed severe nausea and vomiting. Because the symptoms did not remit over time, the patient was sent to the emergency room.

Emergency room staff hypothesized that the symptoms were a reaction to the sedation, but they performed a CT scan of the brain because he had not been previously scanned. The CT images showed a 1 cm well-defined hyperdense lesion at the level of the Foramen of Monro in the midline, most consistent with a colloid cyst, associated with mild hydrocephalus. The left lateral ventricle was more prominent when compared to the right, as shown in Figure 40-1.

A follow-up MRI showed a 1 cm anterior third ventricular lesion, which was relatively isointense on the noncontrast T1 and hypointense on T2-weighted scans. This correlated with the colloid cyst documented on CT. The remainder of the brain showed mild ventricular enlargement and ventricular asymmetry with the left lateral ventricle larger than the right, as shown in Figure 40-2.

Given the low-lying obstructive (impacted) anatomy of the lesion, and the asymmetrically dilated left lateral ventricle, a left transcortical transventricular microsurgical approach was selected by the neurosurgeon as the least likely to cause morbidity and the most likely to attain technical satisfaction. The surgery was done with stealth guidance. An extraventricular drain was

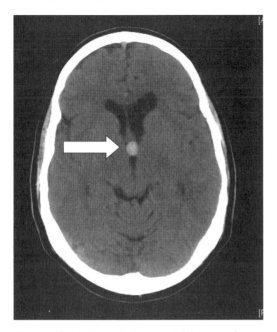

Figure 40-1. Presurgical computed tomography scan of the colloid cyst.

temporarily placed. There were no complications. The surgical pathology was consistent with a colloid cyst.

After a brief stay on the intensive care unit (ICU) and then a Medicine floor, the patient was transferred to the inpatient rehabilitation unit, where he was first evaluated neuropsychologically.

Inpatient Examination

The patient had no reported cognitive deficits prior to surgery. A baseline neuropsychological

evaluation was not ordered. He was working full time as a warehouse supervisor and was fully independent in all of his activities of daily living.

Once on the rehabilitation unit, the patient reported significant cognitive deficits. He felt that he was inattentive with poor memory. He also noted word-finding problems.

He reported that his mood was a little depressed. His sleep was decreased but fair. His appetite was fair with no changes in weight. He was optimistic about his future and denied any suicidal thoughts.

The patient had an additional previous medical history of gastroesophageal reflux disease (GERD) with Barrett esophagitis, a stomach ulcer, and sebaceous cyst. He had no previous psychiatric history. He drank socially, once or twice a week, and reported no recreational drug or tobacco use. The patient had 15 years of education and was a warehouse manager. He was married and had two children.

The patient was evaluated in his room on the rehabilitation unit about 2 weeks postoperatively. He was casually dressed and wore glasses. He was seated in a chair at bedside. His mood appeared dysphoric and mildly anxious with a fair range of affect. He was fidgety. His speech was fluent and of normal rate and rhythm. He appeared mildly fatigued. The patient had significant difficulty retaining task directions, even over brief intervals. He needed them consistently repeated. He was distractible and needed redirection. He also tended to perseverate task directions from one task to another. He was surprised by poor performances and had little insight.

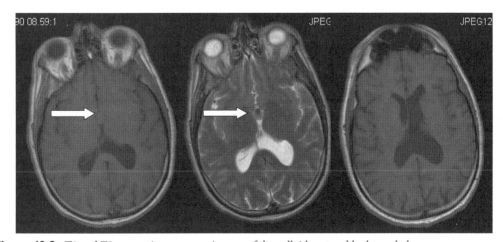

Figure 40-2. T1 and T2 magnetic resonance images of the colloid cyst and hydrocephalus.

He was fatigued but alert. He was oriented to person and year only. He did not know where he was or why he was hospitalized. He had no recall of the cyst or its resection. Please see Table 40 1 for a listing of scores. On the Wechsler Test of Adult Reading (WTAR), the patient's premorbid functioning, as estimated by his reading achievement and demographic factors, was high average.

On attentional measures, his Digit Span was average. His cognitive efficiency (i.e., processing speed) on the Stroop was low average to average. On Trail Making Part A, his efficiency was severely impaired. His cognitive flexibility on Trails B was also severely impaired.

On language measures, the patient's performance on the Boston Naming Test (BNT) was

Table 40-1. Data Summary for the Inpatient Evaluation Two Weeks Postoperatively

WTAR	Raw	Est IQ		BVMT–R		
	43	113		Form: 1	Raw	Percentile
WAIS–III	Raw	SS		Trial 1	1	1
Digits Total	14	8		Trial 2	4	1
Trail Making Test	Sec	T		Trial 3	0	<1
				Trials 1–3	5	<1
Part A	55	26		Learning	3	34
Part B	217	18		Delayed	1	<1
Ratio = 3.94				% Reten	25	<1
Stroop	Raw	T		Rec Hits	6	>16
				Rec FP	6	<1
Color	100	50		Discrim	0	<1
Word	61	40		**RBANS**	Raw	z
Color–Word	15	24–6				
Interference	–21	28–30		Figure Copy	19	.50
HVLT–R				Line Orien	9	–2.13
Form: 4	Raw	T		**WCST**	Raw	%
Trial 1	4			Cat Comp	0	<1
Trial 2	4			Tot Errors	39	1
Trial 3	4			Persev Rsp	33	1
Trials 1–3	12	<20		% CL Rsp	20	1
Delayed	0	<20		Fail Main Set	0	
% Reten	0	<20		Trials to 1st	64	<1
Rec Hits	12			**CLOX**	Raw	
Rec FP	12					
Discrim	0	<20		CLOX 1	9	
MAE	Raw	Percentile		CLOX 2	14	
COWA	13	<1			Raw	
Animal Fluency	Raw	Z		**BDI–II**	9	
Correct	4	–2.5		**BAI**	15	
Boston Naming Test	Raw	Z/MSS				
	32	–5.6				

BAI, Beck Anxiety Inventory; BDI–II, Beck Depression Inventory, Second Edition; BVMT–R, Brief Visuospatial Memory Test; HVLT–R, Hopkins Verbal Learning Test, Revised; MAE, Multilingual Aphasia Examination; RBANS, Repeatable Battery for the Assessment of Neuropsychological Status; WAIS–III, Wechsler Adult Intelligence Scale, Third Edition; WCST, Wisconsin Card–Sorting Test; WTAR, Wechsler Test of Adult Reading.

severely impaired with evidence of decreased word retrieval. He had 32 correct responses with an additional 20 correct with a phonemic cue. His verbal fluencies, both on Controlled Oral Word Association (COWA) and Animal Naming, were moderately to severely impaired.

On the Hopkins Verbal Learning Test, Revised (HVLT-R), the patient's new learning across three trials, delayed free recall, and recognition were all severely impaired. On recognition, he had 12 hits and 12 false positives for 0 discriminability. On the Brief Visuospatial Memory Test, Revised (BVMT-R), the patient's visual new learning, delayed free recall, and recognition were also severely impaired.

With regard to his visual perceptual functioning, on the Repeatable Battery for the Assessment of Neuropsychological Status (RBANS), the patient's Figure Copy was average. His Line Orientation was mildly impaired.

On a clock drawing, he did exhibit executive impairment, leaving off all of the numbers, instead writing in the designated time. His copy of a completed clock was better. On the Wisconsin Card Sorting Test (one deck), his problem solving and reasoning were severely impaired. He completed zero categories and had 39 errors.

On the Beck Depression Inventory, Second Edition (BDI-II), the patient was in the borderline normal range. He endorsed mild anxiety on the Beck Anxiety Inventory (BAI).

Overall, on initial inpatient testing, the patient exhibited psychomotor slowing, impaired cognitive flexibility, impaired word retrieval and fluencies, relatively intact visual perceptual skills, and marked memory and executive impairment. He had mild mood symptoms. Based on his cognitive presentation, it was felt that it was too early for the patient to consider returning to work and he would require 24-hour supervision upon discharge.

Outpatient Reevaluation

The patient returned for an outpatient reevaluation 2 months postoperatively. He was casually dressed and wore glasses. His gait and gross motor functioning were unremarkable. His speech was fluent and of normal rate and rhythm. His mood appeared mildly dysphoric with a fair range of affect. He became overwhelmed at times and was clearly frustrated by poor performances.

The patient struggled to retain some task directions. He was able to provide an appropriate history, to the best of his recollection, but was confabulatory during testing.

On outpatient follow-up, the patient had limited recall of his hospitalization. Since discharge, he had been participating in occupational and speech therapies. The patient and his wife reported that his cognition had progressively improved, but he continued to have a hard time with short-term recall. He forgot appointments and dates, and he still repeated himself. His word finding had improved. His attention was at "fifty percent." He used an alarm clock to facilitate taking his medications and generally remembered. The patient forgot that he was not to drive and drove locally on one occasion without incident. He was in the process of completing a driver's evaluation through occupational therapy. The patient had reportedly started paying bills, but he did not recall having done so. He started going back to work. Though he reported feeling "out of sync," he had performed relatively well.

The patient reported that his mood was "okay," but he could easily get down and frustrated. He was struggling with his recovery. He thought he would be back to baseline within a few months. Sleep was restless. Even when sleep improved, he continued to have bothersome dreams. Appetite was good and his weight was stable. He was concerned about his future, and he felt guilty that he was not providing for his family. He denied suicidal ideation but reported that if he could not go back to work, his family would suffer.

On retesting, the patient was fully alert and oriented to person, place, time, and circumstance. Please see Table 40-2 for his scores. His verbal simple attention span on the WMS-III Digit Span was low average with an average Spatial Span. On Trails A and on the Stroop, his cognitive efficiency (i.e., processing speed) was average to high average with average cognitive flexibility (i.e. set shifting) on Trails B.

Basic divided attention on the Brief Test of Attention (BTA) was average, but he was mildly to moderately impaired on a more complex divided attention task, the Paced Auditory Serial Addition Test (PASAT). Working memory, the capacity to attend to and manipulate information, was average. On the Conners Continuous

Table 40-2. Data Summary for Outpatient Follow-up Evaluation – Two Months Post-Operatively

MAE	Raw	%ile
COWA	44	67

Animals	Raw	Z
Correct	18	-.72

BNT	Raw	Z
	56	.29

Stroop	Raw	T
Word	126	64
Color	85	56
C-W	46	56

Trails	Sec	T
A	28	48
B	49	54
Ratio = 1.75		

WMS-III	Index SS
Aud Immediate	86
Aud Delayed	74
Aud Recog Del	85
Working Mem	102

	Raw	Age-SS
Inf/Orient	14	
Digit Span	13	7
Mntl Ctrl	31	13
LM I	33	9
LM II	8	5
LM %Ret	33	4
LM Recog	24/30	
VRI	95	14
VRII	22	6
VR %Ret	23	5
VR Recog	43	9
VPA I	6	6
VPA II	2	6
VPA %Ret	100	12
VPA Recog	22/24	
L-N Seq	10	10
Sptl Span	15	11

WCST	Raw	%ile
Cat Comp	6	>16
Tot Errors	30	23
Persev Rsp	22	14
% CL Rsp	69	30
FMS	2	6-10
Trials to 1st	15	6-10

RBANS	Raw	Z
Figure Copy	17	-.93
Line Orien	19	1.20

HVLT-R		
Form: 5	Raw	T
Trial 1	5	34
Trial 2	6	26
Trial 3	7	<20
Trials 1-3	18	25
Delayed	0	<20
% Reten	0	<20
Rec Hits	12	
Rec FP	4	
Discrim	8	<20

BVMT-R		
Form: 2	Raw	T
Trial 1	4	39
Trial 2	5	31
Trial 3	6	27
Trials 1-3	15	30
Learning	2	41
Delayed	8	43
% Reten	133	>16%
Rec Hits	5	
Rec FP	0	
Discrim	5	11-16%

CPT-II	Raw	%ile
Om	0	21.49
Comm	6	16.80
Hit RT	409.13	71.59
Hit RT SE	5.14	51.25
Variab	6.82	63.65
Det (d')	1.13	22.72
Resp (B)	.66	49.84
Persev	0	37.35
RT Chng	−.01	35.30
SE Chng	−.04	47.37
RT ISI Ch	.07	82.87
SE ISI Ch	.09	87.68

PASAT	Raw	Z
1	62	-2.79
2	42	-2.32
3	38	-1.66
4	46	- .59

	Raw	%ile
BTA	19	25-74

	Raw	Z
Clox I	13	.35
Clox II	15	.8
BDI-II	21	
BAI	12	

Note. BAI=Beck Anxiety Inventory; BDI-II=Beck Depression Inventory, Second Edition; BNT=Boston Naming Test; BTA=Brief Test of Attention; BVMT-R=Brief Visuospatial Memory Test; CPT-II=Connors Continuous Performance Test; HVLT-R=Hopkins Verbal Learning Test, Revised; MAE=Multilingual Aphasia Examination; PASAT=Paced Auditory Serial Addition Test; RBANS=Repeatable Battery for the Assessment of Neuropsychological Status; WCST=Wisconsin Card Sorting Test; WMS-III=Wechsler Memory Scale, Third Edition.

Performance Test, Second Edition (CPT-II), sustained attention was generally within normal limits, although there was some drop-off in performance with longer interstimulus intervals.

Word finding, on the Boston Naming Test, was average. Verbal fluencies on the COWA and Animal Fluency were average.

On Logical Memory, immediate recall was average with borderline to mildly impaired delayed recall. Delayed recognition was 24/30. On Verbal Paired Associates, immediate and delayed recall were low average. On the HVLT-R, new learning, delayed free recall, and recognition were severely impaired.

The patient was administered two visual memory tasks, Visual Reproduction and the BVMT-R. On Visual Reproduction, his immediate recall was superior with low-average delayed recall. His delayed recognition was average. On the BVMT-R, with multiple learning trials, the patient's new learning was moderately impaired.

His delayed free recall was low average with low-average recognition.

On the RBANS, the patient's Figure Copy was low average. Line Orientation was high average.

The patient's clock drawing was average. On the Wisconsin Card Sorting Test (WCST), a measure of problem solving and reasoning, the patient was slow to develop an initial strategy and was somewhat inconsistent, but he had overall low-average performance.

On brief, face valid screens, the patient endorsed mild anxiety and a mild to moderate level of depression. He endorsed some suicidal thoughts without intent.

Overall, the patient had made a significant improvement in the 2 months postoperatively. Please see Table 40-3 for a score comparison. This was especially true in his cognitive efficiency, cognitive flexibility, language skills, and visual perceptual and executive functioning, with the exception of his complex attention. Memory had

Table 40-3. Score Comparison between Inpatient and Outpatient Evaluations

TEST	Inpatient	Outpatient	BVMT-R		
MAE			Trial 1	1	4
COWA	13	44	Trial 2	4	5
Animals			Trial 3	0	6
Correct	4	18	Trials 1–3	5	15
BNT			Learning	3	2
Correct	32	56	Delayed	1	8
Stroop			% Reten	25	133
Word	100	126	Rec Hits	6	5
Color	61	85	Rec FP	6	0
C-W	15	46	Discrim	0	5
Trail Making			**WCST**	1 deck	2 decks
A	55	28	Cat Comp	0	6
B	217	49	Tot Errors	39	30
HVLT-R			Persev Rsp	33	22
Trial 1	4	5	% CL Rsp	20	69
Trial 2	4	6	FMS	0	2
Trial 3	4	7	Trials to 1st	64	15
Trials 1–3	12	18	**Clox I**	9	13
Delayed	0	0	**Clox II**	14	15
% Reten	0	0	**RBANS**		
Rec Hits	12	12	Figure Copy	19	17
Rec FP	12	4	Line Orien	9	19
Discrim	0	8	**BDI-II**	9	21
			BAI	15	12

BAI, Beck Anxiety Inventory; BDI-II, Beck Depression Inventory, Second Edition; BNT, Boston Naming Test; BVMT-R, Brief Visuospatial Memory Test; HVLT-R, Hopkins Verbal Learning Test, Revised; MAE, Multilingual Aphasia Examination; RBANS, Repeatable Battery for the Assessment of Neuropsychological Status; WCST, Wisconsin Card-Sorting Test.

improved, but he continued to show significant memory impairment with evidence of both decreased new learning and retrieval. He gained greater awareness into his deficits and developed a depression. He was started on Lexapro with a positive response. By his 6-month medical follow-up, the patient was continuing to have some difficulty with his memory and attention, but he was working and completing many of his daily activities independently.

Conclusion

In many ways, the patient's presentation was typical for a patient with a colloid cyst. He was experiencing a worsening headache over a matter of months, and the cyst was only identified after he was scanned when presenting with what were thought to be unrelated symptoms. Findings from CT and MRI were typical. The cyst was located in the third ventricle and was blocking the Foramen of Monro, causing an obstructive hydrocephalus. He underwent a transcortical resection. He initially had marked generalized postsurgical cognitive changes, which over a matter of a few months resolved to isolated deficits in memory and executive functioning (complex attention in this case). The persistent deficits in memory are not surprising in light of the location of the cyst and surgical site proximal to the fornix. There was no reference to forniceal damage in the surgical report and findings may be explained by the cyst location.

There can be significant variability in the long-term cognitive sequelae from surgical resection of a cyst. In this patient's case, there may be long-term residuals, but they are relatively mild and he can continue on with work and other aspects of his life. In other cases, long-term cognitive changes can be more severe and debilitating.

Acknowledgment

Thank you to Jerry Sweet, PhD, for his review and comments of an earlier version of this chapter.

References

Aggleton, J. P., McMackin, D., Carpenter, K., Hornak, J., Kapur, N., Halpin, S., et al. (2000). Differential cognitive effects of the colloid cysts in the third that spare or compromise the fornix. *Brain, 123,* 800–815.

Akins, P. T., Roberts, R., Coxe, W., & Kaufman, B. A. (1996). Familial colloid cyst of the third ventricle: Case report and review of associated conditions. *Neurosurgery, 38(2),* 392–395.

Amy, C. & Walker, E. (2003). Not just another headache: Colloid cyst of the third ventricle. *The Nurse Practitioner, 28(9),* 8-12.

Beems, T., Menovsky, T., & Lammens, M. (2006). Hemorrhagic colloid cyst: Case report and review of the literature. *Surgical Neurology, 65,* 84–86.

Bergsneider, M. (2007). Complete microsurgical resection of colloid cysts with a dual-port endoscopic technique. *Neurosurgery, 60(2),* 33–43.

Brand, M., Kalbe, E., Kracht, L. W., Riebel, U., Munch, J., Kessler, J., et al. (2004). Organic and psychogenic factors leading to executive dysfunctions in a patient suffering from surgery of a colloid cyst of the Foramen of Monro. *Neurocase, 10(6),* 420–425.

Chin, L. (2008). *Colloid cysts.* Retrieved May 27, 2008, from the EMedicine Web site: http://www.emedicine.com/med/topic2906.htm

Desai, K. I., Nadkari, T. D., Muzumdar, D. P., & Goal, A. H. (2002). Surgical anagement of colloid cyst of the third ventricle: A study of 105 cases. *Surgical Neurology, 57,* 295–304.

Friedman, M. A., Meyers, C., & Sawaya, R. (2003). Neuropsychological effects of third ventricle tumor surgery. *Neurosurgery, 52(4),* 791–798.

Grondin, R. T., Hader, W., MacRae, E., & Hamilton, M. G. (2007). Endoscopic versus microsurgical resection of third ventricle colloid cysts. *Canadian Journal of Neurological Sciences, 34,* 197–207.

Hamlat, A., Casallo-Quiliano, C., Saikali, S., Adn, M., & Brassier, G. (2004). Huge colloid cyst: Case report and review of unusual forms. *Acta Neurochirurgica, 146,* 397–401.

Moorthy, R. K., Vinolia, H., Tharyan, P., & Rajshekhar, V. (2006). Assessment of memory and new learning ability following stereotaxy-guided transcortical resection of anterior third ventricular colloid cysts. *Sterotactic andFunctional Neurosurgery, 84,* 205–211.

Morita, A., & Kelly, P. J. (1993). Resection of intraventricular tumors via a computer assisted volumetric stereotactic approach. *Neurosurgery, 32(6),* 920–927.

Motoyama, Y., Hashimoto, H., Ishida, Y., & Iida, J. I. (2002). Spontaneous rupture of a presumed colloid cyst of the third ventricle-A case report. *Neurologica-Medico-Chirurgica (Tokyo), 42,* 228–231.

Moudgil, S. S., Azzouz, M., Abdulkader, A-A., Haut, M., & Gutmann, L. (2000). Amnesia due to fornix infarction. *Stroke, 31,* 1418–1419.

Parwani, A. V., Fatani, I. Y., Burger, P. C., Erozan, Y. S., & Ali, S. Z. (2002). Colloid cyst of the third ventricle: Cytomorphologic features on stereotactic fine-needle aspiration. *Diagnostic Cytopathology, 27*(1), 27–31.

Poreh, A., Winocur, G., Moscovitch, M., Backon, M., Goshen, E., Ram, Z., et al. (2006). Anterograde and retrograde amnesia in a person with bilateral fornix lesions following removal of a colloid cyst. *Neuropsychologia, 44,* 2241–2248.

Sener, R. N. (2007). Colloid cyst: Diffusion MR imaging findings. *Journal of Neuroimaging, 17*(2), 181–183.

Spears, R. C. (2004). Colloid cyst headache. *Current Pain and Headache Reports, 8,* 297–300.

Urso, J. A., Ross, G. J., Parker, R. K., Patrizi, J. D., & Stewart, B. (1998). Colloid cyst of the third ventricle: Radiologic-pathologic correlation. *Journal of Computer Assisted Tomography, 22*(4), 524–527.

41

Anoxic Brain Injury: Two Cases of Anoxic Brain Injury Secondary to Cardiac Arrest

Leslie D. Rosenstein and Paul A. Friedman

Anoxic brain injury occurs after disruption of oxygen supply to the brain for more than 4 to 8 minutes. It often occurs in the context of reduced blood flow (ischemia). Because of the connection to ischemia, patterns of neuronal loss often reflect patterns of blood supply in relation to blood vessel size, with increased likelihood of damage to the so-called watershed areas supplied by smaller blood vessels. Additionally, certain types of neurons as well as certain structures are more susceptible to damage due to oxygen deprivation with resulting metabolic and biochemical changes. These factors combine to increase the likelihood of damage to particular structures (e.g., the hippocampus, neocortex, basal ganglia, cerebellar Purkinje cells, primary visual cortex, frontal regions, and thalamus). See Caine and Watson (2000) and Hopkins and Haaland (2004) for thorough reviews of these issues.

In terms of neuropsychological functioning after anoxia, much has been written about decreased anterograde memory functioning and, less commonly, deficits in retrograde memory. Additionally, many studies have demonstrated that there can oftentimes be changes in executive functioning, drive, and personality, as well as impairments in visual spatial functioning, general cognitive abilities, and motor functions, with some studies documenting language impairments such as word-finding deficits (see Caine & Watson, 2000; Garcia-Molina et al., 2006; Hopkins & Haaland, 2004; Hopkins, Weaver, Chan, & Orme, 2004). Of course, the more prolonged the

anoxic event, the more widespread the damage, with more pervasive deficits.

Factors complicating the study of anoxic encephalopathy and generalizations about neuropsychological outcome include variability in severity and underlying cause (e.g., near drowning, attempted hanging, cardiac arrest, nitrous oxide poisoning, etc.). The underlying cause of the anoxia can affect outcome (see Caine & Watson, 2000). Related, the amount of tissue loss is a critical factor in determining neuropsychological outcome (Hopkins, Tate, & Bigler, 2005), a factor that will vary according to issues such as duration of anoxia or ischemia.

In this chapter, the authors review the cases of two individuals who sustained apparent anoxic brain injuries secondary to cardiac arrest. The first patient, a woman in her early 40s was seen for neuropsychological evaluation on two occasions, at 5½ and 16½ months, respectively. The second patient is a man in his late 50s who was seen for neuropsychological evaluation on one occasion 8 months following his anoxic-ischemic event.

Case Presentations

Patient 1

History and Physical Findings. Patient 1 was a 41-year-old right-handed Caucasian female without known cardiac history, but with a history of smoking and family history of heart disease. On November 21, 2004, she sustained an acute inferolateral myocardial infarction with ventricular fibrillation. At home with her husband, she slumped over, unresponsive. Her husband immediately called EMS and contacted a neighbor, a nurse, who came to the house and performed CPR. EMS arrived within 10 minutes and the patient was shocked with return to spontaneous normal rhythm with a blood pressure. She was intubated and transported to the hospital where blood pressure was 95/40. She remained in a coma for the first 24 hours, gradually becoming more responsive.

Emergent cardiac catheterization revealed occlusion of a very large right coronary artery, with very diminutive circumflex. On November 22, she underwent percutaneous transluminal coronary angioplasty (PTCA) and stent placement.

A computed tomography (CT) scan on November 21 showed no evidence of acute intracranial abnormality. Magnetic resonance imaging (MRI) on November 24 was initially read as showing a subtle punctate area of restricted diffusion just above the right insular cortex, thought possibly to represent a small area of ischemia (See Figure 1). Subtle changes on fluid-attenuated inversion recovery (FLAIR) images were noted within the subarachnoid space and ventricles that may represent blood products or proteinaceous material (See Figure 2). On retrospective review, there is subtle restriction of diffusion at the uncus and hippocampal bodies

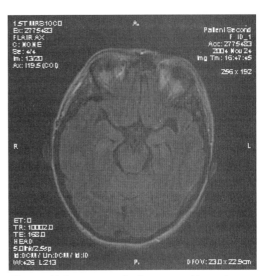

Figure 41-2. Patient 1 fluid-attenuated inversion recovery (FLAIR) magnetic resonance imaging, day 3.

and heads bilaterally. There was no frank infarct. The changes seen on FLAIR images are often seen with patients on high levels of oxygen and are not clinically relevant. A CT scan on November 25 again showed no acute intracranial abnormality, but it did show interval development of sinus inflammatory disease. An electroencephalogram (EEG) on November 24 was abnormal with absence of alpha rhythm. The alpha and beta activity were superimposed on theta range slowing, which may have been a reflection of drug effects. There were no epileptiform discharges seen.

Patient 1 became more alert and responsive, and Physical Medicine and Rehabilitation (PM&R) was consulted. That examination, conducted on November 29, 2004, 8 days after the cardiac arrest episode, showed the patient pleasant, nonobese, and in no acute distress. She was generally cooperative with the examination, and she was able to follow two-stage commands but no three-stage commands. There was prolonged latency for verbal responses. She gave a city and a hospital closer to her residence. When told the correct city, she was able to figure out the correct hospital. She gave the date as November 28 or 29, 2003. She had difficulty registering the names of objects and required multiple repetitions. She was able to recall only one of four objects at 5 minutes. She gave the president

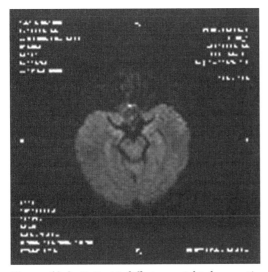

Figure 41-1. Patient 1 diffusion-weighted magnetic resonance imaging, day 3.

as Clinton, but after about 30 seconds gave Bush. When asked why she was in the hospital, she said, "I went to see somebody. Arteries clogged."

Neurological examination was intact except for the presence of mild dystaxia with heel-to-shin, and mild to moderate balance impairment. Patient 1 stood with moderate assist for balance. She was able to take a few short shuffling steps with minimal assist for balance. She was unable to stand on one leg. She was briefly able to stand with feet together and lost balance with closing eyes. Her heart rate and rhythm were regular, and her lungs were clear to auscultation. There was lower sternal tenderness, consequent to resuscitation. There was no leg edema.

Patient 1 was moved to the acute rehabilitation unit on day 7 after the anoxic event. She remained on the unit for 10 days, doing well with ongoing improvement in cognition, memory, balance, and safety. By the time of discharge, she was using a memory log with cueing, latency of responses had normalized, and she was ambulating independently without assistive device.

Her cardiac status remained stable throughout the hospitalization. She was maintained on Plavix and baby aspirin following stenting. She was maintained on lisinopril (10 mg daily) and Lopressor (50 mg twice daily). Blood pressures were often low, in the range of 80/50, and Lopressor was often held. Patient 1 reported several episodes of a fluttering feeling in the chest, without other symptoms. A 24-hour Holter study showed underlying sinus rhythm, with frequent ventricular premature complexes occurring at times in a bigeminal pattern. There was no ventricular tachycardia or atrial tachyarrhythmia, and no significant pauses. Echocardiogram shortly after hospital admission showed ejection fraction of 45%. Medications were adjusted, and she was thought safe for discharge from the cardiac perspective. She was discharged to home with general supervision provided by her husband and family.

Patent 1 was seen for follow-up in the PM&R clinic January 12, 2005, about 1 month after discharge and about 7 weeks after the acute event. Both she and her husband thought that she was improving cognitively. Difficulties were noted particularly with distraction or multitasking. Examination showed the patient alert and conversant, without prolonged latency for responses,

following two- and three-stage commands. She was able to register objects readily, but was only able to recall one of four objects at 5 minutes. She recalled the prior three presidents, but she was unable to recall the fourth. She was able to tandem walk and walk on heels and toes with good balance. She was working with a speech therapist and was on short-term disability from her work as a manager at a department store.

Patient 1 was seen again in the PM&R clinic February 10, 2005, about 11 weeks after the acute event. Electrophysiologic study had shown no inducible sustained monomorphic ventricular tachycardia. It was recommended that she continue with postmyocardial infarction care and surveillance. Examination showed her able to recall four of four words at 5 minutes, with some delay in giving the fourth object. As noted earlier, at the previous visit she recalled only one object. She recalled the previous four presidents, whereas at the previous visit she recalled the previous three. She was reported to be having ongoing cognitive improvement. Speech therapy continued on a decreased frequency, and emphasis was placed on a home program. She was subsequently referred for neuropsychological evaluation, particularly to delineate cognitive disability and prospects for return to work.

First Neuropsychological Evaluation (5½ Months Post Onset).

Past Medical and Psychiatric History. History was obtained from Patient 1 and her husband. She denied past history of hypertension, diabetes, thyroid dysfunction, and traumatic brain injury with loss of consciousness. She also denied past psychiatric treatment.

Family History. The patient denied a family history of known neurological or psychiatric conditions. In terms of cardiovascular history, she did report that her mother underwent open-heart surgery at some point.

Current Medications and Habits. She and her husband reported that her current prescription medications included Plavix, Lopressor, Vytorin, Zestril, Ambien, and aspirin. She also reported that she took vitamins, iron, magnesium, and fish oil. In terms of habits, she reported that she consumed caffeine and related stimulants by way of 4 cups of coffee and 2 glasses of tea per day, as well as occasional Coke. She reported that she quit smoking after her heart attack, having previously smoked some 28 years at a pack per day. She reported that she had not consumed alcohol in the past couple of years, but previously drank only on occasion. She denied illicit drug use.

Sleep. She reported that she usually had delayed sleep onset, though she admitted that she had been sleeping late, until 9 or 10 am daily. She reported that she had good sleep maintenance, and she was not napping during the day. Her husband reported that she did not snore much.

Psychosocial History. She reported her primary and only language to be English. She reported that she had a GED, having left school after the ninth grade due to not doing well and various other factors. She reported that she was a B/C student, never received special education services, and never repeated any grades. She and her husband reported that she had worked waiting tables, cooking, and preparing invoices/statements and customer orders. She reported that she had worked for the previous 5 years at a large department store chain, ultimately working her way up to a supervisory role in the jewelry department. Unfortunately, since being on medical leave (short-term disability), her position had reportedly been eliminated. An additional concern about returning to work related to transportation, as the patient had reportedly not been released to drive and the place of her employment was several miles from home. Patient 1 was living at home with her husband, two additional adult family members, and two small children. Her husband and one of the other adults reportedly traveled together on business, while the other stayed home to care for the children.

Assessment.
Behavioral Observations and Emotional Functioning. Patient 1 was accompanied to the evaluation by her husband. Her grooming and hygiene were noted to be very good. She was pleasant and cooperative throughout the evaluation, and she appeared motivated to perform her best on all tests administered. Good effort was also suggested by her pattern of test performances, good performances on many measures, and performances on embedded measures of effort. Patient 1's mood was appropriate for the situation, and she demonstrated a fairly normal range of affect; she was quiet and reserved, but smiled and laughed appropriately on occasion. Her responses to a questionnaire were indicative of mild depression. Inclusive, she endorsed sadness, anhedonia, loss of interest (including decreased interest in sex), increased restlessness, indecisiveness, decreased energy, increased fatigue, increased sleep, and poor concentration. She denied suicidal ideation.

Adaptive Functions. According to her husband, she was independent with basic self-care, including feeding, toileting, grooming and hygiene, and dressing. She was also reportedly completing domestic chores, including laundry, cooking, and some cleaning. In contrast, he reported that she was unable to drive—she had driven with him in the car in the country, but he noted that she parked crookedly and too close to the garage, and she had reported that she could not tell if she was within her lane. Her husband also reported that his wife had trouble managing the bill paying, reporting that she lost bills. He reported that she put things down and walked away from them. He reported that she had burned herself on the stove while cooking a few times due to apparent inattention. In terms of behavior, he reported that she had little initiative and poor follow through, which he attributed to fatigue. He also reported that she had reduced attention to tasks, generally paying attention to purposeful activities for only up to 10 minutes at a time. Finally, he reported that his wife interacted with others for only short periods of time, and as a passive participant in group activities.

Motor Functions. The patient ambulated independently without apparent difficulty. She did not demonstrate any ideomotor, ideational, or buccofacial dyspraxia per brief assessment and observation. She demonstrated a strong right-hand preference. She demonstrated good hand-eye coordination with respect to speed, bilaterally.

Language. Speech was noted to be fluent, prosodic, and clear, and there were no paraphasic errors noted during conversation. Comprehension of spoken language was noted to be good per observation, and comprehension of written language (i.e., reading) was average per formal assessment.

Visual Spatial Functions. Primary visual perception was noted to be grossly functional per good ability to discriminate small geometric figures. There was also no detectible hemispatial inattention or neglect as demonstrated on a cancellation test. Visual-constructional drawing ability/praxis was found to be very good, with good organization and integration of parts into a whole Gestalt in copying a complex, two-dimensional figure. Finally, with regard to visual spatial functions formally assessed, she was found to be grossly oriented to right and left both intra- and extra-personally per brief assessment. On her self-report, though, it should be noted that she reported difficulty perceiving whether she is within her lane when driving, and her eye movements, per gross observation, appeared disconjugate at times.

Attention and Memory. The patient was alert and she maintained her focus of attention during the 4¼-hour interview, test, and feedback sessions, with only a very brief (< 1 minute) break to stretch her legs; she declined offers for additional or longer breaks. On formal assessment, she demonstrated average span of attention and working memory for auditory verbal stimuli (i.e., forward and reverse digit repetition). She also exhibited average ability to rapidly divide her attention between two competing visual task demands.

In terms of memory, she was found to be oriented to person, place, time, and situation. She had fairly good knowledge of general and personal remote information, and fair knowledge of current events. However, she reported anterograde amnesia following the cardiac arrest, noting that her first recollections are of going home for a day visit just prior to discharge from the rehabilitation unit. In terms of new learning, she demonstrated moderately deficient ability to learn, recall, and retain new verbal information in the form of a word list presented with and without repetition. She did not exhibit significant interference effects during free recall trials, and she demonstrated a positive learning curve with repetition. In regard to visual constructional

memory, average to low-average ability to recall/reproduce new visual spatial/constructional information was demonstrated, with average learning and retention per delayed recognition testing. Finally, though, she demonstrated borderline incidental learning. That is, she was borderline in her ability to incidentally memorize information through copying it repeatedly.

Frontal-Executive Functions. Frontal-executive functions in addition to attention were briefly assessed. She was systematic and organized in her approach to all tasks. She also demonstrated normal processing speed on various tasks. First, she performed within the high-average range on a measure of simple visual scanning speed. As was noted earlier, she performed within the average range on a nearly identical measure that additionally required her to shift her attention rapidly between two competing task demands. Next, she performed within the average range on a measure of grapho-motor copying speed in combination with incidental learning. In contrast to her good organization and processing speed, she demonstrated borderline difficulty with deductive reasoning on a test that required problem solving through concept formation, cognitive flexibility, and set maintenance.

Intellectual Functions. Basic intellectual skills were briefly assessed. She demonstrated average general fund of factual knowledge and superior nonverbal reasoning and pattern analysis.

Applied Academic Skills. The patient demonstrated average reading comprehension per a nontimed test that additionally required word retrieval. She also demonstrated average ability to formulate fluent sentences in writing. Finally, she demonstrated average written calculation skills.

Summary. Patient 1 presented with a history of anoxia secondary to cardiac arrest just 5 months earlier. She continued to exhibit residual deficits in memory functioning. Specifically, she demonstrated impaired ability to learn, recall, and retain new verbal information presented orally with repetition. She additionally demonstrated borderline difficulty with regard to novel problem solving. Her husband also reported problems in adaptive functioning secondary to memory impairment, as well as poor initiative and persistence. However, she demonstrated good language skills, good processing speed, good organization, good motor skills, and academic skills within expectation based on past history. She also performed well on tests of visual spatial skills, though she reported visual perceptual disturbance affecting her driving. Finally, she endorsed symptoms of mild depression, and her behavior at home was consistent with such, though lack of initiative and loss of interest could also have had some degree of neurological basis.

Patient 1 presented with many attributes necessary for successful employment, though her memory impairment and lack of initiative were felt to be potential impediments. It was felt that she needed to develop techniques to compensate for her memory difficulties, and specific techniques were recommended. In addition, transportation was a significant mitigating factor given that she was not able to drive at the time and there were apparently no alternative means of transportation.

The Patient's Second Neuropsychological Evaluation (16½ Months Post Onset). Patient 1 returned for a neuropsychological reevaluation 11 months following the previous evaluation. The purpose of the reevaluation was to further assist with rehabilitation planning and with evaluating her level of disability.

Current History. According to the patient and her husband on this date, she had not returned to work. She reported that she applied for Social Security Disability, which she did receive. She reported that she had improved "a little" in that she was cooking and cleaning. She reported that she was feeling "a little better" emotionally, and that her memory had improved "a little." She reported that she was spending her days cleaning house, straightening out things, playing with her grandson, talking on the phone, and cooking meals. She reported that she was driving a little to the store about two miles from their home in the country using back roads. She reported that she occasionally went to the movies about five miles away, and she felt disoriented in terms of location, though it was a straight shot and there was

no way to get lost. She was not driving further due to the risk of getting lost and because of concerns that she would stop suddenly in front of other drivers if startled by someone driving up behind her quickly. On the country road, there were reportedly few other cars.

Current Medications and Habits. The patient and her husband reported that her current prescription medications included Plavix, Lopressor, Vytorin, Zestril, Lorazepam, and aspirin. She reported discontinuing the Ambien due to awakening in the middle of the night and feeling unusual (i.e., not awake, but not asleep). She also reported that she was taking vitamins, iron, magnesium, and fish oil. In terms of habits, Patient 1 reported that she consumed caffeine and related stimulants by way of 4 cups of coffee, but she generally no longer drank tea or Coke. She remained abstinent of tobacco and alcohol, and she denied history of illicit drug use.

Sleep. She said that she usually had delayed sleep onset, though she admitted that she had continued sleeping late, until 9 or 10 am daily. She reported that she was going to bed at approximately 10 pm and falling asleep approximately 2–3 hours later. She reported that she had good sleep maintenance, and she was not napping during the day. Her husband reported that she does not snore much—just a little bit, stopping when he nudges her with his elbow.

New Psychosocial History. With regard to her previous employment, her husband reported that she was told by her employer that they did not have anybody to be with her to supervise her, and there were concerns about her laying jewelry down and walking off and forgetting it. She reported that she has not attempted other work due to lack of transportation and because her physician had told her she would not be able to go back to work until things got better.

Assessment.

Behavioral Observations and Emotional Functioning. She was again accompanied to the evaluation by her husband. Her grooming and hygiene were again noted to be very good. She was pleasant and cooperative throughout the evaluation, and she appeared motivated to perform her best on all tests administered. Good effort was also suggested by direct assessment of effort, good performances on many measures, and review of embedded measures of effort. Her mood was appropriate for the situation, and she demonstrated a fairly normal range of affect; she was quiet and reserved, but smiled and laughed appropriately on occasion. Her responses to a questionnaire were not indicative of substantial depression. She did endorse discouragement, loss of confidence, decreased enjoyment, some loss of interest, difficulty with decision making, poor concentration, decreased energy, fatigue, and increased sleep. She again denied suicidal ideation.

Adaptive Functions. According to her husband, she was now independent with basic self-care, including feeding, toileting, grooming and hygiene, and dressing. She was also reportedly completing domestic chores, including laundry, cooking, and some cleaning. As noted previously, he reported that she was doing some driving, though not on the highway. Her husband reported that his wife still had trouble managing the bill paying. In terms of behavior, he reported that she had good initiative, self-direction, and attention, and that was an improvement from the previous year. He also reported that she was beginning to do more socially. He denied problem behaviors.

Motor Functions. Ambulation was independent without apparent difficulty. She did not demonstrate any ideomotor, ideational, or buccofacial dyspraxia. Hand-eye coordination was not formally reassessed as she performed normally on a test of hand-eye coordination the previous spring. Handwriting was again noted to be functional.

Language. Speech was again noted to be fluent, prosodic, and clear, and there were no paraphasic errors noted during conversation. Comprehension of spoken language was also again noted to be good per observation, and comprehension of written language (i.e., reading) was average per formal assessment.

Visual Spatial Functions. Primary visual perception was noted to be grossly functional per observation and qualitative review of test performances. There was also no detectible hemispatial inattention or neglect on observation. Visual-constructional drawing ability/praxis was again found to be very good, with good organization and integration of parts into a whole Gestalt in copying a complex, two-dimensional figure. On her self-report, though, it should be noted that she again reported difficulty perceiving whether she is within her lane when driving, and her eyes, per gross observation, were again disconjugate, with ptosis on the right.

Attention and Memory. She was alert and maintained her focus of attention during the 4-hour interview, test, and feedback sessions, with only a very brief restroom break and an intervening 23-minute lunch break (she was actually ready to proceed with testing after a 10-minute lunch break). She declined offers for additional or longer breaks. On formal assessment, on one test of span of attention and working memory for auditory verbal stimuli (i.e., forward and reverse digit repetition) she again performed within the average range. She performed within the low-average range on a second, more complex test of working memory (i.e., number-letter sequencing). She again exhibited average ability to rapidly divide her attention between two competing visual verbal task demands.

In terms of memory, she was found to be oriented to person, place, time, and situation. She had fairly good knowledge of general and personal remote information, though somewhat poor knowledge of current events; she reported that she turns on the news, but does not specifically sit down and watch (i.e., attend to) it. In terms of new learning, she demonstrated borderline deficient ability to learn and recall new verbal information in the form of a list presented orally with repetition, but with moderately deficient retention over delays. She again demonstrated a positive learning curve with repetition, but she had significant forgetting/decay over a delay. On a second measure of verbal memory, the patient demonstrated borderline to mildly deficient ability to learn and recall verbal material presented orally in the form of narratives (i.e., stories) with and without repetition, but this time with good (average) retention of the material over a significant delay. With regard to visual memory, she demonstrated average or better ability to learn, recall/reproduce, and retain new visual spatial/constructional information. Finally, low-average incidental learning was present. That is, she was low average in her ability to incidentally memorize rote information through repeated copying.

Frontal-Executive Functions. Frontal-executive functions in addition to attention were briefly assessed. She was systematic and fairly organized in her approach to all tasks, including the test of rote verbal list learning. She also demonstrated normal processing speed on various tasks. First, she performed within the high-average to superior range on a measure of simple visual scanning speed. As was noted previously, she performed within the average range on a nearly identical measure that additionally required her to shift her attention rapidly between two competing task demands. Next, she performed within the high-average to superior range on a measure of grapho-motor copying speed incombination with incidental learning. During this second evaluation, she performed well on a measure requiring novel problem solving through deductive reasoning, cognitive flexibility, and set maintenance; her performance was better than during the previous evaluation, though practice effects could not be ruled out.

Intellectual Functions. Basic intellectual skills were briefly reassessed. Again she demonstrated average general fund of factual knowledge. She demonstrated average nonverbal reasoning and pattern analysis.

Applied Academic Skills. She demonstrated average reading comprehension per a nontimed test that additionally required word retrieval. She again demonstrated average written calculation skills.

Summary. During this second evaluation, Patient 1 reported that she was feeling better and had experienced some improvement in her memory with regard to daily activities. Her husband reported that she had shown increased initiative and activity level. However, on formal assessment, she continued to exhibit residual deficits in memory functioning. Specifically, she demonstrated impaired ability to learn, recall, and retain new verbal information presented orally with and without repetition. In contrast, she exhibited average or better ability to learn and retain new visual spatial/constructional material. She also again demonstrated functional language skills, good visual spatial skills, good processing speed, fairly good organization (though her husband and she reported difficulty organizing paperwork/bills at home, likely secondary to forgetfulness or misplacing items), and average reading and math skills. On this date, she also demonstrated average divided attention and good cognitive flexibility in her approach to novel problem solving. Consistent with her report that she was feeling better emotionally, she did not endorse symptoms of excessive depression (see Table 41-1).

Patient 1 Follow-Up (21 Months Post Onset). When seen by her primary care physician in August 2006, Patient 1 was not working. She was reportedly having difficulty managing the family checkbook and had written many "hot checks" because she did not remember to record them in her check register. She had developed a system to make cooking easier by placing all her food out on the counter so she would not forget an ingredient. Shopping was reportedly a challenge, even with use of a list, and she would forget items.

Patient 1 Follow-Up (3 Years Post Onset). A follow-up interview was conducted via telephone in late 2007, nearly 3 years following the anoxic event. According to the patient, she was still not working, though she reported that she watches her 4-year-old grandson from 8 a.m. to 5 p.m. during the week. She also reported that circumstances had led her to start driving regularly again. She indicated that she was shopping, cleaning, and preparing meals. She reported that she was still having problems keeping up with bill paying due to poor follow-through related to forgetfulness. She said that she was using notebooks with lists, and found that planners were more trouble. She reported that she was still not smoking or drinking alcohol, but she also reported that she was not exercising. She denied experiencing depression but reported that she was taking Prozac. She noted that she was sleeping well and attributed that to keeping busy during the day with a home project. She reported that her only new medical problem was

Table 41-1. Neuropsychological Test Scores

	Patient 1 First Evaluation	Patient 1 Second Evaluation	Patient 2
WAIS-III Digit Span	SS = 9, 37th percentile	SS = 10, 50th percentile	SS = 9, 37th percentile
Digits Forward	Max = 6, 21st percentile	Max = 7, 43rd percentile	Max = 7, 50th percentile
Digits Backward	Max = 5, 40th percentile	Max = 5, 40th percentile	Max = 3, 5th percentile
Letter-Number Sequencing	—	SS = 7, 16th percentile	—
Information	SS =10, 50th percentile	SS = 9, 37th percentile	SS = 11, 63rd percentile
Matrix Reasoning	SS = 14, 91st percentile	SS = 11, 63rd percentile	SS = 5, 5th percentile
Digit Symbol	SS = 11, 63rd percentile	SS = 13, 84th percentile	SS = 5, 5th percentile
Incidental Learning (IL)	10th percentile	10th–25th percentile	25th percentile
IL Free Recall	1st–2nd percentile	50th percentile	25th percentile
CVLT-2*Total Recall	RS = 31, T = 24	RS = 39, T = 33*	RS = 32, T = 26
Trial 1	3/16, –2.5 SD	4/16, –2 SD*	4/16, –1.5 SD
Trial 2	6/16, –2 SD	6/16, –2 SD*	5/16, –1.5 SD
Trial 3	6/16, –3 SD	8/16, –2 SD*	5/16, –2 SD
Trial 4	7/16, –3 SD	11/16, –1 SD*	5/16, –2 SD
Trial 5	9/16, –2 SD	10/16, –1.5 SD*	7/16, –1.5 SD
B	3/16, –1.5 SD	4/16, –1.5 SD*	3/16, –1.5 SD
Short Delay Free	7/16, –2 SD	9/16, –1.5 SD*	3/16, –2 SD
Short Delay Cued	7/16, –2.5 SD	9/16, –2.5 SD*	5/16, –2 SD
Long Delay Free	5/16, –3.5 SD	6/16, –3.5 SD*	3/16, –1.5 SD
Long Delay Cued	7/16, –3 SD	8/16, –3 SD*	8/16, –1 SD
Recognition Hits	12/16, –4 SD	11/16, –5 SD*	9/16, –3 SD
False Positives	2, .5 SD	0, –5 SD*	11, 2.5 SD
Repetitions	5, 0 SD	15, 2 SD*	1, –1 SD
Free Intrusions	1, 0 SD	3, .5 SD*	2, 0 SD
Cued Intrusions	3, 1 SD	2, 1 SD*	2, 0 SD
WMS-III LM I Total	—	SS = 5, 5th percentile	—
WMS-III LM I 1st Recall	—	SS = 6, 9th percentile	—
Learning Slope	—	SS = 8, 25th percentile	—
WMS-II LM II Recall	—	SS = 7, 16th percentile	—
WMS-III LM % Retention	—	SS = 9, 37th percentile	—
Rey-Osterrieth (RO) Copy	36/36, >16th percentile	36/36, >16th percentile	34/36, >16th percentile
RO Time to Copy	200", >16th percentile	205", >16th percentile	360", 6th–10th percentile
RO 3' Recall	13.5/36, 4th percentile	21.5/36, 50th percentile	18.5/36, 54th percentile
RO 30" Recall	17.5/36, 18th percentile	22.5/36, 58th percentile	11.5/36, 8th percentile
RO Recognition	20/24, 31st percentile	22/24, 73rd percentile	20/24, 38th percentile
Mesulam Left Omissions	RS = 1	—	RS = 0
Mesulam Right Omissions	RS = 1	—	RS = 1
Mesulam Total Time	97"	—	169"
Trail-Making Test A	24", 80th percentile	23", 80th–90th percentile	45", 20th–30th percentile
Trail-Making Test B	67", 30th–40th percentile	62", 50th percentile	97", <20th percentile
WCST Total Categories	3, 6th–10th percentile	6, >16th percentile	0, <1st percentile
WCST Trials to 1st Cat.	11, >16th percentile	11, >16th percentile	Never, 2nd–5th percentile
Failures to Maintain Set	0, >16th percentile	0, >16th percentile	0, >16th percentile
Total Errors	52, 8th percentile	19, 63rd percentile	99, <1st percentile
Percent Perseverative Error	19%, 16th percentile	11%, 58th percentile	53%, <1st percentile
BNT Spontaneous Correct	—	—	58/60
BNT Semantic Cueing	—	—	59/60
BNT Phonemic Correct	—	—	60/60
WJ-III Passage Comp.	Std = 98, 44th percentile	Std = 100, 51st percentile	Std = 114, 82nd percentile
WJ-III Writing Samples	Std = 99, 47th percentile	—	—

Table 41-1. Neuropsychological Test Scores (*Continued*)

	Patient 1 First Evaluation	Patient 1 Second Evaluation	Patient 2
WJ-III Calculations	Std = 103, 59th percentile	Std = 106, 65th percentile	Std = 107, 68th percentile
Grooved Pegboard Dom.	64", 0 SD	—	93", +2.6 SD
Grooved Pegboard Nondom.	66", −.3 SD	—	105", +2.9 SD
BDI-II	RS = 17 (mild)	RS = 12 (minimal)	RS = 13 (minimal)
TOMM (computer) Trial 1	—	RS = 39/50	—
TOMM Trial 2	—	RS = 44/50	—
TOMM Retention	—	RS = 46/50	—
Rey's 15-item Test Total	—	RS = 12/15	—
Rey's 15-item Sets	—	RS = 4/5	—

*CVLT Alternate Form given at second evaluation of Patient 1.

BDI, Beck Depression Inventory; BNT, Boston Naming Test; Cat., Category; CVLT, California Verbal Learning Test; Dom., dominant; RS, raw score; SD, standard deviation; SS, subtest score; Std, standard score; WAIS, Wechsler Adult Intelligence Scale; WCST, Wisconsin Card-Sorting Test; WJ-III, Woodcock-Johnson-III.

a "snapping hip." She said that she benefited from a recent decrease in the number of people living in her home, and she found that resulted in a decrease in her stress.

Patient 2

History and Physical Findings. Patient 2 was a 58-year-old left-handed Caucasian male who had gastric bypass surgery in May 2004 for body mass index of 43. He had reportedly been concerned about increasing obesity-associated health problems, including hypertension, borderline diabetes, and hypercholesterolemia. He had a history of depression, for which he was on Celexa. Patient 2 was described by his wife as having been intelligent and high functioning with a "photographic mind," great fund of knowledge, and excellent mechanical ability. He was a university graduate with a B.A. in Finance. He had been working for a telecommunications company at a computer-based job that he described as pertaining to the management of public telephones. His wife reported that he had taken a great deal of pride in his work.

In the month following his bypass surgery, he reportedly had two episodes of brief loss of consciousness, which were ultimately attributed to hypokalemia. On July 7, 2004, the day after he received that diagnosis, he reportedly suffered cardiac arrest while driving. EMS arrived within 6 minutes and resuscitated him with difficulty.

He was transported to a nearby hospital and then evacuated by helicopter to a larger hospital. He had polymorphic ventricular tachycardia, initial potassium was 2.4, and emergency cardiac catheterization showed right coronary occlusion with hypokinesis of the inferior wall.

At an evaluation by Neurology on July 8, he was comatose, unresponsive to pain, on a ventilator, and had roving eye movements. Later that same day, he developed a tonic-clonic seizure, for which he received Versed and was loaded with fosphenytoin. A CT scan of the head that day showed no acute intracranial abnormality. By July 9, he would arouse and respond to simple commands. He was extubated July 10 and transferred from the cardiac care unit July 12. A pacemaker/defibrillator was placed.

When seen on PM&R consult July 13, he was confused with little meaningful speech. He followed some simple commands. MRI's of the brain July 14, 2004 were unremarkable (See Figure 3, Diffusion Weighted MRI, and Figure 4, T2 Weighted MRI). Note that MRI's were obtained using a rapid scanning technique presumably to compensate for the patient's inability to remain still for the study. He was transferred to the rehabilitation unit July 19 where he improved cognitively and functionally. By the time of discharge July 30, he was able to ambulate with a front-wheeled walker with contact guard up to 200 feet with some cuing and guidance for safety. He required cuing with activities of daily living and was confused at times. Continuous supervision for safety was recommended at discharge. He subsequently received physical, occupational, and speech therapy at home, with a prolonged course of speech therapy. He progressed to ambulation without a device.

Though PM&R follow-up was requested at hospital discharge, he was lost to clinic follow-up until February 9, 2005, about 7 months after the anoxic event. When seen for the first time in clinic by the physician author, his wife reported that he had completed speech therapy by late September 2004. At that time, he had been anxious to go back to work, though he was unable to log into a computer at home. He returned to work part time for 2 weeks, then full time. He came home from work exhausted and frustrated. A person doing similar work in another part of the country came to the office for a week to refresh him in the work and bring him up to speed. This went poorly, though apparently his inability to do his previous work was still not recognized. Once he was left on his own he floundered, continued on the job into November 2004, and was then placed on short-term disability.

When seen in clinic in February 2005, Patient 2 was described by his wife as frustrated and often irritable, with flares of temper. He was described as previously very relaxed and easy going. He complained particularly of memory loss, both

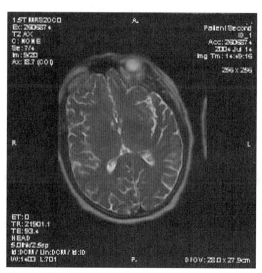

Figure 41-4. Patient 2 T2-weighted magnetic resonance imaging.

short and long term. It was thought that he would be best served with a detailed neuropsychological evaluation particularly to outline cognitive strengths and weaknesses, with recommendations for treatment and compensatory techniques. It was thought that specific documentation would be helpful in the disability process, to assist the patient with his own adjustment, and to allow for appropriate compensatory techniques.

Neuropsychological Evaluation (7½ Months Post Onset).

Current History. He had reportedly shown improvement, but with residual impairments in both anterograde and retrograde memory as well as apathy. He also initially exhibited impaired coordination as demonstrated by illegible handwriting, which had improved somewhat. To date, he had reportedly not suffered any additional seizures.

Past Medical and Psychiatric History. The patient and his wife reported a history of hypertension, hypercholesteralemia, and borderline diabetes. They denied history of traumatic brain injury with loss of consciousness. Patient 2 did reportedly fracture both wrists in a fall in the past. He reportedly underwent surgery at age 7 or 8 for strabismus. In terms of psychiatric history, he had reportedly been treated with antidepressants by his family doctor for the previous 6–7 years.

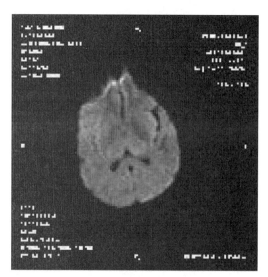

Figure 41-3. Patient 2 diffusion-weighted magnetic resonance imaging.

Family History. He denied family history of psychiatric and neurological conditions. He did reportedly have a strong family history of heart disease.

Current Medications and Habits. The patient and his wife reported that his medications included Metoprolol, Pravachol, and Celexa. He was also reportedly taking sublingual B12 once weekly, daily iron, a multivitamin, and Caltrate. He denied use of herbal remedies. In terms of habits, he consumed caffeine and related stimulants by way of 0 to 3 glasses of tea per day. He denied current use of tobacco products, reporting that he quit a pack-per-day habit in 1974. He reportedly had not consumed alcohol since his gastric bypass and consumed approximately one alcoholic beverage on occasion prior to that. He denied use of illicit drugs.

Sleep. Reportedly he typically had good sleep onset and maintenance. He and his wife reported that he would sleep during the day following a busy day, including that he would stay in bed several hours later than usual. He reportedly only snored lightly and on occasion at the time of the evaluation; prior to his weight loss from the gastric bypass, snoring was reportedly an issue.

Psychosocial History. He indicated that his primary language was English; he was not bilingual. He reported that he had a high school diploma and a Bachelor of Science degree in Finance. He reported that he received A's, B's, and C's in high school, and C's and D's in college. Reportedly he worked in various jobs, including in accounting, supervision, real estate, insurance sales, auto sales, quality assurance, bus driving, and as a stage hand. At the time of the cardiac arrest, he had reportedly been working for a large phone company for 10 years, most recently as a public access support analyst. He was reportedly currently married to his first wife of 30 years. They did not have children.

Assessment.
Behavioral Observations and Emotional Functioning. The patient was accompanied to this evaluation by his wife and their friend. His grooming and hygiene were noted to be very good. He was pleasant and cooperative throughout the long test session, and he appeared motivated to perform his best on all tests administered. Embedded measures of effort (e.g., WCST 8 of 8 perfect matches and 0 failures to maintain set, reliable digit span of 10, and two recognition measures of 83% and 63% correct) were considered. Good effort was suggested by strong performances on some measures, normal performance on most of the embedded measures, and the presence of a consistent pattern of findings. His mood was somewhat bright. His range of affect was mildly restricted at times in that he was somewhat indifferent to, though aware of, his deficits; at other times, his affective response was mildly excessive (e.g., laughter in response to his own jokes). His responses to a questionnaire were not indicative of depression at this time; he endorsed only some guilt, feeling he may be punished, having less energy than he used to, getting more tired or fatigued more easily than usual, having decreased interest in sex, sleeping less, and having decreased appetite (the latter being expected with the gastric bypass).

Adaptive Functions. According to his wife, he was independent with regard to basic skills of daily living, including feeding, toileting, bathing, dressing and undressing, grooming and hygiene, spatial sense of direction, and community mobility. He also reportedly participated in some domestic chores, similar to his level of participation prior to the cardiac arrest. His wife had taken over managing their bank account, though he did continue to handle money, shop, and use banking facilities. While he did not engage in any aggressive, sexually inappropriate, or excessively hyperactive behaviors, he reportedly exhibited apathy, reduced initiative, and reduced persistence. He also reportedly exhibited inflexibility and difficulty completing tasks that were previously easy for him.

Motor Functions. Motor skills were briefly assessed. There was no ideomotor, ideational, or buccofacial dyspraxia per brief formal assessment, and he ambulated without apparent difficulty. He was mildly deficient on a test of hand-eye coordination with respect to speed, bilaterally, though with the expected dominant upper extremity superiority. Handwriting was noted to be legible though somewhat poor and slow in rate.

Intellectual Functions. Per brief assessment, he demonstrated average general fund of factual knowledge. In contrast, he exhibited mildly deficient nonverbal reasoning and pattern analysis.

Language. His speech was noted to be fluent, prosodic, and clear, though somewhat deliberate and slow in rate. However, there were no paraphasic/word substitution errors noted during conversation. On formal assessment, he exhibited good confrontation naming skill/expressive vocabulary for his age and education. Comprehension of spoken language was noted to be good per observation, and reading comprehension was found to be above average.

Visual Spatial Functions. Primary visual perception was noted to be grossly functional per fairly good object recognition. He also did not demonstrate any hemispatial inattention or neglect on formal assessment. He produced a fairly good reproduction on a test of visual constructional drawing ability. Finally, with regard to visual spatial skills assessed, he was found to be well oriented to right and left, both intra- and extra-personally.

Attention and Memory. First, in terms of endurance, within the 1:1 format, the patient completed the 4⅓-hour interview, evaluation, and feedback session with just one brief restroom break; he declined offers for additional breaks. On observation, he was not overly fidgety, and he did not appear to be distracted by extraneous stimuli. He demonstrated average simple span of attention for auditory verbal stimuli (forward digit repetition), but mildly deficient working memory (i.e., reverse digit repetition). He demonstrated average to low-average divided attention.

With regard to memory functioning, he was well oriented to person, place, and situation, and fairly well oriented to time. He had spotty knowledge of general remote information as well as current events, and his wife reported that he had forgotten significant personal remote information (e.g., the death of his mother in 1989—he reportedly thought she was still alive). During today's evaluation, he demonstrated confusion with regard to remote events dating back at least as far as the 1960s (e.g., he reported that Reagan was president when he was in high school in

the 1960s). He also exhibited mildly deficient ability to learn and retain new verbal information presented orally in the form of a list with repetition. He did not exhibit significant interference effects or confabulation during recall trials, though he did exhibit confusion during a recognition trial. With regard to visual spatial memory, he demonstrated average to low-average ability to recall/reproduce and retain new visual constructional material (i.e., ability to draw/recognize a previously copied design from memory). Finally, with regard to memory functioning assessed, he demonstrated average to low-average incidental learning of graphomotor/written information.

Executive Functions. Executive functions in addition to attention were assessed briefly. First, he was fairly systematic and organized in his approach to carrying out a simple cancellation task, and he exhibited the capacity to be organized on an abstract planning task; he was less systematic on more complex tasks. With regard to processing speed, performance was within the average range on a test measuring simple visual scanning/processing speed. He was also average on a nearly identical task that additionally tapped into divided attention, tracking, and set-shifting ability. He performed within the borderline to mildly deficient range on a paper-and-pencil measure of grapho-motor/copying speed in combination with incidental learning. Lastly, cognitive inflexibility and deficient problem-solving skill were noted on a test that required problem solving through concept formation with minimal feedback/assistance, cognitive flexibility, and set maintenance.

Applied Academic Skills. The patient exhibited average to high-average (bright) nontimed reading comprehension, in line with his academic achievement. He demonstrated average to high-average written calculation skills.

Summary. Patient 2 presented with a mild impairment in his ability to learn and retain new verbal information as well as a retrograde memory impairment. He had fairly intact ability to learn new visual material, particularly with hands-on practice copying the material to be learned. While he had intact language and visual spatial skills, he presented with deficient problem-solving skill and cognitive inflexibility. His attentional skills appeared to be intact, though he reportedly exhibited poor initiative and interest in tasks at home. Simple psychomotor/processing speed was found to be intact during the evaluation, while fine motor/hand-eye coordination was mildly to moderately deficient. Though he did have a past history of injury to his wrists, his wife reported a decline in handwriting quality following the anoxic event, suggesting a new impairment. Motor programming was found to be intact. He was not reporting symptoms of significant depression at the time of this evaluation, though, as noted, he had reduced initiative and persistence as well as apathy and a bit of indifference (see Table 41-1).

Patient 2 Follow-Up (10 Months Post Onset). Patient 2 was next seen in the PM&R clinic May 2005, at which time the neuropsychological evaluation and recommendations were discussed with him and his wife. The uncertain disability situation that had been stressful to the patient and his wife in February 2005 had been resolved in a manner favorable to the patient, with early retirement and approval for Social Security disability.

Patient 2 Follow-Up (20 Months Post Onset). At a Neurology evaluation in March 2006, he was noted to have had significant recovery from the ischemic/anoxic insult of July 2004, but he had not returned back to baseline. He was started on a trial of Aricept, up to 10 mg daily, that was then stopped in June 2006 for lack of benefit. He was seen by Psychiatry in July 2006, 2 years after the anoxic injury. The psychiatrist's impression included depression, not otherwise specified, which was noted to have onset before the anoxic encephalopathy, but which probably had been significantly affected by the anoxic injury. He was encouraged to pursue previous hobbies and to exercise. With regard to depression, he was already taking Celexa (60 mg daily). He was noted to have failed to experience benefit with Wellbutrin and Effexor in the past. It was thought that he would benefit from an immediate release medication, and was started on Ritalin (10 mg) in the morning and again at noon. Ritalin was started after communication with the cardiologist; it was noted that he had a pacemaker/defibrillator in

place that would help with any potential cardiac rhythm problems related to medication effects. Subsequently it was thought that some benefit with Ritalin was noted, and this was increased first to 15 mg, then 20 mg twice daily. As of July 2007, he was noted to be more active and social, with improved mood. Issues of motivation and memory persisted, and he was not exercising.

Patient 2 Follow-Up (2 ½ Years Post Onset). Through follow-up interview conducted at 2½ years post event, it was learned that he remained on disability retirement. He reported that he continued to have difficulties with memory, which interfered with his ability to work. He reported that he was otherwise doing fairly well.

Discussion

Both patients demonstrated the often-observed impairments in memory functioning among individuals with anoxic brain injury. In particular, both patients showed impairments in new rote verbal learning and retention, and Patient 2 additionally demonstrated residual retrograde memory impairment. Patient 2 also showed decline in fine motor skills, working memory, nonverbal reasoning, and cognitive flexibility. Both patients reportedly experienced difficulties with poor initiative, though with at least some improvement over time and with medical intervention. Finally, while both patients reportedly became independent with most basic skills of daily living except financial management, neither returned to work.

In closing, it should be noted that both of these patients represent relatively good outcomes, likely due to fairly quick resuscitation and medical intervention. Patient 2 appeared to have slightly worse outcome, particularly in light of his previously high level of functioning. His worse outcome may have related to slightly longer interval before resuscitation. Recovery of individuals with initial successful resuscitation of out-of-hospital cardiac arrest will range from death in the large majority through good recovery in the minority, depending on the length of anoxia/hypoxia and ischemia (see Adrie et el., 2006). As noted earlier, structures that will be affected early in an anoxic/ischemic event typically include those in the watershed areas, while longer periods of deprivation will affect consciousness- and life-sustaining structures throughout the brain. Related, while brain imaging for the present two cases indicated mild or no obvious intracranial abnormality acutely, more severe cases not amenable to formal neuropsychological assessment would likely have more substantial abnormalities on imaging. Moreover, imaging abnormality associated with volume loss would be expected to occur later (see Bulakbasi et al., 2000), while the present cases underwent imaging studies in the first few days following the anoxic event. The present cases, though, do underscore the fact that there can be significant functional impairment even in the face of normal structural imaging.

Acknowledgment

The authors wish to acknowledge and thank Dr. Kenneth D. Williams for his assistance with reviewing MRI findings.

References

Adrie, S., Cariou, A., Mourvillier, B., Laurent, I., Dabbane, H., Hantala, F., Rhaoui, A., Thuong, M., & Monchi, M. (2006). Predicting survival with good neurological recovery at hospital admission after successful resuscitation of out-of-hospital cardiac arrest: The OHCA score. *European Heart Journal, 27*, 2840–2845.

Bulakbasi, N., Pabuscu, Y., Kurtaran, H. K., Tayfun, C., Tasar, M., & Üçöz, T. (2000). Results of acute cerebral anoxia in adults: Is it a reversal sign? *Turkish Journal of Medical Sciences, 30*, 571–577.

Caine, D., & Watson, J. D. G. (2000). Neuropsychological and neuropathological sequelae of cerebral anoxia: A critical review. *Journal of the International Neuropsychological Society, 6*, 86–99.

Garcia-Molina, A., Roig-Rovira, T., Enseñat-Cantallops, A., Sanchez-Carrion, R., Pico-Azanza, N., Bernabeu, M., & Tormos, J. M. (2006). Neuropsychological profile of persons with anoxic brain injury: Differences regarding physiopathological mechanism. *Brain Injury, 20*, 1139–1145.

Hopkins, R. O., & Haaland, K. Y. (2004). Neuropsychological and neuropathological effects of anoxic or ischemic induced brain injury. *Journal of the International Neuropsychological Society, 10*, 957–961.

Hopkins, R. O., Tate, D. F., & Bigler, E. D. (2005). Anoxic versus traumatic brain injury: Amount of tissue loss, not etiology, alters cognitive and emotional function. *Neuropsychology, 19*, 233–242.

Hopkins, R. O., Weaver, L. K., Chan, K. J., & Orme, J. F. (2004). Quality of life, emotional, and cognitive function following acute respiratory distress syndrome. *Journal of the International Neuropsychological Society, 10*, 1005–1017.

42

A Case of Hepatic Encephalopathy in End-Stage Liver Disease Secondary to Alcoholic Cirrhosis

Marc A. Norman

More than 5 million persons in the United States have liver disease and prevalence rates have dramatically increased, so it has become more important that neuropsychologists understand the potential cognitive sequelae related to liver failure. The nature and extent of potential cognitive function/dysfunction secondary to end-stage liver disease (ESLD) varies from normal to severely impaired and is largely related to the underlying etiology, as well as acute or chronic metabolic changes (i.e., hepatic encephalopathy). The liver performs over 500 functions, and proper liver functioning is essential for metabolizing alcohol, toxins, medications, fats, and proteins. Additionally, the liver is critical for clotting factors and bile production in addition to glycogen/glucose storage. Although the liver can regenerate, significant damage may not be reversible. Liver dysfunction can be the result of viral infections (hepatitis B and hepatitis C), metabolic disease (e.g., Wilson disease), biliary dysfunction (e.g., primary biliary sclerosis, primary sclerosing cholangitis), autoimmune hepatitis, and nonalcoholic steatohepatitis (e.g., fatty liver). Especially in early phases of ESLD, these etiologic factors vary in terms of their effect on cognitive functioning.

Alcohol is the leading cause of cirrhosis in the United States, affecting more than 2 million individuals. Chronic alcohol abuse can lead to three types of liver conditions: fatty liver, cirrhosis, and acute or chronic alcoholic hepatitis. Alcohol is absorbed into the bloodstream from the stomach and intestines. The blood goes through the liver before circulating throughout body. Thus, the highest concentration of alcohol is in the blood flowing through the liver. Liver enzymes metabolize alcohol, turning them into water and carbon dioxide, which is then excreted through the urine and lungs. Although obesity is the leading cause of fatty liver, alcohol-related hepatocyte (e.g., liver cell) damage can lead to fatty liver, and this can be reversed with alcohol cessation. Alcohol-related fat accumulation and liver cell inflammation can lead to liver scarring (fibrosis) and cirrhosis (destruction of liver architecture). Medical complications of liver disease are shown in Table 42-1, and several factors may be associated with acute or chronic cognitive impairment, including hepatic encephalopathy.

Hepatic encephalopathy (HE) is potentially life threatening and characterized by impaired mental status, fetor heaticus (a breath odor associated with liver disease), possible slowed electroencephalographic activity and hyperventilation, and motor dysfunction such as asterixis ("flapping tremor"). Asterixis occurs when the arms are held outstretched and the wrists are extended causing a "hand flapping" tremor, appearing much like a bird's wings flapping. Hepatic encephalopathy may occur as an acute, potentially reversible disorder or as a chronic, progressive disorder associated with chronic liver disease. Mild symptoms include irritability and sleep/wake difficulty, but this can progress to worsened mental status, confusion, coma, and death. Patients may present to a hospital setting

Table 42-1. Common Complications of End-Stage Liver Disease

Hepatic Encephalopathy	Hepatorenal Syndrome
Ascites	Hematemesis—portal hypertension
Pruritus	Jaundice (increased bilirubin)
Abdominal pain	Upper GI—esophageal varices, hematemesis
Fatigue	Lower GI—hematochezia, melena
Hepatocellular carcinoma	Spider angiomas
	Palmar erythema

GI, gastrointestinal.

in severe HE in conditions such as fulminant hepatic failure, a condition characterized by acute, severe hepatic failure in an individual with no preexisting hepatic dysfunction(i.e., caused by overdose). Seventy-five percent of individuals die within 3 years of their first HE episode (Bustamonte et al., 1999) and about 80% of individuals with HE-related coma die.

While ammonia is the primary toxic substance associated with HE, manganese and mercaptans may contribute (Zieve, Doizaki, & Zieve, 1974). Serum ammonia level is poorly associated with the degree of HE, leading to the argument that hyperammonemia is not the only factor of HE. This may in part be due to the fact that serum ammonia may not reflect free brain-bound ammonia. As many as one-third of cirrhotic patients may have some degree of mild or subclinical HE (Gitlin, Lewis, & Hinkley, 1986), but HE remains a clinical diagnosis with no definitive tests. Clinical scales of HE include the World Congress of Gastroenterology classification (Ferenci et al., 2002), West Haven Criteria (Atterbury, Maddrey, & Conn, 1978), and Hepatic Encephalopathy Scoring Algorithm (Hassanein, Hilsabeck, & Perry, 2008). The clinical and laboratory variability, subjectivity of clinical measures, as well as the subtlety of mild symptoms make HE difficult to assess, and no gold standard exists. This makes the objective nature of neuropsychological assessment a potentially important tool in assessing HE.

Because the mechanism of HE is likely metabolic, correction of this may lead to improvement.

In a compromised liver, eating too much protein may trigger increased ammonia, but other possible triggers of HE include infections/sepsis, gastrointestinal bleeding, renal disease, alkalosis, low body oxygen, procedures that bypass blood past the liver, and electrolyte abnormalities (especially a decrease in potassium). Among the differentials of HE are alcohol intoxication or withdrawal, sedative overdose, Wernicke-Korsakoff syndrome, subdural hematoma, meningitis, and metabolic abnormalities such as low blood glucose. Common treatments for HE include medications that speed up transit through the bowel, thus lessening the time available for bacteria to metabolize protein into ammonia. Lactulose and some antibiotics (i.e., Rifaximin and neomycin) are typically prescribed, but their effectiveness remains unclear. Many of the relationships among underlying causes of hepatic failure (e.g., alcohol, HCV, etc.) are well discussed in the literature; neuropsychological effects of HE are less studied, but nonetheless important.

The Case of J. M.

The patient is a 68-year-old, left-handed, Caucasian male referred by a Liver Transplant Team as part of a standard transplant candidacy workup. He had ESLD secondary to alcoholic cirrhosis, diagnosed 2 years prior. This gentleman was referred from an outside hospital, so limited medical records were available for this initial transplant evaluation.

This patient reportedly consumed at least 9 to 12 beers daily for more than three decades. He had reportedly been abstinent of alcohol since being diagnosed with ESLD. His primary care physician confirmed this information. He denied any history of alcohol withdrawal. He denied illicit drug use and ceased tobacco use 30 years prior to the time of assessment.

As part of his evaluation he received a complete medical workup. A colonoscopy was performed and found to be negative, and the patient denied viral hepatitis or jaundice. He had lost weight due to multiple paracenteses and diuresis secondary to ascites. Paracentesis is a procedure in which a needle is used to drain abdominal ascitic fluid. High-volume paracentesis may drain more than 10 liters, causing significant weight changes. Fluid may quickly accumulate, causing breathing difficulty, umbilical herniation, and abdominal discomfort. During his transplant hepatology clinic evaluation, he was noted to be alert. He had signs consistent with mild asterixis, mild palmar erythema bilaterally (reddening of the palms), no icterus (yellowing of the skin and eyes), and pitting edema, mostly around the ankles and lower chin. The hepatology team felt that he had grade 2 hepatic encephalopathy, which is generally characterized by decreased attention span and lethargy. The patient had been titrating his lactulose to one bowel movement per day, but the hepatologist increased this lactulose dosing to induce two to three bowel movements per day, with the option of adding neomycin, an additional medication (e.g., antibiotic) to increase bowel movements, at a later time.

J. M.'s medical history was significant for asymptomatic coronary atherosclerosis, massive ascites (with at least four paracenteses), left pleural effusion, anasarca (generalized edema), gastrectomy (34 years prior), back surgery with discectomy (10 years prior), and open cholecystectomy (4 years prior). His symptoms included lower extremity edema and scrotal swelling. His liver function lab tests were elevated, but no ammonia level was reported. An ammonia level approximately 16 months prior revealed a modest elevation (58); however, these levels can quickly change. The patient's medications included spironolactone and furosemide for ascites, and lactulose for reduction of proteins that contribute to his hepatic encephalopathy.

J. M. was a poor historian and had poor insight, and he did not appreciate or recognize that he had cognitive changes. He denied having had experienced symptoms consistent with encephalopathy, but HE had been a documented concern of the treatment team. Unfortunately, he had no close relatives or friends to provide detailed collateral information; however, a friend, who had the patient's power of attorney, reported multiple episodes of confusion. This friend was not with him every day, so he was not closely monitored. The patient denied symptoms consistent with past or present depression, anxiety, or other psychiatric illness. His sleep was poor, with 4 hours per night, and he napped during the day. This pattern is often referred to as sleep/wake reversal and is consistent with mild to moderate HE. His appetite was reportedly poor.

J. M. reported that the attained developmental milestones on time, completed grade 11, and retired from ship construction after 27 years. He served in the military for 3 years, but he was reportedly not involved in combat, exposed to neurotoxins, or experienced a head injury. He was a widower with three children and lived alone.

J. M. was tested two times, 1 month apart. After the first evaluation, there was concern that his poor scores on general cognitive/memory screening measures might be a barrier to transplant outcome. Patients with poor cognitive functioning may have difficulty understanding and following frequently changing immunosupression medication regimens post transplant. Adequate memory functioning is critical to take life-sustaining medications. The importance of cognition and memory becomes more important when patients have little social support, meaning they may be required to self-manage medications. J. M. lived alone and would need to be able to manage his medications post transplant, so greater emphasis was given to memory functioning in the second appointment. Also, the team wanted to determine the potential for his cognitive functioning to have been more permanently affected secondary to an alcohol-related syndrome (i.e., Wernike-Korsakoff, Korsakoff amnesia, alcohol dementia, etc.), and thus less likely that his cognitive impairment would resolve following liver transplant. Consequently, during the second evaluation the California Verbal Learning Test as well as several other learning and memory measures were included. Additionally, a few tests were repeated for comparison.

During the first testing session (Time 1), J. M. was oriented in all spheres but somewhat slow in verbal and motor responding. No asterixis was evident. His affect was flat, and he had poor insight into his cognition and memory. He was unable to appreciate that he had experienced episodes of confusion, although this was noted by the friend who brought him and within his medical chart. No psychotic symptomatology was appreciated. During the second testing (Time 2), J. M. appeared socially more engaged and less lethargic.

Examination Results

The patient was administered an extended neuropsychological screening, in addition to an interview assessing appropriateness for transplant (i.e., compliance, substance use, psychiatric status, social support, etc.). He was administered a broad measure of cognitive functioning, the Repeatable Battery of Neuropsychological Status (RBANS). His scores on indices of Immediate Memory, Visuospatial Construction, Attention, and Delayed Memory were moderately to severely impaired, whereas his Language was low average to mildly impaired.

On psychomotor testing, the patient had bilaterally but equivalently impaired performances on the Grooved Pegboard Test at Time 1. His performances did not change from Time 1 to Time 2 (Table 42-2). His Trail Making Test A performance from Time 1 to Time 2 significantly

improved; however, he was unable to complete Trail Making Test Part B in either evaluation.

His receptive language score, as measured by the Peabody Picture Vocabulary Test-III (PPVT-III), was within the low-average to mildly impaired range. At Time 1, his lexical fluency performance was moderately impaired, with relatively better category fluency. These fluency performances improved by two and one words, respectively, at Time 2; however, this was not a significant improvement. At Time 2, the Boston Naming Test was administered, and his spontaneous naming was considered to be mildly impaired. Additionally, his copy of the Rey-Osterrieth Complex Figure was severely impaired (Figure 42-1).

Table 42-2. J. M.'s Examination Results

RBANS	Testing Date 1		Testing Date 2	
	Index Score	Percentile		
Immediate Memory	61	<1		
Visuospatial/ Constructional	60	<1		
Language	85	16		
Delayed Memory	64	1		
Total Score	62	1		
	Standard Score	Percentile		
PPVT-III	81	10		
	Raw Score	T-Score	Raw Score	T-Score
Lexical Fluency	13	28	15	32
Category Fluency	13	39	14	43
Grooved Pegboard				
Dominant	192 sec	22		22
Nondominant	222 sec	22		22
Trail-Making A	126 sec	20	33 sec	48
Trail-Making B	>300 sec	26	>300 sec	26
Beck Depression Inventory-II	2		3	
WAIS-III Digit Span			SS = 6	9th percentile
Boston Naming Test			41	36
Rey-Osterrieth Complex Copy			15	<20
CVLT–II				
Total Words Trials 1–5				T = 48
Short Delayed Free Recall				z = −.5
Long Delayed Free Recall				z = 0
Recognition Discriminability				

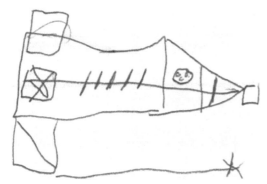

Figure 42-1. Rey-Osterrieth Complex Figure copy.

At Time 2, a more comprehensive memory measure was administered. On a measure of verbal list acquisition and memory, the California Verbal Learning Test-II, J. M.'s performances were not impaired. He scored in the average range on indices of learning and delayed memory, in addition to recognition memory. These scores contrasted dramatically with RBANS memory performances the month prior.

Results of the Beck Depression Inventory–II at Time 1 and Time 2 were not suggestive of depression.

Discussion

This case study highlights several important aspects and challenges of ESLD and the underlying etiological effects. Because of fluctuating course and subjective assessment, it is difficult to assess the degree to which HE contributes to neuropsychological test findings at a given point in time. Alertness, orientation, cognition, and memory may change within the course of hours. It is only when a patient is assessed at another point in time that comparisons can be made. In this example of ESLD the underlying hepatic failure was secondary to alcohol dependence. A clinical diagnosis of chronic, mild HE was made. The patient was known to have mild asterixis and elevated ammonia at times. The amount of elevated ammonia needed to cause HE remains unclear. Moreover, the role of other factors(i.e., mercaptans, manganese, etc.) is unclear and these are not commonly assessed.

At Time 1, the patient's profile suggested diffuse moderately to severely impaired cognition. This finding could be consistent with alcoholic dementia; however, clinically HE was identified and his memory profile at Time 2 was inconsistent with alcoholic dementia. The misattribution of severe cognitive impairment in an individual with ESLD is possible when HE is not considered. Information from the extended memory testing at Time 2 clearly demonstrated that he did not have a significant memory disorder consistent with alcohol dementia, which was considered at Time 1. It is less clear if this finding was reflective of improved HE between Time 1 and Time 2. From Time 1 to Time 2 no performances decreased and Trails A improved beyond what would be expected for practice effects. Other performances, including Trails B and manual dexterity, did not significantly improve. His lexical and semantic fluency pattern did not change from Time 1 to Time 2. In the end, these findings are common in patients with HE. These cases are complex and it is difficult (if not impossible) to definitively separate HE from underlying disease factors and hepatic-related causes.

For most patients, hepatic encephalopathy is episodic and resolves relatively quickly with increased bowel movements. Less frequently the HE is chronic and difficult to control. With mild encephalopathy, patients may experience increased irritability and sleep/wake reversal, but severe encephalopathy is potentially life threatening. In many cases, the metabolic cause is presumed (i.e., high ammonia), and this is treated empirically (i.e., lactulose). Only after empirical treatment has not resolved the encephalopathy is ammonia measured. Because the degree of encephalopathy may quickly fluctuate, ammonia levels are not routinely measured, and the amount of increased ammonia may not directly correspond to cognitive impairment. The influence of HE on cognition remains unclear and inconsistent in mild stages. Even though an ammonia level may assist in assessing an elevated ammonia level, it is often impractical since ammonia levels may rapidly change and a clear relationship between ammonia level and cognitive impairment remains unclear.

Several challenges are apparent as they relate to liver transplantation. This individual had little social support, which is critical for post-transplant care. He will need to consistently take immunosuppression following transplant.

His lack of awareness of his deficits is another challenge. Because HE can occur quickly and it is a potentially life-threatening situation if not effectively treated, this individual is in potential danger of hepatic coma or accidents while in a confused state. The patient could not identify when he experienced increasing confusion so that he could increase his lactulose or seek emergent care. Ideally, this patient should be continually monitored for HE. This monitoring should include the frequency of bowel movements and whether treatment (e.g., lactulose, Rifaximin, etc.) is being titrated to the recommended number of bowel movements. Additionally, assessment of episodic confusion and increased irritability, and sleep/wake reversal is critical in HE assessment and determination about how HE may contribute to neuropsychological test findings.

References

Atterbury, C. E., Maddrey, W. C., & Conn, H. O. (1978). Neomycin-sorbitol and lactulose in the treatment of acute portal-systemic encephalopathy. A controlled, double-blind clinical trial. *American Journal of Digestive Diseases, 23,* 398–406.

Bustamante, J., Rimola, A., Ventura, P. J., Navasa, M., Ciera, I., Reggiardo, V., & Rodes, J. (1999). Prognostic significance of hepatic encephalopathy in patients with cirrhosis. *Journal of Hepatology, 30,* 890–895.

Ferenci, P., Lockwood, A., Mullen, K., Tarter, R., Weissenborn, K., & Blei, A.T. (2002). Hepatic encephalopathy-definition, nomenclature, diagnosis, and quantification: Final report of the working party at the 11th World Congresses of Gastroenterology, Vienna, 1998. *Hepatology, 35,* 716-721

Gitlin, N., Lewis, D. C., & Hinkley, L. (1986). The diagnosis and prevalence of subclinical hepatic encephalopathy in apparently healthy ambulant, non-shunted patients with cirrhosis. *Journal of Hepatology, 3,* 75–82.

Hassanein, T., Hilsabeck, R., & Perry, W. (2008). Introduction to the hepatic encephalopathy scoring algorithm. *Digestive Diseases and Sciences, 53,* 529–538.

Zieve, L., Doizaki, W. M., & Zieve, J. (1974). Synergism between mercaptans and ammonia or fatty acids in the production of coma: A possible role for mercaptans in the pathogenesis of hepatic coma. *Journal of Laboratory Clinical Medicine, 83,* 16–28.

43

Cerebral Neoplasm: Medulloblastoma

Celiane Rey-Casserly and Tanya Diver

Brain tumors are the most common solid tumor of childhood, and medulloblastoma is the most common malignant type diagnosed in childhood (Packer, MacDonald, & Vezina, 2007). It is classified as an embryonal tumor that arises in the cerebellum and fourth ventricle. Medulloblastoma is an aggressive, fast-growing neoplasm that has the potential to disseminate through cerebrospinal fluid (CSF) pathways. Consequently, intensive, multimodality therapy is required for disease control. The peak age of diagnosis is between the ages of 3 and 8 years (El Zein, Bondy, & Wrensch, 2005), a period of active brain development and significant vulnerability to the toxic effects of potentially curative treatments. The challenge in treating the disease is heightened in children diagnosed before 3 years of age due to the increased risk of unacceptable late effects. The standard treatment for medulloblastoma in older children involves surgery, craniospinal radiation, and chemotherapy. Radiation therapy is directed to the brain and spine, and it includes a local boost to the posterior fossa. The overall survival rate is approaching 85% for children without disseminated disease at diagnosis, a substantial improvement compared to only 25 years ago, when survival rates were only 50%–60% (Packer, 2005). A recent European study documents a 10 year overall survival rate of 91% in a cohort of standard risk children (von Hoff et al., 2009). Advances in treatment such as improvements in surgical techniques and care, new methods of radiation therapy, and integration of biological/molecular information

in diagnosis and tailoring of treatment have increased survival rates, and treatment protocols have been modified to reduce toxicity and late effects. The introduction of adjuvant chemotherapy has permitted reductions in craniospinal radiation dose from up to 40 Gy to 18 Gy in some protocols. In infants and very young children, radiation therapy is delayed or omitted with the use of chemotherapy.

Children and adolescents treated for medulloblastoma are at high risk for a range of late effects that affect multiple systems in the body, as well as social-emotional development. These late effects include neurocognitive impairment, endocrine dysfunction, growth retardation, compromised fertility, seizure disorder, hearing loss, neurological deficits, and risk of second malignancy. Factors associated with neuropsychological and physiological late effects include direct effects of the tumor (cerebellar tissue damage), obstructive hydrocephalus, and surgical complications, as well as the toxic effects of treatment on the developing brain (surgery, radiation, chemotherapy). Multimodality tumor directed therapy is associated with a higher risk of psychological adjustment and social functioning problems (Poggi et al., 2005; Vannatta et al., 2008; Vannatta, Gerhardt, Wells, & Noll, 2007). The impact of these risks needs to be evaluated in light of both development and contextual factors. Developmental factors such as earlier age at diagnosis and longer time since diagnosis are associated with a higher risk of neurocognitive impairment (Mulhern et al., 2001; Reimers et al., 2003; Ris, Packer, Goldwein, Jones-Wallace, &

Boyett, 2001). In children, one cannot assume that an injury affecting one domain of functioning will be restricted to that domain over the course of the child's development, and the pattern of impairment may become more diffuse over time (Dennis, Spiegler, Riva, & MacGregor, 2004). Children are more likely to demonstrate a more complex pattern of deficits since an early insult can affect later developing or downstream processes (Bishop, 1997). Additional time-related factors include the era of treatment and the type of care available at the time the child was treated. Protocols are constantly modified as refinements in treatment become available, and these changes are frequently associated with expected improvements in neuropsychological outcomes. For example, proton beam radiation therapy can reduce the dose of radiation received by normal tissues because the maximum dose deposition is focused on the tumor and the exit dose is minimized (Fossati, Ricardi, & Orecchia, 2009; Tarbell, Smith, Adams, & Loeffler, 2000). Although studies of neuropsychological outcomes of children treated with this new modality are yet to emerge, statistical models demonstrate the reduced potential for hearing loss as well as a slower rate of IQ decline for patients with medulloblastoma (Merchant et al., 2008). Social/cultural, psychological, and family factors are critical as well; as has been documented in studies of children with brain injury, family and social factors are key mediators of the impact of insult on outcome (Yeates et al., 2007). Environmental and cultural factors such as access to care, educational support, and community resources can have a substantial role in promoting recovery and optimal adjustment.

Neuropsychological outcomes of children treated for medulloblastoma have been studied extensively (Mulhern, Merchant, Gajjar, Reddick, & Kun, 2004). Early studies documented significant neurocognitive impairment and decline in intellectual ability over time (Hoppe-Hirsch et al., 1990). Children 3 years old or younger who were treated with craniospinal radiation were more likely to have IQ scores below 70 than children treated with focal radiation (Fouladi et al., 2005). Longitudinal studies have demonstrated that a decline in IQ scores is associated with younger age at treatment and higher radiation dose. Children treated at age 7 years or older with 23.4 Gy craniospinal radiation demonstrated a loss of .42 points per year, whereas in children treated with 36–39.6 Gy, IQ loss was 1.56 points per year. For children treated under the age of 7 years, IQ loss per year was 2.41 with 23.4 Gy dose, and 3.71 points per year with the higher dose (Mulhern et al., 2005). The decline in IQ over time following treatment for medulloblastoma appears to be related to failure to acquire information as expected, and not to a deterioration in existing skills (Palmer et al., 2001; Ris et al., 2001). Overall, studies have noted a decline of approximately 2–4 IQ points per year, with a greater decline found early in follow-up, and greater decline in children with higher baseline IQ scores (Kieffer-Renaux et al., 2005; Ris et al., 2001; Spiegler, Bouffet, Greenberg, Rutka, & Mabbott, 2004). Impairments in academic achievement have been documented as well (Mabbott et al., 2005; Mulhern et al., 2005). Declines in cognitive and academic ability appear related to the impact of the disease and its treatment on fundamental psychological processes of attention, information processing, and working memory, which are proposed as core deficits (Mabbott, Penkman, Witol, Strother, & Bouffet, 2008; Palmer, 2008; Palmer, Reddick, & Gajjar, 2007). The underlying pathophysiology of neurocognitive impairments in children treated for medulloblastoma has been presumed to be related to the impact of radiation on developing white matter and ensuing white matter loss (Mulhern et al., 2001; Reddick et al., 2005). Studies have also found reductions in hippocampal volume and hippocampal neurogenesis (Monje et al., 2002; Monje, 2008; Nagel, 2004). Effects of tumor location are important risk factors in neurocognitive outcomes. The role of the cerebellum in cognitive function is increasingly recognized (Dum & Strick, 2003; Middleton & Strick, 1998; Riva & Giorgi, 2000). Several recent studies have documented the impact of damage to the cerebellum as well as obstructive hydrocephalus and postsurgical complications on the neuropsychological outcomes of children with posterior fossa tumors (Cantelmi, Schweizer, & Cusimano, 2008; Mabbott et al., 2008; Roncadin, Dennis, Greenberg, & Spiegler, 2008; Ronning, Sundet, Due-Tonnessen, Lundar, & Helseth, 2005).

We will present two cases of patients treated for medulloblastoma; one was diagnosed at age

6 years, while the other was diagnosed at age 16 years. Both received the same treatment regimen: gross total resection, craniospinal radiation with a focal boost to the posterior fossa, and chemotherapy.

Case Study: Jill

Jill was diagnosed with a medulloblastoma at the age of 6 years after presenting with a 1-week history of acute onset of vomiting and eye deviation. She underwent imaging studies that showed a 3.6 cm by 2.8 cm by 4.0 cm mass in the posterior fossa; there was marked ventriculomegaly but no evidence of a midline shift (Figure 43-1). Following a gross total resection she had persistent nystagmus and cranial nerve VI dysfunction that subsequently improved. She was then treated with a 6-week course of proton beam radiation therapy with concomitant vincristine. Radiation dose was 23.4 Gy craniospinal, with a boost to 54 Gy to the posterior fossa. An audiogram before chemotherapy treatment was initiated revealed normal hearing. Jill was then treated with systemic chemotherapy consisting of cisplatin, vincristine, and CCNU (lomustine). Complications of treatment included poor weight gain, necessitating a G-tube for nutritional supplementation. Her weight fell from the 50th percentile to the 5th percentile during her treatment.

Premorbid History

Jill lives with her parents and older brother. There is no family history of neurological, psychiatric, or learning disorder. Birth history was unremarkable and developmental milestones were acquired as expected. There were no concerns at school; Jill did well mastering academic skills in kindergarten and first grade, although she missed some of first grade due to her treatment. Medical history was unremarkable prior to the diagnosis of medulloblastoma.

Jill was referred for neuropsychological assessment at the age of 7 years. She was completing her chemotherapy treatment. Jill was adjusting to her treatment fairly well, although her parents noted problems with excessive "clinginess" and increased irritability. Jill also had motor coordination issues; she was having some difficulty learning to ride a bicycle and her running was

(a)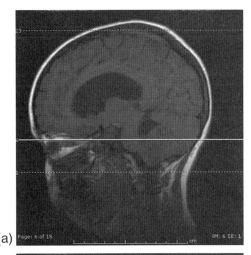

(b)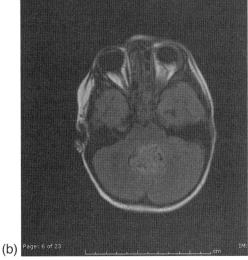

Figure 43-1. Six-year-old female with medulloblastoma: (*a*) Sagittal T1 image showing posterior fossa tumor and ventriculomegaly; (*b*) Axial fluid-attenuated inversion recovery (FLAIR) image showing tumor in posterior fossa.

described as awkward. Her parents reported that she was more subdued and fatigued than before her treatment.

Neuropsychological Examination Results at Age 7

Jill presented as a friendly and engaging youngster. She cooperated readily with the assessment procedures and was very motivated to please. She was alert and oriented, and she was able to direct her attention appropriately. She was easily fatigued and her effort waned as she became tired. She also needed encouragement to tackle less familiar or more challenging tasks. Speech was within normal limits, though at times her speech intonation and pitch were similar to that of a younger child. She is left-handed and her motor coordination issues did not affect her ability to manipulate materials effectively. Subtle eye deviation was noted, and it had been reported to be improving.

Neuropsychological test scores are provided in Table 43-1. On the WISC-III, overall intellectual abilities were within the superior range, with significant discrepancy noted between the average-range Processing Speed Index and the other index scores, which ranged from high average to superior. Jill demonstrated a well-developed fund of knowledge, vocabulary, and verbal learning and memory skills. She was less skilled in identifying verbal concepts and describing relationships among words. Academic achievement measures were at or above expectations for her age. Reasoning and problem-solving abilities were strong. Speed of information processing was noted to be slower than expected on a timed visual scanning task.

Table 43-1. Neuropsychological Data for Jill at Age 7 and 11 Years

General Intellectual Ability

Age 7 WISC-III		Age 11 WISC-IV	
Full Scale	121	Full Scale	102
Verbal Comprehension	114	Verbal Comprehension	106
Perceptual Organization	116	Perceptual Reasoning	102
Freedom from Distractibility	121	Working Memory	107
Processing Speed	109	Processing Speed	85

Domain / Test	Age 7	Age 11
Language / Verbal Memory		
Vocabulary/Naming	Boston Naming Test 44/60 (above average)	Expressive One-Word Vocabulary 106
Verbal Fluency	(NEPSY)	(D-KEFS)
Letters	average	9
Category	average	8
CELF Recalling Sentences	15	11
Children's Memory Scale		
Sequences	14	13
Stories Immediate	10	11
Stories Delayed	10	11
Stories Recognition	13	7
CVLT-C		
Total	T = 70	T = 63
Trial 1	1	−0.5
Trial 5	2	1
Short Delay	2.5	0.5
Long Delay	1.5	0.5
Visual Spatial/Motor		
ROCF Organization-copy	75th percentile	50–75th percentile
Immediate recall	50th–75th percentile	50th–75th percentile
Delayed recall	25th–50th percentile	50th percentile
VMI	104	98
Grooved Pegboard		
Right Hand	within normal limits	within normal limits
Left Hand	within normal limits	within normal limits

Table 43-1. Neuropsychological Data for Jill at Age 7 and 11 Years (*Continued*)

Attention / Executive Control

TEA-Ch		
Sky Search		
Number of Targets	14	11
Time per Target	5	6
Attention Score	8	10
Score	15	6
NEPSY Tower	13	—
CPT-II	—	within normal limits
WCST		
% Errors	—	97
Categories Completed	—	5; >16th percentile
Trials to Complete 1st Category	—	12; >16th percentile
Failure to Maintain Set	—	4; ≤1st percentile
D-KEFS		
Color Naming	—	13
Word Reading	—	10
Inhibition	—	12
Inhibition/Switching	—	8
BRIEF		
Parent:		
Metacognition Index	38	50
Behavioral Regulation Index	42	49
Teacher:		
Metacognition Index	42	—
Behavioral Regulation Index	46	—

Academic Achievement

WJ-III		
Letter-Word ID	119	118
Passage Comprehension	111	99
Calculations	99	111
Reading Fluency	115	83
Math Fluency	107	100

Adaptive/Social Emotional

ABAS		
General Adaptive Composite	—	91
Conceptual	—	95
Social	—	97
Practical	—	88
SIB-R		
Broad Independence	118	—
Motor Skills	115	—
Social/Communication	117	—
Personal Living	104	—
Community Living	115	—
BASC/BASC-2		
Parent		
Externalizing Problems	38	42
Internalizing Problems	48	43
Adaptive Skills	53	49

—test not given/not available.

Formulation: Jill is a 7-year-old girl with high average to superior intellectual abilities, who performs at or above expectation in most domains of functioning. Speed of information processing is relatively slower than expected for her age, and there was some hesitancy noted in her ability to tackle more challenging or unfamiliar tasks. Recommendations included careful monitoring of functioning at school, providing additional time for completing work, particularly as tasks become more complex, and greater emphasis on underlying concepts when teaching new material. Strategies for fostering self-confidence and independence as her treatment course was completed were also discussed with the family.

Neuropsychological Examination Results at Age 11

Jill was referred for follow-up neuropsychological assessment at age 11. Routine imaging had documented no residual or recurrent disease. Jill had developed endocrine dysfunction, including precocious puberty, hypothyroidism, and poor growth velocity. She was being treated with Levoxyl and Lupron. She had poor skeletal growth with a shortened trunk and alopecia secondary to her treatment regimen. She was referred for a nutrition consultation due to weight gain and was working with her family to follow a healthy diet and program of physical activity. Mild bilateral high-frequency hearing loss (6000–8000 Hz range) was diagnosed after completion of chemotherapy. Her parents were concerned about Jill's overly sensitive nature and social immaturity. They noted that she seemed more dependent on her parents than others her age. Jill's parents and teacher reported that she was encountering more difficulty integrating with peers at school, although she had no problems socializing with relatives or in church-sponsored activities. Academic issues emerged in the fifth grade and were characterized by difficulty organizing her thoughts in written work. At the time of assessment Jill was in the sixth grade, and her parents reported increased stress around schoolwork, particularly written assignments and long-term projects.

Jill presented as a friendly young girl who could be quite talkative. She was cooperative and put forth good effort on tasks. Her mood was stable and upbeat. She was able to focus attention effectively on a range of tasks but had trouble sustaining auditory attention. Consistent with previous testing, Jill continued to need encouragement and support to tackle more challenging items. Her approach to problem-solving was methodical, although at times she could lose track of what she was doing. She seemed to do better on tasks that allowed her time to become familiar with what was expected of her.

Neuropsychological data for the assessment at age 11 are shown in Table 43-1. Overall intellectual abilities were now in the average range, and there was a substantial drop in index scores, with the Processing Speed Index in the low average range. The overall decline in performance was likely related to a range of factors, including that lower scores may be expected when a test is revised. Expected index score differences between the WISC-III and the WISC-IV range from 1.5 to 4.5 points, with the least discrepancy seen between the working memory tasks (Williams, Weiss, & Rolfhus, 2003). However, this factor would not account for the degree of decline noted. With increasing age, children are expected to demonstrate integrative skills and to work faster and more efficiently. A decline in test performance may be due to the impact of the tumor and its treatment. Although Jill had continued to acquire new knowledge and skills, she was not progressing at the same rate as her peers, and she demonstrated more compromise in overall speed of information processing and working memory. Verbal learning ability was still above average, although initial auditory attention span length declined. Scores were lower on tests of auditory attention and span such as repeating a list of words, sentences, or digits, and for counting sounds over repeated trials. In the area of executive function, her parents did not report any difficulties on a standardized questionnaire. Problem-solving was methodical, although at times inconsistent. Visual-spatial reasoning skills declined somewhat, though Jill was able to solve visual problems effectively. Visual-motor skills remained fairly stable, although timed scanning and output tasks were generally performed more slowly than expected. For academic achievement, single-word reading was well developed but she demonstrated a decline in reading speed and comprehension. Mastery of math algorithms was progressing well. Socially, Jill was having difficulty integrating with peers. Her father rated her social skills in the "at risk" range on an emotional adjustment questionnaire. Jill expressed concern about her ability to make friends. Adaptive skills were within the normal range, but not as advanced as they had been at age 7.

Formulation: Jill presented with good verbal skills and knowledge but was encountering some difficulties with complex tasks (organizing thoughts on paper), working memory, speed of processing, and social skills. Although her performance on most tasks was in the average range, this represented a decline in skills compared to her prior evaluation. In addition, demands were becoming more complex later in elementary school and Jill was experiencing greater difficulty, particularly when tasks required integration of multiple domains, such as in writing. Given this profile, she would be expected to be less able to mobilize problem-solving strategies and work efficiently in higher grades. Psychological and social adjustment also became an issue. Jill's sensitive nature and lack of confidence contributed to less successful social relationships with her peers. Recommendations included more support in teaching new concepts, allowance for additional time to process information and complete tasks, opportunities for review and previewing to support weaker listening skills, explicit teaching of writing skills, and counseling around social skills and peer relationships. Subsequent to this evaluation, Jill's parents became more concerned about her social experience at school and elected to enroll her in a home schooling program. They considered that this environment would provide more individual attention and support, as well as allow her to work at her own pace. Arrangements were made for social activities through the home schooling program and church functions.

Case Study: John

John presented to a local hospital at age 16 years with a 1-month history of headache, nausea, vomiting, and dizziness. Neuroimaging revealed a posterior fossa mass. He underwent surgical resection; the pathology was consistent with standard risk medulloblastoma. Spinal magnetic resonance imaging (MRI) was negative and there was no evidence of seeding within the central nervous system. John received craniospinal proton beam radiation therapy with a boost to the posterior fossa (craniospinal dose 24 Gy with a total dose of 54 Gy to the posterior fossa), followed by chemotherapy treatment. The chemotherapy regimen consisted of vincristine, cisplatin, and CCNU. When John developed peripheral neuropathy during treatment, the vincristine dose was reduced; he was also treated with Neurontin. John lost more than 20 pounds during his treatment, but he subsequently regained most of this weight. Neuroimaging studies revealed no evidence of tumor recurrence. John developed a mild high frequency (4000–8000 Hz) mixed hearing loss on the left (at age 21).

Premorbid History

John was born 3½ weeks before his due date, weighing 6 pounds, 7 ounces; postnatal complications included jaundice, which was treated with phototherapy. Developmental milestones were attained as expected for speech and language, social, and gross motor skills. Fine motor skills were slow to develop and had never been "an activity of choice." John had trouble with writing assignments as a youngster and had typed his assignments since the second grade. He was diagnosed with attention-deficit/hyperactivity disorder (ADHD), inattentive type at age 8 years. At the time of his diagnosis, he lived with his parents and younger brother. Family history was remarkable for psychiatric issues and left-handedness. John is right-handed.

John was referred for neuropsychological assessment at age 17 years when he was in the 11th grade at a private school and enrolled in several honors level classes. He generally did well academically, although he could become overwhelmed by the multiple demands of the academic setting. He also reported some trouble writing essays, and he had particular difficulty phrasing his ideas so that others could understand them. John was taking complementary medicines and was receiving biofeedback therapy for his attention problems.

Prior to this assessment, John had two neuropsychological evaluations at ages 8 and 11 years. The most recent assessment revealed very superior intellectual functioning on the WISC-III, with similarly well-developed verbal and visual perceptual skills. Speed of information processing was weaker relative to his other skills. John's performance was influenced by his weak executive function skills, including regulation of attention, organization, impulsivity, and cognitive flexibility. He performed better when working with familiar material or when provided with a clear model. While John's academic achievement was significantly above grade level, he made errors that reflected inattention and impulsivity. He also struggled to generate written language independently. This profile was noted to be very similar to that obtained at age 8.

Neuropsychological Examination Results at Age 17

John presented as a very likeable and articulate young man. His mood was generally cheerful and upbeat, and his attention skills were appropriately

mobilized in the testing session. Results from this neuropsychological assessment are presented in Table 43-2. Specifically, administration of the WAIS-III revealed very superior intellectual abilities, with marked discrepancy between John's very superior verbal knowledge and high-average nonverbal problem solving. The Speed of Processing Index was lower than the other index scores.

Overall, test findings reflected John's tendency to review and process information slowly. He also had trouble with motor functioning, particularly fine motor skills. His speed of motor output was often slow, especially when he was required to produce written output. Although such difficulties were longstanding, and reflected by slow fine motor development and by his need for accommodations in early elementary school, John's medical history also had an impact.

Table 43-2. Neuropsychological Data for John at Age 17 and 22 Years

General Intellectual Ability

		Age 17				*Age 22*	
		WAIS-III				**WAIS-III**	
Full Scale		132		Full Scale		132	
Verbal IQ		143		Verbal IQ		137	
Performance IQ		111		Performance IQ		119	
Verbal Comprehension		150		Verbal Comprehension		140	
Perceptual Organization		121		Perceptual Reasoning		133	
Working Memory		119		Working Memory		126	
Processing Speed		96		Processing Speed		106	

Domain / Test	Age 17	Age 22
Language/Verbal Memory		
Vocabulary/Naming (BNT)	59/60; above average	59/60; above average
Verbal Fluency (DKEFS)		
Letter Fluency	16	13
Category Fluency	13	13
Category Switching	15	14
CELF Recalling Sentences	12	12 (21:11 yr norms)
Wechsler Memory Scale-III		
Mental Control	10	10
Logical Memory I	13	11
Logical Memory II	15	13
Stories Recognition	29/30	25/30
CVLT-II		
Total T	T = 56	T = 62
Trial 1	−0.5	0.5
Trial 5	0.5	1.0
Short Delay Free Recall	1.0	1.0
Long Delay Free Recall	0.5	1.0

Table 43-2. Neuropsychological Data for John at Age 17 and 22 Years (*Continued*)

Domain/Test	Age 17	Age 22
Visual Spatial/Motor		
Rey-Osterrieth Complex Figure (RCFT)		
Copy	2–5th percentile	<1st percentile
Immediate Recall	73rd percentile	42nd percentile
Delayed Recall	54th percentile	58th percentile
Grooved Pegboard		
Right Hand (dominant)	within normal limits	within normal limits
Left Hand	below normal limits	within normal limits
Attention/Executive Control		
CPT-II		
No. of Omissions	42	41
No. of Commissions	36	37
Hit Rate	62	56
Variability	38	37
Hit RT Block Change	65	51
WCST		
% Errors	112	—
Categories Completed	>16th percentile	—
Trials to Complete 1st Category	2–5th percentile	—
Failure to Maintain Set	11–16th percentile	—
BRIEF		
Parent/Informant		
Metacognition Index	49	53
Behavioral Regulation Index	42	42
Teacher		
Metacognition Index	42	—
Behavioral Regulation Index	48	—
Self-report		
Metacognition Index	—	53
Behavioral Regulation Index	—	40
WJ-III Achievement		
Letter-Word ID	119	—
Passage Comprehension	129	—
Calculation	130	122
Reading Fluency	104	119
Math Fluency	95	102
WJ-III Cognitive		
Decision Speed	100	112
Adaptive/Social Emotional		
ABAS-Adult Form		
General Adaptive Composite	—	105
Conceptual	—	108
Social	—	118
Practical	—	102
SIB-R		
Broad Independence	123	—
Motor Skills	79	—
Social/Communication	122	—

(*Continued*)

Table 43-2. Neuropsychological Data for John at Age 17 and 22 Years (*Continued*)

Domain/Test	Age 17	Age 22
Adaptive/Social Emotional		
SIB-R		
Personal Living	125	—
Community Living	128	—
BASC		
Parent		
Externalizing Problems	35	—
Internalizing Problems	42	—
Behavioral Symptoms Index	41	—
Adaptive Skills	47	—
BASC/BASC-2		
Self		
Clinical Maladjustment	47	—
School Maladjustment	41	—
Internalizing Problems	—	44
Inattention/Hyperactivity	—	52
Personal Adjustment	57	60
Emotional Symptoms Index	49	44

During chemotherapy treatment, he developed severe neuropathy and imbalance, and residual deficits were evident. John had high expectations for himself, and he was aware of his learning style.

Formulation: Within the context of pre-existing vulnerabilities in attention and fine motor skills, John's profile was consistent with his tumor location and treatment. While he had many strong and well-developed skills, he struggled with rapid processing and production, which affected his ability to demonstrate his knowledge effectively. John was counseled around college selection decisions in light of his learning style and strong verbal skills. He was encouraged to access resources in college around study strategies and time management, and to work with an advisor to plan his course of study. Recommendations for later high school and college included accommodations such as extended time on examinations, continued use of a computer for writing tasks, including access to a computer for in-class examinations and a modified examination schedule.

Interim History

John was seen for neuropsychological reevaluation at age 22. He had been followed regularly at a multidisciplinary brain tumor clinic; neuroimaging findings revealed no evidence of tumor recurrence. Endocrine issues included growth hormone deficiency, hypothyroidism, and low testosterone level, for which he was followed by an endocrinologist. Medications included growth hormone, Levoxyl, and Ritalin.

John was living with his girlfriend and her family in another state at follow-up. He had graduated from college the previous year, and he had studied health and science. John expressed hopes of attending graduate school and was taking prerequisite courses online. He was also volunteering with a local emergency medical technician service and working on two nearby farms.

John reported difficulty recalling highly detailed material and required repetition to recall new terminology, dates, and names. He found visualization and note taking to be helpful strategies. He had less difficulty remembering new concepts than specific details. He reported frustration when his test scores were lower than expected despite his having devoted significant effort and study time. Deadlines posed a significant challenge, particularly when multiple demands had to be met in close proximity. John found it difficult to begin papers; he had no difficulty with the research component, but he struggled to organize his ideas so that others could follow his line of thinking. Furthermore, he had trouble understanding the key points in assignments, noting that there were several instances when he had not answered specific questions accurately. At college, John was provided extra time for assignments; he did not need additional time on examinations. He took Ritalin on the days when he felt increased pressure to be productive, and this helped him manage his writing demands.

John's moods fluctuated, with positive mood observed at reevaluation. He had periods when he felt "down" during college. His parents had divorced in the interim. As noted, he had a girlfriend and he reported solid social supports. At the time of referral, concerns were expressed regarding planning, time and resource management, organization, management of multiple demands, short-term memory, and his inability to see the big picture.

Neuropsychological Examination Results at Age 22

Intellectual abilities, as assessed by the WAIS-III, continued to fall within the very superior range, with nice progress in skill development since his prior assessment. Particular strength was evident in John's verbal knowledge. Ongoing weakness was noted in processing speed. Notably, John's performance reflected greater variability than is typical in the normative population. Specifically, his verbal reasoning and speed of processing discrepancy exceeded that found in greater than 95% of the population. In addition, the nonverbal reasoning and speed of processing discrepancy exceeded that seen in greater than 90% of the population.

John's verbal retention and learning performance was within expectation but less secure than his very strong verbal skills would suggest. His performance on a narrative memory task in particular reflected mild decline relative to previous testing, with average-level recall. John benefited from repetition and utilized an active strategy to facilitate his recall of detailed material. Difficulties with organization, planning, and management of simultaneous demands were also reported.

Formulation: Overall, John continued to demonstrate many competencies and advanced skills.

In fact, he evidenced gains in auditory working memory, memory for detailed verbal information, fine motor speed, and decision-making speed. John was recovering from the effects of chemotherapy at the prior evaluation, which may have affected his performance. He was not taking Ritalin at that time. Recommendations included the need for academic supports at the graduate level, including access to extended time, note-taking support, active planning of examination schedules, and strategies to manage highly detailed material and develop routines to facilitate management of both academic and daily living demands. Ongoing consultation around psychopharmacological intervention of his attention difficulties was also discussed. John was also continuing to consult with his treatment team around fertility issues.

Discussion/Conclusions

We present two cases of patients treated for medulloblastoma under the same protocol, but at different stages in development; assessments were performed at two different time points. Neuropsychological and quality-of-life outcomes are different for these two patients as a function of a range of factors. Neuropsychological interpretation of the pattern of findings and prediction of upcoming risks is informed by an understanding of the disease and its treatment, and by the systemic interactions among brain-related variables, contextual factors, and development (Bernstein, 2000). Predictors of neuropsychological outcomes of children treated for brain tumors include biological, developmental, and reserve variables (Dennis et al., 2004). In this population, outcome domains need to be evaluated over different time periods and assessments of physical, neuropsychological, cognitive, academic/vocational, and psychosocial aspects are needed. Individuals who sustain brain insults in childhood experience changes in developmental trajectory that continue to evolve over time and into adulthood. These two cases highlight the impact of medulloblastoma and its treatment at different stages in development. Brain development is an active, dynamic process that is constrained by genetic and maturational variables, but it is modified by a range of experiential and contextual factors (Stiles, 2008). In Jill's case, she was treated at a young age when significant brain maturation is yet to unfold; brain development in terms of organization of synaptic networks and myelination proceeds into early adulthood (Johnston et al., 2009). The brain's capacity for growth (plasticity) at this stage also makes it more vulnerable to the impact of injury, particularly to treatments that target rapid developing cells or produce oxidative stress (Johnston et al., 2009). With respect to reserve factors, both of these children demonstrated well-developed intellectual abilities and family support systems. Our adolescent patient also had the benefit of a longer period of normal development before his treatment but had some preexisting vulnerabilities affecting attention, organizational skills, and fine motor coordination. His tumor and treatment affected speed and efficiency of information processing. As an adult, these issues affected his ability to demonstrate his superior intellectual abilities. In our younger patient, the tumor and treatment contributed to a decline in intelligence test scores, which implicate compromise of core cognitive functions such as attention, working memory, and speed of processing. Jill will require lifelong monitoring and support for optimal adaptation. Interventions will need to focus on educational as well as social functioning, given the critical role of social support in fostering overall adjustment, health, and well-being (Turner-Cobb, 2002). For children treated for brain tumors, outcomes can be quite heterogeneous given the complex interplay of factors that contribute to functioning across domains. It is the role of the neuropsychologist to integrate data from history, observations, and assessment findings to guide intervention planning and anticipate future risks. For children treated for medulloblastoma, ongoing education, follow-up, and monitoring of adaptation is required.

Acknowledgment

This work was supported in part by the Stop & Shop Pediatric Brain Tumor Program.

References

Bernstein, J. H. (2000). Developmental neuropsychological assessment. In K. Yeates, M. D. Ris & H. Taylor (Eds.), *Pediatric Neuropsychology: Research, Theory, and Practice* (pp. 405–438). New York: Guilford Publications.

Bishop, D. V. M. (1997). Cognitive neuropsychology and developmental disorders: Uncomfortable bedfellows. *The Quarterly Journal of Experimental Psychology, 50A*(4), 899–923.

Cantelmi, D., Schweizer, T. A., & Cusimano, M. D. (2008). Role of the cerebellum in the neurocognitive sequelae of treatment of tumours of the posterior fossa: An update. *The Lancet Oncology, 9*(6), 569–576.

Dennis, M., Spiegler, B. J., Riva, D., & MacGregor, D. L. (2004). Neuropsychological outcome. In D. Walker, G. Perilongo, C. J. A. Punt, & R. E. Taylor (Eds.), *Brain and spinal tumors of childhood* (pp. 213–227). London: Arnold.

Dum, R. P., & Strick, P. L. (2003). An unfolded map of the cerebellar dentate nucleus and its projections to the cerebral cortex. *Journal of Neurophysiology, 89*(1), 634–639.

El Zein, R., Bondy, M., & Wrensch, M. (2005). Epidemiology of brain tumors. In F. Ali-Osman (Ed.), *Contemporary cancer research: Brain tumors* (pp. 3–18). Totowa, NJ: Humana Press.

Fossati, P., Ricardi, U., & Orecchia, R. (2009). Pediatric medulloblastoma: Toxicity of current treatment and potential role of protontherapy. *Cancer Treatment Reviews, 35*(1), 79–96.

Fouladi, M., Gilger, E., Kocak, M., Wallace, D., Buchanan, G., Reeves, C., et al. (2005). Intellectual and functional outcome of children 3 years old or younger who have CNS malignancies. *Journal of Clinical Oncology, 23*(28), 7152–7160.

Hoppe-Hirsch, E., Renier, D., Lellouch-Tubiana, A., Sainte-Rose, C., Pierre-Kahn, A., & Hirsch, J. F. (1990). Medulloblastoma in childhood: Progressive intellectual deterioration. *Child's Nervous System, 6*(2), 60–65.

Johnston, M. V., Ishida, A., Ishida, W. N., Matsushita, H. B., Nishimura, A., & Tsuji, M. (2009). Plasticity and injury in the developing brain. *Brain Development, 31*(1), 1–10.

Kieffer-Renaux, V., Viguier, D., Raquin, M. A., Laurent-Vannier, A., Habrand, J. L., Dellatolas, G., et al. (2005). Therapeutic schedules influence the pattern of intellectual decline after irradiation of posterior fossa tumors. *Pediatric Blood Cancer, 45*(6), 814–819.

Mabbott, D. J., Penkman, L., Witol, A., Strother, D., & Bouffet, E. (2008). Core neurocognitive functions in children treated for posterior fossa tumors. *Neuropsychology, 22*(2), 159–168.

Mabbott, D. J., Spiegler, B. J., Greenberg, M. L., Rutka, J. T., Hyder, D. J., & Bouffet, E. (2005). Serial evaluation of academic and behavioral outcome after treatment with cranial radiation in childhood. *Journal of Clinical Oncology, 23*(10), 2256–2263.

Merchant, T. E., Hua, C.-H., Shukla, H., Ying, X., Nill, S., & Oelfke, U. (2008). Proton versus photon radiotherapy for common pediatric brain tumors: Comparison of models of dose characteristics and their relationship to cognitive function. *Pediatric Blood and Cancer, 51*(1), 110–117.

Middleton, F. A., & Strick, P. L. (1998). The cerebellum: An overview. *Trends in Neurosciences, 21*(9), 367–369.

Monje, M. (2008). Cranial radiation therapy and damage to hippocampal neurogenesis. *Dev Disabil Res Rev, 14*(3), 238–242.

Monje, M. L., Mizumatsu, S., Fike, J. R., & Palmer, T. D. (2002). Irradiation induces neural precursor-cell dysfunction. *Nature Medicine, 8*(9), 955–962.

Mulhern, R. K., Merchant, T., Gajjar, A., Reddick, W. E., & Kun, L. E. (2004). Late neurocognitive sequelae in survivors of brain tumours in childhood. *The Lancet Oncology, 5*(7), 399–408.

Mulhern, R. K., Palmer, S. L., Merchant, T. E., Wallace, D., Kocak, M., Brouwers, P., et al. (2005). Neurocognitive consequences of risk-adapted therapy for childhood medulloblastoma. *Journal of Clinical Oncology, 23*(24), 5511–5519.

Mulhern, R. K., Palmer, S. L., Reddick, W. E., Glass, J. O., Kun, L. E., Taylor, J., et al. (2001). Risks of young age for selected neurocognitive deficits in medulloblastoma are associated with white matter loss. *Journal of Clinical Oncology, 19*(2), 472–479.

Nagel, B. J., Palmer, S. L., Reddick, W. E., Glass, J. O., Helton, K. J., Wu, S., et al. (2004). Abnormal hippocampal development in children with medulloblastoma treated with risk-adapted irradiation. *AJNR. American Journal of Neuroradiology, 25*(9), 1575–1582.

Packer, R. J. (2005). Progress and challenges in childhood brain tumors. *Journal of Neuro-Oncology, 75*(3), 239–242.

Packer, R. J., MacDonald, T., & Vezina, G. (2007). Embryonal tumors. In J. M. Baehring & J. M. Piepmeier (Eds.), *Brain tumors: Practical guide to diagnosis and treatment* (pp. 269–289). New York: Informa Health Care.

Palmer, S. L. (2008). Neurodevelopmental impact on children treated for medulloblastoma: A review and proposed conceptual model. *Developmental Disabilities and Research Reviews, 14*(3), 203–210.

Palmer, S. L., Goloubeva, O., Reddick, W. E., Glass, J. O., Gajjar, A., Kun, L., et al. (2001). Patterns of intellectual development among survivors of pediatric medulloblastoma: A longitudinal analysis. *Journal of Clinical Oncology, 19*(8), 2302–2308.

Palmer, S. L., Reddick, W. E., & Gajjar, A. (2007). Understanding the cognitive impact on children who are treated for medulloblastoma. *Journal of Pediatric Psychology, 32*(9), 1040–1049.

Poggi, G., Liscio, M., Galbiati, S., Adduci, A., Massimino, M., Gandola, L., et al. (2005). Brain tumors in children and adolescents: Cognitive and psychological disorders at different ages. *Psycho-Oncology, 14*(5), 386–395.

Reddick, W. E., Glass, J. O., Palmer, S. L., Wu, S., Gajjar, A., Langston, J. W., et al. (2005). Atypical white matter volume development in children following craniospinal irradiation. *Neuro-Oncology, 7*(1), 12–19.

Reimers, T. S., Ehrenfels, S., Mortensen, E. L., Schmiegelow, M., Sonderkaer, S., Carstensen, H., et al. (2003). Cognitive deficits in long-term survivors of childhood brain tumors: Identification of predictive factors. *Medical and Pediatric Oncology, 40*(1), 26–34.

Ris, M. D., Packer, R., Goldwein, J., Jones-Wallace, D., & Boyett, J. M. (2001). Intellectual outcome after reduced-dose radiation therapy plus adjuvant chemotherapy for medulloblastoma: A Children's Cancer Group study. *Journal of Clinical Oncology, 19*(15), 3470–3476.

Riva, D., & Giorgi, C. (2000). The cerebellum contributes to higher functions during development: Evidence from a series of children surgically treated for posterior fossa tumours. *Brain, 123*(5), 1051–1061.

Roncadin, C., Dennis, M., Greenberg, M. L., & Spiegler, B. J. (2008). Adverse medical events associated with childhood cerebellar astrocytomas and medulloblastomas: Natural history and relation to very long-term neurobehavioral outcome. *Child's Nervous System, 24*(9), 995–1002.

Ronning, C., Sundet, K., Due-Tonnessen, B., Lundar, T., & Helseth, E. (2005). Persistent cognitive dysfunction secondary to cerebellar injury in patients treated for posterior fossa tumors in childhood. *Pediatric Neurosurgery, 41*(1), 15–21.

Spiegler, B. J., Bouffet, E., Greenberg, M. L., Rutka, J. T., & Mabbott, D. J. (2004). Change in neurocognitive functioning after treatment with cranial radiation in childhood. *Journal of Clinical Oncology, 22*(4), 706–713.

Stiles, J. (2008). *The fundamentals of brain development: Integrating nature and nurture.* Cambridge, MA: Harvard University Press.

Tarbell, N. J., Smith, A. R., Adams, J., & Loeffler, J. S. (2000). The challenge of conformal radiotherapy in the curative treatment of medulloblastoma. *International Journal of Radiation Oncology, Biology, Physics, 46*(2), 265–266.

Turner-Cobb, J. M. (2002). Psychosocial and neuroendocrine correlates of disease progression.

In A. Clow, F. Hucklebridge, & P. Evans (Eds.), *Neurobiology of the immune system* (Vol. 52, pp. 358–381). London: Academic Press.

Vannatta, K., Fairclough, F., Farkas-Patenaude, A., Gerhardt, C., Kupst, M., Olshefski, R., et al. (2008, June). *Peer relationships of pediatric brain tumor survivors.* Paper presented at 13th International Symposium on Pediatric Neuro-Oncology, Chicago, IL, USA.

Vannatta, K., Gerhardt, C. A., Wells, R. J., & Noll, R. B. (2007). Intensity of CNS treatment for pediatric cancer: Prediction of social outcomes in survivors. *Pediatric Blood Cancer, 49*(5), 716–722.

von Hoff, K., Hinkes, B., Gerber, N. U., Deinlein, F., Mittler, U., Urban, C., et al. (2009). Long-term outcome and clinical prognostic factors in children with medulloblastoma treated in the prospective randomised multicentre trial HIT'91. *European Journal of Cancer, 45*(7), 1209–1217.

Williams, P. E., Weiss, L. G., & Rolfhus, E. (2003). *WISC-IV technical report #2 psychometric properties.* San Antonio, TX: The Psychological Corporation.

Yeates, K. O., Bigler, E. D., Dennis, M., Gerhardt, C. A., Rubin, K. H., Stancin, T., et al. (2007). Social outcomes in childhood brain disorder: a heuristic integration of social neuroscience and developmental psychology. *Psychological Bulletin, 133*(3), 535–556.

44

Pediatric Epilepsy

Philip S. Fastenau

Childhood-onset epilepsy arises from a variety of causes and is diverse in its presentation and outcomes. An understanding of common neuropsychological deficits, psychosocial comorbidities, and risk factors will equip the neuropsychologist to assess relevant historical variables and neuropsychological functions and to develop more comprehensive intervention strategies.

Overview Of Childhood-Onset Epilepsy

Terminology and Epidemiology

A seizure is a clinical manifestation of abnormal and excessive activity of a set of cortical neurons. Epilepsy is a condition characterized by multiple seizures that are unprovoked (i.e., not due to identifiable acute precipitant, such as fever); some definitions specify that the seizures be separated by more than 24 hours (Hauser, 2001).

Seizures can be classified into several types (CCT-ILAE, 1981). Partial (or "localization-related") seizures originate from a discrete focus in cortex; some of these occur with preservation of awareness (simple partial seizures [SPSs]), whereas others are associated with impaired awareness (complex partial seizures [CPSs]). Within each of these two subtypes, the seizure can remain focal throughout the episode (i.e., without secondary generalization), or it can spread to the contralateral cerebral hemisphere (i.e., with secondary generalization). The second major type is generalized, in which the seizure arises from both cerebral hemispheres simultaneously; these can be further subclassified into generalized absence seizures (characterized by brief staring spells and 3 Hz on electroencephalogram [EEG]) or generalized nonabsence seizures (characterized by various motor symptoms such as tonic, clonic, and myoclonic movements or atonic/"drop" attacks).

Epilepsy can be further classified using a scheme that combines seizure type with other characteristics, including etiology, location of the seizure focus, age of onset, EEG patterns, and prognosis, as well as familial pattern and genetic correlates (CCT-ILAE, 1989). This gives rise to specific syndromes. Some of these arise during infancy and are typically associated with mental retardation, such as Ohtahara syndrome and West syndrome (or "infantile spasms"). Others that appear later are perhaps more likely to come to the attention of the pediatric neuropsychologist. These include Lennox-Gastaut syndrome (or encephalopathic epilepsy with diffuse slow spike waves), Landau-Kleffner syndrome (also known as "acquired epileptic aphasia" because of the arrest or regression of language development induced by seizures), electrical status epilepticus during sleep (ESES; or "continuous spike wave during sleep" [CSWS]), and several absence-related syndromes (childhood absence epilepsy, juvenile absence epilepsy, and juvenile myoclonic epilepsy). Other syndromes that are relatively common are benign epilepsy with centrotemporal spikes (BECTS, or "Rolandic epilepsy") and temporal lobe epilepsy.

With regard to etiology, the majority of children with epilepsy (65%–80%) have idiopathic etiology, which has strong genetic links (Degen, Degen, & Hans, 1991; Degen, Degen, & Koneke, 1993; Segal, Chapman, & Barlow, 1991), or cryptogenic etiology (no clear genetic factor or familial pattern but absence of abnormalities on imaging and neurological exam) (Cowan, Bodensteiner, Leviton, & Doherty, 1989; Theodore et al., 2006). Approximately 20%–35% are symptomatic (i.e., associated with an identifiable structural brain abnormality or neurological condition). In epidemiological studies, common abnormalities include vascular events, intrauterine or perinatal insults (typically with cerebral palsy or mental retardation), trauma, tumors, and brain malformation. Less common abnormalities include neurodegenerative disorders, intracranial infections, chromosomal abnormalities, and neurocutaneous syndromes (especially tuberous sclerosis, neurofibromatosis type 1, Sturge-Weber syndrome) (Cowan et al., 1989; Theodore et al., 2006). Many of the studies documenting structural abnormalities at onset relied heavily on computed tomography (CT). A study by our group using higher resolution magnetic resonance imaging (MRI) among school-aged children identified at least one structural abnormality in 31% of children at the onset of seizures; most common were ventricular enlargement (16%), leukomalacia/gliosis (7%), gray-matter lesions such as heterotopias and cortical dysplasia (4%), volume loss (4%), other white-matter lesions (3%), and encephalomalacia (2%) (Kalnin et al., 2008).

The cumulative incidence of epilepsy is approximately 1% up to age 20. Of these, 10% develop epilepsy before age 1; these are typically severe generalized, symptomatic syndromes accompanied by developmental delays, cerebral palsy, or other neurological deficits. The vast majority of children develop epilepsy after age 1, at which point partial seizures are slightly more common than generalized seizures (Hauser, 2001).

Febrile seizures (seizures provoked by a fever) occur in approximately 2% of children (Hauser, 2001). They are not associated with long-term sequelae if the condition does not evolve into epilepsy (Chang, Guo, Huang, Wang, & Tsai, 2000); however, febrile seizures increase the risk for developing epilepsy, especially when other risk factors are present. Simple febrile seizures (brief, nonfocal, isolated occurrence) increase the risk for developing epilepsy to 2%–3%. Complex febrile seizures (lasting longer than 15 minutes, characterized by focal signs, recurring within 24 hours), when accompanied by a family history of afebrile seizures and neurological abnormalities predating the first febrile seizure, increase the risk of developing epilepsy to 10%–13% (Berg et al., 1992; Tsai & Hung, 1995). Later occurrence of febrile seizures also carry elevated risk for developing epilepsy, with risk increasing after age 3 (Vestergaard et al., 2007) and after age 5 (Voudris et al., 2002). Prolonged febrile seizures have been associated with acute hippocampal changes that can evolve into hippocampal sclerosis (HS; also called mesial temporal sclerosis [MTS]) (Provenzale et al., 2008; Scott et al., 2002). Mesial temporal sclerosis is strongly associated with seizures that are medically refractory ("intractable"), that is, poorly controlled by antiepileptic medications (Grattan-Smith, Harvey, Desmond, & Chow, 1993).

Many children have seizures that are not recognized as such for months or even years prior to diagnosis. Three separate prospective studies (studies characterizing children at the onset of the condition) have consistently found that approximately one-third of children had prior unrecognized seizures before the first seizure was recognized and diagnosed (Austin et al., 2001; Fastenau et al., 2009; Shinnar et al., 1990). That is, among children who are presenting to an emergency department, pediatrician, neurologist, or neuropsychologist for the first time, one in three will have been having these same episodes for months or years without realizing that they were seizures. Those children carry a higher risk of exhibiting behavior problems prior to diagnosis (Austin et al., 2001).

Treatment and Factors Affecting Seizure Control

Seizures can be controlled well by antiepileptic drugs (AEDs) for most children. However, within 3 years of onset 23% of all children with epilepsy (66% of those with early, catastrophic syndromes) meet criteria for being medically refractory (averaging at least one seizure per month for at least 18 months without being seizure-free for 3 consecutive months) after reaching maximum dosing on two AEDs (Berg et al., 2006). After failing to respond to two AEDs, only 3% of individuals achieve seizure freedom on a third AED (Kwan & Brodie, 2000). The rate of medically refractory epilepsy rises to 30% with longer follow-up (across age groups, 9 to 91 years); rates are even higher among those with symptomatic epilepsy (40%) and among those who had more than 20 seizures before starting treatment (51%) (Kwan & Brodie, 2000).

Seizure control can be affected by lifestyle factors. Stress (Reddy & Rogawski, 2002), poor sleep habits or sleep disorders (Malow, 2005), medication nonadherence (Mitchell, Scheier, & Baker, 2000; Sheth & Gidal, 2006), and alcohol consumption (Gordon & Devinsky, 2001) can lead to breakthrough seizures. In women, the menstrual cycle can affect the seizure threshold (Spector, Cull, & Goldstein, 2000). Caffeine, also, has been associated with reduced seizure control (Bonilha & Li, 2004; Kaufman & Sachdeo, 2003). Stress, sleep deprivation, and fatigue rank among the most common precipitants of breakthrough seizures and are highly intercorrelated (Frucht, Quigg, Schwaner, & Fountain, 2000; Spector et al., 2000). Nonadherence has been associated with a variety of adverse clinical and social outcomes among adults (Hovinga et al., 2008).

Some children are prone to status epilepticus (SE), a condition in which the child experiences a prolonged seizure or experiences a rapid succession of seizures without recovering from the prior seizure. This is a medical emergency and requires emergent intervention by paramedics or at the Emergency Department; if there is a history of SE, the child or parent might carry a specific medication to abort the seizure in such circumstances.

The deleterious effects of uncontrolled seizures warrant consideration of alternative treatments, including surgical interventions or the ketogenic diet. Spencer and Huh (2008) conducted a comprehensive review of surgical studies from the past 20 years. They reported that in children neocortical resection results in complete seizure freedom in 59%–70% of children; outcomes are generally better for temporal resection (60%–91% seizure free) compared to resection of nontemporal

cortex (54%–66% seizure free). Factors associated with better seizure control immediately following surgery included unilateral temporal resection, focal lesion on MRI, resection of the lesion and an active region on EEG, and absence of GTCs presurgically. Limited long-term studies suggest that seizure control is relatively stable up to 20 years after surgery; better long-term seizure control is associated with complete resection of the epileptogenic lesion.

With regard to cognitive outcomes following surgery, children tend to stabilize (rather than showing continued deterioration associated with uncontrolled seizures) or even improve. Better developmental and cognitive outcomes have been associated with earlier age at surgery, shorter duration of epilepsy, higher presurgical IQ, and seizure freedom. Declines in verbal memory can be observed following temporal lobectomy, especially with older age at the time of surgery and presence of a structural lesion other than MTS (Spencer & Huh, 2008).

Implantation of a vagal nerve stimulator (VNS) is another surgical option, but it is generally viewed as an alternative for children who are not good candidates for surgical resection (e.g., multilobar or bilateral epileptic foci) (Balabanov & Rossi, 2008; Benifla et al., 2006). Similarly, the ketogenic diet is a well-established nonsurgical option, although not without its own risks (Kossoff & Rho, 2009; Kossoff, Zupec-Kania, Amark, et al., 2009; Kossoff, Zupec-Kania, Rho, et al., 2009).

Comorbidities

Childhood onset of epilepsy is associated with several comorbidities. Mental health problems are very common among children and adolescents with epilepsy (Hermann, 1982). Rates vary across studies, but diagnosable mental health problems have been reported in 26%–29% with uncomplicated epilepsy, which is four to five times higher than observed in general population and 2.5 times higher than observed in other chronic illnesses. Rates are higher when other neurological abnormalities are present (56%–58%). Most common are anxiety disorders (30%–40%), depression (~25%), and attention-deficit/hyperactivity disorder (ADHD; 25%–40% of children with epilepsy) (Davies, Heyman, & Goodman, 2003; Rutter, Graham, &

Yule, 1970). Austin and her colleagues (Austin et al., 2001) demonstrated in a prospective study that behavior problems are evident already at the time of the first identified seizure but that prior unrecognized seizures place children at considerable risk.

Attention-deficit/hyperactivity disorder is more common in epilepsy compared to the general population (38% vs. 6%), but the profiles are different. In the general population two-thirds of adolescents with ADHD have hyperactivity as a significant component of their presentation (e.g., Rohde et al., 1999); however, among adolescents with epilepsy, the vast majority present with predominantly inattentive symptoms (Dunn, Austin, Harezlak, & Ambrosius, 2003; Hermann et al., 2007; Rohde et al., 1999; Sherman et al., 2007). Attention-deficit/hyperactivity disorder occurs with higher frequency in children with more severe conditions (>60%) and is associated with worse quality of life compared to epilepsy without ADHD (Hermann et al., 2007; Sherman et al., 2007). Because behavior problems tend to be internalizing and the ADHD symptoms are mostly inattentive, children and adolescents with epilepsy are at greater risk to be underidentified for services and, thus, undertreated (e.g., Fairbanks, Cunningham, Fastenau, Austin, & Dunn, 2006).

As a group, children with epilepsy perform worse than expected in school. This has been demonstrated in the form of lower grades, lower achievement test scores, more repeated grade levels, more special education placements, and more frequent diagnosis of learning disability (LD) (Farwell, Dodrill, & Batzel, 1985; Fowler, Johnson, & Atkinson, 1985; Mitchell, Chavez, Lee, & Guzman, 1991; Seidenberg et al., 1986). In a recent study of children with chronic epilepsy (on average, about 5 years duration), 48% met psychometric criteria for LD in either writing (38%), math (20%), or reading (13%), with some meeting criteria in more than one domain (Fastenau, Shen, et al., 2008).

Individuals with childhood-onset epilepsy are at significant risk for social problems, especially as they transition through adolescence and into adulthood. Adults with childhood-onset epilepsy are more likely to be unemployed or underemployed, unmarried, and living with parents (Kokkonen, Kokkonen, Saukkonen, & Pennanen, 1997; Sillanpaa, Jalava, Kaleva, & Shinnar, 1998;

Wakamoto, Nagao, Hayashi, & Morimoto, 2000). The greatest disability has been observed in individuals with undercontrolled seizures (Sillanpaa, Haataja, & Shinnar, 2004).

Neuropsychological Functioning

Neuropsychological deficits in children with epilepsy have been documented for many years in chronic populations (e.g., Dodrill & Clemmons, 1984; Farwell et al., 1985; Seidenberg et al., 1988). Many domains have been affected, including attention, psychomotor speed, language, and memory (Deonna, 1993; Dodrill & Clemmons, 1984; Mitchell, Zhou, Chavez, & Guzman, 1992; Piccirilli et al., 1994; Semrud-Clikeman & Wical, 1999; Williams, Griebel, & Dykman, 1998).

Several studies have documented neuropsychological deficiencies close to onset (Hermann et al., 2006; Kolk, Beilmann, Tomberg, Napa, & Talvik, 2001; Oostrom et al., 2003; Stores, Williams, Styles, & Zaiwalla, 1992). Our research team has recently completed a large prospective study following a large cohort of children who had just experienced their first identified seizure ($n = 350$) for 3 years following the first seizure; we also followed a group of healthy sibling controls ($n = 253$) (Fastenau et al., 2009). At onset, 27% of the children with seizures scored at least 1.3 standard deviations below the siblings on one or more neuropsychological domains; this proportion went up to 40% for children with multiple risk factors. Risks associated with deficits at onset included multiple unprovoked seizures (i.e., diagnosis of epilepsy), symptomatic etiology, use of AEDs, and epileptiform activity on the initial EEG; each of these risks individually doubled the risk of having neuropsychological deficits at onset, and the presence of all four risks tripled the risk (Fastenau et al., 2009). In addition, sleep problems, childhood absence epilepsy, and abnormality on neuroimaging (which corresponds with symptomatic etiology) were associated with more neuropsychological deficiencies (Byars et al., 2007; Byars et al., 2008; Fastenau et al., 2009).

Several studies have examined change in cognitive functioning following onset. In one prospective study, deficits were detected at onset, but "group-wise, no changes in cognitive and behavioral differences over time were found" in their small sample over the 4-year follow-up (Oostrom et al., 2005). In our larger study, we found that children with occasional breakthrough seizures (61% of the sample) showed declines or delays in development of processing speed; those with frequent breakthrough seizures (12% of the sample) showed even steeper declines or delays in development of processing speed, as well as less development of memory and executive/attention/construction skills compared to siblings during the 3 years following the first identified seizure. Children with well-controlled seizures continued to develop in all areas at the same rate as their unaffected siblings (Fastenau, Johnson, Dunn, et al., 2008). These findings mirror earlier findings by Bourgeois and colleagues (1983), who observed a decline of 10 or more IQ points in 11% of their prospective cohort during the first 4 years; children who declined were more likely to have persistent seizures or AED levels in the toxic range (which was likely due to higher dosing to control refractory seizures).

Conceptual Model

Fastenau, Dunn, and Austin (2004) constructed a theoretical model to help conceptualize the various factors that affect outcomes following childhood onset of epilepsy. That model illustrates the various factors that have been shown to contribute to the development of neuropsychological deficits and comorbidities in children with epilepsy or, in the case of family functioning, to moderate the impact of neuropsychological deficits on these outcomes (see Fastenau, Shen et al., 2004). The following case study helps to illustrate the contributions of neurological factors, neuropsychological deficits, and the comorbidities described earlier.

Case Presentation

History of Presenting Illness

Melissa was a 12-year-10-month-old, right-handed, Caucasian female referred with a history of medically refractory complex partial seizures. Melissa's history was obtained from interview and from the neurologist's clinic notes. A timeline depicting significant seizure events is presented in Figure 44-1. With regard to developmental history, pregnancy with Melissa was uneventful, and Melissa was delivered vaginally at full term with no complications. Developmental milestones were achieved in timely fashion or

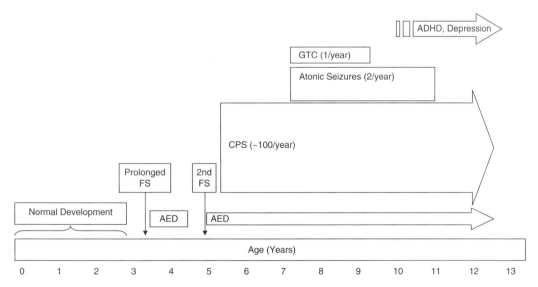

FS = Febrile Seizure, AED = Antiepileptic drug therapy, CPS = Complex Partial Seizure, GTC = Generalized Tonic-Clonic Seizure.

Except where indicated by FS, all seizures were afebrile. Widths of afebrile seizure blocks were intended to grossly convey relative frequency of each seizure type.

Figure 44-1. Timeline of significant events.

earlier than her peers. At age 3, she experienced a prolonged febrile seizure lasting 12 hours; her heart stopped twice while trying to control the seizure. Melissa was placed on an AED (phenytoin) prophylactically, that is, to prevent subsequent seizures; she had no further seizures for a year, at which time it was discontinued. At age 5 she experienced a generalized tonic-clonic seizure ("GTC" or "grand mal"), which was also associated with fever; she was placed on another AED (carbamazepine) at that time.

Shortly thereafter, still age 5, Melissa had her first unprovoked seizure (seizure in the absence of fever or other acute precipitant), which was a complex partial seizure (CPS). This became the primary (or most prevalent) seizure type from that time forward. During these episodes she stared, moved her right arm and hand, drooled, and looked like she was trying to talk but did not say anything; postictally, she became agitated and angry. These seizures occurred approximately two times per week (the most recent one occurred 3 days before the exam) and typically lasted 1–2 minutes. Melissa later developed unprovoked generalized seizures. She had an afebrile GTC at age 7 and a few more since then (the most recent one was 3 years prior to exam). In addition, Melissa had approximately 12 drop attacks and/or episodes of incontinence between the ages of 7 and 11 years.

At school, Melissa did very well in kindergarten; after her first seizure, she was home-schooled for first grade and returned to public school for second grade. She was diagnosed with ADHD at the end of fifth grade. At about that same time she was started on escitalopram for depression. Her father described Melissa as "angry"; he reported discrete episodes when she would become very angry and then not remember the episode later. At the time that Melissa was undergoing a neuropsychological evaluation, she was already scheduled for a consultation with a psychiatrist who specialized in behavioral problems associated with epilepsy in children and adolescents. At the time of this evaluation she was in the seventh grade, excelling at math and spelling but having significant difficulty paying attention; she was in a classroom for children who had mixed diagnoses (LD, ADHD, behavior problems).

Past personal medical history was otherwise unremarkable. There was a distant family history of alcohol dependence and mental illness secondary to lead poisoning; there was no family history of seizures, learning disabilities, or ADHD.

An EEG 4 years earlier showed epileptiform activity in the left temporal region. On an MRI just prior to this exam, the hippocampus was smaller on the left versus the right and was considered by the neuroradiologist to be consistent with MTS. At the time of testing, Melissa was prescribed escitalopram (10 mg qAM) and lamotrigine (300 mg b.i.d.).

Behavior Observations and Validity of Results

During testing, Melissa was cooperative and completed all tasks administered. She stated that she slept only 4–5 hours the night before testing, but she maintained alertness throughout the exam. Throughout testing, she would grit her teeth, pull her hair, pick at her arms and nails, bang her teeth and jaw, and roll her eyes back in her head (especially when frustrated). On Finger Tapping, Melissa showed significant difficulty controlling her right hand and finger. During a test of expressive language functioning (CELF-3 Formulated Sentences), Melissa experienced a seizure. After 30 minutes, she thought she felt back to normal and attempted the JOLO; however, she was still showing signs of agitation, and her performance on the JOLO appeared to be variable so testing was discontinued and the JOLO was deemed to be invalid. Situational and behavioral factors during testing were taken into consideration in the interpretations of the test results. The following results are considered to be reliable and valid unless otherwise qualified.

Test Results

Melissa's test scores are summarized in Table 44-1. She was functioning in the middle of the average range of intelligence overall. Relative deficits were observed in the areas of verbal skills broadly. The WISC-III Verbal Comprehension Standard Score (SS) was 20 points lower than the Perceptual-Organizational SS; the lowest subtest score was on a measure with significant expressive language demands (Vocabulary). Confrontation naming was significantly impaired (BNT).

Table 44-1. Summary of Test Scores

Wechsler Intelligence Scale for Children, 3rd Ed.	Raw	ss	SS-Equivalent
Information	14	7	85
Similarities	22	12	110
Vocabulary	21	5	75
Comprehension	22	8	90
Picture Completion	20	8	90
Picture Arrangement	32	9	95
Block Design	46	10	100
Object Assembly	42	18	140
Arithmetic	20	11	105
Digit Span	15	10	100
Coding	46	7	85
Symbol Search	31	13	115
Verbal Comprehension Index			89
Perceptual Organization Index			109
Freedom from Distractibility Index			104
Processing Speed Index			101

Finger Tapping	Raw	z	SS-Equivalent
Dominant Hand	42.1	0.1	102
Nondominant Hand	37.4	0.5	108

Boston Naming Test	Raw	z	SS-Equivalent
No. Correct	39	−2.4	64

Clinical Evaluation of Language Fundamentals, 3rd Ed.	Raw	ss	SS-Equivalent
Concepts & Directions	26	9	95
Formulated Sentences	Seizure		

Judgment of Line Orientation	Raw	z	SS-Equivalent
No. Correct	Not Valid		

Wide Range Assessment of Memory & Learning	Raw	ss	SS-Equivalent
Story Memory	14	5	75
Verbal Learning (Trials 1–4: 6/9/8/9)	32	9	95
Design Memory	18	3	65
Story Memory Delay	17	Average	WNL
Story Memory Recognition	11	Average	WNL
Verbal Learning Delay	3	Atypical	Atypical
Design Copy (28 Possible Points)	28	WNL	WNL

Rey Auditory Verbal Learning Test	Raw	z	SS-Equivalent
Trial 1	4	−1.8	73
Trial 2	7	−1.1	84
Trial 3	10	−0.2	97
Trial 4	11	−0.2	97
Trial 5	12	0.1	102
Sum 1–5	44	−0.8	88
List B	4	−1.1	84
Trial 6—Raw	6	−2.0	70
Trial 6—% of Trial 5	50		
Delayed Free Recall—Raw	7	−1.6	76
Delayed Free Recall—% of Trial 5	58		
Delayed Recognition T+	15		
Delayed Recognition F+	10		

(Continued)

Table 44-1. Summary of Test Scores (*Continued*)

Extended Complex Figure Test	Raw	z	SS-Equivalent
Copy	20.0	–1.6 *	76
Immediate Recall	7.5	–1.3 *	81
Delayed Recall	7.5	–1.4 *	79
Delayed Recognition (Raw of 6 = Chance)	7	–2.0	70
Matching	8	WNL	WNL

Wisconsin Card-Sorting Test	Raw	T	SS-Equivalent
Total Administered	80		
Total Correct	69		
Percent Errors (Total)	14	65	123
Percent Perseverative Errors	5	73	134
Percent Nonperseverative Errors	9	56	109
Percent Conceptual Level Responses	84	65	122
Categories Completed	6	WNL	WNL
Trials to First Category	13	WNL	WNL
Failure to Maintain Set	1	WNL	WNL
Learning to Learn	2.8	WNL	WNL

Note. For all test scores in the table above, higher scores indicate better performance. See text for descriptions interpretation and qualifications to the results.

*For Rey figure drawings, z scores were generated using preliminary child norms in ECFT Manual (Fastenau, 2003) using the same paradigm (Copy, Immediate Recall, 20- to 30-min Delayed Recall) for direct comparison to Recognition scores. However, the Copy z score is identical to that obtained on a much larger age-matched subgroup ($n = 225$) (Strauss, Sherman, & Spreen, 2006), suggesting that these norms are representative.

SS, standard score ($M = 100$, SD = 15), T = T Score ($M = 50$, SD = 10), ss = Scaled Score ($M = 10$, SD = 3), z = z score ($M = 0$, SD = 1), WNL, within normal limits.

With regard to fine motor manual speed, the right hand showed the appropriate advantage relative to the left hand; however, coordination was much worse on the right hand compared to the left hand. It is also noteworthy that a measure of receptive language was normal (average range); on a measure of expressive syntactical language (CELF-3 FS subtest), Melissa experienced a seizure.

With regard to memory functioning, memory acquisition was deficient for both verbal and spatial information immediately after the stimulus was presented; performance after a delay was nearly identical, suggesting that the forgetting curves are minimal for verbal and spatial information beyond initial acquisition. For verbal learning, acquisition over multiple trials was normal (initial acquisition poor but reaching normal levels by the third trial). However, after Melissa was presented with an alternate list, her recall of the original list dropped to 50% (retroactive interference) and remained at that level after a delay. Furthermore, her recognition performance for

that list was characterized by numerous false-positive endorsements.

The Rey Copy drawing was constructed in a segmented/piecemeal fashion, resulting in a spatially disorganized drawing that suggests lack of appreciation for the gestalt, which was further reflected in her recall for the design. Recognition memory was not significantly different from chance, confirming that the memory trace was never adequately formed (ECFT Recognition, 7 out of 30). This cannot be attributed to deficient visuoperceptual processes because of Melissa's near-perfect score on a subtest of spatial synthesis/construction (Object Assembly) and scores in the average range on other WISC-III spatially taxing subtests. Executive functioning (e.g., abstract thinking, mental flexibility) was very proficient.

Because Melissa could not continue with testing and because surgery was expected, assessment of academic achievement and sustained attention were postponed for the postsurgical evaluation.

Unfortunately, I did not have the opportunity to see her for that evaluation.

Impressions and Recommendations

These neuropsychological results strongly implicate dysfunction of left frontotemporal neural systems. Inasmuch as these findings converge with the left temporal focus identified by EEG, the left temporal/hippocampal abnormality on MRI, and the focal signs in Melissa's behavior during her seizures (speech automatisms and right-side movement), they further support this as the predominant active cerebral focus of Melissa's seizures. The deficiency in spatial memory might be due to spreading activation (especially since the epileptogenic tissue is mesial temporal), given the absence of any other strongly lateralizing signs on the right; however, we cannot rule out a second focus on the right with absolute certainty based on the present results.

1. To the degree that many neuropsychological results converge with other studies to localize the active seizure focus in the area of the left MTS, complete resection of that lesion and seizure focus would carry a good prognosis for seizure reduction from the neuropsychological standpoint. However, a history of GTC seizures can be associated with suboptimal seizure control postsurgically. Melissa's poor spatial memory scores also raise the possibility of a contralateral seizure focus, which would further contribute to a more guarded prognosis with regard to seizure control following resective surgery if confirmed on video EEG.

2. With regard to cognitive prognosis following surgery, the relatively long duration of her condition (7–8 years) and her older age at surgery carry risk for verbal memory decline, but the risk might be offset to some degree by her strong intellectual ability and MTS, especially if complete seizure freedom can be achieved after surgery.

3. In this right-hander whose lesion and seizure disorder appear to have developed after language development was fairly well established, there is a 96%–98% probability that speech and verbal language functions are well supported in the left hemisphere (e.g.,

Knecht et al., 2000; Rasmussen & Milner, 1977). A Wada exam or fMRI could help to ascertain the degree to which the right hemisphere could support language and memory functions following resection.

4. Since surgery will likely involve eloquent cortex (i.e., cortex supporting language functions), language mapping by electrocorticography prior to or during surgery would help to demarcate more clearly the boundaries of functional tissue and to predict the functional consequences with different resection lines.

5. If speech or motor deficits are apparent immediately after surgery, acute rehabilitation should be beneficial to help remediate those deficits.

6. Melissa should have a repeat neuropsychological evaluation 12 months after surgery to identify other residual or resulting cognitive deficits and behavioral issues and to plan psychoeducational and psychiatric interventions to address those challenges.

7. It would be very beneficial to encourage Melissa to establish routines that would maximize her sleep duration and quality. This will be helpful not only in optimizing cognitive and academic functioning but should also improve seizure control.

8. Melissa's anger outbursts (particularly with no recollection or limited memory for the event) are consistent with temporal lobe epilepsy. Better seizure control might incidentally improve control over the anger episodes; however, even after seizures are well managed, children with past seizure histories can continue to have behavioral challenges. Ongoing consultation with a child psychiatrist who specializes in epilepsy would be invaluable for assisting in the management of Melissa's behavioral problems.

Discussion

Melissa illustrates many of the principles of epilepsy as expressed in childhood. These will be summarized and discussed, followed by atypical features to her presentation and to this particular neuropsychological evaluation. Finally, I will provide recommendations for approaching assessment and intervention with this population.

General Features of Childhood-Onset Epilepsy

Melissa was developing normally before she experienced her first seizure, which is characteristic of approximately two-thirds of children with epilepsy, especially those with later onset. Her first unprovoked seizure was a complex partial seizure, which is most commonly associated with temporal lobe origin and the semiology (the signs during the seizure that provide clues to the location of the seizure focus) lateralized to the left hemisphere; Melissa's EEG and MRI both converged with the semiology to implicate left temporal cortex as the source of her primary seizures. Within 2 years, she had a generalized tonic-clonic seizure; it is not uncommon for CPS to be attended by secondary generalization (i.e., spreading of the seizure to the contralateral hemisphere through commissural fibers), but in her case the GTC was believed to be a primary generalized seizure (i.e., an independent seizure type) because it did not start with the same symptoms as her partial seizure. (Video EEG monitoring can help to confirm this as part of a presurgical workup, if both types of seizures can be elicited during the recording period.) Soon thereafter, Melissa developed a third seizure type, atonic epileptic seizures, or "drop attacks" (another subtype of primary generalized seizures); these are much less common, occurring in 1%–3% of children with epilepsy (Duchowny, 1987; Tinuper et al., 1998).

Febrile Seizures

Melissa was having febrile seizures as late as age 5, which increased the probability that she would develop epilepsy. The complex nature of her febrile seizures—prolonged and recurrent—increased the risk not only for developing epilepsy but also for developing MTS, which is associated with medically refractory seizures. These risks likely contributed to the decision to initiate AEDs at that time, especially since the risks of another seizure (even a febrile seizure, given her history of febrile status epilepticus and cardiac arrest) outweighed potential side effects of AEDs. In Melissa's case, all of these risks materialized (epilepsy, refractory seizures, and MTS).

Risk Factors for Early Neuropsychological Deficits and Decline

Melissa possessed many risk factors for developing neuropsychological deficits very early in her condition, including epileptiform activity on her initial EEG, structural abnormality on MRI, symptomatic syndrome, seizure recurrence (i.e., development of epilepsy), and treatment with antiepileptic drugs, as well as a history of ADHD. She also developed persistent seizures very early in the course of her condition, which have been associated with neuropsychological decline.

Sleep, Stress, and Postictal State

Melissa slept only a few hours before traveling to the medical center for her neuropsychological exam. In this sleep-deprived state, she experienced a seizure during a test of expressive language. This illustrates several important points. First, sleep deprivation increases the likelihood of having a seizure, especially in individuals who are stressed or who are not optimally controlled (e.g., those with refractory epilepsy or those who have been nonadherent with AEDs). Second, when seizures occur during neuropsychological testing, often they are correlated with the location of the seizure focus (Helmstaedter, Hufnagel, & Elger, 1992). Finally, following seizures that impair awareness (such as the complex partial seizure that Melissa experienced during testing, but also GTCs), there is a period following the seizure when the individual can experience fatigue, cognitive slowing, and confusion (a "postictal state"); the person might actually sleep for 10 minutes to several hours, but he or she will typically continue to show at least subtle effects for 24 hours (and even several days if the person had several seizures in the same day). As observed on the JOLO with Melissa, even after she felt fine, she showed very obvious cognitive interference on neuropsychological testing. Therefore, it is generally recommended that testing be postponed if the child has had a seizure within 24 hours prior to the evaluation and that testing be discontinued for the day if the child has a seizure during testing.

Lateralizing/Localizing Features

As neuropsychologists, we are often interested in localizing signs, and this is especially important in the child who is being considered for surgical management because the surgical team can place more confidence in a surgical target site if the neuropsychological test results converge with other exams. Melissa's seizures already showed lateralizing features (right arm movement and speech motor activity). In addition, she experienced a seizure during testing while she was completing a test of expressive language (see previous section). Finally, her neuropsychological profile was noteworthy for language deficits (WISC-III VC < PO and very low Vocabulary and BNT) and lack of fine motor control during the right-hand trial of Finger Tapping. Assuming conventional lateralization of verbal aspects of language to the left hemisphere, which is characteristic of 96% of right-handers (Knecht et al., 2000; Rasmussen & Milner, 1977)—as well as 70% of left-handers (Segalowitz & Bryden, 1983)—the formal test results also lateralize to the left for the most part. The equivalent deficiencies on verbal and spatial memory tasks might represent a second seizure focus in the contralateral hemisphere; video EEG can be helpful at determining the extent to which she has characteristic seizures arising from the right.

Cognitive Profiles of Antiepileptic Drugs

Melissa was prescribed one of the newer AEDs, lamotrogine, for which cognitive deficits have not been reported as a common adverse drug reaction. In addition, she was prescribed a level that was in the lower end of the therapeutic range (approximately 4 mg/kg/day). Among the newer AEDs, topirimate has been associated with cognitive difficulties, whereas the others appear to have limited adverse cognitive effects when used in monotherapy and based on group analysis. Among the older AEDs, phenobarbital is most often associated with cognitive side effects, and phenytoin and barbiturates have been implicated to a lesser degree. However, these statements are based largely on studies of monotherapy reported at the group level; any individual child can experience adverse cognitive effects on any AED or

due to interactions among medications; therefore, cognitive complaints must be monitored and clinically correlated with changes in AEDs for each child (Bourgeois, 2004; Ortinski & Meador, 2004).

Comorbidities

Melissa was diagnosed with ADHD (without hyperactivity) and depression 6 years after her first unprovoked seizure; it is possible that these symptoms were present earlier but were undetected, given their internalizing nature. Also, her father described her as angry and reported discrete tirades; because Melissa had no recall for the events afterward, it is possible that these were manifestations of complex partial seizures. This exemplifies an important distinction in epilepsy: Although complex partial seizures are typically defined as involving "loss of consciousness," they are perhaps better described as involving loss of *awareness*. During the seizure the person can continue to carry out some basic automated activities and react to environmental cues in stereotypical fashion (e.g., nodding at someone who is attempting to converse with him or her), but without comprehending or retaining anything during the event. In some cases, the behaviors can be fairly complex and seem intentional (e.g., yelling, striking out), but in truth the person has no awareness. The behavior problems were treated with an antidepressant medication as an adjunct to AEDs, which is recommended but requires special considerations among children and adolescents with epilepsy (Ekinci et al., 2009; Kanner, 2008; Kanner & Dunn, 2004). It is particularly noteworthy that even though she was showing symptoms of ADHD by the fifth grade, she was not identified by the school as needing services for several more years, and it was the behavior problems (not learning concerns) that prompted the services. Underidentification of learning-related problems (e.g., ADHD, LD) is common (Fairbanks et al., 2006). Treatment of ADHD with stimulant medications has been complicated by concerns that stimulants might exacerbate the seizure condition; recent reviews of the evidence suggest that psychostimulants and the nonstimulant atomoxetine are effective and safe with this population (Schubert & Schubert, 2005; Torres, Whitney, & Gonzalez-Heydrich, 2008; Wernicke et al., 2007).

Atypical Features about This Case

Some aspects of Melissa's presentation are less typical, and the approach to testing in the present exam varies in some respects from my recommended outpatient evaluation due to the nature of the referral question and due to testing circumstances. First, although it is not uncommon to have two seizure types (20% of children in our study of children with chronic epilepsy) (Fastenau, Shen et al., 2004), it is rare for a child to have three distinct seizure types. Melissa had CPS as her primary seizure type, together with GTC and atonic seizures.

Second, the approach to testing in the present exam was tailored to a specific referral question and was also limited by testing circumstances. Because Melissa was referred by the epilepsy surgery team, a priority in the evaluation was to determine whether she showed focal features that would lend further support to the other localizing test results and to evaluate current memory and language functioning to assist in forecasting risks associated with surgery. In these circumstances, the test battery was designed to give priority to those goals with the plan to perform a more standard outpatient evaluation after the child recovered from surgery. Also, emotional and behavioral assessment was not administered as part of this specific evaluation because Melissa was already scheduled to be seen in a multidisciplinary child psychiatry clinic; however, behavioral assessment should be an integral part of every evaluation of children with epilepsy, especially when surgery is not imminent.

Considerations for Assessment

When approaching a child with a history of seizures or new onset of seizures, there are many special issues to consider as part of the chart review, interview, testing, and intervention. When taking a history, the neuropsychologist will want to attend to the risk factors enumerated previously (e.g., complex febrile seizures, abnormal EEG or MRI, persistent/refractory seizures) and the comorbidities associated with epilepsy (behavior, academic, and social problems).

Essential to any evaluation will be measures of sustained attention and academic functioning, as well as fundamental skills associated with any academic areas that are deficient (e.g., phonological processing). Processing speed is not only essential to learning and classroom performance but is also predictive of decline in multiple arenas (Fastenau, Johnson, Perkins, et al., 2008). Related to this, when assessing academic skills, it will be beneficial to assess speed of operations (or fluency) in each of the academic domains. In some instances, there will be uniform depression across reading, math, and writing fluency measures with normal achievement of mechanical and conceptual skills, showing the more general (but devastating) impact of processing speed on classroom performance and standardized testing. For nonsurgical or postsurgical evaluations of children with epilepsy, the clinician is advised to approach the evaluation with LD and ADHD in mind, including the component skills required for developing proficiency in any academic domain that appears to be affected (e.g., if reading difficulties are evident, assessing phonological memory/auditory verbal working memory [AVWM], phonological awareness/decoding, rapid automatic naming, vocabulary, etc.). For all academic domains, it is paramount in this population to assess fluency within each domain; the WJ-III (Woodcock, Schrank, Mather, & McGrew, 2007) provides a good platform for systematically assessing fluency in reading, writing, and math for direct comparison to performance on the fundamental/mechanical skills and the applied/conceptual skills using achievement tests that were co-normed on the same standardization sample for ease of direct comparison.

As noted earlier, certain seizure types (e.g., complex partial seizures, generalized nonabsence seizures) often produce fatigue and affect cognition for up to 48 hours after the seizure. Therefore, before beginning testing it is good practice to ask when the child had his or her last seizure and also to ask whether there is a history of status epilepticus and whether the child or parent has abortive medications with them. If a seizure occurs during testing, provide seizure first aid (e.g., see http://www.epilepsyfoundation.org) to keep the child safe during the seizure; involve the parent as soon as it is safe to do so (without leaving the child unattended). If the seizure persists more than 5 minutes (Lowenstein, Bleck, & Macdonald, 1999) or if the child experiences multiple seizures in succession (i.e., status epilepticus), either the parent will need to administer an abortive medication or you will need to call 911.

Intervention and Consultation

In an earlier review of the literature and risk factors for neuropsychological deficits and comorbidities among children with epilepsy, Fastenau, Dunn, and Austin (2004) advocated for a multifaceted approach to intervention. First, it is critical to control the seizures. Neuropsychologists can play a critical role in seizure control by obtaining a detailed history of AEDs and seizure control and educating the child and family about the factors that affect seizure control: taking medications as prescribed with the goal of no missed doses; implementing good sleep habits (e.g., going to bed and waking at the same time every day, removing distractions from the bedroom, avoiding eating or exercising for several hours prior to bedtime); engaging in good stress management activities; and (for individuals of legal age) limiting alcohol consumption to modest levels.

Second, optimize learning and adaptation. The neuropsychological evaluation is critical for identifying cognitive and academic deficiencies; for initiating, informing, and guiding the design of interventions and accommodations in the classroom; and for monitoring progress. Evidence suggests that family intervention to improve emotional support and structure at home can improve outcomes in this population (Fastenau, Shen et al., 2004; Mitchell et al., 1991).

Third, manage behavior problems. The neuropsychological evaluation can play a critical role to characterize the nature of behavior problems; to disentangle the contributions of seizure, cognitive, and emotional factors (e.g., ignoring parents because of brief seizures versus in attention versus defiance); and to arrange for child and family psychotherapy and referral to a psychiatrist (preferably one with expertise in working with people with epilepsy) depending on the nature of the child's needs.

Fourth and finally, educate the family about epilepsy. The Epilepsy Foundation (http://www.epilepsyfoundation.org) has a rich library of resources, ranging from pamphlets to children's books to parent-directed books to videos. In addition, there are regional chapters throughout the United States and either The Epilepsy Foundation or its local chapter can provide information on local meetings and support groups. Outside of the United States, the International League Against Epilepsy (ILAE; http://www.ilae.org) provides similar resources and meetings.

Conclusion

The empirical literature reviewed in conjunction with this case highlights many risk and protective factors for the comorbidities associated with childhood-onset epilepsy, and these factors highlight critical roles for the neuropsychologist in working with this population. First, the neuropsychologist will assess risks for *developing* epilepsy (e.g., brain abnormalities, complex FS, or family history of epilepsy) in a child who is showing symptoms that are suspicious of seizures but who has not been diagnosed. If the child has been diagnosed with epilepsy, that alone carries risk for developing neuropsychological deficits and warrants prompt neuropsychological evaluation; additional risk factors for early cognitive deficits or for cognitive decline should increase the sense of urgency in conducting such an evaluation. As part of the evaluation, it is important to obtain a thorough history of seizures (age of onset, seizure types, seizure frequency, AEDs), factors associated with seizure control (stress, sleep, fatigue, AED nonadherence, menstrual correlates, and alcohol and caffeine use), and potential comorbidities (neuropsychological, academic, behavioral, and social functioning).

The neuropsychological test battery needs to be comprehensive, and processing speed is especially important. Academic testing should include timed and untimed measures to document the potential impact of processing speed on performance in the classroom, even in a child who is mastering the requisite skills. In addition, the neuropsychologist plays an important role in providing or coordinating an array of interventions to improve seizure control (e.g., AED monitoring and adherence), to address neuropsychological deficiencies (e.g., speech, physical, occupational therapy; cognitive rehabilitation; classroom accommodations), and to ameliorate other comorbidities (e.g., psychotherapy or psychiatric consultation for pharmacotherapy, educational interventions, family therapy). Finally, the neuropsychologist who is working with an epilepsy surgery center can play additional roles that are unique to that setting.

Disclosure

Dr. Fastenau is the author of the *Extended Complex Figure Test* (Fastenau, 2003), which was administered as part of the testing in this case study. He receives royalties from the sale of that test. Dr. Fastenau's wife works for Eli Lilly & Co., participates in a stock-based pension, and holds stock options in that company.

References

Austin, J. K., Harezlak, J., Dunn, D. W., Huster, G. A., Rose, D. F., & Ambrosius, W. T. (2001). Behavior problems in children before first recognized seizures. *Pediatrics*, *107*(1), 115–122.

Balabanov, A., & Rossi, M. A. (2008). Epilepsy surgery and vagal nerve stimulation: What all neurologists should know. *Seminars in Neurology*, *28*(3), 355–363.

Benifla, M., Rutka, J. T., Logan, W., Donner, E. J., (2006). Vagal nerve stimulation for refractory epilepsy in children: Indications and experience at The Hospital for Sick Children. *Childs Nervous System*, *22*(8), 1018–1026.

Berg, A. T., Shinnar, S., Hauser, W. A., Alemany, M., Shapiro, E. D., Salomon, M. E., et al. (1992). A prospective study of recurrent febrile seizures. *New England Journal of Medicine*, *327*(16), 1122–1127.

Berg, A. T., Vickrey, B. G., Testa, F. M., Levy, S. R., Shinnar, S., DiMario, F., et al. (2006). How long does it take for epilepsy to become intractable? A prospective investigation. *Annals of Neurology*, *60*(1), 73–79.

Bonilha, L., & Li, L. M. (2004). Heavy coffee drinking and epilepsy. *Seizure*, *13*(4), 284–285.

Bourgeois, B. F. (2004). Determining the effects of antiepileptic drugs on cognitive function in pediatric patients with epilepsy. *Journal of Child Neurology*, *19*(Suppl. 1), S15–S24.

Bourgeois, B. F., Prensky, A. L., Palkes, H. S., Talent, B. K., & Busch, S. G. (1983). Intelligence in epilepsy: A prospective study in children. *Annals of Neurology*, *14*(4), 438–444.

Byars, A. W., Byars, K. C., Johnson, C. S., DeGrauw, T. J., Fastenau, P. S., Perkins, S., et al. (2008). The relationship between sleep problems and neuropsychological functioning in children with first recognized seizures. *Epilepsy and Behavior*, *13*(4), 607–613.

Byars, A. W., deGrauw, T. J., Johnson, C. S., Fastenau, P. S., Perkins, S. M., Egelhoff, J. C., et al. (2007). The association of MRI findings and neuropsychological functioning after the first recognized seizure. *Epilepsia*, *48*(6), 1067–1074.

CCT-ILAE (1981). Proposal for revised clinical and electroencephalographic classification of epileptic seizures. From the Commission on Classification and Terminology of the International League Against Epilepsy. *Epilepsia*, *22*(4), 489–501.

CCT-ILAE (1989). Proposal for revised classification of epilepsies and epileptic syndromes. Commission on Classification and Terminology of the International League Against Epilepsy. *Epilepsia*, *30*(4), 389–399.

Chang, Y. C., Guo, N. W., Huang, C. C., Wang, S. T., & Tsai, J. J. (2000). Neurocognitive attention and behavior outcome of school-age children with a history of febrile convulsions: A population study. *Epilepsia*, *41*(4), 412–420.

Cowan, L. D., Bodensteiner, J. B., Leviton, A., & Doherty, L. (1989). Prevalence of the epilepsies in children and adolescents. *Epilepsia*, *30*(1), 94–106.

Davies, S., Heyman, I., & Goodman, R. (2003). A population survey of mental health problems in children with epilepsy. *Developmental Medicine and Child Neurology*, *45*(5), 292–295.

Degen, R., Degen, H. E., & Hans, K. (1991). A contribution to the genetics of febrile seizures: Waking and sleep EEG in siblings. *Epilepsia*, *32*(4), 515–522.

Degen, R., Degen, H. E., & Koneke, B. (1993). On the genetics of complex partial seizures: waking and sleep EEGs in siblings. *Journal of Neurology*, *240*(3), 151–155.

Deonna, T. (1993). Annotation: Cognitive and behavioural correlates of epileptic activity in children. *Journal of Child Psychology and Psychiatry and Allied Disciplines*, *34*(5), 611–620.

Dodrill, C. B., & Clemmons, D. (1984). Use of neuropsychological tests to identify high school students with epilepsy who later demonstrate inadequate performances in life. *Journal of Consulting and Clinical Psychology*, *52*, 520–527.

Duchowny, M. S. (1987). Atonic seizures. *Pediatrics in Review*, *9*(2), 43–49.

Dunn, D. W., Austin, J. K., Harezlak, J., & Ambrosius, W. T. (2003). ADHD and epilepsy in childhood. *Developmental Medicine and Child Neurology*, *45*(1), 50–54.

Ekinci, O., Titus, J. B., Rodopman, A. A., Berkem, M., Trevathan, E. (2009). Depression and anxiety in children and adolescents with epilepsy: Prevalence, risk factors, and treatment. *Epilepsy and Behavior*, *14*(1), 8–18.

Fairbanks, J. M., Cunningham, N. C., Fastenau, P. S., Austin, J. K., & Dunn, D. W. (2006). ADHD in epilepsy: Discrepant proportions between the CSI/ASI and school classification. *Epilepsia, 47*(Suppl. 4), 133.

Farwell, J. R., Dodrill, C. B., & Batzel, L. W. (1985). Neuropsychological abilities of children with epilepsy. *Epilepsia, 26*(5), 395–400.

Fastenau, P. S. (2003). *Extended Complex Figure Test (ECFT) Manual*. Los Angeles: Western Psychological Services.

Fastenau, P. S., Dunn, D. W., & Austin, J. K. (2004). Pediatric epilepsy. In M. Rizzo & P. J. Eslinger (Eds.), *Principles and practice of behavioral neurology and neuropsychology* (pp. 965–982). New York: Saunders/Churchill Livingstone/Mosby.

Fastenau, P. S., Shen, J., Dunn, D. W., Austin, J. K. (2008). Academic underachievement among children with epilepsy: Proportion exceeding psychometric criteria for learning disability and associated risk factors. *Journal of Learning Disabilities, 41*(3), 195–207.

Fastenau, P. S., Johnson, C. S., Dunn, D. W., Byars, A. W., Perkins, S. M., deGrauw, T. J., et al. (2008). Relationship between seizure control and neuropsychological changes during the first 3 years following seizure onset in children. *Epilepsia, 49*(s7), 494–495.

Fastenau, P. S., Johnson, C. S., Perkins, S. M., Byars, A. W., deGrauw, T. J., Austin, J. K., et al. (2009). Neuropsychological status at seizure onset in children: Risk factors for early cognitive deficits. *Neurology, 73*(7), 526–534.

Fastenau, P. S., Johnson, C. S., Perkins, S. M., Byars, A. W., Dunn, D. W., & Austin, J. K. (2008). Comorbidities associated with declining neuropsychological performance 3 years following first recognized seizure in children. *Journal of the International Neuropsychological Society, 14*(S1), 200–201.

Fastenau, P. S., Shen, J., Dunn, D. W., Perkins, S. M., Hermann, B. P., & Austin, J. K. (2004). Neuropsychological predictors of academic underachievement in pediatric epilepsy: Moderating roles of demographic, seizure, and psychosocial variables. *Epilepsia, 45*(10), 1261–1272.

Fowler, M. G., Johnson, M. P., & Atkinson, S. S. (1985). School achievement and absence in children with chronic health conditions. *Journal of Pediatrics, 106*, 683–687.

Frucht, M. M., Quigg, M., Schwaner, C., & Fountain, N. B. (2000). Distribution of seizure precipitants among epilepsy syndromes. *Epilepsia, 41*(12), 1534–1539.

Gordon, E., & Devinsky, O. (2001). Alcohol and marijuana: Effects on epilepsy and use by patients with epilepsy. *Epilepsia, 42*(10), 1266–1272.

Grattan-Smith, J. D., Harvey, A. S., Desmond, P. M., & Chow, C. W. (1993). Hippocampal sclerosis in children with intractable temporal lobe epilepsy: Detection with MR imaging. *American Journal of Roentgenology, 161*(5), 1045–1048.

Hauser, W. A. (2001). Epidemiology of epilepsy in children. In J. M. Pellock, W. E. Dodson, & B. F. D. Bourgeois (Eds.), *Pediatric epilepsy: Diagnosis and therapy* (2nd ed., pp. 81–96). New York: Demos Medical Publishing.

Helmstaedter, C., Hufnagel, A., & Elger, C. E. (1992). Seizures during cognitive testing in patients with temporal lobe epilepsy: Possibility of seizure induction by cognitive activation. *Epilepsia, 33*(5), 892–897.

Hermann, B. P. (1982). Neuropsychological functioning and psychopathology in children with epilepsy. *Epilepsia, 23*(5), 545–554.

Hermann, B. P., Jones, J. E., Dabbs, K., Allen, C. A., Sheth, R., Fine, J., et al. (2007). The frequency, complications and aetiology of ADHD in new onset paediatric epilepsy. *Brain, 130*(Pt. 12), 3135–3148.

Hermann, B. P., Jones, J. E., Sheth, R., Dow, C., Koehn, M., & Seidenberg, M. (2006). Children with new-onset epilepsy: Neuropsychological status and brain structure. *Brain, 129*(Pt. 10), 2609–2619.

Hovinga, C. A., Asato, M. R., Manjunath, R., Wheless, J. W., Phelps, S. J., Sheth, R. D., et al. (2008). Association of non-adherence to antiepileptic drugs and seizures, quality of life, and productivity: Survey of patients with epilepsy and physicians. *Epilepsy and Behavior, 13*(2), 316–322.

Kalnin, A. J., Fastenau, P. S., deGrauw, T. J., Musick, B. S., Perkins, S. M., Johnson, C. S., et al. (2008). Magnetic resonance imaging findings in children with a first recognized seizure. *Pediatric Neurology, 39*(6), 404–414.

Kanner, A. M. (2008). The use of psychotropic drugs in epilepsy: What every neurologist should know. *Seminars in Neurology, 28*(3), 379–388.

Kanner, A. M., & Dunn, D. W. (2004). Diagnosis and management of depression and psychosis in children and adolescents with epilepsy. *Journal of Child Neurology, 19*(Suppl. 1), S65–S72.

Kaufman, K. R., & Sachdeo, R. C. (2003). Caffeinated beverages and decreased seizure control. *Seizure, 12*(7), 519–521.

Knecht, S., Drager, B., Deppe, M., Bobe, L., Lohmann, H., Floel, A., et al. (2000). Handedness and hemispheric language dominance in healthy humans. *Brain, 123*(Pt. 12), 2512–2518.

Kokkonen, J., Kokkonen, E. R., Saukkonen, A. L., & Pennanen, P. (1997). Psychosocial outcome of young adults with epilepsy in childhood. *Journal of Neurology, Neurosurgery and Psychiatry, 62*(3), 265–268.

Kolk, A., Beilmann, A., Tomberg, T., Napa, A., & Talvik, T. (2001). Neurocognitive development of children with congenital unilateral brain lesion and epilepsy. *Brain and Development, 23*(2), 88–96.

Kossoff, E. H., & Rho, J. M. (2009). Ketogenic diets: Evidence for short- and long-term efficacy. *Neurotherapeutics, 6*(2), 406–414.

Kossoff, E. H., Zupec-Kania, B. A., Amark, P. E., Ballaban-Gil, K. R., Christina Bergqvist, A. G., Blackford, R., et al. (2009). Optimal clinical management of children receiving the ketogenic diet: Recommendations of the International Ketogenic Diet Study Group. *Epilepsia, 50*(2), 304–317.

Kossoff, E. H., Zupec-Kania, B. A., Rho, J. M. (2009). Ketogenic diets: An update for child neurologists. *Journal of Child Neurology, 24*(8), 979–988.

Kwan, P., & Brodie, M. J. (2000). Early identification of refractory epilepsy. *New England Journal of Medicine, 342*(5), 314–319.

Lowenstein, D. H., Bleck, T., & Macdonald, R. L. (1999). It's time to revise the definition of status epilepticus. *Epilepsia, 40*(1), 120–122.

Malow, B. A. (2005). Sleep and epilepsy. *Neurologic Clinics, 23*(4), 1127–1147.

Mitchell, W. G., Chavez, J. M., Lee, H., & Guzman, B. L. (1991). Academic underachievement in children with epilepsy. *Journal of Child Neurology, 6*(1), 65–72.

Mitchell, W. G., Scheier, L. M., & Baker, S. A. (2000). Adherence to treatment in children with epilepsy: Who follows "doctor's orders"? *Epilepsia, 41*(12), 1616–1625.

Mitchell, W. G., Zhou, Y., Chavez, J. M., & Guzman, B. L. (1992). Reaction time, attention, and impulsivity in epilepsy. *Pediatric Neurology, 8*(1), 19–24.

Oostrom, K. J., Smeets-Schouten, A., Kruitwagen, C. L., Peters, A. C., Jennekens-Schinkel, A., & Dutch Study Group of Epilepsy in Childhood. (2003). Not only a matter of epilepsy: Early problems of cognition and behavior in children with "epilepsy only"—A prospective, longitudinal, controlled study starting at diagnosis. *Pediatrics, 112*(6, Pt. 1), 1338–1344.

Oostrom, K. J., van Teeseling, H., Smeets-Schouten, A., Peters, A. C., Jennekens-Schinkel, A., & Dutch Study of Epilepsy in Childhood. (2005). Three to four years after diagnosis: Cognition and behaviour in children with 'epilepsy only'. A prospective, controlled study. *Brain, 128*(Pt. 7), 1546–1555.

Ortinski, P., & Meador, K. J. (2004). Cognitive side effects of antiepileptic drugs. *Epilepsy and Behavior, 5*(Suppl. 1), S60–S65.

Piccirilli, M., D'Alessandro, P., Sciarma, T., Cantoni, C., Dioguardi, M. S., Giuglietti, M., et al. (1994). Attention problems in epilepsy: Possible significance of the epileptogenic focus. *Epilepsia, 35*(5), 1091–1096.

Provenzale, J. M., Barboriak, D. P., VanLandingham, K., MacFall, J., Delong, D., Lewis, D. V., et al. (2008). Hippocampal MRI signal hyperintensity after febrile status epilepticus is predictive of subsequent mesial temporal sclerosis. *American Journal of Roentgenology, 190*(4), 976–983.

Rasmussen, T., & Milner, B. (1977). The role of early left-brain injury in determining lateralization of cerebral speech functions. *Annals of the New York Academy of Sciences, 299*, 355–369.

Reddy, D. S., Rogawski, M. A. (2002). Stress-induced deoxycorticosterone-derived neurosteroids modulate GABA(A) receptor function and seizure susceptibility. *Journal of Neuroscience, 22*(9), 3795–3805.

Rohde, L. A., Biederman, J., Busnello, E. A., Zimmermann, H., Schmitz, M., Martins, S., et al. (1999). ADHD in a school sample of Brazilian adolescents: A study of prevalence, comorbid conditions, and impairments. *Journal of the American Academy of Child and Adolescent Psychiatry, 38*(6), 716–722.

Rutter, M., Graham, P., & Yule, W. (1970). *A neuropsychiatric study in childhood.* Philadelphia: Lippincott Publishers.

Schubert, R. (2005). Attention deficit disorder and epilepsy. *Pediatric Neurology, 32*(1), 1–10.

Scott, R. C., Gadian, D. G., King, M. D., Chong, W. K., Cox, T. C., Neville, B. G. R., et al. (2002). Magnetic resonance imaging findings within 5 days of status epilepticus in childhood. *Brain, 125*(Pt. 9), 1951–1959.

Segal, R. A., Chapman, C., & Barlow, J. (1991). Monozygotic twins with seizures. Shared characteristics. *Archives of Neurology, 48*(10), 1041–1045.

Segalowitz, S. J., & Bryden, M. P. (1983). Individual differences in hemispheric representation of language. In S. J. Segalowitz (Ed.), *Language functions and brain organization* (pp. 341–372). New York: Academic Press.

Seidenberg, M., Beck, N., Geisser, M., Giordani, B., Sackellares, J. C., Berent, S., et al. (1986). Academic achievement of children with epilepsy. *Epilepsia, 27*(6), 753–759.

Seidenberg, M., Beck, N., Geisser, M., O'Leary, D. S., Giordani, B., Berent, S., et al. (1988). Neuropsychological correlates of academic achievement of children with epilepsy. *Journal of Epilepsy, 1*, 23–29.

Semrud-Clikeman, M., & Wical, B. (1999). Components of attention in children with complex partial seizures with and without ADHD. *Epilepsia, 40*(2), 211–215.

Sherman, E. M., Slick, D. J., Connolly, M. B., & Eyrl, K. L. (2007). ADHD, neurological correlates and health-related quality of life in severe pediatric epilepsy. *Epilepsia, 48*(6), 1083–1091.

Sheth, R. D., & Gidal, B. E. (2006). Optimizing epilepsy management in teenagers. *Journal of Child Neurology*, *21*(4), 273–279.

Shinnar, S., Berg, A. T., Moshe, S. L., Petix, M., Maytal, J., Kang, H., et al. (1990). Risk of seizure recurrence following a first unprovoked seizure in childhood: A prospective study. *Pediatrics*, *85*(6), 1076–1085.

Sillanpaa, M., Haataja, L., & Shinnar, S. (2004). Perceived impact of childhood-onset epilepsy on quality of life as an adult. *Epilepsia*, *45*(8), 971–977.

Sillanpaa, M., Jalava, M., Kaleva, O., & Shinnar, S. (1998). Long-term prognosis of seizures with onset in childhood. *New England Journal of Medicine*, *338*(24), 1715–1722.

Spector, S., Cull, C., & Goldstein, L. H. (2000). Seizure precipitants and perceived self-control of seizures in adults with poorly-controlled epilepsy. *Epilepsy Research*, *38*(2–3), 207–216.

Spencer, S., & Huh, L. (2008). Outcomes of epilepsy surgery in adults and children. *Lancet Neurology*, *7*(6), 525–537.

Stores, G., Williams, P. L., Styles, E., & Zaiwalla, Z. (1992). Psychological effects of sodium valproate and carbamazepine in epilepsy. *Archives of Disease in Childhood*, *67*(11), 1330–1337.

Strauss, E., Sherman, E. M. S., & Spreen, O. (2006). *A compendium of neuropsychological tests* (3rd ed.). New York: Oxford University Press..

Theodore, W. H., Spencer, S. S., Wiebe, S., Langfitt, J. T., Ali, A., Shafer, P. O., et al. (2006). Epilepsy in North America: A report prepared under the auspices of the global campaign against epilepsy, the International Bureau for Epilepsy, the International League Against Epilepsy, and the World Health Organization. *Epilepsia*, *47*(10), 1700–1722.

Tinuper, P., Cerullo, A., Marini, C., Avoni, P., Rosati, A., Riva, R., et al. (1998). Epileptic drop attacks in partial epilepsy: Clinical features, evolution, and prognosis. *Journal of Neurology, Neurosurgery and Psychiatry*, *64*(2), 231–237.

Torres, A. R., Whitney, J., & Gonzalez-Heydrich, J. (2008). Attention-deficit/hyperactivity disorder in pediatric patients with epilepsy: Review of pharmacological treatment. *Epilepsy and Behavior*, *12*(2), 217–233.

Tsai, M. L., & Hung, K. L. (1995). Risk factors for subsequent epilepsy after febrile convulsions. *Journal of the Formosan Medical Association*, *94*(6), 327–331.

Vestergaard, M., Pedersen, C. B., Sidenius, P., Olsen, J., Christensen, J. (2007). The long-term risk of epilepsy after febrile seizures in susceptible subgroups. *American Journal of Epidemiology*, *165*(8), 911–918.

Voudris, K. A., Skardoutsou, A., Salapata, M., Servitzoglou, M., Vagiakou, E. A. (2002). Children with onset of febrile seizures after the age of 5 years. *Journal of Child Neurology*, *17*(7), 544.

Wakamoto, H., Nagao, H., Hayashi, M., & Morimoto, T. (2000). Long-term medical, educational, and social prognoses of childhood-onset epilepsy: A population-based study in a rural district of Japan. *Brain and Development*, *22*(4), 246–255.

Wernicke, J. F., Holdridge, K. C., Jin, L., Edison, T., Zhang, S., Bangs, M. E., et al. (2007). Seizure risk in patients with attention-deficit-hyperactivity disorder treated with atomoxetine. *Developmental Medicine and Child Neurology*, *49*(7), 498–502.

Williams, J., Griebel, M. L., & Dykman, R. A. (1998). Neuropsychological patterns in pediatric epilepsy. *Seizure*, *7*(3), 223–228.

Woodcock, R. W., Schrank, F. A., Mather, N., & McGrew, K. S. (2007). *Woodcock-Johnson Psycho-Educational Test Battery—3rd Edition, Normative Update (WJ-III-NU) Brief Battery*. Rolling Meadows, IL: Riverside Publishing.

45

Central Nervous System Germinoma: The Effects of Central Tumors on Neuropsychological Function

Brenda J. Spiegler

Primary intracranial germ cell tumors are relatively rare, accounting for 2%–5% of all childhood central nervous system (CNS) malignancies, and just over half of these (~60%) are germinomas. Germ cell tumors originate from multipotential germ cells and tend to occur in midline structures. Germinomas can be unifocal, generally occurring in the pineal or suprasellar regions, multifocal, or disseminated, but metastases outside the CNS are very rare. There is a predominance of males among those with pineal germinomas, with a sex ratio of about 3:1, but females predominate when the tumor arises in the suprasellar region. The incidence peaks in children between the ages of 10–12 years, with 65% occurring between ages 11–20 years.

Initial clinical presentation depends primarily on the site of the tumor and the presence or absence of raised intracranial pressure (ICP). Pineal germinomas often present with symptoms of raised ICP, including headache, nausea, and vomiting, along with Parinaud syndrome, which is characterized by paralysis of upward gaze, loss of convergence, pupillary dilation with poor reaction to light, and nystagmus. When the tumor is located in the suprasellar region, clinical presentation may be characterized by visual changes due to impingement on the optic pathways (e.g., deficits in visual acuity, failure of pupillary contraction to light, diplopia, and bitemporal hemianopsia) or by endocrine symptoms related to hypothalamic-pituitary axis dysfunction. (e.g., diabetes insipidus, delayed growth, precocious puberty, secondary amenorrhea, panhypopituitarism; Blaney et al., 2006).

Although the characteristic midline location and neuroimaging features are suggestive of the diagnosis, biopsy is required for confirmation. Unlike many other childhood brain tumors (e.g., ependymoma), complete resection does not confer a survival benefit because germinomas are quite sensitive to both chemotherapy and radiotherapy. With appropriate treatment, (e.g., focal and/or craniospinal radiation with or without platinum-based chemotherapy), germinomas have a very favorable prognosis, with up to 95% long-term survival (Blaney et al., 2006). Adjuvant chemotherapy has allowed the dose of craniospinal radiation (CSRT) to be reduced or even eliminated in patients with nondisseminated disease, with the goal of avoiding some of the well-known and problematic late effects of CSRT, including neuropsychological impairment (Fouladi et al., 1998).

There are few long-term studies of neuropsychological outcomes in patients treated for CNS germ cell tumors. Published studies are often descriptive, based on small samples, and/or are limited to quality of life, educational achievement, and intelligence test outcomes. Most commonly, these studies document declining school performance (Mordecai et al., 2000), memory impairment (Carpentieri et al., 2001; Crews, Jefferson, & Barth, 1999; Crucian, Fennell, Maria & Quisling, 2000; Dennis et al., 1991), and/or psychiatric symptoms (emotional lability, obsessive-compulsive symptoms, psychosis

[Mordecai et al., 2000], and anorexia [Damluji & Ferguson, 1987]).

Sutton et al. (1999) assessed quality of life, ability to work, and educational achievement in a group of 22 adolescent and adult patients treated for intracranial germinoma a mean of 10 years after CSRT. According to patient self-report, eight were in or had completed high school, nine were in or had completed college, and five had completed advanced degrees. Nineteen of the 22 described themselves as able to work outside the home and all could drive a car. Survivors rated their quality of life as comparable to controls except for worse physical function and general health. Notably, emotional and psychological function was rated as *better* than the normal population by this group of survivors.

Functional outcome, defined as endocrine and IQ status, was studied in 12 children (age 9–16 at diagnosis) treated with CSRT with a boost to the tumor site (Merchant et al., 2000). IQ scores were obtained for eight patients at diagnosis and compared with re-evaluation a mean of 56 months later (range 13–110 months after baseline). There was no change in IQ over the follow-up period for the group as a whole. One patient did show a precipitous decline (29 IQ points after 56 months), possibly related to multiple endocrinopathies and a visual field defect.

Schmugge and collaborators (Schmugge, Boltshauser, Pluss, & Niggli, 2000) followed 15 patients with primary CNS germ cell tumors, 10 of which were germinomas. At last contact, six of the 15 were attending high school or college, five were serving apprenticeships or working, and four were in programs for mentally disabled adolescents. Nine of the 15 patients, all of whom had been treated with radiation therapy (age range: 3–16 years), reported school difficulties and underwent neuropsychological evaluation between 14 and 157 months after completing treatment. Neuropsychological outcome was considered poor in this subgroup; all patients had mild to severe academic challenges, attention deficits, and "slow" learning rates. Less frequently, fine motor dysfunction ($n = 3$), spatial processing deficits ($n = 2$), and planning/organizational challenges ($n = 4$) were described. Of the six patients who did not report school problems (and so did not undergo neuropsychological

evaluation), four had received radiation. Descriptions of the neuropsychological test battery and specific test results were not provided.

Sands et al. (2001) reported quality of life, intellectual, and academic long-term outcomes in a group of 43 young adults treated in childhood for CNS germ cell tumors. The mainstay of treatment in this group was chemotherapy, with focal radiation (3000 cGy) administered only to those patients who did not achieve a complete response after four cycles of chemotherapy. The 16 patients with CNS germinoma exhibited average performance on measures of Verbal and Full-Scale IQ, reading, spelling, and math. Performance IQ was in the low-average range. Earlier age at diagnosis was associated with lower scores on tests of cognitive function as well as poorer long-term quality of life in the domains of physical and psychosocial functioning.

Strojan and colleagues (Strojan, Zadravec, Anzic, Korenjak, & Jereb, 2006) reported long-term endocrine, somatic, and psychological outcomes in nine patients with CNS germinoma treated with surgery (biopsy, three; partial resection, two; or gross total resection, four), shunting for hydrocephalus ($n = 2$), chemotherapy ($n = 8$), and radiation therapy ($n = 9$). Radiotherapy was restricted to the tumor bed in six of the nine patients. At long-term follow-up (7–14 years post diagnosis), six patients remained alive, the other three having died of recurrent disease or complications of treatment. Psychological evaluation was conducted with five long-term survivors using the Wechsler Bellevue Intelligence Test and the Rorschach Inkblot test. Results were described as reflecting normal or above normal Verbal IQ in four out of five patients and normal or above normal Performance IQ in all five. An estimate of "mental deterioration" (estimated as variance from the population mean) was judged to be significant in three out of five patients. Based on Rorschach responses, emotional disorder was documented in four out of five patients and significant "psycho-organic" syndrome in three out of five. Two patients had graduated from university, two had completed high school, and two had some technical schooling.

Given the absence of comprehensive neuropsychological studies of patients treated with radiation and chemotherapy for CNS germinoma, and the debilitating effect that cranial radiation is known to have on children treated for other pediatric brain tumors (Mulhern, Merchant, Gajjar, Reddick, & Kun, 2004; Palmer, Reddick, & Gajjar, 2007), it is especially important to study this condition from a neuropsychological perspective. The following case study demonstrates the added utility of comprehensive neuropsychological evaluation in identifying the challenges faced by survivors of CNS germinoma. Here we describe focal memory impairment in an adolescent boy diagnosed with bifocal CNS germinoma, his methods of coping, and his long-term outcome.

Case Report: Max

Max, a 14-year-old right handed Caucasian male, presented to our hospital in March of 1999 with a 3-week history of increasingly severe headache accompanied by dizziness and the subsequent onset of blurred vision. On examination, he had papilledema and a computed tomography (CT) scan documented enlarged ventricles and bifocal masses in the pineal and left thalamic regions (see Figure 45-1 for pineal lesion). His endocrine status was normal at diagnosis and thereafter. He was taken to the operating room for a biopsy of the pineal lesion and a third ventriculostomy to treat raised intracranial pressure (ICP), after which his vision returned to normal. Due to a cerebral spinal fluid (CSF) leak and headache, he was readmitted for a repeat third ventriculostomy a few weeks later. Biopsy results confirmed the diagnosis of germinoma, and he went on to receive four courses of platinum-based chemotherapy. Magnetic resonance imaging (MRI) after completion of chemotherapy showed complete resolution of the pineal mass, but no change in the left thalamic mass (see Figure 45-2 for MRI showing thalamic mass). His CSF was positive for malignant cells, so craniospinal radiation was administered in July 1999 (2340 cGy craniospinal dose with a boost of 720 cGy to the thalamic tumor bed).

Premorbid History

Max was the 7 lb, 9 oz product of a normal full-term pregnancy, born by spontaneous vaginal delivery. A nuchal cord and slow progression

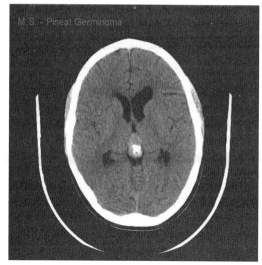

Figure 45-1. Computed tomography: pineal region mass and enlarged ventricles at diagnosis.

through the birth canal were minor complications, but he was discharged home after 4 days as a healthy neonate. Developmental milestones emerged normally and the medical history was entirely benign prior to the diagnosis of CNS germinoma.

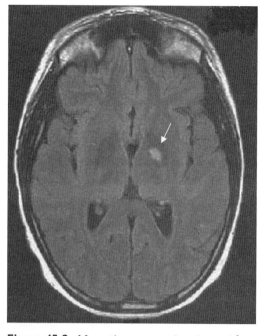

Figure 45-2. Magnetic resonance imaging: axial fluid-attenuated inversion recovery (FLAIR), post chemotherapy, prior to radiation.

At the time of his diagnosis, Max lived with his mother and three younger half-siblings. The family history was complex and although he was only 14 years old, family members treated him as the senior male figure in the household. As a result, his illness and subsequent memory challenges were extremely difficult for the entire family. The family history was significant in that both maternal grandparents died of brain tumors.

Prior to his diagnosis, Max was enrolled in an enriched grade 9 program. He did especially well in math and science, having earned a very high score on a national math competition and he planned to pursue math and science at the university level.

Reason for Referral

Changes in everyday memory were noticeable early in the treatment course. Max asked the same questions repeatedly, and the family began leaving notes all over the house to assist him. This was especially difficult because the family had previously relied on Max for his excellent memory, organization, and judgment. Changes in academic performance were evident immediately upon his return to school in the fall of 1999 (grade 10). Although he understood the concepts being taught and continued to earn very high grades for papers, projects, and assignments (90%–100%), he could not remember what he had studied and did very poorly on tests, where his grades dropped from the 80s to the 60s. He was seen for his first neuropsychological evaluation in December 1999 to address concerns about these memory issues and his declining school performance.

Max presented for neuropsychological evaluation as a pleasant, mature adolescent male who was quite clear and articulate about the changes brought on by his tumor and its treatment. He worked well in the test setting and appeared to be highly motivated. There was some hesitation in his speech, suggestive of mild word-finding problems. He worked more quickly and with greater confidence on nonverbal tasks.

Examination I Results

Results of the 1999 neuropsychological evaluation are shown in Table 45-1. Briefly, this young man's WISC-III Full Scale IQ fell in the Very Superior range, with a marked discrepancy between his Above Average Verbal Comprehension (VCI) score (81st percentile) and Superior to Very Superior scores for Perceptual Organization, Freedom from Distractibility, and Processing Speed (97th–99th percentiles).

Receptive vocabulary (PPVT-III) was commensurate with VCI, in the Above Average range (84th percentile). Mild word-finding difficulties were documented on the Boston Naming Test (raw score = 47). His phonemic verbal fluency (FAS) score of 35 was 1 standard deviation below the mean based on age-appropriate norms.

Visual-spatial processing was excellent. Max earned perfect scores for copying geometric figures (Beery VMI and Rey-Osterrieth Complex Figure; see Figure 45-3). He also performed extremely well on various tests of executive function, including measures of online problem solving and cognitive flexibility (Wisconsin Card Sorting Test, Category Test, Trails B), sustained and divided attention, and working memory.

Consistent with the reported history, Max's performance was impaired on tests of rote verbal memory. While his contextual memory was above average (CMS Story Memory), his ability to memorize a word list or word pairs was markedly impaired (CAVLT-2 and CMS Word Pairs). This impairment stood in stark contrast to both his visual memory (which was average for spatial locations as well as delayed recall of the Rey-Osterrieth figure; see Figure 45-4) and his above-average verbal cognitive level. One should note, however, that his "only" average visual memory may represent a relative impairment for this extremely bright boy.

Coping with Neuropsychological Dysfunction in High School

These results were useful in advocating for Max at his high school, where he was permitted to take open-book examinations, use written notes to support fact retrieval, and be evaluated with extra assignments instead of tests in some classes. He made good use of technology as a memory aid: "I used the Palm Pilot to help remind me of any appointments. I spent a lot of time trying to figure out where I was, why I was there, and where I was supposed to be going, so the Palm

Table 45-1. Test Scores from 1999 and 2008 Evaluations

Test *Age*	1999 *15 yr, 1 mo*	2008 *24 yr, 1 mo*
IQ	**WISC-III**	**WAIS-III**
Verbal Comprehension	113	112
Perceptual Organization	136	130
FDI/WMI	137	130
Processing Speed	129	114
Language		
PPVT-III	115	103
Boston Naming Test	92*	85
FAS SS/raw	84/35‡	95/38‡
Academics		
WRMT-R passage comp	119	95
WRAT3 arithmetic	123	120
Motor - Raw Scores		
Grip strength (R/L)	30/27	40/39
Tapping speed (R/L)	46/39	56/43
Grooved pegs (R/L)	57"/64"	59"/61"
Rey-Osterrieth (SS)		
Copy	112	112
30 minute recall	100	96
Trail-Making Test SS/raw score		
Part A	77/39"	113/19"
Part B	96/54"	114/44"
Wisconsin Card Sorting		
No. of categories (raw)	6	6
Percent perseverative errors (SS)	116	113
Memory	**CAVLT-2**	**CVLT-II**
Immediate Memory Span	74	77
Level of Learning	71	73
Short-delay recall	66	55
Long-delay recall	<60	48
Yes/No recognition hits raw score	13/16	12/16
Yes/No recognition false positive raw score	4/16	6/32
	CMS	**WMS-III**
Immediate Verbal	85	80
Delayed Verbal	82	71
Immediate Visual	103	97
Delayed Visual	100	94
General Memory	89	86
Attn/Concentration	125	124
Delayed Recognition	112	110
TOMM (T1, T2, recall raw scores)		50, 50, 49

Note. All scores are standard scores unless otherwise specified.

*Likely an overestimate as Max's score was compared to norms for 13-year-old children (Yeates, 1994 cited in Baron, 2004).

‡Norms were derived from two different studies and are discontinuous.

Pilot gave me access to my daily schedule." He also used a laptop to take notes in class and was permitted to copy notes from his fellow students. Listening to the teacher and writing notes simultaneously was more than he could manage. While encouraging him to advocate for himself, his mother acted as his external memory in many meetings with teachers and doctors. Max

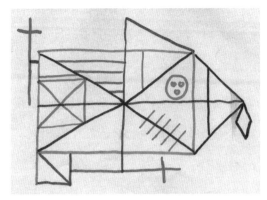

Figure 45-3. Copy of the Rey-Osterrieth Figure, 1999.

explained, "My mom attended all meetings so that she would be my memory. She let me do much of the talking, but when I needed assistance my memory was there sitting right beside me."

Interim History

Max struggled to accept the fact that his previous goal of studying math and science was no longer realistic for him. Max said, "You have to understand that you are now a changed person and that you have to change your life… This is very difficult to deal with as you still have the memory of who you once were. I didn't know the new me and it would take years to establish and accept the new me." After graduating from high school, he enrolled in a University Fine Arts program, to study media and film production. He was determined to be accepted on his actual merit and so did not disclose his neuropsychological

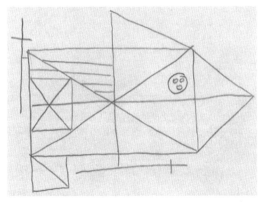

Figure 45-4. Delayed recall of the Rey-Osterrieth Figure, 1999.

condition until he matriculated. When he approached staff at the Office for Student Disabilities at his University, he was told they could not accommodate his memory impairment. Max wrote: "It was hilarious that the Office for Disabilities had their own disability—they had their own wall blocking their ability to think outside the box." He then turned to the dean of his film program who was far more helpful and arranged for him to copy notes from other students.

Max used organization as a major compensatory mechanism to cope with his memory impairment. In Max's words, "Keeping *one* system for organization is important because your life becomes habit driven, not memory driven. You need to be able to access assignment due dates, tests, and appointments." With great effort and determination, Max graduated with a Bachelor of Fine Arts degree. He moved away from home and has begun working in the film industry.

Examination II Results

Max is followed medically at an Oncology Late Effects clinic, where repeat MRIs have remained stable, with no evidence of either the pineal or thalamic mass. In 2008, Max underwent a 9-year follow-up neuropsychological evaluation. Results are reported in Table 45-1, and IQ and memory results from both assessments are directly compared in Figure 45-5. Most notable is the stability in the pattern of strengths and weaknesses. In general, Max has maintained his strengths in visual-spatial processing, attention/working memory, executive function, and math computation. He again produced a perfect copy of the Rey-Osterrieth figure, exhibiting excellent planning and organization by first copying the framework and bisecting lines, then the external components before finally adding the internal details. His incidental memory for the figure accurately portrayed the framework, bisecting lines, and external components but omitted many of the internal details. Max has maintained his excellent executive function, which has largely enabled him to live and work independently. He proceeded through the WCST quickly and efficiently, with absolutely no confusion or perseveration. His performance on the Trail Making Test was also fast and accurate.

Max gave stable but impaired performances on tests of confrontation naming and immediate

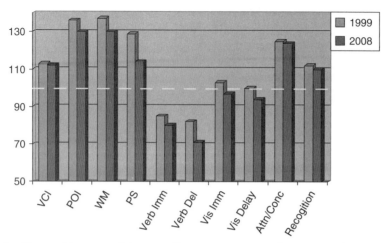

Figure 45-5. Intelligence, Memory and Attention/Concentration scores from 1999 and 2008. For all scores, mean = 100, Standard Deviation = 15.

verbal memory. His verbal fluency (FAS), at the 30th percentile, is considered to be below expectation for a person of his overall intellectual level. Declines were noted on tests of processing speed, receptive vocabulary (PPVT-III), reading comprehension, and delayed verbal memory. His previously documented verbal memory disorder remained painfully apparent.

Coping with Neuropsychological Dysfunction as an Adult:

Max lives independently in a city that is far away from his family. In his current work setting, as a sound editor in the film industry, Max relies on technology, organization, and careful note-taking to manage his work and life responsibilities. Max explains: "So much of what I do now relies on repetition and patterns in my life. It is essential that I do things in whatever normal way I have set up. Doing things outside the box makes me forget to do anything, down to eating a meal." He is tech savvy; his phone syncs with his computer, which syncs with the Internet. He discloses his memory impairment only on a "need to know" basis, now that he has found strategies that work for him.

Discussion

This case demonstrates several important neuropsychological principles and brain–behavior

relationships. Max's initial presentation with severe headache, dizziness, and blurred vision is typical for raised ICP associated with acute hydrocephalus. With treatment for raised ICP via third ventriculostomy, these symptoms resolved.

The location of the two tumor masses, one in the pineal region and the other in the left anterior thalamus is consistent with the symptoms of memory problems. The memory circuitry of the brain, the circuit of Papez, surrounds the third ventricle. The pineal mass caused hydrocephalus by blocking the flow of CSF through the aqueduct of Sylvius; one of the symptoms of acute hydrocephalus can be memory disturbance as the expanded ventricles stretch the white matter fibers in the surrounding regions. Although Max's memory was likely affected for both visual-spatial and verbal material, his verbal memory was far worse and this is understood in relation to the second mass in the left anterior thalamus (Aggleton & Brown, 1999; Linek, Sonka, & Bauer, 2005).

There is a large literature on the neuropsychological late effects of chemotherapy and cranial radiation in children (Moore, 2005; Mulhern & Butler, 2006). Max's chemotherapy did not include methotrexate or steroids, two of the more neurotoxic chemotherapy agents, so it is unlikely that chemotherapy is a primary contributor to his outcome. Factors that predict outcome after cranial radiation include dose, field, age at treatment, and time since treatment. Max received a whole brain dose of 2340 cGy, which is considered moderate, and an additional boost to the left anterior thalamic tumor of 720 cGy. When he was seen in 1999, he had just completed radiation and so it is unlikely that his pattern of deficits at that time was related to radiation since radiation-related impairments tend to emerge over a period of several years (Mulhern et al., 2001; Spiegler, Bouffet, Greenberg, Rutka, & Mabbott, 2004). Therefore, the *changes* in test performance between 1999 and 2008 may be better explained by late radiation effects. It is interesting that declines were noted in the domains of processing speed and delayed verbal memory. Processing speed is a common impairment after whole-brain radiation, but the changes in verbal memory may be specifically related to the tumor location and additional boost applied to the left anterior thalamic nucleus.

There are several aspects of Max's case that are considered to be protective. First, he was in early adolescence at diagnosis and treatment, and it is well accepted that cranial radiation is more damaging to the younger brain (Janzen & Spiegler, 2008; Mulhern et al., 2001). Older children and young adults appear to be less debilitated in the long term. Second, Max's extremely high premorbid cognitive level suggests that he had considerable cognitive reserve upon which to rely. It is certainly the case that he used his excellent reasoning and executive functions to help him adapt and cope. A third protective factor is that Max's family was extremely supportive, providing him with a loving and compassionate environment in which to rediscover his identity. Fourth, Max's tumor was effectively treated; he did not have a recurrence requiring further medical interventions, nor did he have significant medical complications of his treatment (e.g., seizures, stroke endocrinopathy), all of which can impact long-term neuropsychological outcomes (Roncadin, Dennis, Greenberg, & Spiegler, 2008).

Conclusion

This case demonstrates that specific patterns of long-term neuropsychological impairment can best be understood in the context of multiple factors, including medical diagnosis, tumor location, treatment parameters, sociodemographics, and

cognitive reserve. The manner in which Max has understood his condition and coped with adversity provides an important lesson for neuropsychologists working with children and youth. We would do well to learn from Max's experience: "Laughter plays a big role in order to get you through life as so many silly things occur, including being in a totally wrong place and not even knowing how you got there."

Acknowledgments

I would like to thank Max for participating in this project and for allowing me to use his own words to highlight his day-to-day reality and to make his situation come to life. I am also grateful to Dr. Donald Mabbott for his assistance with the imaging and Dr. Laura Janzen for her comments on an earlier version of this paper.

References

Aggleton, J. P., & Brown, M. W. (1999). Episodic memory, amnesia, and the hippocampal-anterior thalamic axis. *Behavioral and Brain Sciences, 22*(3), 425–489.

Baron, I. S. (2004). *Neuropsychological evaluation of the child.* New York: Oxford University Press.

Blaney, S., Kun, L. E., Hunter, J., Rorke-Adams, L. B., Lau, C., Strother, D., & Pollack, I. F. (2006). Tumors of the central nervous system. In D. G. Pizzo (Ed.), *Principles and practice of pediatric oncology* (5th ed., pp. 786–864). Philadelphia: Lippincott Williams & Wilkins.

Carpentieri, S. C., Waber, D. P., Scott, R. M., Goumnerova, L. C., Kieran, M. W., Cohen, L. E., et al. (2001). Memory deficits among children with craniopharyngiomas. *Neurosurgery, 49*(5), 1053–1058.

Crews, W. D., Jr., Jefferson, A. L., & Barth, J. T. (1999). Longitudinal neuropsychological evaluation of a case of pineal tumor occurring in an adolescent girl. *Applied Neuropsychology, 6*(2), 108–114.

Crucian, G. P., Fennell, E. B., Maria, B. L., & Quisling, R.G. (2000). Neuropsychological sequelae of a pituitary germinoma: A case study. *Neurocase, 6,* 65–72.

Damluji, N. F., & Ferguson, J. M. (1987). Pineal gland germinoma simulating anorexia nervosa. *International Journal of Eating Disorders, 6*(4), 569–572.

Dennis, M., Spiegler, B. J., Fitz, C. R., Hoffman, H. J., Hendrick, E. B., Humphreys, R. P., et al. (1991). Brain tumors in children and adolescents. II. The neuroanatomy of deficits in working, associative and serial-order memory. *Neuropsychologia, 29*(9), 829–847.

Fouladi, M., Grant, R., Baruchel, S., Chan, H., Malkin, D., Weitzman, S., et al. (1998). Comparison of survival outcomes in patients with intracranial germinomas treated with radiation alone versus reduced-dose radiation and chemotherapy. *Child's Nervous System, 14*, 596–601.

Janzen, L. A., & Spiegler, B. J. (2008). Neurodevelopmental sequelae of pediatric acute lymphoblastic leukemia and its treatment. *Developmental Disabilities Research Reviews, 14*(3), 185–195.

Linek, V., Sonka, K., & Bauer, J. (2005). Dysexecutive syndrome following anterior thalamic ischemia in the dominant hemisphere. *Journal of Neurological Sciences, 229–230*, 117–120.

Merchant, T. E., Sherwood, S. H., Mulhern, R. K., Rose, S. R., Thompson, S. J., Sanford, R. A., et al. (2000). CNS germinoma: Disease control and long-term functional outcome for 12 children treated with craniospinal irradiation. *International Journal of Radiation Oncology Biology Physics, 46*(5), 1171–1176.

Moore, B. D., 3rd. (2005). Neurocognitive outcomes in survivors of childhood cancer. *Journal of Pediatric Psychology, 30*(1), 51–63.

Mordecai, D., Shaw, R. J., Fisher, P. G., Mittelstadt, P. A., Guterman, T., & Donaldson, S. S. (2000). Case study: Suprasellar germinoma presenting with psychotic and obsessive-compulsive symptoms. *Journal of the American Academy of Child and Adolescent Psychiatry, 39*(1), 116–119.

Mulhern, R. K., & Butler, R. W. (2006). Neuropsychological late effects. In R. Brown (Ed.), *Comprehensive handbook of childhood cancer and sickle cell disease* (pp. 262–274). New York: Oxford University Press.

Mulhern, R. K., Merchant, T. E., Gajjar, A., Reddick, W. E., & Kun, L. E. (2004). Late neurocognitive sequelae in survivors of brain tumours in childhood. *Lancet Oncology, 5*(7), 399–408.

Mulhern, R. K., Palmer, S. L., Reddick, W. E., Glass, J. O., Kun, L. E., Taylor, J., et al. (2001). Risks of young age for selected neurocognitive deficits in medulloblastoma are associated with white matter loss. *Journal of Clinical Oncology, 19*(2), 472–479.

Palmer, S. L., Reddick, W. E., & Gajjar, A. (2007). Understanding the cognitive impact on children who are treated for medulloblastoma. *Journal of Pediatric Psychology, 32*(9), 1040–1049.

Roncadin, C., Dennis, M., Greenberg, M. L., & Spiegler, B. J. (2008). Adverse medical events associated with childhood cerebellar astrocytomas and medulloblastomas: Natural history and relation to very long-term neurobehavioral outcome. *Child's Nervous System 24*(9), 995–1003.

Sands, S. A., Kellie, S. J., Davidow, A. L., Diez, B., Villablanca, J., Weiner, H. L., et al. (2001). Long-term quality of life and neuropsychologic functioning for patients with CNS germ-cell tumors: From the First International CNS Germ-Cell Tumor Study. *Neuro-Oncology, 3*(3), 174–183.

Schmugge, M., Boltshauser, E., Pluss, H. J., & Niggli, F. K. (2000). Long-term follow-up and residual sequelae after treatment for intracerebral germ-cell tumour in children and adolescents. *Annals of Oncology, 11*(5), 527–533.

Spiegler, B. J., Bouffet, E., Greenberg, M. L., Rutka, J. T., & Mabbott, D. J. (2004). Change in neurocognitive functioning after treatment with cranial radiation in childhood. *Journal of Clinical Oncology, 22*(4), 706–713.

Strojan, P., Zadravec, L. Z., Anzic, J., Korenjak, R., & Jereb, B. (2006). The role of radiotherapy in the treatment of childhood intracranial germinoma: Long-term survival and late effects. *Pediatric Blood Cancer, 47*(1), 77–82.

Sutton, L. N., Radcliffe, J., Goldwein, J. W., Phillips, P., Janss, A. J., Packer, R. J., et al. (1999). Quality of life of adult survivors of germinomas treated with craniospinal irradiation. *Neurosurgery, 45*(6), 1292–1298.

Part V

Neurodegenerative Disorders

As the 12 chapters in this section indicate, neurodegenerative disorders are more common among adults, especially in the geriatric age group, but they are also found in children. As neuroscientists discover etiological factors for these progressively deteriorating disorders, neuropsychologists have contributed to defining subtle differences in neurocognition related to these illnesses. It is commonly believed that Alzheimer disease is the most common of these disorders to affect the elderly, but there is greater variation than once thought regarding the underlying neuropathology and resultant subtle cognitive differences across diagnoses.

46

Childhood Multiple Sclerosis

Ben Deery and Vicki Anderson

Multiple sclerosis (MS) is an inflammatory demyelinating condition of the central nervous system (CNS) that primarily targets white matter and most commonly presents between the ages of 20–40 years old (Vukusic & Confavreux, 2001). Multiple sclerosis in childhood is considered to be rare, and diagnosis remains difficult. Many clinicians may be slow to consider a diagnosis of MS in childhood for a variety reasons. Young children may find it hard to describe MS symptoms such as limb weakness or blurred vision, and these may be subtle and difficult for parents to detect. Even clinicians familiar with the diagnosis of MS in childhood may delay diagnosis and find it difficult to identify or predict episodes. Delay in diagnosis when MS is likely is not optimal given early treatment may influence disease course and progression. Although the diagnostic criteria for MS have been recently modified to include a diagnosis in children as young as 10 years of age (McDonald et al., 2001), cases have been documented at younger ages. These children often encounter obstacles because they are diagnosed with a "disease of adulthood."

While the exact prevalence of MS in childhood is unknown, estimates typically vary between 3% and 6%, but they may be as high as 10%–17% depending on the cutoff age (Pinhaus-Hamiel, Barak, Siev-Ner, & Achiron, 1998; Simone et al., 2002). These figures may underestimate the true incidence of childhood MS, with approximately 25% of adults with MS retrospectively reporting knowing something was "wrong"

in adolescence or before (Boston Cure Project, 2004). Overall prevalence of MS varies based on geographical location, becoming more prevalent in temperate climates further away from the equator. One possible explanation for this distribution is the link between sunlight exposure and vitamin D levels (Smolders, Damoiseaux, Menheere, & Hupperts, 2008). Prevalence of childhood MS according to race is unknown. However, anecdotal reports from North America suggest higher rates in minority groups, such as African Americans and Latinos (MacAllister, Christodoulou, Milazzo, & Krupp, 2007). Multiple sclerosis is more common in females, with the approximate 2:1 female to male ratio in adults also mirrored in childhood MS. This ratio varies across age groups, with a lower female predominance in pre-pubescent children (Boiko, Vorobeychik, Paty, Devonshire, & Sadovnick, 2002). Together with a documented spike in gender ratios and prevalence following puberty, these data suggest sex hormones may play an important role in the onset of childhood MS.

Genetic factors also appear to play a major role in MS. Those diagnosed with MS are more likely to carry specific human leukocyte antigens (HLAs), essential elements in immune function (Barcellos et al., 2003). Risk of MS is higher in first-degree relatives than in the general population (5% versus 0.2%) while concordance in monozygotic twins is higher than in dizygotic twins (30% versus 2%–5%), confirming a strong but not exclusive role in the etiology of MS (Compston, 1999; Sadovnick, Dircks, &

505

Ebers, 1999). Studies show that individuals who migrate before puberty or during early adolescence adopt the MS risk of their new country of residence (Compston, 1999). This "age at migration" pattern has led to the hypothesis that environmental exposure in childhood, most likely to some form of viral infection, plays a key etiologic role. This theory implies that there is an "incubation" period before disease onset (Kurtzke, Beebe, & Norman, 1985). However, it fails to adequately explain childhood-onset MS, especially in very young children.

Multiple sclerosis was once thought to involve pathology solely within cerebral white matter. It is now known that damage also occurs to the underlying axons and areas of brain tissue distal from white matter lesions, areas that appear normal on conventional imaging, commonly termed, normal-appearing white matter (NAWM) or normal-appearing brain tissue (NABT). While the exact cause of MS remains a mystery, one popular hypothesis is that of "molecular mimicry," which postulates that CNS myelin proteins share some type of similarity with the MS inciting pathogen. This results in the body's immune system (namely T-cells and B-cells) accidentally mistaking CNS white matter for the pathogen and the body begins "attacking" itself, leading to episodes of inflammation and demyelination (Davies, 1997).

The most common course of MS for both adults and children is a relapsing-remitting course (RRMS), which is characterized by episodes of neurological dysfunction (relapses) with complete or partial recovery and without major progression. However, because recovery may be incomplete, residual disability may accumulate over time. Around 25% of children (compared to 70% of adults) with RRMS will eventually transition to a secondary-progressive MS (SPMS) course, that is, an initial RRMS course followed by progressive neurological impairment (Boiko et al., 2002; Simone et al., 2002). The most severe form of MS, termed *primary-progressive multiple sclerosis* (PPMS), is defined by progressive neurological impairment from the disease onset and is considered rare in childhood (Boiko et al., 2002). Because children with MS typically take longer than adults to reach the stage of irreversible disability, some may consider MS to have a less aggressive course in children. However, Confavreux, Vukusic, and Adeleine (2003) found

that once children reach the PPMS stage they then progress at the same rate as adults. Furthermore, because those with childhood MS are diagnosed at a much earlier age, they are more likely to reach this stage at a younger age.

Initial symptoms in childhood MS are similar to those for adults, including weakness, sensory and visual disturbance, ataxia, speech and swallowing difficulties, bladder/bowel dysfunction, and cognitive/psychological changes. Children are more likely to exhibit systemic symptoms such as headache, vomiting, fever, malaise, and lethargy, followed by poorly localized neurological symptoms. In contrast, adults are more likely to display sensory and motor features. Symptoms typically evolve over days and while recovery can be rapid, they typically resolve over weeks to months. In adults, factors found to influence recovery include degree of recovery from first episode, time between first and second episode, age at onset, and gender (Hammond, McLeod, Macaskill, & English, 2000; Levic et al., 1999). Good neurological recovery is often seen in the initial stages of childhood MS, but factors predictive of a more favorable recovery remain largely unstudied.

No single biological test can confirm a diagnosis of childhood MS. Thus, diagnosis remains a clinical decision involving exclusion of other disorders. Neurological examination, clinical history, and neuroimaging are standard practice, but examination of cerebrospinal fluid (CSF) and visual and somatosensory evoked potentials for evidence of lesions may also be performed (Boutin et al., 1988). Patterns of demyelination in childhood MS are generally similar to those found in adults, involving lesions in the periventricular, juxtacortical, subcortical, infratentorial, and spinal cord white matter (Balassy et al., 2001; Ebner, Millner, & Justich, 1990). Children are more likely to exhibit atypical patterns of demyelination, including large or nodular lesions sometimes mistaken for tumors. Lesion resolution early in the MS course can be complete or partial, indicating that the central nervous system (CNS) has some ability to repair itself, a capacity that appears to become less efficient over time as there may be lesser degrees of remyelination with longer disease duration.

Several conditions may present with features similar to childhood MS, including acute disseminated encephalomyelitis (ADEM), Schilder's disease, Devic's disease or optic neuromyelitis, and Balò's concentric sclerosis. Other conditions that also produce white matter lesions on MRI similar to MS include systemic lupus erythematosus (SLE), primary CNS vasculitis, and sickle cell disease (Banwell et al., 2007). Acute disseminated encephalomyelitis, characterized by a single episode of inflammation and demyelination, is particularly difficult to differentiate from the initial presentation of childhood MS. Approximately one-quarter to one-third of children initially diagnosed with ADEM are diagnosed with MS at a later stage (Hynson et al., 2001; Mikaeloff et al., 2004).

The most common treatment for MS is immunotherapy, which utilizes drugs in an attempt to modify the disease process. These include interferon beta-1a (Avonex or Rebif), interferon beta-1b (Betaseron), and glatiramer acetate (Copaxone). Immunotherapy has been shown to reduce the frequency of relapses, number of lesions seen on magnetic resonance imaging (MRI), disability progression, and rate of brain atrophy (Jacobs et al., 1996; Ruddick, Fisher, Lee, Simon, & Jacobs, 1999). These drugs have not been subjected to randomized studies in childhood MS, but a number of case studies and smaller series indicate they are well tolerated and appear to offer similar benefits (Forrester, Coleman, & Kornberg, 2009; Mikaeloff et al., 2001).

Cognitive deficits in adult MS are well recognized, and they can occur even before the MS diagnosis is confirmed and without any symptoms of marked physical disability (Feinstein, Kartsounis, Miller, Youl, & Ron, 1992). Between 40% and 70% of adults with MS show some form of cognitive impairment, most commonly in information processing, attention, memory, and executive function (Rao, Leo, Bernardin, & Unverzagt, 1991). These cognitive impairments are thought to be caused by disconnection of cortical neural networks (Filippi et al., 2000). Because MS may be seen as less aggressive or severe in children than in adults, this might imply that cognitive deficits will also be milder. A growing body of research into other CNS conditions in childhood, such as traumatic brain injury (Anderson & Moore, 1995), phenylketonuria (Welsh, Pennington, Ozonoff, Rouse, & McCabe, 1990), and hydrocephalus (Fletcher et al., 1996), refute

this hypothesis, suggesting that the immature brain appears to have less opportunity to recover from early brain injury.

The earliest studies of childhood MS that included some form of standardized measure of cognition produced variable findings. Not surprisingly, generalizability of results was limited due to very small sample sizes and reliance on global measures of cognition, for example, intelligence quotients (Bye, Kendall, & Wilson, 1985; Iannetti et al., 1996). A more comprehensive study by Kalb et al. (1999) found a marked degree of subject variability on cognitive measures. As a group, children with MS typically performed within normal ranges, but high rates of specific cognitive and academic impairments were found at an individual level. A more recent study by Banwell and Anderson (2005) showed all 10 children studied had at least one cognitive impairment, with several having deficits in a majority or all areas assessed. Most commonly impaired domains were processing speed, working memory, and executive function. Earlier age of onset and longer disease duration were related to more severe and widespread cognitive impairment. Children in this study were noted to display little evidence of physical disability.

In one of the largest studies conducted in the field, MacAllister et al., (2005) found a variety of cognitive deficits, most commonly in complex attention and memory, in a sample of 37 children with MS. Confrontation naming was also impaired in many, which is in contrast to the normally intact performance reported in adult studies. Around 30% of children required some educational assistance and were classified as having a major cognitive impairment, while almost 50% were diagnosed with a major depressive disorder, an anxiety disorder, or panic disorder. This study highlights the psychological impact of MS in children, which may have both a psychogenic and neurological basis. A 2-year follow-up of these children found cognitive decline was common, and related to baseline neurological impairment and total number of relapses (MacAllister et al., 2007). These findings are supported by our own studies, which have demonstrated impairments in processing speed, basic and complex attentional skills, and inhibition, with deficits in executive functioning and mathematical abilities evolving over time

(Deery, Anderson, Jacobs, Neale, & Kornberg, 2005, 2008). These impairments generally tended to remain stable or worsen over time.

Because children with MS typically show good physical recovery, especially from initial episodes, clinicians may overlook or remain unaware of possible cognitive consequences, and children can often transition back to home and school with unrealistic expectations. It is in this context that the input of a neuropsychologist is important, either in providing a baseline assessment for future comparison or for detecting and managing existing cognitive deficits. This information can be crucial for the child, family, friends, teachers, and other clinicians. The case of S. J., described next, highlights the complexity of this condition and its impact in childhood.

Case Study: S. J.

S. J. is a right-handed, Caucasian male who was referred by his neurologist at age 14 for a baseline cognitive assessment to assist with possible future treatment and management. S. J. was the product of a normal pregnancy and uncomplicated delivery, and his developmental milestones were achieved within normal limits. He has one older and two younger siblings, whose medical histories are unremarkable. There is no family history of any related neurological, psychological, or learning difficulties. Premorbid history was unremarkable, with S. J. described as an average student who did well at sports.

At age 12, S. J. presented to a specialist children's hospital following a fall at school, complaining of nausea and blurred vision which was also "painful." Neurological examination revealed left-sided arm weakness. S. J.'s mother had reported symptoms of a possible chest infection in the month prior to this episode. An MRI revealed scattered areas of demyelination and inflammation in temporal, parietal, and frontal lobes, and a diagnosis of ADEM was made. Approximately 12 months later, S. J. complained of similar symptoms, with a follow-up MRI revealing new areas of demyelination and some resolution of old lesions found on previous imaging. At this stage his diagnosis of ADEM was revised to that suggestive of MS. Six months following his second clinical episode he was referred for a baseline neuropsychological examination.

The serial MRI shown in Figure 46-1 is not that of S. J., which unfortunately was unavailable; however, this series highlights nicely the diagnostic evolution commonly seen in children who are initially diagnosed with ADEM but are later diagnosed with childhood MS, as was the case for S. J.

At interview, S. J.'s parents did not report any significant concerns about his social, emotional, cognitive, or academic functioning, and saw the assessment as important for future planning in the event of possible future relapses. S. J.'s mother described him as "forgetful and distractible" at times, and noted that since beginning high school (shortly following his first episode) he had found school work more challenging than when he was in primary school. S. J. had experienced declining grades over the past couple of years. His mother had interpreted these as related to the onset of adolescence and believed it was a phase that would hopefully pass. S. J. was still actively involved in sports and was described as "physically well."

Examination Results

S. J. presented as a friendly, somewhat sombre young man, who cooperated well on testing but who became frustrated when he found tasks difficult. Conversational speech and language appeared normal, although he did present as somewhat overwhelmed when being interviewed with his parents, when the conversation was more fast paced and included multiple contributors. S. J. fatigued quite quickly after cognitively demanding tests or after a lengthy period of assessment.

S. J. was administered the Wechsler Scale for Children, Fourth Edition (WISC-IV; Wechsler, 2004), Children's Memory Scale (CMS; Cohen, 1997), Trail Making Test A and B (TMT A & B; Army Individual Battery Test, 1944), Test of Everyday Attention for Children (TEA-Ch; Manly, Robertson, Anderson, & Nimmo-Smith, 1999), Rey-Osterrieth Complex Figure (RCF; Anderson, Anderson, & Garth, 2001; Rey, 1964), Controlled Oral Word Association Task (COWAT; Gaddes & Crockett, 1975), Contingency Naming Test (CNT; Anderson, Anderson, Northam, & Taylor, 2000; Taylor, Albo, Phebus, Sachs, & Bierl, 1987), and Wide Range Achievement Test,

Figure 46-1. Capacity for dramatic magnetic resonance imaging (MRI) resolution of white matter lesions in children with multiple sclerosis (MS). (*a*) Axial fluid-attenuated inversion recovery (FLAIR) images of an 8-year-old girl presenting with acute encephalopathy, ataxia, and tremor, diagnosed as acute disseminated encephalomyelitis. Images show ill-defined increased signal in the white matter of the brain stem and cerebellum as well as the deep gray matter. (*b*) Axial FLAIR images of the same child obtained 1 year later. The patient was clinically well. Near-complete resolution of the prior lesions in the brain stem, cerebellum, and deep white matter is noted. No new white matter lesions are present. (*c*) Axial FLAIR images 2 years after her initial presentation demonstrate new lesions in the brain stem (arrow), periventricular white matter, and splenium of the corpus callosum. The patient presented with new neurologic deficits (without encephalopathy) and was diagnosed with MS. (*d*) Axial FLAIR images obtained 4 years after her initial presentation (2 years after the MRI shown in *C*). Although there has been considerable resolution of some of the prior lesions, improvement is not as dramatic as the near-complete MRI lesion resolution noted in *B*, suggesting that remyelination capacity may diminish either with increasing disease duration or with increasing age. The child has experienced four MS relapses, and the MRI shown in *D* was obtained with the child on therapy with glatiramer acetate. (From Banwell et al., 2007. Copyright 2007 by Wolters Kluwer. Reprinted with permission.)

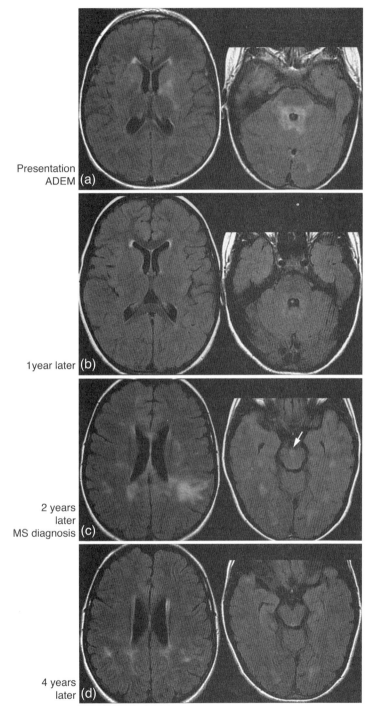

Presentation ADEM (a)

1year later (b)

2 years later MS diagnosis (c)

4 years later (d)

Third Edition (WRAT-3; Wilkinson, 1993). The results are provided in Table 46-1.

Examination found that S. J.'s performances on intellectual assessment were within the average range, with some suggestion of a subtle abstract reasoning difficulty, and relatively weaker processing speed and attention/working memory difficulties. Examination of memory and new learning, and more complex forms of attention and executive functioning, identified significant difficulties.

Memory and Learning

Basic visual memory and that for larger amounts of verbal information were age appropriate. Qualitatively, while S. J.'s story recall included accurate details they were rather disorganized. His ability to learn verbal information without contextual cues in the form of a word list showed a somewhat flattened, inefficient learning curve,

with highly variable organization in his recall and poor recollection after a long delay. Recall of a complex geometric design was quite impaired and appeared influenced by poor planning and organization on the initial copy (Figure 46-2).

Complex Attention

S. J.'s ability to select target information quickly in the presence of distractors was below expectation, while his ability to sustain his attention was acceptable. His ability to switch attention between task demands was impaired, as was his ability to simultaneously divide his attention between competing task demands.

Processing and Executive Skills

S. J.'s speed of information processing and accuracy declined considerably when demands on cognitive flexibility and rule switching were

Table 46-1. S. J.'s Examination Results

WISC-IV	SS	WISC-IV	SS
Information	12	Block Design	11
Vocabulary	13	Matrix Reasoning	8
Similarities	8	Picture Concepts	12
Coding	8	Digit Span	10
Symbol Search	9	Letter Number Sequencing	7
VCI	104	PSI	91
PRI	102	WMI	91
FSIQ	99	TEA-Ch	SS
CMS	SS	Sky Search Final Attention Score	6 / 8
Dots Learning	12	Sky Search Dual Task	5
Dots Delayed	10	CNT	z score
Stories Immediate	11	Trial 1 Time	0.2
Stories Delayed	10	Trial 1 Efficiency	−0.3
Word List Learning	7	Trial 2 Time	0.5
Word List Delayed	6	Trial 2 Efficiency	0.1
RCF	z score	Trial 3 Time	−1.4
Copy	−1.6	Trial 3 Efficiency	−1.2
Recall	−3.6	Trial 4 Time	−2.5
OSS Organization	−1.2	Trial 4 Efficiency	−1.8
Trail-Making Test A	z score	WRAT-3	Std Score
Trails A	0.3	Single word reading	101
Trails B	−1.8	Spelling	90
COWAT	z score	Arithmetic	80
FAS Total	−1.5		
Animals	0.3		

introduced, and his ability to quickly generate words in response to specific letters was also deficient and appeared related to a reduced ability to problem solve and generate possible solutions, rather than simply being due to slow processing speed.

S.J.'s copy of a complex geometric design incorporated the majority of key features, but several minor details were omitted or distorted, affecting his overall score. Perhaps of more clinical significance, its construction was poorly planned and organized; he adopted a piecemeal approach that later appeared to markedly impact his recall (Figure 46-2). As previously noted, abstract thought and reasoning also appeared mildly depressed.

Academic achievement

A brief screen of academic achievement showed good single-word reading and spelling just within the average range. S. J.'s arithmetic skills were lower than anticipated and indicated an academic weakness.

Follow-Up

A neuropsychological reevaluation was scheduled for 1–2 years after initial examination to document S. J.'s ongoing cognitive development and any impact of MS relapses or possible underlying disease processes. Unfortunately, S. J.'s family moved out of the area and could not

be contacted for further follow-up. The family re-presented approximately 18 months later, seeking assistance and advice. Interview at that time revealed that the intervening years since his initial neuropsychological assessment had seen S. J. encounter many challenges and obstacles. S. J. had left school at 16 to take up a trade-oriented study course but dropped out after failing several subjects. He then took a job as an apprentice tradesman, but he had recently left after some difficulties. His employer described S. J. as "sometimes off with the fairies," having "trouble paying attention on the work site," and making "simple mistakes." Around this time S. J. ended a long-standing relationship that followed a period of relationship difficulties. This combination of events had caused significant concern in S. J.'s family and had prompted S. J.'s re-referral.

S. J.'s mother reported that he had experienced several minor relapses since his initial neuropsychological assessment and he had been started on immunotherapy. This involved frequent injections, which S. J. managed independently. His mother described a brief episode in which S. J. hid his medication but pretended to take it. His mother felt this may have been S. J.'s way of having some control over his life or perhaps disagreeing that he needed medication. He recommended therapy after some extra discussions with his treating clinician, and he is now adherent to his treatment regimen. These behavioral aspects of S. J.'s condition highlight the

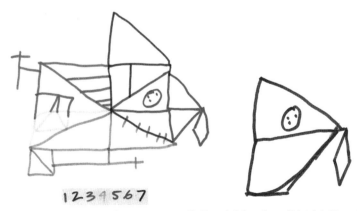

Figure 46-2. S. J.'s Rey-Osterreith Complex Figure copy (*left*) and delayed recall (*right*). Note the very piecemeal and poorly planned/organized approach for his age, which later appears to influence his recall ability.

complexities of chronic and relapsing conditions such as MS for children and adolescents, especially as they transition through key life stages and form their sense of self.

While S. J. did not try to return to his apprenticeship position, on a follow-up phone conversation his mother reported that he had taken up a similar job in a related field with a supportive and informed employer. In this context, he was able to implement some simple and quick accommodations and strategies recommended at re-presentation to assist with his cognitive difficulties. These included strategies such as recording a video of his boss listing required supplies on his mobile phone to replay in the store, using a ruler with a built-in calculator to avoid mental arithmetic, and sending S. J. on frequent errands (e.g., to get water/coffee, supplies), which would help to break up his day and provide him with discrete periods of required concentration interspersed with more physical, less cognitive demanding tasks.

Discussion

Children with MS may be particularly vulnerable to cognitive deficits due to the relative immaturity of their CNS, especially white matter development, which is one of MS's primary targets. The case of S. J. may be considered prototypical of childhood MS. It was chosen to highlight the broad impact on cognitive functioning at different academic and life stages, and to underscore the secondary psychosocial and psychological implications that may result when this condition is diagnosed in childhood; all children may not show the same combination of impairments.

Underlying Neural Processes

Myelin development progresses rapidly during childhood, but its protracted development means it is not fully complete until well into adolescence or early adulthood (Klinberg, Vaidyn, Gabrieli, Moseley, & Heidehus, 1999; Rakic, 1995). White matter damage in childhood leaves cognitive skills at risk by disrupting transmission of impulses between brain networks and regions, potentially resulting in reduced information processing, slowed response speed,

attentional impairments, reduced executive functioning, and learning difficulties. Early CNS insult may also alter or impact on normal white matter development post insult and on cortical connectivity and establishment of cognitive networks, while serial insults have been shown to have cumulative consequences. Taken together, these findings suggest that multiple insults in MS may provide a useful model for the impact of serial injury on the developing brain. Results from animal research (Kolb, 1995) and MS studies, show levels of oligodendrocytes, which later form myelin, increase at lesion sites in recent onset MS but decrease in those who have had MS for many years (Ozawa et al., 1994; Prineas et al., 1993).

Role of Neuroimaging

In any condition that relies heavily on neuroimaging for diagnosis and prognosis, it is important to keep pace with ever-evolving and newer imaging techniques, and this is especially true in the case of MS. Advances, such as diffusion-tensor imaging (DTI) and tractography, and magnetization transfer imaging (MTI), are currently assisting in the identification of potential damage in normal-appearing brain tissue and white matter tracts in people with MS. When combined with functional imaging techniques, such methods have the potential to provide a better understanding of the impact of such conditions on cognitive neural networks, especially in the developing brain.

Impact of Serial CNS "Hits"

Multiple, early insults in childhood MS may leave a child at high risk for a range of cognitive impairments (Banwell & Anderson, 2005; Deery et al., 2005, 2008; MacAllister et al., 2005, 2007), but these cognitive impairments may not become fully apparent until later in childhood when these skills are expected to emerge or become more fully developed. The case of S. J. highlights how some cognitive functions may not be recognized as problematic until demand for such skills increases.

Neuropsychologists need to assess more than global measures of cognition. Attention and executive functioning are particularly pertinent for childhood MS. The case of S. J. shows that IQ measures in isolation do not provide a comprehensive picture, and that information relevant to diagnosis and treatment may be missed. Serial assessment is also important in degenerative conditions such as MS. It is our opinion that all children who experience a single episode of demyelination undergo a baseline assessment to (1) identify any identifiable cognitive deficits in order to assist with possible future management and (2) enable determinations about decline and impairment over time.

Pharmacological Treatments

Immunotherapy drugs have been shown to delay the onset of MS in at-risk patients (Comi et al., 2001) and have a beneficial impact on cognitive deterioration (Fischer et al., 2000). Their use in children with MS, or episodes suggestive of MS, is an important consideration. Case studies and small series have found these drugs to be well tolerated in childhood MS and to reduce relapse rates (Forrester et al., 2009; Mikaeloff et al., 2001), but their potential impact on cognitive function in childhood MS remains unknown. The fact that not all children who experience childhood demyelination and inflammation will be diagnosed with MS makes such decisions difficult for treating clinicians.

Management

Cognitive impairments can occur in children with MS even in the absence of marked physical disability, as documented in adult MS. As a result, the effects of MS in childhood may go unnoticed and lead to unrealistic expectations being placed on the child at home and at school. This may further add to a stressful situation and contribute to emotional difficulties and poor self-esteem. Families, schools, and health professionals need to be aware of the potential cognitive consequences of childhood MS.

Conclusion

The case of S. J. taken together with findings from group studies of childhood MS indicates that younger age at onset is not necessarily a protective factor for cognitive functioning. In fact, children with CNS conditions of "adulthood" may be at increased risk for impairments caused by interruptions to their cognitive, social, and behavioral development, and alterations to typical brain developmental trajectories. Multiple sclerosis in childhood can have a widespread impact on a variety of neuropsychological abilities, such as speed of processing, complex attention, and executive functioning. The full impact of these may not be recognized until years after disease onset, and these limitations have the potential to influence personality, social, behavioral, and academic outcomes. Multiple CNS insults at a young age may produce an additive, synergistic impact on development. Childhood MS remains a relatively "new" diagnosis, with limited research and resources to guide practitioners and allied health professionals regarding the assessment, treatment, management, and follow-up of these children. Future research endeavours and funding opportunities should provide much-needed assistance to increase our knowledge and care for these children and their families.

References

Anderson, P., Anderson, V., & Garth, J. (2001). Assessment and development of organizational ability: The Rey Complex Figure Organizational Strategy Score (RCF-OSS). *The Clinical Neuropsychologist*, *15*, 81–94.

Anderson, P., Anderson, V., Northam, E., & Taylor, H. G. (2000). Standardization of the Contingency Naming Test (CNT) for school-aged children: A measure of reactive flexibility. *Clinical Neuropsychological Assessment*, *1*, 247–273.

Anderson, V., & Moore, C. (1995). Age at injury as a predictor of outcome following pediatric head injury: A longitudinal perspective. *Child Neuropsychology*, *1*, 187–202.

Army Individual Battery Test. (1944). *Manual of directions and scoring*. Washington DC: War Department, Adjunct General's Office.

Balassy, C., Bernet, G., Wober-Bongol, C., Csapo, B., Szeles, J., Fleischmann, D., & Prayer, D. (2001). Long-term MRI observations of childhood-onset relapsing-remitting multiple sclerosis. *Neuropediatrics*, *32*, 28–37.

Banwell, B. L., & Anderson, P. E. (2005). The cognitive burden of multiple sclerosis in children. *Neurology*, *64*, 891-894

Banwell, B. L., Shroff, M., Ness, J. M. Jeffrey, D., Schwid, S., & Weinstock-Guttman, B. (2007).

MRI features of pediatric multiple sclerosis. *Neurology, 68*(Suppl. 2), S46–S53.

Barcellos, L. F., Oksenberg, J. R., Begovich, A. B., Martin, E. R., Schmidt, S., Vittinghoff, E., Goodin, D. S., Pelletier, D., Lincoln, R. R., Bucher, P., Swerdlin, A., Perick-Vance, M. A., Haines, J. L., & Hauser, S. L. (2003). HLA-DR2 dose effect on susceptibility to multiple sclerosis and influence on disease course. *American Journal of Human Genetics, 72*, 710–716.

Boiko, A., Vorobeychik, G., Paty, D., Devonshire, V., & Sadovnick, D. (2002). Early onset multiple sclerosis: A longitudinal study. *Neurology, 59*(7), 1006–1010.

Boston Cure Project. (2004). The path to a cure. Retrieved March 15, 2005, from http://www.acceleratedcure.org/downloads/interview-banwell.pdf

Boutin, B., Esquivel, E., Mayer, M., Chaumet, S., Ponsot, G., & Arthuis, M. (1988). Multiple sclerosis in children: report of clinical and paraclinical features of 19 cases. *Neuropediatrics, 19*, 118–123.

Bye, A. M. E., Kendall, B., & Wilson, J. (1985). Multiple sclerosis in childhood: A new look. *Developmental Medicine and Child Neurology, 27*, 215–222.

Cohen, M. J. (1997). *Children's Memory Scale.* San Antonio, TX: The Psychological Corporation.

Comi, G., Filippi, M., Barkhof, F., Durelli, L., Edan, G., & Fernandez, O. (2001). Effect of early interferon treatment on conversion to definite multiple sclerosis: A randomized study. *The Lancet, 357*, 1576–1582.

Compston, A. (1999). The genetic epidemiology of multiple sclerosis. Philosophical Transactions of the Royal Society of London, Series B-Biological Sciences, 345, 1623–1634.

Confavreux, C., Vukusic, S., & Adeleine, P. (2003). Early clinical predictors and progression of irreversible disability in multiple sclerosis: An amnesic process. *Brain, 126*, 770–782.

Davies, J. M. (1997). Molecular mimicry: Can epitope mimicry induce autoimmune disease? *Immunology and Cell Biology, 75*, 113–126.

Deery, B., Anderson, V., Jacobs, R., Neale, J., & Kornberg, A. (2005). Pediatric MS vs ADEM, more in common than just the letter M? Analysis and comparison of cognitive features. *Journal of the International Neuropsychological Society, 11*(Suppl. 1), A50

Deery, B., Anderson, V., Jacobs, R., Neale, J., & Kornberg, A. (2008). Longitudinal investigation of attention and executive functioning in pediatric multiple sclerosis and acute disseminated encephalomyelitis. *Journal of the International Neuropsychological Society, 14*(Suppl. 1), A3

Ebner, F., Millner, M. M., & Justich, E. (1990). Multiple sclerosis in children: Value of serial MR studies to monitor patients. *American Journal of Neuroradiology, 11*, 1023–1027.

Feinstein, A., Kartsounis, L. D., Miller, D. H., Youl, B. D., & Ron, M. A. (1992). Clinically isolated lesions of the type seen in multiple sclerosis: Cognitive, psychiatric, and MRI follow-up study. *Journal of Neurology, Neurosurgery and Psychiatry, 55*, 869–876.

Filippi, M., Tortorella, C., Rovaris, M., Bozzali, M., Possa, F., Sormani, M. P., Ianucci, G., & Comi, G. (2000). Changes in the normal appearing brain tissue and cognitive impairment in multiple sclerosis. *Journal of Neurology, Neurosurgery, and Psychiatry, 68*, 157–161.

Fischer, J. S., Priore, R. L., Jacobs, L. D., Cookfair, D. L., Rudick, R. A., & Herndon, R. M. (2000). Neuropsychological effects of interferon β-1a in relapsing multiple sclerosis. *Annals of Neurology, 48*(6), 885–892.

Fletcher, J. M., Brookshire, B. L., Landry, S. H., Bohan, T. P., Davidson, K. C., & Francis, D. J. (1996). Attentional skills and executive functions in children with early hydrocephalus. *Developmental Neuropsychology, 12*, 53–76.

Forrester, M. B., Coleman, L., & Kornberg, A. K. (2009). Multiple sclerosis in childhood: Clinical and radiological features. *Journal of Child Neurology, 24*, 56–62.

Gaddes, W. H., & Crockett, D. J. (1975). The Spreen Benton Aphasia Tests: Normative data as a measure of normal language development. *Brain and Language, 2*, 257–279.

Hammond, S. F., McLeod, J. G., Macaskill, P., & English, D. R. (2000). Multiple sclerosis in Australia: Prognostic factors. *Journal of Clinical Neuroscience, 7*, 16–19.

Hynson, J. L., Kornberg, A. J., Coleman, L. T., Shield, L., Harvey, A. S., & Kean M. J. (2001). Clinical and neuroradiologic features of acute disseminated encephalomyelitis in children. *Neurology, 56*, 1308–1312.

Iannetti, P., Marciani, M. G., Spalice, A., Raucci, U., Trasimeni, G., Gualdi, G. F., & Bernardi, G. (1996). Primary CNS demyelinating diseases in childhood: Multiple sclerosis. *Child's Nervous System, 12*, 149–154.

Jacobs, L. D., Cookfair, D. L., Rudick, R. A., Herndon, R. M., Richert, J. R., & Salazar, A. M. (1996). Intramuscular interferon beta-la for disease progression in relapsing multiple sclerosis. *Annals of Neurology, 39*, 285–294.

Kalb, R. C., Di Lorenzo, T. A., La Rocca, N. G., Caruso, L. S., Shawaryn, M. A., Elkin, R., & Dince, W. M. (1999). The impact of early-onset multiple sclerosis on cognitive and psychosocial indices. *International Journal of MS Care, 1*(1), 2–17.

Klinberg, T., Vaidyn, C. J., Gabrieli, J. D. E., Moseley, M. E., & Heidehus, M. (1999). Myelination and organization of the frontal white matter in children: A diffusion tensor MRI study. *NeuroReport, 10,* 2817–2821.

Kolb, B. (1995). *Brain plasticity and behavior.* New Jersey: Erlbaum.

Kurtzke, J. F., Beebe, G. W., & Norman, J. E. (1985). Epidemiology of multiple sclerosis in United-States Veterans. III. Migration and the risk of MS. *Neurology, 35(5),* 672–678.

Levic, Z. M., Dujmovic, I., Pekmezovic, T., Jarebinski, M., Marinkovic, J., Stojsavljevic, N., & Drulovic, J. (1999). Prognostic factors for survival in multiple sclerosis. *Multiple Sclerosis, 5,* 171–178.

MacAllister, W. S., Belman, A. L., Milazzo, M., Weisbrot, D. M., Christodoulou, C., Scherl, W. F., Preston, T. E., Cianciulli, C., & Krupp, L. B. (2005). Cognitive functioning in children and adolescents with multiple sclerosis. *Neurology, 64,* 1422–1425.

MacAllister, W. S., Christodoulou, C., Milazzo, M., & Krupp, L. B. (2007). Longitudinal neuropsychological assessment in pediatric multiple sclerosis. *Developmental Neuropsychology, 32*(2), 625–644.

Manly, T., Robertson, I., Anderson, V., & Nimmo-Smith, I. (1999). *Test of Everyday Attention for Children.* Cambridge, England: Thames Valley Test Company.

McDonald, W. I., Compston, A., Edan, G., Goodkin, D., Hartung, H. P., Lublin, F. D., McFarland, H. F., Paty, D. W., Polman, C. H., Reingold, S. C., Sandberg-Wollheim, M., Sibley, W., Thompson, A., Ven Den Noort, S., Weinshenker, B. Y., & Wolinsky, J. S. (2001). Recommended diagnostic criteria for multiple sclerosis: Guidelines from the international panel on the diagnosis of multiple sclerosis. *Annals of Neurology, 50*(1), 121–127.

Mikaeloff, Y., Moreau, T., Debouverie, M., Pelletier, J., Lebrun, C., Gout, O., Pedespan, J. M., Van Hulle, C., Vermersch, P., & Ponsot, G. (2001). Interferon-β treatment in patients with childhood-onset multiple sclerosis. *The Journal of Pediatrics, 139,* 443–446.

Mikaeloff, Y., Suissa, S., Vallée, L., Lubetzki, C., Ponsot, G., Confavreux, C., Tardieu, M., & the KIDMUS Study Group. (2004). First episode of acute CNS inflammatory demyelination in childhood: Prognostic factors for multiple sclerosis and disability. *Journal of Pediatrics, 144*(2), 246–252.

Ozawa, K., Suchanek, G., Breitschopf, H., Bruck, W., Budka, H., & Jelllinger, K. (1994). Patterns of oligodendroglia pathology in multiple sclerosis. *Brain, 117,* 1311–1322.

Pinhaus-Hamiel, O., Barak, Y., Siev-Ner, I., & Achiron, A. (1998). Juvenile multiple sclerosis: Clinical features

and prognostic characteristics. *Journal of Pediatrics, 132,* 735–737.

Prineas, J. W., Barnard, R. O., Revesz, T., Kwon, E. E., Sharer, L., & Cho, E. S. (1993). Multiple sclerosis: Pathology of recurrent lesions. *Brain, 116,* 681–693.

Rakic, P. (1995). Corticogenesis in human and non-human primates. In M. S. Gazzaniga (Ed.), *The cognitive neurosciences* (pp. 127–145). Cambridge, MA: MIT Press.

Rao, S. M., Leo, G. J., Bernardin, L., & Unverzagt, F. (1991). Cognitive dysfunction in multiple sclerosis: I. Frequency, patterns, and predictors. *Neurology, 41,* 685–691.

Rey, A. (1964). *L'examen clinique en psychologie.* Paris: Presses Universitaires de France.

Rudick, R. A., Fisher, E., Lee, J. C., Simon, J., & Jacobs, L. (1999). Use of the brain parenchymal fraction to measure whole brain atrophy in relapsing-remitting MS. Multiple Sclerosis Collaborative Research Group. *Neurology, 53,* 1698–1704.

Sadovnick, A. D., Dircks, A., & Ebers, G. C. (1999). Genetic counselling in multiple sclerosis: Risks to sibs and children of affected individuals. *Clinical Genetics, 56,* 118–122.

Simone, I. L., Carrara, D., Tortorella C., Liguori, M., Lepore, V., Pellegrini, F., Bellacosa, A., Ceccarelli, A., Pavone, I. & Livrea, P. (2002). Course and prognosis in early onset MS. Comparison with adult-onset forms. *Neurology, 59,* 1922–1928.

Smolders, J., Damoiseaux, J., Menheere, P., & Hupperts, R. (2008). Vitamin D as an immune modulator in multiple sclerosis, a review. *Journal of Neuroimmunology, 194,* 7–17.

Taylor, H. G., Albo, V., Phebus, C., Sachs, B., & Bierl, P. (1987). Post-irradiation treatment outcomes for children with acute lymphoblastic leukemia: Clarification of risks. *Journal of Pediatric Psychology, 12,* 395–411.

Vukusic, S., & Confavreux, C. (2001). Natural history of multiple sclerosis. In S. D. Cook (Ed.), *Handbook of multiple sclerosis* (3rd ed., pp. 433-448). New York: Marcel Dekker.

Wechsler, D. (2004). *Wechsler Intelligence Scale for Children – Australian Edition* (4th ed.). San Antonio, TX: Psychological Corporation.

Welsh, M. C., Pennington, B. F., Ozonoff, S., Rouse, B., & McCabe, E. R. (1990). Neuropsychology of early-treated phenylketonuria: Specific executive function deficits. *Child Development, 61,* 1697–1713.

Wilkinson, G. S. (1993). *Wide Range Achievement Test 3 (WRAT-3) Administration manual.* Wilmington, DE: Wide Range, Inc.

47

Adult Multiple Sclerosis

Darcy Cox

Multiple sclerosis (MS) is the most common neurological disease in young adults (Anderson et al., 1992). The disease is characterized by areas of inflammatory demyelination, or lesions, in the CNS, as well as atrophy of the brain and spinal cord. Peripheral nerves are unaffected. Individuals afflicted with the disorder can develop a wide variety of physical, cognitive, and emotional symptoms depending on the location and extent of the lesions and the extent of CNS atrophy. Common symptoms can include paresthesias and numbness, gait disturbance, weakness, balance disturbance, dizziness, vertigo, visual dysfunction, sexual dysfunction, significant fatigue, pain, depression, and cognitive impairment (Mohr & Cox, 2001). As with most autoimmune disorders, women are more likely to be affected than men (Cooper & Stroehla, 2003; Noonan, Kathma, & White, 2002). The age of onset is usually between 20 and 40 years, although the disease can develop in young children or older adults.

The majority of patients initially experience a relapsing-remitting disease course, consisting of exacerbations, or periods of new symptoms or increased symptom severity lasting more than 24 hours, which then gradually subside (Noseworthy, Lucchinetti, Rodriguez, & Weinshenker, 2000). Many patients experience a complete remission of symptoms between exacerbations particularly during the early years of the disease, but over time, most patients begin to accumulate some persistent symptoms that gradually lead to some level of physical disability. Exacerbations may be related to the development or reactivation of the

inflammatory demyelinating lesions, but the majority of newly developed or reactivated lesions are clinically silent, producing no symptoms noticeable to the patient or detectable on physical exam at the time they develop. At this time, the relapsing-remitting stage of the disease is the most amenable to treatment. In the last 20 years, six medications have been developed that have been shown to reduce the number of exacerbations, reduce the number of new lesions, and slow the progression of disability in patients with relapsing forms of MS (interferon beta-1a IM and SC, interferon beta-1b, glatiramer acetate, mitoxantrone, and natilizumab) (Polman et al., 2006; Rizvi & Agisu, 2004). All of these therapies involve injections, either self-administered subcutaneously or intramuscularly, or intravenous infusions provided in the clinic. Thus, the burden of treatment can be quite high for some patients who are afraid of injections or who have difficulty traveling to their health providers to receive infusions (Mohr, Boudewyn, Likosky, Levine, & Goodkin, 2001). Unfortunately, these treatments are far from perfect. The interferon-betas often produce flu-like side effects and all the medications that are injected subcutaneously can cause injection site reactions. Mitoxantrone can produce cardiotoxicity and blood disorders. Natilizumab can produce progressive multifocal leukodystrophy (PML), an extremely aggressive and potentially fatal viral encephalopathy.

Roughly half of patients who initially present with a relapsing-remitting course will go on to develop secondary progressive disease (Noseworthy et al., 2000). This more advanced stage of the disease is characterized by greater levels of brain and spinal cord atrophy and greater levels of physical and cognitive disability. Natilizimab and mitoxantrone are approved for treatment of patients with secondary progressive MS. While the majority of MS patients have a relapsing course, roughly 10% of patients have primary progressive MS. This disease course is characterized by steady accumulation of disability without exacerbations. Unfortunately, this disease course is less well understood. Currently, there are no treatments that have demonstrated efficacy at slowing this version of the disease.

The FDA-approved disease-modifying treatments are not effective in all patients. Many neurologists use cytotoxic chemotherapy agents, high-dose steroids, or other immunosuppressive treatments as "rescue" treatments for patients who are continuing to accumulate disability while on an approved disease-modifying agent (Frohmann et al., 2005). These medications, particularly high-dose, high-frequency corticosteroids, can have direct negative impacts on cognition and mood. Most patients with MS also require medications to manage their individual MS symptoms. These can include a number of medications for pain, spasticity, and paresthesias that may impact cognitive functioning and mood.

Aside from medication effects and the impact of fatigue and depression, the disease process itself commonly causes cognitive impairment. Cognitive impairment can develop at any point in the disease process, including very early in the course of the disease (Glanz et al., 2007). The estimated point-prevalence of cognitive impairment is 30%–60%, with a lifetime prevalence closer to 50%–75% (Amato, Ponziani, Siracusa, & Sorbi, 2001; Rao, Leo, Bernardin, & Unverzagt, 1991). Cognitive symptoms do not correlate strongly with physical symptoms: individuals who have few or no physical symptoms may have significant cognitive impairment, and individuals who have significant physical disability may be cognitively intact (Amato et al., 2008; Rao, Leo, Bernardin, et al., 1991). However, overall cognitive symptoms appear to be most strongly predicted by the degree of cortical atrophy (Benedict et al., 2002; Morgen et al., 2006). Patients frequently have subtle and diverse findings on

neuropsychological testing, including difficulties with slowed processing speed, reduced working memory, encoding, and recall, and reduced verbal fluency (Zakzanis, 2000). Historically, MS has been characterized as producing a subcortical dementia, but it is important to remember that many different cognitive symptoms can and do develop, and that most patients do not experience symptoms severe enough to meet criteria for a diagnosis of dementia. However, it is reasonable to expect that most patients with significant atrophy will experience slowed processing speed, difficulties with generative naming, and difficulty learning new information. Cognitive dysfunction may well prove a barrier to continued employment or may lead to the need for at least some assistance with personal affairs (Rao, Leo, Ellington, et al., 1991).

Most patients also report and demonstrate significant problems with physical and cognitive fatigue, which further adversely impacts patients' quality of life and ability to maintain paid employment. Fatigue resulting from MS can be worsened by a number of factors, including overheating, exacerbations, and minor infections. Despite fatigue, it is important for MS patients to persist with regular moderate exercise because fatigue tends to worsen significantly in patients who become sedentary.

Depression is also a problem for many individuals with MS. Point-prevalence rates for major depressive disorder in MS are around 20%, and lifetime prevalence may be as high as 50% (Chwastiak et al., 2002; Joffe, Lippert, Gray, Sawa, & Horvath, 1987). This appears to be the result of as yet unidentified factors related to autoimmune dysfunction, rather than a purely psychological response to the particular challenges and losses brought about by the experience of living with MS. However, the uncertainties and challenges associated with living with MS can and do contribute to depression. Depression in MS is rarely self-limiting, but it responds well to both cognitive-behavioral psychotherapy and medication management (Mohr, Boudewyn, Goodkin, Bostrom, & Epstein, 2001; Mohr et al., 2005).

The following case illustrates many of the challenges facing patients with MS who experience cognitive dysfunction and depression secondary to the disease. This case is also illustrative of the coping challenges faced by patients with more aggressive and rapidly progressive disease courses.

Case Study: Mr. A

December 2002

Mr. A was referred by his neurologist in December 2002 to obtain a cognitive baseline and to assess for depression. At the time of his referral, he was 41 years old and had been married for 19 years, with two young children. Prior to his diagnosis, Mr. A had been working as an international marketing executive for a large technology company in Silicon Valley. He reported that over the last 3 years he was noticing increased difficulty with multitasking, a key requirement in his career. He stated that he had started to seek out positions within his company that reduced his responsibility and that allowed him to avoid working on multiple projects simultaneously. Mr. A was laid off from his company in the course of a large workforce reduction. He was diagnosed with MS 1 month later after his wife insisted he see a doctor after he fell while jogging.

Mr. A was the second of three brothers born and raised in Sweden. His family immigrated to the United States when he was 12 years old and he learned English at that time. He has one paternal uncle with MS who lives in Europe. Mr. A earned a partial athletic scholarship to play tennis at an Ivy League university. He earned his BS in Engineering and graduated with the highest academic honors. He then earned his MBA. He and his wife began dating as undergraduates and married while he was in graduate school and she was in law school. After his graduation, he began working in international business development. He and his wife were both very physically active and enjoyed tennis, running, and mountaineering.

At the time of the initial visit, Mr. A reported increasing difficulty jogging (due to foot drop), tingling and pain in his feet, depression, and erectile dysfunction. Cognitively, he reported difficulty multitasking, losing his train of thought during conversations, distractibility, and difficulties with word finding. He stated that his thought processes were a little more concrete and that he had difficulty identifying all the possible alternatives in situations. He also reported feeling extremely guilty about his inability to

find work after he was laid off. However, as a result of wise investments after his company began trading stock publicly, the A family was not in significant financial distress despite the loss of Mr. A's income. While Mr. A was able to acknowledge his family's financial security, he reported intense guilt about the burden that he perceived his illness placed on his wife and his fear that his children would "think less of him" for having MS and being unemployed. He reported sadness, guilt, and passive suicidal ideation. His initial magnetic resonance image (MRI) revealed extensive T-2 lesions throughout his brain, with multiple lesions enhancing with gadolinium. His MRI was also notable for mild atrophy. His neurologist considered his disease to be very active and treated him with cyclophosphamide infusions and interferon beta 1a subcutaneously. His fatigue was severe, requiring two or more rest periods per day.

Mr. A's neuropsychological test results are summarized in Table 47-1. Symptom validity screening did not suggest that Mr. A was suppressing his performance at any point during testing. It was my opinion that his effort was good and test results were valid.

Mr. A's performance on the WAIS-III represented a decline from his estimated premorbid functioning. While his FSIQ was in the high range of general intellectual ability and at the 85th to 90th percentile, his performance demonstrated significant subtest scatter. Some scores were particularly low in the context of Mr. A's engineering and finance background. Mr. A's average score on Arithmetic was considered to be unusual, given his background as a financial executive. His score resulted from difficulty attending to the problems and difficulty generating the solution quickly, as well as a tendency to apply inappropriate strategies to solve the problems. Mr. A's average score on Block Design was also concerning, given his engineering background. This was a result of slowed processing speed and visual-spatial construction deficits, rather than hand weakness or coordination loss. Mr. A's neurologist reported no change in grip strength, finger sensitivity, or motor speed. Mr. A's performance on Similarities was also low. Mr. A demonstrated significant slowing in his processing speed, with his PSI falling in the average range when all other WAIS-III Indices were high

Table 47-1. Mr. A, December 2002

WAIS-III ACSS and Index Scores			
Picture Completion	14	Vocabulary	15
Digit Symbol	9	Similarities	10
Block Design	9	Arithmetic	11
Matrix Reasoning	17	Digit Span	13
Picture Arrangement	13	Information	15
Symbol Search	11	Comprehension	13
VIQ	117	VCI	118
PIQ	116	POI	121
FSIQ	118	WMI	121
		PSI	99

WMS-III ACSS		CVLT-2 Z Scores	
Logical Memory I	10	SDFR	−4
Logical Memory II	10	SDCR	−2
Faces I	7	LDFR	−3
Faces II	9	LDCR	−2
Verbal Paired I	9	Recognition	−2
Verbal Paired II	9	FC Recognition (raw)	16/16/
Visual Rec I	10	TOMM (raw)	50/50/50
Visual Rec II	13		
Auditory Rec	12		
Letter Number	17		
Spatial Span	14		

D-KEFS ACSS			
Trails 1	10	COWAT	45 words
Trails 2	6	Animals	18 words
Trails 3	6	BNT (raw)	50/51/59/60
Trails 4	8	PASAT 3" (raw)	53
Trails 5	11	PASAT 2" (raw)	35
Sorting, CCS	12	SDMT	52 (raw)
		BDI-2 (raw)	23

WCST-64 ACSS	
Total Errors	98
Persev Errors	96

average to superior. Again, this score was not due to motor dysfunction. Mr. A's score on the Symbol Digit Modality Test, a verbal analog of Digit Symbol, was consistent with his performance on Digit Symbol. Mr. A's slowed processing speed was also apparent on the DKEFS Trails tasks, with very low average to mildly impaired performance on processing tasks, but average motor speed and visual scanning.

Mr. A's average processing speed was likely a strong contributor to his day-by-day cognitive difficulties. Mr. A's average performance on most subtests of the WMS-III and his moderately impaired performance on the CVLT-2 was also

concerning. Mr. A demonstrated difficulties with encoding in the face of relatively intact recall. Mr. A did not use a semantic encoding strategy on the CVLT-2. Instead, he attempted to organize the list alphabetically. This strategy was ineffective, but Mr. A did not shift to a semantic organizational strategy on the long delay recall trials even after this was cued on the short delay cued recall trials and his performance improved as a result. He also demonstrated difficulty recognizing items from the list, although he was completely accurate on forced choice testing.

This inability to change his learning strategy when it proved ineffective suggested lack of mental flexibility. However, his performance on the WCST was average for someone of his age with at least 18 years of education. His ability to engage in verbal analog reasoning was average for someone of his age, as was his ability to categorize novel stimuli and to generate novel solutions. Finally, Mr. A's verbal fluency, while within broad normal limits for someone of his age, was not consistent with his educational and occupational history. This finding is complicated because Mr. A learned English in his teens.

Mr. A found the neuropsychological test results to be consistent with his experience of cognitive change and he accepted the diagnosis of depression. Mr. A was unwilling to consider pharmacotherapy for depression due to fears of increased sexual dysfunction. Mr. A elected to enroll in a study examining different psychotherapeutic treatments for depression in MS patients. Unfortunately, he was randomly assigned to a treatment arm that proved to be ineffective. Upon completion of this study without noticeable symptom improvement, Mr. A accepted pharmacotherapy and was treated with 450 mg of bupropion. He reported some improvement in mood and stated that he felt "mentally sharper." He no longer experienced any suicidal ideation.

Over the next 3 years, despite continued aggressive treatment, Mr. A developed spinal lesions and spinal atrophy, as well as additional cortical lesions and cortical atrophy. His gait disturbance worsened and he developed bladder urgency and frequency. He had occasional episodes of bladder incontinence. He engaged aggressively in daily physical therapy and completed an exercise routine developed by a physiotherapist on a daily basis. However, within 18 months, he relied on a single cane for ambulation. He remained unemployed. His fatigue worsened and he required a 2-hour nap most afternoons before his children returned home from school. His lower limb paresthesias worsened and he began gabapentin. He began taking modafinil for fatigue and oxybutynin to manage his bladder symptoms.

October 2005

In the spring of 2005, Mr. A agreed to his neurologist's recommendation to apply for Social Security Disability. His neurologist also recommended follow-up cognitive screening and a reevaluation of worsening depressive symptoms.

Mr. A's cognitive functioning in 2005, summarized in Table 47-2, appeared generally stable when compared to his performance in 2002. His performance on the CVLT-2 was improved, most likely because Mr. A was now using semantic clustering to aid learning. However, Mr. A also needed frequent rehearsal to manage ongoing encoding impairment and continued to struggle with working memory, as revealed by his high number of repetition errors. Mr. A's

Table 47-2. Mr. A, October 2005

Woodcock-Johnson, 3rd Ed. ACSS		CVLT-2–Alternate Z Scores	
Story Memory I	104	SDFR	−.5
Story Memory II	97	SDCR	0
BVMT-R T Scores		LDFR	−1
Immediate	36	LDCR	−.5
Delay	48	Recognition	0
Rec	6/6	FC Rec (raw)	16/16
		Repetitions (raw)	17
Digit Span ACSS	9		
Letter Number ACSS	13	COWAT	45 (words)
Spatial Span ACSS	11	Grocery	18 (words)
SDMT	41 (raw)	BNT (raw)	54/54/60
WCST-64 ACSS		BDI-2 (raw)	18
Total Errors	103		
Perseverative Errors	98		
D-KEFS Sorting, Alternate			
CCS ACSS	16		

ability to attend, concentrate, and process information quickly was also slightly weaker than his performance in these domains in 2002. Mr. A demonstrated worsening visual-spatial memory, with a weaker performance on the BVMT-R than on Visual Reproduction in 2002. His performance on the WCST-64 and the D-KEFS Sorting task was stronger than his performance in 2002 and generally consistent with his estimated premorbid functioning. However, Mr. A reported ongoing concern about his problem-solving abilities. Mr. A readily admitted worsening depression. He stated that he felt guilty for how irritable he was with his wife, but he also felt like she was "constantly nagging" and that she was not supporting his efforts to manage his condition.

I met with Mr. and Mrs. A for an extended interview. The As reported significant martial difficulty. Mr. A described the state of their marriage by saying, "She feels like she has to do everything, and she's probably right." He reported intense anger and frustration when he experienced limitations because of his worsening physical symptoms and profound grief that he was not able to play tennis with his children. He stated that he felt worthless and that both he and his family "would be better off if he were dead" because he "could no longer contribute in any meaningful way." Mr. A continued to engage in daily physical therapy and held himself to a highly restrictive diet. He believed that intensive physical therapy offered him the best chance for preserving his physical functioning. Mr. A had also begun volunteering once a week at a local environmental center. While he verbally disparaged volunteer work as "just filling time," he was insistent that he be available to the center on his regularly scheduled day and time even if it conflicted with other family members' schedules. He later acknowledged that he found volunteer work highly satisfying because his co-workers "didn't know me from before, so they can accept me as I am."

Mrs. A was continuing to work full time. The As had a number of part-time babysitters as well as a housekeeper. However, Mrs. A reported that she felt Mr. A was not "taking the initiative" to do many tasks at home that he could physically perform but that he had not done before his illness, like folding laundry or tidying up. She also felt that he did not set limits on the children's

behavior. Mrs. A found it very frustrating to hear about how engaged her husband was while volunteering or while at physical therapy because at home he was generally irritable and withdrawn. In response to her frustration, Mrs. A increased her efforts to encourage her husband to make changes. She attempted to suggest strategies Mr. A could use to increase his participation in the household and to discipline the children, but Mr. A would "forget" to implement these strategies. Mr. A found these efforts "controlling" and "infantilizing," and he would reply, "I don't need to be told how to father my children." She reported that she could not tell what was the result of true memory failure and what was the result of Mr. A's "unwillingness to compromise." Mr. A agreed with her assessment that some of this "forgetting" in fact represented his refusal to do things in the way she wanted.

Before his diagnosis, Mr. A's primary activities with his children included playing sports and engaging in intense physical activity with them. Due to his extensive travel schedule, he had taken a less active role than his wife in developing and maintaining their daily routines. After he stopped working, he became more involved, but he was more permissive than his wife. When Mr. A perceived his wife as criticizing his parenting style, he would become profoundly angry and frightened. He saw parenting as the only important life role he had left. As his physical disability progressed, he became behaviorally rigid in an attempt to preserve his sense of control and independence. Mrs. A feared that Mr. A's current behavior "could be a personality change due to MS, I heard that can happen if the frontal lobes are involved." She stated that she was afraid "I might never get my husband back."

These difficulties revealed a number of common issues that arise when an MS patient develops cognitive dysfunction and depression, particularly in the context of increased physical disability and fatigue. Mr. A was struggling with a significant change in his self-image and grieving his loss of capability in areas where he had previously excelled. He could no longer completely control either his body or his memory and he responded to his lack of control by developing extremely rigid and controlling behavioral routines. I recommended both individual therapy for Mr. A and couples therapy with a therapist who had extensive experience treating patients with neurological disorders.

Cognitive behavioral, rational-emotive, active coping, and mindfulness techniques were used to help Mr. A manage his intense anger and grief about his diagnosis and disability. Behavioral therapies were also implemented to help Mr. A develop a daily routine that met his goals of physical exercise but that also emphasized the need for regular rest periods, which insured that his fatigue did not become severe. Severe fatigue made it more difficult for him to maintain a positive mood. Mr. A began volunteering as a "class parent" for an hour twice weekly at his children's school in the mornings, which gave him the opportunity to receive ongoing positive feedback about his strengths as a parent. Individual therapy in conjunction with medications was successful and Mr. A's mood improved significantly.

However, couples therapy was complicated by Mr. A's difficulties generating good solutions to complex problems "in the moment." Mr. A would agree to whatever his wife suggested during an argument. Then, when alone, he would ignore the agreement and proceed as he saw fit. Both As found negative affect very difficult to tolerate. As soon as Mr. A's mood improved, they discontinued couples therapy. Mrs. A's concern that some of her husband's difficulties were the result of frontal lobe dysfunction was a potentially valid one. However, Mr. A retained the ability to control his emotional expression and was not demonstrating any problems with disinhibition, apathy, or other frontal behavioral syndromes. It was the view of their couples therapist that while Mr. A was not able to process information quickly, particularly when emotionally upset, Mr. A's cognitive dysfunction was not the primary factor driving the As communication problems.

April 2008

I conducted a screening evaluation of Mr. A for the final time in April of 2008. His most recent MRI was notable for no new lesions but significant cortical atrophy and ventricular enlargement. Mr. A was primarily using an electric wheelchair for ambulation. He transferred independently, and he showered independently using a shower chair. The As had modified one of their vehicles to use hand controls and a wheelchair lift and Mr. A continued to drive. He reported that he felt his depression was "finally really under control," although he continued to participate in occasional booster sessions with his therapist. He continued 450 mg of bupropion. He engaged in water-based physical therapy on most days, but he was no longer angry if the family schedule required that he change his routine. He reported that he needed to be more careful when swallowing and he was awaiting a swallowing evaluation. He continued to have problems with bladder urgency and frequency and paresthenias. He had developed problems with spasticity that he was treating with baclofen. Mr. A had started donepezil in the hope of preserving his cognitive function. He was also was playing games designed to improve "brain fitness" on his personal computer. He continued to volunteer occasionally at the environmental center but he did so less frequently because he found it too physically fatiguing. However, he had increased his involvement in his children's school and he reported that his relationships with his children were close and very satisfying. He stated that he was a better parent as a result of the changes he made in his life to accommodate MS and that he was proud that he could model resiliency for his children. Mr. A reported that he and Mrs. A continued to struggle with him feeling "bossed" and with her feeling overburdened. He also reported some episodes of bladder and bowel dysfunction during sexual activity, which both of them found very embarrassing. However, he stated they were both committed to raising their children together and that they generally enjoyed one another's company.

These results, summarized in Table 47-3, suggest continued worsening of visual-spatial memory, as Mr. A's difficulties on the BVMT-R were not the result of an inability to correctly draw the figures, but difficulty encoding and recalling them. While his performance on the CVLT-2 continued to improve, this improvement appeared to be the result of greater facility with semantic clustering. Mr. A reported that the cognitive puzzles he did on his computer also encouraged the use of this strategy on list-learning tasks. However, his performance on the COWAT did not improve significantly, and his performance on Animal Naming decreased, although Mr. A

Table 47-3. Mr. A, April 2008

		CVLT-2 Z Scores	
WMS-III LM I	10	SDFR	–.5
WMS-III LM II	10	SDCR	–.5
BVMT-R T Scores		LDFR	–.5
Immediate	34	LDCR	0
Delay	32	Recognition	–1
		Repetitions	7
		D-KEFS ACSS	
Digit Span ACSS	14	Trails 1	10
Letter Number ACSS	13	Trails 2	11
Spatial Span ACSS	12	Trails 3	10
SDMT	45 (raw)	Trails 4	8
COWAT	50 (words)	Trails 5	11
Animals	13 (words)	Tower	10
BDI-2	3 (raw)		

reported that he was generating words as part of his computerized therapy program.

Summary

As this case illustrates, cognitive dysfunction can develop quite early in the course of the disease. In Mr. A's case, he had already developed significant cognitive dysfunction before he was diagnosed. These changes were having an adverse impact on his work performance. Mr. A may very well have benefited from workplace accommodations to help manage his difficulties with processing speed and memory. However, it is unlikely that he would have been able to continue in an executive role. If Mr. A had not been laid off, he most likely would have needed to transition to a position that was much simpler and less cognitively taxing than those he held in the past. By October 2005, it was no longer possible for most employers to reasonably accommodate his cognitive and physical disabilities.

Despite his worsening physical symptoms, Mr. A's cognitive symptoms remained fairly stable over a 6-year course. His test performance, while reflecting a significant change from his presumed baseline, remained generally within broad normal limits. During this time, the primary factors adversely impacting Mr. A's quality of life were his depression, his changing self-image, and his interpersonal relationships. As with most patients with MS, Mr. A's depression

responded well to treatment with psychotherapy and pharmacology. In addition, Mr. A was now reporting some benefit-finding, a behavior associated with reduced depression, increased optimism, and active coping (Hart, Vella, & Mohr, 2008). While the As were able to maintain their marriage in a manner that was acceptable to both of them, many couples are unable to negotiate these challenges successfully (King & Arnett, 2005). Despite successfully negotiating the challenges of diagnosis, the As may face additional marital distress when Mr. A becomes more physically disabled and requires more physical assistance from his wife. Mr. A may also be at risk for a relapse of his depression as he becomes more physically dependent.

Mr. A's depression had an impact on a number of domains of cognitive functioning. Research suggests that depression in MS patients can adversely impact working memory, attention, and executive functioning (Arnett et al., 1999; Arnett, Higgenson, & Randolph, 2001; Feinstein, 2006). However, depression alone did not account for the cognitive difficulties Mr. A experienced, and some of these cognitive changes may have made his recovery from depression more challenging. Implementing strategies to manage physical fatigue was also important for Mr. A to improve day-by-day cognitive functioning and to improve mood.

While this case exemplifies the challenges faced by many MS patients, this case is atypical because the As did not need to change their standard of living significantly in response to Mr. A's disability and unemployment. While his disability did alter some of their long-term financial goals, the As were still able to afford an upper middle class lifestyle and to afford uncovered medical expenses, such as extensive physical therapy for Mr. A. Most patients with MS also face financial burdens in addition to the cognitive and physical symptoms of the disease. These financial burdens and concerns can greatly increase the risks of depression and relationship dysfunction.

Neuropsychologists working with patients with MS must be prepared to consider the overlapping influences that depression, fatigue, and neuropathology can have on cognition, and the impact cognitive dysfunction can have on patients' interpersonal relationships, response to treatment, and coping strategies. In addition, neuropsychologists need to address the specific challenges posed by repeated assessments to track progression of disease and assessments occurring in the context of patient requests for Americans with Disabilities Act accommodations from their employers or patients seeking disability benefits. I recommend the use of at least some symptom validity measures when assessing patients with MS, even if limited to reviewing embedded symptom validity indicators. Managing patient fatigue is also important, and it may require multiple assessment sessions. It is also important to specifically consider how patient compensation strategies may impact test scores on repeated measures and the subsequent interpretation of those scores as markers of real-life cognitive functioning. In Mr. A's case, his use of a computerized "brain health" software program may have had some positive impact on some of his test performances, but it may not have had a significant positive impact on his day-by-day functioning (Owen et al., 2010). Multiple sclerosis is a complex disease that leads to a number of burdens for those living with the disease and their families. Neuropsychologists have a great deal to offer to the care of these challenging patients.

References

Amato, M., Ponziani, G., Siracusa, G., & Sorbi, S. (2001). Cognitive dysfunction in early-onset multiple sclerosis: A reappraisal after 10 years. *Archives of Neurology, 58*(10), 1602–1606.

Amato, M., Portaccio, E., Stromillo, M., Goretti, B., Zipoli, V., Siracusa, G., et al. (2008). Cognitive assessment and quantitative magnetic reasonance metrics can help to identify benign multiple sclerosis. *Neurology, 71*, 632–638.

Anderson, D. W., Ellenberg, J. H., Leventhal, C. M., Reingold, S. C., Rodriguez, M., & Silberberg, D. H. (1992). Revised estimate of the prevalence of multiple sclerosis in the United States. *Annals of Neurology, 31*, 333–336.

Arnett, P. A., Higgenson, C. I., & Randolph, J. J. (2001). Depression in multiple sclerosis: Relationship to planning ability. *Journal of the International Neuropsychological Society, 7*, 665–674.

Arnett, P. A., Higgenson, C. I., Voss, W., Wright, B., Bender, W., Wurst, J., et al. (1999). Depressed mood in multiple sclerosis: Relationship to capacity-demanding memory and attentional functioning. *Neuropsychology, 13*(3), 434–446.

Benedict, R., Bakshi, R., Simon, J. H., Priore, R., Miller, C., & Munschauer, F. (2002). Frontal cortex atrophy predicts cognitive impairment in multiple sclerosis. *Journal of Neuropsychiatry and Clinical Neurosciences, 14*(1), 44–51.

Chwastiak, L., Ehde, D., Gibbons, L., Sullivan, M., Bowen, J., & Kraft, G. (2002). Depressive symptoms and severity of illness in multiple sclerosis: Epidemiologic study of a large community sample. *American Journal of Psychiatry, 159*(11), 1862–1868.

Cooper, G., & Stroehla, B. (2003). The epidemiology of autoimmune diseases. *Autoimmunity Reviews, 2*(3), 119–125.

Feinstein, A. (2006). Mood disorders in multiple sclerosis and the effects on cognition. *Journal of the Neurological Sciences, 245*(1–2), 63–66.

Frohmann, E. M., Stuve, O., Havrdova, E., Corboy, J., Achiron, A., Zivadinov, R., et al. (2005). Therapeutic considerations for disease progression in multiple sclerosis. *Archives of Neurology, 62*, 1519–1530.

Glanz, B., Holland, C., Gauthier, S., Amunwa, E., Liptak, Z., Houtchens, M., et al. (2007). Cognitive dysfunction in pateints with clinically isolated syndromes or newly diagnosed multiple sclerosis. *Multiple Sclerosis, 13*, 1004–1010.

Hart, S. L., Vella, L., & Mohr, D. C. (2008). Relationships among depressive symptoms, benefit-findings, optimism, and positive affect in multiple sclerosis patients after psychotherapy for depression. *Health Psychology, 27*(2), 230–238.

Joffe, R. T., Lippert, G. P., Gray, T. A., Sawa, G., & Horvath, Z. (1987). Mood disorder and multiple sclerosis. *Archives of Neurology, 44*, 376–378.

King, K. E., & Arnett, P. A. (2005). Predictors of dyadic adjustment in multiple sclerosis. *Multiple Sclerosis, 11*, 700–707.

Mohr, D. C., Boudewyn, A. C., Goodkin, D. E., Bostrom, A., & Epstein, L. (2001). Comparative outcomes for individual cognitive-behavior therapy, supportive-expressive group psychotherapy, and sertraline for the treatment of depression in multiple sclerosis. *Journal of Consulting and Clinical Psychology, 69*(6), 942–949.

Mohr, D. C., Boudewyn, A.C., Likosky, W., Levine, E., & Goodkin, D.E. (2001). Injectable medication for the treatment of multiple sclerosis: The influence of expectations and injection anxiety on adherence and ability to self-inject. *Annals of Behavioral Medicine, 23*, 125–132.

Mohr, D. C., & Cox, D. (2001). Multiple sclerosis: Empirical literature for the clinical health psychologist. *Journal of Clinical Psychology, 57*, 479–499.

Mohr, D.C., Hart, S. L., Julian, L., Catledge, C., Honos-Webb, L., Vella, L., et al. (2005). Telephone-administered psychotherapy for depression. *Archives of General Psychiatry, 62*(9), 1007–1014.

Morgen, K., Sammer, G., Courtney, S. M., Wolters, T., Melchior, H., Blecker, C. R., et al. (2006). Evidence for a direct association between cortical atrophy and cognitive impairment in relapsing-remitting MS. *Neuroimage*, *30*(3), 891–898.

Noonan, C., Kathma, S., & White, M. (2002). Prevalence estimates for MS in the United States and evidence for an increasing trend for women. *Neurology*, *58*, 136–138.

Noseworthy, J. H., Lucchinetti, C., Rodriguez, M., & Weinshenker, B. G. (2000). Multiple sclerosis. *New England Journal of Medicine*, *343*, 938–952.

Owen, A.M., Hampshire, A., Grahn, J.A., Stenton, R., Dajani, S., Burns, A.S., Howard, R.J., Ballard, C.G. (2010). Putting brain training to the test. *Nature*, *465*, 775–778.

Polman, C., O'Connor, P., Havrdova, E., Hutchinson, M., Kappos, L., Miller, D., et al. (2006). A randomized, placebo-controlled trial of natalizumab for relapsing multiple sclerosis. *New England Journal of Medicine*, *354*(9), 899–910.

Rao, S. M., Leo, G. J., Bernardin, L., & Unverzagt, F. (1991). Cognitive dysfunction in multiple sclerosis. I. Frequency, patterns, and prediction. *Neurology*, *41*, 685–691.

Rao, S. M., Leo, G. J., Ellington, L., Nauertz, T., Bernardin, L., & Unverzagt, F. (1991). Cognitive dysfunction in multiple sclerosis II. Impact on employment and social functioning. *Neurology*, *41*, 692–696.

Rizvi, S. A., & Agius, M. A. (2004). Current approved options for treating patients with multiple sclerosis. *Neurology*, *63*(6), S8–S14.

Zakzanis, K. (2000). Distinct neurocognitive profiles in multiple sclerosis subtypes. *Archives of Clinical Neuropsychology*, *15*(2), 115–136.

48

Progressive Nonfluent Aphasia

Kimberly M. Miller, Sherrill R. Loring, and David. W. Loring

Primary progressive aphasia (PPA) is a neurodegenerative dementia with language disturbance as the prominent initial presenting problem. It was initially characterized as a clinical syndrome by Mesulam and colleagues at the Harvard Neurological Unit in the 1970s. Patients with PPA generally show a progressive agrammatic aphasia without evidence of stroke and without the profound recent memory impairment associated with Alzheimer disease (Mesulam, 2007). In addition to agrammatism, Mesulam (1982) described language impairments, including word-finding difficulties, spelling problems, and poor word comprehension. At initial presentation, cognition other than language is largely unaffected. Mesulam considered language deficits not only to be the most salient cognitive finding in PPA, but he also stated that language must be the most disabling aspect of a patient's presentation for approximately 2 years (Mesulam, 1982). Acalculia and ideomotor apraxia may also accompany the language deficits in the early stages. As the disease progresses, patients with PPA may develop impairments in other domains, such as memory or visuospatial functions, as well as personality changes (e.g., disinhibition, depression, or apathy) and motor or sensory deficits (Amici, Gorno-Tempini, Ogar, Dronkers, & Miller, 2006).

Primary progressive aphasia is an umbrella term referring to a heterogeneous set of neurobehavioral syndromes, often resulting in specific diagnostic challenges. For example, some patients with PPA are fluent with normal prosody and poor comprehension, while others are nonfluent with prominent word-finding difficulties. In terms of presentation, some patients appear to have impairment of more posterior language networks with receptive language difficulty, including understanding the meanings of words, while others may show greater impairment of more anterior language regions and present with more of an expressive aphasia. The various PPA subtypes have been termed *semantic dementia*, *progressive nonfluent (agrammatic) aphasia*, and *logopenic primary progressive aphasia* (Amici et al., 2006; Mesulam, 2007). Further complicating diagnostic precision is the overlap between PPA and frontotemporal lobar degeneration, a group of clinical syndromes that encompasses semantic dementia, PNFA, and frontotemporal dementia due to their similar patterns of neuropathology (Neary et al., 1998). In this chapter, we report the findings of a patient with progressive nonfluent aphasia (PNFA).

Nonfluent aphasia is characterized by spontaneous speech that is hesitant, effortful, and slowed, the most prominent clinical features throughout its course. Current consensus criteria for diagnosis suggest two core clinical features. First, the language impairment must be insidious in onset and show gradual progression. Second, spontaneous speech must be nonfluent with either agrammatism (or telegraphic speech), phonemic paraphasias, or anomia (Neary et al., 1998). Supportive diagnostic criteria may include articulatory errors, impaired repetition, difficulty reading both regular and irregular words, and spelling errors or agrammatism when writing. Knowledge of word meanings is typically intact, although comprehension of complex sentences may be affected. Personality change or interpersonal conduct problems are absent initially, although they may be seen in later stages of the disease and appear similar to those associated with frontotemporal dementia (e.g., perseverative behavior, disinhibition). Other symptoms associated with PNFA may include buccofacial and limb apraxia and contralateral motor symptoms such as tremor or rigidity (Amici et al., 2006; Neary et al., 1998). In late stages of the disease, contralateral primitive reflexes (e.g., rooting) may be present.

Progressive nonfluent aphasia is slightly more common in women (55%–70%) than men (Johnson et al., 2005). The average age of symptom onset is in the early 60s (Johnson et al., 2005), and median survival time following diagnosis is less than 10 years (Ogar, Dronkers, Brambati, Miller, & Gorno-Tempini, 2007). Time of progression from isolated language impairment to a more global dementia is variable. Magnetic resonance imaging (MRI) morphometry studies revealed left anterior insular and posterior frontal atrophy (Ogar et al., 2007). Postmortem histopathologic studies have found PNFA is usually associated with tau pathology, although in some cases focal Alzheimer disease pathology and tau-negative, ubiquitin-positive inclusions have been reported (Ogar et al., 2007).

Neuropsychology's role in evaluating these patients includes taking a careful history of symptom progression since the initial presenting complaint must be a relatively isolated language impairment. Because PNFA patients often have more advanced disease at the time of their neuropsychological evaluation, identifying the relatively isolated language disturbance as the initial cognitive disturbance may be based upon history rather than current neuropsychological findings. It is also crucial to determine whether onset of language impairment was insidious or following neurological insult such as stroke or traumatic brain injury. Medical evaluation should include an extensive language workup in order to make a differential diagnosis between PNFA and other variants of PPA.

The Case of X. M.

Referral Question

X. M. was an 80-year-old, right-handed, Caucasian male who presented with a 2-year history of language disturbance characterized by word-finding difficulties and speech hesitancies. According to the patient and his wife, there were no accompanying memory, behavioral, or personality changes. He was referred for neuropsychological evaluation by his neurologist to help characterize his current cognitive status and to aid in differential diagnosis.

Relevant History

Background history was obtained from separate clinical interviews with X. M. and his wife, who accompanied him to the evaluation. X. M. reported word-finding difficulties of gradual onset beginning approximately 2 years prior to the evaluation. He and his wife were unsure whether these difficulties have worsened over the previous year, although X. M.'s son, who lives in another state, reported a significant change in his father's expressive language problems since he last visited 8 months ago. According to his wife, X. M. frequently demonstrated word substitutions and hesitations while speaking, but his speech is generally coherent and comprehensible. He was able to read books and appears to comprehend them, but he now reads books that are less complex than those to which he was previously accustomed. X. M. was enrolled in his third 3-week session of speech therapy, which he and his wife considered to be helpful.

X. M.'s remote medical history was significant for coronary artery bypass graft and mitral valve repair in 1998. X. M. also underwent atrial defibrillator implantation. He received an appropriate shock for ventricular tachycardia in 2000 but has had no further shocks since this time. Other surgical history includes disc surgery and diverticulitis surgery. He has an intention tremor, which began approximately 3 years ago (L>R). X. M. denied past psychiatric history or treatment. His wife denied any recent personality or behavioral changes in her husband. He has not shown any socially inappropriate behaviors. X. M. has had no changes in weight, appetite, sleeping, or libido over the past year. He has a remote smoking history and currently drank 2–3 ounces of liquor per day. There was no known family history of dementia or movement disorders. X. M.'s current medications included memantine, donepezil, warfarin, atenolol, enalapril, and furosemide.

A computed tomography (CT) scan conducted 8 months previously was interpreted by the current neurologist as showing age-appropriate ischemic demyelination but otherwise no acute abnormalities. An MRI could not be done due to his implanted defibrillator. According to X. M.'s wife, a more recent CT showed interval changes within the frontotemporal region; however, no medical results of this scan were available for review. A carotid ultrasound study conducted 7 months ago found less than 50% stenosis bilaterally, indicating adequate blood flow.

X. M. had been married to his wife for 50 years with three adult children. He had a bachelor's degree and worked in sales for 20 years prior to retiring in the late 1980s. With respect to activities of daily living, X. M.'s wife was responsible for handling household chores, but she had also taken over handling family finances, which represented a change. X. M. continued to drive without recent accidents; however, both he and his wife expressed driving concerns. He reported previously being "a conversation maker" but now felt unable to carry on a conversation. X. M. had withdrawn from some of his previous activities, including the volunteer work that he highly valued, due to his language difficulties.

Behavioral Observations

X. M. was alert and oriented to time, place, and person. He wore glasses and bilateral hearing aids during the assessment. He ambulated independently and showed no apparent gait or balance disturbance. Spontaneous speech was circumlocutory, hesitant, and characterized by articulation errors as well as phonemic and semantic paraphasias. Verbal responses were typically short phrases or single words. X. M. appeared to generally understand task directions during testing, although repetition of instructions was at times necessary. He was friendly during the evaluation and enjoyed joking, and spontaneously initiated conversation despite his

limited verbal expression ability. Mood was euthymic with a normal range of affect. He did not demonstrate overt frustration in response to challenging tasks or his word-finding difficulties. X. M. was engaged in the examination and appeared to put forth full effort. The neuropsychological results were considered valid estimates of his cognitive functioning.

Examination Results

X. M. was administered selected subtests from the Wechsler Adult Intelligence Scales–Third Edition, as is the typical protocol in our neuropsychology dementia clinic. His estimated Full Scale IQ of 97 was in the average range (42nd percentile) with relatively equivalent verbal (VIQ = 97; 42nd percentile) and performance abilities (PIQ = 95; 37th percentile). Premorbid function, estimated using the Wechsler Test of Adult Reading, was in the average range (95, 37th percentile). Taking into account this score as well as the patient's age, PIQ, educational background, and previous occupation, his WAIS-III IQ was not thought to reflect significant decline from previous levels of function. X. M. was generally able to answer test questions through single words or two-to-three word phrases, and his performance across the different WAIS-III subtests was consistently in the average range.

X. M.'s spontaneous speech was nonfluent and consisted of short phrases characterized by hesitancies and circumlocutions. He demonstrated frequent phonemic and semantic paraphasic errors as well as articulation problems. Speech was generally coherent and comprehensible, although occasional instances of slurred words did occur. X. M. was able to express himself adequately through short phrases, which were at times accompanied by hand motions. Volume and prosody were within normal limits, although rate was severely slowed. Auditory comprehension was impaired for complex grammar as well as multipart commands, but intact for simple grammar and one-step commands. He required repetition of test instructions on occasion. Confrontation naming on the Boston Naming Test was relatively preserved (raw score: 52/60). Naming errors were generally semantic in nature (e.g., "bridle" for "muzzle" or "goose" for "pelican"), with only one instance of complete nonresponse.

He showed a strong benefit from phonemic cueing, naming eight additional items with phonemic cues. Responsive naming to auditory description using the Columbia Auditory Naming Task (Hamberger & Seidel, 2003; Miller, Finney, Meador, & Loring, 2008) was within normal limits but characterized by multiple instances of tip-of-the-tongue phenomena. He was able to adequately give word definitions and describe similarities between two items; however, semantic knowledge was variable with borderline performance on Pyramids and Palm Trees, a test requiring matching semantically related pictures. Verbal fluency for both phonetic prompts (C, F, L) and semantic categories (animals, supermarket items, and verbs) was impaired. Oral repetition ability was impaired and characterized by phonemic errors (e.g., when asked to repeat "The spy fled to Greece," X. M. responded, "The fly spread flew to Greece"). Oral sentence and paragraph reading was slowed and characterized by impaired comprehension of content as well as frequent phonemic and graphemic errors. He also frequently omitted words and blended words together (e.g. blending "the girl ran" into "the gran"). In contrast, single-word reading for regular and irregular words, spelling ability, writing to dictation, and paragraph writing were intact.

X. M. demonstrated mild ideomotor apraxia bilaterally. Right-left orientation was normal for identification of locations on his self but was impaired across extrapersonal space with a confronting person deficit noted; however, this difficulty may be due to language comprehension problems since he demonstrated impaired ability to follow multistep commands. Finger localization was bilaterally intact for identification of single fingers with his hands visible and hidden. X. M. had impaired performance for identification of two simultaneously touched fingers with the left hand only. Dyscalculia was assessed using the WRAT-3 Arithmetic subtest. X. M.'s standard score of 105 shows no difficulty performing calculations. Specific performances on measures of language and language-related functions are shown in Table 48-1.

In contrast to impaired language function, X. M. demonstrated intact visuospatial and visuo-constructional abilities. Performance on Judgment of Line Orientation was normal. Construction of simple geometric designs as well as the Rey-Osterrieth Complex Figure was within normal limits. Command and copy drawings of a clock were also normal. Performance on WAIS-III Block Design was normal (SS = 10), as was the ability to determine important missing features in drawings on WAIS-III Picture Completion (SS = 9).

X. M.'s attention, working memory, and processing speed were grossly intact. He demonstrated an auditory span of 7 digits forward (81st percentile) but could repeat only 3 digits backwards (12th percentile). Performance on WAIS-III Letter-Number Sequencing was normal (SS = 8). On Trail Making Test A, he scored in the normal range with respect to completion time and made no errors. Rapid graphomotor processing was normal.

Verbal learning and memory was intact on both story and list-learning tasks, as well as the WMS-R verbal paired associates test. Simple visual memory, assessed using Visual Reproduction (Wechsler, 1945), was normal upon immediate delay, but at the 4th percentile for delayed recall with impaired recognition memory (2/4). Similarly, recall of the Rey-Osterrieth Complex Figure was below the 1st percentile for both immediate and delayed recall, in the context of a normal copy of the figure. Recognition of the figure items was also impaired. In sum, X. M. demonstrated intact verbal memory but impaired visual memory.

On tests of abstract reasoning and concept formation, including WAIS-III Similarities and the Wisconsin Card Sorting Test, X. M. scored in the normal range. In contrast, he had difficulty with tasks requiring cognitive flexibility. Performance on the WMS-III Mental Control was at the 1st percentile, and on Trail Making Test Part B he made five errors. Rapid, verbal-motor cognitive set shifting was impaired with errors noteworthy for perseverations of activity and semantically related errors. Crossed response inhibition and manual motor sequencing (fist, edge, palm) were moderately impaired bilaterally. Writing of recursive m and n's and loops was normal.

X. M. did not endorse a clinically significant amount of symptoms on the Geriatric Depression Inventory (total score = 6/30). This is consistent with his high-spirited and energetic presentation during the interview and assessment. X. M. and

Table 48-1.

Test	Score	Percentile/Performance Classification
Boston Naming Test	52/60	37th percentile
No. correct with phonemic cues	8/8	
Pyramids and Palm Trees	48/52	Borderline
WAIS-III Similarities	SS = 11	63rd percentile
WAIS-III Vocabulary	SS = 9	37th percentile
Letter Fluency (C, F, L)	14	5th percentile
Animal Fluency	8	1st percentile
Supermarket Fluency	11	Impaired
Verb Fluency	9	Impaired
Test for the Reception of Grammar (TROG)		
Total Score	73/80	1st percentile
Simple Grammar	16/16	61st percentile
Plurals	8/8	66th percentile
Negatives	16/16	61st percentile
Locations	11/12	1st percentile
Complex Grammar	10/16	1st percentile
Gray Oral Reading Test (GORT-2)		
Oral Reading Quotient	58	<1st percentile
Reading Rate	SS = 6	9th percentile
Reading Accuracy	SS = 4	2nd percentile
Reading Comprehension	SS = 3	1st percentile
WRAT-3 Reading (single word)	Stand. Score = 99	47th percentile
WRAT-3 Spelling	Stand. Score = 106	66th percentile
Boston Diagnostic Aphasia Examination (selected subtests)		
Commands	2/5	Impaired
Complex Ideational Material	7/8	Normal
Sentences to Dictation	10/12	Normal
Writing Sample (Cookie Theft)	5/5	Normal
Florida Token Test	10/10	Normal
Sentence Repetition	7/10	Impaired
Brief Praxis Assessment	4/6 Right; 4/6 Left	Bilaterally Impaired

SS, scaled score; WAIS-III, Wechsler Adult Intelligence Scales, Third Edition.

his wife were both given questionnaires inquiring about his symptoms and their severity. There was minimal discrepancy between their responses, indicating that X. M. is fully aware of his problems.

Discussion

X. M.'s neuropsychological evaluation results revealed language impairment characterized by prominent word-finding difficulty, articulatory problems, and phonemic as well as semantic paraphasic errors. Comprehension was impaired for complex grammar and reading of sentences and paragraphs, while comprehension of simple grammar and verbal commands was intact. Phonemic and semantic fluency were impaired. X. M.'s naming was generally intact, although there was an increased delay in responding with frequent "tip of the tongue" responses, particularly in the auditory modality. Sentence repetition and praxis were impaired. In contrast, writing ability was intact. Outside of the domain of language, X. M.'s Full-Scale IQ was in the average range, which was not thought to reflect a decline from a previously higher level of functioning. His visuospatial and visuoconstruction abilities were intact. Attention and processing speed were also intact. X. M.'s memory was normal for verbal material, but impaired for visual material. He displayed significant impairments on multiple measures of frontal /executive function, including poor motor programming and difficulty changing response sets. Scores on self-report mood measures were within normal limits.

These results raise several differential diagnosis possibilities. Because X. M.'s onset of language problems was insidious in nature and CT scans showed no evidence of obvious infarct, it is unlikely his deficits are due to focal stroke. X. M.'s presenting complaint was disturbance in language, not memory, suggesting a nonamnestic type of dementia, primary progressive aphasia (PPA). The subtypes of PPA to be ruled out are semantic dementia, progressive nonfluent aphasia, and logopenic primary progressive aphasia. Frontotemporal dementia is another type of nonamnestic dementia to consider due to X. M.'s impairments on multiple measures of executive function.

Prior to neuropsychological testing, it was clear that X. M.'s speech output was nonfluent. His responses often were single words or two-to-three-word phrases. Although sparse, his words appropriately conveyed his meaning. This presentation is not consistent with a diagnosis of semantic dementia, in which speech is fluent, but loss of word meaning leads to "empty" or vague speech. In contrast, word-finding difficulties, dysfluent speech, and intact knowledge of single words are characteristic of both progressive nonfluent aphasia (PNFA) and logopenic PPA (Amici et al., 2006). Performance on neuropsychological measures of language is useful for distinguishing between these two diagnoses. Gorno-Tempini and colleagues (2004) found that compared to PNFA patients, those with logopenic PPA show impaired comprehension for even syntactically simple constructions, impaired visual confrontation naming performance (with a strong benefit from multiple-choice recognition cuing), and are more likely to display dyscalculia. Because X. M. had intact comprehension for simple sentence constructions, intact confrontation naming

ability, and no difficulty performing calculations, his clinical presentation is most consistent with PNFA. A diagnosis of frontotemporal dementia was deemed unlikely because X. M. showed no changes in personality, mood, or socially appropriate behaviors. These features are often present very early in the course of frontotemporal dementia, whereas with PNFA behavioral changes are not typically seen until late stages of the disease (Neary et al., 1998).

One neuropsychological finding was inconsistent with PNFA. He displayed impairment in visual memory, and thus his deficits were not purely restricted to the domain of language during the 2 years since his problems first began. It is possible that X. M.'s language disturbance actually began longer than 2 years ago, as it is difficult for family members to pinpoint when subtle changes began to occur, and at the time of evaluation his dementia had begun to progress into other domains. Another possibility is that X. M.'s poor visual memory simply represents a premorbid area of weakness unrelated to his clinical diagnosis. There is considerable intraindividual variability on neuropsychological test performance even in healthy older adults (Schretlen, Munro, Anthony, & Pearlson, 2003). In considering various diagnoses, we considered the overall clinical picture since patients often do not fit perfectly into established diagnostic schemes. Mesulam wrote that his 2-year diagnostic criteria for PNFA in which language impairment must be the most salient feature "was meant to be interpreted with considerable latitude" (Mesulam, 2007). This underscores the importance of developing a case conceptualization based on the global pattern of neuropsychological test findings.

After determining X. M.'s profile was most consistent with PNFA, a feedback session with X. M. and his family was scheduled. During this session, the diagnosis and its course were explained. X. M.'s family was eager to learn ways to slow down the progression of his PNFA. Unfortunately, there are presently no medications shown to be effective in clinical trials. Since X. M. and his wife felt that speech therapy had benefited him thus far, he was encouraged to continue this therapy. Other patients with PNFA may find it helpful to use communication enhancement devices or hand gestures to convey their ideas.

The neuropsychologist plays an important role in establishing the diagnosis and characterizing the pattern of impaired and preserved functions of patients with PNFA and other types of PPA, since neuroimaging and neurological examination results alone cannot distinguish between subtypes of PPA. Through comprehensive language assessment, the neuropsychologist can develop an understanding of the patient's neuropsychological profile, then compare how this profile fits with known syndromes. Additionally, neuropsychologists can be helpful to concerned family members by providing an explanation of the diagnosis and guiding them toward appropriate resources concerning further evaluations if needed (e.g., speech evaluation or safe driver evaluation), treatment options, education and planning for the future.

References

Amici, S., Gorno-Tempini, M. L., Ogar, J. M., Dronkers, N. F., & Miller, B. L. (2006). An overview on primary progressive aphasia and its variants. *Behavioural Neurology, 17*(2), 77–87.

Gorno-Tempini, M. L., Dronkers, N. F., Rankin, K. P., Ogar, J. M., Phengrasamy, L., Rosen, H. J., et al. (2004). Cognition and anatomy in three variants of primary progressive aphasia. *Annals of Neurology, 55*(3), 335–346.

Hamberger, M. J., & Seidel, W. T. (2003). Auditory and visual naming tests: Normative and patient data for accuracy, response time, and tip-of-the-tongue. *Journal of the International Neuropsychological Society, 9*(3), 479–489.

Johnson, J. K., Diehl, J., Mendez, M. F., Neuhaus, J., Shapira, J. S., Forman, M., et al. (2005). Frontotemporal lobar degeneration: Demographic characteristics of 353 patients. *Archives of Neurology, 62*, 925–930.

Mesulam, M. M. (1982). Slowly progressive aphasia without generalized dementia. *Annals of Neurology, 11*(6), 592–598.

Mesulam, M. M. (2007). Primary progressive aphasia: A 25-year retrospective. *Alzheimer Disease and Associated Disorders, 21*(4), S8–S11.

Miller, K. M., Finney, G. R., Meador, K. J., & Loring, D. W. (submitted). Auditory description versus visual confrontation naming in dementia.

Neary, D., Snowden, J. S., Gustafson, L., Passant, U., Stuss, D., Black, S., et al. (1998). Frontotemporal lobar degeneration: A consensus on clinical diagnostic criteria. *Neurology, 51*(6), 1546–1554.

Ogar, J. M., Dronkers, N. F., Brambati, S. M., Miller, B. L., & Gorno-Tempini, M. L. (2007). Progressive nonfluent aphasia and its characteristic motor speech deficits. *Alzheimer Disease and Associated Disorders, 21*(4), S23–S30.

Schretlen, D. J., Munro, C. A., Anthony, J. C., & Pearlson, G. D. (2003). Examining the range of normal intraindividual variability in neuropsychological test performance. *Journal of the International Neuropsychological Society, 9*(6), 864–870.

Wechsler, D. (1945). A standardized memory scale for clinical use. *Journal of Psychology, 19*, 87–95.

49

Early-Onset Alzheimer Disease

Ruth E. Yoash-Gantz

Early-onset Alzheimer disease (EAD) is defined as onset prior to age 65. As reported in 2007, incidence of early-onset dementias in the United States, including EAD was 200,000 to 500,000 people (Alzheimer's Association, 2007). Harvey, Skelton-Robinson and Rossor (2003) report a prevalence figure for EAD (45–64 age group) as 35 per 100,000 people based on an epidemiological catchment area prevalence survey in several London boroughs. These rates are comparable to those obtained in the Northern Health Region study (34.6; Newens et al., 1993), the Framingham study (31.8; Kokmen, Beard, Offord, & Kurland, 1989), and Finland (32.7; Sulkava et al., 1985).

Neuropsychological profile differences between EAD and late-onset Alzheimer disease (LAD) remain unclear. Studies in the 1980s and 1990s, prior to genetic and neuropathology discoveries, generally concluded there were clinically distinct profiles. Filley, Kelly, and Heaton (1984) noted greater impairment in Verbal IQ than Performance IQ. Loring and Largen (1985) found that an EAD group had greater deficits on age-adjusted tests of sustained concentration and mental tracking than did an LAD group. Others (Jacobs et al., 1994; Kono, Kuzuya, Yamamoto, & Endo, 1994; Seltzer & Sherwin, 1983) found that EAD had more frequent language impairment, consistent with Filley et al. (1986). Noted focal degenerative changes included naming, praxis, calculation (left hemisphere; Haxby et al., 1990), executive dysfunction and behavior dysregulation (frontal lobes; Johnson, Head, Kim, Starr, &

Cotman, 1999), and visuospatial loss (right parietal lobe; Benson, Davis, & Snyder, 1988).

More recent comparative findings of cognitive profiles in EAD and LAD have been mixed. Caine and Hodges (2001) found that cortical visuospatial functions are more impaired in EAD than in LAD. Suribhatla et al. (2004) found that after adjusting for overall dementia severity and premorbid IQ, there was greater frontoparietal/right hemisphere involvement in EAD and greater temporal/left hemisphere involvement in LAD and they hypothesized these differences may be related to age of onset of AD and corresponding genetic risk profiles. Licht, McMurtray, Saul, and Mendez (2007) compared EAD with very LAD and found preferentially impaired verbal fluency and motor-executive deficits in the LAD group, but differences disappeared when age was considered. They did not find disproportionate language or visuospatial deficits in EAD compared with LAD.

Mendez (2006) discussed three potential diagnostic errors in early-onset dementias. Although EAD is the predominant cause of early onset dementia, there are numerous other causes. Secondly, the traditional model of LAD is characterized by prominent memory difficulty and word-finding problems, but EAD may have predominant cognitive deficits other than memory loss. Finally, EAD may present with greater neuropsychiatric than cognitive deficits.

Several studies have noted different progression rates for EAD than for LAD. These studies have found a greater rate of decline in EAD than in LAD (Jacobs et al., 1994; Kono et al., 1994; Seltzer & Sherwin, 1983). More recently, Greicius, Geschwind, and Miller (2002) reported that disease progression in EAD is sometimes more rapid than in LAD.

Consensus on the clinical diagnosis of Alzheimer disease was reached in 1984 with the development of the NINCDS-ADRDA criteria (McKhann et al., 1984), and these criteria continue to be applied in the diagnosis of both EAD and LAD. Advances in neuroimaging and neuropathology have been useful in increasing diagnostic accuracy. Positron emission tomography (PET) scans and neuropathology suggest more severe deficits in parietal areas in EAD than in LAD (Frisoni et al., 2005; Kemp et al., 2003). Due to these and other scientific advances in neuropathology and neuroimaging, proposed new guidelines have recently been published (Dubois et al., 2007). The goal of the proposed guidelines is to define the clinical, biochemical, structural, and metabolic presence of AD, rather than relying on traditional functional measurement and effort to determine etiology.

Genomics has uncovered differences between EAD and LAD. Cases of EAD are more likely to have a genetic etiology than are cases developing after age 65 (Lleo et al., 2002), which are mostly comprised of sporadic occurrence (no genetic risk factor). Three genes have been associated with EAD, each seeming to correspond with a somewhat different age of onset (Lovestone, 1999). The presenelin-1 (PS-1) gene on chromosome 14 has been associated with onset between ages 30 and 40 years, and mutations in this gene were found in 95 of 101 cases with onset before age 35 (Filley et al., 2007). The amyloid precursor protein (APP) gene on chromosome 21 is associated with onset between ages 40 and 50 years. Finally, the presenelin-2 (PS-2) gene on chromosome 1 is associated with onset between ages 50 and 65 years.

The Case of Mr. Smith

Mr. Smith was referred for evaluation by his primary care provider following concerns raised by his wife regarding declining memory. At the time of evaluation, Mr. Smith was a 65-year-old, married, right-handed, Caucasian male with 16 years of formal education. He was a minister

for many years, retiring early due to cognitive deficit the year prior to this evaluation; he was unable to write or deliver sermons. He was living at home with his full-time employed wife, and they had four adult children assisting in care. Mrs. Smith provided most of his personal history; he was unable to recall most of his adult life, including his 30+ years as a minister. Mr. Smith had normal developmental milestones as reported by his wife. He was honorably discharged from 2 years of noncombat service in the Army.

Mr. Smith's medical diagnoses at time of evaluation included diabetes mellitus (treated with oral hypoglycemic) and essential tremor. He had no history of head injury or other insult to the brain. Cognitive decline began 5 years prior to the current evaluation. He had undergone dementia evaluation 2 years prior to this exam and magnetic resonance image (MRI) of the brain at that time was negative. He was placed on Aricept, became weak, and the medication was discontinued. Those outside records were not available. Mrs. Smith reported his strong family history of "memory loss," including his mother, two maternal aunts, and a recently deceased brother. Mr. Smith was receiving ongoing primary care. Medications at the time of evaluation included paroxetine, glyburide, propranolol, and buspirone.

Mr. Smith had no history of psychiatric diagnosis, treatment, or hospitalization. He denied auditory or visual hallucinations. He denied depression or mania. He reported occasional anxiety and confusion "once in a great while." He had no history of alcohol or other substance use, including tobacco. Mrs. Smith reported he had a gun at home but neither of them knew its location.

Mr. Smith was independent in four out of six activities of daily living (ADLs) at the time of evaluation. He needed reminders to bathe as his personal hygiene had declined, and he needed assistance in dressing. In the prior year, he had developed balance instability and began stumbling and falling, but there was no report of injury to the head. He was dependent on others for almost all instrumental activities of daily living (IADLs). He was no longer driving. He spent his days at home alone and called his wife at work approximately 10 times per day, asking where she was (despite having called her work phone number). Mrs. Smith reported that often she returned home from work to find things broken or missing. He was able to do light house-keeping only, but no cooking. He used a gas heater but tended to leave it on and unattended. Mrs. Smith reported that he was beginning to become increasingly confused toward the latter part of the day, often changing into pajamas in the late afternoon.

On interview and observation, Mr. Smith appeared to be physically fit, was dressed in casual clean clothing, and his hygiene was good. He carried two broken pairs of glasses in his pockets. He did not wear hearing aids. He ambu-lated independently and gait appeared normal. He had poor ability to do alternating movements and was unable to maintain balance during tandem walking. Mr. Smith was polite during testing despite becoming increasingly uncoop-erative. He often stopped answering questions, stood up, and left the testing room. Testing was eventually discontinued. He fatigued easily. Mood was euthymic and affect was quite labile. He appeared quite anxious at times and seemed to cover his confusion with attempts at humor. Spontaneous language was fluent without para-phasic/dysarthric speech error. There was sig-nificant word-finding difficulty. He had poor ability to attend to tasks, was very easily con-fused, and had poor ability to maintain a mental set or understand test instructions. He was ori-ented to name only. He stated his age was "230," then "62." He was unable to recall date of birth. He did not recall attending 4 years of college or working lifelong as a minister. Instead, he stated he worked in a steel mill, an occupation he held prior to entry in the military. He stated he had

six children instead of four, and he could not remember their names or ages. He was unable to name any U.S. Presidents since 1960. He was unable to recall any current events.

Mr. Smith was administered the following tests: Repeatable Battery for the Assessment of Neurop-sychological Status (RBANS), Boston Naming Test, Controlled Oral Word Association Test (COWA), Greek Crosses, Clock Test, Wechsler Memory Scale–Revised (WMS-R, Mental Control only), Stroop Test, Trail Making Test (TMT), Finger Tapping Test (FTT; unwilling), Hand Dynamometer (HD; unwilling), Geriatric Depression Scale (GDS), Clinical and Caregiver Interviews, and Review of Records.

Test Findings

Mr. Smith's behavior and functional level limited the extent of testing. (see Table 49-1).

Given Mr. Smith's presentation during the clinical interview, it was clear that dementia was the likely diagnostic category (obvious learning/memory impairment, obvious impairment in another cognitive domain, obvious functional decline). The goal of testing was to document level of severity and to determine type of demen-tia. The RBANS was selected as an initial screen-ing measure due to its normative base and because the patient was college educated. The Dementia Rating Scale was considered; however, there were concerns that the patient may hit the ceiling on several of the subtests, thus obfuscat-ing results.

Mr. Smith had overall moderately severe cere-bral dysfunction of a diffuse nature on the focused test battery. He refused motor testing (Finger Tapping and Hand Dynamometer); thus,

Table 49-1. Test Scores

Test	Score	Test	Score
RBANS (Index Scores)		BNT	$z = -11.92$
Total Scale	SS = 45	COWA	$z = -2.99$
Immediate Memory	SS = 40	WMS-R Mental Control	$z = -0.73$
Visuoconstruction	SS = 50	Greek Crosses	T = 00
Language	SS = 57	Clock Test (Sunderland system)	Raw = 4
Attention	SS = 60	Stroop-Word	T < 20
Delayed Memory	SS = 40	Color	T < 20
TMT-Part A	T < 20	Color/Word	T = 20
Part B	T < 18	GDS	Raw = 2

information regarding possible hemispheric lateralization was not available. Although it is unlikely to see such lateralization with EAD, it is preferable that testing include brief evaluation of motor/sensory testing to rule out diagnoses associated with lateralized deficits (e.g., cerebrovascular disease in this case).

Mr. Smith's RBANS performance was markedly impaired; Attention and Language domains were least impaired. Learning (RBANS, List Learning, Story Memory) was severely impaired; he lost set on Story Memory and began telling a story about a girl he knew in school. On retrieval tasks (RBANS, List Recall, Story Recall, Figure Recall), he demonstrated the rapid rate of initial forgetting characteristic of Alzheimer disease. Recognition memory was fraught with false-positive responses, another memory characteristic typical for Alzheimer disease. Because these patients have minimal memory storage, and little ability to retrieve from storage, they tend to respond in the affirmative when given a yes/no format.

Mr. Smith's expressive language functioning was also markedly impaired. Word-finding difficulty was noted during the interview. Confrontation naming (Boston Naming Test) was severely impaired, with a raw sore of 25/60 ($z = -11.92$), including 24 spontaneous correct responses and one additional from stimulus cue. Errors included "octopus" for helicopter, "crutches" for stilts, "gallatin" for noose, and "an active tar" for volcano. Category fluency (RBANS, Animal Naming, ($z = -3.40$) was moderately severely impaired and letter fluency (COWA, $z = -2.99$) was moderately impaired.

Mr. Smith had severely impaired visuospatial performances. He performed within the severely impaired range on a test of constructional praxis (Greek Crosses, see Figure 49-1). When asked to draw a clock face, he drew a circle and inserted seven two-digit numbers in the area of the clock face from 3:00–7:00. Then, he drew the numbers 15 to 20 outside the clock (Clock Test, see Figure 49-2). This was a severely impaired performance.

Mr. Smith's executive functioning was also severely impaired. He performed within this range on tests of perceptual set shifting (Stroop Test) and efficiency in following new sequential procedures (Trail Making Test). He was unable to establish or maintain a mental set. Although overlearned social judgment was adequate early in testing, his confusion and paranoia quickly led to disinhibition, agitation, and impulsivity. He demonstrated poor novel judgment and insight.

Mr. Smith did not endorse symptoms of depression on the GDS, consistent with his history. He was somewhat suspicious of the testing environment due to his confusion.

Discussion

The pattern of Mr. Smith's test performances together with his medical history and family history indicate likely EAD. His frequent falls and mild bilateral upper extremity tremor are not inclusive or exclusive signs of AD. His severely impaired visuospatial and memory functions and moderately to severely impaired language functions were consistent with AD. Furthermore, the progression of his ADL/IADL decline was quite steep and consistent with the presenile (prior to age 65) form of AD.

Efforts to schedule the feedback session via telephone to the Smith home resulted in Mr. Smith disconnecting the call, either due to suspicion or to impaired procedural memory regarding use of the phone. Mrs. Smith was contacted at work to arrange the appointment. Mr. Smith was very defensive, denied memory

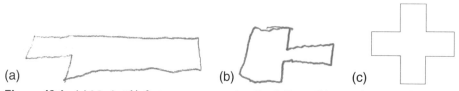

Figure 49-1. (*a*) Mr. Smith's first attempt at copying Greek Cross, (*b*) second attempt, (*c*) and copy of Greek Cross stimuli.

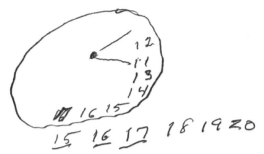

Figure 49-2. Mr. Smith's drawing of a clock face from memory. Note the loss of set with numbers advancing beyond those found on a clock, and extending outside the border of the clock.

problems, and became easily agitated when diagnosis was presented. He was taken to another room to chat with the technician so that the examiner could focus attention on educating Mrs. Smith and discussing recommendations. Recommendations included refraining from driving, removing all guns from the home, removing the gas heater from the basement, routinely assessing home environment for needed modifications to ensure safety, removing all medications (including those for pets) to a safe location, monitoring morning glucose by Mrs. Smith before leaving for work, obtaining Safe Return Kit and caregiver support from the Alzheimer's Association, referral to VAMC Eldercare Team for ongoing monitoring and assistance, consideration of trial of another cholinesterase inhibitor, and getting legal affairs in order (powers of attorney, Living Wills, etc.). Note that there was no recommendation for brief written notes and reminders; Mr. Smith's level of confusion would negate benefit from these measures and could add to disruptive behavior.

Mr. Smith's rate of decline continued over the next year. An MRI of the brain 1 month after evaluation noted moderately pronounced atrophy and mild microvascular white matter disease. Mr. Smith entered the home of an elderly female neighbor and was hostile toward her, accusing her of conspiring against him. Trials of other cholinesterase inhibitors were ineffective. Mr. Smith began wandering from the home and flagging down passing cars, looking for his wife. He became incontinent. He had two brief adult daycare placements that failed due to agitation. Mr. Smith was intolerant of nonfamily care pro-

viders and they did not qualify for VA Aid and Attendance for Mrs. Smith to be the primary paid caregiver. The daughters provided care when they were not working. Mrs. Smith pursued guardianship.

Mr. Smith was admitted to the VA dementia care unit within 14 months of the evaluation. He was 67 years old. On admission, motor agitation and aggression were noted to increase across the course of the day. Within 6 months, he was nonambulatory and dysphagic, was oriented to name only, was unable to respond to Scripture passages, and was dependent for all ADLs. Family continued to be very involved in his care. Aggressive behavior continued and multiple medication trials were attempted. Nutritional status became compromised with significant loss of weight. Expressive language ceased. He succumbed to several respiratory infections. He expired 4 years and 8 months after diagnosis at the age of 70.

Conclusion

Mr. Smith's case is considered prototypical of EAD. Symptoms began at approximately age 60 with a reverse chronological loss of autobiographical information. He had a strong family history of "memory loss" in two first-degree and two second-degree relatives. The rate of decline rapidly increased over time and was significantly complicated by psychiatric and behavioral disruptions. Mr. Smith was physically robust at the time he was admitted for long term-care at age 67, but his paranoia had become increasingly problematic at home. While such behavioral disturbances are common causes of institutionalization of most dementia patients, EAD patients are generally physically stronger, thus creating tougher management issues for the caregiver.

Mr. Smith's pattern of cognitive decline is consistent with EAD. At the time of this evaluation, reportedly 5 years after onset, he no longer recalled much of his adulthood. Verbal fluency measures noted the typical "cortical dementia" pattern with greater category/semantic impairment than letter/phonemic impairment. This is believed to be due to the loss of acetylcholine affecting "memory for words," which are generally stored semantically rather than phonemically.

Mr. Smith's visuospatial performance was also severely impaired with inability to produce fairly simple geometric figures (Greek Crosses). His loss of mental set and lack of recall of a clock face on the Clock Test is also consistent with AD.

Mr. Smith's learning and memory pattern is consistent with AD. He demonstrated very poor acquisition of new verbal information and a rapid rate of initial forgetting. He was unable to recall any information following the delay, and recognition memory was replete with false-positive responding. Visual memory was also characterized by loss of all information; often these patients will deny that they were exposed to the stimuli.

Executive performance among EAD patients is typically fraught with inability to maintain a mental set. Mr. Smith completed Trails A slowly but without error. He was unable to complete Trails B; after numerous clarifications by the examiner, he was able to complete only six connections in 8 minutes. He was unable to respond correctly to any items on the Stroop Color/Word task. He refused motor testing, and had this been completed, it is likely that there would have been no lateralized deficit to either hemisphere on motor tasks.

Mr. Smith's rapid physical decline from ages 67–70 is also consistent with EAD. He became nonambulatory and dysphagic. Nutritional intake was compromised and expressive language ceased. He died less than 5 years after diagnosis.

References

Alzheimer's Association. (2007, March 20). Alzheimer's disease prevalence rates rise to more than five million in the United States. *Alzheimer News*. Chicago: Author.

Benson, D. F., Davis, R. J., & Snyder, B. D. (1988). Posterior cortical atrophy. *Archives of Neurology*, 45, 789–793.

Caine, D., Hodges, J.R. (2001). Heterogenity of semantic and visuospatial deficits in early Alzheimer's disease. *Neuropsychology, 15(2),* 155-164.

Dubois, B., Feldman, H. H., Jacova, C., DeKosky, S. T., Barberger-Gateau, P., Cummings, J. et al. (2007). Research criteria for the diagnosis of Alzheimer's disease: Revising the NINCDS–ADRDA criteria. *Lancet Neurology*, 6, 734–746.

Filley, C. M., Kelly, J., & Heaton, R. K. (1986). Neuropsychologic features of early- and late-onset Alzheimer's disease. *Archives of Neurology*, 43, 574–576.

Filley, C. M., Rollins, Y. D., Anderson, A., Arciniegas, D. B., Howard, K. L., Murrell, J. R., et al. (2007). The genetics of very early onset Alzheimer Disease. *Cognitive and Behavioral Neurology, 20(3)*, 149–156.

Frisoni, G. B., Testa, C., Sabattoli, F., Beltramello, A., Soininen, H., & Laakso, M. P. (2005). Structural correlates of early and late onset Alzheimer's disease: Voxel based morphometric study. *Journal of Neurology, Neurosurgery and Psychiatry*, 76, 112–114.

Greicius, M. D., Geschwind, M. D., & Miller, B. L. (2002). Presenile dementia syndromes: An update on taxonomy and diagnosis. *Journal of Neurology, Neurosurgery, and Psychiatry*, 72, 691–700.

Harvey, R. J., Skelton-Robinson, M., & Rossor, M. N. (2003). The prevalence and causes of dementia in people under the age of 65 years. *Journal of Neurology, Neurosurgery, and Psychiatry*, 74, 1206–1209.

Haxby, J. V., Grady, C. L., Koss, E., Horwitz, B., Heston, L., Schapiro, M., et al. (1990). Longitudinal study of the cerebral metabolic asymmetries and associated neuropsychological patterns in early dementia of Alzheimer type. *Archives of Neurology*, 47, 753–760.

Jacobs, D., Sano, M., Marder, K., Bell, K., Bylsma, F., Lafleche, G., et al. (1994). Age at onset of Alzheimer's disease: Relation to the pattern of cognitive dysfunction and rate of decline. *Neurology*, 44, 1215–1220.

Johnson, J. K., Head, E., Kim, R., Starr, A., & Cotman, C. W. (1999). Clinical and pathological evidence for a frontal variant of Alzheimer disease. *Archives of Neurology*, 56, 1233–1239.

Kemp, P. M., Holmes, C., Hoffmann, S. M., Bolt, L., Holmes, R., Rowden, J., et al. (2003). Alzheimer's disease: Differences in technetium-99m HMPAO SPECT scan findings between early onset and late onset dementia. *Journal of Neurology, Neurosurgery, and Psychiatry*, 74, 715–719.

Kokmen, E., Beard, C. M., Offord, K. P., & Kurland, L. T. (1989). Prevalence of medically diagnosed dementia in a defined United States population: Rochester, Minnesota, January 1, 1975. *Neurology*, 39(6), 773–776.

Kono, K., Kuzuya, F., Yamamoto, T., & Endo, H. (1994). Comparative study of cerebral ventricular dilation and cognitive function in patients with Alzheimer's disease of early versus late onset. *Journal of Geriatric Psychiatry and Neurology, 7*, 39–45.

Licht, E. A., McMurtray, A. M., Saul, R. E., & Mendez, M. F. (2007). Cognitive differences between early- and late-onset Alzheimer's disease. *American Journal of Alzheimer's Disease and Other Dementias*, 22, 218–222.

Lleo, A., Blesa, R., Queralt, R., Ezquerra, M., Molinuevo, H. L., Pena-Casanova, et al. (2002). Frequency of mutations in the presenilin and amyloid precursor protein genes in early-onset Alzheimer disease in Spain. *Archives of Neuroogy*; *59*(11),1759–1763.

Loring, D. W., & Largen, J. W. (1985). Neuropsychological patterns of presenile and senile dementia of the Alzheimer type. *Neuropsychologia*; *23 (3),* 351-357.

Lovestone, S. (1999). Early diagnosis and the clinical genetics of Alzheimer's disease. *Journal of Neurology*, *246*, 69–72.

McKhann, G., Drachman, D., Folstein, M., Katzman, R., Price, D., & Stadlan, E. M. (1984). Clinical diagnosis of Alzheimer's disease: Report of the NINCDS–ADRDA Work Group under the auspices of Department of Health and Human Services Task Force on Alzheimer's Disease. *Neurology, 34*, 939–944.

Mendez, M. F., (2006). The accurate diagnosis of early-onset dementia. *International Journal of Psychiatry in Medicine, 36(4),* 401–412.

Newens, A. J., Forster, D. P., Kay, D. W., Kirkup, W., Bates, D., & Edwardson, J. (1993). Clinically diagnosed presenile dementia of the Alzheimer type in the Northern Health Region: Ascertainment, prevalence, incidence and survival. *Psychological Medicine*, *23*(3), 631–644.

Seltzer, B., & Sherwin, I. (1983). A comparison of clinical features in early-and late-onset primary degenerative dementia. One entity or two? *Archives of Neurology, 40*, 143–146.

Sulkava, R., Wikstrom, J., Aromaa, A., Raitasalo, R., Lehtinen, V., Lahtela, K., et al. (1985). Prevalence of severe dementia in Finland. *Neurology, 35*(7), 1025–1029.

Suribhahatla, S., Baillon, S., Dennis, M., Marudkar, M., Muhammad, S., Munro, D., et al. (2004). Neuropsychological performance in early and late onset Alzheimer's disease: Comparisons in a memory clinic population. *International Journal of Geriatric Psychiatry, 19(12),* 1140–1147.

50

Looking into the Crystal Ball of Mild Cognitive Impairment: I See Alzheimer Disease

Jim Andrikopoulos

The detection of early Alzheimer's disease (AD) was introduced into the neurology literature 30 years ago. In 1979, Leonard Berg, from Washington University in St. Louis, Missouri, partnered with colleagues in the Department of Psychology, primarily Martha Storandt, to submit a National Institutes of Health grant to study early AD. Thus, the first large-scale systematic effort to distinguish early AD from normal aging began (Morris & Landau, 2007). They produced in the 1980s the first series of papers on the diagnosis of early AD. There have since been advances in neuroimaging, genetics, potential biomarkers, and the introduction of constructs to characterize the transition from normal aging to AD. The practical relative yield of this research has been marginal insofar as diagnosis of early AD still rests on one factor: the knowledge and experience of the individual clinician. Alzheimer's disease is unique in that it is primarily a disorder of cognition, making the role of the neuropsychologist paramount. This role is partially hampered by some research that seems to have paradoxically undermined the ability of the neuropsychologist to focus on what is clinically critical versus what may be popular and intellectually appealing.

Via the case presentation method, the purpose of this chapter is to highlight the clinically critical issues that will allow the neuropsychologist to make a diagnosis of AD before the dementia is obvious. While it is the rule rather than the exception that a case presentation be unusual, interesting, and diagnostically challenging, the objective of this case presentation will be to go "back to the basics" by presenting a prototypical case of a patient with early AD. In meeting this objective I will draw on my clinical experience and a database of consecutive patients personally examined between 1991 and 2003. In this writer's opinion, clinical neuropsychology is not primarily about the data (i.e., cognitive testing), but the disease. A disproportionate amount of time will be spent on conceptualizing incipient AD, and not the testing or case itself. Finally, implied in any casebook presentation is that the personal experiences and anecdotes of the writer might be of some use to the reader.

The detection of AD prior to developing manifest dementia cannot fully be explored without a selective and critical review of mild cognitive impairment (MCI). Selective because it is not possible to cover the whole of the MCI literature in this chapter because there is no single topic in clinical neurology that has been researched more. For this the reader is referred to three textbooks (Burns & Morris, 2008; Peterson, 2003; Tuokko & Hultsch, 2006). Critical because MCI is not without controversy (Whitehouse & Brodaty, 2006). The issue at hand is identifying incipient AD. There is a patently obvious transitional period from normal aging to AD. If coining a construct, namely MCI, to describe this transition helps identify and treat patients before they develop obvious AD, then the construct has served a clinical purpose. The following overview argues the construct of MCI has failed in this regard. The review will focus on aspects of MCI that need to be reframed in the mind of the clinician in order to direct the focus on what is clinically critical in diagnosing incipient AD.

After the modern-day use of the term MCI was introduced into the literature (Flicker, Ferris, & Reisberg, 1991), the next seminal event was a paper by Ronald Peterson and the Mayo Clinic AD group that set forth the definition of MCI and popularized the term (Petersen et al., 1999). They defined MCI as patients with *(a)* a memory complaint, *(b)* normal activities of daily living, *(c)* normal general cognitive function, *(d)* abnormal memory for age, and *(e)* not demented. The crux of the problem is the two main clinical features that define MCI, the memory complaint and the memory impairment. From a neuropsychological standpoint, they are at odds with basic psychometric principals and clinical tenets that are essential to the detection of developing AD. The very definition of MCI hampers early detection. First is the issue of a memory complaint in which critical importance is not attached to who is complaining: the patient, physician, or family member. When the construct of MCI came to my attention in 2001, I was struck by the irrelevance placed on the source of the memory complaint. In a general outpatient neurology practice, the neuropsychologist encounters two types of patients, those that think they have a memory problem, and those that actually have one. In 1991 a colleague, Nils Varney, summarized for me how to conceptualize the memory complaint. When the patient complains of a memory problem, send the patient to a psychiatrist. When the family complains, send the patient to a neurologist. While the axiom had rarely failed to apply in my experience with AD patients, I nevertheless had to second-guess my clinical approach to AD in light of the MCI criteria. I had a student conduct a literature search to look at the clinical significance of memory complaints. The preponderance of the articles collected suggested that patient memory complaints are a function of an underlying emotional state versus neurologic condition. This was found in an epidemiological study by the Mayo AD group (Smith, Petersen, Ivnik, Malec, & Tangalos, 1996) and cited in their 1999 MCI paper. With the advent of the MCI criteria the memory complaint has been subjected to additional research. Some have suggested, contrary to prior research, it portends a dementia (Barnes, Schneider, Boyle, Bienias, &

Bennett, 2006). As the literature on the significance of memory complaints is too large to deal with here, I will address this issue via the case example in the discussion section.

The second issue regarding the memory complaint is that when present there is no attempt to characterize it. A memory complaint to a neuropsychologist is what a tremor is to a movement disorders specialist. Both are the most common presenting symptom for each respective profession. In contrast to the memory complaint in MCI, the tremor complaint triggers a series of questions in the mind of the neurologist. When was the onset of the tremor? Is it a resting or an intention tremor? Who in the patient's family has it? What medication is the patient on? Is there any rigidity, akinesia, or postural instability? Is this a precursor to Parkinson's disease, or an atypical initial presentation of a Parkinson-plus syndrome? Carrying out this line of questioning in regard to tremor may lead to a diagnosis. Finally, what is the base rate of a memory complaint in an elderly population? At a time when the concept of age-associated memory impairment was popular, Koivisto et al. (1995) found that in a randomly selected normal population between 60 to 78 years of age, a memory complaint was present in 76%. Documenting the mere presence of a symptom with such a high base rate in the normal population is an exercise in diagnostic futility.

The second problematic definition of MCI is that the patient must score at least 1.5 SD below the mean on a standardized memory test. In 1991, during my first full year of clinical practice as a VA employee I had written a proposal to obtain pilot money to develop a recognition paradigm for a memory test. To norm it, I proposed using an IQ of 85 or lower as a means of ruling out patients with neurologic disease. Laird Cermack at the Boston VA, who reviewed the proposal, reminded me that non-neurological patients can score below 85, and poor test performance is not synonymous with neurological disease. Edgar Miller (1983) best illustrates the prevailing neuropsychological assessment fallacy of the day:

If damage to structure X is known to produce a decline in performance on test T, it is tempting to argue that any new subject or group of subjects having a relatively poor performance on T must have a lesion in X. In fact, the logical status of this argument is the same as arguing that because a horse meets the test of being a large animal with four legs, that any newly encountered animal with four legs must be a horse. A newly encountered specimen could of course be a cow or hippopotamus and still meet the same test. Similarly, new subjects who do badly on T may do so for reasons other than having a lesion at X. (p. 131)

Continuing the earlier line of reasoning, what is the base rate of such a memory score in normal elderly? Four memory tests yielding eight standard scores were administered to older adults (55–87 years; N = 550) as part of the Wechsler Memory Scale–III standardization sample. Of the sample, 26% had one or more scores at or below 1.5 SD below the mean (Brooks, Iverson, Holdnack, & Feldman, 2008). The balance of the MCI criteria, normal activities of daily living, and no dementia are interrelated. Their presence means dementia, precluding the need for the term MCI.

Case Presentation

The patient is an 80-year-old, right-handed, widowed, Caucasian female with 17 years of education culminating in a Masters of Education degree. Her internist referred her to rule out a dementing illness. Medical history was positive for hypertension, gastroparesis, allergies, depression, and esophageal ulcer. Her medication included Benicar, Celexa, Lyrica, Reglan, Zebeta, and Ambien. Bentyl, Claritin, and Tylenol were taken as needed. Her internist considered adding Cymbalta, but decided to wait until after the neuropsychological evaluation. Family history was positive for hypertension, endometrial cancer, and stroke, but no history of memory loss in any first-degree relatives. Her mother died of cancer at 99 and her father of a stroke at 87. There was a history of depression in her father and posttraumatic stress disorder in one brother secondary to his World War II service. Notable is that her husband had multiple sclerosis for 30 years. Half of that time was spent in a nursing home until he died at 67. Her internist ordered a computed tomography (CT) of the brain and laboratory work that included B12 and a thyroid level. All were normal.

Cognitive Testing

She was oriented to month and day of the month but missed the day of the week by one day.

She knew the time within 30 minutes. This is considered intact. She named the last three Presidents of the United States in order. She named the town in which she lived, gave her mailing address, age, birth date, the name of the city in which she was currently being examined, and the name of the hospital at which she was being tested. The Geriatric Depression Scale (GDS) revealed no depression. Her test results and the typical AD battery we use are outlined in Table 50-1.

Family Interview

The patient's daughter indicated that the onset of the patient's memory difficulty has been over the last two years, with the most significant change over the last six months. Her family thinks she has been hiding some of the difficulties. She is a person that very much wants to be in control of her affairs. When asked for examples of memory loss, the daughter indicated two months ago there was an incident where they had to explain to her the rules to a card game that she always knew. She lost at Scrabble recently, which is rare for her. She used to work 1000-piece puzzles, and now she cannot work a 100-piece puzzle. There was an incident where she insisted that her nephew was born at a certain place that he was not. She forgets appointments. When they left to come to the appointment with me, she asked where they were going. She was told two days earlier. She called one of their dogs by the wrong name, calling it after a dog they had as children. Others have noticed problems. This includes her son-in-law, granddaughter, and sister. Her long-term memory is fine. Over the last two months they have noticed worsening word-finding difficulty. It is hard for her to get out the words. Now she seems to refer to items as "that thing." Her daughter was asked about any personality change. The patient's granddaughter used to help her clean the house when the patient lived alone. In the past, the patient would follow her around to make sure she did everything right. The patient eventually became apathetic, not caring how her granddaughter cleaned. The daughter denied any irritability or depression. She had severe bouts of depression when younger due to her husband's multiple sclerosis. She seems to be "living in the past" nowadays. She thinks a lot about her sister, who had passed away as well as

Table 50-1. Case Presentation Test Summary

Intelligence

WAIS-R	Raw Score	Scaled Score
Information	22	14
Similarities	27	15
Vocabulary	61	17
Digit Span	15	10
Block Design	34	14
Picture Completion	21	15
Matrix Reasoning	20	17
		Standard Score
Verbal Comprehension	46	131
Perceptual Organizational	46	135

Memory

RAVLT		Scaled Score
Total 1–5	27	5
List B	4	11
Trial 6	2	5
Delayed Recall	1	6
Recognition	9	7
Wechsler Memory Scale-III		Scaled Score
Logical Memory I	32	11
Logical Memory II	3	6
Visual Reproduction I	61	10
Visual Reproduction II	0	5

Attention

WMS-III-Working Memory		
Spatial Span	7	6
Letter-Number Sequencing	12	15
		T-Score
Trail-Making A	42	44
Trail-Making B	101	46

Language		Percentile
Visual Naming	56	64
Controlled Oral Word	28	18

Visuocognitive

Judgment of Line Orientation	23	40
Facial Recognition Test	45	51

Psychological

Geriatric Depression Scale	7	

her husband. She sleeps quite a bit. She used to quilt, but has dropped that activity. She does not do any activities at church. About five years ago she probably would read about "five books a week," but now she reads none. There are some questionable problems with activities of daily living. One thing that they discovered when she moved in with her son was that her daughter-in-law, who is a physician, noticed she was not taking her medication correctly, skipping some days. The patient has not felt safe to drive anymore so she stopped driving a month ago. She indicated, "I feel fuzzy. I should not be driving." Recently she forgot to record some check numbers in her checkbook. Prior to moving in with her son, she did all her activities of daily living. The daughter denied that the patient had difficulties cooking, and the patient still manages her own financial affairs.

Patient Interview

When asked why she was here, she replied, "I really do not know, I did what they told me." After she thought a minute, she indicated that there is a memory problem "to some degree." She denied it was any worse than other people her age, or that it produces problems with activities of daily living. She denied feeling sad or unhappy. She still enjoys quilting. When asked why she moved in with her son this past year, she indicated that the family felt that they would like to have her close to better care for her.

Discussion

The diagnosis was early AD, and the following recommendations were made. In the early stages, when memory is the sole deficit, the diagnosis is less certain than when other deficits accompany the memory problem. In such circumstances, a follow-up may be indicated depending on the progression of symptoms over the next year. If after a year it is obvious she has gotten worse, then another evaluation would not be necessary. For the family I recommended the book *The Thirty-Six Hour Day*. I did not feel she was clinically depressed but that her symptoms reflected neurovegatative signs of AD. It is not necessary to add another antidepressant. I recommended she be placed on an acetylcholinesterase inhibitor. Her current living circumstance is sufficient in terms of the level of supervision, but her financial affairs should be supervised. As my clinical practice has always operated as a consultation service to other health-care professionals, these results are communicated not to the patient or family, but to the referral source.

On the cognitive testing the patient demonstrates the prototypical profile of early AD. There is generally preserved cognitive function except for memory. The Mayo AD group now refers to this as the amnestic variant of MCI (Petersen et al., 2006). The borderline performance on Spatial Span likely reflects a false-positive finding owing to the intact performance on more sensitive measures of attention. It might be reasonable to conclude that the memory testing might have been far worse in a person with a lower or even average IQ. This illustrates the cognitive reserve hypothesis (Roe, Xiong, Miller, & Morris, 2007). Highly educated individuals are not as likely to manifest clinical symptoms of dementia versus less-educated individuals. It is important to emphasize that the disease process does not pay homage to the educated. Education is not neuroprotective per se. Instead it makes diagnosing early AD more difficult. The clinician must decide whether that educated patient crossed a threshold that reflects a decline as opposed to the less educated patient.

Before moving on to the crux of the examination, the family interview, let me highlight some aspects of the cognitive testing. Arthur Benton and his students developed many of the tests we employ (Benton, Sivan, Hamsher, & Varney, 1994). Temporal Orientation is administered to every patient. Impaired orientation predicts impaired memory but not vice versa. In the case of early AD, this is likely to be intact. In our database, 39% of AD patients (N = 326) have no worse than low-normal orientation. One in five (21.5%) are perfectly oriented. They know the date, day of the week, and time within 30 minutes. For memory, we administer the Rey Auditory Verbal Learning Test. If delayed recall is nil, there is no need to give additional memory testing unless there is evidence to suggest a false-positive result. This impaired delayed recall must be corroborated by the family interview. When a borderline score is obtained, the additional memory tests listed in Table 50-1 are given. We give two language (Controlled Oral Word and

Visual Naming) and two visuocognitive tests (Facial Recognition and Judgment of Line Orientation). We find that both language tests are equally failed, while in the visuocognitive domain, Judgment of Line Orientation, primarily a measure of parietal lobe function, is failed more often. One of the earliest positron emission tomography (PET) studies showed that hypoperfusion in the posterior parietal lobes of AD patients was twice that of other areas (Foster et al., 1984). Sensitive measures of attention (i.e., Letter Number Sequencing and Trail Making Part B) must also be included. Finally, the tests most sensitive to the effects of early AD are given in the first 90 minutes of the examination, before the first break. This is done in order to make a preliminary assessment at the break regarding the possibility of AD so as to begin the interview with the family once the patient returns to the testing with the psychometrician. Normal testing will shorten the family interview.

In early AD, where there is an absence of concomitant neurological signs, the only other diagnostic tool aside from the cognitive testing is the family interview. In other dementing conditions, the presence of neurological signs lessens the contribution of the interview. Additionally, more so than any other neurological disorder, it is the interview of the family, and not the patient that is the sine qua non of early diagnosis. A competent evaluation of early AD cannot be done without the interview of a collateral source. The reader should now glance at the family interview questions in Table 50-2 in order to follow the rationale of the family interview that is explained later. I cannot emphasize enough the importance of the collateral interview. I had an opportunity in October 2008 to visit the Washington University AD group. The informant interview has been the cornerstone of their approach. In the research arm of their clinic, a neurologist determines the presence of dementia via a brief mental status examination, a patient interview, and a semistructured 10-page interview with an informant. Patient and family interviews are taped so another neurologist can rate them. In the research arm of their clinic, the AD diagnosis is made independent of the neuropsychological testing. What I learned from my visit is to structure my current family interview even more.

Table 50-2. Suggested Family Interview Questions

1) Do you notice a problem with the patient's memory?
2) Do you think that the patient's memory is worse than other people of his/her age?
3) Was the onset of the memory problems sudden or gradual? Sudden means it began over the course of a day or days, was related with a hospitalization, illness, or stressor.
4) Since the memory problem began, is it getting better, same, or worse?
5) Can you provide the most severe instances of memory loss you have noticed in the last week or month? These should be instances that worried you, not just misplacing keys.
6) Have you noticed any problem with word finding? Does he/she have difficulty coming up with the right word, use a wrong word, or call something by the wrong name?
7) Have you noticed any personality changes?
8) Are there difficulties with activities of daily living, such as getting lost in familiar and unfamiliar surroundings, taking medication incorrectly, or managing finances?
9) Have others noticed these difficulties independently of you?
10) Have others provided examples of what they observed that you can share?
11) Have others suggested the patient should see a doctor for these problems?
12) Who first raised the issue with his/her doctor regarding being referred for memory problems? Did you discuss this with his/her doctor, the patient, or another person?
13) Of the difficulties the patient is having (i.e., memory, language problems, a personality change, or difficulties with daily living problems) what problem troubles you most?
14) Of the difficulties that you describe, which symptom did you notice first, followed by the next one that appeared, and so on?

First, the patient and the family must be interviewed separately. In our database, 25.2% (N = 301) of patients have psychosis. One cannot expect a family member to feel comfortable detailing the patient's delusions in their presence. While psychosis is not an issue in early AD, anosognosia is. The patient resents the person who relays problems the patient thinks he or she does not have. Families are grateful that the interviews are conducted separately. Most interviews, regardless of the condition or circumstance, are not conducted at the beginning of the testing. In our work setting, an outpatient neurology clinic, we have a sufficient amount of medical records and background information to know the diagnostic issues. Should an issue arise after the interview, additional testing can be done.

Over the years I have found that families and patients seem to form clusters based on how they respond to the interview. This admittedly idiosyncratic classification system is outlined in Table 50-3. It serves to provide the reader with a roadmap of what to expect. I group the family interviews into three categories, the *leaders*, *misleaders*, and *leaderless*. The leaders constitute roughly 85% of families. The case presentation illustrates the leaders category. These are families

Table 50-3. Classifying the Family and Patient Interviews

Family Interview	Patient Interview
Leaders	No
Misleaders	Yes, but no
a) Mistaken onset	Yes, I am worried
b) Mistaken diagnosis	
i) Mistaken doctor	
ii) Mistaken family	
Leaderless	

that give you a chronological detailed history of the patient's problems in such a way as to make the diagnosis straightforward. The misleaders, about 10%, form two groups. The first of the misleaders is the *mistaken onset* group. Anybody who has examined enough AD patients has heard how the patient's cognitive decline began after the hip or bypass surgery, or some other medical event that could not possibly explain the current clinical presentation. The patient's pre-existing dementia came to light because that medical event served to exacerbate what was already there. The brain has already been compromised by one form of brain disease: AD. It does not have the cognitive reserve to withstand a second insult: a concomitant delirium. This marked behavior change draws the attention of the family, yet once it resolves, which by definition it must, the patient does not seem like "the same person they once were." Not only that but the patient seems to be getting worse.

The second group of misleaders is the *mistaken diagnosis* group. These families fall into two subgroups, depending on who is incorrect about the AD diagnosis, the doctor or family. These I term the *mistaken doctor* versus the *mistaken family*. The first scenario has the family saying the doctor is mistaken. The patient does not have AD. Between the media, the Internet, and possibly having seen another family member or friend suffer from it, families may have some awareness of AD. In this situation the testing shows obvious impairment, yet the family fails to provide an example of any substance that helps to corroborate your test findings. When they do provide an example, they immediately dismiss it: "He is not working so he has no reason to know what month it is." These families sense the diagnostic road you are on, but they are silently saying, "You are mistaken doctor." Commonly it is a spouse in denial, a denial that is confirmed by a phone call placed to one of the patient's children. If a phone call is not possible, a 1-year follow-up is recommended in order to document the decline that the family member could not understandably relay.

In the second mistaken diagnosis scenario we have the reverse. The doctor saying the family is mistaken about the diagnosis. As noted above, memory complaints in the neurological outpatient likely reflects worried well behavior, and not neurological disease. There is no reason to believe that the vocal complaint of the family member in regard to the patient might not be a reflection of that family member's emotional and psychological makeup. These spurious complaints are met by annoyance on the part of the patient who accurately perceives his or her memory is fine. Commonly this concern is precipitated when the family member has read, heard, or seen on television something regarding AD. Asking the informant whether others have independently observed a memory problem and having the informant provide an example guard against the false-positive reporting of the well-meaning but alarmist family member.

This leaves us with about 5% of families that fall into the *leaderless* category. These families have no insight about the patient. In the absence of another family member who can shed some light on the situation, a presumptive diagnosis of AD is made based on the cognitive testing, and the ruling out of other causes via a neurological examination. Rarely is a reversible cause for the patient's presentation uncovered. The patient is seen a year later to document any cognitive decline to confirm the diagnosis.

While most questions in Table 50-2 are self-explanatory, and some have been touched upon, let me elaborate on a few. It is never acceptable to only ask whether a memory problem is present, but to then ask whether it is worse than other people his or her age. This requires some judgment on the part of the interviewee. One way to tease this out is to ask the spouse to compare the patient's memory with that of her own siblings or the patient's siblings. The child of the patient is asked to compare the memory of one parent versus the patient. The question of onset is straightforward with the exception of the aforementioned caveats. The most critical aspect about examining the memory complaint is that the family member must provide narratives of incidents in which the patient's memory has failed. It is simply not enough for the family member to say that the patient repeats or misplaces things. The more uncertain the diagnosis based on the cognitive results, the more narratives are needed. While memory is the most critical, narratives should be sought out for all the major categories (i.e., memory, language, personality, and daily living skills). The second most important interview category is personality changes (e.g., apathy, irritability, relinquishing of hobbies).

Early in the experience of the Washington University AD group, they found the collateral source reported "depressive symptoms" in their AD research subjects, despite enrollment criteria excluding subjects with affective disorders. It became apparent that organic neurovegatative symptoms of AD and not clinical depression was being described. In fact, they found depression to be rare in their AD subjects (Burke, Rubin, Morris, & Berg, 1988). Many AD patients have a loss of interest, meeting one of the two core criteria for clinical depression. The other criterion of depressed mood is rarely met. The GDS has been factor analyzed for both mood and neurovegetative symptoms. In our database, about 40% of AD patients have a GDS in the depressed range (N = 244). Looking at mood versus vegetative symptoms of depression, on average 90% of AD patients denied mood symptoms, while nearly half reported vegetative symptoms. In response to the question, "Do you feel happy most of the time?" 92% of our AD sample responded yes.

While the interview of the family may take as long as an hour in early onset, borderline, or complicated cases, the patient interview takes half the time. Before the patient is interviewed we have reviewed outside medical records, often have a complete medical workup, the cognitive testing, and the family interview at our disposal. With this information, there is nothing that the patient is likely to say that will shed any light on the diagnosis. In the event the cognitive testing is negative, the patient interview might identify emotional factors. If the workup is positive for early AD, all you will likely get is a patient interview characterized by a lack of insight. As in our case presentation, the interview served to document this lack of insight more than anything else.

I also group the patient interviews into three categories, the *no, yes but no*, and *yes I am worried*. These are the answers you get from the patient when you ask about their memory. There are patients that will say no to the presence of memory difficulty. There are those that will say yes, but no worse than others their age. This constitutes 90% of incipient AD patients. The yes I am worried group admits to memory impairment, sees it as being worse than others their age, is worried about a dementia, and the testing confirms their fears. In my experience, this scenario is very rare. If this happens, more common is the following situation. There is nothing to preclude the lifelong worried well or chronic psychiatric patient from developing AD. The AD patient reporting memory impairment judges it to be worse than others his or her age and has always been worried about one medical condition or other. This patient's correct analysis is not insight, but coincidental somatization that has been ever-present. This is the "boy that cried wolf" scenario. The patient interview is concluded by inquiring about any problems with personality changes, activities of daily living, mood, and the presence of stressors.

There are few differential diagnoses in early AD. The most common is depression versus dementia. The family often feels the patient is depressed. In the context of a memory complaint and depression, the physician commonly entertains "pseudodementia" as a diagnosis. The myth surrounding the term is that the cognitive deficits of an elderly depressed patient are equal or somehow can be confused with the level of impairment found in early AD. Pseudodementia can be dismissed on two counts. First, clinical depression is uncommon in early AD. Second, the level of cognitive impairment seen in early AD is not equivalent to that found in geriatric depressed outpatients. The term *pseudodementia* is a pseudoterm adopted by medicine, as they have no method for distinguishing the two conditions: namely cognitive testing. A neuropsychological evaluation typically makes for a more straightforward differential diagnosis (Lamberty & Bieliauskas, 1993).

A second differential diagnosis is a frontal lobe dementia. In this case a predominately apathetic variant of frontal lobe dementia, as opposed to the prototypical inappropriate behavior variant might mimic the early neurovegetative symptoms in AD. First, cognitive testing is beneficial. Relatively spared memory in the presence of frontal lobe dysfunction might suggest a frontal lobe dementia. While the family may report a memory change, the examples are not compelling. For frontal lobe tests, we add the Stroop, animal fluency, Ruff Figural Fluency, and the Nelson Modification of the Wisconsin Card Sorting Test. Additionally, a personality change that precedes the memory impairment would suggest a frontal lobe dementia. The questions in Table 50-2 regarding what symptoms the informant considers salient and the order in which they appear in the patient help tease this out.

There is a final differential to consider. In the world of differential diagnosis, when the competent doctor is stumped, it generally means one of three things. The diagnosis is not readily appreciated because what the patient has is rare, not real, or it is an atypical presentation of a typical disease. A cursory Medline search with the words *heterogeneity, subtype, subgroups,* and *asymmetry* in reference to AD will yield a plethora of studies. Researchers at the National Institutes of Health initially observed this heterogeneity (Friedland et al., 1988). They used functional imaging to demonstrate that asymmetrical hypoperfusion correlated with the cognitive testing. Early in the course of AD a patient may present with disproportionate language impairment relative to visuocognitive abilities and vice versa. The dissociation can be so striking as to suggest a stroke. The diagnostic confusion occurs when the patient has pronounced language impairment with an equal or lesser degree of memory impairment. This might suggest a primary progressive aphasia. This can be teased out by giving visual memory tests to document the presence of memory impairment independent of language. The family is asked what came first, the language or memory problem. Additionally, the presence of primary progressive aphasia has to, by definition, precede other cognitive impairment by two years (Mesulam, 2001).

To make appropriate recommendation readers should be familiar with criteria for AD (McKhann et al., 1984) and the American Academy of Neurology (AAN) dementia guidelines (Knopman et al., 2001). All AD workups should include a CT or magnetic resonance image (MRI) of the brain, thyroid and B_{12} testing. The AAN MCI guidelines are less useful (Petersen et al., 2001). While neuropsychological testing and screening instruments (e.g., MMSE) are considered a guideline, the interview of an informant and brief focused cognitive tests (e.g., clock drawing) are optional. A MMSE examination in the case presentation would have yielded normal results. Per the MCI practice guidelines, the patient's performance on clock drawing is weighted the same as obtaining information that is obligatory to the diagnosis of AD. The definition of AD is a progressive decline in cognitive function sufficient to interfere with activities of daily living. Who but an informant is going to provide a history of progressive cognitive decline? A final recommendation is treatment.

Acetylcholinesterase inhibitors should be recommended in patients with early AD even if the full AD criteria are not met. The goal of the MCI concept was to facilitate early diagnosis that would translate into early treatment so as to delay conversion to AD. To date, donepezil, galantamine, and rivastigmine are three acetylcholinesterase inhibitors that are FDA approved for the treatment of mild to moderate AD. All have failed in MCI clinical trials (Feldman et al., 2007; Petersen et al., 2005; Winblad et al., 2008). This lack of success is because (a) MCI is a faulty concept, (b) cognitive instruments used in MCI trials are not sufficiently sensitive to detect progression and thus conversion to AD, (c) MCI patients cannot meet the primary outcome measure of these studies, conversion to AD, since MCI is early AD, and (d) acetylcholinesterase inhibitors do not work in patients with MCI. I think a combination of the first three likely accounts for the failed trials

Conclusions

MCI researchers are canvassing clinics and communities for elderly to enroll in epidemiological, clinical, and treatment studies. The memory complaint and memory score of these subjects do not constitute a clinical entity, but a statistical anomaly. To remedy this situation, knowledgeable and experienced clinicians are needed to diagnose incipient AD at the memory impairment stage and to call it what it is: early AD. No doubt this can be difficult at times. However, coining a construct to alleviate the collective diagnostic angst of the medical community will not advance the science. Part of the remedy for this problem can be found in clinical neuropsychology. With the possible exception of identifying the "psychogenic" patient, there is probably no condition in adult clinical neurology in which the diagnostic role of the clinical neuropsychologist is more critical than the detection of early AD.

References

Barnes, L. L., Schneider, J. A., Boyle, P. A., Bienias, J. L., & Bennett D. A. (2006). Memory complaints are related to Alzheimer disease pathology in older persons. *Neurology*, 67, 1581–1585.

Benton, A. L., Sivan, A. B., Hamsher, K., & Varney, N. R. (1994). *Contributions to neuropsychological assessment: A clinical manual* (2nd ed.). New York: Oxford University Press.

Brooks, B. L., Iverson, G. L., Holdnack, J. A., & Feldman, H. H. (2008). The potential for misclassification of mild cognitive impairment: A study of memory scores on the Wechsler Memory Scale-III in healthy older adults. *Journal of the International Neuropsychological Society, 14,* 463–478.

Burke, W. J., Rubin, E. H., Morris, J. C., & Berg, L. (1988). Symptoms of "depression" in dementia of the Alzheimer type. *Alzheimer's Disease and Associated Disorders, 2,* 356–362.

Burns, J. M., & Morris, J. C. (2008). *Mild cognitive impairment and early Alzheimer's disease. Detection & diagnosis.* New York: Wiley.

Feldman, H. H., Ferris S., Winblad, B., Sfikas, N., Mancione L., He, S et al. (2007). Effect of rivastigmine on delay to diagnosis of Alzheimer's disease from mild cognitive impairment: The InDDEx study. *Lancet Neurology, 6,* 501–512.

Flicker, C., Ferris S. H., & Reisberg, B. (1991). Mild cognitive impairment in the elderly: Predictors of dementia. *Neurology, 41,* 1006–1009.

Foster NL, Chase TN, Mansi L, Brooks R, Fedio P, Patronas NJ & Di Chiro G. (1984). Cortical abnormalities in Alzheimer's disease. Annals of Neurology, 16, 649-54.

Friedland, R. P., Koss, E., Haxby, J. V., Grady C. L., Luxenberg, J., Schapiro, M. B., et al. (1988). NIH conference. Alzheimer disease: Clinical and biological heterogeneity. *Annals of Internal Medicine, 109,* 298–311.

Knopman, D. S., DeKosky, S. T., Cummings, J. L., Chui, H., Corey-Bloom, J., Relkin, N. et al. (2001). Practice parameter: Diagnosis of dementia (an evidence-based review). Report of the Quality Standards Subcommittee of the American Academy of Neurology. *Neurology, 56,* 1143–1153.

Koivisto, K., Reinikainen, K. J., Hänninen, T., Vanhanen, M., Helkala, E. L., Mykkänen L., et al. (1995). Prevalence of age-associated memory impairment in a randomly selected population from eastern Finland. *Neurology, 45,* 741–747.

Lamberty, G. J., & Bieliauskas, L. A. (1993).Distinguishing between depression and dementia in the elderly: A review of neuropsychological findings. *Archives of Clinical Neuropsychology, 8,* 149–170.

McKhann, G., Drachman, D., Folstein, M., Katzman, R., Price D., & Stadlan, E. M. (1984). Clinical diagnosis of Alzheimer's disease: Report of the NINCDS-ADRDA Work Group under the auspices of Department of Health and Human Services Task Force on Alzheimer's Disease. *Neurology, 34,* 939–944.

Mesulam, M. M. (2001). Primary progressive aphasia. *Annals of Neurology, 49,* 425–432.

Miller, E. (1983). A note on the interpretation of data derived from neuropsychological tests. *Cortex, 19,* 131–132.

Morris, J. C., & Landau, W. M. (2007). Leonard Berg, M.D. (1927-2007): In Memoriam. *Neurology, 69,* 1206–1207.

Peterson, R. C. (Ed.). (2003). *Mild cognitive impairment: Aging to Alzheimer's disease.* New York: Oxford University Press.

Petersen, R. C., Parisi, J. E., Dickson, D. W., Johnson, K. A., Knopman, D. S., Boeve, B. et al. (2006). Neuropathologic features of amnestic mild cognitive impairment. *Archives of Neurology, 63,* 665–672.

Petersen, R. C., Smith, G. E., Waring, S. C., Ivnik, R., J., Tangalos, E. G., & Kokmen, E. (1999). Mild cognitive impairment: Clinical characterization and outcome. *Archives of Neurology, 56,* 303–308.

Petersen, R. C., Steven, J. C., Ganguli, M., Tangalos, E. G., Cummings, J. L., & DeKosky, S. T. (2001). Practice parameter: Early detection of dementia: Mild cognitive impairment (an evidence-based review). Report of the Quality Standards Subcommittee of the American Academy of Neurology. *Neurology, 56,* 1133–1142.

Petersen, R. C., Thomas, R. G., Grundman, M., Bennett, D., Doody, R., Ferris, S., et al. (2005). Vitamin E and donepezil for the treatment of mild cognitive impairment. *New England Journal of Medicine, 352,* 2379–2388.

Roe, C. M., Xiong, C., Miller, J. P., & Morris, J. C. (2007). Education and Alzheimer disease without dementia: Support for the cognitive reserve hypothesis. *Neurology, 68,* 223–228.

Smith, G. E., Petersen R. C., Ivnik, R. J., Malec, J. F., & Tangalos, E. G. (1996). Subjective memory complaints, psychological distress, and longitudinal change in objective memory performance. *Psycholology and Aging, 11,* 272–279.

Tuokko, H. A., & Hultsch, D. F. (Eds.). (2006). *Mild cognitive impairment: International perspectives.* New York: Taylor & Francis.

Whitehouse, P., & Brodaty, H. (2006). Mild cognitive impairment. *Lancet, 17,* 367.

Winblad, B., Gauthier, S., Scinto L., Feldman, H., Wilcock, G. K., Truyen, L., et al. (2008). Safety and efficacy of galantamine in subjects with mild ognitive impairment. *Neurology, 70,* 2024–2035.

51

Clinical and Neuropathologic Presentation of Dementia with Lewy Bodies

Tanis J. Ferman

It is now well established, based on sensitive immunostaining techniques on autopsy tissue, that dementia with Lewy bodies (DLB) is the second most common cause of neurodegenerative dementia. Alzheimer disease (AD) is the most common neurodegenerative dementia. In 2005, the third International Workshop meeting on DLB resulted in publication of revised consensus diagnostic criteria for DLB (McKeith et al., 2005). These criteria are presented in Table 51-1.

Identifying the presence of dementia requires the clinician to determine whether the day-to-day cognitive problems are interfering with activities of daily living (ADLs). Moreover, patients and their caregivers may complain of memory difficulties, but careful inquiry may reveal whether the problem is actually a breakdown of attention (i.e., trouble keeping track of details, losing attentional set), word finding, or even visuospatial difficulties (i.e., getting lost, trouble finding objects among other objects).

The neurocognitive evaluation is helpful in assisting with the differential diagnosis of DLB, but it requires a good clinical history. Establishing whether the patient has a history of rapid eye movement (REM) sleep behavior disorder (dream enactment behavior during sleep), motor features suggestive of parkinsonism, fully formed visual hallucinations, and fluctuating abilities that resemble delirium is relevant. Also determining the presence of somnolence, visual misperceptions, history of exposure to neuroleptics, sensitivity/responsiveness to medication, cur-

rent medication doses and reactions to them, ongoing stressors, and drug/alcohol use are a vital part of the dementia evaluation.

Parkinsonism/Visual Hallucinations/Fluctuations

When parkinsonism is present in DLB, it is typically symmetric, involves gait difficulty, rigidity, and bradykinesia. Resting tremor is less common but postural/static tremor is fairly common. Visual hallucinations in DLB must be fully formed and are generally people or animals (though sometimes may be objects), and they tend to occur within the first 5 years of DLB (Ferman et al., 2003). In AD, they tend to occur in the advanced stages as demonstrated by results from autopsy-confirmed samples (Hope, Keene, Fairburn, Jacoby, & McShane, 1999; Perry et al., 1990; Rockwell, Choure, Galasko, Olichney, & Jeste, 2000). Fluctuations resemble signs of delirium without identifiable precipitants of such mental status changes. Caregivers may describe periods when the patient cannot do tasks that he or she can later do (e.g., may be unable to figure out the microwave, remote control, or how to make a sandwich, but can later do these things easily). The Mayo Fluctuations Scale requires the presence of at least three of the four features to reliably distinguish DLB fluctuations from those in AD: *(a)* daytime drowsiness and lethargy despite getting enough sleep the night before; *(b)* daytime sleep of 2 or more hours before 7pm; *(c)* stares into space for long periods (but is

Table 51-1. Revised Criteria for the Clinical Diagnosis of Dementia with Lewy Bodies (DLB)

Central Feature (essential for diagnosis of possible or probable DLB)
- Dementia
  - ○ Progressive cognitive decline of sufficient magnitude to interfere with normal social or occupational function.
  - ○ Prominent or persistent memory impairment may not necessarily occur in the early stages but is usually evident with progression.
  - ○ Deficits on tests of attention, executive function, and visuospatial ability may be especially prominent.

Core Features (Two core features are sufficient for diagnosis of probable DLB, or one for possible DLB)
- Fluctuating cognition with pronounced variation in attention and alertness
- Recurrent visual hallucinations that are well formed and detailed
- Spontaneous features of parkinsonism

Suggestive Features (One or more in the presence of one or more core features, then a diagnosis of probable DLB can be made. In the absence of any core features, one or more suggestive features is sufficient for possible DLB)
- REM sleep behavior disorder
- Severe neuroleptic sensitivity
- Low dopamine transporter uptake in the basal ganglia demonstrated by single-photon emission computed tomography or positron emission tomographic imaging

Source. From McKeith et al. (2005)

responsive); and *(d)* times when flow of ideas seems disorganized, unclear, or illogical (Ferman et al., 2004). Cognitive fluctuations have also been demonstrated on formal testing whereby DLB is associated with greater variability with attention, vigilance, and reaction time relative to AD (Ballard, Walker, O'Brien, Rowan, & McKeith, 2001; Ferman et al., 1999; Walker et al., 2000).

REM Sleep Behavior Disorder

In 2005, REM sleep behavior disorder (RBD) was added to the diagnostic criteria for DLB. The presence of dementia plus RBD alone is now sufficient for a diagnosis of possible DLB, and RBD plus a core feature represents probable DLB (see Table 51-1) (McKeith et al., 2005). REM sleep behavior disorder involves the loss of normal muscle atonia during rapid eye movement sleep. As a result, muscle activity is augmented during dream sleep. This may be represented by subtle movements or may be quite vigorous and involve pantomiming complex behavioral sequences while asleep. Examples of RBD include running, fighting, defending oneself or one's family, kicking the dog off the porch, playing sports, or engaging in combat during the war. Some patients

and their bedpartners sustain injuries that may be rather minor (e.g., hair pulling, bruises) to quite severe (lacerations, broken bones). The muscle movements must be associated with a dream (and is not somnambulism, which occurs in NREM stage 3–4 sleep) and cannot be a single flailing of a limb (e.g., that may be observed with sleep apnea) and does not constitute sleep-talking (which can occur in any stage of sleep).

Case Report

The patient's first encounter with our clinic was at the age of 81. He was a right-handed retired post-office supervisor with 12 years of formal education. He was accompanied by his wife. Prior to coming to our clinic, this patient had obtained a diagnosis of AD, but was interested in a second opinion.

At about the age of 75, he developed dream enactment behavior during sleep. He would typically have dreams that involved trying to defend himself or somebody else. For example, he dreamed that he was trying to grab at a boy who was walking toward a fire while calling out to him in an effort to save him. and he actually grabbed his wife's hair and pulled it while frantically yelling "No! Stop!". His movements during sleep appeared to mimic dream content. He did not have a history of snoring or restless legs syndrome. He was initially treated with clonazepam (0.5 mg) for his REM sleep behavior disorder, but this was eventually discontinued as the symptoms lessened over time.

At about age 77, he developed a gradual and progressive decline in his thinking skills. The first symptoms included slowed mentation, a tendency to lose his train of thought and trouble fixing things around the house (e.g., hanging a door correctly, fixing the commode), which was a change for him since he had always been exceptionally talented with mechanical tasks. He was experiencing episodes when he seemed "spaced out," drowsy and lethargic and he would get easily distracted, stare into space (though did respond when spoken to), and would say things that were out of context but grammatical. He described feeling "swimmy headed" or "woozy". An electroencephalogram (EEG) was carried out and findings revealed mild slowing but no sharp waves or epileptiform discharges. It was during these times that his abilities tended to deteriorate, and then at other times, he was much more alert and attentive and more nearly normal with a better ability to carry out mechanical tasks or get his points across. At times he would forget what his wife told him, though would typically recognize the information when reminded. He was not initiating new activities on his own, but was happy to comply with any task when asked. He was hesitant with word finding but did not substitute the wrong words during conversation.

At age 80, he was started on a cholinesterase inhibitor and his wife reported a rather dramatic improvement in attention, processing speed, initiation and reduced intensity of fluctuations.

At around the age of 81, excessive daytime sleepiness became a major issue. Despite getting 9 hours of sleep at night, and despite the absence of snoring, apnea, or restless legs syndrome, he was dozing on and off in the daytime. Nonetheless, when his wife asked him to do things, he was still willing to get up and do them.

By age 81, he was still taking care of the pool, yard work, did the grocery shopping, laundry, some driving and sharing the finances though his wife was managing his medication. Nonetheless, his attention problems worsened and he

developed much greater and more consistent trouble carrying out mechanical tasks. For example, he had trouble snapping a seatbelt, using a key to lock/unlock a door, and fixing things such as car maintenance.

By age 82, he developed fully formed, recurrent visual hallucinations that included a little girl, tents in the neighbor's yard, an escaped convict, a neighbor, books on the floor he was trying to pick up, pieces of trash that were not there, and some bugs. He had visual misperceptions, such as mistaking a pattern on the floor for spilled water or insects. There were a few episodes where he thought he heard a noise outside that was not there, but he never heard voices or music. He did not experience visual misidentification or Capgras phenomena.

By age 83, he was no longer initiating conversation much. His wife described his overall level of functioning as "peaks and valleys" with times where he was reasonably attentive and able to follow what was happening around him, and other times when he was mixed up, incoherent and had trouble staying awake. At this point, he became unable to independently figure out many mechanical tasks, such as the microwave, his electric razor, how to operate the lawnmower, how to hang a picture, how to check the chlorine level in the pool, and he had increasing difficulty finding objects in a cluttered area (e.g., looking for an item in the refrigerator, or on a crowded table). His wife had now taken over medications, finances, driving, cooking, pool maintenance, and all other household responsibilities.

By the age of 85, his visual hallucinations persisted and he developed occasional false beliefs (delusions) that accompanied the hallucinations he was experiencing. For example, he routinely saw five women whom he thought appeared smart, and so he presumed they were running for President and would ask about that. He never experienced paranoia or suspiciousness and was not fearful of the images. He did not develop visual misidentification of family or Capgras (reduplicative) phenomena.

Neurologic Examination/Imaging

At age 81, neurologic examination revealed very mildly reduced facial expression, slight hypophonia, absent arm swing when walking, mild stiffness when turning, bilateral mild static/ postural tremor, mild micrographia, but intact toe walking, tandem gait and no problem with postural stability. Reflexes were symmetric, toes were downgoing, and there was a positive glabellar tap. A diagnosis of very mild parkinsonism was made, but symptoms were very mild and not deemed necessary to treat. His evaluation at age 82 revealed slower alternating movements, mild bilateral limb rigidity that had progressed since age 81, and slight worsening of the static/ postural tremor in both hands. Nonetheless, he was able to handle buttons and laces, and had no trouble turning over in bed. By age 83, posture was slightly stooped, gait was mildly unsteady with mild shuffling, slight difficulty with turns but no falls (mild postural instability), speech was lower in volume and more difficult for others to hear, and handwriting was more micrographic. He had full eye movements and no evidence of apraxia.

Magnetic resonance imaging (MRI) of the brain obtained at age 80 and 81 revealed no evidence for infarction or hemosiderin deposits. There was evidence of multiple punctate foci of T2 signal abnormality in the periventricular and subcortical white matter in both cerebral hemispheres, as well as generalized mild cerebral and cerebellar atrophy. At age 77 and again at age 80, an electroencephalogram (EEG) indicated mild slowing but no sharp waves or epileptiform discharges.

Medical History/Family History/ Medications

His past medical history includes a history of melanoma, prostate surgery, kidney stones, and cataract surgery. Family history included memory difficulty in his mother that began in her 80s, and she died at age 92; his father died of a kidney problem at age 69 but had no neurologic problems.

Medications during course of illness included 10 mg of donepezil (initiated at age 80), 10 mg b.i.d. of memantine (initiated at age 83), and 0.5 mg of clonazepam (initiated at age 81, and discontinued at age 83). He was offered levodopa-carbidopa by age 83, but the family opted to avoid it because his extrapyramidal symptoms were mild.

Neurocognitive Evaluations

Four neurocognitive evaluations spanning the course of 5 years are provided in Table 51-2. His initial evaluation revealed difficulty with divided attention, visual perception and visual problem solving with preserved memory and naming. In subsequent years, slowed processing speed and slowed fluency became more evident while his attention and visual perceptual skills worsened. Memory and naming remained relatively preserved, though his list learning was affected by his attention difficulties. At the advanced stage of his disease, he demonstrated an extremely low level of performance on a global measure of functioning (Dementia Rating Scale = 68) and limited ability to manage complex activities of daily living. Nonetheless, his memory for story material and object naming continued to fall within normal limits for his age. With each evaluation, he was aware of his symptoms and his cognitive difficulties and was frustrated by them, but he did not present with signs or symptoms of depression or anxiety.

Clinical Diagnosis

When we saw this patient, it was felt that his difficulties with mechanical tasks, his trouble organizing his day, and his problems handling his medications were significant and interfered with his day-to-day functioning. As such, at his initial evaluation (after 4 years of reported change of function), the cognitive presentation plus his history of probable REM sleep behavior disorder, fluctuations, and mild parkinsonism was sufficient for a diagnosis of probable DLB. Given the preservation of memory at the initial and subsequent neurocognitive evaluations, this was not deemed to represent AD. Initially he had a fairly dramatic improvement to donepezil, which improved his attention and reduced the frequency and intensity of his fluctuations.

Neuropathology Examination and Final Diagnosis

After an estimated duration of illness of 8 years, the patient passed away 1 month after his last neurocognitive evaluation at the age of 85. He underwent brain autopsy, which revealed no

Table 51-2. Longitudinal Neurocognitive Evaluation

	Age at Evaluation (Years)			
	81	82	83	85
Neurocognitive Tests (raw)				
MMSE	28/30	23/30	15/30	10/30
Dementia Rating Scale	132/144	118/144	109/144	68/144
Neurocognitive Tests (age-adjusted scaled scores)[*]				
WRAT-3 reading	104	—	—	—
Digit Span	9	6	5	2
Block Design	5	6	2	2
Picture Completion	6	3	—	—
Rey Complex figure copy	2	2	2	2
Judgment of Line Orientation	6	2	2	2
Stroop Color Word Task (word, color, c/w)	8,2,2	—	5,2,5	2,2,2
Trail-Making A and B	7,2	2,2	2,2	2, 2
Logical Memory I and II	12,13	14,12	10,9	7, 8
Auditory Verbal Learning Task (delayed recall)	12	6 (raw = 8)	6 (raw = 0)	6 (raw = 0)
		(raw = 0)		
Auditory Verbal Learning Task (raw recognition hits, false positives)	12	8 (raw = 14,4)	10 (raw = 11,3)	10 (raw = 12,4)
		(raw = 12,8)		
Letter Fluency	10	8	6	5
Semantic Fluency	7	4	4	4
Boston Naming Test	9	13	9	13

Wechsler Adult Intelligence Scale–III, Wechsler Memory Scale–Revised.

[*]Mayo Older American Normative Sample.

neurofibrillary tangles (NFT) in the cortex and only sparse neurofibrillary tangle pathology in the hippocampus (NFT Braak stage III). The basal nucleus of Meynert had severe neuronal loss with numerous Lewy bodies (alpha-synuclein positive neuronal inclusions) and Lewy neurites (alpha-synuclein positive inclusions in cell processes). Lewy body and Lewy neurite pathology was present in the brain stem regions (including substantia nigra, raphe nucleus, pontomedullary region, and locus ceruleus), limbic, and cortical regions. The substantia nigra exhibited mild neuronal loss and Lewy bodies in the remaining neurons. The hippocampus had normal neuronal population, but there were many dystrophic Lewy neurites in the CA2/3 region and mild Lewy body density in the end-plate. Cortical Lewy body pathology was greatest in the temporal lobe and parahippocampal gyrus, and least in the parietal and occipital lobes. Amyloid plaque pathology was present in the neocortex, but it was predominantly without tau-positive neurites and without an amyloid core indicative of diffuse amyloid deposits often observed in normal aging (Dickson et al., 1992). There was no detectable amyloid angiopathy and only minimal atherosclersis (<25% stenosis) in the large vessels. The final neuropathologic diagnosis was diffuse Lewy body disease.

Discussion

The patient's initial evaluation revealed a pattern of impaired attention and visual spatial/perceptual difficulties with preserved naming and memory. Although his memory for list material worsened over time and after the initial evaluation fell within the impaired range, this may be accounted for by the attentional demands of the task. In contrast, memory for paragraph material showed a decline but remained well preserved over the course of his illness. This pattern of disproportionate attention and visual perceptual deficits in early DLB, with worse naming and memory in AD, has repeatedly been demonstrated across studies (Calderon et al.,

2001; Ferman et al., 2002, 2006; Hamilton et al., 2008; Salmon et al., 1996).

In DLB the visual difficulties are not due solely to problems with executive function or speed. Mori and colleagues (2000) examined this issue eloquently, and they found deficits in elementary visual perception in DLB but not in AD. Also, perceptual deficits may be more severely affected (or at least affected earlier) than spatial localization in DLB, based on greater impairment on the former than the latter (Mosimann et al., 2004). This may be related to the heavier distribution of Lewy bodies in temporal versus parietal regions, though often as the disease progresses, both regions become affected and visual perceptual and spatial difficulties may be apparent.

Memory difficulties, when present in early DLB, tend to be mild and stand in contrast to the pronounced amnestic disturbance of AD (Ferman et al., 1999, 2006; Salmon et al., 1996). Not uncommonly, patients do poorly on list learning, but they may manage fairly well on tasks of story recall. Some patients with DLB may demonstrate evidence of rapid forgetting, especially as the disease progresses. Given that co-occurring Alzheimer pathology is not uncommon in DLB, this may be a contributing factor in some cases.

REM sleep behavior disorder precedes the onset of neurodegenerative disease by many years and often by decades (Boeve et al., 1998). It is more often observed in the synucleinopathies (i.e., LBD, Parkinson disease, Multiple System Atrophy) than in the tauopathies (e.g., AD, frontotemporal dementia) (64% vs. 3%) (Boeve et al., 2003, Boeve, Silber, Ferman, Lucas, & Parisi, 2001). There are two published case reports of idiopathic RBD (without any core features of DLB) who have come to autopsy and results demonstrated brainstem Lewy body pathology (Boeve et al., 2007; Uchiyama et al., 1995). A history of RBD increases the risk of developing a neurodegenerative disease with a 10 year risk of 40.6% (Postuma et al., 2009). RBD with dementia and no parkinsonism or visual hallucinations, was cognitively indistinguishable from DLB matched in dementia severity, and within 6 years, a subset of the RBD/dementia group developed parkinsonism and/or visual hallucinations indicating an eventual conversion to

DLB (Ferman et al., 2002). We followed 8 patients with Mild Cognitive Impairment (MCI) to autopsy which revealed Lewy pathology, and all 8 had early features of attention and/or visuoperceptual difficulties and 7 had RBD (Molano et al., 2010). Others have shown that patients with RBD without dementia performed significantly more poorly on attention and/or visual construction tasks (Terzaghi et al., 2008, Gagnon et al., 2009, Ferini-Strambi et al., 2004), and RBD is associated with worse cognitive performance in patients with PD who do not have dementia (Vendette et al., 2007). These results indicate that RBD with dementia may be the very earliest stage of DLB.

The extrapyramidal signs in our patient remained relatively mild throughout the course of his illness. Some patients with DLB have rather prominent parkinsonism but others do not have this feature. Indeed, 25% of our autopsy-confirmed cases of DLB do not have clinical parkinsonism (despite nigral Lewy body pathology). Thus, even if the parkinsonism is mild or absent, it is still important to consider DLB as a clinical diagnosis.

Our patient's family was extremely conservative in their use of medications, and they never tried levodopa-carbidopa (L-dopa). Overall, patients with DLB tend to have their parkinsonism suboptimally treated due to largely inadvertent concerns of worsening cognitive or behavioral function. Although dopamine agonists do exacerbate DLB symptoms, L-dopa is well tolerated, with beneficial effect on motor function (Bonelli et al., 2004) and no reported adverse cognitive, neuropsychiatric or sleep effects (Molloy et al., 2006, Molloy et al., 2009).

Distinguishing DLB from AD has implications from a treatment standpoint, and one goal of proper diagnosis is to help avoid iatrogensis. For example, medications with dopamine D2 receptor antagonism (e.g., traditional neuroleptics and some atypical neuroleptics) can precipitate or exacerbate extrapyramidal signs leading to varying degrees of neuroleptic sensitivity (McKeith et al., 1992, Piggott et al., 1998). In addition, DLB has been associated with profound cholinergic neuronal loss and severe depletion of choline acetyltransferase levels early in the disease course, whereas AD and normal controls often show little drop in such levels until the advanced stages of dementia (Davis et al., 1999; Perry et al., 1993; Perry et al., 1994; Tiraboschi et al., 2002). Exposure to medications with anticholinergic properties often worsens cognitive and neuropsychiatric symptoms in patients, and it is important to consider dose-response effects, and medications that would not traditionally be considered anticholinergic (Chew et al., 2008). On the other hand, proper diagnosis may provide earlier exposure to beneficial treatment. Cholinesterase inhibitors have been associated with improvement in cognition and a reduction in intensity of psychiatric symptoms, sometimes dramatically in DLB (McKeith et al., 2000). The patient presented in this report benefitted tremendously from a cholinesterase inhibitor early on, and he was maintained on it throughout the course of his illness. His neuropathologic findings are consistent with diffuse Lewy body disease and a low NFT Braak stage. Lewy bodies and Lewy neurites were documented, and the latter has shown to be more resilient to macrophages following neuronal loss and may be better markers (due to prolonged presence) as opposed to Lewy bodies.

The patient came to our clinic for a second opinion after receiving a full workup from another center and a diagnosis of AD. The family reported that the diagnosis of DLB seemed to "fit" him better. Early detection and differential diagnosis of DLB from AD is important for the provision of education and support for the family. It helps to demystify some of the challenging behaviors and may help with better overall care and improved understanding of how to manage the symptoms, medically and behaviorally.

Acknowledgments

The neuropathology examination was performed and interpreted by Dennis W. Dickson, MD. Supported by National Institutes of Health grant R01 – AG15866 and P50 AG16574. Cognitive test administration and scoring was carried out by Sonya Prescott, BS.

References

Ballard, C., Walker, M., O'Brien, J., Rowan, E., & McKeith, I. (2001). The characterization and impact of "fluctuating" cognition in dementia with Lewy bodies and Alzheimer's disease. *International Journal of Geriatric Psychiatry, 16*, 494–498.

Boeve, B. F., Dickson, D. W., Olson, E. J., Shepard, J. W., Silber, M. H., Ferman, T. J., et al. (2007). Insights into REM sleep behavior disorder pathophysiology in brainstem-predominant Lewy body disease. *Sleep Medicine, 8*, 60–64.

Boeve, B. F., Silber, M. H., Ferman, T. J., Kokmen, E., Smith, G. E., Ivnik, R. J., et al. (1998). REM sleep behavior disorder and degenerative dementia: An association likely reflecting Lewy body disease. *Neurology, 51*, 363–370.

Boeve, B. F., Silber, M. H., Ferman, T. J., Lucas, J. A., & Parisi, J. E. (2001). Association of REM sleep behavior disorder and neurodegenerative disease may reflect an underlying synucleinopathy. *Movement Disorders, 16*, 622–630.

Boeve, B. F., Silber, M. H., Parisi, J. E., Dickson, D. W., Ferman, T. J., Benarroch, E. E., et al. (2003). Synucleinopathy, pathology and REM sleep behavior disorder plus dementia or parkinsonism. *Neurology, 61*, 40–45.

Bonelli, S.B., Ransmayr, G., Steffelbauer, M., Lukas, T., Lampl, C., Deibl, M. (2004). L-Dopa responsiveness in dementia with Lewy bodies, Parkinson disease with and without dementia. *Neurology, 63*, 376–378.

Calderon, J., Perry, R. J., Erzinclioglu, S. W., Berrios, G. E., Dening, T. R., & Hodges, J. R. (2001). Perception, attention and working memory are disproportionately impaired in dementia with Lewy bodies compared with Alzheimer's disease. *Journal of Neurology, Neurosurgery and Psychiatry, 70*, 157–164.

Chew, M.L., Mulsant, B.H., Pollock, B.G., Lehman, M.E., Greenspan, A., Mahmoud, R.A., Kirshner, M.A., Sorisio, D.A., Bies, R.R., Gharabawi, G. (2008). Anticholinergic activity of 107 medications commonly used by older adults. *Journal of the American Geriatrics Society, 56*, 1333–1341.

Davis, K. L., Mohs, R. C., Marin, D., Purohit, D. P., Perl, D. M., Lantz, M., et al. (1999). Cholinergic markers in elderly patients with early signs of Alzheimer disease. *Journal of the American Medical Association, 281*, 1401–1406.

Dickson, D. W., Crystal, H. A., Mattiace, L. A., Masur, D. M., Blau, A. D., Davies, P., et al. (1992). Identification of normal and pathological aging in prospectively studied nondemented elderly humans. *Neurobiology of Aging, 13*, 179–189.

Dickson, D.W., Feany, M.B., Yen, S.H., Mattiace, L.A., Davies, P. (1996). Cytoskeletal pathology in non-Alzheimer degenerative dementia: new lesions in diffuse Lewy body disease, Pick's disease and corticobasal degeneration. *Journal of of Neural Transmission, 47*, 31–46.

Ferman, T. J., Boeve, B. F., Smith, G. E., Silber, M. H., Kokmen, E., Petersen, R. C., & Ivnik, R. J. (1999). REM sleep behavior disorder and dementia: Cognitive differences when compared to Alzheimer's disease. *Neurology, 52,* 951–957.

Ferman, T.J,, Dickson D.W,, Graff-Radford, N., Arvanitakis, Z., DeLucia, M.W., Boeve, B.F., Parfitt, F., Duara, R., Barker, W., Waters, C., Jimison, P.G., Brassler, S.J. (2003) Early onset of visual hallucinations in dementia distinguishes pathologically-confirmed Lewy body disease from AD. *Neurology, 60,* A264.

Ferman, T. J., Boeve, B. F., Smith, G. E., Silber, M. H., Lucas, J. A., Graff-Radford, N. R., et al. (2002). Dementia with Lewy bodies may present as dementia and REM sleep behavior disorder without parkinsonism or hallucinations. *Journal of the International Neuropsychological Society, 8,* 907–914.

Ferman, T. J., Smith, G. E., Boeve, B. F., Graff-Radford, N. R., Lucas, J. A., Knopman, D. S., et al. (2006). Neuropsychological differentiation of dementia with Lewy bodies from normal aging and Alzheimer's disease. *The Clinical Neuropsychologist, 20,* 623–636.

Ferman, T. J., Smith, G. E., Boeve, B. F., Ivnik, R. J., Petersen, R. C., Knopmann, D., et al. (2004). DLB fluctuations: Specific features that reliably differentiate DLB from AD and normal aging. *Neurology, 62,* 181–187.

Ferini-Strambi, L., Gioia, D., Castropnovo, V., Oldani, A., Zucconi,M., Cappa, S.F. (2004). Neuropsychological asessment in idiopathic REM sleep behavior disorder (RBD). Does the idiopathic form of RBD really exist? *Neurology, 62,* 41–45.

Gagnon, J.F., Vendette, M., Postuma, R.B., Desjardins, C., Massicotte-Marquez, J., Panisset, M., Montplaisir, J. (2009). Mild cognitive impairment in rapid eye movement sleep behavior disorder and Parkinson's disease. *Annals of Neurology, 66,* 39–47.

Hamilton, J., Salmon, D., Galasko, D., Raman, R., Emond, J., Hansen, L. A., et al. (2008). Visuospatial deficits predict rate of cognitive decline in autopsy-verified dementia with Lewy bodies. Neuropsychology, 22, 729–737.

Hope, T., Keene, J., Fairburn, C. G., Jacoby, R., & McShane, R. (1999). Natural history of behavioral changes and psychiatric symptoms in Alzheimer's disease. A longitudinal study. *British Journal of Psychiatry, 174,* 39–44.

Kaufer, D. I. (2002). Pharmacologic therapy of dementia with Lewy bodies. *Journal Geriatric Psychiatry and Neurology, 15,* 224–232.

McKeith, I., Del Ser, T., Spano, P., Emre, M., Wesnes, K., Anand, R., et al. (2000). Efficacy of rivastigmine in dementia with Lewy bodies: A randomized, double-blind, placebo-controlled international study. *Lancet, 356,* 2031–2036.

McKeith, I. G., Dickson, D. W., Lowe, J., Emre, M., O'Brien, J. T., Feldman, H., et al. (2005). Diagnosis and management of dementia with Lewy bodies: Third report of the DLB consortium. *Neurology, 65,* 1863–1872.

McKeith, I., Fairbairn, A., Perry, R., Thompson, P., & Perry E. (1992). Neuroleptic sensitivity in patients with senile dementia of Lewy body type. *British Medical Journal, 205,* 673–678.

Molano, J., Boeve, B., Ferman, T., Smith, G., Parisi, J., Dickson, D., Knopman, D., Graff-Radford, N., Geda, Y., Lucas, J., Kantarci, K., Shiung, M., Jack, C., Silber, M., Pankratz, V.S., Petersen, R.. (2010). Mild cognitive impairment associated with limbic and neocortical lewy body disease: a clinicopathological study. *Brain, 133,* 540–56.

Molloy, S., Minett, T., O'Brien, J.T., McKeith, I.G., Burn, D.J. (2009). Levodopa use and sleep in patients with dementia with Lewy bodies. *Movement Disorders, 24,* 609–612.

Molloy, S.A., Rowan, E.N., O'Brien, J.T., McKeith, I.G., Wesnes, K., Burn, D.J. (2006). Effect of levodopa on cognitive function in Parkinson's disease with and without dementia and dementia with Lewy bodies. *Journal of Neurology, Neurosurgery and Psychiatry, 77,* 1323–1328.

Mori, E., Shimomura, T., Fujimori, M., Nobutsugu, H., Toru, I., Mamoru, H., et al. (2000). Visuoperceptual impairment in dementia with Lewy bodies. *Archives of Neurology, 57,* 489–493.

Mosimann, U. P., Mather, G., Wesnes, K. A., O'Brien, J. T., Burn, D. J., & McKeith, I. G. (2004). Visual perception in Parkinson disease dementia and dementia with Lewy bodies. *Neurology, 63,* 2091–2096.

Perry, E. K., Haroutunian, V., Davis, K. L., Levy, R., Lantos, P., Eagger, S., et al. (1994). Neocortical cholinergic activities differentiate Lewy body dementia from classical Alzheimer's disease. *Neuroreport, 5,* 747–749.

Perry, E. K., Irving, D., Kerwin, J. M., McKeith, I. G., Thompson, P., Collerton, D., et al. (1993). Cholinergic transmitter and neurotrophic activities in Lewy body dementia: Similarity to Parkinson's and distinction from Alzheimer disease. *Alzheimer Disease and Associated Disorders, 7,* 69–79.

Perry, E., Marshall, E., Perry, R., Irving, D., Smith, C. J., Blessed, G., & Fairbairn, A. F. (1990). Cholinergic and dopaminergic activities in senile dementia of the Lewy body type. *Alzheimer Disease and Associated Disorders, 4,* 87–95.

Piggott, M. A., Perry, E. K., Marshall, E. F., McKeith, I. G., Johnson, M., Melrose, H. L., et al. (1998).

Nigrostriatal dopaminergic activities in dementia with Lewy bodies in relation to neuroleptic sensitivity: Comparisons with Parkinson's disease. *Biological Psychiatry, 44,* 765–774.

Postuma, R. B., Gagnon, J. F., Vendette, M., Fantini, M., Massicotte-Marquez, J., & Montplasir, J. (2009). Quantifying the risk of neurodegenerative disease in idiopathic REM sleep behavior disorder. *Neurology, 72,* 1296–1300.

Rockwell, E., Choure, J., Galasko, D., Olichney, J., & Jeste, D. V. (2000). Psychopathology at initial diagnosis in dementia with Lewy bodies versus Alzheimer's disease: Comparison of matched groups with autopsy-confirmed diagnoses. *International Journal of Geriatric Psychiatry, 15,* 819–823.

Salmon, D. P., Galasko, D., Hansen, L. A., Masliah, E., Butters, N., Thal, L. J., et al. (1996). Neuropsychological deficits associated with diffuse Lewy body disease. *Brain and Cognition, 31,* 148–65.

Terzaghi, M., Sinforiani, E., Zuccella, C., Zambrelli, E., Pasotti, C., Rustioni, V., & Raffaele M. (2008). Cognitive performance in REM sleep behavior disorder as a possible early marker of neurodegenerative disease. *Sleep Medicine, 9,* 341–342.

Tiraboschi, P., Hansen, L. A., Alford, M., Merdes, A., Masliah, E., Thal, L. J., & Corey-Bloom, J. (2002). Early and widespread cholinergic losses differentiate dementia with Lewy bodies from Alzheimer disease. *Archives of General Psychiatry, 59,* 946–951.

Uchiyama, M., Isse, K., Tanaka, K., Yokota, N., Hamamoto, M., Aida, S., et al. (1995). Incidental Lewy body disease in a patient with REM sleep behavior disorder. *Neurology, 45,* 709–712.

Vendette, M., Gagnon, J. B., Decary, A., Massicotte-Marquez, J., Postuma, R. B., Doyon, J., et al. (2007). REM sleep behavior disorder predicts cognitive impairment in Parkinson's disease without dementia. *Neurology, 69,* 1843–1849.

Walker, M. P., Ayre, G. A., Perry, E. K., Wesnes, K., McKeith, I. G., Tovee, M., et al. (2000). Quantification and characterization of fluctuating cognition in dementia with Lewy bodies and Alzheimer's disease. *Dementia and Geriatric Cognitive Disorders, 11,* 327–35.

52

A Case of Corticobasal Syndrome

John A. Lucas

Corticobasal degeneration (CBD) is a neurodegenerative disease characterized by progressive asymmetric rigidity and apraxia. First described in 1967 by Rebeiz and colleagues, the early descriptions of CBD focused primarily on the neurologic manifestations of the disorder. Initial studies suggested that "mental faculties" in CBD patients were relatively well preserved, although some patients developed dementia late in the course of the disease (Rebeiz et al., 1967; Riley, Lang & Lewis, 1990; Rinne, Lee, Thompson, & Martin, 1994). Over the past decade, however, there has been increased recognition of the cognitive and behavioral manifestations of CBD (Kertesz, Martinez-Lage, Davidson, & Munoz, 2000; Graham, Bak, & Hodges, 2003; Boeve, 2005; McMonagle, Blair, & Kertesz, 2006). Specifically, recent studies have demonstrated the onset of cognitive difficulties early in the disease course, with a subset of patients demonstrating measurable cognitive changes prior to the onset of motor symptoms.

Corticobasal degeneration is a rare disorder. The exact prevalence and incidence rates are unknown, but the estimated incidence ranges from 0.02 to 0.92 per 100,000 per year. Incidence estimates of corticobasal syndrome (described later) are higher and range from 4.9 to 7.3 per 100,000 per year (Togasaki & Tanner, 2000). Corticobasal degeneration is reportedly more prevalent in women. Disease onset is most often seen in patients from age 60 to 80 years, although autopsy-confirmed CBD has been seen in patients as young as age 45. Medications do not appear to alter the neurodegenerative process, and the disease typically progresses to death within 6–9 years of diagnosis.

Differential diagnosis of CBD in clinical settings is challenging because the disease shares pathology and phenotypic expression with other closely related disorders, including progressive supranuclear palsy (PSP) and frontotemporal dementia (FTD) (Boeve, Lang, & Litvan, 2003). Corticobasal degeneration and PSP are both akinetic-rigid syndromes in the Parkinson spectrum and both can present with cognitive symptoms of progressive aphasia and/or executive dysfunction similar to the clinical presentation of FTD. Patients with CBD may also develop features of posterior cortical atrophy (PCA). Moreover, patients without movement disorder who initially present with signs of nonfluent aphasia, FTD, or PCA may subsequently develop CBD symptoms. Postmortem studies confirm that patients diagnosed with CBD based on clinical presentation during life commonly show a wide range of etiologies, including PSP, frontotemporal lobar degeneration, Pick disease, Creutzfeldt-Jakob disease, Alzheimer disease (AD), motor neuron disease inclusion dementia, neurofilament inclusion body disease, and nonspecific neurodegeneration (Dickson et al., 2002).

Given that the clinical phenotype of CBD is not disease specific, some have suggested that the diagnosis of corticobasal *syndrome* (CBS) be used to describe patients who demonstrate the characteristic clinical constellation of CBD symptoms during life, and that the diagnosis of

"CBD" be reserved for neuropathologically confirmed cases. This convention will be used in the case study presented here.

Neurologic Symptoms

The neurologic presentation of patients with CBS is strikingly asymmetric. Early in the disorder, patients may present with asymmetric limb rigidity and bradykinesia reminiscent of idiopathic Parkinson disease. Lack of responsiveness to levodopa and presence of additional cortical symptoms, however, typically lead to reconsideration of the diagnosis.

A hallmark feature of CBS is the presence of unilateral ideomotor limb apraxia. Limb kinetic apraxia, ideational apraxia, and buccofacial apraxia may be present in addition to ideomotor apraxia, but they are less commonly seen. In some cases, patients may develop an "alien limb syndrome," with the affected limb performing involuntary, often semi-purposeful, movements either in addition to or instead of a planned or willed movement. The patient is usually aware of the movement but is unable to control it. Patients may complain that their arm and/or leg "misbehaves," fails to do what is intended, or feels as if it belongs to someone else.

Other common motor features include limb myoclonus, asymmetric postural limb tremor, limb dystonia, dysphagia, and dysarthria (Boeve, 2005). Vertical gaze difficulty, severe postural instability, backward falls, cerebellar signs, and features of dysautonomia are not typically seen in CBS and may help differentiate the disorder from other akinetic-rigid syndromes such as PSP and multiple system atrophy (MSA).

Tactile perception of light touch and pinprick sensation remains intact in CBS, but evidence of cortical sensory loss is typically present. Formal examination typically reveals unilateral extinctions to double simultaneous stimulation and evidence of dysgraphesthesia and astereognosis.

Neuroradiologic Features and Gross Pathology

On magnetic resonance imaging (MRI), patients with autopsy-proven CBD typically demonstrate: (1) atrophy of the posterior frontal cortex, superior parietal cortex, and middle portion of the corpus callosum on T1-weighted images, (2) hypointense signal changes in the putamen on T1-weighted images, and (3) hyperintense signal changes in the motor cortex or subcortical white matter on T2-weighted images (Josephs et al., 2004). Asymmetric findings may be observed with greater atrophy contralateral to the affected limb, but this is not always the case. When compared to PSP patients, MRI findings in CBD patients reveal greater cortical atrophy and less subcortical involvement (Josephs et al., 2008).

Asymmetric hypoperfusion and hypometabolism involving frontoparietal cortices (with or without basal ganglia involvement) have been reported on single-photon emission computed tomography (SPECT) and positron emission tomography (PET), respectively (Eckert et al., 2005; Koyama et al., 2007); however, these findings are not considered sufficiently sensitive or specific to CBD.

Upon postmortem examination, gross pathology shows narrowing of cortical gyri, most notable in the superior frontal and superior parietal cortices (Dickson et al., 2002). Temporal and occipital lobes are relatively spared in cases where there were no clinical signs of dementia or aphasia. Patients with significant cognitive and language symptoms, however, often demonstrate additional involvement of inferior frontal and temporal lobes on autopsy. Additional findings on gross pathology may include volume loss of the cerebral white matter in the affected areas, thinning of the corpus callosum, and attenuation of the anterior limb of the internal capsule. There may be flattening of the head of the caudate; the thalamus may appear smaller than usual. The substantia nigra virtually always shows significant pigmentation loss. The pons and medulla remain relatively well preserved on gross inspection.

Histopathology

Swollen "achromatic" or "ballooned" neurons are important histopathological markers of CBD and are commonly found in the superior frontal and parietal cortices. Tau immunostaining reveals a range of neuronal lesions in CBD, including (a) neurofibrillary lesions (i.e., "corticobasal bodies") in the locus ceruleus and substantia nigra, (b) glial thread-like processes in the neuropil of affected gray and white matter, *(c)* argyrophilic inclusions (i.e., "coiled bodies") in oligodendroglia, and *(d)* neocortical astrocytic plaques with a distinct annular array of tau-immunoreactive processes (Dickson et al., 2002).

Cognitive and Neurobehavioral Features

The constellation of cognitive symptoms typically observed in patients presenting with CBS is largely consistent with the known distribution of cortical and subcortical neuropathology. Handwriting, drawing, copying, and other visuospatial construction abilities are typically compromised due in part to apraxia. It is also common, however, for patients to demonstrate impairment on visuospatial tasks that have no significant motor demands (Graham, et al., 2003).

As with most parkinsonian disorders, frontal-executive dysfunction is typically observed on formal neuropsychological evaluation. Studies demonstrate impaired performances on measures such as the Wisconsin Card Sorting Test, Trails B, Stroop Interference, and verbal fluency tasks (Pillon et al., 1995; Van Voorst et al., 2008). The frontal deficit in CBS, however, is typically not as severe as that seen in PSP.

Patients with corticobasal syndrome may initially present with anomia and progressive non-fluent aphasia, including slow speech rate, prolonged intervals between syllables and words, decreased articulatory accuracy, phonological substitutions, agrammatism, and/or telegraphic language output (McMonagle et al, 2006). A recent study by Murray and colleagues (2007) reported that nearly one-half of autopsy-proven CBD patients demonstrated effortful speech upon initial examination and one-third demonstrated evidence of word-finding problems on formal testing. Nearly 90% of all patients in this series developed signs of anomia and nonfluent aphasia during the subsequent course of illness.

Patients with CBS may also demonstrate progressive spelling impairments that are unrelated to handwriting difficulty. Early in the disease, spelling errors tend to be phonologically plausible, whereas later in the illness errors are more likely to be phonologically implausible (Graham et al., 2003). There are also several reports in the literature regarding the presence of calculation deficits. In a series of autopsy-proven CBD cases, approximately one-fourth of patients presented with acalculia at the time of diagnosis (Murray et al., 2007). Those without initial difficulty, however, did not go on to develop calculation problems later in the illness.

Basic attention span and episodic memory remain relatively well preserved in CBS. When memory deficits are observed, they are typically seen later in the disease process and are generally mild in comparison to those of patients with AD. The nature of memory problems in CBS appears to reflect poor use of strategic processes during encoding and retrieval, and thus tend to be more suggestive of frontal-subcortical system involvement rather than medial temporal lobe dysfunction (Graham et al., 2003).

Depression, apathy, irritability, and agitation are common features of CBS. A recent archival study of patients with pathologically confirmed CBD found evidence of three distinct neurobehavioral syndromes, including depression, obsessive-compulsive behaviors, and a frontal-type behavioral disorder characterized by impulsivity and disinhibition (Geda et al., 2007). Visual hallucinations were not present in any of the patients studied and can help differentiate CBS from Lewy body dementia, where visual hallucinations are common.

The Case of D. L.

A 58-year-old, right handed, white female with 12 years of formal education was referred by her primary care physician to evaluate complaints of memory and expressive language difficulties. The patient and her husband had been noticing a mild progression of these difficulties for 2 years. Her words would often "come out wrong," either in a stutter or with incorrect pronunciation. Although initially infrequent and limited to long or low-frequency words, by the time she presented for evaluation the problem was occurring more often and affecting more common words. She also reported feeling less attentive and less able to remember things that people told her.

In the year following the onset of her cognitive symptoms, the patient also began to notice the gradual onset of motor difficulties. She complained of occasional lack of control of the right hand, stating that it would "misbehave" and do something other than what she intended it to do. Her handwriting had also become progressively slower and less fluid. By the time she presented for evaluation, she had begun to use her left hand for tasks that she would have normally performed with her right hand. She felt slower and less steady in her gait, but had not suffered any falls. She reported no tremor, urinary incontinence, or visual hallucinations at the time of the evaluation.

With regard to activities of daily living, the patient reported giving up some of her responsibilities in managing the household finances because of difficulty writing checks and performing math calculations. She was managing her medications independently and driving without significant difficulty, although her husband had noticed some slowing in her reaction time.

Appetite was unchanged and she reported normal nighttime sleep, with no evidence of apneic episodes, dream enactment behavior, or abnormal movements during sleep. She reported having good energy in the morning, but she would typically become fatigued as the day progressed. Her symptoms worsened in parallel with increased fatigue, but there were otherwise no reported fluctuations in her cognitive abilities.

She reported being in good spirits at the time of the assessment, but her husband noted a 1–2 year history of increased apathy. He stated that the patient had once been "the life of the party" but was no longer initiating conversation or activities. Although she would interact with others at their initiation, she no longer seemed motivated to seek out interpersonal contact.

The patient's past medical history included hypertension and high cholesterol, both of which were well controlled. Medications included Plavix and Lipitor. Family history was negative for dementia, movement disorder, or vascular disease.

Prior to her neuropsychological assessment, the patient was evaluated by a staff neurologist who found evidence of mild, largely asymmetric motor and sensory deficits in the right upper extremity, including limb rigidity, bradykinesia, action myoclonus, agraphesthesia, astereognosis, and extinctions to double simultaneous stimulation. No resting tremor, gross muscle weakness, axial rigidity, postural instability, or gaze abnormality was noted. The radiologist read

the MRI as unremarkable; however, the neurologist noted evidence of left greater than right posterior frontal lobe atrophy.

On the day of her neuropsychological evaluation, the patient presented as a neatly dressed, well groomed, alert, and fully oriented woman who appeared her stated age. Verbal output during conversation was mildly slow and hesitant, with occasional imprecision in articulation (e.g., "fish" for "fist"). Casual gait revealed reduced arm swing on the right, with the arm held extended at the elbow. Mild lack of coordination was observed in the right hand during writing, drawing, and manual tasks and at times she would switch to using her left hand. Response times were slow. Vision and hearing appeared adequate to perceive test stimuli. She was pleasant throughout the session and did not appear concerned by cognitive or motor difficulties. She appeared to put forth adequate effort and results were considered valid estimates of her current cognitive status.

Examination Results

General intellectual functioning was low average for the patient's age, as measured by the third edition of the Wechsler Adult Intelligence Scale (WAIS-III; Table 52-1). Verbal intellectual ability was average for her age and consistent with premorbid estimates based on demographic variables and word reading skill. Nonverbal intellectual ability was impaired and represents a cognitive weakness, with the magnitude of the observed 19-point discrepancy between VIQ and PIQ being found in less than 10% of the WAIS-III standardization sample. Examination of WAIS-III factor scores revealed average verbal knowledge, low-average working memory, borderline perceptual organization ability, and impaired processing speed.

The remainder of the neuropsychological test results are presented in Table 52-2. On language assessment, the patient was able to follow single and multiple-step auditory verbal commands accurately on the Token Test. Expressive vocabulary was average on the WAIS-III. Mild slurring, hesitancy, and phonemic substitutions were observed on repetition of multisyllabic words and longer sentences from the Boston Diagnostic Aphasia Examination (BDAE-3). Performance on

Table 52-1. Premorbid and Intellectual Functioning

Wechsler Test of Adult Reading (WTAR)		
Standard Score	95	
Demographics-Predicted Score	99	
Estimated VIQ	96	
WAIS-III		
VIQ = 91	**VC** = 94	
PIQ = 72	**PO** = 78	
FSIQ = 80	**WM** = 88	
	PS = 69	
	Raw	Age SS
Vocabulary	35	9
Similarities	16	8
Arithmetic	8	6
Digit Span	18	11
Information	16	10
Letter-Number Sequencing	7	7
Picture Comp	16	8
Digit Symbol	14	3
Block Design	13	5
Matrix Reasoning	5	6
Symbol Search	12	5

the Boston Naming Test was low average for her age and education (51/60), with seven additional correct responses produced when phonemic cues were provided. Occasional phonological substitution/transposition errors were noted in her BNT responses (e.g., "agraspagrus" for *asparagus*, "ornicron" for *unicorn*). On both repetition and naming tasks, the patient would readily recognize when she was making errors and she would spontaneously attempt to correct them. Generative naming to phonological cues and semantic categories was impaired.

She demonstrated low-average performance on the WAIS-III Picture Completion subtest and mild difficulty judging the spatial orientation of lines. Clock drawing was intact, both to command and copy. Her copy of a complex figure, however, was impaired, with evidence of poor organization and mild spatial distortion.

Cognitive processing speed was variable. Speeded word reading and color naming on the Color-Word Interference subtest of the Delis-Kaplan Executive Function Scales (D-KEFS) were within normal limits, whereas speeded word generation on verbal fluency tasks was impaired. Performances on WAIS-III Symbol Search and

Digit Symbol subtests were impaired. On the D-KEFS Trail-Making subtest, visuomotor sequencing speed fell in the low-average to mildly impaired range.

Auditory-verbal attention span was average. Her ability to mentally arrange sequences of numbers and letters was low average. In contrast, she demonstrated impairment on measures of mental calculation, divided attention (D-KEFS Trail Making Condition 4), and inhibition of a prepotent response (D-KEFS Color-Word Interference Condition 3).

She demonstrated mild learning inefficiency on the California Verbal Learning Test (CVLT-II). She freely recalled 8/16 words following a 20-minute delay, which was also mildly impaired, but reflected relatively intact retention as compared to her performance on the final learning trial (9/16) and her short-delayed free recall (8/16). On recognition testing, she correctly identified 11/16 target words, with no false-positive errors. Immediate and delayed memory for Logical Memory stories and Visual Reproduction figures on the Wechsler Memory Scale (WMS-III) were average for her age, with above-average retention over time.

Table 52-2. Neuropsychological Test Data

	Raw	Percentile
Token Test	44/44	75
Boston Naming Test	51/60	18
COWAT	20	5
Semantic Fluency	29	9
Judgment of Line Orientation	15/30	4
Clock Drawing		wnl
Rey-Osterreith copy	22/36	1
DKEFS Trail Making		
Condition 1	33	9
Condition 2	60	9
Condition 3	55	16
Condition 4	164	2
Condition 5	51	16
DKEFS Color-Word Interf.		
Condition 1	35	16
Condition 2	25	37
Condition 3	80	9
Condition 4	119	1
Wisconsin Card Sorting		
Perseverative Responses	12	55
Categories = 4	4	11–16
Set Losses = 4	4	≤1
Frontal Assessment Battery		
Similarities	3/3	N/A
Lexical Fluency	1/3	N/A
Motor Series Programming	1/3	N/A
Conflicting Instructions	3/3	N/A
Go-No-Go	3/3	N/A
Environmental Control	3/3	N/A
Total	14/18	N/A
Wechsler Memory Scale		
Logical Memory I	37	50
Logical Memory II	22	63
Percent Retention	85	75
Visual Reproduction I	76	37
Visual Reproduction II	63	75
Percent Retention	83	84
CVLT–2		
Trial 1–5	37	8
Short Delay Free	8	16
Short Delay Cued	8	7
Long Delay Free	8	7
Long Delay Cued	8	7
Recognition Hits	11	1
False Positives	0	16
BDI–2	3	

Verbal abstract reasoning on WAIS-III Similarities was low average for her age. Nonverbal conceptualization as measured by WAIS-III Matrix Reasoning was mildly impaired. She scored in the borderline range on the Frontal Assessment Battery, with points lost for reduced lexical fluency and difficulty acquiring Luria's 3-step hand sequence. She demonstrated difficulty maintaining cognitive set on the Wisconsin Card Sorting test.

The patient denied clinically significant symptoms of depression, obtaining a score of 3 on the Beck Depression Inventory (BDI-II).

Discussion

Results of this neuropsychological examination reveal a pattern of cognitive deficits that are largely consistent with subcortical and frontal system dysfunction. Namely, there is evidence of psychomotor slowing, retrieval difficulties on naming and list-learning tasks, and executive deficits on D-KEFS subtests, Wisconsin Card Sorting Test, and Rey-Osterrieth copy (i.e., poor organization). Behaviorally, the patient's husband reported reduced spontaneity and initiation, and the patient did not appear distressed by her problems during the test session, suggesting some degree of anosognosia.

In addition to her frontal-subcortical deficits, the patient also demonstrates language expression difficulties, both during conversation and on repetition and naming tasks. The quality of her impairments suggests a mild apraxia of speech and/or progressive nonfluent aphasia.

The patient's cognitive dysfunction was of insidious onset and progressed gradually for 2 years prior to her neuropsychological evaluation, and she developed an asymmetric extrapyramidal and cortical sensory disorder over this period of time. Taken together, the patient's clinical presentation, neurologic exam, neuroimaging results, and frontal-subcortical features of the neuropsychological profile suggest a neurodegenerative disorder in the Parkinson spectrum. The constellation of symptoms and the report of speech/language disturbance as an initial feature are consistent with a clinical diagnosis of CBS. The diagnosis would be further supported if the patient proves unresponsive to a trial of levodopa.

With regard to other Parkinson-spectrum disorders outside the corticobasal syndrome, the absence of hallucinations, fluctuating alertness, REM-sleep behavior disorder, or characteristic visual spatial impairments on neuropsychological testing argues against a diagnosis of Lewy body dementia. Likewise, the absence of prominent cerebellar or autonomic symptoms lowers the likelihood of MSA. Patients with frontotemporal dementia with parkinsonism associated with mutation on chromosome 17 (FTDP-17) may present with apathy and (less commonly) signs of dystonia such as demonstrated by this patient; however, the hallmark behavioral change of marked disinhibition is not present. Moreover, the absence of FTD-type dementia and/or parkinsonism in the patient's first-degree relatives effectively rules out this hereditary disease.

Given the clinical features of this case, it is tempting to go beyond the "CBS" nomenclature and consider a more specific diagnosis of "CBD." With the extrapyramidal signs being asymmetric rather than symmetric and the absence of vertical supranuclear gaze palsy or backward falls, one might feel confident in ruling out PSP as an etiology. Similarly, the patient's parkinsonism, intact memory retention, and absence of muscle wasting may be considered sufficient evidence to rule out disorders such as frontotemporal lobar degeneration, Alzheimer disease, and motor neuron disease, respectively. As noted earlier, however, there is significant neuropathologic heterogeneity underlying the classic "CBD" phenotype, resulting in poor positive predictive value for underlying CBD pathology when the diagnosis is based on clinical presentation alone. As such, we cannot confidently rule out PSP or other disorders within the CBS spectrum, as any number of pathologies may ultimately be identified upon postmortem examination.

Beyond diagnostic decision making, the neuropsychological assessment provides valuable information for the practical management of the patient's symptoms. The patient's slowing and executive dysfunction suggest that driving safety may be compromised. If she is reluctant to voluntarily abstain from driving, an objective driving evaluation would be recommended through a local rehabilitation facility or department of motor vehicles office.

With regard to medication management, she should be supervised to ensure that she is taking her medications in accordance with her prescribed regimen. She may also benefit from changes in her medication from pills to elixirs if she develops swallowing difficulty as her disease progresses.

Referral for evaluation by a speech and language therapist may help attenuate the patient's deteriorating communication skills. Recent studies of patients with progressive nonfluent aphasia suggest that speech and language therapies may provide some protective benefit and slow the progression of anomia over time. Treatment efforts are most beneficial early in the disease, when semantic knowledge and episodic memory are relatively well preserved and can support new learning. As the disease progresses, speech and language therapies may be implemented to teach the patient alternate means of functional communication (e.g., augmentative communication devices, functional communication boards).

The need for positive supportive measures should also be evaluated. Assessment of the home environment, evaluation of physical and occupational therapy needs, benefits of exercise programs, and other measures to optimize the patient's level of functioning should be explored through appropriate referrals.

Given the relatively poor prognosis associated with a diagnosis of CBS, counseling is recommended for the patient's family and care providers. The patient's apathy and possible anosognosia, as reported by her husband and observed during the neuropsychological assessment, can be beneficial to her, but her husband and family will likely need help adjusting to and coping with the diagnosis. Education regarding the cognitive and behavioral changes associated with the patient's clinical syndrome, as well as discussion of effective strategies for managing these changes will be essential in helping the patient and her family. Referral for practical education for managing physical changes associated with disease progression would also be helpful. Information about national support organizations (Association for Frontotemporal Dementias, Worldwide Education and Awareness for Movement Disorders, etc.) and local caregiver support groups should be provided.

Finally, repeating the neuropsychological studies annually can help gauge the momentum of disease progression over time, revisit functional recommendations, and guide decisions regarding the level of care required by the patient.

References

Boeve, B., Lang, A., & Litvan, I. (2003). Corticobasal degeneration and its relationship to progressive supranuclear palsy and frontotemporal dementia. *Annals of Neurology, 54*, S15–S19.

Boeve, B. (2005). Corticobasal degeneration: The syndrome and the disease. In I. Litvan (Ed.), *Atypical Parkinsonian disorders* (pp. 309–334). Totawa, NJ: Humana Press.

Chand, P., & Litvan, I. (2008). Progressive supranuclear palsy and corticobasal degeneration: Similarities and differences. *Future Neurology, 3*, 299–307.

Dickson, D., Bergeron, C., Chin, S., Duyckaerts, C., Horoupian, D., Ikeda, K., Jellinger, K., Lantos, P. L., Lippa, C. F., Tabaton, M., Vonsattel, J. P., Wakabayashi, K., & Litvan, I. (2002). Office of rare diseases neuropathologic criteria for corticobasal degeneration. *Journal of Neuropathology and Experimental Neurology, 61*, 935–946.

Eckert, T., Barnes, A., Dhawan, V., Frucht, S., Gordon, M. F., Feigin, A. S., Eidelberg D. (2005). FDG PET in the differential diagnosis of parkinsonian disorders. *Neuroimage. 26*, 912–921.

Geda, Y. E., Boeve, B. F., Negash, S., Graff-Radford, N. R., Knopman, D. S., Parisi, J. E., Dickson, D. W., Petersen R. C. (2007). Neuropsychiatric features in 36 pathologically confirmed cases of corticobasal degeneration. *Journal of Neuropsychiatry & Clinical Neurosciences. 19*, 77–80.

Graham, N. L., Bak, T. H., & Hodges, J. R. (2003).Corticobasal degeneration as a cognitive disorder. *Movement Disorders, 18*, 1224–1232.

Graham, N. L., Zeman, A., Young, A.W., Patterson, K., & Hodges, J.R. (1999). Dyspraxia in a patient with corticobasal degeneration: the role of visual and tactile inputs to action. *Journal of Neurology, Neurosurgery, & Psychaitry. 67*, 334–344.

Josephs, K. A., Tang-Wai, D. F., Edland, S. D., Knopman, D. S., Dickson, D. W., Parisi, J. E., Petersen, R. C., Jack, C. R., Jr., Boeve, B. F. (2004). Correlation between antemortem magnetic resonance imaging findings and pathologically confirmed corticobasal degeneration. *Archives of Neurology, 61*(12), 1881–1884.

Josephs, K.A.. Whitwell, J. L., Dickson, D. W., Boeve, B. F., Knopman, D. S., Petersen, R. C., Parisi, J. E., Jack, C. R. Jr. (2008). Voxel-based morphometry in autopsy proven PSP and CBD. *Neurobiology of Aging. 29*, 280–289

Kertesz, A., Martinez-Lage, P., Davidson, W., & Munoz, D. G. (2000). The corticobasal degeneration syndrome overlaps progressive aphasia and frontotemporal dementia. *Neurology, 55*, 1368–1375).

Koyama, M., Yagishita, A., Nakata, Y., Hayashi, M., Bandoh, M., Mizutani, T. (2007). Imaging of corticobasal degeneration syndrome. *Neuroradiology. 49*, 905–912.

McMonagle, P., Blair, M., & Kertesz, A. (2006). Corticobasal degeneration and progressive aphasia. *Neurology, 67*, 1444–1451.

Murray, R., Neumann, M., Forman, M. S., Farmer, J., Massimo, L., Rice, A., Miller, B. L., Johnson, J. K., Clark, C. M., Hurtig, H. I., Gorno-Tempini, M .L., Lee, V. M-Y., Trojanowski, J. Q. Grossman, M. (2007). Cognitive and motor assessment in autopsy-proven corticobasal degeneration. *Neurology. 68*, 1274–1283.

Pillon, B., Blin, J., Vidailhet, M., Deweer, B., Sirigu, A., Dubois, B., & Agid, Y. (1995). The neuropsychological pattern of corticobasal degeneration. *Neurology, 45*, 1477–1483.

Rebeiz, J., Kolodny, E., & Richardson, E. (1967). Corticodentatonigral degeneration with neuronal achromasia: A progressive disorder of late adult life. *Transactions of the American Neurological Association, 92*, 23–26.

Riley, D. E., Lang, A. E., Lewis, A. (1990) Cortical-basal ganglionic degeneration. *Neurology, 40*, 1203–1212

Rinne, J.O., Lee, M.S., Thompson, P.D., & Marsden, C.D. (1994). Corticobasal degeneration: A clinical study of 36 cases. *Brain, 117*, 1183–1196.

Togasaki, D. M., & Tanner, C. M. (2000). Epidemiologic aspects. *Advances in Neurology, 82*, 53–59.

Van Voorst, W. A., Greenaway, M. C., Boeve, B. F., Ivnik, R. J., Parisi, J. E., Ahlskog, E., Knopman, D. S., Dickson, D. W., Petersen, R. C., Smith, G. E., Josephs, K. A. (2008) Neuropsychological findings in clinically atypical autopsy confirmed corticobasal degeneration and progressive supranuclear palsy. *Parkinsonism & Related Disorders. 14*, 376–378.

53

Serial Neuropsychological Assessment in a Case of Huntington Disease

David E. Tupper

Named after George Huntington (1850–1916), who first described the clinical manifestations of a hereditary chorea that involved twisting and grimacing (Huntington, 1872; Lanska, 2000), Huntington disease is a degenerative neurogenetic disorder. Huntington disease has been found all over the world, prevalence estimates range from about 5–8 per 100,000, and there is no cure, with relentless progression of symptoms. It has been seen variously as a subcortical dementia, as a movement disorder, or as a neuropsychiatric disorder, depending upon its presentation and primary manifestations. However, toward the later stages of the disorder, many if not most individuals with Huntington disease will commonly demonstrate the prominent triad of choreic involuntary movements, marked cognitive impairments, and some type of affective or psychiatric disturbance (Folstein, 1989).

As an example of the remarkable scientific advances in our understanding of neurogenetic disorders, more than 100 years after being described as familial by Huntington, the gene responsible for Huntington disease was localized to the tip of the short arm of chromosome 4 in the 4p16.3 region in 1983, and it is now identified by having an excessive number of trinucleotide (CAG: cytosine, adenosine, guanine) repeats in the IT-15 gene. Exon 1 of the gene contains a stretch of the uninterrupted CAG trinucleoide repeats, which encode a protein called huntingtin, whose function is presently unknown.

Huntington disease shows an autosomal dominant inheritance pattern, such that each child of an afflicted parent has a 50% chance of inheriting the gene, and all gene carriers will develop the illness if they live long enough. Normal or asymptomatic individuals have 35 or fewer CAG repeats, whereas Huntington disease is caused by expansions of 36 or more CAG repeats. There is an inverse relationship between CAG repeat number and age of onset, such that a greatly expanded gene is associated with earlier onset of illness, as well as more rapid progression. A simple and accurate genetic blood test for the CAG repeat length abnormality in Huntington disease is available and is considered definitive for the diagnosis, although the ultimate diagnosis of Huntington disease in an individual—because it is such a significant life event—should be considered carefully and ethically, preferably with the support and assistance of a comprehensive assessment of relevant genetic, neurologic, emotional, and psychosocial factors (Nance & Westphal, 2002).

The age of onset for Huntington disease is most commonly during midlife with symptoms typically beginning during the age range of 35 to 50 years, although both younger and older variants are seen. Adult-onset Huntington disease typically manifests as a triad of symptoms, including a choreic movement disorder, cognitive disturbance, and psychiatric or behavioral disorder, although each of these components separately may be the earliest presenting characteristic. Chorea is common in adults with Huntington disease, and the motor component is characterized by brief, irregular, nonrhythmic involuntary movements, particularly of the extremities, as well as variable oral motor dysfunction (dysarthria, dysphagia, or drooling). Clinically, although chorea is frequently the defining characteristic of Huntington disease, it is often accompanied or preceded by a cognitive disorder that shows prominent memory and executive dysfunction, as well as by mood disturbance and other psychiatric features such as apathy, irritability, and obsessive-compulsive characteristics.

Huntington disease is a disorder that especially involves the basal ganglia and regions in the cerebral cortex (Kremer, 2002). Neuropathologically, Huntington disease demonstrates diffuse and regional cerebral atrophy, which is most dramatic in the caudate nuclei and, to a lesser extent, the putamen. Loss of small, spiny, GABA-ergic neurons in the dorsomedial aspects of the head of the caudate are noted early in the disease progression, and later the putamen and complete caudate become involved. Postmortem examinations have revealed that as many as 80% of Huntington disease brains display atrophy of the frontal lobes, and the cerebellum and globus pallidus also show changes. As with some other trinucleotide repeat diseases, neurons show intraneuronal aggregates (inclusions) in nuclei and neuronal processes that are composed of truncated glutamine derivatives of the mutant huntingtin protein.

The neuropsychological presentation of Huntington disease is varied, depending upon the age of the individual, the age at onset of clinical manifestations, the advancement of the disease, and the severity of the genetic mutation (Brandt & Butters, 1996). Neuropsychological assessment can assist in the initial diagnosis and functional characterization of individuals with Huntington disease, as well as to help track cognitive and other changes over time (Nance & Westphal, 2002). Recently, large-scale studies of the early neuropsychological presentation of individuals with gene-positive but undiagnosed Huntington disease have assisted in clarifying the early neurocognitive changes seen in this disorder and will likely lead to development of predictive batteries for clinical and research use (Paulsen et al., 2006).

Cognitive impairments in Huntington disease may actually represent greater functional impairment for individuals than the motor symptoms, and the severity of the cognitive disorder has been correlated with the disease duration, extent of subcortical (especially caudate) atrophy, and striatal glucose metabolism rate (Brandt, 1991; Paulsen & Mikoś, 2008). Intellectual and mental status decline is associated with progression and duration of the illness, but the dementia of Huntington disease is frequently described as a subcortical dementia profile and lacks traditional localizing features such as aphasia and agnosia (Folstein, Brandt, & Folstein, 1990). Executive dysfunction is prominent and is often attributed to interruption of prefrontal cortex pathways as a result of dorsomedial caudate degeneration. The memory dysfunction present is characterized by deficits in the retention of new information, and improved performance is sometimes seen with cuing and on recognition tasks. Attention-demanding cognitive operations are often the first to deteriorate in Huntington disease, and complex attention tasks are among the most sensitive measures in early stages. Clinically significant aphasia is rarely seen, but dysarthria and dysprosodia are common, and impaired fluency, naming, and narrative expression are often seen. Psychiatrically, prominent emotional or behavioral symptoms are noted in many individuals with Huntington disease, with mood disturbance and depression most common, and suicidal ideation frequently reported. Apathy, irritability, and inertia are common psychiatric characteristics in Huntington disease, and some individuals develop significant obsessive-compulsive characteristics, cognitive inflexibility, or even psychotic features (Woodcock, 1999).

Case Study: H. D.

History

H. D. was a 42-year-old female when she was first referred for neuropsychological evaluation. She had a family history of Huntington disease in her father, who died the year before H. D.'s initial evaluation when he was in his late 60s, and in an older brother, who was described at that time as having significant movement and speech problems for many years (he subsequently also died). H. D. was sent to a comprehensive Huntington disease clinic for formal neurological and neuropsychological evaluation after having received a confirmatory genetic test for Huntington disease (CAG repeats = 44) several weeks earlier at a local medical clinic. A head computed tomography (CT) scan completed at an outside facility was described as within normal limits. Her workup for Huntington disease was initiated subsequent to concerns at her job, as she was suspended for not getting her work done in a timely manner about 2 weeks prior to the assessment.

With regard to her background, H. D. is in the middle in her family and also has a younger sister who does not have Huntington symptomatology. At the time of her initial assessment, she had been married to her husband for 21 years and they had no children. H. D. had a high school education, with no learning problems identified in school, and she also attended a vocational school for 2.5 years. She had worked prior to her assessment in a medium-sized manufacturing company providing computer assistance for 5 years, and she had worked since her education in similar jobs, with no previous vocational difficulties. Past medical history was basically unremarkable otherwise, with no major medical or psychiatric concerns; she had fainted once due to heat and wore eyeglasses for nearsightedness. She took no regular medications. H. D. spent most of her free time in activities with her husband, she walked and exercised frequently, and she liked to be active outdoors. She and her husband also lived in a rural setting, and she had a special interest in presenting show animals.

H. D. underwent a reasonably comprehensive initial evaluation and completed an interview as well as performance-based testing in a number of neuropsychological domains. The presenting complaint, as she and her husband reported it, was that she had recently been diagnosed with Huntington disease, and that it was causing problems for her at work. Her husband stated that he suspected her of showing changes consistent with Huntington disease several years earlier, and the changes he noted included slight twitching in her fingers, difficulty making decisions, and sometimes mixing up her words when talking. H. D. was described as being very functional and capable overall, with very subtle changes only. She was described as very independent and accepting of her disorder. No major functional concerns were described at home, although she was reported to be perhaps slightly more passive. H. D. presented with slightly choppy speech, with bursts of language, but otherwise showed no visible physical limitations or other problems in casual interactions.

Results of H. D.'s assessment included low-average to mildly impaired intellectual capabilities, which were considered reduced from premorbid expectations. She showed well-preserved verbal vocabulary skills, with no overt language problems in most of the testing, but some difficulties with complex verbal reasoning. Motor testing revealed average bilateral grip strength, with marked reduction in motor speed and dexterity, and she was observed to demonstrate mild involuntary choreic movements with no evidence of voluntary movement disorder seen in apraxia testing. H. D. showed problems with simple and divided attention, practical judgment, and overall organization and implementation of more complex actions and sequences. Memory and learning for both verbal and visual information were moderately to severely impaired with difficulties in both acquisition and retention of information. Low-average planning and variable executive capabilities were noted, with some evidence of perseverative responding. No overt psychopathology was identified in either interview or by self-report endorsements, although H. D. reported very mild depressive tendencies.

H. D.'s evaluation results were thought to suggest evidence of moderate intellectual impairment relative to premorbid levels, as well as more specific deficits in coordinated motor activities, learning and memory, and executive capabilities. She showed a rather unusual pattern of greater verbal than nonverbal dysfunction for an individual with Huntington disease, and this was interpreted as indicative of her problems with expressive language skills, fluency, and verbal memory. Her results were felt to be consistent with early-stage Huntington disease, and her impairments in memory and motor skills in particular were felt to present notable difficulties for her in her job performance. It was thought that she would not be capable of returning to her previous job, and that it may be difficult to develop a modified position that could completely accommodate her deficits and needs. Based on the genetic confirmation of H. D.'s Huntington disease, as well as the neuropsychological documentation of her functional disabilities and her job performance problems (particularly slowness in task completion), she was considered disabled from her job.

Following the evaluation, H. D. remained living with her husband, who provided supervision for her on an informal basis, although he also worked a full-time job. H. D. and her husband continued to live together in a rural home, and they tried to participate in activities that optimized her quality of life, such as frequent traveling together. H. D. did not have very close contact with her other family members, so her husband was her major support system. She did not leave her home very often without him, and she spent most of her time caring for their show animals. When questioned about her usual activities, H. D. basically reported fairly

repetitive and stereotyped daily activities, and otherwise she stated that she spent most of her time alone reading.

Serial Assessments

In rather unusual circumstances, H. D. has access to partial salary continuation as part of a long-term disability insurance plan that her company had and that she had purchased prior to becoming symptomatic. However, that program requires documentation of her continuing functional vocational disability on an annual basis, which has occurred with neuropsychological reevaluation. Beginning approximately 41 months after her initial assessment, H. D. returned to complete annual neuropsychological evaluations, which have taken place for about 10 consecutive years since then. Thus, H. D. has been evaluated 11 different times to date, over a time frame of about 13½ years, as she has aged from 42 to 56 years.

Table 53-1 presents the data from select neuropsychological measures for all of the evaluations H. D. has completed to the present time.

Table 53-1. Longitudinal Findings for Select Neuropsychological Measures in Case H. D.

Evaluation Number	1	2	3	4	5	6	7	8	9	10	11
H. D.'s Age at Testing (Years)	42	47	48	49	50	51	52	53	54	55	56
Intellectual Skills (WAIS-R, WASI)											
Full Scale IQ	84	85	98	89	100	83	87	92	87	88	77
Verbal IQ	82	87	100	92	103	77	80	88	90	86	81
Performance IQ	87	84	95	89	96	93	98	97	87	94	77
Complex Attention and Sequencing (Trail-Making Test, completion time in seconds)											
Trails A	44	41	48	60	65	73	108	87	89	77	81
Trails B	140	172	142	294	202	192	214	172	287	300	300
Manual Dexterity (Grooved Pegboard, completion time in seconds)											
Right Hand	98	97	128	99	106	110	125	106	181	159	141
Left Hand	94	114	105	117	105	123	137	189	184	195	163
Verbal Expressive Fluency (COWA, no. of words)											
Letter Fluency	33	25	21	10	19	13	27	22	11	16	9
Category Fluency	15	13	10	15	8	8	10	9	6	7	7
Constructional Skills (Rey-Osterreith Complex Figure)											
Copy Score	21.0	26.5	22.5	22.5	21.0	14.0	19.5	27.0	23.0	20.0	12.5
Visual Memory (Rey Complex Figure)											
Delayed Recall Score	11.5	7.0	7.0	8.0	4.0	3.5	9.5	13.0	8.0	11.5	6.0

(Continued)

Table 53-1. Longitudinal Findings for Select Neuropsychological Measures in Case H. D.(*Continued*)

Evaluation Number	1	2	3	4	5	6	7	8	9	10	11
Verbal Memory (CVLT/CVLT-II)											
Trials 1-5 Total Score	22	39	31	27	22	23	13	21	18	24	22
LDFR	2	6	4	3	2	4	2	2	2	5	1
Executive Function/Mental Shifting (Wisconsin Card-Sorting Test)											
Perseverative Responses	32	80	13	16	17	-	21	17	47	60	46

Note. Raw or calculated scores are provided to emphasize actual performances, with standardized scores as appropriate

The measures in the table provide consistent quantitative information about a number of neuropsychological domains and, although some variations in exact test versions have been used from time to time, there has been fairly good consistency in the results obtained. The data in the table are provided in raw (or calculated) score form, to demonstrate the actual level of performances by H. D. over time.

Perusal of the table suggests that H. D. has shown a great deal of variability in her performances over time, although there is a general downward trend (that is, poorer performances) for many but not all of the measures included. Thus, H. D. has shown relatively stable overall intellectual capabilities, as reflected in her Full Scale, Verbal, and Performance IQ scores on the Wechsler scales; this stability probably represents the fact that these scores are for more "crystallized" or well-learned capabilities, and also that H. D. actually showed some intellectual compromise compared to premorbid expectations in her initial assessment. Clearly, any measures that are dependent on motor skill, speed, or verbal expression (e.g., COWA, Trail Making Test, Grooved Pegboard, Copy of Rey Complex Figure) have been impaired in all assessments but show generally progressive decline longitudinally, with slower motor performances and greater impairment in fluency of verbal or manual expression. Memory is also a domain notably affected for H. D., and both verbal and visual memory are poor and have progressively deteriorated. Objective evidence of problems with mental shifting as a component of executive dysfunction is noted in H. D.'s increasing problems with divided attention on Trails B and increased perseverative responding on the Wisconsin Card Sorting Test.

Aside from the neuropsychological documentation of her condition over time, several other factors have potentially impacted the manifestations of her Huntington disease during this 10-year time frame. H. D.'s husband died suddenly and unexpectedly between the time of her fifth and sixth evaluations. Because of their very close, and obviously dependent relationship, and the fact that she was living independently with his assistance, it was anticipated by clinic staff that she would need additional support and possibly an out-of-home placement. Interestingly, H. D. has been able to maintain her own home with the assistance of several very devoted and kind neighbors who have assisted her. For several years after her husband's death, H. D. visited the home of a close friend and neighbor and assisted in a home-based sales business on a regular, almost daily, basis, which provided her a way to remain active and productive, and also to receive informal assistance and supervision for her own needs. This was not a formal relationship but served H. D.'s needs for several years until her friend moved away and the business went bankrupt. Unfortunately, H. D. does not have similar close relationships with others (including family), and she has increasingly remained alone in her own home, as she does not leave the house on her own very frequently and does not often socialize. She reports that she continues to drive, although it is only during the summer months, and only to go to the store.

In addition to H. D.'s increasingly precarious psychosocial situation soon after her husband died, she self-initiated alternative treatments consisting of herbal drinks, vitamins, and monthly acupuncture. H. D. has become increasingly stuck on the idea that these alternative treatments not only are helping her, but have essentially stopped the progression of her Huntington disease symptomatology, in spite of the fact that others note continued progression of her disorder.

Comparison between Initial and Most Recent Evaluations

The first and most recent evaluations for H. D. can be compared to show perhaps more qualitatively the overall deterioration evident in her findings. Table 53-2 shows the complete evaluation data from H. D.'s first and eleventh neuropsychological assessments, with all test data included. For additional qualitative perspective, Figure 53-1 provides examples of H. D.'s performances for the copy trials of the Rey Complex Figure during both evaluations, and Figure 53-2 shows examples of her current writing and copying capabilities during the most recent assessment.

A review of Table 53-2 clearly demonstrates that H. D. has shown substantial change over time in several domains of functioning, such as her verbal expressive skills, motor speed and dexterity, visuospatial organization and visual memory, retention of both verbal and visual information, and aspects of conceptual and executive functioning. In formal testing, H. D. demonstrates impairments in any type of speeded activity, such as on the Trail Making Test, where her simple sequencing time on Part A doubled, and her Part B performance, reflective of the additional divided attentional component, not only became slower but she ultimately was unable to complete the task within the time limit and made three sequencing errors. Memory retention has decreased significantly over time, and now H. D. is only able to correctly recall several words from the CVLT-II list after a delay and has limited accurate recall (less than 50%) of the Rey figure over time. She has become increasingly perseverative over time, and she now is more limited in her conceptual capabilities and practical judgment, as reflected in her limited category attainment on the WCST and her poorer performance on the Cognitive Estimation test. As previously, H. D. denied any significant symptomatology on her completion of the Symptom Checklist-90 Revised and the Frontal Systems Behavioral Examination, while a neighbor endorsed mild problems with working memory and shifting her behavior.

Table 53-2. Comparisons between Initial (#1) and Most Recent (#11) Evaluation Results in Case H. D. (Conducted 13 Years apart)*

	Evaluation #1	Evaluation #11
General Cognitive/Intelligence		
WAIS–R/WASI		
FSIQ	84	77
VIQ	82	81
PIQ	87	77
Vocabulary	10	6
Similarities	7	7
Block Design	7	7
Matrix Reasoning	—	4
Attention		
WAIS–R/WAIS–III		
Digit Span	9 (7F, 3B)	6 (5F, 3B)
Trail Making Test (in seconds)		
Part A	44 (T = 33)	81 (T = 26)
Part B	140 (T = 27)	300+ (T = 9)
Language		
Controlled Oral Word Association (no. of words)		
Letter Fluency	33	9
Category Fluency	15	7
Memory		
CVLT/CVLT–II		
Trials 1–5 Total	22 (T = 5)	22 (T = 21)
SDFR	4 (–4)	3 (–3)
SDCR	4 (–5)	4 (–4)
LDFR	2 (–5)	1 (–4)
LDCR	3 (–5)	2 (–4)
Recognition Hits	11 (–4)	3 (–5)
False Positives	4 (+1)	0 (–1)
Rey Complex Figure		
Copy Score	21.0	12.5
Immediate Recall	11.0	5.0
Delayed Recall	11.5	6.0
Recognition Total	—	15
Motor/Visuo–Motor		
Dynamometer (grip strength in kg)		
Right Hand	36 (T = 59)	—
Left Hand	34 (T = 58)	—
Finger Tapping Test (mean no. of taps)		
Right Hand	42 (T = 44)	21 (T = 24)
Left Hand	35 (T = 41)	19 (T = 17)

(Continued)

Table 53-2. Comparisons between Initial (#1) and Most Recent (#11) Evaluation Results in Case H. D. (Conducted 13 Years apart)*(*Continued*)

	Evaluation #1	Evaluation #11
Grooved Pegboard (completion time in seconds)		
Right Hand	98 (T = 21)	141 (T = 20)
Left Hand	94 (T = 30)	163 (T = 25)
Apraxia Screening (maximum = 18)	18	18
Conceptual/Executive		
Tinkertoy Test (complexity score)	4	3
Cognitive Estimation Test (deviation score)	6	10
Porteus Mazes (Test Quotient)	82	—
DKEFS Tower (achievement)	—	9
Wisconsin Card-Sorting Test		
Categories achieved	6	1
Errors	51	74
Perseverative responses	32	46
Behavioral/Emotional Ratings		
Frontal Systems Behavioral Examination (FrSBe)– self and informant ratings		
Symptom Checklist– 90–Revised		

*Raw or calculated scores are listed, with standardized scores (SS, T, z) as appropriate.

At the time of this most recent evaluation, H. D. by observation also showed more prominent choreic movements than during her earlier assessments, and these have begun to affect her writing and drawing skills (see the repeated patterns copying, for example, in Figure 53-2). Interestingly, H. D. does not appear to demonstrate any clear apraxia or voluntary movement difficulties, as seen in her basically intact performance for a brief quantitative screening measure, but her involuntary movements have increased in frequency and intensity and affect her motor coordination, dexterity, and speed.

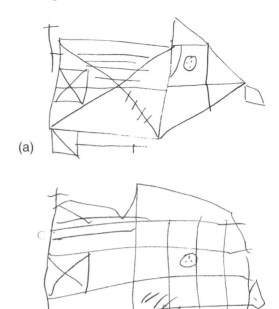

(a)

(b)

Figure 53-1. Copy of the Rey-Osterreith Complex Figure by Case H. D. during the initial (*a*) and most recent (*b*) evaluations.

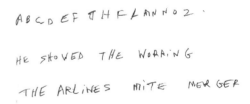

(a)

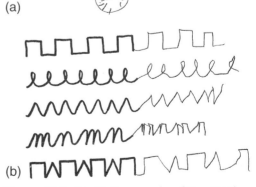

(b)

Figure 53-2. Qualitative examples of Case H. D.'s graphomotor skills (*a*) and repeated patterns (*b*) during the most recent evaluation (#11).

However, H. D. does show delayed responses and problems in motor initiation, noted by observation and during testing. No unusual motor asymmetries have been detected throughout her various assessments. In addition, H. D. is noted to be showing increasing dysarthria, which has made completion of some of her verbal testing rather difficult. She currently speaks in shorter bursts of language than she did during earlier assessments, and she is only about 50%–75% intelligible overall, although there are some times in which she has perfectly clear speech for brief durations. To help compensate, she sometimes subvocalizes a response repetitively before producing it in louder form. Her prominent motor difficulties therefore are increasingly affecting not only her manual activities and gait but also her verbal communication.

Psychologically, H. D. has been demonstrating increasing concerns. During the interview as part of her most recent assessment, she directly denied any increasing symptoms, including any of the motor, cognitive, or other changes that were notable to the examiner who had worked with her in previous assessments. H. D. appeared to downplay the significance of her pronounced symptoms at this more progressed point and stated that she had no safety issues living by herself. Although frequently seen in individuals with Huntington disease, H. D. has consistently denied any depression or suicidal ideation. Her affect—although difficult to assess accurately—was rather flat, and she had rigid facial expression. Repetitive actions such as repeatedly looking into her mailbox were described by her neighbor for her, although H. D. denied similar concerns. As noted previously, H. D. has become mentally stuck on the idea that her symptoms have been stopped with her alternative treatments, and her cognitive inflexibility is apparent in her denials of current concerns.

H. D. is currently in the mid to later stages of the progression of her Huntington disease. She currently continues to live independently but is rather precarious, and she could be considered somewhat of a recluse. At the time of this most recent assessment, it was felt that she showed further advancement in the progression of her Huntington disease, and that she was moderately to severely disabled by the combination of impairments she demonstrated. Greater risk of safety-related problems was felt to be present, with H. D. advancing to the point where she would soon need greater daily supervision and assistance, and where independent living may soon not be possible.

Comments

H. D. may be one of the most regularly evaluated individuals with Huntington disease in the world. The clinical presentation and progression of her Huntington disease demonstrates notable variability, but yet a course of steady decline over the years. H. D. has been evaluated neuropsychologically during the early and middle stages of the progression of her disorder and has shown both objective quantitative changes consistent with advancing Huntington disease and qualitative motor and psychological changes that are typical in this condition. H. D. was mildly to moderately disabled at the time of her initial neuropsychological assessment, and she had a family history and genetic testing evidence of the presence of Huntington disease. Thus, the serial neuropsychological evaluations conducted for H. D. have not been for diagnostic purposes, but rather for descriptive purposes to document the progression of her disorder. To date, although she has continued to live fairly independently, H. D. will soon be advancing to the later stages of the disorder, which will create more significant functional disability in her daily life and may lead to loss of her ability to live on her own.

H. D. has demonstrated the triad of motoric, cognitive, and psychological impairments that is frequently seen in individuals with Huntington disease. Her dementia would be considered a subcortical dementia as she shows a combination of attentional, memory, and executive dysfunction, along with her involuntary movement disorder, but has less affected crystallized intellectual skills. Formal neuroimaging has not been completed recently for H. D., but the usual neuropathological changes in striatal structures and connections would be expected for her, along with likely developing cortical pathology. It is anticipated that H. D. will soon become more difficult to assess quantitatively, so additional comprehensive neuropsychological evaluations may not occur.

References

Brandt, J. (1991). Cognitive impairments in Huntington's disease: Insights into the neuropsychology of the striatum. In F. Boller & J. Grafman (Eds.), *Handbook of neuropsychology* (Vol. 5, pp. 241–264). Amsterdam: Elsevier.

Brandt, J., & Butters, N. (1996). Neuropsychological characteristics of Huntington's disease. In I. Grant & K. M. Adams (Eds.), *Neuropsychiatric assessment of neuropsychiatric disorders* (2nd ed., pp. 312–341). New York: Oxford University Press.

Folstein, S. E. (1989). *Huntington's disease: A disorder of families*. Baltimore: Johns Hopkins University Press.

Folstein, S. E., Brandt, J., & Folstein, M. F. (1990). Huntington's disease. In J. L. Cummings (Ed.), *Subcortical dementia* (pp. 87–107). New York: Oxford University Press.

Huntington, G. (1872). On chorea. *Medical and Surgical Reporter, 26*, 317–321.

Kremer, B. (2002). Clinical neurology of Huntington's disease: Diversity in unity, unity in diversity. In G. Bates, P. S. Harper, & L. Jones (Eds.), *Huntington's disease* (3rd ed., pp. 28–61). Oxford, England: Oxford University Press.

Lanska, D. J. (2000). George Huntington (1850–1916) and hereditary chorea. *Journal of the History of the Neurosciences, 9*(1), 76–89.

Nance, M. A., & Westphal, B. (2002). Comprehensive care in Huntington's disease. In G. Bates, P. S. Harper, & L. Jones (Eds.), *Huntington's disease* (3rd ed., pp. 475–500). Oxford, England: Oxford University Press.

Paulsen, J. S., Hayden, M., Stout, J. C., Langbehn, D. R., Aylward, E., Ross, C. A., Guttman, M., Nance, M., Kieburtz, K., Oakes, D., Shoulson, I., Kayson, E., Johnson, S., Penziner, E., & the Predict-HD Investigators of the Huntington Study Group. (2006). Preparing for preventive clinical trials: The Predict-HD study. *Archives of Neurology, 63*(6), 883–890.

Paulsen, J. S., & Mikoś, A. (2008). Huntington's disease. In J. E. Morgan & J. H. Ricker (Eds.), *Textbook of clinical neuropsychology* (pp. 616–635). New York: Taylor & Francis.

Woodcock, J. H. (1999). Behavioral aspects of Huntington's disease. In A. B. Joseph & R. R. Young (Eds.), *Movement disorders in neurology and neuropsychiatry* (2nd ed., pp. 155–160). Malden, MA: Blackwell Science.

54

Two Neuropsychologists with Huntington Disease

Jason Brandt and Barnett Shpritz

Notwithstanding its limitations as a source of generalizable knowledge, the case study forms the bedrock of both cognitive and clinical neuropsychology (Code, Wallesch, Joanette, & Lecours, 1996, 2003). It has been argued that the case study permits an interrogation of neurocognitive mechanisms in a way that no group study ever can (Caramazza & McCloskey, 1988). Moreover, the case study compels an appreciation of the patient's unique characteristics and life circumstances that is fundamental to the clinical practice of psychiatry and psychology (Jaspers, 1997; McHugh & Slavney, 1998).

There is often something especially compelling about case studies where the subjects are themselves health professionals (see Kapur, 1997). These narratives are particularly poignant when the subject has cared for patients with the very disorder with which he/she has become afflicted.

This chapter presents two case studies of clinical neuropsychologists who developed Huntington disease (HD), a relatively rare neurodegenerative disease, but one which has made a disproportionate contribution to the neuropsychological literature (or at least is disproportionately represented; Grant, 2008). Huntington disease presents in mid-life with a movement disorder (primarily dystonia and chorea), emotional alterations (primarily depression, irritability, and apathy), and a "subcortical"-type dementia (primarily cognitive slowing, and spatial and executive impairment) (Brandt & Butters, 1986; Folstein, 1989; Harper, 1996). It has

been appreciated since George Huntington's initial description of the illness in 1872 that HD is inherited as an autosomal dominant trait. However, its genetic locus was not identified until 1983 (Gusella et al., 1983), and the specific DNA mutation responsible was discovered 10 years later (Huntington's Disease Collaborative Research Group, 1993). The mutation, named *huntingtin*, consists of an abnormally expanded CAG trinucleotide repeat coding for glutamine at 4p16.3. There is now strong evidence that abnormally long polyglutamine tracts aggregate within neurons and ultimately cause selective cell death (Ross, 2002; Ross & Margolis, 2001; Walker, 2007).

An extensive clinical literature has documented the neurocognitive changes that accompany HD (for reviews, see Brandt, 2008; Paulsen & Conybeare, 2005; Zakzanis, 1998). Similar but extremely mild abnormalities are occasionally found in mutation carriers who do not yet meet criteria for disease diagnosis ("presymptomatic" cases) (Brandt, Shpritz, Codori, Margolis, & Rosenblatt, 2002; Brandt et al., 2008; Kirkwood et al., 1999; Paulsen et al., 2001; Snowden, Craufurd, Thompson, & Neary, 2002; Solomon et al., 2007). But can standardized neuropsychological tests—even those most sensitive to HD-yield meaningful data when the patient is a neuropsychologist? Does intimate knowledge of neuropsychological procedures make these tests invalid for clinical assessment or disease monitoring? The case studies presented here may shed light on this issue.

The two patients described in this chapter underwent neuropsychological testing on multiple occasions in the context of their participation in research in the Baltimore Huntington's Disease Project (BHDP) at the Johns Hopkins University School of Medicine. This National Institutes of Health (NIH)-funded research center, first established in 1982, has supported both neurobiological and clinical research on HD, including a Longitudinal Cohort Study of the neurological, psychiatric, brain morphometric, and neuropsychological course of the disease. Patients afflicted with HD, presymptomatic persons who carry the HD mutation, and mutation-negative offspring of HD patients (control subjects) are examined and tested annually, have periodic brain magnetic resonance imaging (MRI) scans, and are asked to agree to brain autopsy for neuropathological study upon their demise.

Several publications from our research group have described the longitudinal changes in cognition in participants with clinical HD (e.g., Brandt et al., 1996; Ward et al., 2006) and presymptomatic subjects (e.g., Brandt et al., 2002, 2008; Campodonico et al., 1998). The two patients described here are not necessarily representative HD patients; quite the contrary, the fact that they are neuropsychologists makes them extraordinary. They are presented here to illustrate the presentation and course of a particular neurodegenerative disease in health professionals with expertise in dementia, and the applicability of neuropsychological methods to those with intimate knowledge of those methods.

Since the clinical neuropsychology community is still relatively small, special attention has been paid to safeguarding the anonymity of these patients. Nonessential, potentially identifying details of their histories were altered or omitted for the sake of confidentiality.

Case T. Q.

History

T. Q. was born in 1951 and adopted as a young child. His biological mother reportedly was diagnosed with HD at age 42 and died at age 57. A maternal aunt was affected as well. T.Q.'s maternal grandfather died when he fell off a roof,

leading to some suspicion that he might have been the source of the HD gene. The patient has a half-sister 14 years his junior who reportedly is well.

The patient's early developmental history was unremarkable. He completed high school without any difficulty and then attended university, where he majored in psychology. He then went on to obtain his doctorate in clinical neuropsychology from a well-established and respected program. From 1984 to 1988, he worked as a pediatric neuropsychologist on the staff of a university-affiliated hospital. In 1988, he left this position and established an independent practice in neuropsychological evaluation and consultation. Dr. Q reported that his practice was quite successful and he enjoyed his work a great deal.

When he was 30 years old, the patient sought out the circumstances of his adoption and discovered that his biological mother had HD. By this time, he had married and fathered a child.

The patient's medical history prior to the onset of HD was relatively unremarkable. He experienced an episode of possible carbon monoxide exposure in 1979, but he never sought medical evaluation and had no apparent sequelae. He experienced an episode of low mood, anergia, loss of interest, fleeting thoughts of suicide, and increased sleep while in graduate school. The patient was treated with psychotherapy and the episode remitted within 4–6 months. He subsequently had occasional periods of depression which never lasted very long or caused serious life disruption.

Dr. Q first exhibited increased clumsiness and mild involuntary movements at age 41. He was evaluated by a neurologist who was unable to render a diagnosis. An MRI scan of the brain at that time (1992) was reportedly normal. The patient's symptoms progressed over the next few years, and he developed apathy, irritability, dysarthria, poor concentration, and impaired spatial judgment (the latter objectified by his putting several "dings" in his car). In February 1996, Dr. Q had his first BHDP evaluation at Johns Hopkins. He described his mood as "fine" and he appeared cheerful but anxious. Dr. Q related difficulty concentrating at work and trouble completing clinical reports on his patients. Neurologic exam revealed slightly jerky pursuit eye movements, mild motor impersistence, dyscoordinated tongue movements, dysdiadochokinesis, and mild chorea which worsened under the stress of mental arithmetic. Dr. Q's score on the Quantified Neurological Exam (Folstein, Jensen, Leigh, & Folstein, 1983) was 16. (Scores on this standardized exam of the motor system can range from 0 to 123, with most neurologically normal people scoring below 5, and just-diagnosable patients with HD typically scoring in the high teens.) The patient was told that his exam was probably indicative of HD, and blood was drawn for genetic confirmation. DNA testing for the HD mutation revealed that Dr. Q had 43 CAG repeats. Since repeat lengths ≥36 are abnormal, the diagnosis of HD was confirmed. Dr. Q discontinued his practice of clinical neuropsychology in July 1996.

A repeat brain MRI scan in 2001 revealed only a small focus of decreased signal in the left aspect of the pons thought to be a capillary telangiectasia (an asymptomatic and benign vascular malformation) and subcortical and periventricular small vessel ischemic changes. Clinical reading of the MRI scan did not comment on any atrophy of the head of the caudate nucleus or putamen.

Neuropsychological Findings

No neuropsychological evaluation was performed on Dr. Q's initial clinic visit, nor on his follow-up visit 13 months later. However, his motor impairment, psychiatric condition, and functional abilities worsened considerably over this interval (see Table 54.1). In July 1998, Dr. Q enrolled in the Longitudinal Cohort Study, which includes annual neuropsychological testing. There was some discussion among the BHDP staff as to whether Dr. Q's neuropsychological test data would be meaningful, since he was familiar with most of the tests and, in fact, used many of them frequently in his practice. However, it was decided to collect the data first and interpret them later.

As seen in Table 54-1, Dr. Q's HD had progressed quickly. His score on the QNE was 42 on his 1998 visit, indicating moderately advanced disease. His scores on scales rating irritability, apathy, and depression were more than 3 SDs higher than those of mutation-negative control subjects of comparable age and education. Dr. Q had clear impairments in instrumental activities of everyday living (HD-ADL scale; Rothlind,

Bylsma, Peyser, Folstein, & Brandt, 1993). Of note, his score on the Mini-Mental State Exam (MMSE) was no lower than on his first BHDP visit, when he was minimally affected.

Neuropsychological testing in July 1998 revealed pervasive impairments. Dr. Q performed more than 3 SDs below his peers on tests requiring rapid processing of visual and auditory information (Symbol Digit Modalities Test [SDMT], Stroop Color-Word Test, Brief Test of Attention), as well as new learning and memory for both a word list (Hopkins Verbal Learning Test; HVLT) and spatial locations (Hopkins Board). His performance on the WAIS-R Vocabulary subtest was excellent, while his Block Design score was below average. Dr. Q commented spontaneously that he was very familiar with, and had often administered, the SDMT, Controlled Oral Word Association Test (COWAT), Trail Making Test (TMT), and Wisconsin Card Sorting Test (WCST). He was severely impaired on the first two of these and performed normally on the second two.

Dr. Q did not return for another study visit until February 2001. At that time, his QNE had increased to 67, and his MMSE had declined to 22. With a single exception, his performance on every neuropsychological test had declined, some markedly so. On the WCST, the patient's performance remained unimpaired. In fact, he required six fewer cards to complete the six sorts than on his prior visit.

Dr. Q's last study visit was in April 2002. He was brought in by his family in a wheelchair, "seated in a fetal position." He was able to walk but had constant flailing movements of all four extremities. He could not stand still and had sustained many falls. His QNE score was 88. Dr. Q was unable to speak intelligibly due to dyskinetic movements of the mouth and tongue, and he was unable to be administered the Longitudinal Cohort Study's neuropsychological test battery. He was placed on hospice care in 2003 and survived 3 more years. Dr. Q died the day after his 55th birthday in 2006.

Neuropathology

As prearranged, and with the consent of Dr. Q's family, an autopsy limited to the brain was performed approximately 6 hours after death.

Table 54-1. Clinical Ratings and Neuropsychological Exam Scores for Patient T. Q.

	February 1996	March 1997	July 1998	February 2001	April 2002
Age	44	45	46	49	50
Quantified Neurological Exam	16	38	42***	67	88
Mini-Mental State Exam	27	25	27*	22	
HD-ADL Scale[1]	1	14	22***	30	
Irritability Scale[2]	11	22	25***	27	
Apathy Scale[2]	10	13	13***	29	
Hamilton Depression Scale	0	4	4***	4	
NEUROPSYCHOLOGICAL EXAMINATIONS					
WAIS-R Vocabulary, age-corrected scaled score			16	Not	
WAIS-R Block Design, age-corrected scaled score			7**	administered	
WAIS-R estimated I.Q.			111	(per protocol)	
Grooved Pegboard Test					
Dominant hand time			N/A	216	
Nondominant hand time			N/A	335	
Symbol Digit Modalities Test (written trial)			20***	12	
Brief Test of Attention			8***	6	
Controlled Oral Word Association Test			23***	8	
Developmental Test of Visual-Motor Integration, raw			14**	9	
Hopkins Verbal Learning Test					
Total of Recall Trials			16***	13	
Delayed Recall[3]			N/A	6	
Recognition Discrimination			10**	7	
Hopkins Board[4]					
Errors to Criterion			15***	25	
Trials to Criterion			10**	10	
Delayed Recall of Items			9	6	
Delayed Recall of Locations			7	5	
Trail Making Test					
Part A time			39*	54	
Part B time			51	194	
Stroop Color-Word Test					
Word T-score			20***	17	
Color T-score			23***	13	
Color-Word T-score			32**	19	
Interference T-score			55	48	
Wisconsin Card Sorting Test					
Cards Used			76	70	
Sorts Achieved			6	6	
Inefficiency (Cards/Sort)			12.67	11.67	

Note. The patient's first neuropsychological exam, on entry to the Longitudinal Cohort Study, was in July 1998. His scores from this visit are compared to a group of six mutation-negative control subjects matched in age (+ 3 years) and education (all college graduates or more).

[1]Rothlind et al. (1993).

[2]Burns et al. (1990)

[3]Prior to November 1998, the original Hopkins Verbal Learning Test (HVLT) (Brandt, 1991) was administered. This version did not include delayed recall; the yes/no recognition trial followed immediately the third free recall trial. After November 1998, the HVLT-R (Brandt & Benedict, 2001) was administered .

[4]Brandt et al. (2005).

*1 SD below average for age and education.

**2 SD below average for age and education.

***3 SD below average for age and education.

The brain was of normal weight at 1250 grams. Gross examination revealed no significant cortical atrophy and no evidence of hemorrhage. Serial coronal sections of the cerebral hemispheres revealed the cortical and subcortical gray and white matter to be of normal configuration, without hemorrhages, infarctions, or mass lesions. The medial surface of the head of the caudate nucleus was moderately atrophied; the tail of the caudate nucleus was not visible, but it was identified microscopically. Mild atrophy of the putamen and globus pallidus was also evident. Histological examination of the striatum revealed marked neuronal loss and glial proliferation. Immunohistochemical staining for ubiquitin revealed abundant intranuclear inclusions in the mid-frontal gyrus and striatum, and moderate inclusions in the amygdala. All these findings are consistent with Huntington disease, Vonsattel grade 2 (out of 4) (Vonsattel et al., 1985).

Commentary

The course of Dr. Q's HD was fairly typical, if a bit rapid. He was diagnosed at age 44, around the same age his mother was. Age of onset of HD is negatively correlated with CAG repeat length, and the median age of onset for someone with 43 repeats is 44 (95% CI = 42–45) (Brinkman, Mezei, Theilmann, Almqvist, & Hayden, 1997). The time from Dr. Q's first clinical signs until his death was 14 years, though he may have been symptomatic for few years longer.

Several observations can be made regarding the neurocognitive assessment of this gentleman. First, serial testing of Dr. Q illustrates clearly the insensitivity of the MMSE in early HD (Brandt, Folstein, & Folstein, 1988; Rothlind & Brandt, 1993). Even as his neurological symptoms worsened considerably (from 1996 to 1998), his MMSE score remained unchanged. More detailed neuropsychological testing revealed pervasive cognitive deficits. In fact, the only tests that were performed entirely within the normal range were the WAIS-R Vocabulary subtest, TMT, and WCST. Dr. Q was highly familiar with these tests, having administered them many times as a clinical neuropsychologist. However, he displayed clear deficits on many tests he used regularly, including WAIS-R Block Design subtest, the SDMT, and the COWAT.

The WAIS-R Vocabulary subtest, which assesses crystallized semantic knowledge, is well known to hold up in HD (and many other basal ganglia disorders) (Josiassen, Curry, Roemer, DeBease, & Mancall, 1982; Ward et al., 2006; Zakzanis, 1998). The TMT is typically sensitive in HD, but Dr. Q's presumed frequent use of this instrument (it is one of the most frequently used neuropsychological tests [Guilmette, Faust, Hart, & Arkes, 1990; Rabin, Barr, & Burton, 2005]) may have allowed him to rely on overlearned knowledge and well-practiced procedures for its execution. While the WCST has been shown to be sensitive in some studies of HD (Josiassen, Curry, & Mancall, 1983; Rebok, Bylsma, Keyl, Brandt, & Folstein, 1995), it is a test whose utility depends on it being novel. That is, once you know the sorting rules, it is no longer a test of concept acquisition, set maintenance, and shifting in response to feedback.

From his very first visit to the BHDP, Dr. Q was reported to have increased irritability and apathy, and he shortly thereafter developed significant depressive symptoms. Again, this is fairly typical, as irritability, apathy, and depression are the most prevalent neuropsychiatric phenomena in HD (Burns, Folstein, Brandt, & Folstein, 1990; Chatterjee, Anderson, Moskowitz, Hauser, & Marder, 2005; Paulsen, Ready, Hamilton, Mega, & Cummings, 2001). Treatment of these states includes both pharmacological and behavioral/environmental interventions (Naarding, Kremer, & Zitman, 2001; Rosenblatt, Ranen, Nance, & Paulsen, 1999).

Case I. G.

History

I. G. was a 17-year-old high school student when he first contacted the BHDP for information and counseling regarding HD. His family was part of a large kindred that was very well known to the BHDP staff; there were no fewer than 17 members affected with HD in three generations. I. G.'s mother, age 40, had HD with very significant psychiatric symptomatology, but she did not acknowledge that anything was wrong with her.

Dr. G's contact with the clinic staff became more frequent as his mother's psychiatric symptoms of HD worsened. She had become verbally and physically abusive and explosively violent; she once chased Dr. G and his brother with a butcher knife, attempting to kill them. She had several brief psychiatric hospitalizations but remained extremely unstable and threatening, prompting the patient and his brother to move in with their paternal grandmother.

I. G. graduated high school and then moved out of state to attend a major state university. He was a good student and obtained his bachelor's degree in psychology. After working 2 years as a research assistant, he enrolled in a clinical psychology Ph.D. program, with specialization in neuropsychology.

In 1992, at the age of 25, Dr. G contacted the BHDP for the purpose of pursuing presymptomatic genetic testing. His mother now had severe choreiform movements, was unable to walk, and resided in a nursing home. Dr. G had married a young woman, also a psychologist-in-training. The couple had no children. He sought counseling and genetic testing because he felt his future was "ambiguous," causing him significant anxiety. He and his wife also wanted to make decisions about childbearing. Dr. G had been in psychotherapy for 2 years for depressed mood and to mitigate the emotional trauma of growing up with a severely psychiatrically ill and abusive parent. Dr. G was neurologically normal upon entry into the presymptomatic testing program; he received a score of 0 on the QNE. Based on a standardized psychiatric interview, he was diagnosed with an adjustment disorder with depressed mood.

After several counseling sessions, some with his wife, over 4 months, Dr. G underwent genetic testing in 1993. At the time, only linkage testing for a genetic marker was available (Brandt et al., 1989). Blood samples from multiple affected and unaffected family members were obtained, and the DNA haplotype segregating with HD in the family was established. Dr. G had a positive test, with an estimated 99% probability of inheriting the HD mutation. The patient and his wife were clearly distressed by the news, but not distraught. They were assigned a therapist in the BHDP for ongoing psychological care and support. (Re-analysis of Dr. G's DNA sample for the actual gene mutation when such testing became available confirmed that he did have the mutation, with 50 CAG repeats.)

At 3 months after disclosure of his test results, Dr. G stated, "I'm doing pretty good overall. I was depressed for 3 months, but now things are starting to pick up, especially when I'm not alone." He had just completed his comprehensive exams and felt confident of his performance. He went on to complete the course work for his doctoral degree and took an externship at an inpatient psychiatric facility.

At his June 1994 follow-up visit, Dr. G obtained a score of 2 on the QNE, well within the normal range. He had been diagnosed with chronic fatigue syndrome and tested positive for the Epstein-Barr virus. Dr. G's marriage was conflict-ridden, but, in spite of this, he reported bright spirits. He was about to start his full-time clinical internship, with a very strong emphasis on neuropsychological assessment.

By the next year, cognitive, emotional, and relationship problems began to emerge. Dr. G and his wife had divorced. In addition, he was described by his internship director as apathetic and uninterested, and it seemed "as if he never had a course in psychology." Matters appeared to improve somewhat after the patient disclosed to his supervisors and peers that he had received a positive genetic test for HD. Nevertheless, his condition remained precarious. His QNE score at his April 1995 visit was 5.

Dr. G returned to the BHDP for reevaluations in 1996 and 1997. His mother died of HD in March 1997, causing him a combination of sadness, anger, and guilt. He continued to work on his Ph.D. dissertation, but he reported being inefficient and distracted by worry about HD. Dr. G had a new girlfriend, and although he was very interested in eventually having children with her, she was understandably reluctant. His QNE score was 12 at both of these visits, reflecting mild choreiform movements under stress. However, he was judged by neuropsychiatrists expert in HD to not yet meet diagnostic criteria, in part because he was functioning reasonably well. Although it was a struggle for him, Dr. G completed his Ph.D. in 1997. He acquired a position as a clinical psychologist specializing in neuropsychological assessment at a state hospital.

Dr. G did not return for his next follow-up until February 1999. He continued to work full time performing psychological and neuropsychological assessments. He reported that he received good evaluations at work, and he denied any impairment in adaptive functioning. (He was unaccompanied to this visit, and no informant was available for confirmation.) Dr. G received 10 points on the QNE at this visit and entered the Longitudinal Cohort Study. By the time he returned for a study visit the following year (September 2000), he had stopped working due to cognitive, motor, and emotional symptoms. He obtained a QNE score of 12, had marked impairments in adaptive functioning (according to his father), and was diagnosed formally as affected with HD at this visit. He was 33 years old.

Brain MRI scans in April 1995 and September 2000 were both read as normal. Single-photon emission computed tomography (SPECT) imaging in April 1995 revealed no perfusion abnormalities.

Neuropsychological Findings

Dr. G had five brief neuropsychological exams as a presymptomatic person before entering the Longitudinal Cohort Study (see Table 54-2). The first of these (August 1992) was before he received the results of his genetic test, and the next four were after disclosure. Performance on the SDMT declined monotonically over these assessments, and there was a downward trend on several other tests requiring rapid processing (e.g., part A of the TMT, word and color-word trials of Stroop Color-Word Test). It is noteworthy that even as Dr. G's QNE score increased over these exams, his manual speed and dexterity (assessed with the Grooved Pegboard Test) remained stable.

On entering the Longitudinal Cohort Study in 1999, Dr. G reminded the staff that he was a psychologist and "would probably do better on all the testing than anyone tested so far." Because he was extremely well versed in the Wechsler intelligence scales, the decision was made to forgo administration of the WAIS-R Vocabulary and Block Design subtests. In retrospect, this was an unfortunate decision; as seen in the case of T. Q., even intimate knowledge of the Block Design subtest may not be sufficient to compensate for the spatial and constructional impairment caused by HD (Mohr et al., 1991; Strauss & Brandt, 1986). Nonetheless, very severe impairments

(3 SDs below age- and education-matched mutation-negative control subjects) were observed on tests of memory. On the HVLT-R, Dr. G displayed extremely poor delayed recall. On the Hopkins Board (Brandt, Shpritz, Munro, Marsh, & Rosenblatt, 2005), which allows the subject multiple trials to learn the location of nine stimulus items, Dr. G also displayed a profound visuospatial learning impairment. He made more errors and required more trials to meet the learning criterion than healthy peers. His 20-minute delayed recall of the items was normal, but his delayed recall of their locations was impaired. Dr. G also gave impaired performances on the SDMT and HVLT-R yes/no recognition trial, whereas the BTA, COWAT, Developmental Test of Visual-Motor Integration (VMI), and WCST were all performed within normal limits.

On his September 2000 exam, Dr. G was reported by his father to be displaying marked irritability, apathy, and depression. Among his cognitive test results, most notable are his continued decline on the SDMT, slower performance on both parts of the TMT, and slower word reading score on the Stroop Color-Word Test. Performance on the WCST remained normal on all study visits.

Commentary

Although Dr. G had an unambiguously abnormal neurocognitive exam in February 1999, there are indications of worsening cognitive/motor performance even before that. His monotonic decline in performance on the SDMT was particularly striking, and similar to that reported in early symptomatic cases (Ho et al., 2003). This patient was not formally diagnosed until September 2000, although it is clear that he had been displaying subtle motor abnormalities for at least 4 years.

Dr. G's first Longitudinal Cohort Study testing (February 1999) was at a time when his QNE was only 10 and he was not yet formally diagnosed as affected. Nonetheless, he displayed striking impairments in new learning and memory. This is consistent with the findings of Solomon and colleagues (2007) from a multi-center cohort of mutation-positive and very mildly symptomatic, but not-yet-diagnosed mutation-carriers. Other research, including a meta-analysis by Zakzanis (1998), also suggests that HD patients differ most

Table 54-2. Clinical Ratings and Neuropsychological Exam Scores for Patient I. G.

	August 1992	June 1994	April 1995	October 1996	October 1997	February 1999	September 2000
Age	25	27	28	29	30	32	33
Quantified Neurological Exam	0	2	5	12	12	10	12
Mini-Mental State Exam	29	30	28	28	29	29	30
HD-ADL Scale[1]							24
Irritability Scale[2]							23
Apathy Scale[2]							22
Hamilton Depression Scale						1	6
NEUROPSYCHOLOGICAL EXAMINATIONS							
Grooved Pegboard Test							
Dominant hand time	59	52	59	56	60	62	66
Nondominant hand time	59	59	64	60	60	76*	79
Symbol Digit Modalities Test (written trial)	49	44	42	42	33	33**	32
Brief Test of Attention	20	18	19	19	15	18	18
Controlled Oral Word Association Test						38	36
Developmental Test of Visual-Motor Integration, raw						22	23
Hopkins Verbal Learning Test							
Total of Recall Trials	26	24	30	31	31	27*	25
Delayed Recall[3]	N/A	N/A	N/A	N/A	N/A	8***	9
Recognition Discrimination	11	10	12	11	12	10**	11
Hopkins Board[4]							
Errors to Criterion						3***	5
Trials to Criterion						6***	6
Delayed Recall of Items						9	9
Delayed Recall of Locations						7***	7
Trail-Making Test							
Part A time	19	17	26	27	27	25	31
Part B time	59	54	69	82	45	64	77
Stroop Color-Word Test							
Word T-score	43	37	40	39	36	37*	31
Color T-score	37	41	39	38	37	33*	32
Color-Word T-score	48	46	46	40	40	40*	46
Interference T-score	56	54	54	49	51	52	61
Wisconsin Card-Sorting Test							
Cards Used	71	73	70	73	74		73
Sorts Achieved	6	6	6	6	6		6
Inefficiency (Cards/Sort)	11.83	12.17	11.67	12.17	12.33		12.17

Note. The patient's first five neuropsychological exams were as a participant in the Presymptomatic Genetic Testing Study. His positive genetic test result was disclosed in April 1993, he entered the Longitudinal Cohort Study in February 1999, and was diagnosed with Huntington disease in September 2000. The two research studies have overlapping, but nonidentical neuropsychological protocols. His scores from the 1999 visit are compared to a group of 21 mutation-negative control subjects matched in age (+ 3 years) and education (all college graduates or more).

[1]Rothlind et al. (1993).

[2]Burns et al. (1990).

[3]Prior to November 1998, the original Hopkins Verbal Learning Test (HVLT) (Brandt, 1991) was administered. This version did not include delayed recall; the yes/no recognition trial followed immediately the third free recall trial. After November 1998, the HVLT-R (Brandt & Benedict, 2001) was administered & Benedict, 2001) was administered.

[4]Brandt et al. (2005).

*1 SD below average for age and education.

**2 SD below average for age and education.

***3 SD below average for age and education.

from normal subjects in delayed recall and memory acquisition.

Dr. G also performed 2 SDs below normal on the yes/no recognition trial of the HVLT-R. This finding is consistent with data from several studies that call into question the widely held belief that recognition performance is intact in HD and other subcortical dementias (Brandt, Corwin, & Krafft, 1992; Lang, Majer, Balan, & Reischies, 2000; Montoya et al., 2006). Dr. G also displayed greater impairment in recall of spatial locations than recall of items on the Hopkins Board. This pattern is typical of HD and is unlike that seen in normal aging, Alzheimer disease, or Parkinson disease (Brandt et al., 2005). It may suggest greater parietal lobe dysfunction in HD, either directly or indirectly, than generally appreciated.

Patient I. G. had a long history of emotional difficulties that preceded the emergence of motor signs of HD. This can undoubtedly be attributed in large part to the extremely adverse circumstances of his early childhood and the severe physical and emotional abuse he endured (Duisterhof, Trijsburg, Niermeijer, Roos, & Tibben, 2001). However, affective disturbance in the offspring of HD patients may also be a very early manifestation of the disease itself (Folstein, Franz, Jensen, Chase, & Folstein, 1983). Consistent with most studies, there was no indication that I. G.'s cognitive or emotional well-being was affected adversely by disclosure of his genetic test results in the context of our highly structured research protocol (Codori & Brandt, 1994; Codori, Slavney, Young, Miglioretti, & Brandt, 1997; Duisterhof et al., 2001; Wiggins et al., 1992).

Discussion

The two patients described here were both neuropsychologists with considerable knowledge of the construction and performance requirements of neuropsychological tests, as well as actual test stimuli. Each had years of experience in test administration, scoring, and interpretation. Nonetheless, they both displayed very considerable performance deficits on many tests that are typically performed poorly by the average HD patient. Although we did not systematically assess the extent of T.Q.'s or I. G.'s familiarity or experience with each of the tests in our protocols, it appears that some very widely used neuropsychological tests, such as WAIS-R Block Design, SDMT, and Stroop Color-Word Test, retain their ability to detect cognitive decline even in experienced neuropsychologists. Common among these tests is their demand on speed of processing (although the same could be said of the TMT, which was less sensitive). Memory tests that are less universally known, such as the HVLT-R and Hopkins Board, are also extremely sensitive in early HD (Brandt et al., 1992, 2005; Solomon et al., 2007) and revealed deficits in both our patients. The WCST was performed normally by both patients at all study visits. The fact that performance on this test does not decline in longitudinal studies of HD (Ho et al., 2003; Snowden, Craufurd, Griffiths, Thomspons, & Neary, 2001; Ward et al., 2006) is consistent with the notion that the WCST's utility depends on its being encountered for the first time.

The cases of T. Q. and I. G. illustrate the difficulty in deciding when a person who is gradually becoming symptomatic from a neurodegenerative disease actually meets criteria for diagnosis. This may be particularly difficult in a disease like HD, where persons who carry the disease-causing genetic mutation can be identified and subjected to intense clinical scrutiny. Although standardized neurological exams, such as the QNE and the Unified Huntington's Disease Rating Scale (Huntington Study Group, 1996) have been developed and allow reliable elicitation and scoring of motor abnormalities, there are no agreed-upon criteria for caseness. The decision to make the diagnosis of HD remains a clinical judgment that considers life circumstances and the performance of role responsibilities in addition to signs and symptoms. The patients described here first showed minor motor signs of the illness 3–4 years prior to their receiving the diagnosis of HD.

Patient I. G. had a longer *huntingtin* mutation (50 CAG repeats) than patient T. Q. (43 repeats), and he also had earlier onset (age 33 at diagnosis versus age 44). This is consistent with the well-established negative correlation between size of the CAG expansion and age of clinical onset of HD (Andrew et al., 1993; Claes et al., 1995; Duyao, Ambrose, & Myers, 1993; Kieburtz et al., 1994; Stine et al., 1993). There is also mounting evidence that longer repeat length is associated with more rapid progression of illness (Brandt et al., 1996; Illarioshkin et al., 1994; Mahant, McCusker, Byth, Graham, & the Huntington Study Group, 2003). However, not all studies find this relationship (Kieburtz et al., 1994; Ward et al., 2006), and of the two cases described here, the patient with the *shorter* repeat length (T. Q.) appears to have had a more rapidly progressive course.

Among the other lessons that these case studies illustrate is that routine, clinical readings of brain MRI scans often fail to reveal abnormalities in early-stage HD (Walker, 2007). This is in spite of the fact that studies of brain morphology using quantitative MRI scans, and positron emission tomography (PET) and functional magnetic resonance imaging (fMRI) studies of brain metabolic activity, reveal unambiguous striatal, cortical, and white matter changes in early HD and in some presymptomatic cases (Aylward et al., 2004; Ciarmiello et al., 2006; Paulsen et al., 2004; Rosas, Feigin, & Hersch, 2004; Rosas et al., 2005). Clinical brain imaging in early HD is probably most valuable in ruling out other neuropathological entities.

The two neuropsychologists with HD described in this chapter exemplify many of the clinical features of this neurodegenerative disease. Their serial neurocognitive testing reveals the clinical utility of these assessment procedures even in patients with extensive knowledge of, and experience in, clinical neuropsychological methods.

Acknowledgments

The authors gratefully acknowledge the collaboration of the many faculty and staff of the Baltimore Huntington's Disease Project at the Johns Hopkins University School of Medicine (Christopher Ross, M.D., Ph.D., principal investigator). This work was supported by grant NS16375 from the National Institute on Neurological Disorders and Stroke, and a Center of Excellence Award from the Huntington's Disease Society of America.

Disclosure

Dr. Brandt receives royalty income from Psychological Assessment Resources, Inc. on sales of the Hopkins Verbal Learning Test-Revised, one of the neuropsychological tests described in this chapter. This relationship is managed by the Johns Hopkins University in accordance with its conflict of interest policies.

References

Andrew, S. E., Goldberg, Y. P., Kremer, B., Telenius, H., Theilmann, J., Adam, S., et al. (1993). The relationship between trinucleotide (CAG) repeat length and clinical features of Huntington's disease. *Nature Genetics, 4,* 398–403.

Aylward, E. H., Sparks, B. F., Field, K. M., Yallapragada, V., Shpritz, B. D., Rosenblatt, A., et al. (2004). Onset and rate of striatal atrophy in preclinical Huntington disease. *Neurology, 63,* 66–72.

Brandt, J. (1991). The Hopkins Verbal Learning Test: Development of a new memory test with six equivalent forms. *The Clinical Neuropsychologist, 5,* 125–142.

Brandt, J. (2008). Huntington's disease. In I. Grant & K. Adams (Eds.), *Neuropsychological assessment in neuropsychiatric disorders* (3rd ed., pp. 223–240). New York: Oxford University Press, 2009.

Brandt, J., & Benedict, R. H. B. (2001). *The Hopkins Verbal Learning Test—Revised professional manual.* Odessa, FL: Psychological Assessment Resources, Inc.

Brandt, J., & Butters, N. (1986). The neuropsychology of Huntington's disease. *Trends in Neuroscience, 9,* 118–120.

Brandt, J., Bylsma, F. W., Gross, R., Stine, O. C., Ranen, N., & Ross, C. A. (1996). Trinucleotide repeat length and clinical progression in Huntington's disease. *Neurology, 46,* 527–531.

Brandt, J., Corwin, J., & Krafft, L. (1992). Is verbal recognition memory really different in Alzheimer's and Huntington's disease? *Journal of Clinical and Experimental Neuropsychology, 14,* 773–784.

Brandt, J., Folstein, S. E., & Folstein, M. F. (1988). Differential cognitive impairment in Alzheimer's disease and Huntington's disease. *Annals of Neurology, 23,* 555–561.

Brandt, J., Inscore, A. B., Ward, J., Shpritz, B., Rosenblatt, A., Margolis, R. L., & Ross, C. A. (2008). Neuropsychological deficits in Huntington's disease gene carriers and correlates of early "conversion". *Journal of Neuropsychiatry and Clinical Neurosciences 20,* 466–472.

Brandt, J., Quaid, K. A., Folstein, S. E., Garber, P. A., Maestri, N. E., Abbott, M. H., et al. (1989). Presymptomatic diagnosis of delayed-onset disease with linked DNA markers: The experience in Huntington's disease. *Journal of the American Medical Association, 261,* 3108–3114.

Brandt, J., Shpritz, B., Codori, A. M., Margolis, R., & Rosenblatt, A. (2002). Neuropsychological manifestations of the genetic mutation for Huntington's disease in presymptomatic individuals. *Journal of the International Neuropsychological Society, 8*, 918–924.

Brandt, J. Shpritz, B., Munro, C.A., Marsh, L., & Rosenblatt, A. (2005). Differential impairment of spatial location memory in Huntington's disease. *Journal of Neurology, Neurosurgery and Psychiatry, 76*, 1516–1519.

Brinkman, R. R., Mezei, M. M., Theilmann, J., Almqvist, E., & Hayden, M. R. (1997). The likelihood of being affected with Huntington's disease by a particular age, for a specific CAG size. *American Journal of Human Genetics, 60*, 1202–1210.

Burns, A., Folstein, S., Brandt, J., & Folstein, M. (1990). Clinical assessment of irritability, aggression, and apathy in Huntington's and Alzheimer's disease. *Journal of Nervous and Mental Disease, 178*, 20–26.

Campodonico, J. R., Aylward, E., Codori, A. M., Young, C., Krafft, L., Magdalinski, M., Ranen, N., Slavney, P., & Brandt, J. (1998). When does Huntington's disease begin? *Journal of the International Neuropsychological Society, 4*, 467–473.

Caramazza, A., & McCloskey, M. (1988). The case for single-patient studies. *Cognitive Neuropsychology, 5*, 517–528.

Chatterjee, A., Anderson, K. E., Moskowitz, C. B., Hauser, W. A., & Marder, K. S. (2005). A comparison of self-report and caregiver assessment of depression, apathy, and irritability in Huntington's disease. *Journal of Neuropsychiatry and Clinical Neurosciences, 17*, 378–383.

Ciarmiello, A., Cannella, M., Lastoria, S., Simonelli, M., Frati, L., Rubinsztein, D. C., & Squiteri, F. (2006). Brain white-matter volume loss and glucose hypometabolism precede the clinical symptoms of Huntington's disease. *Journal of Nuclear Medicine, 47*, 215–222.

Claes, S., van Zand, K., Legius, E., Dom, R., Malfoid, M., Baro, F., et al. (1995). Correlations between triplet repeat expansion and clinical features in Huntington's disease. *Archives of Neurology, 113*, 749–753.

Code, C., Wallesch, C-W., Joanette, Y., & Lecours, A. R. (Eds.). (1996). *Classic cases in neuropsychology.* East Sussex, England.: Psychology Press.

Code, C., Wallesch, C-W., Joanette, Y., & Lecours, A. R. (Eds.). (2003). *Classic cases in neuropsychology* (Vol. 2). East Sussex, England.: Psychology Press.

Codori, A. M., & Brandt, J. (1994). Psychological costs and benefits of predictive testing for Huntington's disease. *American Journal of Medical Genetics, 54*, 174–184.

Codori, A. M., Slavney, P. R., Young, C., Miglioretti, D. L., & Brandt, J. (1997). Predictors of psychological adjustment to genetic testing for Huntington's disease. *Health Psychology, 16*, 36–50.

Duisterhof, M., Trijsburg, R. W., Niermeijer, M. F., Roos, R. A. C., & Tibben, A. (2001). Psychological studies in Huntington's disease: Making up the balance. *Journal of Medical Genetics, 38*, 852–861.

Duyao, M. P., Ambrose, C. M., & Myers, R. H. (1993). Trinucleotide repeat length: Instability and age of onset in Huntington's disease. *Nature Genetics, 4*, 387–392.

Folstein, S. E. (1989). *Huntington's disease: A disorder of families.* Baltimore: Johns Hopkins University Press.

Folstein, S. E., Franz, M. L., Jensen, B. A., Chase, G. A., & Folstein, M. F. (1983). Conduct disorder and affective disorder among the offspring of patients with Huntington's disease. *Psychological Medicine, 13*, 45–52.

Folstein, S. E., Jensen, B., Leigh, R. J., & Folstein, M. F. (1983). The measurement of abnormal movement: Methods developed for Huntington disease. *Neurobehavioral Toxicology and Teratology, 5*, 605–609.

Grant, I. (2008, February 8). *On the emerging role of neuropsychology in understanding brain effects of medical illnesses: Example of HIV.* Presidential address to the Annual Meeting of the International Neuropsychological Society, Waikoloa, Hawaii.

Guilmette, T. J., Faust, D., Hart, K., & Arkes, H. R. (1990). A national survey of psychologists who offer neuropsychological services. *Archives of Clinical Neuropsychology, 5*, 373–392.

Gusella, J. F., Wexler, N. S., Conneally, P. M., Naylor, S. L., Anderson, M. A., Tanzi, R. E., et al. (1983). A polymorphic DNA marker genetically linked to Huntington's disease. *Nature, 306*, 234–238.

Harper, P. S. (1996). *Huntington Disease.* London: W.B. Saunders.

Ho, A. K., Sahakian, B. J., Brown, R. G., Barker, R. A., Hodges, J. R., Ane, M. N., et al. (2003). Profile of cognitive progression in early Huntington's disease. *Neurology, 61*, 1702–1706.

Huntington's Disease Collaborative Research Group. (1993). A novel gene containing a trinucleotide repeat that is expanded and unstable on Huntington's disease chromosomes. *Cell, 72*, 971–983.

Huntington Study Group. (1996). Unified Huntington's Disease Rating Scale: Reliability and consistency. *Movement Disorders, 11*, 136–142.

Illarioshkin, S. N., Igarashi, S., Onodera, O., Markova, E. D., Nikolskaya, N. N., Tanaka, H., et al. (1994). Trinucleotide repeat length and rate of progression of Huntington's disease. *Annals of Neurology, 36*, 630–635.

Jaspers, K. (1997). *General psychopathology*. (J. Hoenig & M. W. Hamilton, Trans.). Baltimore: Johns Hopkins University Press.

Josiassen, R. C., Curry, L. M., & Mancall, E. L. (1983). Development of neuropsychological deficits in Huntington's disease. *Archives of Neurology, 40*, 791–796.

Josiassen, R. C., Curry, L., Roemer, R. A., DeBease, C., & Mancall, E. L. (1982). Patterns of intellectual deficit in Huntington's disease. *Journal of Clinical Neuropsychology, 4*, 173–183.

Kapur, N. (Ed.). (1997). *Injured brains of medical minds: Views from within*. Oxford, England: Oxford University Press.

Kieburtz, K., MacDonald, M., Shih, C., Feigin, A., Steinberg, K., Bordwell, K., et al. (1994). Trinucleotide repeat length and progression of illness in Huntington's disease. *Journal of Medical Genetics, 31*, 872–874.

Kirkwood, S. C., Siemers, E., Stout, J. C., Hodes, M. E., Conneally, P. M., Christian, J. C., & Foroud, T. (1999). Longitudinal cognitive and motor changes among presymptomatic Huntington disease gene carriers. *Archives of Neurology, 56*, 563–568.

Lang, C. J. G., Majer, M., Balan, P., & Reischies, F. M. (2000). Recall and recognition in Huntington's disease. *Archives of Clinical Neuropsychology, 15*, 361–371.

Mahant, N., McCusker, E. A., Byth, K., Graham, S., & the Huntington Study Group. (2003). Huntington's disease: Clinical correlates of disability and progression. *Neurology, 61*, 1085–1092.

McHugh, P. R., & Slavney, P. R. (1998). *The Perspectives of Psychiatry* (2nd ed.). Baltimore: Johns Hopkins University Press.

Mohr, E., Brouwers, P., Claus, J. J., Mann, U. M., Fedio, P., & Chase, T. N. (1991). Visuospatial cognition in Huntington's disease. *Movement Disorders, 6*, 127–132.

Montoya, A. Pelletier, M., Menear, M., Duplessis, E., Richer, F., & Lepage, M. (2006). Episodic memory impairment in Huntington's disease: A meta-analysis. *Neuropsychologia, 44*, 1984–1994.

Naarding, P., Kremer, H. P. H., & Zitman, F. G. (2001). Huntington's disease: A review of the literature on prevalence and treatment of neuropsychiatric phenomena. *European Psychiatry, 16*, 439–445.

Paulsen, J. S., & Conybeare, R. A. (2005). Cognitive changes in Huntington's disease. *Advances in Neurology, 96*, 209–225.

Paulsen, J. S., Ready, R. E., Hamilton, J. M., Mega, M. S., & Cummings, J. L. (2001). Neuropsychiatric aspects of Huntington's disease. *Journal of Neurology, Neurosurgery and Psychiatry, 71*, 310–314.

Paulsen, J. S., Zhao, H., Stout, J. C., Brinkman, R. R., Guttman, M., Ross, C. A., et al. (2001). Clinical markers of early disease in persons near onset of Huntington's disease. *Neurology, 57*, 658–662.

Paulsen, J. S., Zimbelman, J. L., Hinton, S. C., Langbehn, D. R., Leveroni, C. L., Benjamin, M. L., et al. (2004). fMRI biomarker of early neuronal dysfunction in presymptomatic Huntington's disease. *American Journal of Neuroradiology, 25*, 1715–1721.

Rabin, L. A., Barr, W. B., & Burton, L. A. (2005). Assessment practices of clinical neuropsychologists in the United States and Canada: A survey of INS, NAN, and APA Division 40 members. *Archives of Clinical Neuropsychology, 20*, 33–65.

Rebok, G. W., Bylsma, F. W., Keyl, P. M., Brandt, J., & Folstein, S. E. (1995). Automobile driving in Huntington's disease. *Movement Disorders, 10*, 778–787.

Rosas, H. D., Feigin, A. S., & Hersch, S. M. (2004). Using advances in neuroimaging to detect, understand, and monitor disease progression in Huntington's disease. *NeuroRx, 1*, 263–272.

Rosas, H. D., Hevelone, N. D., Zaleta, A. K., Greve, D. N., Dalat, D. H., & Fischl, B. (2005). Regional cortical thinning in preclinical Huntington disease and its relationship to cognition. *Neurology, 65*, 745–747.

Rosenblatt, A., Ranen, N. G., Nance, M. A., & Paulsen, J. S. (1999). *A physician's guide to the management of Huntington's disease*. New York: Huntington's Disease Society of America.

Ross, C. A. (2002). Polyglutamine pathogenesis: Emergence of unifying mechanisms for Huntington's disease and related disorders. *Neuron, 35*, 819–822.

Ross, C. A., & Margolis, R. L. (2001). Huntington's disease. *Clinical Neuroscience Research, 1*, 142–152.

Rothlind, J. C., & Brandt, J. (1993). A brief assessment of frontal and subcortical functions in dementia. *Journal of Neuropsychiatry and Clinical Neurosciences, 5*, 73–77.

Rothlind, J. C., Bylsma, F. W., Peyser, C., Folstein, S. E., & Brandt, J. (1993). Cognitive and motor correlates of everyday functioning in early Huntington's disease. *Journal of Nervous and Mental Disease, 181*, 194–199.

Snowden, J., Craufurd, D., Griffiths, H., Thompson, J., & Neary, D. (2001). Longitudinal evaluation of cognitive disorder in Huntington's disease. *Journal of the International Neuropsychological Society, 7*, 33–44.

Snowden, J. S., Craufurd, D., Thompson, J., & Neary, D. (2002). Psychomotor, executive, and memory function in preclinical Huntington's disease. *Journal of Clinical and Experimental Neuropsychology, 24*, 133–145.

Solomon, A. C., Stout, J. C., Johnson, S. A., Langbehn, D. R., Aylward, E. A., Brandt, J., Ross, C. A., et al. (2007). Verbal episodic memory declines prior to diagnosis in Huntington's disease. *Neuropsychologia, 45*, 1767–1776.

Stine, O. C., Pleasant, N., Franz, M. L., Abbott, M. H., Folstein, S. E., & Ross, C. A. (1993). Correlation between onset age of Huntington's disease and the length of the trinucleotide repeat in IT-15. *Human Molecular Genetics, 2*, 1547–1549.

Strauss, M. E., & Brandt, J. (1986). Attempt at preclinical identification of Huntington's disease using the WAIS. *Journal of Clinical and Experimental Neuropsychology, 8*, 210–218.

Vonsattel, J. P., Myers, R. H., Stevens, T. J., Ferrante, R. J., Bird, E. D., & Richardson, E. P., Jr. (1985). Neuropathological classification of Huntington's disease. *Journal of Neuropathology and Experimental Neurology, 44*, 559–577.

Walker, F. O. (2007). Huntington's disease. *Lancet, 369*, 218–228.

Ward, J., Sheppard, J-M., Shpritz, B., Margolis, R. L., Rosenblatt, A., & Brandt, J. (2006). A four-year prospective study of cognitive functioning in Huntington's disease. *Journal of the International Neuropsychological Society, 12*, 445–454.

Wiggins, S., Whyte, P., Huggins, M., Adam, S., Theilmann, J., Bloch, M., et al. (1992). The psychological consequences of predictive tetsting for Huntington's disease. *New England Journal of Medicine, 327*, 1401–1405.

Zakzanis, K. K. (1998). The subcortical dementia of Huntington's disease. *Journal of Clinical and Experimental Neuropsychology, 20*, 565–578.

55

Cognitive and Behavioral Impairment in Amyotrophic Lateral Sclerosis

Beth K. Rush

Amyotrophic lateral sclerosis (ALS) is a primary neurodegenerative disease affecting both upper and lower motor neurons. In the United States, approximately 5600 people are diagnosed with ALS each year, with up to 30,000 people carrying the diagnosis of ALS at any one point in time. Amyotrophic lateral sclerosis most commonly strikes between the ages of 40 and 70 years, with average age of disease onset at age 55. Mean survival time is 2 to 5 years from diagnosis, with considerable interperson variability in disease course. The majority of ALS cases are sporadic. Only 5%–10% of all cases in the United States are familial or hereditary. Several causative genes are linked to hereditary ALS, but the most frequently observed genetic marker associated with familial ALS is the SOD1 mutation.

In 60% of cases, ALS onset is heralded by muscle weakness in the upper or lower limbs, or in the muscles supporting speech, swallowing, and breathing. Speech intelligibility can diminish as a function of degeneration of upper motor neuron speech areas, progressive weakness of bulbar muscles, and/or as a function of diminished air resonance owing to respiratory muscle weakness. Advancing disease can result in dyspnea, hypoxemia, and eventual ventilatory failure. Motor impairments, communication limitations, and deteriorating pulmonary function result in increasing functional dependence with disease progression. As such, there is greater reliance on caregivers and assistive devices over time.

Patients with ALS are frequently told that the disease usually spares cognition (e.g., Abe, 2000; Leavitt, 2002). An association between ALS and cognitive impairment was first proposed in the 1800s, but only recently have studies consistently documented the possibility of progressive cognitive impairment in parallel to progressive motor impairment (Murphy, Henry, & Lomen-Hoerth, 2007). The prevalence of cognitive impairment in ALS is difficult to calculate as estimates vary depending on whether cases of cognitive impairment without dementia are considered in addition to cases manifesting fully developed dementia. The most liberal estimates suggest a prevalence of cognitive impairment in up to 50% of patients with ALS, with sporadic and familial cases equally affected.

Executive functions are commonly compromised, but a continuum of cognitive and behavioral impairments has been observed, implicating disturbance in both the frontal and temporal lobes of the brain (Murphy, Henry, & Lomen-Hoerth, 2007). The cognitive impairment of ALS appears to share the same variability as the cognitive impairment associated with frontal temporal lobar degeneration (FTLD; Neary et al., 1998) and can include behavioral variant, semantic dementia (SD), and progressive nonfluent aphasia (PNFA) subtypes of FTLD. In a study specifically investigating dementia subtypes in 23 ALS patients, 6 patients met criteria for a dementia syndrome (Murphy et al., 2007). One of these six cases demonstrated cognitive deficits consistent with Alzheimer dementia, and five of these cases demonstrated cognitive deficits consistent with FTLD. Interestingly, of the five cases revealing FTLD-like deficits, two met criteria for behavioral variant, two met criteria for the SD variant, and one met criteria for PNFA variant. Thus, the cognitive and behavioral impairment observed in ALS may not be exclusively associated with a behavioral variant syndrome.

It is only recently that neuropsychologists have become involved in ALS patient care (Miller et al., 2009). Neuropsychologists are now asked to screen for cognitive impairment in ALS and to make recommendations to the patient care team at different stages of the illness on the basis of the type of cognitive deficits revealed with each screening evaluation. The role of the neuropsychological evaluation in ALS patient care is of both scientific and clinical importance. Scientifically, frontal temporal cognitive impairment likely has implications for disease progression and how to understand phenotypes of both ALS and FTLD. Practically, it remains controversial as to whether the presence of cognitive impairment in ALS suggests a different course of disease progression. The presence of cognitive impairment has important implications for patient independence, patient care decisions, and family education and management of the patient's condition. A "one-size fits all" approach to ALS care and intervention frequently frustrates patients, families, and care providers. Appropriate screening of cognitive status in ALS is essential to understanding the extent of the illness and to dynamically tailoring interventions for the patient, family, and the ALS patient care team as the patient's illness advances. This can ultimately minimize frustration for the patient as well as the entire care team surrounding the patient.

The Case of Mr. Doe

A neurologist specializing in neuromuscular disease consulted the author for a neuropsychological evaluation of Mr. Doe, who was undergoing diagnostic evaluation following a 2-year history of progressive speech and swallowing difficulty. At the time of the neuropsychological evaluation, Mr. Doe was a 55-year-old, right-handed, Caucasian man with 12 years of education. He and his son owned a custom construction business. Mr. Doe described a 6–12-month history of progressive short-term memory decline.

He would ask his son the same questions repeatedly throughout the day. He set out to do multiple errands in a day and forgot to complete half of what he intended. Over the prior 18 months, he had developed a slur in his speech and was having more difficulty finding his words in conversation. Although he remained independent with most activities and continued to work full time in his business, his wife was beginning to question his judgment with driving. There had been a few occasions when Mr. Doe tried to pull out in front of an oncoming car without recognition of his poor timing.

Mr. Doe had a 20-year history of upper extremity fasiculations. Interestingly, his son, 30 years his junior, demonstrated similar upper extremity fasiculations that had also been present for several years. Although the fasiculations remained relatively stable over time for Mr. Doe, over the prior 24 months, he began demonstrating weakness and "tremors" in his hands, as well as cramping in both arms and in his left leg and foot. Fortunately, he had not had any falls. He reported that his nighttime sleep was restful, although he was fatigued during the day. His wife commented that he seemed to "sign and moan" during sleep and that on a few occasions he had such severe coughing spells that he could not seem to catch his breath. Also in the prior 24 months, Mr. Doe had developed reduced appetite secondary to swallowing difficulty. Typically, he was regurgitating during most meals and most recently he had begun to experience coughing spells after eating. He was seen in an emergency room for this problem and was prescribed Clonazepam because his coughing spells were thought to represent panic attacks.

Mr. Doe denied depression or anxiety at the time of the evaluation, but he was very concerned about his illness. Over the last year, he had been evaluated at several outside medical institutions by several neurologists. He was becoming increasingly concerned about his capacity to work. He had no prior history of depression or other psychiatric symptoms. He was concerned not just for himself but also for the prognosis of his son.

Mr. Doe had two maternal aunts with myasthenia gravis but no other known family medical history of similar symptoms. He had been told by outside neurologists that his differential diagnosis included motor neuron disease, Kennedy's disease, and myasthenia gravis. His presentation was somewhat unusual for ALS in that he had a 20-year history of relatively stable (nonprogressive) upper extremity fasiculations. Only recently had the quality of his fasiculations started to change and did Mr. Doe begin to experience associated cramping in his upper extremities. Genetic testing for Kennedy's disease was negative. A few days prior to his neuropsychological evaluation, Mr. Doe underwent a comprehensive neurologic exam, an electromyelogram (EMG), a magnetic resonance imaging (MRI) study, and a positron emission tomography (PET) scan. He also underwent genetic testing for the SOD-1 mutation. The neurologic exam revealed fasiculations, muscle atrophy and weakness compatible with lower motor neuron disease, and bilateral Hoffman signs compatible with upper motor neuron disease. The EMG documented lower motor neuron disease. The MRI revealed age-disproportionate, mild cortical atrophy, nonspecific white matter change in the bilateral frontal, parietal, and occipital lobes, yet there were no abnormalities noted in the pyramidal tract. The PET scan was interpreted as a normal study with no focal areas of atypical metabolism. Mr. Doe was negative for the SOD-1 mutation.

Examination Results

During the neuropsychological evaluation, Mr. Doe was grossly oriented to person, place, time, and the purpose of the evaluation. The patient's longstanding level of cognitive function was estimated to be high average using the Reading Recognition subtest of the Wide Range Achievement Test–3 (WRAT-3).

Given that this was an initial evaluation, and that results would likely serve as a baseline to judge all future comparisons, the Mattis Dementia Rating Scale–2 (DRS-2) was administered to evaluate Mr. Doe across several cognitive domains commonly affected in the context of dementia.[1] Mr. Doe's overall score on the DRS-2 was mildly impaired. He had the greatest difficulty on the subtests requiring verbal fluency, attention, and memory.

There was variability evidenced across subtests of attention administered (Digit Span, Arithmetic, and Picture Completion subtests from the WAIS-3). He demonstrated slowed processing with numerical sequencing on Trails A.

Clear evidence of executive dysfunction resulted from the administration of Trails B, the Wisconsin Card Sorting Test (WCST), and the Frontal Assessment Battery (FAB). Speed of alternation and mental flexibility on Trails B was slowed. He struggled to achieve three categories on the WCST and tended to perseverate on problem-solving strategies despite receiving feedback to alternate his approach. On the FAB, he lost points for abstract verbal reasoning, phonemic fluency, learning a motor program, and withholding a previously relevant motor response.

Although confrontation naming and praxis were intact on language testing, verbal fluency was markedly slow, regardless of whether he generated with lexical or semantic cues.

Visual spatial and visual constructional skills were largely intact as evidenced by Judgment of Line Orientation and WAIS-3 Block Design performances. His reproduction of the Rey-Osterrieth Complex Figure reflected an accurate account of the gestalt with accurate placement of details, but his approach to the drawing was disorganized and piecemeal, suggesting significant difficulties with planning his approach to the task.

Although there was evidence of subtle problems with learning on the CVLT-2 and WMS-3 Logical Memory, there was no evidence for difficulty with memory retention or memory retrieval.

Mr. Doe acknowledged concern about his medical situation and cognitive symptoms, but he denied the presence of clinical depression, suicidal ideation, or suicidal intent when completing the Beck Depression Inventory–2.

Discussion

Mr. Doe's neuropsychological profile revealed mild to moderate impairments in problem solving, mental flexibility, and speeded word retrieval with slight inefficiencies in attention and processing speed. In contrast, memory retention, visual spatial skills, visual constructional skills, and naming skills were well preserved. Although Mr. Doe and his family were concerned about his memory, evaluation findings suggested that rather than rapid forgetting, subjectively reported "memory" problems were likely the result of difficulty maintaining mental set, diminished problem-solving ability, and difficulty remaining flexible with thinking during the day.

Mr. Doe's cognitive performance was clearly below estimates of his longstanding level of function. This, taken with his report of a progressive cognitive decline over the prior year, suggested a neurodegenerative etiology to his cognitive impairment. At the time of the evaluation, Mr. Doe remained independent with all activities of daily living and continued to work full time in his own business. For this reason, he did not meet clinical criteria for a dementia. That said, the neuropsychological profile was worrisome and suggested a prodrome of dementia with prominent frontal systems features.

Mr. Doe's presentation was explained to the patient, his family, and the ALS care team, including the neurologist, the speech language pathology team, the physical therapist, the occupational therapist, and the respiratory therapist. Given Mr. Doe's swallowing problems and evolving speech fluency problems, a consultation with Speech Language Pathology was recommended to review the range of compensatory strategies available that could increase safety with swallowing and maintain the functionality of Mr. Doe's expressive communication over time. Because Mr. Doe's wife had started to observe some changes in judgment while Mr. Doe was driving, a formal driving evaluation was recommended to ensure safe operation of a motor vehicle. Mr. Doe was encouraged to continue working, but to do so with oversight and collaboration from his son as to ensure that he appreciated any nuances of the work and could conduct the work safely (without harm to himself or to others). Mr. Doe was encouraged to make daily to-do lists that involved breaking up tasks with multiple steps into smaller tasks to complete throughout the day. The prodrome of dementia was discussed with the family at length. Mr. Doe and his family were encouraged to complete advanced directives, a living will, and to document other important preferences reflecting Mr. Doe's values so that the care team could remain respectful of his wishes throughout the course of his illness. The family was also provided with additional caregiver education resources through the ALS Association,

the Muscular Dystrophy Association, and The Association for Frontal Temporal Dementias.

In this case, as in other cases of other neurodegenerative disease, repeat neuropsychological evaluation was recommended in 6 to 9 months to further document cognitive trajectory and to revisit functional recommendations. Given that ALS disease course is accelerated compared to other neurodegenerative diseases resulting in dementia, traditional serial assessment intervals for tracking dementia course (such as 12 to 18 months in Alzheimer dementia) should be abbreviated in evaluation of ALS patients to ensure capture of dynamic changes in cognition and behavioral presentation that can markedly impact ALS care and intervention.

Although this case reflects a prodrome of a predominantly behavioral variant frontal temporal dementia, it is important to understand that cognitive impairment in the context of ALS can be quite variable. In many cases, it becomes important to screen for spelling errors, writing errors, and comprehension deficits, in addition to executive functions as progressive nonfluent aphasia and semantic dementia subtypes have also been observed in ALS cases. Quite often, these cognitive problems surface in the context of a care-related intervention with the patient. For example, a patient may be having unanticipated difficulty learning how to use an alternative augmentative communication (AAC) device in speech therapy, or the patient may decline to accept respiratory or feeding recommendations made by the care team even if the interventions are in line with the patient's wishes regarding long-term supportive care. Many times, care providers and family will inadvertently attribute these problems to depressive withdrawal or adjustment-related reactions to illness when the real problems are attributable to underlying language impairment or impairments in judgment and reasoning. It becomes important to use empirical testing through neuropsychological evaluation to generate clinical impressions of ALS patients so that cognitive and behavioral problems are not overlooked or misattributed to psychiatric factors.

Opportunities are abundant for neuropsychological evaluation of ALS patients. Routine and serial screening of cognitive and behavioral status in ALS patients can contribute to scientific

Table 55-1. Neuropsychological Test Data

Estimate of Premorbid Intellectual Function

WRAT–3 Reading (Wilkinson, 1993)

	Standard Score	Percentile
	111	77

Global Cognitive Function

Dementia Rating Scale (Lucas et al., 1998)

	Raw Score	MOANS SS
Attention	32/37	6
Initiation/Perseveration	30/37	4
Construction	6/6	10
Conceptualization	34/39	8
Memory	21/25	6
Total Score	123/144	5

Orientation/Attention/Processing Speed

WMS–3 Orientation: 13/14

WAIS–3 (Wechsler, 1997)	Raw Score	ACSS	Percentile
Digit Span	11	7	16
Arithmetic	15	11	63
Picture Completion	15	7	16
Trails A (Heaton et al., 2004)	42s; 0 err		16

Executive Function

	Raw Score	Percentile
Trails B (Heaton et al., 2004)	111s; 1 err	14

WCST (Heaton et al., 1993)	Raw Score	Percentile
Categories	3	6 - 10
Perseverative Responses	49	4
Set Failures	2	>16
Correct	62	
Errors	66	

Frontal Assessment Battery (Dubois et al., 2000)

	Raw Score
Similarities	1/3
Lexical Fluency	1/3
Motor Series Programming	2/3
Conflicting Instructions	3/3
Go-No-Go	1/3
Environmental Control	3/3
Total	11/18

Language Function

	Raw Score	Percentile
Boston Naming Test (Heaton et al., 2004)	56	62
COWAT (Tombaugh et al., 1999)	12	<1
Semantic Fluency (Monsch et al., 1994)	28	4
BDAE Praxis		
Natural Gestures	12/12	
Conventional Gestures	12/12	

(*Continued*)

Table 55-1. Neuropsychological Test Data (*Continued*)

Language Function

Use of Pretend Objects	24/24
Bucco-Facial/Respiratory Movements	12/12

Visual Spatial Function
Judgment of Line Orientation (Benton et al., 1983)

Raw Score	Percentile
30	86+

Rey Osterrieth Complex Figure (Meyers & Meyers, 1995)

Raw Score	Percentile
31.5	11–16

WAIS–3 Block Design (Wechsler, 1997)

Raw Score	Percentile
12	75

Memory Function
WMS–3 (Wechsler, 1993)

	Raw Score	ACSS
VR I	91	13
VR II	44	10
VR % Retention	48	9
LM I	28	7
LM II	17	9
LM % Retention	77	10

CVLT–2 Short Form (Delis et al., 2000)

3/7/6/6

	Raw Score	Percentile
Trial 1–4	22	16
L.D. Free Recall	6	50
Recognition Hits	9	69
False Positives	0	

Emotional Function

	Raw Score
BDI–2 (Beck, 1996)	9

understanding about the disease and its course. Information from a neuropsychological evaluation of an ALS patient can have an important impact on the direction and trajectory of ALS care and intervention at various stages of the advancing disease and illness.

Note

1. The lowest age of the Mayo Older Adult Normative Studies (MOANS) standardization group for the DRS-2 is age 56, so the MOANS DRS scores included in the test summary are actually based on a 56-year-old (Lucas et al., 1998).

References

Abe, K. (2000). Cognitive function in amyotrophic lateral sclerosis. *ALS and Other Motor Neuron Disorders, 1*, 343–347.

Beck, A. (1996). *Beck Depression Inventory—II.* New York: The Psychological Corporation.

Benton, A. L., Hamsher, K. D., Varney, N. R., & Spreen, O. (1983). *Contributions to neuropsychological assessment: a clinical manual.*

Delis, D. C., Kramer, J. H., Kaplan, E., & Ober, B. A. (2000). *California Verbal Learning Test—Second Edition (CVLT-II).* San Antonio, TX: Psychological Corporation.

Dubois, B., Slachevsky, A., Litvan, I., & Pillon, B. (2000). A frontal assessment battery at bedside. *Neurology* 55: 1621–1626.

Heaton, R. K., Chelune, G. J., Talley, J. L., Kay, G. G., & Curtiss, G. (1993). *Wisconsin Card Sorting Test Manual: Revised and expanded*. Odessa, FL: Psychological Assessment Resources.

Heaton, R. K., Miller, S. W., Taylor, M. J., & Grant, I. (2004). Revised comprehensive norms for an expanded Halstead–Reitan battery. Odessa, Florida: Psychological Assessment Resources.

Leavitt, B. K. (2002). Hereditary motor neuron disease caused by muations in the ALS2 gene: "The long and short of it." *Clinical Genetics, 62*, 265–269.

Lucas, J. A., Ivnik, R. J., Smith, G. E., Bohac, D. L., Tangalos, E. G., Kokmen, E., Graff-Radford, N. R., & Petersen, R. C. (1998). Normative data for the Mattis Dementia Rating Scale. *Journal of Clinical and Experimental Neuropsychology, 20,* 536–547.

Meyers, J. E., & Meyers, K. R. (1995). *Rey Complex Figure Test and Recognition Trial: Professional manual.* Odessa, Florida: Psychological Assessment Resource.

Miller, R. G., Jackson, C. E., Kasarskis, E. J., England, J. D., Forshew, D., Johnston, W., Kalra, S., Katz, J. S., Mitsumoto, H., Rosenfeld, J., Shoesmith, C., Strong, M. J., Woolley, S. C. & the Quality Standards Subcommittee of the American Academy of Neurology. (2009). Practice parameter update: The care of the patient with amyotrophic lateral sclerosis: Multidisciplinary care, symptom management, and cognitive/behavioral impairment (an evidence-based review): Report of the Quality Standards Subcommittee of the American Academy of Neurology. Neurology, 73, 1227–1233.

Miller, R. G., Rosenberg, J. A., Gerlinas, D. F., Mitsumoto, H., Newman, D., Sufit, R., Borasio, G. D., Bradley, W. G., Bromberg, M. B., Brooks, B. R., Kasarskis, E. J., Munsat, T. L., and

Oppenheimer, E. A. (1999). Practice parameter: The care of the patient with amyotrophic lateral sclerosis (an evidence-based review): Report of the Quality Standards Subcommittee of the American Academy of Neurology. *Neurology* 52: 1311–1329.

Monsch, A.U., Bondi, M.W., Butters, N., Paulsen, J.S., Salmon, D.P., Brugger, P., & Swenson, M.R. (1994). A comparison of category and letter fluency in Alzheimer's disease and Huntington's disease. *Neuropsychology* 8: 25–30.

Murphy, J. M., Henry, R. G., Langmore, S., Kramer, J. H., Miller, B. L., & Lomen-Hoerth, C. (2007). Continuum of frontal lobe impairment in amyotrophic lateral sclerosis. *Archives of Neurology, 64,* 530–534.

Murphy, J., Henry, R., & Lomen-Hoerth, C. (2007). Establishing subtypes of frontal lobe impairment in amyotrophic lateral sclerosis. *Archives of Neurology, 64,* 330–334.

Neary, D., Snowden, J. S., Gustafson, L., Passant, U., Stuss, D., Black, S., Freedman, M., Kertesz, A., Robert, P. H., Albert, M., Boone, K., Miller, B. L., Cummings, J., & Benson, D. F. (1998). Frontotemporal lobar degeneration: A consensus on clinical diagnostic criteria. *Neurology, 51,* 1546–1554.

Tombaugh, T. N., Kozak, J., & Rees, L. (1999). Normative data stratified by age and education for two measures of verbal fluency: FAS and animal naming. *Archives of Clinical Neuropsychology* 14: 167–177.

Wechsler, D. (1993). *WMS-III administration and scoring manual.* San Antonio, TX: The Psychological Corporation.

Wechsler, D. (1997). *WAIS-III administration and scoring manual.* San Antonio, TX: The Psychological Corporation.

Wilkinson, G. S. (1993). *The Wide Range Achievement Test: Manual.* Third Edition. Wilmington, DE: Wide Range; 1993.

56

Progressive Supranuclear Palsy

Alexander I. Tröster and Rebecca C. Williams

Progressive supranuclear palsy (PSP), also known as Steele-Richardson-Olszewski syndrome, was first described in 1964 (Steele, Richardson, & Olszewski, 1964), with little modification since to its original clinical description. Its symptoms often lead to a misdiagnosis of Parkinson disease (PD). Indeed, it was recently suggested that there are two clinical phenotypes of PSP (Williams et al., 2005): one called Richardson syndrome (characterized by early gait instability and falls, supranuclear vertical gaze palsy, and cognitive dysfunction), and another called PSP-parkinsonism, closely resembling Parkinson disease (with asymmetric onset of motor symptoms, tremor, and moderate initial response to levodopa). Traditionally, PSP's defining clinical features include postural instability, in which the patient presents with seemingly inexplicable falls that happen in the first year of symptom onset; axial rigidity; slowing of vertical saccades and vertical supranuclear gaze palsy (downgaze is affected before upgaze); and pseudobulbar palsy (e.g., dysphagia, dysarthria, and paroxysmal movements of the tongue or jaw, pseudobulbar affect) (Lubarsky & Juncos, 2008; Pearce, 2007; Santacruz, Uttl, Litvan, & Grafman, 1998). Survival is reported to be only 6–7 years from onset (Santacruz et al., 1998), with few patients living beyond 14 years.

Progressive supranuclear palsy involves tau protein deposition and neurofibrillary tangle formation in the brain's subcortical regions (including, but not limited to, subthalamic nucleus, globus pallidus, substantia nigra, midbrain, and pontine reticular formation), in association with neuronal loss in the dentate nucleus of the cerebellum and superior cerebellar peduncle. In some cases, pervasive neurofibrillary tangles have also been found in the cortex, hippocampus, and brain stem (Lubarsky & Juncos, 2008; Pearce, 2007). The diencephalic and cortical regions affected in PSP include caudate, putamen, mediodorsal thalamic nucleus, nucleus accumbens, and nucleus basalis of Meynert. Positron emission tomography (PET) has revealed hypometabolism in the caudate, brain stem, and midfrontal regions and hypermetabolism in cortical motor areas, thalamus, and parietal cortex (Eckert et al., 2005). Frontal atrophy on magnetic resonance imaging (MRI) has been linked to cognitive deficits in PSP (Cordato et al., 2002)

Progressive supranuclear palsy has a prevalence of about 5–7 per 100,000, with symptom onset occurring after age 40 and peaking at approximately age 63 (Lubarsky & Juncos, 2008). Although signs of PSP may be evident as early as age 40, formal diagnosis typically occurs after age 60, though one study reported peak incidence rates after age 80 (Bower, Maraganore, McDonnell, & Rocca, 1997). Most cases of PSP are sporadic. Familial cases have been reported, but the notion that some forms of familial PSP (usually atypical in presentation) relate to tau gene mutations (chromosome 17) remains controversial, with some advocating that such cases are better referred to as familial tauopathies than PSP (Wszolek et al., 2001).

Dementia is reported to occur in 50%–80% of patients, though some consider this to be an overestimate related to patient bradyphrenia, visual disturbance, and behavioral issues such as apathy and depression (Tröster & Fields, 2008). Patients with PSP often have early and prominent executive dysfunction, and they perform poorly on tests such as card sorting, verbal fluency, and execution of graphic sequences (Dubois, Pillon, Legault, Agid, & Lhermitte, 1988; Pillon et al., 1995). Indeed, frontal dysfunction mediated cognitive and behavioral changes may be among the first signs of PSP in a subgroup (about 20%) of patients (Kaat et al., 2007). Impaired verbal fluency is often seen in PSP, but language is typically thought to be preserved. However, one study found PSP patients to show similar impairments to Alzheimer disease patients on a visual confrontation naming test (Boston Naming Test), with 44% of the PSP patients scoring in the impaired range(van der Hurk & Hodges, 1995). In addition, PSP can present resembling primary progressive aphasia (PPA) (Boeve et al., 2003; Mochizuki et al., 2003). Episodic memory impairments (e.g., in prose, word list, and paired associate recall) are observed in PSP (Litvan, Grafman, Gomez, & Chase, 1989; Pillon, Dubois, Lhermitte, & Agid, 1986; Pillon et al., 1995), but the impairment is less severe than that in Alzheimer disease (Aarsland, Hutchinson, & Larsen, 2003; Pillon et al., 1986; Pillon, Dubois, Ploska, & Agid, 1991). Patients with PSP do poorly on procedural learning tasks but show intact priming (Grafman, Litvan, & Stark, 1995).

Apathy, depression, and loss of inhibition are common behavioral disturbances, with apathy predominating over other neurobehavioral aberrations (Litvan, 2004; Litvan, Paulsen, Mega, & Cummings, 1998; Lubarsky & Juncos, 2008; Santacruz et al., 1998). Neurobehavioral symptoms may actually worsen in response to levodopa treatments, and such changes should be noted clinically.

Due to the multifaceted presentation of symptoms in PSP, a comprehensive, individualized treatment plan is optimal when considering patient therapy. Physical and speech therapy, appropriate modifications to accommodate specific visual complaints, antidepressants, and support groups for patients and caregivers are all valuable approaches to treatment.

Case Study: A. B.

Background

A. B., a 70-year-old white man with 15 years of education was referred for neuropsychological evaluation by his neurologist given concerns that he was displaying bradyphrenia, irritability, and heightened emotionality. He was foreign born but had lived in the United States for over 40 years and was fluent in English. Until retirement he had been a successful businessman buying and selling ships and a corporate upper-level executive. He had seen the same primary care physician for 7 years at the time the patient first mentioned signs of a possible movement disorder. At that visit, A. B. complained of occasional unsteadiness of gait for the past year. A. B.'s wife reported her husband to be bumping into things more frequently, to occasionally fall backwards when arising from a chair, and to have become more irritable. Medical records showed that increased irritability had first been mentioned about 3 or 4 years prior to diagnosis, but this had been attributed to possible mild depression in reaction to retirement and medical illness (pneumonia and collapsed lung). The patient's wife also noted that friends visiting had inquired of her what was "wrong" with her husband, because he seemed different. At the visit with his primary care physician, A. B. demonstrated diminished facial expression, eye blink and spontaneous movements, and monotonic speech. At that time, A. B. also noted that he had recently begun experiencing mild difficulty with word finding but no changes in memory. His primary care physician referred A. B. to a neurologist with expertise in movement disorders.

At his first neurologic evaluation (about a year after he first noticed symptoms of movement disorder), A. B. reported that he found it increasingly difficult to get into and out of the car. His wife commented that, in retrospect, she may have noticed subtle changes in A. B.'s movement (stiffness and unsteadiness when arising) as much as 2 years before. He also struck her as being slower in thinking, despite having been quick witted in the past. Depression and change in personality (irritability) had occurred 3–4 years previously, and the couple had seen a marital counselor. Also revealed was a remote history of alcohol abuse. Neurologic history was significant for Bell palsy and shingles. Although he had attended marital counseling, there was no prior formal diagnosis of depression or psychiatric treatment. A. B. had a history of tobacco and alcohol abuse, and current alcohol consumption (aside from a recent 6-month period of sobriety) was estimated at three to four glasses of wine daily. He had been a heavy smoker and had a history of chronic obstructive pulmonary disease (COPD).

Neurologic examination revealed intact cranial nerves, normal sensation (temperature, light touch, pinprick, vibration, and position), normal reflexes with no Romberg sign, and normal muscle tone and bulk. Strength was intact, although the left interosseous muscle was weaker than the right, and left shoulder shrug was diminished compared to the right. Facial expression was masked and the patient was said to have an "icy stare." Speech was hypophonic and voice was raspy. Saccades were moderately to severely impaired and vertical gaze was similarly severely impaired. Dysdiadochokinesis was evident bilaterally, with rapid alternate movements more impaired on the left than right. Finger tapping was similarly more impaired on the left than the right. Bradykinesia was limited to the left upper extremity. He had mild rigidity in the neck and

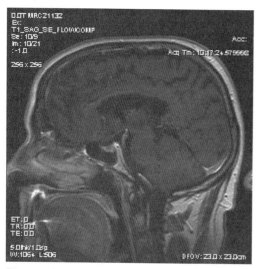

Figure 56-1. Sagittal T1-weighted magnetic resonance imaging scan revealing possible mild tegmental thinning and mild frontal cortical atrophy (obtained near time of diagnosis of progressive supranuclear palsy).

bilaterally in the upper (but not lower) extremities. There was no tremor, dyskinesia, dystonia, or myoclonus. Posture was normal and the patient arose from a chair without difficulty. Tandem walking was normal and stride length was long. Armswing was diminished bilaterally. A. B. required four steps to make a 360-degree turn. Noted also was pseudobulbar affect.

Diagnosis of PSP was confirmed by two other neurologists specializing in movement disorders within 6 months of the initial neurologic evaluation resulting in provisional diagnosis of PSP. Treatment with levodopa was minimally beneficial, and in fact, at one point, lead to dyskinesias. Ancillary services, such as speech therapy, were not pursued by the patient. A. B. had expired within 4 years after diagnosis, though the exact circumstances of his death were unknown.

Neuropsychological Evaluation

A. B. underwent neuropsychological evaluation about 3 months after provisional diagnosis of PSP, at which time he had experienced symptoms of movement disorder (e.g., falling backwards occasionally when arising, difficulty getting into and out of a car, pseudobulbar affect) for 1–2 years. The patient acknowledged mild word-finding problems that were not of concern to him but otherwise denied cognitive impairment and mood disturbance. His wife provided a timeline of changes she had noticed: depression and egocentricity about 3–4 years prior to diagnosis of PSP. About 1 year prior to diagnosis, friends had remarked how different A. B. seemed to them: he monopolized conversation, seemed disinterested in others, and appeared apathetic in general. His thought and speech seemed slower to others than in the recent past. About a year before diagnosis he had several falls while walking and arising from chairs. In the year of diagnosis, A. B.'s wife perceived her husband to be even slower in thought and movement, and she described her husband, previously characterized as systematic and sequential in action and thought, as having problems with information synthesis and analysis and maintaining focus. Visuoperceptual and possibly praxis problems had also become evident in that the patient buttoned his shirt in a lopsided manner and had difficulty threading his belt through all belt loops. He restricted his driving of a car to the immediate vicinity of his home because his wife had discouraged him from driving because he had in the past seemed to drift from one lane to another. He was otherwise independent in physical and instrumental activities of daily living at the time of evaluation.

On presentation at neuropsychological evaluation, A. B.'s gait was only slightly slowed and he had no tremor or dyskinesia. His brow was raised, and he had a startled facial expression which changed little over time. He had no color blindness or visual field cut, but on screening had impaired saccades and markedly impaired vertical gaze, especially downward gaze. Hearing was adequate for participation in the evaluation. He was alert and oriented, and generally attentive. A. B.'s spontaneous speech was halting, and word-finding appeared slowed especially for nouns and proper names, but paraphasic errors were not observed. Oral language comprehension appeared grossly intact. Memory for personal historical information and current events was grossly intact. Thought process at times was tangential and circumstantial but generally linear and goal directed. Though polite, A. B. demonstrated poor conversational turn-taking skills and sometimes monopolized conversation, aggrandizing his accomplishments. He cooperated with testing initially, but when confronted by tasks he found difficulty, for example, verbal fluency, he tended to minimize his difficulty by stating that he had never been good at such tasks, or that the tasks were irrelevant or "obnoxious." As testing progressed, his mood became more mercurial and effort waned. Consequently, testing was completed over two sessions and a memory test, on which he seemed to put forth suboptimal effort on the first occasion, was repeated using an alternate form on the second occasion with more success.

Formal testing (see Table 56-1 for results) was begun with a cognitive screening examination for several reasons: *(a)* to enlist the cooperation of the patient by using a task on which he would probably have several successful experiences and encounter only minor difficulty; *(b)* to determine whether the patient would be able to complete visual tasks and to what extent visual and motor impairments might necessitate modification to standard test administration procedures; *(c)* to obtain an estimate of A. B.'s frustration tolerance; and *(d)* to identify areas of cognition to be prioritized for more detailed evaluation. On the screening examination (Mattis Dementia Rating Scale; DRS-2) his total score fell into the mildly impaired range, below expectations for age and his educational and occupational background. The poorest performance was identified on the DRS-2's Initiation/ Perseveration subtest (26/37): 12 points were lost on the supermarket verbal fluency task (8/20), and A. B. was unable to carry out correctly the manual pronation/supination, extension/flexion, or finger tapping task (largely due to impairment of the movements with the left hand). Drawing of ramparts was intact, but he did self-correct an error when asked to draw a series of "X"s and "O"s (see Figure 56-2). His score on the Construction subtest was below average, and he failed to reproduce the unevenly spaced lines, and he self-corrected spontaneously his incorrect drawing of a diamond within a box (see Figure 56-2).

A Full-Scale IQ could not be meaningfully derived from his performance on the third edition of the Wechsler Adult Intelligence Scale (WAIS-III) because of the 28-point discrepancy between his borderline Performance IQ and his average Verbal IQ. This 28-point discrepancy was both statistically meaningful ($p < .05$), meaning it was unlikely due to chance, and clinically meaningful, in that a similar or larger discrepancy had occurred in only about 1% of the test standardization sample. Two subtests (Letter Number Sequencing and Symbol Search) were not administered. The much lower PIQ than VIQ reflects both the patient's visual problems (gaze palsy) and motor problems, though visuoperceptual task performance was below expectations regardless of whether subtests made motor demands (e.g., Matrix Reasoning and Picture Arrangement were similarly below average). Visuoperceptual problems were also evident from broken configurations on the Block Design task (score in the impaired range), requiring the patient to assemble two-colored blocks into patterns illustrated two-dimensionally on stimulus cards (see Figure 56-3).

Auditory attention was adequate (maximum digit span was six forward and foour backward). Performances on tasks requiring visual attention, information processing speed, and visual

Table 56-1. Neuropsychological Test Scores Obtained by A. B. within 3 Months of Diagnosis of Progressive Supranuclear Palsy (and about 1–2 Years after Movement Symptom Onset)

Test		Raw Score	T-score (or Percentile)
Dementia Rating Scale–2			
Attention	(/37)	36	53
Initiation/Perseveration	(/37)	26	27
Construction	(/16)	5	40
Conceptualization	(/39)	39	60
Memory	(/25)	23	47
Total	(/144)	129	37
Wechsler Adult Intelligence Scale–III			
Subtest Scores			
Vocabulary		50	57
Similarities		24	57
Arithmetic		11	47
Digit Span		14	47
Information		19	53
Comprehension		23	53
Picture Completion		11	40
Coding		25	33
Block Design		8	30
Matrix Reasoning		6	40
Picture Arrangement		4	40
IQ			
Full Scale		90	25th percentile
Verbal		103	58th percentile
Performance		75	5th percentile
Trail-Making Test			
Part A		130"	16
Part B		289"	23
Stroop Color and Word Test			
Word Score		39	<15
Color Score		24	15
Color-Word Interference Score		9	24
Wisconsin Cart Sorting Test–64			
Total Errors		33	37
Perseverative Responses		20	42
Perseverative Errors		18	41
Nonperseverative Errors		15	38
Conceptual Level Responses		22	35
Categories Completed	(/6)	1	11th–16th percentile
Trials to Complete 1st Category		52	2nd–5th percentile
Failure to Maintain Set		0	
Frontal Systems Behavior Scale (Family Rating)			
Before Illness Onset			
Apathy		22	46
Disinhibition		30	65
Executive Dysfunction		29	50
Total		81	47
After Illness Onset			
Apathy		39	72
Disinhibition		41	93
Executive Dysfunction		53	84
Total		133	79

Table 56-1. Neuropsychological Test Scores Obtained by A. B. within 3 Months of Diagnosis of Progressive Supranuclear Palsy (and about 1–2 Years after Movement Symptom Onset) (*Continued*)

Test		Raw Score	T-score (or Percentile)
Verbal Fluency			
FAS		9	17
Animals		6	18
Boston Naming Test	(/60)	48	39
Finger Tapping Test			
Dominant Han		42	36
Nondominant Hand		23	19
Grooved Pegboard			
Dominant Hand		142	29
Non-dominant Hand		*Discontinued*	
California Verbal Learning Test–II			
Trial 1	(/16)	3	35
Trial 2		3	30
Trial 3		2	20
Trial 4		4	30
Trial 5		6	35
Trials 1–5		18	28
Trial B		3	40
Short-Delay Free Recall		4	35
Short-Delay Cued Recall		5	30
Long-Delay Free Recall		3	30
Long-Delay Cued Recall		5	30
Semantic Clustering		0.1	45
Serial Clustering Forward		0	45
Yes/No Recognition Total Hits		14	50
Total False Positives		13	80
Total Recognition Discriminability		1.4	35
Total Intrusions (All Recall Trials)		0	50
Total Repetitions (All Recall Trials)		4	40
Wechsler Memory Scale–III Abbreviated			
Subtest Scores			
Logical Memory I	(/75)	40	57
Logical Memory II	(/50)	19	43
Family Pictures I	(/64)	25	43
Family Pictures II	(/64)	12	30
Composite Scores		*Standard Scores*	
Immediate Memory		99	47th percentile
Delayed Memory		87	19th percentile
Total Memory		92	30th percentile
Profile of Mood States			
Tension-Anxiety		14	66
Depression		17	67
Anger-Hostility		18	79
Vigor-Activity		18	44
Fatigue-Inertia		4	45
Confusion		10	66
Total Mood Disturbance		45	65
Beck Depression Inventory–II	(/063)	9	
Beck Anxiety Inventory	(/63)	2	

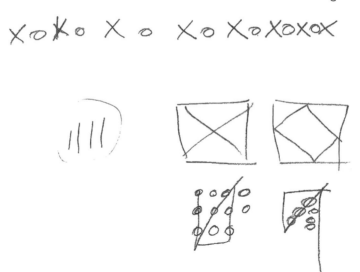

Figure 56-2. Selection of A. B.'s drawings from the Mattis Dementia Rating Scale.

scanning were uniformly poor. On the Trail Making Test, the patient made no errors on the first part of the tasks, which emphasize psychomotor speed, visual scanning, and numeric sequencing, but performance was slow and the score was in the severely impaired range. On the second part of this test, also requiring alphanumeric sequencing and attentional set shifting, A. B.'s score fell into the moderately to severely impaired range and he had one set loss error and took considerable time to recover from this error. The patient's poor performance on the Stroop tasks, a visual selective attention test also requiring the inhibition of a prepotent verbal response, and during the Color-Word interference task could not be attributed to poor attentional control because performance was impaired on all three parts of the tests, suggesting the impairment might be attributable largely to the downward gaze palsy instead.

Executive dysfunction was evident on a card-sorting task demanding of conceptualization and

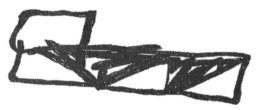

Figure 56-3. Illustration of a broken 2 x 2 configuration on WAIS-III Block Design.

cognitive flexibility in response to verbal feedback (Wisconsin Card Sorting Test, 64-card version). The patient took 52 trials to complete the first category (impaired for age and education) and only completed that one category (borderline to low average). Perseverative tendency was only mildly elevated for age and education but noteworthy (18 perseverative errors). Overall, given the lack of failures to maintain set, the test findings suggest slowness in conceptualization coupled with a mild tendency to persevere with a given strategy in the face of feedback that the strategy is incorrect. Executive dysfunction was also inferred from his wife's report on a rating scale (Frontal Systems Behavior Scale) that addresses the frequency with which she observed in her husband behaviors possibly related to frontal dysfunction, both before and after illness onset about 1 year previously. On that instrument, A. B.'s wife indicated that her husband had shown mild signs of disinhibition before illness onset, but that since illness he had developed behaviors consistent with marked apathy, disinhibition, and executive dysfunction.

A. B.'s performance on language tests was variably impaired, and, as one might expect in a frontal-subcortical disorder, verbal fluency was much more severely affected than visual confrontation naming. During the letter fluency task, mild disinhibition was evident from the patient's generation of expletives. However, no perseverative or intrusive tendency was observed.

Further indication that the patient's impoverished performance on expressive language tasks was due to problems with initiation and deployment of efficient word retrieval strategies rather than loss of word knowledge or degradation of semantic networks is that he benefitted from phonemic cuing on the visual confrontation naming test (BNT: 48/60; 6 correct after phonemic cues).

Motor test performance, as might be predicted, was impaired, more so on the left (consistent with motor examination findings during neurological evaluation). Thus, on finger tapping, performance with the right hand was mildly impaired, whereas performance with the left hand was severely impaired. On the Grooved Pegboard, demanding of fine visuomotor coordination, dexterity, and speed, performance was moderately impaired with the right hand, and the task had to be discontinued for the left hand because the patient persisted in aiding left hand performance with the right hand.

A. B.'s performance on memory tests was variably impaired. Consistent with prior observations in Parkinson disease and other forms of parkinsonism, his performance was poorest on a word list learning task especially demanding of self-initiation and deployment of efficient learning strategies, and less so on a task that provided external structure to the recall task (prose recall). On the CVLT-II (second administration about a month after initial performance was deemed flawed by suboptimal effort), immediate recall across the five learning trials revealed slow learning (slope was below average) and probable use of a passive learning strategy and reliance on short-term memory (slightly lower than average clustering and an exaggerated recency but diminished primacy effect). There was no indication of unduly rapid forgetting, and delayed recall (especially with cues) was generally commensurate with performance on the last trial of immediate recall. Provision of a recognition format versus free recall was not helpful. Although the patient on yes-no recognition testing identified 14/16 targets, he also made a large number of false-positive errors (13), revealing impaired recognition discriminability. However, during all recall trials, there were no significant numbers of intrusion (4) or repetition errors (0) made. Prose recall (Logical Memory) was average.

Although recall of pictured scenes (Family Pictures) was average immediately after presentation of pictures, delayed recall was poor, but it was felt that this was not due to rapid forgetting but rather due to weak effort and a strong "don't know" response tendency rather than error-prone responding.

Self-report of mood state was somewhat inconsistent: the patient denied depression and anxiety during interview and on the Beck Depression Inventory and beck Anxiety Inventory, but he reported above-average depressive and anxious symptoms on the Profile of Mood States, on which he also endorsed anger and cognitive inefficiency for the week prior to evaluation relative to a geriatric normative group.

Discussion

Patient A. B., seen for neuropsychological evaluation about 1–2 years after symptom onset and 3 months after initial provisional diagnosis of PSP, demonstrated a mild decline in overall level of cognitive functioning. Relatively preserved were simple attention and language comprehension and use. In contrast, he demonstrated marked impairments on tests of executive function and motor speed and dexterity. These impairments are consistent with his wife's report, revealing her husband's increasing apathy and disinhibition (perhaps even predating motor symptoms) and executive dysfunction and motor impairment. Verbal fluency, unlike visual confrontation naming and provision of word definitions, was impaired, and this finding is consistent with slowed speech noted by family and friends in conversations. Although his mild dysarthria might have contributed to poor verbal fluency, a collapse of efficient word retrieval strategies seems a more plausible primary etiology. Provision of phonemic cues during naming elevated performance to levels more consistent with expectations. Poor and slow use of learning and retrieval strategies probably also underlies A. B.'s poorer performance on a list-learning task in comparison to the externally structured prose recall task. Overall, his pattern of cognitive strengths and weaknesses corresponds to that described in a fairly sparse literature pertaining to neuropsychological findings in PSP with prominent frontal systems abnormalities.

Given A. B.'s possible early behavioral changes, including depressive symptoms, irritability, apathy, and egocentricity, a possible differential diagnosis of frontal temporal dementia (FTD) should be considered. However, his visual and motor findings, speech changes, and pseudobulbar affect are atypical for FTD. The very rapid deterioration in motor and executive functions is also more typical of PSP than FTD.

A. B. followed up with his neurologists for about another year after diagnosis but never participated in recommended speech therapy. Not unexpectedly, levodopa provided only minimal benefit in ameliorating motor symptoms. Indeed, it was associated with dyskinesias and increased sleepiness. A. B. was placed on an antidepressant (paroxetine), which somewhat improved irritability. He did not return for neuropsychological consultation, so it was unclear whether he followed recommendations to use a personal digital assistant to remind him of appointments and medication schedules, and to use elaborative mnemonic strategies. Similarly, it was unknown whether he guided his behavior by written plans detailing steps toward their execution. Unfortunately, autopsy findings were not available, but it became known that A. B. passed away within 4 years of diagnosis of PSP, a fairly typical course of illness per descriptions in the literature (about 6 years between symptom onset and death). He had had pulmonary complications from COPD and recurrent lung infections, but their role in his death were not known.

References

Aarsland, D., Hutchinson, M., & Larsen, J. P. (2003). Cognitive, psychiatric and motor response to galantamine in Parkinson's disease with dementia. *International Journal of Geriatric Psychiatry, 18*(10), 937–941.

Boeve, B., Dickson, D., Duffy, J., Bartleson, J., Trenerry, M., & Petersen, R. (2003). Progressive nonfluent aphasia and subsequent aphasic dementia associated with atypical progressive supranuclear palsy pathology. *European Neurology, 49*(2), 72–78.

Bower, J. H., Maraganore, D. M., McDonnell, S. K., & Rocca, W. A. (1997). Incidence of progressive supranuclear palsy and multiple system atrophy in Olmsted County, Minnesota, 1976 to 1990. *Neurology, 49*(5), 1284–1288.

Cordato, N. J., Pantelis, C., Halliday, G. M., Velakoulis, D., Wood, S. J., Stuart, G. W., et al. (2002). Frontal atrophy correlates with behavioural changes in progressive supranuclear palsy. *Brain, 125*(Pt 4), 789–800.

Dubois, B., Pillon, B., Legault, F., Agid, Y., & Lhermitte, F. (1988). Slowing of cognitive processing in progressive supranuclear palsy. A comparison with Parkinson's disease. *Archives of Neurology, 45*(11), 1194–1199.

Eckert, T., Barnes, A., Dhawan, V., Frucht, S., Gordon, M. F., Feigin, A. S., et al. (2005). FDG PET in the differential diagnosis of parkinsonian disorders. *Neuroimage, 26*(3), 912–921.

Grafman, J., Litvan, I., & Stark, M. (1995). Neuropsychological features of progressive supranuclear palsy. *Brain and Cognition, 28*(3), 311–320.

Kaat, L. D., Boon, A. J., Kamphorst, W., Ravid, R., Duivenvoorden, H. J., & van Swieten, J. C. (2007). Frontal presentation in progressive supranuclear palsy. *Neurology, 69*(8), 723–729.

Litvan, I. (2004). Update on progressive supranuclear palsy. *Current Neurology and Neuroscience Reports, 4*(4), 296–302.

Litvan, I., Grafman, J., Gomez, C., & Chase, T. N. (1989). Memory impairment in patients with progressive supranuclear palsy. *Archives of Neurology, 46*(7), 765–767.

Litvan, I., Paulsen, J. S., Mega, M. S., & Cummings, J. L. (1998). Neuropsychiatric assessment of patients with hyperkinetic and hypokinetic movement disorders [published erratum appears in Arch Neurol 1998 ; 55(12):1591]. *Archives of Neurology, 55*(10), 1313–1319.

Lubarsky, M., & Juncos, J. L. (2008). Progressive supranuclear palsy: A current review. *Neurologist, 14*(2), 79–88.

Mochizuki, A., Ueda, Y., Komatsuzaki, Y., Tsuchiya, K., Arai, T., & Shoji, S. (2003). Progressive supranuclear palsy presenting with primary progressive aphasia – clinicopathological report of an autopsy case. *Acta Neuropathologica (Berlin), 105*(6), 610–614.

Pearce, J. M. (2007). Progressive supranuclear palsy (Steele-Richardson-Olszewski syndrome): A short historical review. *Neurologist, 13*(5), 302–304.

Pillon, B., Dubois, B., Lhermitte, F., & Agid, Y. (1986). Heterogeneity of cognitive impairment in progressive supranuclear palsy, Parkinson's disease, and Alzheimer's disease. *Neurology, 36*(9), 1179–1185.

Pillon, B., Dubois, B., Ploska, A., & Agid, Y. (1991). Severity and specificity of cognitive impairment in Alzheimer's, Huntington's, and Parkinson's diseases and progressive supranuclear palsy. *Neurology, 41*(5), 634–643.

Pillon, B., Gouider-Khouja, N., Deweer, B., Vidailhet, M., Malapani, C., Dubois, B., et al. (1995).

Neuropsychological pattern of striatonigral degeneration: Comparison with Parkinson's disease and progressive supranuclear palsy. *Journal of Neurology, Neurosurgery, and Psychiatry, 58*(2), 174–179.

Santacruz, P. M. A., Uttl, B. P., Litvan, I. M. D., & Grafman, J. P. (1998). Progressive supranuclear palsy: A survey of the disease course. *Neurology, 50*(6), 1637–1647.

Steele, J. C., Richardson, J. C., & Olszewski, J. (1964). Progressive supranuclear palsy. A heterogeneous degeneration involving the brain stem, basal ganglia and cerebellum with vertical gaze and pseudobulbar palsy, nuchal dystonia and dementia. *Archives of Neurology, 10*, 333–359.

Tröster, A. I., & Fields, J. A. (2008). Parkinson's disease, progressive supranuclear palsy, corticobasal degeneration, and related disorders of the frontostriatal system. In J. E. Morgan & J. H. Ricker (Eds.), *Textbook of clinical neuropsychology* (pp. 536–577). New York: Psychology Press.

van der Hurk, P. R., & Hodges, J. R. (1995). Episodic and semantic memory in Alzheimer's disease and progressive supranuclear palsy: A comparative study. *Journal of Clinical and Experimental Neuropsychology, 17*(3), 459–471.

Williams, D. R., de Silva, R., Paviour, D. C., Pittman, A., Watt, H. C., Kilford, L., et al. (2005). Characteristics of two distinct clinical phenotypes in pathologically proven progressive supranuclear palsy: Richardson's syndrome and PSP-parkinsonism. *Brain, 128*(Pt. 6), 1247–1258.

Wszolek, Z. K., Tsuboi, Y., Uitti, R. J., Reed, L., Hutton, M. L., & Dickson, D. W. (2001). Progressive supranuclear palsy as a disease phenotype caused by the S305S tau gene mutation. *Brain, 124*(Pt. 8), 1666–1670.

57

Pick Disease

Shane S. Bush and Thomas Myers

Pick disease (PiD), named after its discoverer, Arnold Pick, is a progressive form of frontotemporal dementia (FTD) characterized by focal degeneration of the frontal and temporal brain regions, and/or the presence of argyrophilic globular inclusions (Pick bodies) and swollen, achromatic neurons (Pick cells) (Kertesz, 1998). Pick originally described the clinical symptoms of the disorder and their associated frontotemporal cerebral atrophies in a series of case studies that included progressive aphasia and behavioral disturbances (Pick, 1892). His descriptions of the brain were based on gross examinations without the benefit of microscopic analysis. Alzheimer (1911) later defined PiD on the basis of histology, noting the presence of the Pick bodies and Pick cells, as well as the absence of amyloid (senile) plaques and neurofibrillary tangles.

Pick bodies are typically found in several cerebral locations, including the following: dentate gyrus, pyramidial cells of the CA1 section and subiculum of the hippocampus, hypothalamic lateral tuberal nucleus, dorsomedial region of the putamen, globus pallidus, locus ceruleus, mossy fibers and monodendritic brush cells in the granule cell layer of the cerebellum, and frontal and temporal neocortex (Braak, Arai, & Braak, 1999; Wang, Zhu, Feng, & Wang, 2006; Yamakawa, 2006).

In addition to having an affinity for fairly specific anatomical locations, the Pick bodies in the neocortex are located in the II and IV layers of the cortex, which project within the cortex and to thalamic synapses, respectively. Although cortical

layers III and V have few, if any, Pick bodies, they tend to sustain marked neuronal atrophy. The straight, fibrous appearance of tangled tau proteins found in Pick bodies differs substantially from the paired and coiled construction of the neurofibrillary tangles found in Alzheimer disease (Wang et ., 2006; Yancopoulou et al., 2003).

The *Diagnostic and Statistical Manual of Mental Disorders-Fourth Edition Text Revision* (*DSM-IV-TR*) lists diagnostic criteria for PiD based on the criteria for dementia due to a general medical condition with the presence of behavioral (personality) disturbances and language impairment (American Psychiatric Association, 2000). However, as with Alzheimer disease, histological analysis for definitive diagnosis requires a biopsy of the brain and therefore is typically not performed in vivo.

Although some investigators and clinicians restrict the use of the term *Pick disease* to cases with confirmed histopathological findings, others have argued for use of the more diverse and comprehensive term *Pick complex* (PC), which incorporates overlapping clinical syndromes such as primary progressive aphasia (PPA), fontal lobe dementia and FTD, semantic dementia, corticobasal degeneration, and other related conditions (Kertesz, 1998; Twamley & Bondi, 2003). These disorders share many symptoms seen in PiD, and histopathological evidence (Pick cells and Pick bodies) has been found in cases of progressive aphasia, semantic dementia, and FTD with primarily behavioral changes and executive dysfunction (Grossman, 2002).

Evidence of a progression of histopathological changes from a first syndrome or variant (e.g., FTD-behavioral variant) to a second syndrome (e.g., corticobasal degeneration) and a third syndrome supports overlapping pathology and the concept of the Pick complex (Kertesz, McMonagle, Blair, Davidson, & Munoz, 2005).

Using the histological method of diagnosis, PiD is quite rare, with a prevalence of 30 to 60 cases per 100,000 in the general population, or between 1 and 5 per 1000 cases of Alzheimer disease (AD) (Boller & Muggia, 1999). Other studies found that PiD comprises approximately 2% of cases seen in a memory disorders unit, compared to 63% of cases diagnosed with AD (Binetti, Locascio, Corkin, Vonsattel, & Growdon, 2000). Viewing the collection of these disorders as part of the PC, Kertesz (1998) reported prevalence rates equivalent to vascular dementia, with a ratio of 1 PC to 4 AD.

Miller et al. (1998) reported that 50% of PiD patients present with greater left hemisphere involvement, while 20% have greater right hemisphere pathology. Patients with greater right hemisphere involvement are more likely to display psychiatric symptoms and come to the attention of psychiatry, whereas patients with primarily left hemisphere involvement tend to display language difficulties suggestive of neurologic dysfunction. In contrast to these general trends, Waddington and colleagues (1995) reported a case study of a woman with a clinical diagnosis of schizophrenia who displayed increasing affectivity and cognitive deficits. Upon biopsy, all the neuropathological signs of PiD were present, along with left frontotemporal atrophy, left Sylvian fissure abnormalities, and enlargement of the anterior and temporal horns of the left lateral ventricle.

Although frontotemporal regions are the most commonly affected areas in PiD, lesions may be present in other areas, with corresponding clinical manifestations. For example, Tsuchiya et al. (2001) found that in a sample of six Japanese cases with neuropathologically verified PiD, lesions were multicentrically placed. They reported that two patients with speech apraxia had lesions in the primary motor area. A patient with depression showed widespread lesions in the orbitofrontal region. The remaining three patients showed lesions in the parietal area, including the postcentral gyrus. Another case study of a PiD patient with progressive aphemia and agrammatism presented with restricted cortical atrophy in the frontal operculum, as well as considerable neuronal loss in premotor cortex and the anterior half of the precentral gyrus (Sakurai et al., 1998).

Because of the similarities between PiD and FTD, much of the research on FTD can be utilized to describe PiD, and the terms are used interchangeably in some studies (McKhann et al., 2001). Gustafson (1993) reported that approximately 50% of FTD patients have a family history of dementia. Reports from the UCLA Alzheimer's Disease Center state that about 20% of FTD patients have a first-degree relative with either dementia or motor neuron disease (Miller et al., 1995). With Pick disease specifically, an inherited mutation in the tau gene increases the risk of developing the disease; however, the vast majority of cases arise spontaneously with no known genetic or environmental link. The onset of PiD is most common between the ages of 40 and 65, with an average age of 54 years. Although the incidence of AD increases significantly with age, it is rare to have an onset of FTD after age 75 (McKhann et al., 2001). The average life expectancy following diagnosis of FTD ranges from 4–6 years, although persons with the frontal variant have a median survival of just 3 years following diagnosis (Hodges, Davies, Xuereb, Kril, & Halliday, 2003; Rascovsky et al., 2005).

The Work Group on FTD and PiD described two core clinical phenotypes (McKhann et al., 2001). The first phenotype involves gradual, progressive changes in behavior. Early changes in social and personal conduct are noted, with little or no regard for the social environment. A lack of inhibition often results in impulsive and inappropriate behaviors such as swearing, outbursts of frustration, or lack of social tact. As the disease progresses, patients may make poor financial decisions or engage in more impulsive acts such as grabbing things that are not theirs, shoplifting, or engaging in inappropriate sexual behavior. Repetitive or compulsive behaviors also sometimes occur, resulting in patients repeating specific personal acts or physical actions. Diet and hygiene are also noted to change. Overeating may occur, or patients may eat only certain foods. Patient with FTD typically lack insight regarding their behaviors and show little concern for their actions (McKhann et al., 2001).

The second type of FTD presentation suggested by the work group involves a change in language functioning, with relative sparing of other cognitive domains. Language disturbances may involve expression, including word usage and naming. Difficulties in reading and writing also develop. Expressive language abilities generally deteriorate until the patient eventually becomes mute. Despite these changes, word meaning and comprehension remain intact. This form of FTD is referred to as primary progressive aphasia by some researchers and clinicians (McKhann et al., 2001). Another group of FTD patients present with difficulty understanding word meaning.

These language symptoms, although primary, may be followed by behavioral changes (McKhann et al., 2001). In one case, a PiD patient displayed symptoms of aphasia for 9 years before developing mild behavioral disturbances (Scheltens, Hazenberg, Lindeboom, Valk, & Wolters, 2000). Serial neuroimaging studies revealed progressive bilateral temporal atrophy. Graff-Radford and colleagues (1990) reported a case of PiD in a 59-year-old man with primary problems involving learning and retrieving names. In this case neuronal loss and gliosis were most prominent in left anterior temporal cortices.

Although research in the area has grown over the years, FTD is commonly mistaken as AD by clinicians (McKhann et al., 2001). In an attempt to improve diagnostic methods, six patients with PiD in whom the presence of Pick bodies was verified were compared to a group of patients with AD. On neuroimaging, patients with PiD showed either marked frontal or temporal pole atrophy, allowing them to be clearly differentiated from patients with AD. With neurocognitive testing, patients with PiD produced a pattern characterized by relatively intact recent memory but marked impairment of executive functions (Knopman et al., 1989). With regard to neurotransmitter systems, frontotemporal dementias affect serotonin and dopamine systems but leave the acetylcholine system relatively intact (Huey, Putnam, & Grafman, 2006). Complicating the diagnostic picture is recent postmortem evidence of multiple pathologies, including AD pathology in 17% of patients who have received

clinical diagnoses of frontotemporal lobar degeneration (Forman et al., 2006).

The initial clinical presentation and rate of decline may also be distinguishing factors between PiD and AD. Binetti and colleagues at the Memory Disorders Unit of Massachusets General Hospital compared 44 patients with PiD to 123 patients with AD (Binetti et al., 2000). The mean age of patients at initial evaluation did not differ, but the age at disease onset was significantly lower for patients with PiD. In terms of the initial symptoms of the disease, speech (word finding) and personality changes (apathy, agitation, depression, irritability, appetite change, disinhibition, and euphoria) were more prevalent in PiD patients. Although memory loss was the most commonly reported first symptom in both groups, it was more prevalent in AD patients. PiD patients were also found to have greater impairment in activities of daily living (ADLs). Rate of decline was found to be significantly greater in PiD on language tests such as the Boston Naming Test and semantic verbal fluency tests, as well as on measures of ADLs. Most other measures of cognitive functioning declined at the same rate, despite PiD patients performing better on a test of delayed story recall (Binetti et al., 2000).

Mendez, Selwood, Mastri, and Frey (1993) identified five clinical features present in PiD that can distinguish it from AD. These distinguishing features included presenile onset (i.e., prior to age 65), an initial personality change, hyperorality, disinhibition, and roaming behavior. These authors also reported that PiD patients have greater speech disturbances than do AD patients, and they also engage in reiterative speech. Positron emission tomography (PET) has also been found to differentiate PiD from AD. In PiD, glucose metabolism may be reduced in frontal and temporobasal regions, the hippocampus, and the caudate nucleus (Szilies & Karenberg, 1986).

Additional neuropsychological dysfunction was found in a longitudinal case study of a 67-year-old man (Hodges & Gurd, 1994). Initially, anterograde memory was severely impaired, while remote memory remained intact. The patient showed selective difficulty in retrieving contextually rich and time-specific personal memories and in dating personal and public memories. Remote memory deteriorated with the progression of the disease. Both phonemic (lexical) and semantic (categorical) fluency were impaired to an equal degree.

Case Report

Mrs. A, a 58-year-old, right-handed, Caucasian female, was referred for a neuropsychological evaluation by her neurologist to clarify the nature and extent of neurocognitive and behavioral changes that emerged during the past 3 years. She had no prior history of neurological injuries or other significant injuries or illnesses, nor did she report significant psychiatric problems or treatment.

Mrs. A was accompanied to the appointment by her husband, Mr. A, who provided much of the history because Mrs. A does not believe that she has experienced any noteworthy changes in recent years. Mr. A stated that his wife has experienced multiple, significant changes in her personality, behavior, and memory in the past 3 years. With regard to personality and behavior changes, he reported that Mrs. A began smoking 4 years ago, gained a substantial amount of weight, has reduced investment in grooming and hygiene, and had very little interest in their daughter's wedding or the birth of their first grandchild. She is also impulsive; careless with money, resulting in debt; attempts to cover up problems and lies or forgets about financial problems; is careless with cigarettes; and is forgetful. Additionally, she is quieter, gets lost often, sleeps more than usual, watches television much of the time, and does puzzles. All of these traits and behaviors are uncharacteristic of Mrs. A's behaviors and interests throughout most of her life. In contrast to the observations and reports of family members, Mrs. A stated that she feels fine and is the same person that she was 5 or 10 years ago. She does not think that she has any problems.

Mrs. A reportedly underwent a recent magnetic resonance imaging (MRI) and electroencephalogram (EEG) of the brain, both of which were normal. Lab tests revealed a significant vitamin B12 deficiency. A PET scan is planned. Results of a Mini-Mental State Exam administered by the referring neurologist were a perfect 30 out of 30.

Mrs. A's father died of pneumonia at 80; he had had a 5-year history of dementia, including memory deficits, aggression, and mutism. He had

been a resident in a nursing home until he became aggressive and was then transferred to a local hospital. He became mute approximately 2 years before he died. Mrs. A was responsible for monitoring his care. There are no other relatives known to have had dementia.

Mental Status and Behavioral Observations

Mrs. A was alert and oriented, with the exception of the exact date. During the interview, she frequently turned to Mr. A for answers regarding dates, medications, and other information. In addition, Mr. A at times corrected inaccurate information provided by Mrs. A. Mrs. A's receptive language was adequate for basic questions and instructions. Her speech was fluent. Her thoughts were goal directed. There was no evidence of hallucinations or delusions, and none was reported. Her affect generally appeared neutral or mildly annoyed; however, she became tearful when discussing the poor health of extended family members. As the testing progressed, brighter affect was observed. Although she did not believe that the evaluation was needed, she agreed to undergo the evaluation, to try her best, and to respond honestly. Her behavior was appropriate. She was pleasant, cooperative, and appeared to try her best. She was able to work for extended periods, taking just a couple of brief breaks.

Procedures

- Clinical interviews of Mr. and Mrs. A
- Behavioral observations
- Neuropsychological Symptom Checklist
- Neuropsychological tests and functions assessed:
  1. Boston Naming Test (BNT): Confrontation naming
  2. California Verbal Learning Test–Second Edition (CVLT-II): Verbal learning and recall of semantically related words
  3. Complex Ideational Material (CIM): Auditory comprehension
  4. Conner's Continuous Performance Test-II (CPT-II): Sustained attention/ vigilance, reaction time, impulsivity
  5. Double Simultaneous Stimulation: Sensory extinction

6. Lafayette Grooved Pegboard Test (GP): Speeded fine motor coordination

7. North American Adult Reading Test (NAART): Reading of irregularly spelled words; estimate of premorbid intellectual ability

8. Rey Complex Figure Test (RCFT): Visuospatial construction ability and visual memory

9. Reynolds Intellectual Assessment Scales (RIAS): Intellectual functioning and cognitive factors that comprise intelligence, such as verbal and nonverbal reasoning

10. Stroop Color and Word Test (SCWT): Processing speed; selective attention, cognitive flexibility, and response inhibition

11. Trail Making Test (TMT), Parts A & B: Visual search and sequencing and mental set shifting. Scoring is based on completion time.

12. Verbal Fluency: Speeded word generation and animal naming

13. Wechsler Adult Intelligence Scale–Third Edition (WAIS-III), Working Memory Index subtests: Working memory

14. Wide Range Achievement Test–Fourth Edition (WRAT4): Academic achievement in the areas of word reading, spelling, and arithmetic

15. Wisconsin Card Sorting Test (WCST): Executive functions, including reasoning, conceptual tracking, and mental set shifting

16. Word Memory Test (WMT): Test-taking effort/response validity

Test Results

See Appendix Table 57-1 for a list of test scores. For consistency throughout the report, T scores are used. The following interpretive ranges from the RIAS manual are provided for reference.

Verbal Descriptor	Standard Score	T Score	Percentile
Significantly Below Average	≤69	≤29	≤2
Moderately Below Average	70–79	30–36	3–8
Below Average	80–89	37–42	9–23
Average	90–109	43–56	24–73
Above Average	110–119	57–62	74–90
Moderately Above Average	120–129	63–69	91–97
Significantly Above Average	≥130	≥70	≥98

Effort/Validity. Mrs. A's performance on symptom validity tests and indicators embedded within neurocognitive tests was consistent with sufficient effort. In addition, her MMPI-2 responses reflected a forthright approach. Thus, her overall approach to the neuropsychological evaluation was considered valid.

Estimated Premorbid Level. A measure of word reading, the "best performance" method, and consideration of demographic variables were used to estimate Mrs. A's optimal level of predecline functioning. Based on these methods, her prior level of intellectual/cognitive functioning is estimated to have been in the Average range. Scores falling 2 standard deviations below this range were considered impaired.

Intellectual Functioning. Mrs. A's overall level of intellectual functioning was in the Average range (RIAS Composite Intelligence Index T = 44). The difference between her Verbal Intelligence Index and Nonverbal Intelligence Index was not significant, indicating that her visually based intellectual abilities are generally consistent with her verbally based abilities.

Within the Verbal domain, Mrs. A scored in the Average range on a task that required the integration of vocabulary and receptive language development with deductive reasoning and general knowledge (Guess What T = 45). She scored in the Below-Average range on a measure of verbal reasoning (Verbal Reasoning T = 40). Within the Nonverbal domain, Mrs. A scored in the Average range on a measure of nonverbal analogical reasoning, spatial ability, and visual imagery (Odd-Item Out T = 45). She also scored in the Average range on a measure that required the integration of visual-perceptual skills with spatial and nonverbal reasoning to deduce a solution (What's Missing T = 47).

Attention and Concentration (Working Memory). Mrs. A scored in the Average range on the WAIS-III Working Memory Index. Subtests included mental arithmetic, repeating strings of digits (six digits forward, three in reverse sequence), and repeating letter-number sequences. On the RIAS Verbal and Visual Memory subtests, which assess immediate recall/working memory, she scored in the Average range. On a measure of sustained attention/vigilance, reaction time, and impulsivity (CPT), she scored in the Average range.

Processing Speed. Mrs. A's scores ranged from the Below-Average range to the Average range in this domain. While her performance on a test of speeded visual search and sequencing (TMTA) was in the Average range, her performances on measures of speeded word reading and speeded color naming (SCWT) were in the Below-Average range.

Sensory and Motor Functions. Mrs. A's auditory and visual sensory functions appeared to be adequate for basic questions and instructions. She performed accurately with tactile-hand and visual discrimination to unilateral and bilateral simultaneous stimulation. However, she demonstrated left-sided suppressions to unilateral and bilateral stimulation, suggesting decreased hearing in her left ear of peripheral origin.

Mrs. A is right handed. On a measure of upper extremity fine motor coordination (GP), she scored in the Average range with her dominant (right) hand but in the Below-Average range with her nondominant hand.

Language. Receptively, Mrs. A demonstrated no difficulty understanding information conveyed in the relatively quiet, distraction-free evaluation setting. However, on a measure of her ability to understand sentence- and paragraph-length information (CIM), she scored in the Moderately Below-Average range.

Expressively, Mrs. A's speech was fluent. There was no evidence of dysarthria or paraphasia in her spontaneous speech. On a measure of her ability to name pictured objects (BNT), she performed in the Below-Average range and produced multiple semantic paraphasic errors.

Visuospatial Skills. Visuospatial skills involve awareness of visual detail, the ability to copy designs, the ability to manipulate items or objects mentally or manually, and visual reasoning. Mrs. A scored in the Average range on a measure of nonverbal analogical reasoning, spatial ability, and visual imagery (RIAS OIO). In contrast, she performed in the Moderately Below-Average range on a measure of graphomotor reproduction (drawing/copying) of a complex figure (RCFT).

Learning and Memory. Mrs. A's performance was impaired in this domain. On a test of verbal learning and memory (CVLT-II), she scored in the Moderately Below-Average range after hearing the list once and in the Significantly Below-Average range after five learning trials. She also scored in the Significantly Below-Average range following both short and long delays, and she did not benefit from categorical cues. Her ability to identify words from the list and discriminate them from distractors was also in the Significantly Below-Average range. Thus, her performance on the CVLT-II revealed greatest impairment with storage of new verbal information.

On a measure of her ability to recall a complex design that she had previously drawn/copied (RCFT), she scored in the Significantly Below-Average range following a 3-minute delay with interference and in the Significantly Below-Average range following a 25-minute delay. Her recognition score was artificially elevated by endorsement of designs that were not part of the original figure. Thus, her performance on the RCFT revealed impaired ability to store new visual information.

Executive Functions. Executive functions generally include the ability to control one's actions, through intentional initiation and inhibition of behavior; the ability to shift from one cognitive activity to another; planning and organization; and reasoning skills. Mrs. A's performance in this domain varied somewhat but was generally lower than her estimated premorbid level of functioning.

On a measure of visual reasoning and the ability to shift response sets in response to changing demands (WCST), Mrs. A scored in the Moderately Below-Average range for overall number of errors and in the Significantly Below-Average range for the number of nonperseverative errors. She performed in the Below-Average range on a measure of speeded conceptual tracking and mental flexibility (TMTB). She scored in the Average range on a test requiring inhibition of one response option in order to respond to another option (SCWT). On measures of speeded verbal fluency (phonemic and semantic), she scored in the Below-Average range with phonemic prompts and in the Average range with semantic prompts.

Additionally, Mrs. A produced a significant number of intrusive responses (reporting words that were not from the list) on the CVLT-II and endorsed a significant number of false-positive designs on the RCFT recognition component. In addition, she evidenced poor planning and organization on the RCFT.

Psychological and Behavioral Functioning. On the MMPI-2, Mrs. A's responses indicated that she is not experiencing psychological distress. She did not endorse a significant number of symptoms of depression, anxiety, or other psychiatric disorders. Her responses were consistent with those of women who tend to reject traditional female roles and pursue interests that are stereotypically more masculine. Women with such traits tend to be active, assertive, competitive, aggressive, and dominating. They are seen by others as coarse, rough, and tough. They are typically outgoing, uninhibited, and self-confident, as well as logical and calculated in their behavior. They are relatively unemotional and are seen as unfriendly by others. According to Mrs. A's family, these traits are substantially different from the traits that characterized her personality throughout most of her life.

Summary

Mrs. A has been observed by family to be forgetful and to have experienced significant personality changes in the past 3 years. There was no observed or detected acute medical, neurological, or psychosocial event immediately preceding the onset of her symptoms.

The results of the present neuropsychological evaluation revealed cognitive functioning in the Below-Average to Average range for most domains, including overall level of intellectual functioning, attention and concentration, processing speed, most aspects of language, and some aspects of executive functioning. In contrast, comprehension of complex information, visuospatial constructions, and aspects of executive functioning fell in the Moderately Below-Average range. In addition, decreased hearing in her left ear was detected. However, the most significant finding was her impaired performance on memory tests, with poor retention of new verbal and visual information. Also, aspects of executive functioning that involve planning and problem solving were impaired. Psychologically, although Mrs. A is not experiencing emotional distress, significant changes in her personality have been observed in recent years.

The level and pattern of Mrs. A's neuropsychological impairments is most consistent with dementia due to Pick disease, the essential features of which include changes in personality early in the course, deterioration of social skills, emotional blunting, behavioral disinhibition, and language abnormalities. Memory impairment is also a prominent symptom but tends to emerge after the personality changes. Pick disease is a progressive, degenerative disease of the brain that primarily affects the frontal and temporal lobes. Although vitamin B12 deficiency can affect neurocognitive functioning, Mrs. A's examination results appear to be more consistent with Pick disease than with B12 deficiency alone.

Conclusions

Pick disease is one of a number of conditions that comprise the Pick complex. As the case of Mrs. A illustrates, personality change is a classic early symptom of Pick disease. Clinically, a careful history and consideration of the presenting problems as described by family members may be as diagnostic as neurocognitive test results, particularly early in the disease process. However, impaired test results associated with disrupted frontal and temporal lobe functioning are also commonly evident and become increasingly pronounced as the disease progresses.

Consideration is often given to medications to address neurocognitive and/or behavioral problems. Because frontotemporal dementias, such as PiD, affect serotonin and dopamine neurotransmitter systems and leave the acetylcholine and system relatively intact, medications commonly used to maximize memory in Alzheimer disease (e.g., anticholinesterase agents) are used less frequently with individuals with PiD (Huey, Putnam, & Grafman, 2006). In contrast, there is some evidence of abnormal glutamate signaling in the cerebral cortex of

Appendix Table 57-1. Neuropsychological Test Scores

	T Score		T Score
NAART		*LEARNING CHARACTERISTICS*	
FSIQ	48	Semantic clustering	45
RIAS		Serial clustering	55
VIX	44	Percent Recall primacy	55
NIX	46	Percent Recall middle	25
CIX	44	Percent Recall recency	65
CMX	50	Total Learning Slope Trials 1–5	35
WCST-64		*RECALL CONTRAST*	
Total Errors	32	Proactive Interference B v. trial 1	55
PSV resp.	39	Retroactive Int, SDFR v. trial 5	55
PSV errors	38	Long Retention LDFR v. SDFR	40
NonPSV errors	27	*RECALL ERRORS*	
Percent conceptual level responses	33	Total Repetitions	40
Categories completed (3)	34–37	Total Intrusions	65
Trials to complete first category (56)	30–33	Total Recall Discriminability	25
SCWT		*DELAYED RECOGNITION*	
W	38	Y/N Recognition Hits	30
C	41	Y/N Recognition False Positives	70
CW	44	Total recognition discriminability	25
Int	44	Total Response Bias	55
TMT		Forced-Choice Recogition	15/16
A	50	*RECALL/RECOGNITION CONTRAST*	
B	38	Recog Discrim v. LDFR	60
GP		**WAIS-III**	45
Dominant	50	WMI	45
Nondominant	42	**CPT II**	
CIM	34	Omissions	43
BNT	42	Commissions	44
Letter Fluency (FAS)	41	Hit RT	45
Category Fluency (Animals)	54	**MMPI-2**	
RCFT (retrieval profile)		Fp	73
Copy	34–37	Mf	89
Time to copy	>40	Noother scales elevated above 65	
Immediate Recall	<20	**WMT**	
Delayed Recall	23	IR	98%
Recognition	42	DR	100%
CVLT-II		CNS	98%
LEVEL OF IMMEDIATE RECALL			
List A Trial 1	35	**DSS**: Tactile-hand: no errors or	
Trial 5	20	suppressions	
Trials 1–5	32	Visual: no errors or suppressions	
List B	40	Auditory: 4/4 left-side suppressions	
LEVEL OF DELAYED RECALL		to unilateral stimulation	
List A short-delay free recall	25		
short-delay cued	10		
long-delay free	15		
long-delay cued	20		

persons with PiD (Dalfo, Albasanz, Rodriguez, Martin, & Ferrer, 2005), which may prove promising for symptom relief with NMDA receptor antagonists. Antidepressants, particularly selective serotonin reuptake inhibitors (SSRIs), have been found to be effective with helping to manage behavior changes associated with PiD (Lippa, 2006). Education and support are often important services that neuropsychologists can provide or facilitate for persons with PiD and their families.

References

Alzheimer, A. (1911). Uber eigenartige Krankheits-falle des spateren Alters. *Zeitschrift fur die Gesamte Neurologie und Psychiatrie, 4,* 356–385.

American Psychiatric Association (APA). (2000). *Diagnostic and statistical manual of mental disorders* (4th ed., Text rev.). Washington, DC: Author.

Binetti, G., Locascio, J. J., Corkin, S., Vonsattel, J. P., & Growdon, J. H. (2000). Differences between Pick disease and Alzheimer disease in clinical appearance and rate of cognitive decline. *Archives of Neurology, 57,* 225–232.

Boller, F., & Muggia, S. (1999). Non-Alzheimer dementias. In G. Denes & L. Pizzamiglio (Eds.), *Handbook of clinical and experimental neuropsychology* (pp. 747–775). Hove, East Sussex, England: Psychology Press.

Braak, E., Arai, K., & Braak, H. (1999). Cerebellar involvement in Pick's disease: Affliction of mossy fibers, monodendritic brush cells, and dentate projection neurons. *Experimental Neurology, 159,* 153–163.

Dalfo, E., Albasanz, J. L., Rodriguez, A., Martin, M., & Ferrer, I. (2005). Abnormal group I metabotropic glutamate receptor expression and signaling in the frontal cortex in Pick disease. *Journal of Neuropathology and Experimental Neurology, 64,* 638–647.

Forman, M. S., Farmer, J., Johnson, J. K., Clark, C. M., Arnold, S. E., Coslett, H. B., et al. (2006). Frontotemporal dementia: Clinicopathological correlations. *Annals of Neurology, 59,* 952–962.

Graff-Radford, N. R., Damasio, A. R., Hyman, B. T., Hart, M. N., Tranel, D., Damasio, H., et al. (1990). Progressive aphasia in a patient wit Pick's disease: A neuropsychological, radiologic, and anatomic study. *Neurology, 40,* 620–626.

Grossman, M. (2002). Frontotemporal dementia: A review. *Journal of the International Neuropsychological Society, 8,* 566–583.

Gustafson, L. (1993). Clinical picture of frontal lobe degeneration of non-Alzheimer type. *Dementia, 6,* 1–8.

Hodges, J. R., Davies, R., Xuereb, J., Kril, J., & Halliday, G. (2003). Survival in frontotemporal dementia. *Neurology, 61,* 349–354.

Hodges, J. R., & Gurd, J. M. (1994). Remote memory and lexical retrieval in a case of frontal Pick's disease. *Archives of Neurology, 52,* 742–743.

Huey, E.D., Putnam, K.T., & Grafman, J. (2006). A systematic review of neurotransmitter deficits and treatments in frontotemporal dementia. *Neurology, 66,* 17–22.

Kertesz, A. (1998). Pick's disease and Pick complex: Introductory nosology. In A. Kertesz & D. G. Munoz (Eds.), *Pick's disease and Pick complex* (pp. 1–12). New York: Wiley-Liss, Inc.

Kertesz, A., McMonagle, P., Blair, M., Davidson, W., & Munoz, D. G. (2005). The evolution and pathology of frontotemporal dementia. *Brain, 128,* 1996–2005.

Knopman, D. S., Christensen, K. J., Schut, L. J., Harbaugh, R. E., Reeder, T., Ngo, T., et al. (1989). The spectrum of imaging and neuropsychological findings in Pick's disease. *Neurology, 39,* 362–363.

Lippa, C. F. (2006). An individualized approached to treatment for Alzheimer's disease, Pick's disease, and other dementias. *American Journal of Alzheimer's Disease and Other Dementias, 21,* 354–359.

McKhann, G. M., Albert, M. S., Grossman, M., Miller, B., Dickson, D., & Troganowski, J. Q. (2001). Clinical and pathological diagnosis of frontotemporal dementia. Report of the work group on frontotemporal dementia and Pick's disease. *Archives of Neurology, 58,* 1803–1809.

Mendez, M. F., Selwood, A., Mastri, A. R., & Frey, W. H. (1993). Pick's disease versus Alzheimer's disease: A comparison of clinical characteristics. *Neurology, 43,* 289–292.

Miller, B. L., Boone, K., Mishkin, F., Swartz, J. R., Koras, N., & Kushi, J. (1998). Clinical and neuropsychological features of frontotemporal dementia. In A. Kertesz & D. G. Munoz (Eds.), *Pick's disease and Pick complex* (pp. 23–32). New York: Wiley-Liss.

Pick, A. (1892). Uber die Beziehungen der senilen hirnatrophie zur aphasie. *Pragen Medizinischen Wochenschrift 17,* 165–167.

Rascovsky, K., Salmon, D. P., Lipton, A. M., Leverenz, J. B., DeCarli, C., Jagust, W. J., et al. (2005). Rate of progression differs in frontotemporal dementia and Alzheimer disease. *Neurology, 65,* 397–403.

Sakurai, Y., Murayama, S., Fukusako, Y., Bando, M., Iwata, M., & Inoue, K. (1998). Progressive aphemia in a patient with Pick's disease: A neuropsychological and anatomic study. *Journal of the Neurological Sciences, 159,* 156–161.

Scheltens, P., Hazenberg, G. J., Lindeboom, J., Valk, J., & Wolters, E. C. (2000). A case of progressive aphasia without dementia: "Temporal" Pick's disease? *Journal of Neurology, Neurosurgery, and Psychiatry, 53,* 79–80.

Szilies, B., & Karenberg, A. (1986). Disorders of glucose metabolism in Pick's disease. *Fortschritte der Neurologie- Psychiatrie, 54,* 393–397.

Tsuchiya, K., Ikeda, M., Hasegawa, K., Fukui, T., Duroiwa, T., Haga, C., et al. (2001). Distribution of cerebral cortical lesions in Pick's disease with Pick bodies: A clinicopathological study of six autopsy cases showing unusual clinical presentations. *Acta Neuropathologica, 102,* 553–571.

Twamley, E. W., & Bondi, M. W. (2003). The differential diagnosis of dementia. In J. H. Ricker (Ed.), *Differential diagnosis in adult neuropsychological assessment* (pp. 276–326). New York: Springer Publishing Co.

Waddington, J. L., Youssef, H. A., Farrell, M. A., & Toland, J. (1995). Initial 'schizophrenia-like' psychosis in Pick's disease: Case study with neuroimaging and neuropathology, and implications for frontotemporal dysfunction in schizophrenia. *Schizophrenia Research, 18,* 79–82.

Wang, L. N., Zhu, M. W., Feng, Y. Q., & Wang, J. H. (2006). Pick's disease with Pick bodies combined with progressive supranuclear palsy without tuft-shaped astrocytes: A clinical, neuroradiologic and pathological study of an autopsied case. *Neuropathology, 26,* 222–230.

Yamakawa, K., Takanashi, M., Watanabe, M., Nakamura, N., Kobayashi, T., Hasegawa, M., Mizuno, Y., Tanaka, S., & Mori, H. (2006). Pathological and biochemical studies on a case of Pick disease with severe white matter atrophy. *Neuropathology, 26,* 586–591.

Yancopoulou, D., Crowther, R. A., Chakrabarti, L., Gydesen, S., Brown, J. M., & Spillantini, M.G. (2003). Tau protein in frontotemporal dementia linked to chromosome 3 (FTD-3). *Journal of Neuropathology and Experimental Neurology 62,* 878–882.

Part VI

Vascular Disorders

Vascular disorders probably represent one of the most important "teaching tools" for students and practitioners of neuropsychology. Many forms of vascular disorders result in discrete or localized cerebral damage, with corresponding focal or selective loss of cognitive function. These relatively specific cognitive profiles, particularly secondary to strokes, have provided fundamental knowledge about the "behavioral geography" of the brain; that is, much of what is known about lateralized brain functions and specific brain regions has been learned from cases of vascular pathology. The five chapters that follow provide the clinician with examples of many of these specific brain–behavior relationships.

58

Neuropsychological Assessment in a Case of Left Middle Cerebral Artery Stroke

Erin D. Bigler

Blood supply to the cerebral hemispheres is divided into the anterior and posterior cerebrovascular systems. Just above its entrance into the cranial vault, the internal carotid artery branches into the middle and anterior cerebral arteries (MCA and ACA, respectively), which form the anterior distribution. With an entrance ascending the lower brain stem, the two vertebral arteries come together to form the basilar artery with the top of the basilar bifurcating into the two posterior cerebral arteries (PCA), which form the posterior distribution. The anterior and posterior systems are integrated via connections of communicating arteries that form the circle of Willis. This chapter deals with only the neuropsychological sequelae of an MCA cerebrovascular accident (CVA) or stroke. *Stroke* and *CVA* are terms used interchangeably in this chapter. Superimposed on a coronal magnetic resonance imaging (MRI) scan, see Figure 58-1; see also the color figure in the color insert section presents a schematic illustrating the distribution of the three main cerebral arteries, and as clearly shown, the MCA covers the largest territory. The MCA is the largest both in size and extent of vascular supply to each hemisphere. If the reader would place the palm of each hand over each ear, and fan out the fingers while clasping the side of the head, this represents the general coverage of the MCA as to its vascular input to the brain. Cerebrovascular accident is one of the most common neurological events, which represents the second most common cause of death and a major cause of disability constituting one of the most frequent disorders seen by

neuropsychologists (Donnan, Fisher, Macleod, & Davis, 2008). Because of its size and extent of hemispheric distribution, MCA strokes are commonplace (Reeves et al., 2008; Towfighi, Saver, Engelhardt, & Ovbiagele, 2008).

Using MRI technique that measures water diffusion, Figure 58-2 shows the degree of damage that accompanies MCA occlusion in an acute CVA, demonstrating the evolution of an extensive infarction that includes a large sector affecting much of the left hemisphere as shown in the figure. This figure also shows how different MRI sequences can identify the extent of the structural damage following a stroke. Such extensive damage not only disrupts the entirety of the intrahemispheric networks of the brain but also disrupts interhemispheric communication. Because MCA strokes tend to be unilateral, hemispheric specific changes are typically present when an MCA stroke occurs (Reeves et al., 2008; Towfighi et al., 2008). Regardless of hemisphere affected, because the MCA provides the blood supply to the lateral surface of the pre- and postcentral region of the brain that controls motor and somatosensory function, MCA strokes often will affect contralateral motor and somatosensory function, which was the circumstance for the case in Figure 58-2. Large or strategically placed MCA infarcts may also produce visual field defects in the contralateral visual field. From a cognitive impairment perspective, however, MCA strokes typically produce very different neuropsychological patterns of impairment depending on which hemisphere is affected and

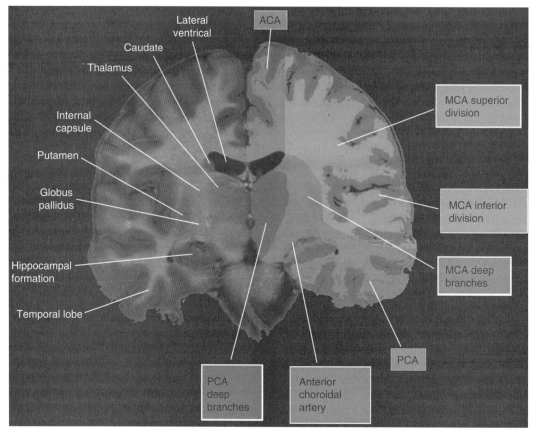

Figure 58-1. Coronal image through the midsection of the thalamus showing different major brain structures and the distribution of the three main cerebral arteries: anterior cerebral artery, blue; middle cerebral artery, mustard yellow; posterior cerebral artery, red-flesh tone. Note the extensiveness of the distribution of the middle cerebral artery, which covers a larger territory than any other cerebral artery.

where in the MCA distribution the stroke has occurred. In right-handed individuals left MCA strokes typically are disruptive of language-based cognitive functions, whereas right MCA strokes are more likely to selectively impair nonverbal, visuospatial, and visuoconstructive abilities (Bigler & Clement, 1997; Bornstein & Matarazzo, 1982; Hutsler & Galuske, 2003; Lezak, Howieson, & Loring, 2004; Morgan & Ricker, 2008). Indeed, much of the earlier work on hemispheric specialization that has consistently demonstrated this was based on MCA cases with lateralized hemispheric damage (Hutsler & Galuske, 2003). As for the case presented in Figure 58-2, this patient was globally aphasic with a right-side paralysis. When such extensive damage is present, the neurocognitive deficits are typically dramatic, unmistakable where impairments are demonstrated

with even the most cursory of exams. With less complete CVAs, neuropsychological impairment nonetheless will typically develop along the general dichotomy of left MCA stroke more likely compromising language-based cognitive functions, whereas right MCA stroke is more likely to affect visuospatial, visuomotor, and nonverbal abilities in right-handed individuals. Regardless of whether the stroke is either a left- or right-hemisphere CVA, infarction along more middle-to-anterior MCA segments will produce motor (in the contralateral upper extremity most likely) and executive impairments, whereas more posterior-to-middle MCA segments are likely to affect motor and sensory functioning combined with impaired spatial and perceptual abilities.

Saver (2006) provides some astonishing insights at the histological level into the effects of stroke

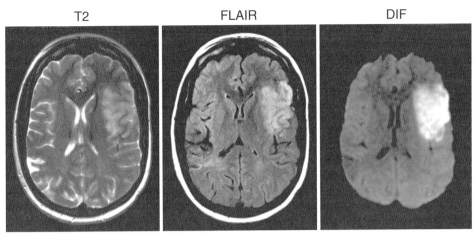

Figure 58-2. T2, fluid attenuated inversion recovery (FLAIR) and diffusion weighted (DWI abbreviated as DIF) axial magnetic resonance imaging studies all at approximately the same level and within 18 hours of acute symptom onset of aphasia and right-side hemiplegia in a 20-year-old patient with known clotting disorder (thrombocytopenia). The DWI sequence is particularly sensitive to the signal changes in parenchymal water content associate with stroke and, as can be visualized, a large area of infarction has begun. The patient's initial presentation of dense right hemiplegia combined with a global aphasia is characteristic of a large middle cerebral artery stroke. The images are presented in radiological perspective where right is on the viewer's left. The extensive areas of damage are shown in the left hemisphere of this patient.

on a typical brain that should always be kept in mind by the neuropsychologist performing an assessment on a patient who has suffered a stroke. The average duration of a large-vessel ischemic stroke, like the one shown in Figure 58-2, is approximately 10 hours (range 6 to 18 hours), where 120 million neurons, 830 billion synapses, and 447 miles of myelinated fibers are lost each hour. Saver estimates that the typical patient loses 1.9 million neurons each minute in which stroke is untreated. Given this kind of information, it is important for the neuropsychologist to understand the extent of structural damage as shown on neuroimaging studies as well as the duration of the patient's acute neurological presentation, to have some clinical insight into how extensive the cortical and subcortical damage from a CVA can be.

As will be explained later, case selection for this chapter on the neuropsychological presentation of an MCA stroke focused on a patient with more subtle residual neuropsychological impairments in the subacute to chronic phase. The more severe MCA strokes produce distinctive clinical syndromes of contralateral hemiplegia and hemi-somatosensory deficit and may also include aphasia, neglect, and hemianopia, as already

mentioned. When present, these "hard" neurological signs of cortical damage in someone with a CVA are considered pathognomic for contralateral MCA stroke and can be straightforwardly identified, requiring minimal neuropsychological assessment methods. For the typical right-handed individual with left-hemisphere MCA stroke, the aphasia can be marked and level of deficit preclude administration of many of the standardized neuropsychological measures that would be typically given. Likewise, right-hemisphere MCA stroke can produce marked left-side neglect along with profound deficits in perceptual-motor function that again would preclude administration of many of the non-verbal standardized neuropsychological tests. These more global cases of pathology associated with MCA stroke are fully discussed in traditional literature of clinical assessment in neuropsychology (Bigler & Clement, 1997; Lezak et al., 2004; Morgan & Ricker, 2008).

Case Presentation

The case selected is from a relatively young individual (age 40 at the time of the left MCA stroke) specifically selected to avoid other cardiovascular and cerebrovascular confounds and risk factors. Older age and cardiovascular risk factors (hypertension, hypercholesteremia, diabetes mellitus, obesity, *etc.*) are major predictors of stroke, but such disorders usually affect the brain in other ways as well in addition to whatever focal effects occur from the stroke (Lawes, Vander Hoorn, & Rodgers, 2008). Presence of these other cerebrovascular risk factors increases the likelihood of getting mixed, and nonlateralized findings, even in the presence of a focal MCA stroke. For this case, selecting a younger individual with an MCA stroke secondary to injury to the carotid artery with resultant MCA stroke provides a more pure case of just the effects of the MCA stroke without the adverse influence of concomitant cardiovascular or cerebrovascular risk factors. While the patient was involved in a high-speed front-end collision, he was seatbelted in a heavy-duty pick-up truck, did not lose consciousness, had no amnesia when assessed in the field or emergency room (ER), had a negative initial computed tomography (CT) scan of the brain, and was not diagnosed with a head injury. However, after first assessed and being monitored in the ER he began to have a change in mental status, which then rapidly progressed to the clinical presentation of a global aphasia and right-side hemiplegia and hemisensory loss, including a right hemianopia, a classic presentation of an evolving large MCA stroke. While in the ER, another round of radiological studies was undertaken, which again were initially unremarkable. Over the course of the next few days, however, it was determined that he had suffered a left carotid artery dissection, likely a result of trauma to the neck, resulting in the left MCA infarction as shown in see Figure 58-3; see also the color figure in the color insert section and 58-4. Note that on this CT the most prominent findings are out in the periphery of the superior MCA distribution, a so-called watershed infarction (Momjian-Mayor & Baron, 2005). Prior to the neuropsychological consultation that is discussed later in this chapter, the patient had been involved in both intense inpatient and outpatient rehabilitation therapy, including speech and language, occupational, and physical therapies. He was now 5 months post injury, which represents another selection factor for this case: to assess the more striking effects of lateralized

damaged from an MCA stroke, a patient needs to be assessed early on because of the adaptive mechanisms that occur as a consequence of recovery, restitution, and compensation often mask over time the initial focal effects of a lateralized lesion (Carey & Seitz, 2007). At the time of assessment, he was still receiving speech and language therapy and was in a physical conditioning program.

Premorbidly, the patient had just retired from the military, where he was an officer. He had a college degree and a distinguished service career in the military. He was physically fit and had recently participated in a marathon run, testament to his fitness prior to the injury and stroke. In high school and college, he was a skilled athlete playing competitive sports. He reportedly was an above-average student, with no history of learning disability. There was no prior history of any neurological and neuropsychiatric disease or disorder and no family history for CVA. As such, no premorbid limitations were present and premorbid cognitive ability level for the purposes of the neuropsychological examination was assessed to likely be at least a standard deviation above the mean across all cognitive domains assessed.

Table 58-1 summarizes neuropsychological test results. As with any neuropsychological assessment, validity of test performance must be the first issue addressed. On the forced-choice Test of Neuropsychological Malingering (Pritchard, 1998), the patient achieved 100% accuracy, which was also reflected in his performance on the standard Rey 15-Item Test. Likewise, recognition recall on the CVLT-II was 15/16 for free recall and 16/16 for the forced-choice component. The patient's WRMT was impaired, as would be expected in a patient with this type of history, which would affect cerebral pathways critical for normal memory function, but considerably above chance levels, supporting the veracity of neuropsychological test performance. Another aspect of validity comes from the expected "pattern" of impairment (see Table 58-1). In this case, non-language-based executive function measures such as Halstead's Category Test and the WCST would be expected to be minimally to not affected. In contrast, language-based tasks like word fluency were impaired, along with suppressed verbal

Table 58-1. Left Cerebrovascular Accident: Neuropsychological Findings

NAME:		AGE:	**41**	DOB:		DOI:		GENDER:		**Male**
ETHNICITY:	**Caucasian**	EDUCATION:	**16**	PSYCHOMETRIST:			DATE:			
PRESENTING PROBLEM/HISTORY:			Left MCA							

Repeatable Battery for the Assessment of Neuropsychological Status (RBANS)						
IMMEDIATE MEM	69	LANGUAGE	95	DELAYED MEMORY	98	
VISUOSPACIAL	96	ATTENTION	94	TOTAL SCALE	86	

MOTOR TESTS

Motor:	Right:	Left:	Lateral Dominance	
Grip:	55	56.6	Hand:	**Right**
Tap:	61.8	52.8	Eye:	**Right**
			Foot:	**Right**
			Writing Hand:	**Right**

SENSORY-PERCEPTUAL TESTS

Reitan – Klove SENSORY-PERCEPTUAL EXAMINATION
Right visual field extinction to double simultaneous visual stimulation right side errors on finger recognition.

Smell Test: 3   **Out of 3 correct**

VERBAL-LANGUAGE TESTS

REITAN-INDIANA APHASIA SCREEN		WIDE RANGE ACHIEVEMENT TEST-3rd Edition				WORD FLUENCY (FAS) 1 minute	
2 errors, 17*3=31; Troubles naming cross,			St. Score	%ile	Grade	F	7
Called (+) or (t) even when told starts with "C"		Reading	83	13	8th	A	7
BOSTON NAMING SCORE:	58/60	Spelling	85	16	8th	S	10
Speech Sounds	3 ERROR	Math	88	21	7th	Mean:	8
Seashore Rhythm	3 ERROR						

VISUAL-SPATIAL		VALIDITY MEASURES			
Hooper Visual Organization Test	28 (T=47)	TNM	100%	Rey 15 Item	15/15

MEMORY TESTS

California Verbal Learning Test-2				Rey Osterreith (Lezak Scoring)					
Trial	Raw Score	Trial	Raw Score	Copy	36				
T1	4	Short Delay Free	5	15' Recall	15.5				
T2	9	Short Delay Cued	10	Comments:	**Slow 4:47 on copy; 4:34 recall**				
T3	11	Long Delay Free	8	Benton Visual Retention Test-R: Form C					
T4	12	Long Delay Cued	11		Observed		Expected		
T5	13	Total 1-5 T-Total	49	Correct	6	LF	1	8	IQ:	95-109
LIST B	2	Total 1-5 T-Score	49	Errors	4	RF	3	2	Age:	15-49
		Recognition	15	Warrington Recognition Memory					
		Forced Choice Recog	16 of 16	Verbal Raw Score	39	Percentile	5-10		
		# False Positive	2	Visual Raw Score	35	Percentile	<5		

Wechsler Memory Scale-III		INTELLECTUAL/COGNITIVE/EXECUTIVE					
Auditory Immediate	80	Trail Making Test					
Visual Memory	109	Trails A	Sec	31	Errors	0	
Immediate Memory	93	Trails B	Sec	102	Errors	1	
Auditory Delayed	89	Category Test (Standard Computer)					
Visual Delayed	106	Errors	26		T-Score	48	
Aud Recog Delayed	110	W.C.S.T					
General Memory	100	# of Categories:		6			
Working Memory	93	# of PSV Errors	8	# of PSV Responses	8		
		WASI					
		VIQ	98	PIQ	111	FSIQ	104

PERSONALITY/EMOTIONAL FUNCTIONING						
SYMPTOM CHECKLIST 90-R		BDI		11		
		BAI		12		
SOM	73	ANX	62	PSY	69	
OC	≥80	HOS	74	GSI	74	
IS	70	PHOB	48	PSDI	64	
DEP	73	PAR	69	PST	71	

intellectual and verbal memory performance, expected deficits in a right-hand dominant individual with lateralized left-hemisphere damage (see Table 58-1). Presence of a lesion anywhere within the declarative memory and language pathways of the brain can affect working memory (see Martin & Ayala, 2004), which was also suppressed in this individual (see Table 58-1, Working Memory Index on the Wechsler Memory Scale and the Attention scale on the RBANS). Inefficient working memory also contributes to the cognitive impairments displayed by any individual with a neurological disorder or injury anywhere in the brain because of the ubiquitous nature of working memory subserving all cognitive processing (see Weiskrantz, 1990).

On motor examination, interestingly his finger oscillation speeds were within normal limits but an occupational therapy evaluation just 6 weeks prior to the neuropsychological assessment had revealed continued right-side motor slowing. It should be recalled that he was originally hemiplegic and the right-side weakness and motor dexterity had been a major focus of his therapy. The patient continued to complain of "clumsiness" and "lack of coordination" on the right. Nonetheless, the finger oscillation findings demonstrated good recovery of function. Diminished right-side weakness was demonstrated on strength of grip testing, where his nondominant hand outperformed his dominant. Most telling, however, was a right visual field inattention to double simultaneous visual stimulation and a tendency to make right visual field visual retention errors on the BVRT. Somatosensory processing was generally intact, but right-side finger recognition errors were noted on the Reitan-Klove Sensory-Perceptual Examination. These motor and sensory-perceptual findings are clearly lateralized and when present, such as in this case, are considered pathognomonic indicators of lateralized hemispheric damage.

Emotional testing demonstrated some endorsement of depression. He was not diagnosed with clinically significant depression and was on no antidepressant or psychoactive medications at the time of the assessment.

Discussion/Conclusions

As can be seen from Figures 58-3 and 58-4 for the left MCA clinical case selected, extensive damage to the left hemisphere was present, with the damage occurring predominantly in what is described as the watershed distribution of the left hemisphere. As would be expected from this type of brain injury, consistent changes in neuropsychological performance reflective of residual impairment in language-based functions is evident as shown in Table 58-1. Recalling that this patient had a college education, he should have had little difficulty performing in the above-average range on basic academic tasks as assessed by the WRAT-3. Likewise, his Verbal IQ score was nearly a standard deviation below his Performance IQ, another observation commonly observed in patients with left-hemisphere MCA stroke.

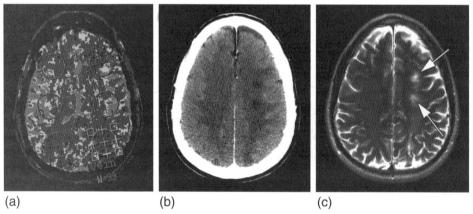

(a)   (b)   (c)

Figure 58-3. All scans are in radiological perspective where the left is on the viewer's right, with the computed tomography (CT) being done 2 days post symptom onset and the magnetic resonance imaging 1 year post stroke. (*a*) Perfusion CT showing subtle asymmetry of blood flow, consistent with ischemia in the left the middle cerebral artery (MCA). (*b*) CT scan showing focal areas of ischemia (dark regions) and reduced density within the white matter of the left hemisphere (note the central white matter of the left hemisphere is darker, reflecting less density). (*c*) T2-weighted focal left hemisphere signal abnormalities (arrows) reflective of old ischemic changes associated with the history of left MCA infarction. Notice the subtle signal differences throughout the entirety of the central white matter of the left hemisphere. Also note that the areas of chronic infarction in the left hemisphere match very closely with the acute areas of infarction.

TRUE INVERSION RECOVERY   FLAIR

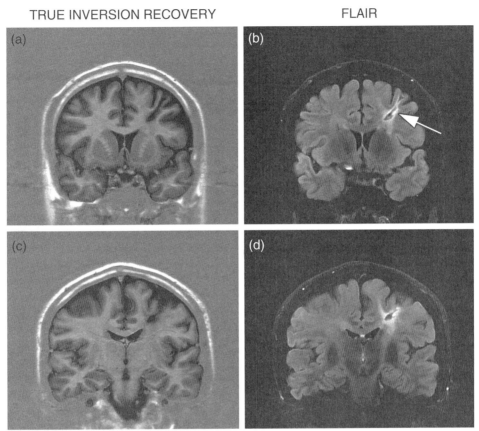

Figure 58-4. Coronal magnetic resonance imaging views demonstrating the anatomical distribution of the middle cerebral artery (MCA) infarction from a left carotid artery dissection. The true inversion sequences as shown in *a* and *c* demonstrates a deep white matter infarction with a large wedge-like defect in the posterior frontal lobe. Note that there is some generalized cortical atrophy of the left frontal region, with greater prominence of cortical sulci. The fluid-attenuated inversion recovery (FLAIR) sequence (*b* and *c*) show extensive white matter signal changes in the central white matter of the left hemisphere, again consistent with the type of cerebral infarction that comes from ischemic changes in the distribution of the MCA of the left hemisphere.

While the effects of the lateralized damage affect verbal-based functions, it is also clear that some nonverbal abilities have also been compromised, especially with regard to memory. An interesting study by Schooler and colleagues (2008), who examined veterans with penetrating brain injuries from the Vietnam war, showed that the key element disrupting memory was presence of a lesion, with the location of the lesion not being the determiner of memory impairment. This makes sense in regard to current conceptualizations of integrated human brain function, where the key is on connectivity of brain regions and their disruption when injury/damage occurs,

rather than the focal location of an injury (see Grefkes et al., 2008; Hagmann et al., 2007, 2008). The disruption of function in one hemisphere can affect the "intact" hemisphere (see Rumiati, 2005; Schallert, Fleming, & Woodlee, 2003) and clearly, that had occurred in the current case study. This study also demonstrates preservation of areas function, such as executive function and the ability to efficiently perform Halstead's Category Test and the WCST.

Emotionally, the patient at the time of this assessment was doing about as well as could be expected given the circumstance and residual impairments at the time of assessment.

MCA stroke can be associated with higher incidence of neurogenic depression (Chemerinski & Levine, 2006; Newberg, Davydow, & Lee, 2006). The patient did display mild elevations on the depression scale of the SCL-90 and the BDI. Elevations on the Somatization and Obsessive-Compulsive (O-C) subscales were also evident on the SCL-90, but these are commonplace in neurological patients reflecting the loss of physical function with the O-C elevations reflective of the need to rehearse information and routines because of the memory/cognitive problems present (Aben, Verhey, Lousberg, Lodder, & Honig, 2002).

The case described above is from a patient with focal left-hemisphere infarction secondary to left-carotid dissection. It does reflect a typical presentation of left-hemisphere damage that is revealed by neuropsychological techniques. How would this contrast with a right-handed patient who sustained a right MCA stroke? Right-hemisphere MCA stroke often preserves language-based cognitive functions with greater deficits in visuospatial functioning. This would result in a pattern of deficits that generally would be opposite of what is presented in Table 58-1, where language functions would be preserved and nonverbal, visuospatial, and visuoconstructive abilities would likely be the most affected. However, working memory effects occur with right-hemisphere stroke as well, which can have a prominent effect on all types of cognitive tasks (Malhotra et al., 2005; Mansueti, de Frias, Bub, & Dixon, 2008).

Also, returning to Figure 58-1, the vascular distribution of the MCA covers extensive territory, and therefore the types of neuropsychological findings are going to vary depending on the exact locale of the lesion(s) from the stroke. Fortunately, with today's imaging capabilities, this can be exquisitely shown, meaning that every neuropsychologist dealing with patients who have suffered a MCA stroke need to be intimately familiar with the neuroimaging findings because they will be the best source for demonstrating where gross pathology has occurred.

References

Aben, I., Verhey, F., Lousberg, R., Lodder, J., & Honig, A. (2002). Validity of the beck depression inventory, hospital anxiety and depression scale, SCL-90, and hamilton depression rating scale as screening instruments for depression in stroke patients. *Psychosomatics, 43*(5), 386–393.

Bigler, E. D., & Clement, P.F. (1997). Diagnostic clinical neuropsychology. In Austin: University of Texas Press.

Bornstein, R. A., & Matarazzo, J. D. (1982). Wechsler VIQ versus PIQ differences in cerebral dysfunction: A literature review with emphasis on sex differences. *Journal of Clinical Neuropsychology, 4*(4), 319–334.

Carey, L. M., & Seitz, R. J. (2007). Functional neuroimaging in stroke recovery and neurorehabilitation: Conceptual issues and perspectives. *International Journal of Stroke, 2*(4), 245–264.

Chemerinski, E., & Levine, S. R. (2006). Neuropsychiatric disorders following vascular brain injury. *Mt Sinai Journal of Medicine, 73*(7), 1006–1014.

Donnan, G. A., Fisher, M., Macleod, M., & Davis, S. M. (2008). Stroke. *Lancet, 371*(9624), 1612–1623.

Grefkes, C., Nowak, D. A., Eickhoff, S. B., Dafotakis, M., Kust, J., Karbe, H., et al. (2008). Cortical connectivity after subcortical stroke assessed with functional magnetic resonance imaging. *Annals of Neurology, 63*(2), 236–246.

Hagmann, P., Cammoun, L., Gigandet, X., Meuli, R., Honey, C. J., Wedeen, V. J., et al. (2008). Mapping the structural core of human cerebral cortex. *PLoS Biology, 6*(7), e159.

Hagmann, P., Kurant, M., Gigandet, X., Thiran, P., Wedeen, V. J., Meuli, R., et al. (2007). Mapping human whole-brain structural networks with diffusion MRI. *PLoS ONE, 2*(7), e597.

Hutsler, J., & Galuske, R. A. (2003). Hemispheric asymmetries in cerebral cortical networks. *Trends in Neuroscience, 26*(8), 429–435.

Lawes, C. M., Vander Hoorn, S., & Rodgers, A. (2008). Global burden of blood-pressure-related disease, 2001. *Lancet, 371*(9623), 1513–1518.

Lezak, M. D., Howieson, D., & Loring, D.W. (2004). *Neuropsychological assessment* (4th ed.). New York: Oxford University Press.

Malhotra, P., Jager, H. R., Parton, A., Greenwood, R., Playford, E. D., Brown, M. M., et al. (2005). Spatial working memory capacity in unilateral neglect. *Brain, 128*(Pt. 2), 424–435.

Mansueti, L., de Frias, C. M., Bub, D., & Dixon, R. A. (2008). Exploring cognitive effects of self reported mild stroke in older adults: Selective but robust effects on story memory. *Neuropsychology, Development, and Cognition. Section B, Aging and Cognition, 15*(5), 545–573.

Martin, N., & Ayala, J. (2004). Measurements of auditory-verbal STM span in aphasia: Effects of item, task, and lexical impairment. *Brain and Language, 89*(3), 464–483.

Momjian-Mayor, I., & Baron, J. C. (2005). The pathophysiology of watershed infarction in internal carotid artery disease: Review of cerebral perfusion studies. *Stroke, 36*(3), 567–577.

Morgan, J. E., & Ricker, J. H. (Eds.). (2008). *Textbook of clinical neuropsychology.* New York: Taylor & Francis.

Newberg, A. R., Davydow, D. S., & Lee, H. B. (2006). Cerebrovascular disease basis of depression: Post-stroke depression and vascular depression. *International Review of Psychiatry, 18*(5), 433–441.

Pritchard, D. A. (1998). Tests of Neuropsychological Malingering (Version 2.0) [computer software]. New York: CRC Press.

Reeves, M. J., Bushnell, C. D., Howard, G., Gargano, J. W., Duncan, P. W., Lynch, G., et al. (2008). Sex differences in stroke: Epidemiology, clinical presentation, medical care, and outcomes. *Lancet Neurol, 7*(10), 915–926.

Rumiati, R. I. (2005). Right, left or both? Brain hemispheres and apraxia of naturalistic actions. *Trends in Cognitive Science, 9*(4), 167–169.

Saver, J. L. (2006). Time is brain–quantified. *Stroke, 37*(1), 263–266.

Schallert, T., Fleming, S. M., & Woodlee, M. T. (2003). Should the injured and intact hemispheres be treated differently during the early phases of physical restorative therapy in experimental stroke or parkinsonism? *Physical Medicine and Rehabilitation Clinics of North America, 14*(Suppl. 1), S27–S46.

Schooler, C., Caplan, L. J., Revell, A. J., Salazar, A. M., & Grafman, J. (2008). Brain lesion and memory functioning: Short-term memory deficit is independent of lesion location. *Psychonomic Bulletin and Review, 15*(3), 521–527.

Towfighi, A., Saver, J. L., Engelhardt, R., & Ovbiagele, B. (2008). Factors associated with the steep increase in late midlife stroke occurrence among US men. *Journal of Stroke and Cerebrovascular Disease, 17*(4), 165–168.

Weiskrantz, L. (1990). Problems of learning and memory: One or multiple memory systems? *Philosophical Transcripts of the Royal Society of London, Part B Biological Sciences, 329*(1253), 99–108.

59

Language Impairments following Basal Ganglia Stroke: Hold and Release Functions in Cognition

Alyssa J. Braaten, Anna Bacon Moore, Eileen L. Cooley, and Anthony Y. Stringer

The basal ganglia, a cluster of nuclei embedded deep within the cerebral hemispheres, are estimated to be affected in up to 60% of patients with intracerebral hemorrhagic stroke (Su, Chen, Kwan, & Guo, 2007). Hence, the basal ganglia are likely to be compromised in many of the stroke patients evaluated by neuropsychologists. While long considered to be a primary motor center within the brain, neuropsychological studies have drawn increasing attention to the role of the basal ganglia in cognition (Crosson, Benjamin, & Levi, 2007). As will be seen, the basal ganglia do not directly mediate cognitive function, but rather play a regulatory role, inhibiting some cognitive activities while enhancing others. This chapter explores the cognitive functions of the basal ganglia in the context of a patient with a left basal ganglia hemorrhagic stroke. An appreciation of the anatomy and circuitry of the basal ganglia is necessary to understand the specific impact of the basal ganglia on cognition. We begin, therefore, with an anatomical overview and present a neuropsychological model of basal ganglia circuitry as a prelude to our discussion of the clinical case.

Basal Ganglia Anatomy and Function

Figure 59-1 shows the gross anatomy of the basal ganglia. (Not all structures described in the text are shown in Figure 59-1. For a more detailed depiction of basal ganglia anatomy, please see Blumenfeld, 2002.) Although anatomists vary slightly in their descriptions, the basal ganglia are typically subdivided into the striatum, globus pallidus, and the subthalamic nucleus (the latter structure is not shown in Figure 59-1). The striatum consists of the caudate nucleus, the putamen (which together comprise the "neostriatum"), the nucleus accumbens, and the olfactory tubercle (not shown). The globus pallidus can be subdivided into medial and lateral segments. The putamen and globus pallidus are sometimes grouped together under the term "lenticular" or "lentiform" nucleus because of their lens shape. The middle cerebral artery is the primary artery feeding the basal ganglia; however, blood is also supplied by the anterior cerebral, anterior choroidal, and the posterior cerebral arteries. The middle cerebral artery is the most common blood vessel involved in stroke, which is likely the reason the basal ganglia are so frequently affected.

Considering the consequences of basal ganglia pathology, few would debate the importance and contribution of the basal ganglia for motor behavior. Both Parkinson disease and Huntington disease are pathological conditions of the basal ganglia that prominently affect motor function. Individuals suffering from Parkinson disease exhibit rigidity and motor slowing, while

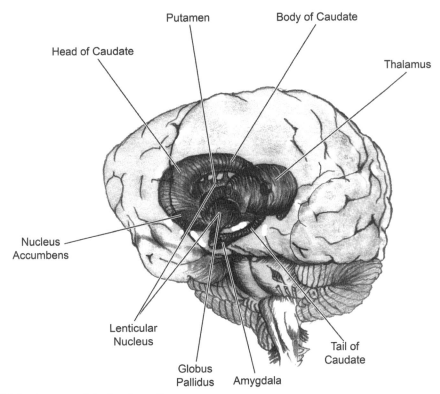

Head of Caudate

Putamen

Body of Caudate

Thalamus

Nucleus
Accumbens

Lenticular
Nucleus

Globus
Pallidus

Amygdala

Tail of
Caudate

Figure 59-1. Anatomy of the basal ganglia.

those with Huntington disease show involuntary choreoathetoid movements. Similarly strokes of the basal ganglia typically impair motor function, producing hemiparesis, hypotonia, gait disturbance, and tremor (Ghika-Schmid, Ghika, Regli, & Bogousslavsky, 1997; Inagaki, Koeda, & Takeshita, 1992). Despite the motor effects of basal ganglia disease, these structures do not actually generate movements (Mink, 1996). Instead, in the healthy brain, the basal ganglia regulate movement by enhancing selected motor output, while suppressing competing or irrelevant motor output (Mink, 1996; Penney & Young, 1986). Similarly, the basal ganglia enhance and suppress neuronal output relevant to cognition.

Basal Ganglia Cognitive Circuitry

The basal ganglia participate in five parallel, but largely discrete frontal-subcortical circuits that have been referred to as the motor, occulomotor, dorsolateral prefrontal, lateral orbitofrontal, and anterior cingulate circuits (Alexander, DeLong, & Strick, 1986). These circuits originate and

terminate in frontal cortical regions, including the supplementary motor cortex, the frontal eye fields, the dorsolateral prefrontal cortex, the orbitofrontal cortex, and the anterior cingulate, respectively (Akkal, Dum, & Strick, 2002; Alexander et al., 1986; Cummings & Trimble, 2002; Inase, Tokuno, Nambu, Akazawa, & Takada, 1999; Strick, Dum, & Picard, 1995). Other important basal ganglia circuits originate in the primary motor cortex, ventral premotor cortex, dorsal premotor cortex, and pre-supplementary motor area (Crosson et al., 2007). All circuits include portions of the striatum, globus pallidus, substantia nigra, thalamus, and cortex. Although these circuits follow distinct paths, they converge in the striatum and globus pallidus (Alexander et al., 1986).

As noted earlier, the basal ganglia do not directly mediate cognitive function. Instead, similar to their regulatory function with regard to movement, they play an important role in regulating the processing and use of cognitive information. More specifically, the basal ganglia enhance target cognitive activities while suppressing competing

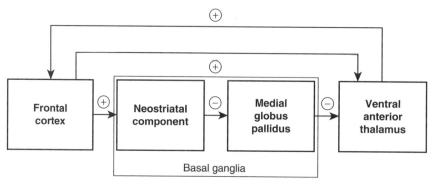

Figure 59-2. Frontal cortex-basal ganglia-thalamic circuit direct loop.

activity (Crosson et al., 2007). This enhancement of cognitive activity may be conceptualized as a "release" function, in that it permits activity to occur. The suppression of competing activity may be conceptualized as a "hold" function in that activity is prevented from occurring. The presupplementary motor area, dorsolateral prefrontal, lateral orbitofrontal, and anterior cingulate circuits are most involved in these hold and release functions that regulate cognition.

The Crosson Model

Crosson proposed a model in which each basal ganglia circuit is composed of direct, indirect, and hyperdirect loops (Crosson et al., 2003; Nambu et al., 2000; Nambu, Tokuno, & Takada, 2002). Figures 59-2, 59-3, and 59-4 provide a simplified illustration of the three loops within a circuit that originates in the frontal cortex. A more detailed description of this circuit may be found in Crosson et al. (2003). As detailed next, each circuit includes excitatory and inhibitory components that underlie basal ganglia hold and release functions.

In the direct loop of the circuit (Figure 59-2), the frontal cortical component sends excitatory (glutatamate) projections to the neostriatum, which in turn sends inhibitory gamma-aminobutyric acid (GABA) projections to medial globus pallidus. Normally, using GABA, the medial globus pallidus inhibits the ventral anterior thalamus. Hence, by inhibiting the inhibitory output of the globus pallidus, this component of the loop releases the ventral thalamus, allowing it to send an excitatory signal back to frontal cortex (again

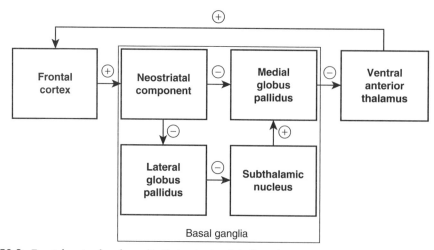

Figure 59-3. Frontal cortex-basal ganglia-thalamic circuit indirect loop.

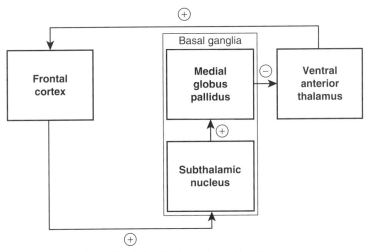

Figure 59-4. Frontal cortex–basal ganglia–thalamic circuit hyperdirect loop.

via glutamate). In this manner, the direct loop in Crosson's model underlies the release function of the basal ganglia. In other words, this component underlies the basal ganglia's ability to facilitate activity initiated in the cortex.

The indirect loop (Figure 59-3) includes additional basal ganglia structures, as well as portions of the direct loop that now serve a different function. The frontal cortical projection to the neostriatum inhibits the lateral globus pallidus, which in turn inhibits the subthalamic nucleus (both utilizing GABA). The net effect of this loop is to increase excitatory input from the subthalamic nucleus to the medial globus pallidus, allowing it to increase inhibition to the thalamus. The indirect loop is part of the hold function of the basal ganglia. If we conceptualize the direct loop as releasing a target behavior, the indirect loop suppresses or holds competing behaviors.

The hyperdirect loop (Figure 59-4) similarly suppresses or holds competing behavior. In this component of the circuit, frontal cortex sends excitatory projections directly to the subthalamic nucleus, which in turn, sends excitatory projections to the medial globus pallidus (both using glutamate). The medial pallidal component then inhibits the thalamus via GABA. This decreases excitatory thalamic output to the cortex. Again, however, the decrease is in competing behavior. The thalamus continues to facilitate target behavior via the activity of the direct loop.

Nambu et al. (2000) reported data supporting Crosson's model in primates. Basal ganglia activity was recorded after electrical stimulation of the primary motor cortex. Shortly after the stimulation, a wave of excitatory input hit the medial globus pallidus (via the hyperdirect loop). When excited the medial globus pallidus increased its inhibition of the thalamus that, in turn, dampened thalamocortical activity. Thus, consistent with the model, this wave of excitation to the medial globus pallidus suppresses or holds actions. The initial wave of suppression essentially "resets" the basal ganglia circuitry in preparation for changing to a new activity (Nambu et al., 2002).

Subsequently, a wave of inhibitory activity arrives at the medial globus pallidus (via the direct loop). This second wave frees thalamocortical projections from pallidal inhibition, thereby enhancing or releasing thalamocortical activity. Finally, a wave of excitation affects the medial globus pallidus via both the hyperdirect and indirect loops. This excitation suppresses thalamocortical activation by increasing pallidal inhibition of its thalamic target (Crosson et al., 2007; Nambu et al., 2002).

Thus, data from primates support Crosson's model of the three loops underlying the basal ganglia's hold and release functions with regard to motor behavior. Crosson's model also makes comparable predictions about the basal ganglia's role in cognition that have been supported in healthy human studies using functional neu-roimaging (Crosson et al., 2003).

The Model's Predictions for Cognition

With disruption of frontal-subcortical circuits due to injury or disease, the excitatory and inhibitory functions of the basal ganglia are affected. Crosson's model predicts that regard-less of whether the involved basal ganglia circuits predominantly govern motor behavior or cogni-tion, damage will cause an imbalance in the direct, indirect, and hyperdirect loops affecting one's ability to hold unwanted actions or cogni-tions, and release target actions or cognitions. Thus, a patient with basal ganglia dysfunction may be unable to hold unwanted responses, making errors of commission on tasks which require spontaneous generation. Alternatively, basal ganglia patients may struggle to overcome inhibition, resulting in a decrease in cognitive output. In addition, since these basal ganglia circuits terminate in frontal areas, measures assessing frontal lobe functions (i.e., measures of problem solving, reasoning, and overall execu-tive functioning) will be negatively affected.

The following case of a patient with a left basal ganglia hemorrhagic stroke illustrates the cogni-tive functions of the basal ganglia as conceptual-ized in the Crosson model. Upon evaluation, the patient demonstrated significant difficulty with measures of language, memory, and executive functioning, despite relatively good motor func-tion. We examine the specific role of the basal ganglia in these cognitive functions with respect to the frontal-subcortical circuits and model just described.

Case Report

History

J. K. was a 70-year-old, right-handed, bilingual, Middle Eastern male with a doctorate in a highly specialized field.[1] He spoke English as a second language since elementary school, completed graduate training in English-speaking countries, and practiced his profession in the United States for more than 40 years. He had no history of developmental learning or attention disorder and excelled in his academic training.

J. K. presented to the emergency room with aphasia and right hemiparesis. Computerized tomography (CT) and magnetic resonance imag-ing (MRI) (see Figure 59-5) revealed an 11.5 mm left basal ganglia hemorrhage centered over the lentiform nucleus with resulting vasogenic edema and mass effect. Such a lesion could potentially affect direct, indirect, and hyperdi-rect loops in the fronto-subcortical circuits of Crosson's model. J. K. remained in intensive care for 9 days, was hospitalized in a medical surgical unit an additional week and then received inpa-tient rehabilitation (physical, occupational, and speech therapy) for 2 weeks. Following dis-charge, he participated in outpatient speech therapy, which was ongoing when he was referred for neuropsychological testing.

Medical history was significant for hyperten-sion, diabetes, hyperlipidemia, and coronary artery disease. One month before his stroke, he underwent his second cardiac catheterization (his first was 4 years earlier) and stent placement. J. K. was taking medications for his hypertension and heart disease (amlodipine besylate, valsar-ton hydrochlorothiazide, and aspirin), diabetes (glucotrol), and hyperlipidemia (simvastatin). There was no known psychiatric history and no current report of psychiatric symptoms, includ-ing depression and anxiety. No other medical problems were identified.

General Neuropsychological Results

J. K. was referred in the last weeks of his speech therapy to determine his potential to resume his professional activity. He was examined 4 months from the onset of his stroke. At the time of testing, J. K.'s speech was fluent and free of para-phasic errors. Articulation, grammar, syntax, and comprehension during the interview appeared intact, although he reported impaired word-finding ability and memory. He was not aware of any other cognitive problems and tended to minimize those he did report. Optimal test conditions were maintained, rapport was easily established and sustained during testing, and the patient was cooperative and pleasant through-out the evaluation. He persisted throughout test-ing and appeared to put forth his best effort. The Reliable Digit Span index (Greiffenstein, Gola, & Baker, 1995) (i.e., the sum of longest forward

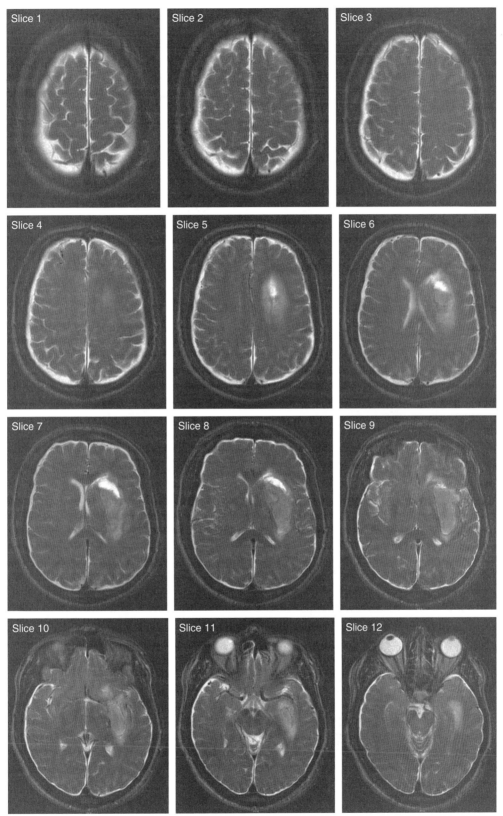

Figure 59-5. Magnetic resonance imaging scans of patient J. K. showing left basal ganglia hemorrhage centered over the lentiform nucleus.

and backward digit span score) has been used to identify patients exhibiting poor effort. The adequacy of J. K.'s effort is thus supported by his reliable digit span of 7 and his accuracy score of 93.8% on the forced-choice recognition trial of the California Verbal Learning Test–Second Edition (Delis, Kramer, Kaplan, & Ober, 2000).

Neuropsychological results are presented in Table 59-1. The table includes tests administered, associated scores, and impairment ranges.[2] J. K. displayed mildly impaired vigilance and moderately impaired ability to simultaneously track and reverse digit sequences. In contrast, his forward digit span and forward and reverse spatial span remained intact. As can be seen in Table 59-1, visual perception, spatial perception, and stimulus recognition abilities were intact. J. K. displayed moderately to severely impaired psychomotor strength, speed, and dexterity bilaterally, with slightly greater impairment in his right hand. He was mildly impaired in his ability to copy simple and more complex geometric figures with his right hand. In the language domain, despite intact ability to describe a pictured scene, to comprehend basic commands, and to repeat words and phrases, J. K. had moderately impaired phonemic and semantic word generation and moderately impaired confrontation naming. On the Boston Naming Test (Kaplan, Goodglass, & Weintraub, 1983), J. K. often described the target word, but he was unable to come up with the proper name, making a total of 26 errors in 60 trials. J. K.'s incorrect responses were often semantically related to the proper name. For example, when presented with the item "palette" J. K. responded with "paint brush." With phonemic cues, J. K. was able to report the correct name on 11 of the 26 incorrect trials. Other components of speech and language appeared grossly intact, although some scores were lower than expected given his background.

With verbal information, J. K. was moderately impaired in his ability to learn with repetition and very severely impaired in his ability to retain verbal information. In fact, after both a short and longer (20 minute) delay on a list-learning task, J. K. had no recollection of the information even when presented with category cues. J. K. showed a highly elevated number of repetition and intrusion errors (greater than 4 standard deviations from the mean). (The nature of these intrusions will be discussed in more detail later.) During a verbal recognition memory trial, he endorsed nearly as many distracter items as target items. Despite his severe verbal memory impairment, his score on a forced-choice recognition trial was within normal limits. As noted previously, this finding suggests good effort. In contrast to his severe verbal memory impairment, J. K. was consistently within normal limits in his ability to learn visuospatial information with repetition and to retain this information after a 15-minute delay.

J. K. displayed severely impaired problem-solving abilities, with severe perseveration evident in his performance. He obtained a Full-Scale IQ of 85 on the Wechsler Abbreviated Scale of Intelligence (The Psychological Corporation, 1999). Overall, his intellectual functioning was in the Low-Average range and fell at the 16th percentile. His demographic background and reading score on the Wechsler Test of Adult Reading (WTAR; The Psychological Corporation, 2001) suggest that his premorbid intellectual functioning was at least average. However, it should be noted that he made several errors during reading, sometimes substituting visually similar words for the target word (e.g., "gunt" for gnat and "*equal*" for *ethereal*) and rotating letters within words (e.g., "p" for b). His current intellectual functioning represents a significant decline from the WTAR estimate, but it is also likely that the WTAR estimate is decreased as an artifact of his language impairment.

Language Impairments Associated with the Basal Ganglia

As noted earlier, phonemic and semantic fluency were significantly below expectation given J. K.'s educational background. After a 30-second delay in which he produced no responses, he was able to identify only two words beginning with the letter "F." Across all three letters on which he was tested, he produced an average of only one correct response per 15-second interval. In addition, J. K. failed to maintain set on multiple occasions. This was particularly striking when he was asked to alternate between fruits and furniture. In the category of fruit, J. K. produced "cucumber," "frankfurter," and "lazy chair."

Table 59-1. J. K.'s Neuropsychological Examination Results

Attention and Mental Tracking	Score	Impairment Range
Digit Vigilance[a]		
—No Distracter Baseline Errors	4	−1
—Conversational Noise Errors	1	WNL
Wechsler Memory Scale–Third Edition[b]		
Total Digits Forward	5	WNL
Total Digits Backward	2	−2.07
Spatial Span Forward	6	WNL
Spatial Span Backward	6	WNL

Stimulus Awareness and Visual Perception	Score	Impairment Range
Visual Field Errors[c]	0	WNL
Unilateral and Bilateral Simultaneous Stimulation Errors[c] (all sensory modalities)	0	WNL
Visual Acuity[d] (with corrective lenses)—Right Eye	20/30	WNL
—Left Eye	20/20	WNL
Line Bisection[e]—Percent Deviation	−2.44	WNL
Ishihara Test for Colour Blindness[f]	15	WNL
Visual Object and Space Perception Battery[g] Test 3: Object Decision	16	WNL
Benton Facial Recognition Test[h]	49	WNL

Spatial Perception and Stimulus Localization	Score	Impairment Range
Randot Stereotests[i] (Binocular Disparity Judgment)—Arc Seconds	70	WNL
Benton Judgment of Line Orientation Test[h]	33	WNL
Visual Object and Space Perception Battery		
Test 7: Number Location	10	WNL
Test 8: Cube Analysis	10	WNL
Luria Mental Rotation[a]	8	WNL

Stimulus Recognition	Total Correct	Impairment Range
Recall of Colors of Familiar Objects[a]	8	WNL
Recognition of Object Drawings[a]	6	WNL
Recognition of Famous Faces (Presidents)[a]	6	WNL
Recognition of Drawings of Fingers[a]	5	WNL
Recognition of Famous Landmarks[a]	5	WNL

Psychomotion	Score	Impairment Range
Hand Dynamometer[c] (Kilograms)—Right Hand	*discontinued*	
—Left Hand	23.5	−2
Finger Tapping[c] (Average Taps) —Right Hand	22.4	−1
—Left Hand	20.4	−1
Grooved Pegboard[j]		
—Right Hand Total Time (in seconds)	164	−3
—Right Hand Drops	0	WNL
—Left Hand Total Time (in seconds)	138	−3
—Left Hand Drops	1	WNL
Sequential (Fist/Edge/Palm) Movements[a]		
—Initial Hand (Right/Left)	Right	
—Guidance Required (Nonverbal/Verbal)	Nonverbal	
—Right Hand (Total Correct)	10	WNL
—Left Hand (Total Correct)	10	WNL

(*Continued*)

Table 59-1. J. K.'s Neuropsychological Examination Results (*Continued*)

Psychomotion	Score	Impairment Range
Tandem Reciprocal Movements[a]		
—Guidance Required (Nonverbal/Verbal)	Nonverbal	
—Shift Trial (Perseverative) Errors	0	WNL
—Nonshift Trial (Disinhibited/Echopraxic) Errors	0	WNL
Triple Loops[a] (Extra Loops in Ten Trials)	0	WNL
Reaching for Targets[a] (Number Correct)—Right Hand	12	WNL
—Left Hand	12	WNL
Praxis Errors[k]		
Buccofacial Pantomime	0	WNL
Right Hand Pantomime	2	WNL
Ideomotor Left-Hand	2	WNL
Pantomime Ideational	0	WNL
Drawing Errors[a] (Square, Cross, Triangle)—Right Hand	3	−1
—Left Hand	1	WNL
Drawing Errors (Cube)—Dominant (Right) Hand	2	WNL
Tombaugh-Taylor Complex Figure Copy Trial[l]	57	−1.86

Language and Calculation	Score	Impairment Range
Boston Naming Test[m]	34	−2.67
Western Aphasia Battery[k]–Oral Language Subtests		
Fluency	10	WNL
Comprehension	8.75	WNL
Repetition	9.6	WNL
Naming	9.7	WNL
Western Aphasia Battery–Written Language Subtests		
Reading Aloud	10	WNL
Reading Comprehension	10	WNL
Spelling of Simple Words	10	WNL
Alphabet Writing	12	WNL

Cognitive Fluency	Score	Impairment Range
Delis-Kaplan Executive Function System[n]–Verbal Fluency Test		
Letter Fluency	3	−2.33
Category Fluency	4	−2
Category Switching Accuracy Score	1	−3
Set Loss Error	8	WNL
Repetition Error	11	WNL

Anterograde Learning and Memory	Score	Impairment Range
Tombaugh-Taylor Complex Figure		
Trial 1 Recall	33.3	WNL
Trial 2 Recall	54.4	WNL
Trial 3 Recall	71.9	WNL
Trial 4 Recall	71.9	WNL
Delayed Recall	70.2	WNL
California Verbal Learning Test–Second Edition[o]		
Trial 1 Recall	3/16	−1.5
Trial 2 Recall	5/16	−1
Trial 3 Recall	4/16	−2
Trial 4 Recall	4/16	−2
Trial 5 Recall	5/16	−2
List B Recall	4/16	WNL

Table 59-1. J. K.'s Neuropsychological Examination Results (*Continued*)

Anterograde Learning and Memory	Score	Impairment Range
California Verbal Learning Test–Second Edition[o]		
Short-Delay Free Recall	0	–3
Short-Delay Cued Recall	0	–3.5
Long-Delay Free Recal	0	–2.5
Long-Delay Cued Recall	0	–3.5
Total Repetitions	10	–1.5
Free Recall Intrusions	17	–4.5
Cued Recall Intrusions	17	–4
Recognition Hits	14/16	WNL
False-Positive Errors	12	–2
Forced-Choice Recognition (percent)	93.8	

Ideation and Problem Solving	Score	Impairment Range
Wisconsin Card Sorting Test[a] (Emory Short Form)		
Correct Strategies Identified before Start	3	WNL
Correct Strategies Identified at Midpoint	2	–1
Correct Strategies Identified at End	2	–1
Erroneous Strategies Reported at All Intervals	2	WNL
Completed Sorts	1	–3
Total Errors	36	–3
Perseverative Errors	28	–3
Percent Perseverative Errors	77.8	–3
Impulsive (Failure to Maintain Set) Errors	1	–1

Intellectual Functioning	Score	Impairment Range
Wechsler Test of Adult Reading[p]–Demographic and Reading Based Estimated Premorbid Full-Scale IQ	106	WNL
Wechsler Abbreviated Scale of Intelligence[q] (two subtests)		
Vocabulary	10	WNL
Matrix Reasoning	4	–2
Full Scale Intelligence Quotient	85	–1

Note. Impairment ranges are *z*-scores whenever available. Operationally, 1–2 standard deviations below the mean = mildly impaired,; 2–3 standard deviations below the mean = moderately impaired; 3 or more below the mean = severely impaired; WNL, within normal limits.

[a] Stringer, 1996.

[b] Wechsler, 1997.

[c] Reitan & Wolfson, 1993.

[d] Hart & Hopkins, 2003.

[e] Schenkenberg, Bradford, & Ajax, 1980.

[f] Ishihara, 1992.

[g] Warrington & James, 1991.

[h] Benton, Hamsher, Varney, & Spreen, 1983.

[i] Rothstein & Sacks, 1972.

[j] Klove, 1963.

[k] Kertesz, 1982.

[l] Tombaugh, Schmidt, & Faulkner, 1992.

[m] Kaplan et al., 1983.

[n] Delis, Kaplan, & Kramer, 2001.

[o] Delis et al., 2000.

[p] The Psychological Corporation, 2001.

[q] The Psychological Corporation, 1999.

Notably only one of these set loss errors was from the alternate category (furniture), while the other two were from extraneous food categories.

Memory Impairments Associated with the Basal Ganglia

As noted previously, J. K.'s performance on the short and long delayed recall trials of the California Verbal Learning Test–Second Edition (Delis et al., 2000) was very severely impaired. The CVLT-II Standard Form consists of five learning trials of a 16-word list, presentation of a 16-word distracter list, and short- and long-delayed spontaneous and cued recall trials, followed by a recognition trial. The list that the patient is to acquire consists of the names of furniture, vegetables, ways of traveling, and animals. J. K.'s mistakes included a significant number of semantically and phonemically unrelated intrusions. For example, across the initial learning trials, J. K. produced such extraneous, unrelated words as "callaway," "straight," "repair," and "lawn." He also demonstrated significant intrusions following a distracter trial. These intrusions included both words from the distracter list and completely unrelated intrusions (e.g., "argue" and "bargain price"). These errors continued despite the provision of semantic cues. He was unable to spontaneously recall any of the target words, and he did not profit from the use of cues. In fact, cues led to additional intrusion errors (e.g., when cued to recall furniture from the list, J. K. responded in the following order "arms," "leg," and "tall buildings").

Problem-Solving Impairments Associated with the Basal Ganglia

Problem-solving impairments were also noted in J. K.'s evaluation. For example, he demonstrated significant impairment on an abbreviated version of the Wisconsin Card Sorting Test (Stringer, 1996). This version of the test utilizes only the cards that do not share multiple attributes (e.g., the same shape and color), yielding a total of 24 cards in each of two decks. The traditional instructions are given to the patient; however, after the key cards are placed on the table, the patient is asked to name ways in which the cards can be sorted. The patient is asked the same question after the first 24 cards, and again at the end of the test. The sorting strategy is changed after every sixth correct match, as opposed to the traditional 10, due to the reduced number of cards. J. K. was able to identify all three sorting strategies each time he was asked, which excludes the possibility that his poor performance was secondary to an inability to identify strategies. However, despite his ability to identify sorting strategies, he was able to successfully complete only one sort secondary to significant perseveration (Table 59-1).

Discussion

Summary of Findings Relevant to Crosson's Model.

The case presented highlights the similarity between the well-known motor impediments and the lesser-known cognitive consequences of basal ganglia pathology. According to Crosson's model, damage to the basal ganglia can lead to an imbalance in the direct, indirect, and hyperdirect loops, which affects the ability to hold or suppress unwanted cognitions while releasing target cognitions. The extent of this imbalance in hold and release functions may be related to the size of the lesion and the specific basal ganglia pathways and nuclei affected. Given a sufficiently large lesion, a patient with basal ganglia dysfunction will be unable to inhibit unwanted responses and will therefore make intrusion errors. In addition, the patient will simultaneously demonstrate difficulty releasing target responses. These hold and release deficits are likely to be especially evident with regard to tasks that require the spontaneous generation of responses, such as fluency and free recall tasks.

The current case presented with a sizeable 11.5 mm basal ganglia lesion affecting the globus pallidus, caudate, and putamen (i.e., lentiform nucleus). As the direct, hyperdirect, and indirect pathways run through the globus pallidus, errors secondary to the disruption of these pathways are likely. Hence, we expect to see the imbalance in hold and release functions that the Crosson model predicts in J. K.'s neuropsychological performance.

The predicted pattern was evident both in J. K.'s language and memory test performance.

With regard to language, J. K.'s limited phonemic fluency (i.e., an average of 1 response every 15 seconds) and prolonged latency (e.g., a 30-second delay to respond) appear consistent with difficulty overcoming the inhibitory or hold function of the basal ganglia. In addition, he made striking set loss errors (e.g., reporting "frankfurter" in the fruit category), suggesting an inappropriate release (or failure to inhibit) of extraneous but semantically related responses.

During memory performance, J. K. again produced extraneous responses. This included both semantically related and unrelated words. One example, in particular, appears to illustrate the imbalance in hold and release functions. As noted earlier, when cued with the memory category "furniture," J. K. responded "arms," "leg," and "tall buildings." Some items of furniture have arms and legs; hence, these errors may be semantically related. However, "tall buildings" is clearly a categorically unrelated error. Cognitively, J. K. is attempting to release responses in the furniture category, but he appears unable to hold activation discretely to the target category. Activation spreads to other categories, and the resulting responses are not inhibited. Thus, again we see a pattern of errors consistent with an imbalance in the hold and release functions of the basal ganglia.

Given that J. K.'s lesion is confined to the left basal ganglia, we did not expect, and did not find, analogous problems with visuospatial abilities. Motor impairment was evident and more severe contralateral to the left basal ganglia lesion and consisted of both weakness and slow performance. In addition, problem-solving impairment was evident on a shortened version of the Wisconsin Card Sorting Test. Despite J. K.'s ability to identify sorting strategies, he perseverated throughout the test, never shifting from his initial sorting category. Problem-solving deficits may arise following basal ganglia lesions due to the reciprocal connections between the frontal lobes and the basal ganglia. It is possible that the same imbalance in hold and release functions accounts for the failure to shift and perseveration during problem solving. However, unlike J. K.'s highly distinct pattern of language and memory errors, his pattern of problem-solving performance may not be specific to the basal ganglia as it may be seen with lesions in other brain regions.

Limitations

While J. K.'s cognitive performance is consistent with Crosson's model, findings from a single case do not provide a scientific test of the model. Furthermore, structural radiologic scans do not have sufficient resolution to discretely identify direct, indirect, and hyperdirect basal ganglia pathways. We can only infer the involvement of these pathways from the gross anatomical areas identified in J. K.'s MRI scans. In addition, J. K.'s 11.5 mm hemorrhage is large enough to produce a lesion zone that extends beyond the discrete frontal-subcortical pathways in Crosson's model. Nonetheless, our case illustration provides neuropsychological support for the Crosson model and the predicted parallels between basal ganglia motor and cognitive impairments.

Implications for Assessment Practices

It is important to assess, quantitatively and qualitatively, basal ganglia hold and release functions that impact cognition. Appropriate measures for doing so will require the spontaneous generation of responses within and between semantic categories and should allow quantification of the degree of intrusion or slippage between categories. Current measures appropriate to this task include tests of word and design fluency, naming, memory cued by semantic or visual categories, and set holding and shifting during Stroop tasks (Stroop, 1935) or problem solving. Unfortunately, existing measures were not designed for the express purpose of quantifying hold and release errors in basal ganglia patients. There is both a need and an opportunity for neuropsychologists to expand upon current procedures.

Future measures should quantify the distance between categories in order to capture the extent of basal ganglia impairment. For example, the categories "fruits" and "vegetables" are semantically closer than "fruits" and "tools." Hence, patients with a lesser degree of basal ganglia involvement might be more likely to show release errors between more closely related categories while patients with a greater deficit (such as J. K.) might show errors even between disparate categories. In a parallel manner, visual categorization might be impacted by right basal ganglia lesions and hence measures that quantify errors based on visual similarity may also be helpful in assessing these patients. Future tests may also be enhanced by incorporating current experimental tasks shown to be sensitive to basal ganglia function. This includes priming and ambiguous sentence tasks requiring inhibition of competing responses (Chenery, Angwin, & Copland, 2008; Copland, Chenery, & Murdoch, 2000).

With improved assessment methods, neuropsychologists have the potential to increase understanding of the basal ganglia's role in cognition. More importantly, with improved cognitive assessments, neuropsychologists will contribute substantially to the clinical care of the estimated 60% of stroke patients who present with basal ganglia dysfunction.

Notes

1. To preserve anonymity, we are limiting the details about the patient's education and work history.
2. Operationally, we label scores that are 1–2 standard deviations below the mean as mildly impaired, scores that are 2–3 below the mean as moderately impaired, and scores that are 3 or more below the mean as severely impaired.

References

Akkal, D., Dum, R. P., & Strick, P. L. (2002). Cerebellar and basal ganglia inputs to the presupplementary area. *Society for Neuroscience Abstract Viewer/Itinerary Planner*, Online, Program No. 462.14.

Alexander, G., DeLong, M., & Strick, P. (1986). Parallel organization of functionally segregated circuits linking basal ganglia and cortex. *Annual Review of Neuroscience, 9*, 357–381.

Benton, A. L., Hamsher, K. de S., Varney, N., & Spreen, O. (1983). *Contributions to neuropsychological assessment: A clinical manual.* New York: Oxford University Press.

Blumenfeld, H. (2002). *Neuroanatomy through clinical cases.* Sunderland, MA: Sinauer Associates.

Chenery, H., Angwin, A., & Copland, D. (2008). The basal ganglia circuits, dopamine, and ambiguous word processing: A neurobiological account of priming studies in Parkinson's disease. *Journal of International Neuropsychological Society, 14*, 351–364.

Copland, D. A., Chenery, H. J., & Murdoch, B. E. (2000). Persistent deficits in complex language function following dominant nonthalamic subcortical lesions. *Journal of Medical Speech-Language Pathology, 8*, 1–15.

Crosson, B., Benefield, H., Cato, M., Sadek, J., Moore, A., Wierenga, C., et al. (2003). Left and right basal ganglia and frontal activity during language generation: Contributions to lexical, semantic, and phonological processes. *Journal of the International Neuropsychological Society, 9*, 1061–1077.

Crosson, B., Benjamin, M., & Levy, I. (2007). Role of the basal ganglia in language and semantics: Supporting cast. In J. Hart, Jr. & M. Kraut (Eds.), *Neural basis of semantic memory* (pp. 219–243). New York: Cambridge University Press.

Cummings, J. L., & Trimble, M. R. (2002). *Neuropsychiatry and behavioral neurology.* Arlington, VA: American Psychiatric Publishing, Inc.

Delis, D. C., Kaplan, E., & Kramer, J. H. (2001). *Delis-Kaplan Executive Function System, examiner's manual.* San Antonio, TX: The Psychological Corporation.

Delis, D. C., Kramer, J. H., Kaplan, E., & Ober, B. A. (2000). *California Verbal Learning Test – Second Edition (CVLT-II).* San Antonio, TX: Psychological Corporation.

Ghika-Schmid, F., Ghika, J., Regli, F., & Bogousslavsky, J. (1997). Hyperkinetic movement disorders during and after acute stroke: The Lausanne stroke registry. *Journal of Neurological Sciences, 146*, 109–116.

Greiffenstein, M. F., Gola, T., & Baker, W. J. (1995). Validation of malingered amnesic measures with a large clinical sample. *Psychological Assessment, 6*, 218–224.

Hart, A. C., & Hopkins, C. A. (2003). *International classification of diseases, 9th revision, clinical modification* (Vol. 1, 6th ed.). Salt Lake City, UT: Ingenix.

Inagaki, M., Koeda, T., & Takeshita, K. (1992). Prognosis and MRI after ischemic stroke of the basal ganglia. *Pediatric Neurology, 8*, 104–108.

Inase, M., Tokuno, H., Nambu, A., Akazawa, T., & Takada, M. (1999). Corticostriatal and corticosubthalamic input zones from the presupplementary motor area in the macaque monkey: Comparison with the input zones from the supplementary motor area. *Brain Research, 833*, 191–201.

Ishihara, S. (1992). *Ishihara's Test for Colour Blindness.* Tokyo, Japan: Kanehara & Company.

Kaplan, E. F., Goodglass, H., & Weintraub, S. (1983). *The Boston Naming Test* (2nd ed.). Philadelphia: Lea & Febiger.

Kertesz, A. (1982). *Western Aphasia Battery Test manual.* Orlando, FL: Grune & Stratton.

Klove, H. (1963). Clinical neuropsychology. In F. M. Forster (Ed.), *The medical clinics of North America.* New York: Saunders.

Mink, J. (1996). The basal ganglia: Focused selection and inhibition of competing motor programs. *Progress in Neurobiology, 50*, 381–425.

Nambu, A., Tokuno, H., Hamada, I., Kita, H., Imanishi, M., Akazawa, T., et al. (2000). Excitatory cortical inputs to pallidal neurons via the subthalamic nucleus in the monkey. *Journal of Neurophysiology, 84*, 289–300.

Nambu, A., Tokuno, H., & Takada, M. (2002). Functional significance of the cortico subthalamopallidal "hyperdirect" pathway. *Neuroscience Research, 43*, 111–117.

Penney, J. B., Jr., & Young, A. B. (1986). Striatal inhomogeneities and basal ganglia function. *Movement Disorders, 1*, 3–16.

Reitan, R. M., & Wolfson, D. (1993). *The Halstead-Reitan Neuropsychological Test Battery*. Tucson, AZ: Neuropsychology Press.

Rothstein, T. B., & Sacks, J. G. (1972). Defective stereopsis in lesions of the parietal lobe. *American Journal of Ophthalmology, 73*, 281–284.

Schenkenberg, T., Bradford, D. C., & Ajax, E. T. (1980). Line bisection and unilateral visual neglect in patients with neurologic impairment. *Neurology, 30*, 509–517.

Strick, P. L., Dum, R., & Picard, N. (1995). Macro-organization of the circuits connecting the basal ganglia with the cortical motor areas. In J. C. Houk, J. L. Davis, & D. G. Beiser (Eds.), *Models of information processing in the basal ganglia* (pp. 117–130). Cambridge, MA: MIT Press.

Stringer, A. Y. (1996). *A guide to adult neuropsychological diagnosis*. Philadelphia: F. A. Davis Company.

Stroop, J. R. (1935). Studies of interference in serial verbal reactions. *Journal of Experimental Psychology, 18*, 643–662.

Su, C., Chen, H., Kwan, A., Lin, Y., & Guo, N. (2007). Neuropsychological impairment after hemorrhagic stroke in the basal ganglia. *Archives of Clinical Neuropsychology, 22*, 465–474.

The Psychological Corporation. (1999). Wechsler Abbreviated Scale of Intelligence manual. San Antonio, TX: Author.

The Psychological Corporation. (2001). Wechsler Test of Adult Reading. San Antonio, TX: Author.

Tombaugh, T. N., Schmidt, J. P., & Faulkner, P. (1992). A new procedure for administering the Taylor Complex Figure: Normative data over a 60 year span. *Clinical Neuropsychologist, 6*, 63–79.

Warrington, E. K., & James, M. (1991). *The Visual Object and Space Perception Battery manual*. Bury St. Edmunds, England: Thames Valley Test Company.

Wechsler, D. (1997). *Wechsler Memory Scale-III administration and scoring manual*. San Antonio, TX: The Psychological Corporation.

60

Vascular Dementia

Nikki H. Stricker, Joseph R. Sadek, and Kathleen Y. Haaland

Vascular dementia is the second leading cause of dementia in the elderly following Alzheimer's disease. Prevalence estimates in pathologic studies suggest that vascular dementia accounts for roughly 11% of dementia cases (Jellinger, 2008), with clinical estimates ranging from 4.5% to 39% (Kase, 1991). Prevalence estimates vary widely due to the heterogeneous nature of vascular dementia, sampling bias, the high prevalence of mixed neuropathology, and the existence of multiple classification systems (*DSM, ICD-10,* NINDS-AIREN, ADDTC; see Haaland & Swanda, 2008 for review) that are not interchangeable (Gold et al., 2002). Multiple mechanisms of cerebrovascular disease can have differing clinical presentations, and several subtypes of vascular dementia have been proposed (Erkinjuntti, 2007), including strategic infarct dementia (see Roman et al., 1993), subcortical vascular dementia (also known as small-vessel dementia or subcortical ischemic vascular dementia), and multi-infarct dementia (also known as cortical vascular dementia or post-stroke dementia).

Multi-infarct dementia (Hachinski, Lassen, & Marshall, 1974) is often viewed as the prototypical vascular dementia syndrome, characterized by multiple cortical or subcortical infarcts that can be visualized by neuroimaging, sudden onset of symptoms with stepwise progressive deterioration, focal neurologic signs, and neuropsychological deficits that are related to specific sites of damage. The cognitive deficits associated with multi-infarct dementia are fairly heterogeneous,

depending on lesion location. Although historical views of vascular dementia were based on multi-infarct dementia, it is now recognized that cognitive deficits associated with cerebrovascular disease are much broader than that captured by multi-infarct dementia. Although multi-infarct dementia is often considered the type of vascular dementia most frequently encountered by neuropsychologists (Lezak, Howieson, & Loring, 2004), and as such was chosen for the current case study, this may not be the case. A recent magnetic resonance imaging (MRI) study revealed that subcortical vascular dementia, specifically small-vessel vascular dementia, accounted for 74% of 706 vascular dementia cases based on *DSM-IV* and NINDS-AIREN criteria, MRI, and neurological and neuropsychological evaluation (Staekenborg et al., 2008), although without neuropathological data it cannot be determined whether additional early Alzheimer pathology may also have contributed.

The cognitive and behavioral changes in subcortical vascular dementia are more homogeneous than those in multi-infarct dementia due to their association with a particularly significant disruption of prefrontal-subcortical circuits. These changes are often more insidious and are characterized by predominant executive dysfunction, psychomotor slowing, and changes in gait, urinary functioning, affect, and mood (see Roman, Erkinjuntti, Wallin, Pantoni, & Chui, 2002 for review). Clinically significant deficits associated with cerebrovascular mechanisms often do not meet traditional criteria for dementia. For example, the *DSM-IV* requires cognitive impairment in two or more domains, one of which must be memory. Such traditional dementia criteria are largely based on the clinical presentation of Alzheimer's disease, wherein the hallmark symptom is early memory impairment. Only one of the previously mentioned dementia classification symptoms (ADTTC; Chui et al., 1992) does *not* require memory impairment for a diagnosis of vascular dementia, although multiple researchers have argued against the memory criteria (Benisty et al., 2008; Bowler, 2003; Hachinski et al., 2006; Roman et al., 2004).

Alternatives to the highly debatable term "vascular dementia," such as *vascular cognitive impairment* (VCI; Hachinski, 1994) and *vascular cognitive disorder* (VCD; Sachdev, 1999; see O'Brien et al., 2003 for review), have been proposed in an effort to capture a wider range of cognitive impairment resulting from various causes of cerebrovascular disease and to allow for early identification of this impairment (Bowler, 2002). There are a multitude of vascular risk factors that are associated with vascular cognitive impairment, including arterial hypertension, diabetes, hypercholesterolemia, history of stroke or transient ischemic attack, smoking, atrial fibrillation, myocardial infarction, coronary heart disease, and generalized atherosclerosis (Erkinjuntti, 2007; Roman et al., 2004). It has been shown that vascular risk factors also increase one's risk of developing Alzheimer's disease (Jin, Ostbye, Feightner, Di Legge, & Hachinski, 2008) and some researchers have argued that vascular dementia and Alzheimer's disease may share a common etiology (Casserly & Topol, 2004; de la Torre, 2002; Zlokovic, 2004). The differential diagnosis of vascular dementia from Alzheimer's disease is often part of the neuropsychological referral question. This distinction can be difficult and is confounded by the high prevalence of co-occurring vascular and Alzheimer neuropathology (see Jellinger & Attems, 2007 for review). Several studies have suggested that whereas episodic memory impairment is the most significant cognitive deficit in Alzheimer's disease, greater executive dysfunction relative to other cognitive domains is the hallmark of vascular dementia (Desmond, 2004; Graham, Emery, & Hodges, 2004), although some studies do not support the specificity of executive dysfunction (Reed et al., 2007).

The following case study was selected because it exemplifies a multi-infarct dementia, with MRI evidence of both cortical and subcortical involvement that corresponds to the patient's clinical presentation.

Case Study

The patient is a 58-year-old, left-handed, single, Caucasian male with 12 years of education and a history of multiple strokes (1973, 2006). He has never been married, has no children, denied any history of learning disability, and worked in a medical facility for 40 years, most recently in medical records. He was referred by his physician because the family and attorney had concerns that the patient's cognitive deficits had resulted in bankruptcy.

The history was obtained from the patient, his sister, and hospital records. The patient had two cerebrovascular accidents that required hospitalization. The first in 1973 was associated with persisting deficits in peripheral vision, and impairment in speed of processing, divided attention and switching tasks, and topographic orientation. The second in 2006 was reportedly associated with additional persisting deficits that included left homonymous hemianopsia, decreased sensory perception on the right side of the body, spastic gait, additional psychomotor slowing, bradykinesia, slurred speech, decreased writing legibility, and decreased short-term memory. There was urinary incontinence and retention following the stroke that partially resolved. His most recent neurological exam also noted hyperreflexia and mildly increased tone in the patient's extremities. These deficits negatively affected his ability to function at his job and he subsequently retired.

An MRI of the brain (see Figure 60-1) 2 days following the 2006 stroke revealed moderate diffuse cerebral volume loss, multiple bilateral infarcts in the occipital and frontal lobes, left cerebellar infarct, small lacunar infarcts in the left putamen and bilateral thalami, and mild to moderate periventricular white matter changes. In addition, diffusion weighted images showed punctate areas of restricted diffusion on the periphery of the left occipital infarct consistent

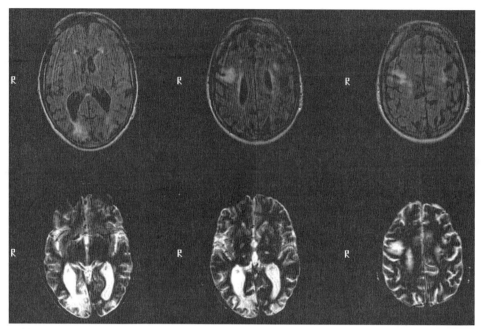

Figure 60-1. Magnetic resonance imaging. (*Top row*) Axial slices of fluid-attenuated inversion recovery (FLAIR) sequence that is complicated by motion artifact. (*Bottom row*) Axial slices of T2-weighted sequence.

with new small areas of infarction, located at the posterior temporal occipital junction.

The patient reported that he was currently filing for bankruptcy due to outstanding credit card debt and loss of his job following the 2006 stroke. The patient's sister has had durable power of attorney for his finances since that time. Although the patient reported some decrease in function, he did not seem to appreciate the full significance of his deficits. He lives alone and reported no functional impairment except that he has not driven since the last stroke. The patient's sister, however, reported impairments in several instrumental activities of daily living (e.g., finances, cooking, shopping).

Other medical history included a 40-year history of hypertension and one pack per day of cigarette smoking, a remote history of heavy alcohol use, and a strong family history of vascular risk factors, including congenital heart problems and factor V Leiden deficiency (genetic disorder that increases the risk of blood clots). The patient scored 12 out of a possible 13 points on Rosen's modification of the Hachinski Ischemic Score (HIS; Rosen, Terry, Fuld, Katzman, & Peck, 1980) due to the presence of the following characteristics: abrupt onset, "stepwise" decline, somatic complaints, hypertension history, stroke history, focal neurological symptoms, and focal neurological signs. Even on this briefer ischemic scale, the patient's score is well above the suggested 7-point cut-off suggestive of multi-infarct dementia based on Hachinski's original scale. The patient denied any significant psychiatric history. Medications included Finasteride (5 mg) and Tamsulosin (0.4 mg) daily for benign hypertrophy of the prostate, Hydrochlorothiazide (25 mg) and Metoprolol (25 mg daily) for hypertension, and Warfarin (8 mg daily) for thrombosis prevention.

The patient was pleasant, responsive to questioning, and he cooperated with all aspects of the evaluation. He ambulated with the assistance of a walker but could move without it when needed. He exhibited occasional word-finding difficulty, and his speech was slow and dysarthric, but of normal volume and prosody. He demonstrated good attention, understood test instructions, and appeared to put forth adequate effort. His response latency was slow. His affect was full range, stable, and consistent with euthymic mood. The neuropsychological evaluation was considered valid.

Test Results

Please refer to Table 60-1 for raw scores and normative test data. Estimated premorbid intelligence (Shipley) and simple auditory attention were in the average range. Working memory was impaired as evidenced by his inability to perform more than two digits backward and missing two calculations on serial sevens. He showed slight evidence for left hemifield neglect on line bisection, although he seemed to adequately compensate for this on other tasks. Although his slowed motor speed, visual field cut and possible neglect likely contributed to his moderately to severely impaired performance on two psychomotor tasks (Trails A and Digit Symbol), his slowness in reciting familiar sequences and his long response latencies throughout the exam suggest that he has deficits in processing speed that cannot be explained by motor or visual impairment.

Learning and memory skills were characterized by mildly impaired encoding and retrieval without evidence of rapid forgetting. On a word list learning task (CVLT-II), he recalled 4/16 words on trial 1 (mildly impaired, –1.5 SD) and 10/16 words by trial 5 (average range, –0.5 SD). Short- and long-delay free recall were within the average range (8/16 and 7/16 words, respectively), and he did not benefit from cues. He showed poor self-monitoring across the learning

Table 60-1. Neuropsychological Test Scores (Raw and Normative Values)

Cognitive Domain/Test	Raw Score	Normative Score
General Cognition		
Estimated Premorbid Intellectual Functioning		
Shipley Institute of Living Scale		
Vocabulary	28	48 T
Abstraction	12	46 T
Estimated WAIS-R IQ = 102		
Screening Measure		
Mini Mental Status Exam	25	
Attention / Working Memory / Processing Speed		
Digit Span (WAIS-III)	11	7 SS
Longest digit span forwards	6	68 cum.%
Longest digit span backwards	2	98.5 cum%
Digit Symbol Coding (WAIS-III)	9	2 SS
Mental Control (WMS-III)	13	5 SS
Trail-Making Test Part A	247	14 T
Line Bisection	slight evidence for left hemifield neglect	
Memory		
California Verbal Learning Test–Second edition		
Learning/Acquisition (Trials 1–5 Total)	34	40 T
Trial 1	4	–1.5 z
Trial 5	10	–0.5 z
List B	3	–1.5 z
Short-delay Free Recall	8	–0.5 z
Short-delay Cued Recall	6	–1.5 z
Long-delay Free Recall	7	–0.5 z
Long-delay Cued Recall	6	–1.5 z
Total Recognition Discriminability	1.8	–1.0 z
Rey-Osterreith Complex Figure Test		
Immediate Recall	0.5	< 20 T

(Continued)

Table 60-1. Neuropsychological Test Scores (Raw and Normative Values) (*Continued*)

Cognitive Domain/Test	Raw Score	Normative Score
Language		
Letter Fluency (FAS)	21	32 T
Semantic Fluency (animals)	16	43 T
Boston Naming Test	51	42 T
Perceptual Errors	3	
Constructional and Visuospatial Abilities		
Rey-Osterreith Complex Figure Test		
Copy	0.5	<1%
Time to Copy	540	<1%
Block Design (WAIS-III)	16	5 SS
Hooper Visual Orientation Test	10	moderate
Judgment of Line Orientation (Benton)	21	low aver.
Executive Functions		
Wisconsin Card-Sorting Test-64		
Perseverative Responses	39	27 T
Categories Achieved	2	11%–16%
Halstead-Reitan Trail-Making Test (Part B)	>300	13 T
Sensory/Perceptual Skills		
Visual Field Errors		
Right visual field	0/24	
Left visual field	17/24	
Tactile Finger Recognition Errors		
Dominant Left Hand	12/20	
Nondominant Right Hand	12/20	
Finger Tip Writing Errors		
Dominant Left Hand	9/20	
Nondominant Right Hand	6/20	
Motor Skills		
Halstead-Reitan Finger Tapping		
Dominant Left Hand	18.4	9 T
Nondominant Right Hand	23	12 T
Grooved Pegboard		
Dominant Left Hand	193	19 T
Nondominant Right Hand	unable to perform	
Emotional Functioning		
Beck Depression Inventory	11	

WAIS-R, Wechsler Adult Intelligence Scale–Revised; WAIS-III, Wechsler Adult Intelligence Scale–Third revision; WMS-III, Wechsler Memory Scale–Third revision.

and recall trials, with an excessive number of intrusions (12 intrusions, 1.5 SD). His performance on yes/no recognition was within the low average range, consistent with his recall performance. His recall of a complex design after a 3-minute delay was qualitatively similar to his copy, suggesting that he was able to retain the limited amount of material he encoded initially (both were similarly distorted and impaired as will be discussed later).

Language skills were generally intact for confrontation naming, and there was also no obvious difficulty with language comprehension. The patient's performance was mildly to moderately impaired on a task that required rapid generation of words within phonetic categories, likely due to executive dysfunction (i.e., impaired initiation). His performance improved to the low average range when asked to rapidly generate words within a semantic category.

The patient showed marked deficits in visuospatial skills due to impaired organization and planning rather than frank spatial deficits. Perception of line orientations and his ability to copy simple figures were largely intact, but his ability to copy a highly complex geometric design was severely impaired (see Figure 60.2; see also the color figure in the color insert section). His approach was disorganized and piecemeal. He drew a distorted outline of the figure and did not appear to appreciate the gestalt. He drew some of the details of the design, but they were distorted and misplaced. He also showed moderately impaired performance on block constructions and when asked to integrate cut-up objects and perceive how the pieces fit together (Hooper Visual Organization Test). He frequently focused on one detail of the cut-up object without integrating the rest of the pieces. For example, he perceived a cup as a purse, likely because he focused on the cup handle, and he perceived a table as a shelf because he failed to integrate the legs.

There was other clear evidence of executive dysfunction, including difficulty with flexibility of thinking, problem-solving skills, ability to respond to feedback, perseverative responding, and sequencing. He committed a high number of errors and perseverative responses on a card-sorting task (WCST-64) indicative of difficulty

developing solutions to the task, shifting between target sets, learning from previous mistakes, self-monitoring, and verbal control of his behavior. For example, he continued to perseverate to form even though he verbalized that the current principle was color. Although he demonstrated impairment on a test requiring rapid alternation between numbers and letters (Trails B), he did not make any errors and he was similarly slow on a numeric sequencing task that did not require alternation (Trails A). As noted previously, his ability to rapidly generate words beginning with a target letter was mildly to moderately impaired and his ability to copy a complex figure was severely impaired, consistent with an overall pattern of disorganization and inefficient planning.

Fine motor dexterity (Grooved Pegboard) and simple motor speed (Finger Tapping) were severely impaired bilaterally, especially in the right nondominant hand for dexterity. Sensory perceptual testing confirmed his left visual field cut. He had difficulty distinguishing between his fingers bilaterally on a test of tactile finger recognition (finger agnosia), and there was evidence of graphesthesia bilaterally. The patient's finger agnosia and graphesthesia may be related to old thalamic infarcts in the absence of left parietal involvement, but the presence of diffuse damage makes any precise neuroanatomical correlates difficult.

Self-report was indicative of mild depression, but the symptoms he endorsed were related to physical changes from stroke, such as low energy

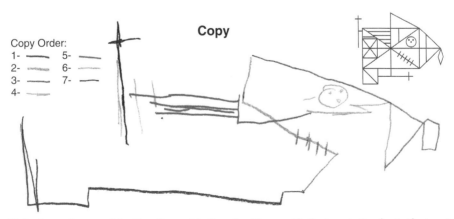

Figure 60-2. Patient's copy of the Rey-Osterreith Complex Figure with the target stimulus in the top right corner.

and physical barriers to activities. Therefore, depression did not appear to significantly contribute to his impaired performance.

Discussion

This patient's performance on neuropsychological evaluation was in the moderately impaired range overall, which represented a decline from his estimated average premorbid level of functioning. While his language, simple spatial skills, and learning and memory skills were largely intact, he demonstrated deficits that were consistent with his history of multiple bilateral strokes and periventricular white matter abnormalities. His neuropsychological profile was characterized by (1) greatest impairment in executive functions, including lack of awareness of his deficits, impaired working memory, perseverative responding, impaired flexible problem solving, spatial organization, rapid word generation, sequencing and speed of information processing, which were consistent with documented infarcts, lacunes, and periventricular white matter changes, (2) mildly impaired encoding and retrieval without evidence of rapid forgetting, (3) bilateral motor deficits, worse on the right, and (4) functional impairment. The patient's MMSE score of 25 was not in the impaired range. Because this widely used screening measure is relatively insensitive to executive dysfunction, it frequently overestimates the patient's general level of cognitive functioning when executive deficits are predominant. It is often helpful to point this out in clinical reports for the benefit of other providers.

The referral question of whether his cognitive status may have contributed to his debt accrual cannot be confidently answered because his debt was acquired prior to the 2006 stroke and one cannot reliably conclude what his cognitive abilities and functional capacities were during that period, although subcortical white matter changes that accumulate gradually over time may have contributed. The patient's marked deficit in executive functions and his lack of insight into his deficits suggest that he currently does not have the capacity to make financial decisions, and it is appropriate that his sister continue to manage his finances and retain power of attorney. The sister's participation in medical appointments was encouraged to help the patient remember and implement any medical recommendations.

This patient's clinical presentation is consistent with a diagnosis of vascular dementia. First, he has multiple vascular risk factors and a history of two frank strokes. There is documented MRI evidence of these events, other silent infarcts, and microvascular ischemic disease. Second, his neuropsychological profile is consistent with these vascular insults, particularly the subcortical involvement, with relatively greater impairments in executive function, attention and psychomotor speed relative to his largely intact language, simple spatial skills, and memory. In addition, there was evidence of stepwise cognitive decline and focal neurological signs (e.g., visual field cut) that correspond to the two frank cerebrovascular accidents. This corresponds to his high score on Rosen's modification of the HIS that is well within the range suggestive of vascular dementia. Third, there is evidence of functional decline, which is a necessary component of any dementia diagnosis. Finally, these deficits cannot be explained by psychiatric factors or another degenerative condition. Specifically, dementia of the Alzheimer's type (DAT) can be ruled out given the patient's relatively young age and the absence of significant memory deficits, including rapid forgetting, a hallmark feature of DAT.

This case is a prototypical example of multi-infarct dementia. However, there are a few aspects of this case that are not necessarily required for a diagnosis of other vascular dementia subtypes, specially subcortical vascular dementia. Although a stepwise decline and a fluctuating course are often considered a key feature of the clinical course in vascular dementia, this is only the case if there are frank cerebrovascular accidents with obvious functional impairment, such as hemiparesis or sudden onset of aphasia. Often, the patient presents with insidious cognitive and functional decline that corresponds with silent strokes or progression of microvascular ischemic disease. In addition, the patient's chief cognitive complaint is often "memory problems," which can lead other providers to suspect early Alzheimer's disease.

However, on neuropsychological testing, these "memory problems" are often related to executive dysfunction and problems with retrieval. In these more insidious onset cases, it is important to have documentation of cerebrovascular disease on neuroimaging, other explanations for cognitive impairment such as psychiatric disorders and other types of dementia need to be ruled out, and there must be evidence of functional decline in order to diagnose vascular dementia.

References

Benisty, S., Hernandez, K., Viswanathan, A., Reyes, S., Kurtz, A., O'Sullivan, M., et al. (2008). Diagnostic criteria of vascular dementia in CADASIL. *Stroke*, *39*(3), 838–844.

Bowler, J. (2003). Epidemiology: Identifying vascular cognitive impairment. *International Psychogeriatrics*, *15*(Suppl. 1), 115–122.

Bowler, J. V. (2002). The concept of vascular cognitive impairment. *Journal of Neurological Sciences*, *203–204*, 11–15.

Casserly, I., & Topol, E. (2004). Convergence of atherosclerosis and Alzheimer's disease: Inflammation, cholesterol, and misfolded proteins. *Lancet*, *363*(9415), 1139–1146.

Chui, H. C., Victoroff, J. I., Margolin, D., Jagust, W., Shankle, R., & Katzman, R. (1992). Criteria for the diagnosis of ischemic vascular dementia proposed by the State of California Alzheimer's Disease Diagnostic and Treatment Centers. *Neurology*, *42*(3 Pt. 1), 473–480.

de la Torre, J. C. (2002). Vascular basis of Alzheimer's pathogenesis. *Annals of the New York Academy of Science*, *977*, 196–215.

Desmond, D. W. (2004). The neuropsychology of vascular cognitive impairment: Is there a specific cognitive deficit? *Journal of Neurological Sciences*, *226*(1–2), 3–7.

Erkinjuntti, T. (2007). Vascular cognitive deterioration and stroke. *Cerebrovascular Disorders*, *24*(Suppl. 1), 189–194.

Gold, G., Bouras, C., Canuto, A., Bergallo, M. F., Herrmann, F. R., Hof, P. R., et al. (2002). Clinicopathological validation study of four sets of clinical criteria for vascular dementia. *American Journal of Psychiatry*, *159*(1), 82–87.

Graham, N. L., Emery, T., & Hodges, J. R. (2004). Distinctive cognitive profiles in Alzheimer's disease and subcortical vascular dementia. *Journal of Neurolgy, Neurosurgery, and Psychiatry*, *75*(1), 61–71.

Haaland, K. Y., & Swanda, R. M. (2008). Vascular dementia. In J. E. Morgan & J. H. Ricker, (Eds.), *Textbook of clinical neuropsychology* (pp. 384–391). New York: Psychology Press.

Hachinski, V. (1994). Vascular dementia: A radical redefinition. *Dementia*, *5*(3–4), 130–132.

Hachinski, V., Iadecola, C., Petersen, R. C., Breteler, M. M., Nyenhuis, D. L., Black, S. E., et al. (2006). National Institute of Neurological Disorders and Stroke-Canadian Stroke Network vascular cognitive impairment harmonization standards. *Stroke*, *37*(9), 2220–2241.

Hachinski, V. C., Lassen, N. A., & Marshall, J. (1974). Multi-infarct dementia. A cause of mental deterioration in the elderly. *Lancet*, *2*(7874), 207–210.

Jellinger, K. A. (2008). The pathology of "vascular dementia": A critical update. *Journal of Alzheimers Disease*, *14*(1), 107–123.

Jellinger, K. A., & Attems, J. (2007). Neuropathological evaluation of mixed dementia. *Journal of Neurological Sciences*, *257*(1–2), 80–87.

Jin, Y. P., Ostbye, T., Feightner, J. W., Di Legge, S., & Hachinski, V. (2008). Joint effect of stroke and APOE 4 on dementia risk: The Canadian Study of Health and Aging. *Neurology*, *70*(1), 9–16.

Kase, C. S. (1991). Epidemiology of multi-infarct dementia. *Alzheimer Disease and Associated Disorders*, *5*(2), 71–76.

Lezak, M. D., Howieson, D. B., & Loring, D. W. (2004). *Neuropsychological assessment*. New York: Oxford University Press, Inc.

O'Brien, J. T., Erkinjuntti, T., Reisberg, B., Roman, G., Sawada, T., Pantoni, L., et al. (2003). Vascular cognitive impairment. *Lancet Neurology*, *2*(2), 89–98.

Reed, B. R., Mungas, D. M., Kramer, J. H., Ellis, W., Vinters, H. V., Zarow, C., et al. (2007). Profiles of neuropsychological impairment in autopsy-defined Alzheimer's disease and cerebrovascular disease. *Brain*, *130*(Pt. 3), 731–739.

Roman, G. C., Erkinjuntti, T., Wallin, A., Pantoni, L., & Chui, H. C. (2002). Subcortical ischaemic vascular dementia. *Lancet Neurology*, *1*(7), 426–436.

Roman, G. C., Sachdev, P., Royall, D. R., Bullock, R. A., Orgogozo, J. M., Lopez-Pousa, S., et al. (2004). Vascular cognitive disorder: A new diagnostic category updating vascular cognitive impairment and vascular dementia. *Journal of Neurological Sciences*, *226*(1–2), 81–87.

Roman, G. C., Tatemichi, T. K., Erkinjuntti, T., Cummings, J. L., Masdeu, J. C., Garcia, J. H., et al. (1993). Vascular dementia: Diagnostic criteria for research studies. Report of the NINDS-AIREN International Workshop. *Neurology*, *43*(2), 250–260.

Rosen, W. G., Terry, R. D., Fuld, P. A., Katzman, R., & Peck, A. (1980). Pathological verification of ischemic score in differentiation of dementias. *Annals of Neurology, 7,* 486–488.

Sachdev, P. (1999). Vascular cognitive disorder. *International Journal of Geriatric Psychiatry, 14*(5), 402–403.

Staekenborg, S. S., van Straaten, E. C., van der Flier, W. M., Lane, R., Barkhof, F., & Scheltens, P. (2008). Small vessel versus large vessel vascular dementia: Risk factors and MRI findings. *Journal of Neurology, 255*(11), 1644–1651.

Zlokovic, B. V. (2004). Clearing amyloid through the blood-brain barrier. *Journal of Neurochemistry, 89*(4), 807–811.

61

Large Right-Hemisphere Hemorrhagic Stroke

Ellen M. Crouse and Brad L. Roper

Extensive damage to either cerebral hemisphere is typically associated with severe and ongoing neurocognitive impairments that differ depending on the hemisphere affected. Because language and communication difficulties are so easily noticed, clinicians may be more familiar with patterns commonly seen in left-hemisphere (LH) damage. However, widespread right-hemisphere (RH) damage may be equally debilitating both neurocognitively and neuropsychiatrically. In this case report, we briefly review hemorrhagic stroke as it is relevant to the case, followed by a more extensive but necessarily brief review of the typical neurocognitive and neuropsychiatric manifestations of RH damage. Following presentation of the case, our discussion focuses on practical implications and on broader issues that arise when considering the case.

Intracranial hemorrhage can have dramatically different effects on the brain depending on the point of origin. Acute extraparenchymal bleeds may involve both cerebral hemispheres and can result in a rapid increase in intracranial pressure and eventual death if not treated quickly. Intraparenchymal hemorrhage, particularly hemorrhage arising from hypertension, may present more insidiously, allowing time for bleeding to exert mass effect on surrounding structures, causing edema and crossing the normal boundaries of vascular territories. Hypertension is the most common cause of intraparenchymal hemorrhage and most often affects smaller vessels such as the lenticulostriate arteries. The basal ganglia (typically putamen) are the most frequently affected structures in hypertensive hemorrhage, followed in descending order by the thalamus, cerebellum, and pons (Blumenfeld, 2002). A recent meta-analysis by Feigin, Lawes, Bennet, and Anderson (2003) reveals that, while ischemic events are far more prevalent causes of stroke than hemorrhagic events, the latter are much more likely to result in fatality within the first month post stroke, regardless of whether the hemorrhage is subarachnoid or intraparenchymal. Of relevance to the current case, there also appears to be an increased risk for subsequent myocardial infarction in individuals who have experienced a stroke (Dhamoon et al., 2007; Rincon et al., 2008). In regard to unilateral stroke, research suggests that higher prevalence rates for LH stroke likely are related to treatment seeking rather than to true differences in incidence. That is, because symptoms of LH stroke are more likely to be recognized by patients and/or their families within the first few hours, these patients have a higher probability of treatment during the emergent phase (Ito, Kano, & Ikeda, 2008).

One of the first inklings of a functional division by hemisphere was Broca's (1865) discovery of an area in the left frontal lobe that was intimately connected to motoric aspects of speech production, with no analogous region evident in the RH. Thus, the classic view of differences between the two hemispheres focuses on stimuli type or content, describing the LH as being specialized for processing verbal stimuli and the RH for processing visuospatial stimuli. Much of current research continues to support this broad conceptualization. For example, with regard to attentional processes that occur very rapidly after stimulus presentation, the RH seems to be primed for attending to visual information, while the LH is more attuned to verbal stimuli (Rossion, Joyce, Cottrell, & Tarr, 2003). Similarly, patients with RH damage, particularly in the supramarginal gyrus, produce more visuospatial errors on a clock-drawing task, while those with LH injury tend to make time-placement errors (Tranel, Rudrauf, Vianna, & Damasio, 2008). However, other research suggests that a content-driven explanation of function by hemisphere is not entirely accurate. For example, Evans and Federmeier (2007, 2008) suggest that while the LH may dominate the encoding of words, the RH also plays an important role in the process. Thus, the two hemispheres appear to interact and collaborate with each other to a greater extent than the traditional content-driven view of brain lateralization implies. Understanding that lateralization of function is relative rather than absolute, we now briefly review the impairments that are more typically seen in RH damage.

Visuoperceptual, visuoconstructional, visuospatial, and hemiattentional impairments are common in RH stroke. Regarding visuoperceptual abilities, typically impairments in determining line orientation are associated with RH damage (Farah, 2003). Prosopagnosia or impaired recognition of familiar faces is usually seen with bilateral lesions, but several cases stemming from unilateral RH damage have been reported (Bauer & Demery, 2003). Recognition of individual faces appears to rely heavily on the right fusiform gyrus, although bilateral occipitoparietal regions are also involved in the task (Coolican, Eskes, McMullin, & Lecky, 2008; Minnebusch, Suchan, Koster, & Daum, 2008). Some degree of left spatial inattention is common in RH damage (Heilman, Watson, & Valenstein, 2003). Clinicians should be aware that people with RH stroke can exhibit spatial neglect in the absence of visual field defects. Patients may also miss the more "global" aspects of visual images in favor of a focus on more "local" details (Robertson, Lamb, & Knight, 1988). The loss of gestalt is also reflected in visuoconstructional impairments associated with RH damage, in which the overall shape of, for example, a copied figure is impaired, whereas fine detail is less impaired (McFie & Zangwill, 1960).

When hemispatial neglect is present, several additional impairments may be seen, with a poorer functional outcome post stroke (Lee et al., 2008). Individuals with RH damage (especially in the putamen, pulvinar nucleus, caudate nucleus, or superior temporal gyrus) may produce drawings in which elements in the left visual field are missing or are crowded onto the right side of the drawing, or they may ignore people or objects in the left hemispace (Karnath, Himmelbach, & Rorden, 2002). A disruption in reading secondary to neglect, termed *neglect dyslexia*, is common in posterior RH damage and reflects failure to recognize letters located on the left side of words or words toward the left of the page (Coslett, 2003). Left neglect and visuospatial impairments from posterior nondominant lesions may lead to a disruption of writing known as spatial agraphia (Roeltgen, 2003). Finally, dressing apraxia may occur secondary to a combination of visuoperceptual deficits, visual neglect, and/or inattention (Sunderland, Walker, & Walker, 2006).

The RH has also been associated with mental imagery, and one recent case study suggests that the connection between the right thalamus and temporal lobe is critical to our ability to generate mental images (Gasparini et al., 2008). Neuroimaging research and regional blood flow studies provide support for these findings. In a study of changes in blood flow in the middle cerebral artery, performance of neuropsychological tasks that tap visuospatial attention and mental manipulation (e.g., visual searching and 3-D puzzles) resulted in marked increases in RH circulation (Vingerhoets & Stroobant, 1999). Taken as a whole, these findings suggest that careful attention should be given to assessment of visuoperceptual, visuoconstructional, and hemiattentional functions in patients with RH damage, as such functions are often impaired.

Although language impairments are most strongly associated with LH lesions, over the last several decades a growing body of evidence suggests that important aspects of language also may be affected by RH lesions. Of note, RH language impairments are less conspicuous than those observed in LH stroke and may be difficult to pin down without formal evaluation.

Recent neuroimaging supports a role for the RH in language function. For example, the right superior temporal sulcus (STS) and surrounding region, as well as the right anterior fusiform gyrus and temporal pole, appear to be involved in speech comprehension, possibly due to these regions' roles in the integration of visual and auditory speech stimuli (Crinion & Price, 2005; Sharp, Scott, & Wise, 2004; Szycik, Tausche, & Munte, 2008). Problems with speech comprehension also may be due to a combination of difficulty sustaining attention to speech and to limited ability to infer the speaker's attitude or motive (Saldert & Ahlsén, 2007). In regard to expressive language, conversational speech after RH damage is likely to be more tangential and egocentric than the speech of healthy adults, as well as being characterized by either unusual verbosity or paucity (Lehman Blake, 2006). In addition, RH involvement has been associated with impaired speech prosody, both receptive (Harciarek, Heilman, & Jodzio, 2006) and expressive (Geschwind & Iacoboni, 2006). In sum, a large RH stroke may result in some degree of language impairment, particularly when the temporal lobe, superior temporal sulcus, and fusiform gyrus are affected.

Research on memory function generally suggests material-specific decrements based on affected hemisphere, such that individuals with RH damage, particularly in the temporal region, perform more poorly on visual than on verbal recall tasks (Jones-Gotman, 1986), although verbal working memory and efficiency of verbal encoding also may be affected (Cherney & Halper, 2007; Wagner, Sziklas, Garver, & Jones-Gotman, 2009). In keeping with these findings from neuroimaging research, patients with large RH strokes have a higher probability of word-recall impairment than healthy controls, in addition to more difficulty with visual recall (Gillespie, Bowen, & Foster, 2006; Lee et al., 2008). However, difficulty with recall may be significantly influenced by the inability to perceive and coherently organize the overall gestalt of the visual material to be remembered (Lunge, Waked, Kirschblum, & DeLuca, 2000).

As many of the memory problems noted in RH stroke appear to be affected by encoding difficulties, the question of impaired attention naturally arises. Indeed, a recent case study report from Lazar and colleagues (2007) suggests that

RH stroke can have profound effects on attention, working memory, and the ability to multi-task in daily life, even in the absence of frank evidence of frontal-lobe involvement. Murine models of RH stroke suggest that cholinergic dysfunction may result in problems with attention that affect other aspects of cognition (Hoff, van Oostenbrugge, Liedenbaum,Steinbusch, & Blokland, 2007). In keeping with these findings, human research reveals that disruption to pathways involved in attention plays a central role in visuospatial neglect (Shimozaki, Kingstone, Olk, Stowe, & Eckstein, 2006), possibly due to the tendency for most people to attend more to stimuli presented in the left visual fields (Siman-Tov et al., 2007). Right-hemisphere regions involved in attention and alertness include the frontal dorsolateral cortex, anterior cingulate, inferior parietal cortex, thalamus, and basal ganglia, as well as brainstem structures (Siman-Tov et al., 2007; Sturm et al., 2004). Not surprisingly, inattention affects working memory, and RH strokes that affect subcortical white matter tracts are likely to result in visual memory deficits and slowed processing speed (Berryhill & Olson, 2008; Habekost & Rostrup, 2007). Regarding other aspects of executive functioning, the RH frontostriatal circuit appears to play a central role in visuospatial planning and analysis (Ricker & Millis, 1996), a point particularly relevant to the current case. Yehene, Meiran, and Soroker (2008) posit that the basal ganglia are critical components in the frontosubcortical system in task switching, action selection, and inhibition of irrelevant stimuli.

Regarding general mental status, research suggests that LH versus RH injury has little differential effect. Rather, mental status is influenced more by total lesion load (Viswanathan et al., 2007), premorbid functioning (Appelros, 2005), and location of lesion in the mediodorsal thalamic nucleus (Kumral, Gulluoglu, & Dramali, 2007) or in frontal subcortical pathways (Nagaratnam, Bou-Haidar, & Leung, 2003). In addition, Spaletta et al. (2002) note an interaction between depression and laterality, such that impairment in general mental status is greatest in people with a combined history of LH stroke and depression.

Regarding psychiatric disturbances, although depression is traditionally considered to be more common in LH damage, it may be found in milder forms in RH stroke, particularly when there is a previous history of mood disorder (Beblo, Wallesch, & Herrmann, 1999; Caeiro, Ferro, Santos, & Figueira, 2006). Cummings (1997) has provided a comprehensive review of psychiatric factors in RH damage. Depression is less likely to occur when lesions are located in the anterior parietal cortex and motor strip. Although less common than depression and more common in head injury than stroke, neurologically acquired mania has been reported almost exclusively in RH injury. Psychosis can also occur after stroke, particularly when the temporoparietal region is affected, but there is little evidence of hemispheric predominance. Additionally, individuals with RH damage often have difficulty recognizing and interpreting emotional aspects of communication, whether the source of information is visual, as in facial expression, or auditory, as in speech prosody (Adolphs, Damasio, Tranel, Cooper, & Damasio, 1996; Harciarek et al., 2006). The RH appears to be specialized for recognizing negative affect, suggesting that individuals with RH stroke would have more difficulty perceiving sadness or irritation in those around them than in picking up on more positive emotions (Adolphs, Jansari, & Tranel, 2001). As such, RH patients may present clinically as alexithymic (Schäfer et al., 2007), and their caregivers frequently report an inability on the part of such patients to empathize with the ways in which the stroke has affected other family members. Finally, in regard to awareness of deficits, patients with RH stroke frequently either blatantly deny obvious problems, such as left hemiplegia, or tend to downplay or underestimate their functional impact (Peskine & Azouvi, 1991).

Case Presentation

G. H. is a 52-year-old, right-hand-dominant, African American man with a history of essential hypertension (HTN) since his mid 20s. He experienced a major RH stroke, with resultant dense left hemiplegia 10 months prior to our neuropsychological evaluation. Although images were not available, report of head computed tomography (CT) 1 week post stroke indicated a hemorrhage to the right basal ganglia and adjacent white

matter with surrounding edema and mass effect. Assessment of cranial nerve function 3 months post stroke revealed asymmetric nasal labial fold and smile, with continuous drooling on the right side. The tongue and uvula were at the midline. The patient showed severely diminished corneal reflex for the left eye, as well as difficulty closing the eye. All other oculomotor and pupillary reflexes were normal bilaterally, and the patient showed no nystagmus. Sensation of light touch was diminished in left face from the forehead to the chin. Pinprick, light touch, and vibration sense were diminished in the left extremities and the trunk. Motor testing was notable for hyperreflexia, hypertonicity, and clonus in the left upper and lower extremities, with absent shoulder shrug on the left. There were no abnormal cerebellar findings on neurologic exam. Gait and motor strength could not be evaluated secondary to dense hemiplegia and hypertonicity.

During acute recovery, G. H. showed language disturbance that was not well characterized in available records. He also showed dysphagia. He participated fully in physical therapy (PT) and speech therapy (ST) in the months following his stroke. At 9 months post stroke, he continued to have problems with his left leg buckling and needed at least minimal assist with transfers. At that time, ST notes indicate no residual dysphagia or language impairments but continuing cognitive impairments, which the patient failed to acknowledge.

In regard to other medical issues, as of 9 months post stroke, G. H.'s systolic blood pressure was frequently in the 140s to 150s, with diastolic BP in the upper 90s, an improvement over prior systolics in the 170s. Other relevant medical history included hyperlipidemia and onset of chest pain 3–4 months post stroke. Subsequent cardiac evaluation and catheterization noted cardiomyopathy, with atherosclerosis of the distal right coronary artery and ejection fraction of 35%. Both the stroke and cardiomyopathy were attributed to his history of HTN. Family medical history reportedly included hypertension, stroke, MI, and aneurysm.

Regarding childhood history, G. H. denied any complications at birth or with early developmental milestones. He reported problems with reading comprehension and attention throughout school but denied ever being diagnosed with a learning disability or repeating a grade. He described himself as "always curious and learning" and as learning information best with a "hands on" approach. He graduated from high school and completed about 2 years of college education, after which he served in the U.S. Navy for 20 years as a mechanic. Following an honorable discharge, he worked as manager at a large distribution company for 16 years. G. H. reported being married to his current wife for 27 years and having two adult children with whom he had close relationships.

When asked about current mood, G. H. indicated that he occasionally felt "down" but that his mood had improved since he began PT. He stated that he felt a sense of pride about being able to walk with rail assist in PT and expressed a belief that he would eventually walk again. He attributed mood problems to disagreements with his wife rather than to the effects of his stroke, describing frustration with what he felt were unreasonable limitations imposed by his wife. Specifically, he believed that he could drive safely with an adapted vehicle and be more independent. He denied current suicidal ideation, plan, or intent. He denied any history of abuse of alcohol or illicit substances. He reportedly quit smoking cigarettes about 4 months prior to his stroke, with a smoking history of 12 pack years. Family history of psychiatric disorder was denied.

When asked about current cognitive problems, G. H. indicated a desire to regain his abilities and independence. He noted mild problems with expressive language and occasional difficulty following conversations, particularly when more than one person is talking at a time. He did not spontaneously mention loss of left motor function, but when asked directly, he acknowledged that left hemiplegia precluded walking currently, adding confidently that he would be able to walk again in the future. He voiced a strong desire to return to driving, stating that he hoped results of evaluation would confirm that he is able to drive. He denied having any significant problems with visuospatial skills, memory, attention, concentration, processing speed, problem solving, or reasoning. In contrast, G. H.'s wife expressed particular concern about his safety, due to behavioral changes (primarily impulsivity and mild emotional lability) and his lack of awareness of deficits, as she was working full time outside the home. She also described her husband as less sensitive to her emotions and to the stress she was facing than he would have been prior to his stroke.

G. H. was referred at 10 months post stroke for evaluation of current level of cognitive functioning and to provide recommendations for enhancing rehabilitation and managing his behavior. He was tested over two sessions due to a tendency to fatigue quickly. He arrived for the evaluation in a motorized wheelchair, which he had difficulty navigating through tight turns and doorways, a problem he attributed to having recently received and being in the process of learning to use the wheelchair, although he actually had been in possession of it for 2 months. He wore casual clothing appropriate to setting and season and had good grooming and hygiene. He appeared anxious initially, with mildly diminished eye contact, but he gradually relaxed, and eye contact improved as the interview progressed. Affect was somewhat blunted, with subtle left facial hemiparesis evident. Social comportment was superficially intact on initial interactions. However, during the evaluation he demonstrated mild impairments in social reciprocity. Speech was notable for frequent pauses, as well as evidence of mild word-finding difficulty, aprosody, and dysarthria. Thought processes were logical and coherent although occasionally tangential. No evidence of formal thought disorder was noted. Regarding awareness of deficits, G. H. could superficially describe changes (e.g., "I need a wheelchair until I can walk again"), but he lacked awareness of the effects and implications of his impairments (e.g., believing that he could drive safely even though he was unable to maneuver a wheelchair without running into objects). He was alert and oriented to person, place, and situation, but he was only grossly oriented to time. He was cooperative and appeared to make good effort throughout the evaluation, and results were deemed to provide an accurate reflection of his abilities.

The reader is referred to Table 61-1 for detailed report of test scores. Overall, G. H.'s performance suggested greater decrements in visuospatial versus verbal abilities since his stroke. Across the evaluation, he demonstrated broadly intact performance in terms of verbal reasoning skills, social judgment, and contextual verbal memory.

Table 61-1. Test Scores

Folstein Mini Mental State Exam (MMSE)	21/30
Wechsler Adult Intelligence Scale–III (WAIS-III)	IQ Scores
Verbal IQ	**82**
Performance IQ	**67**
Full-Scale IQ	**73**
	Index Scores (Age-Scaled Scores)
Verbal Comprehension Index	**86**
Vocabulary	6
Similarities	8
Information	8
Perceptual Organization Index	**70**
Picture Completion	6
Block Design	4
Matrix Reasoning	5
Working Memory Index	**73**
Arithmetic	6
Digit Span	6
Letter-Number Sequencing	5
Processing Speed Index	—
Digit Symbol-Coding	3
Symbol Search	N/A
Other Subtests	
Comprehension	8
Picture Arrangement	5
Digit Span (Maximum Spans)	Raw Scores
Digits Forward	5
Digits Backward	3
Token Test	Percentile
Raw Score = 34/44	<1
Wechsler Memory Scale–III (WMS-III)	Scaled Scores
Logical Memory I	10
Logical Memory II	11
California Verbal Learning Test–II (CVLT-II)	T and z-scores
Acquisition (4, 7, 6, 8, 7 words)	$T = 38$
Trial B (2)	$z = -2.0$
Short-Delay Free / Cued Recall (7 / 8)	$z = -0.5$
Long-Delay Free / Cued Recall (6 / 7)	$z = -1.0$
Recognition Correct/False + (9 / 0)	$z = -3.0$
Forced-Choice Trial = 16	WNL
Rey-Osterrieth Complex Figure Test (ROCF):	Percentiles
Copy (22.0 points)	<1
Immediate Recall (7.0 points)	<1
Delayed Recall (6.0 points)	<1
Judgment of Line Orientation (JoLO):	Percentile
Raw Score = 8/30	<1.5
Hooper Visual Organization Test (HVOT):	T-Score
Raw Score = 25.5/30	50

Table 61-1. Test Scores (*Continued*)

Trail-Making Test:	T-Scores
Trails A (96", 0 errors)	20
Trails B (214", 3 errors)	37
Booklet Category Test (BCT):	Raw Scores
Subtest I	0
Subtest II	0
Subtest III	31
Subtest IV	32
Subtests V–VII	N/A

WNL, within normal limits.

Note. N/A denotes items or tests not administered due to G. H.'s frustration with task and/or fatigue.

Expressive language problems were evident in his weaker expressive vocabulary performance, apparently related to an unelaborative approach to the test. Auditory-verbal working memory was borderline impaired. Additionally, he had some difficulty in following more complex commands involving tokens that appeared to be related to working memory difficulties. Memory for short paragraphs was intact. His ability to learn and recall word lists following several trials was low average, with relatively good retention of the material over time. In contrast, memory for visuospatial material was severely impaired.

Evidence of greater impairment of RH-mediated functions was noted across most tasks on the evaluation. For example, G. H.'s performance on visuoperceptual tasks was notably worse when the stimuli used were more purely visual and less amenable to verbal mediation (i.e., impaired Block Design and Judgment of Line Orientation but intact Hooper Visual Organization Test). Regarding his performance on the latter, he benefited from identifying small segments or elements of the figures as familiar rather than relying on mentally "reassembling" the pieces. His performance on the Rey-Osterrieth Complex Figure was noteworthy for a consistent pattern of initiating the drawings at the right of the page and progressing across toward the left. He tended to draw single elements of the design in a piecemeal fashion rather than capturing the overall gestalt and using this as an organizing framework (see Figures 61.1, 61.2; see also the color figure in the color insert section, and 61-3).

As shown in Table 61-2, on the MMPI-2, G. H. showed an unusual pattern of elevations on validity scales. His somewhat elevated L scale reflected a tendency to deny minor character flaws, consistent with his denial of cognitive or emotional problems on interview. He showed a similar mild elevation on the F scale. His Back F was elevated despite only one elevation among content scales, and his Infrequency Psychopathology scale ($F_{(p)}$) was most elevated of all validity indicators, whose elevation was enhanced by his endorsement of three items shared by L and reflecting denial. Other endorsed items on $F_{(p)}$ reflect acknowledgement of actual physical limitations secondary to stroke, as well as some endorsement of unusual psychiatric symptoms, the "core" construct of $F_{(p)}$. Because of his denial, the MMPI-2 profile may underestimate everyday psychiatric symptoms, as he tended to present himself as free of emotional problems. Generally speaking, his MMPI-2 clinical profile was within normal limits with the exception of slightly elevated somatic symptoms, a finding common in patients with CVA that is understandable in light of his motor limitations. Based on these results, G. H. presented as being free of ongoing problems

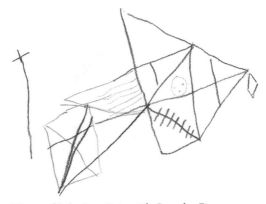

Figure 61-1. Rey-Osterrieth Complex Figure copy drawing.

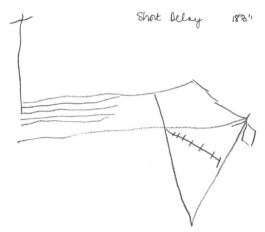

Figure 61-2. Rey-Osterreith Complex Figure 3-minute delay drawing.

with mood, anxiety, or other psychiatric symptoms. However, the MMPI-2 is less sensitive to alexithymia and personality changes that may be seen in RH damage.

Discussion/Conclusions

The case of G. H. is emblematic of many of the problems typically observed in people who have experienced a large RH stroke. Noteworthy points in his case include dense left hemiplegia, marked deficits in visuospatial skills and visual memory, problems with tracking and comprehending others' speech, and evidence of a substantial lack of insight into his difficulties. In addition, both he and his wife described problems in their relationship since his stroke. G. H.'s attribution of relationship difficulties to the restrictions that his wife

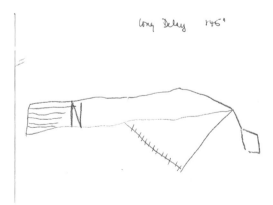

Figure 61-3. Rey-Osterreith Complex Figure 30-minute delay drawing.

Table 61-2. MMPI-2 Results

Minnesota Multiphasic Personality Inventory, 2nd Ed. (MMPI-2)	T Scores
? Cannot Say	Raw = 0
L	78
F	76
K	60
Back F	92
F(p)	99
1 (Hs)	70
2 (D)	57
3 (Hy)	61
4 (Pd)	54
5 (Mf)	42
6 (Pa)	64
7 (Pt)	55
8 (Sc)	67
9 (Ma)	51
0 (Si)	53

placed on his mobility (e.g., no driving) highlights his limited awareness of changes in function post stroke. His wife's report of decreased empathy on the part of her husband provides a vivid example of typical concerns often felt but not always expressed by loved ones. As family members may be hesitant to speak up about such observations out of a sense of guilt or shame, it is important for clinicians working with this population to provide an environment in which caregivers feel secure in talking about these concerns and to ask direct questions about the possibility of such issues.

In G. H.'s case, a central concern was safety. His visuospatial impairments and limited insight significantly elevate the risk for falls and other injuries. Similarly, his strongly stated desire to return to driving made it critical to communicate with other health providers about associated risks. Healthcare providers who have less experience with patients with RH stroke history might be fooled by G. H.'s ability to "talk a good line" and make plausible but inaccurate excuses for small accidents, such as running the edge of his wheelchair into the doorframe. Such incidents are important red flags when considering the safety needs of RH stroke patients. Thus, clear recommendations were made regarding his inability to drive and other safety issues. Finally, in thinking through recommendations for such patients, it is valuable to consider the real-life implications of problems with communication. One of the simplest recommendations made to care providers and family was to routinely ask G. H. to restate important new information in his own words. Doing so provides a means to ensure that he has clearly understood the information, as well as potentially enhancing future recall.

Extending the discussion beyond the current case, widespread RH involvement may produce a range of deficits that lead to unique clinical presentations and associated challenges for both family members and healthcare professionals. Because language is so central to everyday interaction, the obvious impairments in communication typically seen in LH stroke may openly advertise patients' deficits and alert others to their needs. Indeed, speech or communication difficulties may lead casual observers to overpathologize and assume that patients have severe and global impairments, with a failure to appreciate areas of spared function. In contrast, the relatively preserved basic language abilities seen in a patient with RH stroke may lead others to assume that the person is cognitively intact. Unfortunately, such assumptions may also be made by healthcare providers. Such impressions may be accentuated by the characteristic denial of any cognitive problems seen in RH patients.

In contrast to the "stealth" presentation of some RH patients in superficial interactions, family members caring for such patients may be painfully aware of a loved one's impairments, limitations, and personality changes. Visuospatial impairments may manifest in everyday activities, as in dressing apraxia, requiring daily assistance with such activities. Although difficulties with spatial orientation may occur even within the home, more subtle deficits may manifest as route-finding difficulties in less familiar settings, resulting in obvious safety concerns. Hemiattentional impairments may exacerbate the effects of visuoperceptual deficits and may require creative solutions, such as physically positioning the patient such that important environmental stimuli are within the preserved attentional hemifield.

Although visual-perceptual, hemiattentional, and other neurocognitive impairments may be burdensome to family members, they may experience more stress in response to the social and emotional changes that often accompany RH damage. Loss of emotional perception, expression, and awareness may have a devastating effect on relationships between family members and patients. Patients may lack any sense of intimacy with or social connection to those individuals with whom they previously enjoyed the closest of personal bonds. Family members may understand that ability impairments are associated with the stroke, while emotional impairments may be interpreted as reflecting callousness, disinterest, or disdain. Frequently added to this unfortunate recipe is patients' lack of awareness of both neurocognitive and emotional impairments. As such, patients may show little, if any, appreciation for the sacrifices others make on their behalf. Additionally, patients may fail to appreciate the limitations placed on them and may openly challenge such limitations, increasing conflict with family and presenting special safety concerns as noted previously. Obviously, in light of these challenges, neuropsychologists may play an important role beyond mere assessment to include consultation with other providers and interventions with patients and family members.

Practical considerations aside, the impairments shown by patients with RH damage are often very intellectually engaging. Such patients may reveal deficits in those abilities that normally operate implicitly, with minimal conscious awareness of "doing" or "thinking." For example, in such patients we gain an understanding of how our brain models the space around us and our position in it, and we palpably experience the behaviors that manifest when those spatial and attentional models no longer function. Likewise, common deficits in RH damage may include social perception, expression, and awareness. The emotional processing deficits seen in RH patients bring us a greater awareness of the implicit emotional monitoring and expression in which we all engage in our interactions with others. The breadth, utility, and importance of emotional processing underscores our status as social animals designed to navigate environments of great social complexity. Finally, in RH damage we often observe a striking lack of insight that may include awareness of cognitive deficits, the external world, or even one's own body. All of these examples carry important implications from the standpoint of consciousness and conscious experience. Perhaps one of the central conceits of our history as a species has been the certainty with which we form our own individual perceptions of the world and our place in it. The deficits in awareness seen in RH damage may provide a useful vantage point from which to reflect upon the gaps in our own individual perceptions.

References

Adolphs, R., Damasio, H., Tranel, D., & Damasio, A. R. (1996). Cortical systems for the recognition of emotion in facial expressions. *The Journal of Neuroscience: The Official Journal of the Society for Neuroscience, 16*(23), 7678–7687.

Adolphs, R., Jansari, A., & Tranel, D. (2001). Hemispheric perception of emotional valence from facial expressions. *Neuropsychology, 15*(4), 516–24.

Appelros, P. (2005). Characteristics of Mini-Mental State Examination 1 year after stroke. *Acta Neurologica Scandinavica, 112*(2), 88–92.

Bauer, R. M., & Demery, J. A. (2003). Agnosia. In K. M. Heilman & E. Valenstein (Eds.), *Clinical neuropsychology* (4th ed., pp. 236–295). New York: Oxford University Press.

Beblo, T., Wallesch, C. W., & Herrmann, M. (1999). The crucial role of frontostriatal circuits for depressive disorders in the postacute stage after stroke. *Neuropsychiatry, Neuropsychology, and Behavioral Neurology, 12*(4), 236–246.

Berryhill, M. E., & Olson, I. R. (2008). The right parietal lobe is critical for visual working memory. *Neuropsychologia, 46*(7), 1767–1774.

Blumenfeld, H. (2002). *Neuroanatomy through clinical cases.* Sunderland, MA: Sinauer Associates, Inc.

Broca, M. P. (1865). Sur la siege de la faculte´ langage articule. *Bulletin of the Society of Anthropology, 6*, 377–396.

Caeiro, L., Ferro, J. M., Santos, C. O., & Figueira, M. L. (2006). Depression in acute stroke. *Journal of Psychiatry and Neuroscience, 31*(6), 377–383.

Cherney, L. R., & Halper, A. S. (2007). Performance on the California Verbal Learning Test following right hemisphere stroke: A longitudinal study. *Topics in Stroke Rehabilitation, 14*(1), 21–25.

Coolican, J., Eskes, G. A., McMullen, P. A., & Lecky, E. (2008). Perceptual biases in processing facial identity and emotion. *Brain and Cognition, 66*, 176–187.

Coslett, H. B. (2003). Acquired dyslexia. In K. M. Heilman & E. Valenstein (Eds.), *Clinical neuropsychology* (4th ed., pp. 108–125). New York: Oxford University Press.

Crinion, J., & Price, C. J. (2005). Right anterior superior temporal activation predicts auditory sentence comprehension following aphasic stroke. *Brain, 128*(12), 2858–2871.

Cummings, J. L. (1997). Neuropsychiatric manifestations of right hemisphere lesions. *Brain and Language, 57*, 22–37.

Dhamoon, M. S., Tai, W., Boden-Albala, B., Rundek, T., Paik, M. C., Sacco, R. L., et al. (2007). Risk of myocardial infarction or vascular death after first ischemic stroke: The Northern Manhattan Study. *Stroke, 38*(6), 1752–1758.

Evans, K. M., & Federmeier, K. D. (2007). The memory that's right and the memory that's left: Event-related potentials reveal hemispheric asymmetries in the encoding and retention of verbal information. *Neuropsychologia, 45*(8), 1777–1790.

Evans, K. M., & Federmeier, K. D. (2008). Left and right memory revisited: Electrophysiological investigations of hemispheric asymmetries at retrieval. *Neuropsychologia,* 2008 September 4 [Epub ahead of print].

Farah, M. J. (2003). Disorders of visual-spatial perception and cognition. In K. M. Heilman & E. Valenstein (Eds.), *Clinical neuropsychology* (4th ed., pp. 146–160). New York: Oxford University Press.

Feigin, V. L., Lawes, C. M. M., Bennett, D. A., & Anderson, C. S. (2003). Stroke epidemiology: A review of population-based studies of incidence, prevalence, and case-fatality in the late 20th century. *Lancet Neurology, 2*(1), 43–53.

Gasparini, M., Hufty, A. M., Masciarelli, G., Ottaviani, D., Angeloni, U., Lenzi, G. L., et al. (2008). Contribution of right hemisphere to visual imagery: A visual working memory impairment? *Journal of the International Neuropsychological Society, 14*(5), 902–911.

Geschwind, D. H., & Iacoboni, M. (2006). Structural and functional asymmetries of the human frontal lobes. In B. Miller & J. Cummings (Eds.), *The human frontal lobes: Functions and disorders.* (pp. 68–91). New York: Guilford Press.

Gillespie, D., Bowen, A., & Foster, J. (2006). Memory impairment following right hemisphere stroke: A comparative meta-analytic and narrative review. *Clinical Neuropsychologist, 20*(1), 59–75.

Habekost, T., & Rostrup, E. (2007). Visual attention capacity after right hemisphere lesions. *Neuropsychologia, 45*(7), 1474–1488.

Harciarek, M., Heilman, K. M., & Jodzio, K. (2006). Defective comprehension of emotional faces and prosody as a result of right hemisphere stroke: Modality versus emotion-type specificity. *Journal of the International Neuropsychological Society, 12*(6), 774–781.

Heilman, K. M., Watson, R., & Valenstein, E. (2003). Neglect and related disorders. In K. M. Heilman &

E. Valenstein (Eds.), *Clinical Neuropsychology* (4th ed., pp. 296–346). New York: Oxford University Press.

Hoff, E. I., van Oostenbrugge, R. J., Liedenbaum, M., Steinbusch, H. W. M., & Blokland, A. (2007). Effects of right-hemisphere cortical infarction and muscarinic acetylcholine receptor blockade on spatial visual attention performance in rats. *Behavioural Brain Research*, *178*(1), 62–69.

Ito, H., Kano, O., & Ikeda, K. (2008). Different variables between patients with left and right hemispheric ischemic stroke. *Journal of Stroke and Cerebrovascular Diseases*, *17*(1), 35–38.

Jones-Gotman, M. (1986). Right hippocampal excision impairs learning and recall of a list of abstract designs. *Neuropsychologia*, *24*, 659–670.

Karnath, H., Himmelbach, M., & Rorden, C. (2002). The subcortical anatomy of human spatial neglect: putamen, caudate nucleus and pulvinar. *Brain*, *125*(Pt. 2), 350–360.

Kumral, E., Gulluoglu, H., & Dramali, B. (2007). Thalamic chronotaraxis: Isolated time disorientation. *Journal of Neurology, Neurosurgery, and Psychiatry*, *78*(8), 880–882.

Lazar, R. M., Festa, J. R., Geller, A. E., Romano, G. M., & Marshall, R. S. (2007). Multitasking disorder from right temporoparietal stroke. *Cognitive and Behavioral Neurology*, *20*(3), 157–162.

Lee, B. H., Kim, E., Ku, B. D., Choi, K. M., Seo, S. W., Kim, G., et al. (2008). Cognitive impairments in patients with hemispatial neglect from acute right hemisphere stroke. *Cognitive and Behavioral Neurology*, *21*(2), 73–6.

Lehman Blake, M. (2006). Clinical relevance of discourse characteristics after right hemisphere brain damage. *American Journal of Speech-Language Pathology*, *15*(3), 255–267.

Lunge, D., Waked, W., Kirschblum, S., & DeLuca, J. (2000). Organizational strategy influence on visual memory performance after stroke: Cortical/subcortical and left/right hemisphere contrasts. *Archives of Physical Medicine and Rehabilitation*, *81*, 89–94.

McFie, J. & Zangwill, O. L. (1960). Visual constructive disabilities associated with lesions of the left cerebral hemisphere. *Brain*, *83*, 243–260.

Minnebusch, D.A., Suchan, B., Koster, O., & Daum, I. (2008). A bilateral occipitotemporal network mediates face perception. *Behavioral Brain Research*, 2008 Nov 11. [Epub ahead of print].

Nagaratnam, N., Bou-Haidar, P., & Leung, H. (2003). Confused and disturbed behavior in the elderly following silent frontal lobe infarction. *American Journal of Alzheimer's Disease and Other Dementias*, *18*(6), 333–339.

Peskine, A., & Azouvi, P. (1991). Anosognosia and denial after right hemisphere stroke. In G. P. Prigatano & D. L. Schacter (Eds.), *Awareness of deficit after brain injury* (pp. 198–214). New York: Oxford University Press.

Ricker, J. H., & Millis, S. R. (1996). Differential visuospatial dysfunction following striatal, frontal white matter, or posterior thalamic infarction. *The International Journal of Neuroscience*, *84*(1–4), 75–85.

Rincon, F., Dhamoon, M., Moon, Y., Paik, M. C., Boden-Albala, B., Homma, S., et al. (2008). Stroke location and association with fatal cardiac outcomes: Northern Manhattan Study (NOMAS). *Stroke*, *39*(9), 2425–2431.

Robertson, L. C., Lamb, M. R., & Knight, R. T. (1988). Effects of lesions of temporal-parietal junction on perceptual and attentional processing in humans. *The Journal of Neuroscience*, *8*(10), 3757–3769.

Roeltgen, D. P. (2003). Agraphia. In K. M. Heilman & E. Valenstein (Eds.), *Clinical neuropsychology* (4th ed., pp. 126–145). New York: Oxford University Press.

Rossion, B., Joyce, C. A., Cottrell, G. W., & Tarr, M. J. (2003). Early lateralization and orientation tuning for face, word, and object processing in the visual cortex. *NeuroImage*, *20*(3), 1609–1624.

Saldert, C., & Ahlsén, E. (2007). Inference in right hemisphere damaged individuals' comprehension: The role of sustained attention. *Clinical Linguistics and Phonetics*, *21*(8), 637–655.

Schäfer, R., Popp, K., Jörgens, S., Lindenberg, R., Franz, M., & Seitz, R. J. (2007). Alexithymia-like disorder in right anterior cingulate infarction. *Neurocase*, *13*(3), 201–208.

Sharp, D. J., Scott, S. K., & Wise, R. J. S. (2004). Retrieving meaning after temporal lobe infarction: The role of the basal language area. *Annals of Neurology*, *56*(6), 836–846.

Shimozaki, S., Kingstone, A., Olk, B., Stowe, R., & Eckstein, M. (2006). Classification images of two right hemisphere patients: A window into the attentional mechanisms of spatial neglect. *Brain Research*, *1080*(1), 26–52.

Siman-Tov, T., Mendelsohn, A., Schonberg, T., Avidan, G., Podlipsky, I., Pessoa, L., et al. (2007). Bihemispheric leftward bias in a visuospatial attention-related network. *The Journal of Neuroscience*, *27*(42), 11271–11278.

Spalletta, G., Guida, G., De Angelis, D., & Caltagirone, C. (2002). Predictors of cognitive level and depression severity are different in patients with left and right hemispheric stroke within the first year of illness. *Journal of Neurology*, *249*(11), 1541–1551.

Sturm, W., Longoni, F., Weis, S., Specht, K., Herzog, H., Vohn, R., et al. (2004). Functional reorganisation in patients with right hemisphere stroke after training of alertness: A longitudinal PET and fMRI study in eight cases. *Neuropsychologia, 42*(4), 434–450.

Sunderland, A., Walker, C. M., & Walker, M. F. (2006). Action errors and dressing disability after stroke: An ecological approach to neuropsychological assessment and intervention. *Neuropsychological Rehabilitation, 16*(6), 666–683.

Szycik, G. R., Tausche, P., & Münte, T. F. (2008). A novel approach to study audiovisual integration in speech perception: Localizer fMRI and sparse sampling. *Brain Research, 1220*, 142–149.

Tranel, D., Rudrauf, D., Vianna, E. P. M., & Damasio, H. (2008). Does the Clock Drawing Test have focal neuroanatomical correlates? *Neuropsychology, 22*(5), 553–562.

Vingerhoets, G., & Stroobant, N. (1999). Lateralization of cerebral blood flow velocity changes during cognitive tasks. A simultaneous bilateral transcranial Doppler study. *Stroke, 30*(10), 2152–2158.

Viswanathan, A., Gschwendtner, A., Guichard, J., Buffon, F., Cumurciuc, R., O'Sullivan, M., et al. (2007). Lacunar lesions are independently associated with disability and cognitive impairment in CADASIL. *Neurology, 69*(2), 172–179.

Wagner, D. D., Sziklas, V., Garver, K. E., & Jones-Gotman, M. (2009). Material-specific lateralization of working memory in the medial temporal lobe. *Neuropsychologia, 47*(1), 112–122.

Yehene, E., Meiran, N., & Soroker, N. (2008). Basal ganglia play a unique role in task switching within the frontal-subcortical circuits: Evidence from patients with focal lesions. *Journal of Cognitive Neuroscience, 20*(6), 1079–1093.

62

Ruptured Aneurysm of the Anterior Communicating Artery

Marykay Pavol and Rashmi Rastogi

An aneurysm is a small, thin-walled blister protruding from an artery, typically at a bifurcation or branching (Adams & Victor, 1993). Most aneurysms are believed to result from developmental defects, although an alternate theory suggests they may result from damage to the vessel from hemodynamic forces (Adams & Victor, 1993; Agrawal et al., 2008). Risk factors for aneurysm and hemorrhage include female gender, pregnancy, hypertension, cigarette smoking, age (40–60 years old), family history of aneurysm, and certain genetic diseases (Vates, Zabramski, Spetzler, & Lawton, 2004; Weir, 2002). Patients are usually asymptomatic prior to the aneurysm rupture. When the rupture occurs, blood is forced into the subarachnoid space; the patient may complain of a severe headache, sometimes reported as the "worst headache of (his or her) life," and often loses consciousness. Seizures are common. If the hemorrhage is extensive, the patient may die suddenly or become comatose. The patient's neurological status following the hemorrhage is often graded according to a rating scale published by Hunt and Hess in 1968 (Table 62-1) (Vates et al., 2004). See Cullum, Rilling, Saine, and Samson, (2008) and Brown, Lazar, and Delano-Wood (2008) for recent reviews of intracranial hemorrhage and cerebral aneurysms.

The anterior communicating artery (ACoA) is a small artery at the anterior portion of the Circle of Willis that connects the left and right anterior cerebral arteries (Waxman, 1996). According to The International Cooperative Study on the Timing of Aneurysm Surgery, the anterior communicating artery is the most common aneurysm site, representing 34% of total aneurysms (Vates et al., 2004). Anterior communicating artery aneurysms also result in the greatest morbidity, among anterior circulation aneurysms (Agrawal et al., 2008).

Once the patient has been hospitalized following symptom onset, workup includes a head computed tomography (CT) scan, which usually reveals hemorrhage. Angiogram typically confirms the aneurysm. Occasionally, no aneurysm is found or, conversely, multiple aneurysms may be identified (Vates et al., 2004). Due to the high risk of rebleeding in a ruptured aneurysm, most patients undergo surgery to reduce the likelihood of further hemorrhage. The surgery may include the placement of a clip ("clipping") at the base of the aneurysm, to prevent new bleeding (Cullum et al., 2008; Levy et al., 2004). An alternate procedure involves the insertion of a thin platinum thread into the aneurysm ("coiling" or "coil embolization"). The thread is made into a coil, which prompts the formation of a clot in the aneurysm, thus preventing further bleeds. (Cullum et al., 2008; Levy et al., 2004). There are many branching vessels coming off the ACoA that supply blood to several important areas (Serizawa et al., 1997). Preservation of these vessels is both surgically challenging and important in reducing morbidity (Agrawal et al., 2008).

The outcome data following surgery (e.g., rebleeding rates, vasospasm, risk of shunt-dependent hydrocephalus) are varied, with some studies

Table 62-1. Hunt and Hess Clinical Grading Scale

Grade 1. Asymptomatic, mild headache, slight nuchal rigidity

Grade 2. Moderate to severe headache, nuchal rigidity, no neurologic deficit other than cranial nerve palsy

Grade 3. Drowsiness/confusion, mild focal neurologic deficit

Grade 4. Stupor, moderate–severe hemiparesis

Grade 5. Coma, decerebrate posturing

supporting better outcome with clipping, other studies finding better outcome with coiling, and still others with mixed findings or no significant differences (de Oliveira et al., 2007a; de Oliveira et al., 2007b; Hoh et al., 2004; Jartti et al., 2008; Mitchell et al., 2008; Rabenstein et al., 2003; Salary, Quigley, & Wilberger, 2007; van der Schaaf et al., 2005). With regard to cognition, the findings are also somewhat mixed. Tidswell, Dias, Sagar, Maves, and Battersby (1995) reported that clipping resulted in higher family reports of cognitive deficit. Chan, Ho, and Poon (2002) and Proust et al. (2009) reported significantly fewer deficits in memory and executive function in patients who underwent coiling compared to clipping. This difference was posited to result from the coil's pliability, smaller size, and reduced tendency to disrupt ACoA perforating branches as compared to the clipping, making the coil less invasive. However, Brown et al. (2008) presented several studies finding minimal or no differences in cognitive outcome between clipping versus coiling treatment groups.

The two most common complications following aneurysm bleed and surgery are hydrocephalus and vasospasm (Adams & Victor, 1993; Cullum et al., 2008). Hydrocephalus may require a temporary ventriculostomy or, if substantial hydrocephalus persists, a permanent shunt. Triple-H (hypertensive, hypervolemic, hemodilution) therapy is the standard of care for vasospasm prophylaxis (Lee, Lukovits, & Friedman, 2006). Both complications have been associated with cognitive deficit (Heuer, Smith, Elliot, Winn, & LeRoux, 2004; Stenhouse, Knight, Longmore, & Bishara, 1991; Tidswell et al., 1995). The Hunt and Hess score (a correlate of bleed severity) and age have also been associated with cognitive outcome (Salary et al., 2007).

Beyond the risks of cognitive deficit associated with the bleed, surgery, and complications of aneurysm repair in any location, there is evidence that the location of the ACoA may present particular risks for cognitive impairment. As was noted earlier, there are several small branching vessels from the ACoA. These perforating branches may perfuse a wide variety of areas, including the hypothalamus, anterior commissure, anterior cingulate, septum pellucidum, genu of the corpus callosum, portions of the fornices, optic chiasm, and the basal forebrain region (Alexander & Freedman, 1984; Bottger, Proseigel, Steiger, & Yassouridis, 1998; Gade, 1982; Serizawa et al., 1997; Vincentelli et al., 1991). The basal forebrain, an area of particular importance, is defined as the region at the base of the frontal lobes including the nucleus basalis of Meynert, the diagonal band of Broca, and the septal nuclei, providing a major source of cholinergic input to the cortex and medial temporal lobes (Everitt & Robbins, 1997; Loring, 1999). The areas perfused by these perforating branches have been linked to memory, initiation/motivation, personality, and electrolyte balance (Bottger et al., 1998; Brand & Markowitsch, 2003; Brust & Chamorro, 2004; Cavazos, Wang, Sitoh, Ng, & Tien, 1997; Crosson, 1992; Damasio, Graff-Radford, Eslinger, Damasio, & Kassell, 1985; Devinsky, Morrell, & Vogt, 1995; Everitt & Robbins 1997; Hadland, Rushworth, Gaffan, & Passingham, 2003; Vincentelli et al., 1991; Wright, Boeve, & Malec, 1999). Disruptions of these perforating branches due to bleeding and surgery in the area surrounding the ACoA may involve a variety of different areas, depending on which perforating vessels are involved. Variability across patients may also arise from vascular anomalies and differences in the number of perforating branches (Serizawa et al., 1997; Vincentelli et al., 1991). Additionally, infarction due to the hemorrhage and/or surgery may produce damage to other areas not served by the perforating branches, including basal ganglia and frontal regions (Brust & Chamorro, 2004; Deluca & Diamond, 1995; D'Esposito, Alexander, Fischer, McGlinchev-Berroth, & O'Connor, 1996; Diamond, DeLuca, & Kelley, 1997; Irle, Wowra, Kunert, Hampl, & Kunze, 1992; Wright et al., 1999).

Much has been published on the cognitive deficits associated with ACoA aneurysm bleeds.

Reports of memory deficit following surgery for ACoA aneurysms date back to 1953 (Gade, 1982). Alexander and Freedman (1984) described amnesia and personality change after repair of ACoA aneurysm bleed and referred to the changes as the "ACoA syndrome." In a now classic review, Deluca and Diamond detailed the evidence for an "ACoA syndrome" (Deluca & Diamond, 1995). They drew on the work of Alexander and Freedman (1984), Damasio et al. (1985), Deluca (1992), Gade (1982), and Volpe and Hirst (1983), among many others. Deluca and Diamond remarked on the significance of the amnesia in the ACoA patients, as dense memory deficits had typically been associated with diencephalic/mesial temporal lobe damage and the ACoA patients demonstrated amnesia without damage to these regions. Instead, the ACoA patients shed light on the role of the basal forebrain in memory. Their literature review led them to define three major behavioral changes: *(1)* confabulation (related to frontal lobe pathology); *(2)* amnesia (related to basal forebrain pathology); and *(3)* personality change, including lack of spontaneity, reduced initiation, decreased self-control, and apathy (related to frontal lobe dysfunction). Their review of the neuropsychological literature also revealed that intellectual, attention, visuospatial, implicit memory, and language skills were relatively spared following ACoA aneurysm rupture/repair. In contrast, delayed recall, retrograde memory, mental flexibility, and concept formation were usually areas of substantial impairment. Akinesia and "alien hand" were also reported in some cases. The case for an ACoA syndrome has since been supported by Beeckmanns, Vancoille, and Michiels (1998), Chan et al. (2002), Myers et al. (2008), and Wright et al. (1999).

Other studies, however, failed to find a profile *specific* to ACoA aneurysm rupture and repair. Tidswell et al. (1995) and Hutter, Kreitschmann-Andermahr, and Gilsbach (2001) found cognitive impairment in the ACoA aneurysm groups, but the impairments were not significantly different from those patients with aneurysm ruptures in other locations. Similarly, in a review of cognitive outcome following aneurysm hemorrhage, Brown et al. (2008) presented studies suggesting that all subarachnoid hemorrhages tend to produce a diffuse profile of deficits as opposed to specific profiles associated with particular hemorrhagic locations. Bottger et al. (1998) found too wide a variety of cognitive deficits in their ACoA patients to be consistent with a particular ACoA profile. Cullum et al. (2008), upon reviewing the mixed findings regarding presence of executive dysfunction in ACoA patients, observed that the interindividual variability in this population (even among patients with similar imaging findings) underscores the importance of the neuropsychological exam.

Nonetheless, there remains evidence that damage to basal forebrain and/or frontal regions (as is frequently reported with ACoA rupture) produces particular types of memory deficits. Myers et al. (2002, 2008) reported that, compared to subjects with medial temporal lobe damage, the ACoA patients had slowed learning for a task but, once the task was learned, showed better generalization. Diamond et al. (1997) described that, unlike patients with mesial temporal lobe damage, ACoA patients benefitted from organizational strategies for recall, did not show accelerated rates of forgetting, and had a greater discrepancy in recall versus recognition. O'Connor and Lafleche (2004) reported that ACoA patients showed less severe retrograde memory impairments than patients with temporal lobe damage.

The Case of C. E.

C. E. was a 51 year-old, right-handed male who was admitted to an inpatient rehabilitation unit for treatment of deficits following anterior communicating artery aneurysm bleed. C. E. was observed to have a seizure at home 3 weeks earlier. After the seizure he was alert and oriented, complaining of headache. He was hospitalized and workup (head CT, angiogram) revealed a subarachnoid hemorrhage due to a ruptured anterior communicating artery aneurysm (4 mm in size). He developed hydrocephalus with declining neurological status (Hunt & Hess score declined from 2 to 3) and a ventricular drain was placed. The following day (Day 3) he underwent clipping of the aneurysm via right frontal craniotomy. He was started on triple-H for vasospasm prophylaxis. The ventricular drain was removed on Day 5. Periodic head CTs over the following 7 months continued to show mild communicating hydrocephalus as well as damage in the right frontal lobe (basal forebrain region), extending inferiorly to the level of the gyrus rectus, and in the corpus callosum. The right basal ganglia were less affected with only mild volume loss. After the aneurysm clipping he was unresponsive but by Day 14 he began to appear more alert, confused, and combative at times. A feeding tube was placed due to poor oral intake. Medical history was also significant for hypertension, IV drug abuse (heroin), human immunodeficiency virus (HIV), hepatitis B, and hepatitis C.

C. E. was single and lived in public housing. He had no family contacts; thus, a limited social history was provided by a friend and by a community social worker. C. E. had done odd jobs in the past and worked for a community agency at the time of his hospitalization. He did not smoke or drink and had been on methadone for many years. Psychiatric history was otherwise negative. Prior to admission, he reportedly had a pleasant, joking demeanor and was well liked by other housing residents and staff. Additional background information was not available.

Upon admission to rehabilitation, C. E. was lethargic and required cues for arousal, with intermittent motor restlessness/agitation. His behavior was treated with environmental modifications (quiet private room, low lights, frequent rest breaks) and monitored with the Agitated Behavior Scale (Corrigan, 1989). Attention was poor, response speed was severely slow, and he frequently did not respond at all to questions/directions. His status prohibited formal assessment; thus, an unstructured approach was utilized with maximum cuing as needed. He was oriented to name only. He followed 1–2-step commands inconsistently and followed no 3-step commands. Comprehension of simple yes-no questions was impaired. He denied emotional distress, but his answers were of questionable reliability. In therapies, C. E. typically needed total assistance for self-care. He was able to briefly stand with the assistance of two people. Some staff stated a belief that he was willfully ignoring questions and possibly feigning impairment. The neuropsychologist educated the staff about possible abulia resulting from involvement of mesial frontal/anterior cingulum areas and

provided evidence as to why malingering was unlikely.

Approximately 5 weeks later, his attention had increased to 20 minutes in a functional task and he was oriented to self and grossly to place (hospital). He no longer showed frequent signs of agitation, although rare agitation/dyscontrol occurred in response to environmental stressors. He required cues or calendar for orientation to date and hospital name. Response speed improved and he responded to all questions. Staff no longer voiced concerns about feigned impairment. He required only supervision (no physical assistance) to complete self-care tasks and walked safely with one staff member gently guiding him. He answered simple yes-no questions accurately (20/20) but was more impaired for complex questions (16/20). He was eating more food but intake remained suboptimal. He was observed to have poor recall of recent events. Formal testing revealed impairments in orientation to date and hospital name, mental and manual sequencing, time estimation, immediate and delayed memory, visuospatial/constructional skill, coding speed, complex language comprehension, and reasoning for hypothetical problem situations (see Table 62-2). Auditory attention (Digit Span) was low average and basic language was within normal limits.

Over the course of the next month, C. E. continued to make gains in therapies and needed only supervision for self-care and walking. Appetite improved to normal. Attention improved to 30 minutes in a functional activity. He remained oriented to self and grossly to place only, despite therapist attempts to improve orientation to date and hospital name. He retained no information beyond a few minutes. He was unable to learn formal compensatory memory strategies, although he learned to look at a wall calendar for the date and hospital name. Social skills were intact. He was generally calm but became briefly agitated at times due to his wish to leave the unit. He also developed agitation when placed with a roommate who yelled continually but this behavior resolved after a room change. Thereafter he remained calm, showing little initiative to leave his room or perform hygiene (he was cooperative when asked to do so). At 5 months post-ACoA rupture, C. E. required no physical assistance or supervision for his basic self-care

Table 62-2. Two Months post ACoA Rupture

Cognitive Log	7/30	Impaired

Repeatable Battery for the Assessment of Neuropsychological Status

Subtest	Raw Score
List Learning	9
Story Memory	7
	Immediate Memory Index Score = 44, < 0.1 percentile
Figure Copy	12
Line Orientation	2
	Visuospatial/ Constructional Index Score = 53, 0.1 percentile
Picture Naming	10
Semantic Fluency	12
	Language Index Score = 82, 12th percentile
Digit Span	8
Coding	13
	Attention Index Score = 60, 0.4 percentile
List Recall	0
List Recognition	11
Story Recall	1
Figure Recall	0
	Delayed Memory Index Score = 40, < 0.1 percentile

Neurosensory Center Comprehensive Examination of Aphasia

Token Test	113/163	Impaired

Cognitive Competency Test

Verbal Reasoning	5/20	Impaired

and walking but continued to manifest severe functional memory deficits.

His memory impairments, absence of family support, and lack of deficits in self-care and ambulation complicated discharge planning; thus, C. E. remained on the rehabilitation unit for 9 months. He learned to recognize staff faces but did not learn any names. He did not initiate movement out of his room and continued to need some guidance to find his way around the small rehabilitation unit. The following results reflect formal reassessment 8 months after the rupture and clipping of the ACoA aneurysm (see Table 62-3). C. E. remained oriented to self and grossly to place only, not hospital name or date. Mental flexibility and time estimation were impaired. He continued to show profound memory deficits, poor visuomotor coding speed, and borderline (but improved) visuospatial skills. Results suggest a decline in language, but he did not otherwise show signs of language impairment. Digit span remained stable and low average. C. E. was discharged to a skilled nursing facility soon after this evaluation. Anecdotal reports indicated that, shortly after admission to the nursing facility, C. E. became agitated, had an altercation with an aide, and was transferred to a psychiatric facility. He was since lost to follow-up.

Table 62-3. Eight Months post ACoA Rupture

Cognitive Log	13/30	Impaired

Repeatable Battery for the Assessment of Neuropsychological Status

Subtest	Raw Score
List Learning	12
Story Memory	12
	Immediate Memory Index Score = 61, 0.5 percentile
Figure Copy	16
Line Orientation	13
	Visuospatial/ Constructional Index Score = 78, 7th percentile
Picture Naming	8
Semantic Fluency	9
	Language Index Score = 64, 1st percentile
Digit Span	8
Coding	19
	Attention Index Score = 64, 1st percentile
List Recall	0
List Recognition	13
Story Recall	1
Figure Recall	3
	Delayed Memory Index Score = 44, < 0.1 percentile

Discussion

Given the uncertainty about whether ACoA aneurysm rupture and repair produces a specific cognitive profile, it is difficult to say whether this patient is typical of the disorder. The timing of the assessment appears to be important, as was also observed by Deluca and Diamond (1995) and Haug et al. (2007). Immediately following the rupture and surgery, C. E.'s severe abulia and slowed responses resulted in a more global pattern of deficits. As the abulia and response speed improved, a more specific pattern emerged, fairly consistent with reports of the ACoA syndrome. The features of the purported ACoA syndrome manifested by C. E. included severe deficits in memory, reasoning, initiation and, at times, impulse control. He showed relative strengths in auditory attention, visuospatial, and language skills. Sentence comprehension, visual construction, functional attention, and social interaction improved over time. Most striking after 9 months, he showed no ability to retain new declarative information and initiated very little behavior. The minimal evidence of new learning he demonstrated (recognizing faces, learning use of the orientation board) suggested the operation of nondeclarative memory systems. This patient differed from some reports of the ACoA syndrome in that he did not show confabulation.

The case of C. E. raises some interesting issues, particularly from a rehabilitation perspective. C. E. demonstrates a case of significant discrepancy between progress in occupational and physical therapies (good) with cognitive recovery (poor). This complicated discharge planning, as C. E.'s intact self-care and ambulation skills made him inappropriate for admission to most subacute rehabilitation programs. His cognitive deficits prohibited him from living independently and he had no family or friends who could provide a supervised home environment. The implications and treatment of these types of deficits have been studied by Mills, Karas, and Alexander (2006). The facility that finally admitted C. E. was not familiar with management of behavioral disturbances, resulting in an unfortunate (and likely inappropriate) admission to a psychiatric facility. C. E.'s rare (but significant) agitated/aggressive outbursts may be tied to decreased "self-control" as was noted by Steinman

and Bigler (1986). Awareness of this potential may help in understanding why a generally calm patient with little initiation may become agitated. The combination of C. E.'s memory and reasoning deficits with his reduced capacity for self-control (more prominent early in his recovery) may have left him ill-equipped to deal with the stresses of a new facility and unfamiliar staff. The role of the neuropsychologist was important throughout C. E.'s rehabilitation admission but most especially in the early phase, when members of the rehabilitation team misinterpreted the abulia/slowed response speed as evidence for malingered/factitious disorder. Follow-up neuropsychological assessment was also useful for discharge planning in documenting the severity of cognitive impairment as compared to his intact basic activities of daily living.

In summary, rupture and surgery of ACoA aneurysms may result in a wide range of outcomes. Outcome may be influenced by surgery type, complications (primarily hydrocephalus and vasospasm), degree of involvement of ACoA perforating branches, as well as degree of infarction to other areas. With this number of potential variables, it is not surprising that we fail to find uniformity in the deficit profiles. Rupture and surgery of an ACoA aneurysm may result in minimal deficits, moderate impairment, or, as in the case of C. E., profound memory and behavior disturbance. Involvement of basal forebrain regions, as seen in C. E., appears to be of particular importance for memory outcome.

References

Adams, R. D., & Victor, M. (1993). *Principles of neurology* (5th ed.). New York: McGraw Hill Inc.

Agrawal, A., Kato, Y., Chen, L., Karagiozov, K., Yoneda, M., Imizu, S., Sano, H., & Kanno, T. (2008). Anterior communicating artery aneurysms: An overview. *Minimally Invasive Neurosurgery, 51*, 131–135.

Alexander, M. P., & Freedman, M. (1984). Amnesia after anterior communicating artery aneurysm rupture. *Neurology, 34*, 752–757.

Beeckmans, K., Vancoillie, P., & Michiels, K. (1998). Neuropsychological deficits in patients with anterior communicating artery syndrome: A multiple case study. *Acta Neurological Belgium, 98*, 266–278.

Bottger, S., Prosiegel, M., Steiger, H. J., & Yassouridis, A. (1998). Neurobehavioural disturbances, rehabilitation outcome, and lesion site in patients after rupture and repair of anterior communicating artery aneurysm. *Journal of Neurology, Neurosurgery, and Psychiatry, 65*, 93–102.

Brand, M., & Markowitsch, H. J. (2003). Amnesia: Neuroanatomic and clinical issues. In T. E. Feinberg & M. J. Farah (Eds.), *Behavioral neurology and neuropsychology* (pp. 431–443). New York: McGraw Hill Inc.

Brown, G. G., Lazar, R. M., & Delano-Wood, L. (2008). Cerebrovascular disease. In I. Grant & K. M. Adams (Eds.), *Neuropsychological assessment of neuropsychiatric disorders* (3rd ed.). New York: Oxford University Press.

Brust, J. C. M., & Chamorro, A. (2004). Anterior cerebral artery disease. In J. P. Mohr, D. W. Choi, J. C. Grotta, B. Weir, & P. A. Wolf (Eds.), *Stroke pathophysiology, diagnosis and management* (pp. 101–122). Philadelphia: Churchill Livingstone.

Cavazos, J. E., Wang, C. J., Sitoh, Y. Y., Ng, S. E., & Tien, R. D. (1997). Anatomy and pathology of the septal region. *Neuroimaging Clinics of North America, 7*, 676–678.

Chan, A., Ho, A., & Poon, W. S. (2002). Neuropsychological sequelae of patients treated with microsurgical clipping or endovascular embolization for anterior communicating artery aneurysm. *European Neurology, 47*, 37–44.

Corrigan, J. D. (1989). Development of a scale for assessment of agitation following traumatic brain injury. *Journal of Clinical and Experimental Neuropsychology, 11*, 261–277.

Crosson, B. (1992). *Subcortical functions in language and memory*. New York: The Guilford Press.

Cullum, C. M., Rilling, L. M., Saine, K., & Samson, D. (2008). Intracranial hemorrhage, vascular malformations, cerebral aneurysms, and subarachnoid hemorrhage. In J. E. Morgan & J. H. Ricker (Eds.), *Textbook of clinical neuropsychology* (pp. 392–410). New York: Taylor & Francis.

Damasio, A. R., Graff-Radford, N. R., Eslinger, P. J., Damasio, H., & Kassell, N. (1985). Amnesia following basal forebrain lesions. *Archives of Neurology, 42*, 263–271.

Deluca, J. (1992). Cognitive dysfunction after aneurysm of the anterior communicating artery. *Journal of Clinical and Experimental Neuropsychology, 14*, 924-934.

Deluca, J. & Diamond, B. J. (1995). Aneurysm of the anterior communicating artery: A review of neuroanatomical and neuropsychological sequelae. *Journal of Clinical and Experimental Neuropsychology, 17*, 100–121.

D'Esposito, M., Alexander, M. P., Fischer, R., McGlinchev-Berroth, R., & O'Connor, M. (1996). Recovery of memory and executive function following anterior communicating artery rupture. *Journal of the International Neuropsychological Society, 2*, 565–570.

de Oliveira, J., Beck, J., Setzer, M., Gerlach, R., Vatter, H., Seifert, V., & Raabe, A. (2007a). Risk of shunt-dependent hydrocephalus after occlusion or ruptured intracranial aneurysms by surgical clipping or endovascular coiling: A single-institution series and meta-analysis. *Neurosurgery, 61*, 924–934.

de Oliveira, J. G., Beck, J., Ulrich, C., Rathert, J., Raabe, A., & Seifert, V. (2007b). Comparison between clipping and coiling on the incidence of cerebral vasospasm after aneurismal subarachnoid hemorrhage: A systematic review and meta-analysis. *Neurosurgical Review, 30*, 22–30.

Devinsky, O., Morrell, M. J., & Vogt, B. A. (1995). Contributions of anterior cingulated cortex to behaviour. *Brain, 118*, 279–306.

Diamond, B. J., DeLuca, J., & Kelley, S. M. (1997). Memory and executive functions in amnestic and non-amnestic patients with aneurysms of the anterior communicating artery. *Brain, 120*, 1015–1025.

Everitt, B., & Robbins, T. (1997). Central cholinergic systems and cognition. *Annual Review of Psychology, 48*, 649–684.

Gade, A. (1982). Amnesia after operations on aneurysms of the anterior communicating artery. *Surgical Neurology, 18*, 46–49.

Hadland, K. A., Rushworth, M. F., Gaffan, D., & Passingham, R. E. (2003). The effect of cingulate lesions on social behaviour and emotion. *Neuropsychologia, 41*, 919–931.

Haug, T., Sorteberg, A., Sorteberg, W., Lindegaard, K. F., Lundar, T., & Finset, A. (2007). Cognitive outcome after aneurismal subarachnoid hemorrhage: Time course of recovery and relationship to clinical, radiological, and management parameters. *Neurosurgery, 60*, 649–656.

Heuer, G. G., Smith, M. J., Elliott, J. P., Winn, H. R., & LeRoux, P. D. (2004). Relationship between intracranial pressure and other clinical variables in patients with aneurismal subarachnoid hemorrhage. *Journal of Neurosurgery, 101*, 408–416.

Hoh, B. L., Topcuoglu, M. A., Singhal, A. B., Pryor, J. C., Rabinov, J. D., Rordorf, G. A., Carter, B. S., & Ogilvy, C. S. (2004). Effect of clipping, craniotomy, or intravascular coiling on cerebral vasospasm and patient outcome after aneurismal subarachnoid hemorrhage. *Neurosurgery, 55*, 779–786.

Hutter, B. O., Kreitschmann-Andermahr, I., & Gilsbach, J. M. (2001). Health-related quality of life after aneurismal subarachnoid hemorrhage: Impacts of bleeding severity, computerized tomography findings, surgery, vasospasm, and neurological grade. *Journal of Neurosurgery, 94*, 241–251.

Irle, E., Wowra, B., Kunert, H. J., Hampl, J., & Kunze, S. (1992). Memory disturbances following anterior communicating artery rupture. *Annals of Neurology, 31*, 473–480.

Jartti, P., Karttunen, A., Isokangas, J. M., Jartti, A., Koskelainen, T., & Tervonen, O. (2008). Chronic hydrocephalus after neurosurgical and endovascular treatment of ruptured intracranial aneurysms. *Acta Radiologica, 49*, 680–686.

Lee, K. H., Lukovits, T., & Friedman, J. A. (2006). "Triple-H" therapy for cerebral vasospasm following subarachnoid hemorrhage. *Neurocritical Care, 4*, 68–76.

Levy, E. I., Kim, S. H., Bendok, B. R., Boulos, A. S., Xavier, A. R., Yahia, A. M., Qureshi, A. I., Guterman, L. R., & Hopkins, L. N. (2004). Interventional neuroradiologic therapy. In J. P. Mohr, D. W. Choi, J. C. Grotta, B. Weir, & P. A. Wolf (Eds.), *Stroke pathophysiology, diagnosis and management* (pp. 1475–1520). Philadelphia: Churchill Livingstone.

Loring, D. W. (1999). *INS dictionary of neuropsychology*. New York: Oxford University Press.

Mills, V. M., Karas, A., & Alexander, M. P. (2006). Outpatient rehabilitation of patients with chronic cognitive impairments after ruptured anterior communicating artery aneurysms reduces the burden of care: A pilot study. *Brain Injury, 20*, 1183–1188.

Mitchell, P., Kerr, R., Mendelow, A. D., & Molyneux, A. (2008). Could late rebleeding overturn the superiority of cranial aneurysm coil embolization over clip ligation seen in the International Subarachnoid Aneurysm Trial? *Journal of Neurosurgery, 108*, 437–442.

Myers, C. E., Bryant, D., DeLuca, J., & Gluck, M. A. (2002). Dissociating basal forebrain and medial temporal amnesic syndromes: insights from classical conditioning. *Integrative Physiological and Behavioral Science, 37*, 85-102.

Myers, C. E., Hopkins, R. O., Deluca, J., Moore, N. B., Wolansky, L. J., Sumner, J. M., & Gluck, M. A. (2008). Learning and generalization deficits in patients with memory impairments due to anterior communicating artery rupture or hypoxic brain injury. *Neuropsychology, 22*, 681–686.

O'Connor, M. G., & Lafleche, G. M. (2004). Retrograde amnesia in patients with rupture and surgical repair of anterior communicating artery aneurysms. *Journal of the International Neuropsychological Society, 10*, 221–229.

Proust, F., Martinaud, O., Gerardin, E., Derrey, S., Leveque, S., Bioux, S., Tollard, E., Clavier, E., Langlois, O., Godefroy, O., Hannequin, D., & Freger, P. (2008). Quality of life and brain damage after microsurgical clip occlusion or endovascular coil embolization for ruptured anterior communicating artery aneurysms: Neuropsychological assessment. *Journal of Neurosurgery, 110*, 19–29.

Rabenstein, A. A., Pichelmann, M. A., Friedman, J. A., Piepgras, D. G., Nichols, D. A., Melver, J. I., Toussaint, L.G., III, McClelland, R. L., Fulgham, J. R., Meyer, F. B., Atkinson, J. L., & Wijdicks, E. F. (2003). Symptomatic vasospasm and outcomes following aneurismal subarachnoid hemorrhage: A comparison between surgical repair and endovascular coil occlusion. *Journal of Neurosurgery, 98*, 319–325.

Salary, M., Quigley, M. R., & Wilberger, J. E., Jr. (2007). Relation among aneurysm size, amount of subarachnoid blood, and clinical outcome. *Journal of Neurosurgery, 107*, 13–17.

Serizawa, T., Saeki, N., & Yamaura, A. (1997). Microsurgical anatomy and clinical significance of the anterior communicating artery and its perforating branches. *Neurosurgery, 40*, 1211–1218.

Steinman, D. R., & Bigler, E. D. (1986). Neuropsychological sequelae of ruptured anterior communicating artery aneurysm. *International Journal of Clinical Neuropsychology, 8*, 135–140.

Stenhouse, L. M., Knight, R. G., Longmore, B. E., & Bishara, S. N. (1991). Long-term cognitive deficits in patients after surgery on aneurysms of the anterior communicating artery. *Journal of Neurology, Neurosurgery and Psychiatry, 54*, 909–914.

Tidswell, P., Dias, P. S., Sagar, H. J., Maves, A. R., & Battersby, R. D. (1995). Cognitive outcome after aneurysm rupture: relationship to aneurysm site and perioperative complications. *Neurology, 45*, 875–882.

van der Schaaf, I., Algra, A., Wermer, M., Molyneux, A., Clarke, M., van Gijn, J., & Rinkel, G.. (2005). Endovascular coiling versus neurosurgical clipping for patients with aneurismal subarachnoid haemorrhage. *Cochrane Database of Systematic Reviews, 19*, Issue 4. Art. No.: CD003085. DOI: 10.1002/14651858. CD003085.pub2.

Vates, G. E., Zabramski, J. M., Spetzler, R. F., & Lawton, M. T. (2004). Intracranial aneurysms. In J. P. Mohr, D. W. Choi, J. C. Grotta, B. Weir, & P. A. Wolf (Eds.), *Stroke pathophysiology, diagnosis and management* (pp. 1279–1335). Philadelphia: Churchill Livingstone.

Vincentelli, F., Lehman, G.., Caruso, G.., Grisoli, F., Rabehanta, P., & Gouaze, A. (1991). Extracerebral course of the perforating branches of the anterior communicating artery: Microsurgical anatomical study. *Surgical Neurology, 35*, 98–104.

Volpe, B. T. & Hirst, W. (1983). Amnesia following rupture and repair of an anterior communicating artery aneurysm. *Journal of Neurology, Neurosurgery, and Psychiatry, 46,* 704–709.

Waxman, S. G. (1996). *Correlative neuroanatomy* (23rd ed.). Stamford, CT: Appleton & Lange.

Weir, B. (2002). Unruptured intracranial aneurysms: A review. *Journal of Neurosurgery, 96,* 3–42.

Wright, R. A., Boeve, B. F., & Malec, J. F. (1999). Amnesia after basal forebrain damage due to anteriorcommunicating artery aneurysm rupture. *Journal of Clinical Neuroscience, 6,* 511–515.

Subject Index

Note: Page numbers followed by "*f*" and "*t*" denotes figures and tables, respectively.